Psychiatry and Neuroscience Update – Vol. V

Pascual Ángel Gargiulo
Humberto Luis Mesones-Arroyo
Editors

Psychiatry and Neuroscience Update – Vol. V

Addiction: From Laboratory and Anthropology to Clinical Practice

Springer

Editors
Pascual Ángel Gargiulo
Laboratory of Neurosciences and Experimental Psychology,
Latin American Technological Corporation Foundation (FUCOTEL),
Cathedra of Psychopathology
Catholic University of Argentina,
Area of Pharmacology, Department of Pathology, National University of Cuyo,
CONICET
Guaymallén, Mendoza, Argentina

Humberto Luis Mesones-Arroyo
Laboratory of Neurosciences and Experimental Psychology,
Latin American Technological Corporation Foundation (FUCOTEL),
Cathedra of Psychopathology
Catholic University of Argentina,
Area of Pharmacology, Department of Pathology, National University of Cuyo,
CONICET
Guaymallén, Mendoza, Argentina

ISBN 978-3-031-72221-9 ISBN 978-3-031-72219-6 (eBook)
https://doi.org/10.1007/978-3-031-72219-6

This Springer imprint is published by the registered company Springer Nature Switzerland AG
The registered company address is: Gewerbestrasse 11, 6330 Cham, Switzerland

Foreword

The present volume of Psychiatry and Neuroscience Update is dedicated to the many advances already made in neurobiological investigation and the also many different pathways explored. But drug addiction is a problem that exceeds the limits of laboratory, metabolism and genetics. Psychiatry, psychology and sociology must be asked to contribute. Penal legislation and international cooperation are already challenged by organized crime.

How drugs of abuse affect the limbic system, and how they alter neurotransmission is evident, and how this emotional circuit affects emotion, reason and social behaviour is also well demonstrated. Epidemiology also has shown the relation between social, "recreational", consumers and those who become addicted. In a number of cases, serious psychiatric disorders and permanent consequences can be expected. But abnormal blood flow in the prefrontal cortex, amygdala and thalamus treated with SSRIs, MAOI or Tricyclic antidepressants do not fulfil the need to prevent and treat a disorder that has become a pandemic.

Much more has to be done to alert parents, teachers and society of the danger involved in accepting as fashionable to make reunions in which marihuana, cocaine, amphetamines or similar are nice experiences of escaping from reality for a short time. And without consciousness of being responsible for paying narco-traffic and becoming accomplices of delinquency.

Much can be done if from our profession we are prepared to make known these truths through social media.

Science explores nature and anthropology studies biology, psychology and sociology. A fourth dimension is out of reach, *ta meta physika*, spiritual. But medicine is more than a natural science, it is a human science and answers the needs of human being seeking for help. Vocation to aid, heal and shelter those who suffer is basic in medicine.

Learning more means exploring, researching and acquiring technical skills. Staying up to date in one of the many medical specialties is a difficult task to achieve and requires time to read, have access to conferences and courses.

Springer is a leader in Updates such as this new volume, very complete and timely, achieved through joint work with the tireless Pascual Ángel Gargiulo.

Buenos Aires, Argentina — Humberto Luis Mesones-Arroyo

Preface

The main objective of this update is to provide readers with a contribution with an updated, clear and scientifically based position regarding the consumption of illegal drugs and its main consequences. However, the additional objectives are not forgettable. The role of education and its relevance in prevention is clearly postulated in this section and other parts of this book. Furthermore, the importance of education and social concerns in treatment is formally sustained. Along these lines, some significant cultural and social facts, particularly linked to the work of Huxley and his followers, are analysed here in detail, dedicating a special chapter to them. This is due to the importance they had, especially in the 1960s, in the spread of drug use.

In many cases, some contents may be repetitive. But it is our intention to present them from different points of view and frame, since this allows a more complete approach to the subject. Likewise, different approaches to the same topic can coexist. This, far from constituting a difficulty, we understand that it allows the reader to know different points of view, and not a rigid vision of the problem. We see in this an invitation to the meditative "fair play" of each person who addresses our book.

As in previous updates, the book is divided into four main sections. The first section is dedicated to epistemological considerations about the study of normal and abnormal behaviours. The second section develops mainly areas of translational neurosciences to the human brain. The third section is dedicated to neurosciences, learning, teaching and the role of social environment. The fourth section is developed for explaining human pathological behaviours, following a line from brain disorders and projecting to psychopathology.

The first section aims to start anthropological frames of reference to the topic. The first section starts with the chapter of Dr Francesca Brencio. In it she shows how phenomenology and hermeneutics can allow us to understand and develop clinical encounters in terms of intersubjectivity. An attempt is also made to decipher the role of this intersubjectivity in the field of medication prescription. The history of phenomenology is briefly reconstructed. Some recent adaptations to neurosciences and cognitive sciences are mentioned. The clinical encounter is analysed from the perspective of intersubjectivity. Finally, the impact of medications on the intersubjective encounter is analysed. This is a rigorous and illuminating chapter which leads to the clarification of the context in which the medication is prescribed.

In Chap. 2, Prof. Dr Juan Ernesto Calderón highlights the need for a multidisciplinary approach to the problem of addictions. In this context, he raises the possibility of an approach to addiction from multiple perspectives. He develops the concept of discipline and its relevance in scientific practice. He considers that the disciplinary matrix is the way of seeing the world. This way conditions consequent actions, which are influenced not only by the understanding of the object but also by the application of treatments and therapies as interventions linked to the disciplinary matrix. Throughout the chapter, he proposes an organization of disciplines in order to respond to the problems that arise from interdisciplinarity. This bright epistemic approach highlights the relevance of the review of previous concepts regarding action.

In Chap. 3, written by Luis Echarte, Augusto Pascual Ítalo Gargiulo and Pascual Ángel Gargiulo, we analyse mainly the essay of Aldous Huxley in the novel *Brave New World*. We consider this work by Huxley to be still an original and valuable tool in the field of the study of addictions and their treatment. In this chapter, we analyse the theoretical framework related to approaches in research and treatment of addictions. We study here the social factors involved, and the solutions proposed in the novel. Other works, such as *The Doors of Perception*, among others, are analysed in this chapter within the aforementioned context. This chapter represents an attempt to socially and historically contextualize the phenomenon of addictions.

In Chap. 4, Miriam Dolly Arancibia de Calmels studies the search for vital sense. The interference of hedonism versus pain is raised here. The requirement of a pause in everyday life is also matter of proposals and developments. Difficulties surging from hyper-digitization, acceleration, violence and frivolity are here considered. The relevance and imposition of social standards are presented as difficulties in this process. Attitudes are here presented and considered, mainly facing pain and happiness, searching for vital sense. In this chapter, searching for existing ways for a deep reflection on one's own vital sense is the main objective. A personal definition of the sense of the own life is the final goal. The role of pain and happiness is here considered closely related to this goal. This chapter constitutes an interesting and deep reflection about sense of life, raised from the topic of addictions.

In Chap. 5, Lucas Marcelo Rodriguez, Santiago Alejandro Resett and María José Zinoni develop the study of the relationship between the meaning of life and permissiveness in the use and abuse of substances during adolescence. They focus on the maturation of cognitive structures in this period and its relation with existential questions, reason for living and meaning of life. They develop a relationship between meaning of life and moral judgement (permissiveness and penalization) in this age and context. The authors focus particularly on substance using and abusing, particularly alcohol, cannabis and cocaine. They sustain that empirical results show a higher meaning of life related to greater penalization of the consumption of drugs, such as alcohol, cannabis and cocaine. They postulate a higher meaning of life in the population of less permissive adolescents to the consumption of cannabis. Existential emptiness is matter of interesting considerations. Consequences and corollaries are widely and interestingly discussed.

Chapter 6 is dedicated to epistemic competencies related to philosophy in therapeutic praxis. This chapter, written by Prof. Dr María Teresa Gargiulo, constitutes a lucid and deep analysis of Pedro Laín Entralgo's writings. This author conceives the epistemic competences of philosophy both in the field of a comprehensive theory of disease and of the sick man and its natural projection in the field of medical practice. The multiple influences of philosophy on the ontological assumptions of medicine are highlighted. The author states that the interest of these topics is related to how philosophical inquiry directly affects human health and illness and remains valid. This chapter constitutes a deep approach to medical anthropology, and constitutes a historical contextualization in the areas of epistemic status of medical practice. As the author postulates, this chapter is a message, in which it is postulated that medical anthropology invites philosophy to intervene directly in the healing process itself. It implies that medical anthropology is the window to open the real and existential process of the patient.

In Chap. 7, Prof. Dr Rocco Genaro addresses the topic of free will, addiction and the feeling of self-control. In a dense, rigorous and deep chapter, he focuses firstly in analysis of addiction as strong appetites. He defines compulsion as an overwhelming and intense desire. It leads, in this proposition, to immediate action. This action seems to crowd out other impulses and mental states. It is due to the fact that one's attention is preponderantly focused on acquiring and taking a drug. The relation with *self-control* is here clearly established. The author explores the relationship between free will-determinism, addiction, compulsion and self-control. This chapter constitutes an interesting dialogue between different positions regarding all mentioned variables, introspection and consciousness. The present study constitutes a reference piece regarding nuclear items of philosophy of mind.

In Chap. 8, Dr Ricardo Aranovich postulates the beginning of consumption as antidepressant self-medication, a way to reach a well-being state or a way to escape from discomfort. He points that young people are in a vulnerable situation in terms of their moods. Adolescence is here defined as a state in which adult needs suddenly arise in a child without having the resources to satisfy them. The author enumerates a lot of historical and social factors that may induce an uncertainty state. These factors may be inducing a facilitation to consume as a way to avoid these uncertainty feelings, disorientation and anxiety. The introspection and the vocation discovery are proposed as a correct mode of overcoming these negative and unresolved states. They facilitate resources to face existence. This chapter constitutes an interesting analysis of existential variables linked to addiction and valid tools to overcome existential disorientation.

Chapter 9 is dedicated by Prof. Dr Ricardo Jorge Llanque Ferrufino to transcultural studies regarding the cocaine use in miners. The present study seeks to identify some sociocultural factors in the ritual named "coca leaf *pijcheo*" by Bolivian miners in the Cerro de San José, in the city of Oruro, Bolivia. This ethnographic work was carried out in a mining cooperative in this city. The *pijchu* is a ritual act where a part of one's energy is offered to the pre-colonial mining deity *Tío* (*Uncle*). This ritual is limited to the Andean logic of *urku* (masculine) and *uma* (feminine) in the ingestion of alcohol and coca. It also allows strengthening the ties between the miners and this Andean deity, in addition to psychologically preparing the miner for his work. Here, during the working day, the *pijchu* becomes a symbolic banquet where the worker becomes transubstantiated and manages to obtain resistance at work, becoming immune to fatigue and hunger, since he absorbs the energies that give him powers from chewing the coca leaf. A profuse imagery, arising from original pieces from the Museum of Anthropology of the Technical University of Oruro, adorns this chapter, actually interesting from the historical, anthropological and cross-cultural perspectives. It is a culturally notable and striking work.

The second section develops mainly areas of translational neurosciences to the human brain, especially in the field of addictions. It is initiated by Chap. 10, in which Manuel Alejandro Guevara, a veterinary doctor with extensive experience in translational models, coordinated an international team studying and reviewing ontogenetic-phylogenetic evolution of corticostriatal pathways. This chapter reviews the structure and function of these pathways, recalling first of all their ontogeny and phylogeny, in order to point out possible animal models to carry out various translational approaches, with particular emphasis on those proposed by our research team. Parallels and divergences between the different species, with the aim of legitimizing or ruling out possible animal models, are here displayed. In this context, we describe and analyse here the conformation of the brain and the corticostriatal pathways in amniotes (reptiles, birds and mammals), pointing its absence in anamniotes (fish and amphibians). A special relevance is given to glutamatergic transmission. Finally, a review of the nosological entities in which these brain structures are involved is developed. It is the case of Parkinson's syndrome and disease, Gilles de la Tourette syndrome, Huntington's Chorea and Amyotrophic Lateral Sclerosis (ALS). In this sense, and in psychiatric pathology, dysfunction of the same pathways has been reported in a group of disorders, such as attention deficit disorder (ADHD), autism, obsessive compulsive disorder (OCD) and schizophrenia. This chapter is a paradigmatic example of possibilities offered by translational models.

In Chap. 11, José E. Burgos and Santiago Castiello define and develop the concept of *Pavlovian impulsivity*. They consider connectionist predictions, with implications for addiction. These authors define impulsivity as the preference for a small reward after a short delay versus a large reward after a long delay. This is closely related to possible underlying addictive behaviour. Translational studies in animals have focused on operant conditioning. In this scheme, reinforcement depends on the response. The authors in this chapter uses a sophisticated existing neural network conditioning model to predict a new, empirically testable phenomenon. This phenomenon is defined here as *Pavlovian impulsivity*. It is an impulsive behaviour that arises from Pavlovian (response-independent) reinforcement. This work arises from a complex computer simulation. In this chapter, implications for a better understanding of impulsive behaviour are discussed.

Chapter 12 is an interesting approach to a bridging between biological to psychological dynamics in the field of addictions. Marcela Schumacher and Osvaldo Agamennoni proposes that the use of substances may be considered a way to produce transient feelings of pleasure. It leads, posteriorly, to the development of dependence. This very interesting approach starts from the fact that drug consumption has a number of stages from the initiation to the pathological state known as addiction considered a chronic disorder. This chapter is particularly dedicated to cannabinoid substances, but in general, it is oriented to establish correlations between biological and psychological variables. In a transdisciplinary study, the dynamics of the vicious cycle of an addict is described. Additionally, this chapter tends to validate mindfulness as an appropriate therapy destined to help to get out of it. This chapter constitutes a valid attempt to establish relations between biology and psychotherapy approaches.

Chapter 13, written by Valeria Teresa Pedrón and Graciela Noemi Balerio, is dedicated to show sex differences and the role of the $GABA_B$ receptors in morphine addiction. This study starts from the fact that clinical and preclinical studies have interestingly shown a higher analgesic response to morphine administration in males when compared to females. Additionally, clinical studies have shown the fact that women need higher doses of morphine for an analgesic effect, and that they also have higher risks of developing addiction. Sex differences have also been observed in preclinical studies. Female mice are more sensitive to the rewarding effects of morphine and, on the other hand, present a lower intensity in somatic and motivational manifestations during morphine withdrawal. Additionally, the possible target role of $GABA_B$-receptors is here analysed, and preliminary results of baclofen are here discussed. Both thematics should be relevant for clinical and preclinical research.

In Chap. 14, Professor Michel Bourin develops the topic of the neurobiology of addictions. He describes in detail the brain reward system and its relationship with the mesolimbic dopaminergic pathway and its destination, the Nucleus Accumbens Septi (NAS) or ventral striatum. He explains how with the repetition of rewarding stimuli lasting neurobiological changes are caused within the reward circuit and associated regions. This is evident, particularly, with drugs of addiction. The stimulation and consequent positive reinforcement are more intense with addictive drugs than with more common rewards. Neural adaptations occur, mainly in reward circuits and connected brain areas, which tend to be perpetuated. This explains the generation of complex changes in psychological and behavioural functions, linked to these neuroadaptations. This chapter constitutes a sample of knowledge and teaching capacity for transmission, updating and didactics.

Chapter 15 is dedicated by Prof. Dr Michel Bourin to animal models of addiction. He highlights the relevance of early management of addictive activity of molecules. It leads to techniques adequately adjusted to this purpose. Animal models constitute an accepted method designated to searching for these characteristics of new potentially addictive compounds. The acquisition of drug self-administration behaviour constitutes a valid animal model of addiction initiation. Consequently, the resumption of this behaviour after its extinction constitutes an animal model of relapse or “Craving”. Using these techniques, researchers developed new theories of addiction based primarily on knowledge of drugs that act on neurobiological substrates. This knowledge clarified the knowledge of the mechanisms and neuronal structures involved in these phenomena. These results, observed in animals, were translationally extrapolated to human conditions. It was a huge benefit in terms of research strategy. These findings also helped guide criteria for the design of clinical trials that evaluate possible compounds linked to drug dependence.

Prof. Dr Michel Bourin dedicates Chap. 16 to cocaine addiction. He initially highlights its consequences. These consequences may influence public health and economy. He establishes here the differences between recreational and controlled use of drugs of addiction. He distinguishes successive pathophysiological steps in addiction. In this process, the first stage results from an activation of brain's reward circuit. It is induced by the substance consumed. It may be also induced by a practice performed. Reward circuit is mediated by dopamine. The pathway involved is the mesolimbic dopaminergic pathway, which originates in the midbrain and projects to the NAS. If the consumption is repeated, it will induce a conditioning by a Pavlovian learning. Biologically, dopamine discharges will be gradually released in an anticipated manner. It constitutes a prediction of reward arrival. A new consumption is so promoted, reproducing the situation. The consumption (and related cues) promotes new consumptions, and when stopping consumption starts, withdrawal symptoms can emerge. This chapter constitutes an additional example of update and didactic abilities.

Chapter 17 is also dedicated by Prof. Dr Michel Bourin to benzodiazepine addiction. He considers it a difficult story. He considers benzodiazepines (BZD) as low-toxicity drugs. They act on $GABA_A$ receptors. These drugs have a very high therapeutic index. However, they exert some undesirable effects at therapeutic doses. These undesirable effects are more frequent in the elderly population. The main of them are memory and behavioural problems. It has been postulated that, regardless of age, the use of benzodiazepines also carries risks of abuse and psychological and physical dependence. Likewise, the existence of a withdrawal syndrome when stopping treatment has been affirmed. Furthermore, some evidences validated the idea of a withdrawal syndrome. It may arrive after discontinuation of planned or even unplanned treatment. The author considers very relevant at this point the fact that this condition is recognized within the DSM-V. This chapter is, again, a fusion of update and didactic abilities.

In Chap. 18 Professor Dr Walter Manucha and Virna Martín Giménez develops some interesting ideas about Phyto-, synthetic and endogenous cannabinoids as theoretical possibilities for therapeutic molecules in the treatment of addictions. They describe addiction as an emotional dysfunction accompanied by other symptoms like inadequate behaviour, difficulties in managing abstinence with high desires for consumption, loss of self-knowledge orientation and difficulties in the treatment with others. Their proposal consists mainly of new usable drugs. They consider certain phytocannabinoids (synthetic and endogenous), as possible acting agents as therapeutic molecules. Its use in these pathologies may be mediated through its action linked to multiple receptors. The authors also postulate that type 1 and 2 cannabinoid receptors may be used as targets for treatment in anti-addictive procedures. They postulate a possible role in treating addictions like alcohol, opioid, methamphetamine, cocaine and nicotine addictions.

In Chap. 19, Professor Dr. Walter Manucha and Virna Martín Giménez propose new nanotechnological approaches conceived as theoretical treatment possibilities in the addiction's treatment. The authors sustain that the science of nanomaterials has relevant possibilities in biological therapy. Nanoformulation promises to be a relevant topic for the development of new pharmacological approaches to therapeutics. This procedure may be an attractive tool optimizing the advantage of beneficial properties of drugs, minimizing their undesirable side effects. The idea is to influence pharmacodynamic and pharmacokinetic behaviour of drugs modifying physicochemical characteristics. It may improve therapeutic compliance of patients. Loading cannabinoids in nanoformulations is postulated. It may lead to greater efficacy and less toxicity. It may induce also a more controlled/prolonged release than cannabinoids in free form. A special attention is paid to summarize the main findings in the area to the applications of encapsulated cannabinoids to nanomedical strategies and applications. It must be remarked that the authors are referring here to potential therapeutic uses of cannabinoid derivates.

Prof. Dr Michel Bourin dedicates Chap. 20 to cannabis as a drug of addiction. The author rescues the popular conviction that cannabis derivatives are not *dangerous*, that they are a *soft* drug. This conception, more or less popular and more or less widespread, has led to an undervaluation of the risks of its consumption. Among other arguments, pointed out by the author, would be the claim that cannabis products do not lead to a physical withdrawal syndrome, unlike alcohol, opiates or benzodiazepines. Against this, Professor Bourin opposes the fact that we can be dependent without the need for the presence of a physical withdrawal syndrome. And this happens even if its presence is, in other cases, an aggravating factor. On the other hand, addiction always results in particularly evident discomfort when attempting suppression. The fact that a percentage of consumers end up addicted is relevant, even more so in the case of daily consumers. Today a withdrawal syndrome is recognized with states of irritability, insomnia, dysphoria and anxiety. The presence of a state of *craving*, such as an uncontrollable need to consume, has also been referred to. Last but not least, cannabis use has been identified as a pathway to the emergence of psychotic disorders. It is not clear whether it is cannabis that leads to schizophrenia or it is psychosis that leads to cannabis use. This chapter constitutes a demystification of the concept of the idea that cannabis, because it is a *natural* drug, does not generate health consequences.

In Chap. 21, the group directed by Carlos Alberto Tomaz and integrated by Asghar Alejafar, Saeid Charsouei, Ali Amadalipour and Adel Kashefi, deeply describes endocannabinoid system and postulates that it is a relevant cross-talk mechanism relating neurosciences and psychiatry. The endocannabinoid system is postulated as one of the main components of the nervous pathways involved in various physiological and mental functions. Like all neurotransmission systems, it integrates endogenous cannabinoids or endocannabinoids, their receptors and the enzymes involved in their degradation and biosynthesis. The activation of this system can be produced by *exogenous cannabinoids*. These are many compounds derived from *Cannabis sativa*. These compounds have been used since ancient times, both for recreational and medicinal purposes. This chapter reviews the functions of this system, as well as the theory of clinical endocannabinoid deficiency (CECD). The relationship between this system and various psychiatric conditions is exposed, and the possible role of this system with probiotic disorders is also studied. The possibility is raised here that the function of endocannabinoid signalling represents an important mechanism of many processes, both physiological and pathological. This chapter concludes that this system can be considered a potential target for future research on many mental disorders. This contribution stands out for its originality and broad points of observation. The authors link this system to several psychiatric entities, like depression, psychosis, epilepsy, stress and addiction.

Chapter 22 is dedicated to melatonin and the chronobiology of drug abuse. Professor Daniel Cardinali starts his chapter with the consideration that drug dependence is a multifactorial biological and behavioural disorder. According to it, he proposes psychosocial and pharmacological interventions. Unfortunately, these treatments do not usually have the expected results. In this chapter, he analyses the possibilities of melatonin to modify some aspects of addiction. Thus, evidence arising from research in experimental animal models and clinical trials in human beings is presented. Studies carried out in various areas of the brain, mainly associated with reward and emotionality, have yielded interesting results. Thus, the effectiveness of melatonin supplementation has been proven in various behavioural schemes. In the area of behaviour, this is the case of controlling drug-seeking behaviour and behavioural sensitization. At the cellular and molecular level, actions on neuroplasticity, prevention of autophagy, apoptosis, oxidative stress and mitochondrial neurotoxic lesions were observed. Given the interaction between the circadian system and drug addiction, the use of melatonin in addicted people may work well as a successful chronobiological strategy. This chapter is the result of years of experience and research work by the author.

In Chap.23, the relationship between sleep and psychotropic substances is developed by Dr. Vinicius Dokkedal Silva. The action of stimulants, depressants and hallucinogens is here deeply studied. Sleep may be interfered by this drug in a different manner. Different drugs acting on sleep are available in the market. These drugs act on sleep and behaviour by a multitude of mechanisms and pathways. The particularities of each drug need to be considered. It is very important in the case of assessing sleep in recreational substance users. The author mentions some special cases. Examples of this are hidden insomnia due to cocaine use and benzodiazepine withdrawal symptoms. For this reason, the author carries out an exhaustive analysis of the main substances with effects on sleep, focusing on the most recent findings. This leads to paying particular attention to the decisive role that sleep plays in the treatment of patients with substance use disorder. This is a truly up-to-date chapter on the topic, written by a renowned researcher on the subject.

In Chap. 24, Dra. Ana Sofía Vallés and Dr Francisco Barrantes focus on describing the role of acetylcholine receptors in drug addiction. For the writing of this chapter, they put into play their own extensive career in researching the topic. The need to recognize the circuits involved in addictions, considered as chronic neuropsychiatric disorders, is postulated. Various cholinergic receptors are described and classified, and those expressed in the mammalian brain are identified. Particular attention is paid to nicotinic acetylcholine receptors (nAChR). They assert that these receptors play a very relevant role in various addictive disorders. The receptor subtypes present great combinatorial diversity. This would have, as a behavioural correlate, a great functional diversity in drug-induced responses in different brain areas. Authors present a solid and documented development of the topic with its own findings.

In Chap. 25, links between neurobiological basis and behavioural features of craving are described. The chapter, written by Augusto Pascual Ítalo Gargiulo, Antonela Ariela Trovato, Ana Paula Colombini and Ángel José Martín Gargiulo, constitutes an interesting approach to pathophysiology of craving and, in a wider sense, a relevant example of neurobehavioural correlations. The authors affirm that craving has been a crucial concept in the topic of addictions since the 1990s. Given that its conceptualization is very relevant to the topic, and that there are no agreements on it, an attempt is made to give form to the idea and relate it to the underlying neurobiological mechanisms. This proposal is based on post-Skinnerian behaviourism, neuroscience and neural networks. Post-Skinnerian behaviourism integrates initial behaviourism and new knowledge of verbal behaviour, explained through relational framework theory. The triggers of desire and the way the brain processes this information are presented. The neurotransmitters and neural circuits involved are included. All this allows a more complete explanation of this phenomenon, with its clinical and therapeutic consequences. This is an actualized and complete update chapter on a central theme in the topic.

Chapter 26 is dedicated to the psychoneurobiology of dopaminergic pathways and the reward system. The authors, Dr Gustavo Tafet and Tomás Ortiz Alonso, provide an exhaustive description of the neurobiological mechanisms of reward and positive emotions. The mesolimbic (M-L), nigrostriatal (N-S) and mesocortical (M-C) dopaminergic pathways are described. The Nucleus Accumbens Septi (NAS) is mentioned, with other limbic structures. Its integrative role of dopaminergic impulses coming from the ventral tegmental area (VTA) and excitatory pathways coming from the prefrontal cortex (PFC) and the hippocampal formation is analysed here. A circuit of projections involved in salience and valence is proposed, which, associated with reward information, allows the detection and anticipation of the reward. The M-L is proposed as a "reward pathway". The N-S pathway acts by projections on the ventromedial Medial Prefrontal Cortex (MPC) influencing goal directed behaviours. These circuits are also involved with developing active coping strategies. This is a chapter of great interest in the correlations between brain structures and addictive and non-addictive behaviours.

In Chap. 27, Dr Adel Kashefi and Prof. Dr Carlos Alberto Tomaz focus on methylphenidate (MPH) and reward. They review the functional role of neurotransmitters in drug-seeking behaviour and relapse process. The authors recognize the important use of the psychostimulant MPH in hyperactivity disorder (ADHD) and narcolepsy. However, prolonged use of MPH may produce brain damage and long-term neuropsychiatric effects. It is the case of impaired cognitive function, changes in brain's reward circuit and, consecutively, addiction. Considering related structures, NAS and orbitofrontal cortex are recognized as two important regions involved in dopaminergic action, reward and appetitive conditioning. Regarding involved neurotransmitters, MPH acts on dopamine and noradrenaline inhibiting catecholamines reuptake. Behaviourally, MPH increases reward-seeking behaviours. Additionally, it also enhances motivation to self-administer amphetamine. MPH injections induce dopamine release. This fact activates signal transduction pathways that may modify learning-related molecular changes. The authors mention other neurotransmitter systems involved in reward. In this chapter, the authors comment and discuss their most recent findings on the topic of MPH conditioned place preference (CPP) test. His experiments have been carried out on both rodents and monkeys. They have found long-lasting rewarding drug effects with MPH. The authors propose the role of numerous mechanisms and neurotransmitters involved in both drug reward and relapse. They conclude by relating the regions involved in dependency with the structures linked to associative learning. Furthermore, the authors present possible reward pathways, changes in the intensity of neurotransmitter signalling, intracellular signalling and ultimately mechanisms and regions involved in drug reward and relapse. The inference from the literature mentioned in this review is that regions involved in central representations of predictive reward are a subset of those actually involved in associative learning.

The authors dedicate Chap. 28 to neurosteroids and their relationship with carcinogenesis and drug use, and the impact on the reproductive axis of drug abuse. Dra. Myriam Raquel Laconi, Antonella Rosario Ramona Cáceres, María de los Ángeles Sanhueza and Daniela Alejandra Cardone present the original results of their team. The authors describe the neuroesteroids' role, their association with carcinogenesis and the effects of drug abuse on them. They also analyse the impact of drug abuse on the reproductive axis. Neurosteroids play an essential role in the regulation of the hypothalamic-pituitary-gonadal axis. They are involved in the activities of reproductive physiology. It is the case of hypothalamic and sex hormone release, and the physiological variables involved in reproduction (ovulation, folliculogenesis, luteogenesis and male and female sexual response). Psychological variables (anxiety, memory, stress and depression) are also influenced by them. The authors describe biosynthesis and mechanisms of action, inducing fast and slow responses. In this chapter, the authors focus mainly on progesterone, allopregnanolone, pregnenolone and dehydroepiandrosterone. It is very interesting that the authors highlight that these neurosteroids may influence the effects induced by drugs such as cocaine and cannabis. By the inverse way, these drugs can affect serum levels of neurosteroids. The authors here discuss findings on interactions between neurosteroids and drugs of abuse, in animals and humans. They comment also their experiences with allopregnanolone, considering it an interesting molecule related to psychiatric and neurological pathologies. This chapter is an interesting integration between physiology end endocrine and psychiatric pathology.

The international group coordinated by Dr Manuel Alejandro Guevara presents Chap. 29. The main topic is ketamine actions. The action of ketamine, from anaesthesia to its addictive properties, is compiled here, including some mention of its antidepressant properties. This chapter reviews the effects of ketamine as a drug of abuse. Its recreational use was reliably documented in 1965. It occurred three years after its synthesis. Starting from that moment, its use as a street drug became rapidly diffused. The motive was due to several factors. These were its low cost, its rapid onset of action, its short duration of action and, particularly, its psychotropic effects. Among the psychotropic effects is the possibility of inducing states of psychosis as a glutamate antagonist. Some translational models based on this antagonist effect, which is pharmacologically specific, are reviewed here. Translational models of psychosis are reviewed, particularly in relation to the proposed pathophysiology of schizophrenic illnesses. At this point, evidence arising from findings from our laboratory is analysed. Finally, its uses are pointed out, from the classic one as an anaesthetic to the more recent ones, as a "recreational" drug. The risk of developing psychosis and brain damage is detailed.

The third section covers the topics of learning, teaching and the role of social environment. Its first section, Chap. 30 addresses issues related to executive functions, mainly working memory. In this chapter, written by us and Prof. Dra. Mirta Ison, we develop the theme of executive functioning. We postulate here the importance to think about contextualized ways to evaluate executive functions. It provides greater ecological validity. Executive functions (EFs) may be defined as cognitive skills. They are involved in activities that are novel to the individual. These activities require a creative solution. The evaluation of executive functioning performance should tend to reflect the actions that a person has in their daily life. This evaluation should reflect how to approach the exploration and measurement of executive functions. It challenges us to continue developing innovative and integrative evaluation proposals. Finally, we conclude that the most valid way to evaluate EF is by including and considering the characteristics and specificities of the individual's specific sociocultural context.

In Chap. 31, Prof. Dr Eric Wainright developed the theme of screen technology abuse and stress. Despite positive elements, recent technological advances have presented unexpected difficulties. It is the case of the existence of cell-phone addiction, and to other portable technologies. There is no agreement in the interpretation, the delimitation and the criteria regarding this disorder. The COVID-19 pandemic led to an exponential worldwide increase of internet use. Many businesses and home office activities operated during confinement, maintaining their continuity. Furthermore, these technological advances have allowed education to continue almost normally. However, behavioural changes in children related to excessive time of portable screen technologies worried educators and parents. Researchers highlight also the effects on normal people and mental health patients. The fact that the use of social media has also increased strikingly during the lockdown has been interpreted as a way to mitigate the psychological consequences of isolation in various populations. Cell phone abuse has been associated with other elements. It is the case of problems in impulse control disorders. It may also be the case of persons with extremely high self-esteem and extroverted. In both types of abuse, an association with stress, anxiety and depression has been found. Sleep disturbances have also been observed. Additionally, substance abuse like tobacco and alcohol has been linked to problematic cell phone use. This is a chapter of high interest in current living conditions.

Chapter 32 continues the theme of the previous chapter. The group integrated by Santiago Resett, María Emilia Oñate and Belén Mesurado presents the problem of addiction, mainly in adolescents and young people. They introduce the idea of "phubbing". This new concept refers to the act of ignoring others you are with, paying exclusive attention to the cell phone. Authors start noting benefits of information and communication technologies, highlighting more democratic access to knowledge, social connection and entertainment. On the other hand, they point out negative behaviours. It is the case of cyberbullying, trolling, grooming and phubbing. Because of the psychosocial costs it entails, phubbing attracted researcher's attention in a prevalent manner. Phubbing implies a disturbance in interpersonal communication due to a cell phone addiction. Its scientific study is incipient, mainly in Latin American countries. In this chapter, addiction to new technologies is conceptualized. Subsequently, the origin and evolution of the term "phubbing" is studied. Finally, scientific tools are detailed for measuring this new reality in adolescents and young people in Argentina. The authors end the chapter with guidelines for its detection and prevention. The present study illustrates in an interesting way a very recent disorder.

In Chap. 33, the thematic of social networks addiction in adolescents and young people is displayed. The effects of these behaviours and the possible approaches are here interestingly reviewed by the team directed by Elisa María Martínez Canales. They defined social networks addiction as uncontrolled and continued use of digital sites such as Twitter, Instagram or Facebook. These addicts lose control of using and, additionally, they avoid normal course of life. The authors propose a criterion for abuse of social networks, consisting of a time greater than 6 hours a day. If so, the person shows dependence on them. A state of euphoria prevails when using social networks, without considering the long-lost time and its consequences. Negative effects occur, such as difficulties working normally, sedentary lifestyle, social isolation and social withdrawal. Some health problems induced by abusive use of social networks are anxiety, depression, sleep disorders, withdrawal syndrome and low self-esteem. The authors define "nomophobia" as an anxiety for connecting to social networks. They can be text messages with WhatsApp or they can feel "dead" due to the impossibility of connecting to cyberspace. Finally, they propose some basic criteria to identify social networking addiction. It is, like the previous chapter, an interesting description of new social problems related to the use of new technologies.

Prof. Virginia Leonor Herbas Pacheco coordinated, in Chap. 34, an international-wide group in the area of educational procedures for patients with alcohol addiction. It has relevant content for medicine and nursing. The relevance of consequences of alcohol abuse starts this chapter. Consequences on individual and social mental health are here detailed. The alcoholism role creating risks for consumers as well as for the whole society is here studied. The role of alcoholism favouring the development of conflicts and other consequences are here also considered. There is a consensus reviewing articles that show that the biggest consumers, statistically, are adolescents and young adults. If they start alcohol consumption very early, the situation constitutes an actual public health problem. This chapter has a clear objective, trying to establish a criterion with the aim of promoting health education as a main pillar of public health. Doctors and nurses maintain active interaction with the individual, their family and the community. It is due to the type of constant care they carry out, aiming to help healthy and sick people. It plays an important role in positive influences. They consist in motivating favourable changes. These changes are present in lifestyle, and are exerted through teaching about the harmful effects of alcohol abuse and its deleterious consequences. The main thematic is related to present elements describing alcoholism and its consequences regarding self-care, autonomy, capacity for responsibility and the relevant individual's own resolution. A brief review and the corresponding evaluation of previous prevention intervention studies and suggested treatment activities are made. This chapter is an interesting prevention study in the field of alcoholism.

The next Chap. 35 is coordinated also by Prof. Virginia Leonor Herbas Pacheco, dedicated to foetal alcohol spectrum disorders (FASD). It is the result of a new coordination of an international team. This chapter starts considering the fact that alcohol consumption is a currently widespread and permissively habit for both men and women. However, it implies some risks, mainly in the pregnant women. In these women, alcohol represents a risk in the embryonic/foetal stage. Habits are previous to pregnancy. FASD constitute a wide range of diseases. They could occur as a consequence of consumption of alcohol during pregnancy. It would favour the presence of behavioural disorders along life. However, foetal alcohol spectrum disorders are absolutely preventable. The main form of intervention is the educational awareness. It should be directed to pregnant and non-pregnant women reducing risk and prevent harm. An important number of topics are here analysed. It is the case of neurocognitive findings and behavioural profile of the foetal alcohol spectrum disorder. It is also the case of neuropsychological disorders of FASD and autism. Other very important related topics are here studied. It is the case of alcohol as a teratogen, the animal models of FASD, preventive care procedures and suggested therapeutic approaches and complementary diagnostic methods. It is concluded that there is a need to increase information about the consequences of this consumption in order to prevent these disorders.

The fourth section is dedicated to explain human diseases and pathological behaviours. In it we group the chapters in which it is proposed a cerebral causality relationship with the observed disorder.

The first chapter in this section is Chap. 36. In it, Prof. Dr Guilherme Messas and Prof. Dr Maria Julia Soares raise the relevance of values in the decision-making process in the treatment of alcohol abuse disorders. The authors point that this involves bringing together complex and conflicting values linked to the patient. The fact that there are several possible treatments, both pharmacological and psychotherapeutic, allows for choices and, in this way, adaptation to the individual case as closely as possible. This has implications for the decision-making process. The authors maintain and highlight the need for the final objectives of therapy to be individualized for each case, for each patient. In some cases, it can lead to abstinence. In other treatments focused on generating harm, reduction can be carried out. Shared decisions are necessary to design an individualized treatment that focuses on the patient's own values. There must be intelligence between the clinical team, the patient and his family. A stronger therapeutic alliance is thus established. Treatment is better adjusted to needs and they can be better led to assume their responsibilities. All this is essential to structure the treatment in an effective way.

The second chapter of this section, Chap. 37, is led and coordinated by Prof. Dr Jorge Herrera. It is directed to study in a detailed manner the neuropsychological instruments for the evaluation of alcohol abuse disorders (AAD). This nosological entity constitutes a public health problem. It is due to the psychosocial and interpersonal disturbances originated in it. Additionally, it is also related to various medical illnesses and the personal costs it generates. Acute and chronic consequences of alcohol abuse on cognitive and adaptive functioning are here analysed and related to evaluation instruments. These are designed in order to study the patients with a history of this disorder with specific batteries. The authors provide here information on neuropsychological tools used to assess individuals with this condition. An extent number of tests are here detailed, with a brief comment of its use in recent publications. In this way, the tests are presented with a few examples of recent use, that are mentioned in each case. Measurement instruments cited in research studies led to demonstrate its use measuring the effects of alcohol abuse on specific cognitive functions. The chapter constitutes a solid contribution of a team working in the field since an important time ago.

In Chap. 38, our group, integrated by Norman Lopez, Jorge Herrera, Yuliana Flórez, César Castellanos and me, develops a chapter dedicated to the neurocognitive effects of substance abuse and their measurement using neuropsychological tests. Given that regular and intensive consumption of drugs of abuse brings severe consequences at a brain and functional level, abnormalities can be observed in neuropsychological tests. This is because consumption, by affecting various brain structures, can generate disorders of cognition and behaviour. An extensive number of tests are here studied. They are: Repeatable neuropsychological status assessment battery (RBANS), Mini-Mental State Examination, Rey Auditory Verbal Learning Test, Controlled Word Association Test, Halstead Category Test, Wisconsin Card Sorting Test, STROOP Colours and Words Test, Rey-Osterrieth Complex Figure Test, Benton Visual Retention Test, Symbols and Digits Test and the Halstead-Reitan Tracing Test. In all cases, it is done a review of the current state of knowledge and some recent publications using them are commented after it. These tests allow us to evaluate the neuropsychological effects of chronic drug use. This chapter analyses the main substances that have the potential to affect brain function and mental processes, especially executive functions. This is an effort to update the main tools for studying impairment induced by drugs of abuse.

In Chap. 39, Dra. Marcela Waisman campos and Dr Pablo Bagnati focus on cognitive dysfunctions in addictions. They start their chapter considering that progress in research on drug abuse has allowed today to a better understanding of the cellular and molecular mechanisms related to the positive and the negative reinforcing effects. Most reinforcement models were based on primary hedonic effects. They were induced by consumption of addictive substances. It is the case of conditioned place preference, paradigms of self-administration and intracranial self-stimulation, among others.

These animal models have inherent limitations that have been matter of critical considerations. Extrapolation of results is always difficult and has limitations. Application of such a knowledge implies a transferring of basic scientific results obtained in the lab to the daily medical practice. It is an actual challenge. In all cases, a singularization adjusted to the patient is necessary. By this reason, it is necessary to study the link between substance use disorders (SUD) and the cognitive function of the patient. This link has been studied in the case of alcohol, but now other substances that need to be studied have arisen. The authors describe the importance of a thorough and efficient evaluation of the patient's cognitive domains. The types of deficits found must also be assessed, establishing a relationship with consumption patterns. The influence that these cognitive deficits have must also be assessed, both at an acute functional level and in continued use. This chapter is an interesting example of interface between basic research and clinical practice.

Chapter 40 is dedicated to the face recognition as a tool in neuropsychiatric studies. The authors, Prof. Dra. María Clotilde Tavares, Prof. Dr Carlos Alberto Tomaz and Prof. Dra. Jessica Méndez de Souza, point out the importance of face perception study. It allows us particularly to study perception of emotional state and intentions. This capacity is confirmed in primates, but, particularly, in humans. In this sense, the human being has a great capacity to recognize innumerable faces. This ability is essential for human being in multiple aspects of everyday life. It is the case of socialization but also when impaired by neuropsychiatric disorders like autism, prosopagnosia and schizophrenia. The processing of faces and the brain areas involved in these processes are important tools for studying brain mechanisms and psychoses. This ability has been used for research purposes. It may be applied to human and non-human primates research. This chapter constitutes a very interesting link between basic and clinical research.

In Chap. 41, Luis Antón-Toro et al.'s review present conception of alcohol binge drinking in adolescents. With an interesting and provocative title, they raise the approach by asking the who, the how and the why. Last years, alcohol binge drinking (BD) has attracted attention because its increasing health and social concern. It is very relevant in adolescent population. This phenomenon is characterized by the ingestion of a large quantity of alcohol in brief intervals of time. The goal is achieving alcohol intoxication for leisure purposes. Prevalence is increasing rapidly in adolescents. This fact represents a potential health disorder considering that the vulnerability is greater in the adolescent brain. It is due to the fact that along adolescence, the brain goes through intense changes, in a process of maturation and refinement of its anatomical and functional properties. Structures such as fronto-subcortical and prefrontal circuits can be affected or damaged by early alcohol consumption. This fact would later facilitate the lack of inhibitory control of alcohol consumption. Additionally, decision-making may be worsening, facilitating careless intake. Numerous neuropsychological and neuroimaging studies have shown consequences of BD practice. Longitudinal studies are necessary to understand the conditions that would make some individuals at risk of behaviours like BD. This chapter constitutes a wide overview of state of the art of BD along adolescence.

Chapter 42 is dedicated to the distinctive features of magnetoencephalography (MEG) and electroencephalography (EEG) of healthy and pathological ageing. Written by a large team, the first author is Dr Brenda Nadia Chino-Vilca, and the team is led by Prof. Dr Fernando Maestú. The field studied is the electrical neurophysiology of normal ageing and pathological processes. In the brain, as in the whole organism, the accumulation of small alterations over time leads to loss of function. Along the ageing process, this phenomenon is observed in healthy and pathological conditions. In the brain, it is correlated to significant alterations in the brain oscillatory activity. Inside the brain, weak magnetic and electric fields are generated by electric currents, and they may be detected by two non-invasive techniques, magnetoencephalography (MEG) and electroencephalography (EEG). These techniques allow studies of resting or task-based states. These procedures may be used for the study of ageing and brain damage, but also to study the influence of lifestyle in the prevention and promotion of health. This chapter should be considered as a relevant milestone in the study of the brain and its alterations.

Dr. Nicolás Fayed and his team offer Chap. 43, referring to a historical approach to brain imaging. This group, integrated also by Dra. Alicia Fayed and Dr Humberto Morales, review the techniques that allowed us to understand the human brain, following a sequential path. They describe the course of advances from the time of Ramón y Cajal to the present day. They postulate that efforts to understand the brain are very important, and are necessary to improve the understanding of our origins and future pathways of evolution. The authors describe multiple advances of the neurosciences. They mention the role of multiple new subdivisions, aiming to incorporate new realities regarding brain structure and function. They mention the well-recognized disciplines, like neuroanatomy, neurophysiology and neuropharmacology. However, they postulate that today it is necessary to incorporate other emerging subdisciplines, like neuro-genetic or computational neuroanatomy. Fayed et al. describe the successive moments of brain study, starting from the initial studies of Ramón y Cajal, following for other techniques and conceptions like cortex cartography and studies of blood flow. They finally end describing recent imaging techniques. This is an extremely interesting chapter, with extensive reference to the study of the brain in its historical face and up to the present day.

Chapter 44, written by the same team and with Dr Humberto Morales as first author, is dedicated to neuroimaging in drug and substance abuse. As a continuation of the previous chapter, in this review application of image studies to the effect of drugs is presented. Starting from drug abuse as a public health problem, the authors affirm that cannabis is the most consumed drug. Heroin is the elected opiate, and alcohol is a legal drug but its chronic abuse is associated with demonstrated morbidity. The most common complications of illicit drug abuse are hypoxic-ischemic injuries or cerebrovascular diseases. They consider that on imaging studies, the prevalent findings include intracranial haemorrhage, stroke, infectious changes, chronic leuko-encephalopathy and atrophic changes. More detailed post-mortem examinations exhibit an extensive damage in the brain. It seems to be very relevant and more diffuse in grey and white matter. The vasculature and the blood-brain barrier are affected by drug effect. It has been reported that Parkinson's disease can be associated with drug abuse. Neuroimaging is today offering findings not only in acute events but also in chronic processes due to neurological consequences of drug abuse. This chapter constitutes a continuation of the previous, focusing in the application of neuroimages to drug abuse.

In Chap. 45, Dr Ricardo Marcos Pautassi and his team propose drinking to cope as a vulnerability factor to alcohol use disorder. They invoke evidence from clinical and preclinical research. They posit alcohol use disorder (AUD) as a chronic condition in which the patient continues to drink despite recognizing the consequences, such as the association with negative occupational, social and health consequences. The authors maintain that there are factors that promote and determine risky alcohol consumption and AUD. For this reason, it may be considered vulnerability factors and protective factors. In turn, these factors can be described as distal. This means that they interact with other closer factors, such as the reasons for drinking. The pharmacological effects of ethanol and individual sensitivity to it also play a role as close factors. The phenomenon of the appearance of signs or "clues" related to alcohol is not minor. This chapter represents a rigorous approach to some very core facts of alcoholism.

Prof. Dra. María José Polache and her team, integrated by Sandra Fernández-Rodríguez, María José Cano-Cebrián and Teodoro Zornoza, explore, in Chap. 46, the neurobiology of the ethanol relapse and its prevention. They study the role of N-Acetyl-cysteine in these treatment possibilities. They start from the affirmation that alcohol use disorder (AUD) has a high relapse rate. It makes this disorder a very complex and chronic illness. The authors propose the resumption of alcohol consumption after a long period of abstinence as one of the most serious situations of this pathology. For this reason, relapse has been particularly studied in this pathology. Particular attention has been paid to the underlying mechanisms. To this end, several preclinical models have been used. Here they are analysed, evaluating their advantages and drawbacks. The authors analyse what they consider a very interesting model, with high translational power, and based mainly on the alcohol deprivation effect (ADE). This model is also the most used preclinical approach to relapse. This form is accepted given its facial, ecological and predictive validity. The authors describe their results, commenting the effects of N-acetylcysteine (NAC) as a possible substance for relapse preventing. This chapter describes with brightness relapse mechanisms and their possible treatment.

Chapter 47 is dedicated to the effects of psychoactive drugs on the brain. The author, Prof. Dr. Raúl Gagliardi, a recognized scientific leader in Europe and Argentina, proposes a variety of mechanisms involved in acute and chronic brain responses to drugs. In this schedule, addiction is considered as a chronic disease. It needs time to develop and overcome with difficulty. These psychoactive drugs can have long-term effects producing addiction. This addiction phenomenon needs consume persistence, even after abstinence periods. The negative effects on the addict are here detailed. Consequences on the individual addict, his family and the social environment are here mentioned. Two different positions regarding personal responsibility are here described by the author. He describes that some studies focus on individual responsibility, while others in social environment. It is mentioned, finally, that some studies consider the role of the addict's genetic. The interference of drugs on brain's communication system is here developed. Brain areas involved in development of addictions are here deeply studied. The role of psychoactive drugs altering the reward centre function modifying the action of neurotransmitters, mainly dopamine, is here widely and clearly explained. Drug-induced epigenetic modifications are here explained in a bright manner. In this chapter, very distant perspectives are interestingly integrated. It constitutes a wide view of multiple interrelated variables.

Chapter 48 constitutes a new and interesting approach to addiction. In this chapter, Prof. Dr. Raúl Gagliardi addresses the issue of drug abuse in adolescents. He considers that it is a widespread situation, with a very high number of consequences, involving problems with the law and existential limitations. In some cases, death is the consequence. The author remarks that cessation of the addiction phenomenon does not start with a simple intention. Changes in the brain are related to compulsive abuse. Risks of developing drug addiction are here presented in an interesting way. Factors influencing it include biological constitution, social environment and age or stage in which these processes are initiated. The most frequent drugs used by adolescents are alcohol and marijuana. Alcohol, cocaine and methamphetamines may induce violent behaviours, and some drugs increase the suicide risk. Overdoses are a dangerous fact that induces a very high number of deaths worldwide. The author points out that a responsible attitude towards oneself and others is a fundamental element to avoid drug consumption. The entire family and educators can recognize drug abuse and can help the adolescent stop using it. Addiction is defined as a profound transformation of the processes of autopoiesis (self-building), homeorhesis (dynamic systems that allow an individual's life possible) and homeostasis (changes in stability). This chapter is a new interesting and transcendent contribution of the author to biology and consequences of addiction.

In Chap. 49, Dr Ralph Meyers brings in his chapter 30 years of psychiatric clinical experience on the subject of early detection and treatment options for psychosis in transition from childhood to adolescence. He remembers that in the 1980s they worked with young adults with psychosis. Very often they had a history of drug abuse. They worked with limited medications, and there were concepts that were not clearly established. They decided to start with a systemic therapy concept. This took place in a room with psychotic patients aged 18 to 30 years. A training programme was established to bring them closer to a healthier life. At that time, there was no experience combining individual therapies and education for the patient's family. These and other limitations of adult psychiatry led the author to dedicate himself to child and adolescent psychiatry. In this subspecialty, family therapy was used to make diagnoses earlier and improve the results obtained in adult psychiatry. In this chapter, Dr Meyers provides a case list of patients from his interesting personal experience. He also introduces the importance of detecting siblings with psychosis, and establishes individual relationships with drug consumption. He mentions a Canadian study and another German study on psychosis and drug use. Relationships between adult psychiatry and child and adolescent psychiatry are proposed. This is a chapter of high clinical value written by an experienced professional.

Chapter 50 is dedicated to the diagnosis and the management of attention-deficit/hyperactivity disorder (ADHD) in patients with comorbid substance use disorder. The author, Prof. Dra. Betsy BUSCH, is an active clinical researcher in the field. She postulates that ADHD must be considered a common precursor and a comorbidity in treatment of substance use disorders (SUDs). This statement would be supported by the fact that up to one in four patients presenting SUD may have a comorbid ADHD. Furthermore, the author postulates common neurobiological features for both disorders. Clinically, both have a chronic course and severe functional impairments. She adds that untreated childhood ADHD may lead to comorbidities SUD+ADHD, that worse the prognostic of SUDs, and that treatment of comorbid ADHD may improve it. In this context, the screening and diagnosis of ADHD seems to be very important, and a specific treatment may improve significantly the course of the disorder. It should be realized using a double schedule: pharmacological and psychotherapeutic. The second one would be cognitive-behavioural psychotherapy (CBT). This would be better in the form of specifically adapted ADHD-specific skills training, i.e. "integrated CBT". ADHD treatment have shown benefit to patients suffering SUD+ADHD. This chapter is a broad set of arguments about the advantages of combining both treatments in SUD+ADHD, made by a prominent specialist with extensive experience in clinical research and consultation.

In Chap. 51, written by the group of Prof. Dr Miriam Melis, and integrated by Claudia Sagheddu and Giuseppe Virdis, the authors review the stigma to therapy. They develop the evolution of psychiatry in substance use disorders (SUDs). The authors consider that drug addiction has been considered a mind disorder. It implies that it has factors underlying this phenomenon of lack of willpower and moral failing. It has been proposed that these factors may be psychological, economic and social factors. Since the term addiction still has a negative connotation, there are still prejudices about drug addicts today. They are considered weak individuals, responsible for their fragility. This can lead to social exclusion and lack of attendance. Finally, these situations can be elements that make it impossible or prevent a change in attitude. Stigma prevails over the possibilities of help individuals with SUDs. By this reason, important efforts have been developed in the past century aiming to study the biological bases of SUDs. It is currently accepted that SUD is a chronic, recurring brain disease, characterized by a wide range of symptoms that lead to loss of control leading to drug seeking and ingestion, ignoring the consequences. Different chemicals lead to brain alterations in circuits involved with emotions, motivation and, finally, behaviour. For all this, SUD is considered today a brain disease. This conceptual modification has led to the reduction of subjective moral judgment. It has also modified the position of the addict. Finally, it has led to a development of pharmacological and psychotherapeutic therapies that, together, have led to a better therapeutic approach. The authors provide, in this chapter, deep elements for a wide an interesting positions reconsideration in this area.

In a very original Chap. 52, an original and amazing proposal is drawn by Javier Bernacer, Julia Velez-Ramos and José Ignacio Murillo. They suggest the addiction as a rigid disposition towards akratic actions. They consider that classical theories of SUDs addiction suppose that the addicted person is not able to control his tendencies to drug consumption. However, the authors cite evidences of an intentional and free behaviour affronting drugs by the consumers. The new models interpret substance addiction as an akratic behaviour. This fact could be interpreted as an amazing interdisciplinary effort destined to the comprehension of the phenomenology of these disorders. They define akratic behaviour as an action against reason, even knowing the best course of action according to reason. The authors conceive addiction as a rigid habit that leads to akratic actions. They first cite and present the studies of Heather, conceiving addiction as an akrasia. In a second moment, they present platonic and Aristotelian notions of akrasia. In this point, positions of Amelie Rorty and Alfred Mele are analysed. In third place, authors explain their personal position about habits. They explain the Aristotelian notion of habits, and they postulate that addiction and akrasia could be understood as habits. In this way, they adopt the criterion to distinguish good habits (those that are flexible) of bad habits (those that are rigid). This criterion is the cognitive enrichment. The authors argue that since addiction is acquired through cognitively impoverished actions, addiction can be considered a bad habit that leads the person towards acratic actions. In this context, it is considered that a certain deliberative capacity is preserved. But the rigid and automatic nature generated by addiction clearly conflicts with entirely intentional behaviour. The authors conclude that the relationship between addiction and akrasia is illuminated by the Aristotelian notion of habit. The present interpretation constitutes an amazing renovation in the field of addictive behaviours, and the whole chapter becomes in this manner a very relevant point of view in the interpretation of this kind of behaviour.

Chapter 53 is dedicated by María Contreras, José Víctor Orón and Francisco Güell, to the relationships between attachment and pornography addiction. The authors draw attention to the fact that in societies with free access to the Internet, a significant increase in the consumption of pornography is being observed. Many consider their own consumption as problematic, and refer to it for its consequences. These include loneliness, family disturbances, work inadaptations, interpersonal difficulties and mental health problems. All of them would be related to isolation and feelings of loneliness. There has been much discussion about whether to consider pornography addiction within psychiatric disorders. In fact, this addiction has been included within the symptoms of hypersexual disorder (HSD). All this makes this topic relevant. Different theorizations have been proposed to address this problem. Recently, a relationship between this addiction and attachment style has been proposed. It has been suggested that its development would originate and begin in interpersonal difficulties with the main attachment figures. In this way, the possibility is supported that these people have this type of behaviour in order to alleviate unresolved conflicts of early affectivity. This is an original and innovative chapter, which opens a new panorama for the interpretation of addictive behaviours, relating them to early experiences.

Guayamallén, Mendoza, Argentina Pascual Ángel Gargiulo

Contents

Part II From Basic Neurosciences to Human Brain

The original version of the book has been revised. A correction to this book can be found at https://doi.org/10.1007/978-3-031-72219-6_54

Contributors

Andrés Acuña Laboratorio de Neurociencias y Psicología Experimental, Fundación Corporación Tecnológica Latinoamericana (FUCOTEL), Cátedra de Psicopatología, Facultad de Humanidades y Ciencias Económicas, Universidad Católica Argentina (UCA), Área de Farmacología, Facultad de Ciencias Médicas, Universidad Nacional de Cuyo (UNCuyo), Consejo Nacional de Investigaciones Científicas y Técnicas (CONICET), Mendoza, Argentina

Osvaldo Agamennoni Laboratorio de Desarrollo en Neurociencias Cognitivas (CIC—UNS), Universidad Nacional del Sur—Depto. de Ingeniería Eléctrica y de Computadoras, Instituto de Investigaciones en Ingeniera Eléctrica (IIIE—UNS CONICET), Comisión de Investigaciones Científicas de la Provincia de Buenos Aires, Bahía Blanca, Argentina

Pascual Jiménez Aguilar Carrera de Enfermería. Facultad Ciencias de la Salud, Universidad Técnica de Oruro, Universidad Técnica de Oruro (UTO), Oruro, Bolivia

Ali Ahmadalipour Research Center of Psychiatry and Behavioral Sciences, Tabriz University of Medical Sciences, Tabriz, Iran

Asghar Alejafar Faculty of Medicine, Department of Neurology, Tabriz University of Medical Sciences, Tabriz, Iran

Luis Echarte Alonso Humanities and Medical Ethics Unit, School of Medicine, University of Navarra, Pamplona, Spain

Vida Amiri Jahed Research Center of Psychiatry and Behavioral Sciences, Tabriz University of Medical Sciences, Tabriz, Iran

Luis Fernando Antón-Toro Department of Experimental Psychology, Complutense University of Madrid (UCM), Madrid, Spain

Center for Cognitive and Computational Neuroscience (C3N), University Complutense of Madrid (UCM), Madrid, Spain

Faculty of Health, Department of Psychology, University Camilo José Cela (UCJC), Madrid, Spain

Miriam Dolly Arancibia Cátedra de Filosofía Social, Departamento de Sociología, Facultad de Ciencias Sociales, Universidad Nacional de San Juan, San Juan, Argentina

Ricardo Aranovich Fundación Acta, Ciudad de Buenos Aires, Argentina

Ana María Arias Carrera de Enfermería. Facultad Ciencias de la Salud, Universidad Técnica de Oruro (UTO), Oruro, Bolivia

Ruth Ávila Herbas Carrera de Enfermería, Facultad Ciencias de la Salud, Universidad Técnica de Oruro, Universidad Técnica de Oruro (UTO), Oruro, Bolivia

Pablo M. Bagnati Department of Cognitive Neurology, Neuropsychiatry and Neuropsychology, Instituto de Investigaciones Neurológicas "Raúl Carrea", Fundación para la Lucha contra las Enfermedades Neurológicas de la Infancia (FLENI), Buenos Aires, Argentina

Graciela Noemí Balerio Facultad de Farmacia y Bioquímica, Cátedra de Farmacología e Instituto de Investigaciones Farmacológicas (ININFA-UBA-CONICET), Universidad de Buenos Aires, Ciudad Autónoma de Buenos Aires, Argentina

Francisco J. Barrantes Biomedical Research Institute (BIOMED), UCA-CONICET, Buenos Aires, Argentina

Iker Barrutieta Arberas LaNCE-Neuropharm Research Group, Facultad de Medicina y Enfermería, Department of Neurosciences, University of the Basque Country (UPV-EHU), Leioa, Spain

Iker Barrutieta-Arberas LaNCE-Neuropharm Research Group, Facultad de Medicina y Enfermería, Dep Neurosciences, University of the Basque Country (UPV-EHU), Leioa, Spain

Javier Bernacer Mind-Brain Group, Institute for Culture and Society (ICS), University of Navarra, Pamplona, Spain

International Center for Neuroscience and Ethics (CINET), Fundación Tatiana, Madrid, Spain

Michel Bourin Neurobiologie de l'anxiété et de la dépression, Université de Nantes, Nantes, France

Neurobiology of Anxiety and Mood Disorders, University of Nantes, Nantes, France

Adrián J. Bravo Department of Psychological Sciences, William & Mary, Williamsburg, VA, USA

Francesca Brencio Member of the Research Group "Filosofía Aplicada: Sujeto, Sufrimiento, Sociedad," Andalusian Research Plan, Code: PADI-HUM-018, University of Seville, Seville, Spain

José E. Burgos Universidad de Guadalajara, Centro de Estudios e Investigaciones en Comportamiento, Guadalajara, Jalisco, Mexico

Betsy Busch Tufts University School of Medicine, Boston, MA, USA

Antonella Rosario Ramona Cáceres Laboratorio de Fisiopatología ovárica, Instituto de Medicina y Biología Experimental de Cuyo IMBECU-CONICET, Mendoza, Argentina

Cátedra de Fisiología y Biofísica. Facultad de Ingeniería y Facultad de Ciencias Médicas, Universidad de Mendoza, Mendoza, Argentina

Juan Ernesto Calderón Faculty of Philosophy and Letters, Facultad de Filosofía y Letras, Department of Philosophy, Universidad Nacional de Cuyo, Centro Universitario, Mendoza, Argentina

Nicole Caldichoury Departamento de Ciencias Sociales, Universidad de Los Lagos, Los Lagos, Chile

M. José Cano-Cebrián Faculty of Pharmacy, Department of Pharmacy and Pharmaceutical Technology and Parasitology, University of Valencia, Valencia, Spain

Daniel P. Cardinali Faculty of Medical Sciences, Pontificia Universidad Católica Argentina, Buenos Aires, Argentina

Daniela Alejandra Cardone Laboratorio de Fisiopatología ovárica, Instituto de Medicina y Biología Experimental de Cuyo IMBECU- CONICET, Mendoza, Argentina

Cátedra de Fisiología y Biofísica. Facultad de Ingeniería y Facultad de Ciencias Médicas, Universidad de Mendoza, Mendoza, Argentina

Cesar Castellanos Instituto Dominicano para el Estudio de la Salud Integral y la Psicología Aplicada (IDESIP), Santo Domingo, República Dominicana

Santiago Castiello Department of Experimental Psychology, University of Oxford, Oxford, UK

Saeid Charsouei Faculty of Medicine, Department of Neurology, Tabriz University of Medical Sciences, Tabriz, Iran

Brenda Chino Center for Cognitive and Computational Neuroscience (C3N), Complutense University of Madrid, Madrid, Spain

Institute of Neuroscience, Autonomous University of Barcelona (UAB), Barcelona, Spain

Achucarro Basque Center for Neuroscience, Leioa, Spain

Ana Paula Colombini Laboratorio de Neurociencias y Psicología Experimental. Fundación Corporación Tecnológica Latinoamericana (FUCOTEL). Cátedra de Psicopatología. Facultad de Humanidades y Ciencias Económicas. Universidad Católica Argentina (UCA). Área de Farmacología. Facultad de Ciencias Médicas, Universidad Nacional de Cuyo (UNCuyo). Consejo Nacional de Investigaciones Científicas y Técnicas (CONICET), Mendoza, Argentina

Centro Integral de Salud Mental Argentino (CISMA), Buenos Aires, Argentina

Hospital Bernardino Rivadavia, Buenos Aires, Argentina

María Contreras Mind-Brain Group, ICS, University of Navarra, Pamplona, Spain

Faculty of Education and Psychology, University of Navarra, Pamplona, Spain

Juan Carlos Coronado Facultad de Ciencias de la Salud, Universidad Católica de Temuco, Araucanía, Chile

Ángeles Correas Department of Experimental Psychology, Complutense University of Madrid (UCM), Madrid, Spain

María de los Ángeles Sanhueza Laboratorio de Fisiopatología ovárica, Instituto de Medicina y Biología Experimental de Cuyo IMBECU- CONICET, Mendoza, Argentina

Jaisalmer de Frutos Lucas Center for Cognitive and Computational Neuroscience (C3N), Complutense University of Madrid, Madrid, Spain

Department of Experimental Psychology, Complutense University of Madrid, Madrid, Spain

Centre for Precision Health, Edith Cowan University, Joondalup, WA, Australia

Alberto del Cerro León Department of Experimental Psychology, Complutense University of Madrid (UCM), Madrid, Spain

Faculty of Health, Department of Psychology, University Camilo José Cela (UCJC), Madrid, Spain

Luis Enrique Echarte Alonso Humanities and Medical Ethics Unit, School of Medicine, University of Navarra, Pamplona, Navarra, Spain

Luis Enrique Echarte Humanities and Medical Ethics Unit, School of Medicine, University of Navarra, Pamplona, Navarra, Spain

Maryam Farrahizadeh Faculty of Advanced Technologies in Medicine, Department of Neuroscience, Iran University of Medical Sciences, Tehran, Iran

Alicia Fayed Department of Hematology, Hospital Miguel Servet, Zaragoza, Spain

Nicolás Fayed Department of Radiology, Section of Neuroradiology, Quirónsalud Hospital, Zaragoza, Spain

Sandra Fernández-Rodríguez Faculty of Pharmacy, Department of Pharmacy and Pharmaceutical Technology and Parasitology, University of Valencia, Valencia, Spain

Yuliana Flórez Yuliana Departamento de Ciencias Sociales, Universidad de La Costa, Barranquilla, Colombia

Departamento de Ciencias Sociales, Universidad de La Costa, Barranquilla, Colombia

Raul Gagliardi International Center for Migrations, Health, and Development, Geneva, Switzerland

Luis Miguel García-Moreno Department of Psychobiology and Methodology in Behavioral Sciences, Complutense University of Madrid (UCM), Madrid, Spain

Ángel José Martín Gargiulo Laboratorio de Neurociencias y Psicología Experimental. Fundación Corporación Tecnológica Latinoamericana (FUCOTEL). Cátedra de Psicopatología. Facultad de Humanidades y Ciencias Económicas. Universidad Católica Argentina (UCA). Área de Farmacología. Facultad de Ciencias Médicas, Universidad Nacional de Cuyo (UNCuyo). Consejo Nacional de Investigaciones Científicas y Técnicas (CONICET), Mendoza, Argentina

Centro Integral de Salud Mental Argentino (CISMA), Buenos Aires, Argentina

Facultad de Medicina, IBCN (Instituto de Biología Celular y Neurociencias)-CONICET, UBA (Universidad de Buenos Aires), Buenos Aires, Argentina

Augusto Pascual Ítalo Gargiulo Laboratorio de Neurociencias y Psicología Experimental. Fundación Corporación Tecnológica Latinoamericana (FUCOTEL). Cátedra de Psicopatología. Facultad de Humanidades y Ciencias Económicas. Universidad Católica Argentina (UCA). Área de Farmacología. Facultad de Ciencias Médicas, Universidad Nacional de Cuyo (UNCuyo). Consejo Nacional de Investigaciones Científicas y Técnicas (CONICET), Mendoza, Argentina

Centro Integral de Salud Mental Argentino (CISMA), Buenos Aires, Argentina

Marcos Constantino Josué Gargiulo Laboratorio de Neurociencias y Psicología Experimental. Fundación Corporación Tecnológica Latinoamericana (FUCOTEL). Cátedra de Psicopatología. Facultad de Humanidades y Ciencias Económicas. Universidad Católica Argentina (UCA). Área de Farmacología. Facultad de Ciencias Médicas, Universidad Nacional de Cuyo (UNCuyo). Consejo Nacional de Investigaciones Científicas y Técnicas (CONICET), Mendoza, Argentina

Centro Integral de Salud Mental Argentino (CISMA), Buenos Aires, Argentina

María Teresa Gargiulo Departamento de Filosofía, Facultad de Filosofía y Letras, Universidad Nacional de Cuyo/CONICET, Mendoza, Argentina

Mercedes María Lucrecia Gargiulo Laboratorio de Neurociencias y Psicología Experimental. Fundación Corporación Tecnológica Latinoamericana (FUCOTEL). Cátedra de Psicopatología. Facultad de Humanidades y Ciencias Económicas. Universidad Católica Argentina (UCA). Área de Farmacología. Facultad de Ciencias Médicas, Universidad Nacional de Cuyo (UNCuyo). Consejo Nacional de Investigaciones Científicas y Técnicas (CONICET), Mendoza, Argentina

Centro Integral de Salud Mental Argentino (CISMA), Buenos Aires, Argentina

Pascual Ángel Gargiulo Laboratory of Neurosciences and Experimental Psychology, Latin American Technological Corporation Foundation (FUCOTEL), Cathedra of Psychopathology, Catholic University of Argentina, Area of Pharmacology, Department of Pathology, National University of Cuyo, CONICET, Guaymallén, Mendoza, Argentina

Rocco J. Gennaro Department of Political Science and Philosophy, LAC 3055, University of Southern Indiana, Evansville, IN, USA

Francisco Güell Mind-Brain Group, ICS, University of Navarra, Pamplona, Spain

Manuel Alejandro Guevara Laboratorio de Neurociencias y Psicología Experimental. Fundación Corporación Tecnológica Latinoamericana (FUCOTEL). Cátedra de Psicopatología. Facultad de Humanidades y Ciencias Económicas. Universidad Católica Argentina (UCA). Área de Farmacología. Facultad de Ciencias Médicas, Universidad Nacional de Cuyo (UNCuyo). Consejo Nacional de Investigaciones Científicas y Técnicas (CONICET), Mendoza, Argentina

Evelina Haralanova Department of Psychiatry and Medical Psychology, Medical University of Sofia, Sofia, Bulgaria

First Psychiatric Clinic, University Hospital for Neurology and Psychiatry "St. Naum", Sofia, Bulgaria

Svetlozar Haralanov Department of Psychiatry and Medical Psychology, Medical University of Sofia, Sofia, Bulgaria

First Psychiatric Clinic, University Hospital for Neurology and Psychiatry "St. Naum", Sofia, Bulgaria

Virginia Leonor Herbas Pacheco Carrera de Enfermería. Facultad Ciencias de la Salud, Universidad Técnica de Oruro (UTO), Oruro, Bolivia

Ruth Ávila Herbas Carrera de Enfermería. Facultad Ciencias de la Salud, Universidad Técnica de Oruro (UTO), Oruro, Bolivia

Jorge Herrera College of Medicine Florida International University, FL, USA

Maryam Homaei Research Center of Psychiatry and Behavioral Sciences, Tabriz University of Medical Sciences, Tabriz, Iran

Leila Hosseinzadeh Anvar Department of Neurology, Faculty of Medicine, Tabriz University of Medical Sciences, Tabriz, Iran

Mirta Susana Ison Zintilini Human, Social and Environmental Science Institute of the National Scientific and Technical Research Council (INCIHUSA—CONICET), Technological Scientific Centre (CCT Mendoza-CONICET), Mendoza, Argentina

Faculty of Psychology, Aconcagua University, Mendoza, Argentina

Pascual Jiménez Aguilar Carrera de Enfermería. Facultad Ciencias de la Salud, Universidad Técnica de Oruro (UTO), Oruro, Bolivia

Adel Kashefi Laboratory of Neuroscience and Behavior, Institute of Biology, University of Brasília, Brasilia, DF, Brazil

Laboratory of Neurosciences and Behavior, Department of Physiological Sciences, University of Brasilia, Brasília, Brazil

Laboratory of Learning and Memory, Research Center and Department of Physiology, School of Medicine, Semnan University of Medical Sciences, Semnan, Iran

Myriam Raquel Laconi Laboratorio de Fisiopatología ovárica, Instituto de Medicina y Biología Experimental de Cuyo IMBECU- CONICET, Mendoza, Argentina

Cátedra de Fisiología y Biofísica. Facultad de Ingeniería y Facultad de Ciencias Médicas, Universidad de Mendoza, Mendoza, Argentina

José Vicente Lafuente Sánchez LaNCE-Neuropharm Research Group, Dep Neurosciences, Facultad de Medicina y Enfermería, University of the Basque Country (UPV-EHU), Leioa, Spain

José Vicente Lafuente LaNCE-Neuropharm Research Group, Facultad de Medicina y Enfermería, Department of Neurosciences, University of the Basque Country (UPV-EHU), Leioa, Spain

Adriana Inés Landa de Gargiulo Laboratorio de Neurociencias y Psicología Experimental. Fundación Corporación Tecnológica Latinoamericana (FUCOTEL). Cátedra de Psicopatología. Facultad de Humanidades y Ciencias Económicas. Universidad Católica Argentina (UCA). Área de Farmacología. Facultad de Ciencias Médicas, Universidad Nacional de Cuyo (UNCuyo). Consejo Nacional de Investigaciones Científicas y Técnicas (CONICET), Mendoza, Argentina

Andrés Ledezma Centro de Investigación en Gerontología Aplicada (CIGAP), Facultad de Salud, Universidad Santo Tomas, Antofagasta, Chile

Escuela de Kinesiología, Facultad de Salud, Universidad Santo Tomás, Antofagasta, Chile

Luis Hernán Llano Laboratorio de Neurociencias y Psicología Experimental, Fundación Corporación Tecnológica Latinoamericana (FUCOTEL), Cátedra de Psicopatología, Facultad de Humanidades y Ciencias Económicas, Universidad Católica Argentina (UCA), Área de Farmacología, Facultad de Ciencias Médicas, Universidad Nacional de Cuyo (UNCuyo), Consejo Nacional de Investigaciones Científicas y Técnicas (CONICET), Mendoza, Argentina

Ricardo Jorge Llanque Ferrufino Antropólogo, Carrera de Antropología, Universidad Técnica de Oruro, Oruro, Bolivia

Norman Darío López Velásquez Centro de Investigación e Innovación en Gerontología Aplicada (CIGAP), Facultad de Salud, Universidad Santo Tomas, Temuco, Chile

Carrera de Kinesiología, Facultad de Salud, Universidad Santo Tomás, Temuco, Chile

Norman López Escuela de Kinesiología, Facultad de Salud, Universidad Santo Tomás, Temuco, Chile

Centro de Investigación en Gerontología Aplicada (CIGAP), Universidad Santo Tomas, Temuco, Chile

Fernando Maestú Department of Experimental Psychology, Complutense University of Madrid (UCM), Madrid, Spain

Center for Cognitive and Computational Neuroscience, Complutense University of Madrid, Madrid, Spain

Instituto de Investigación Sanitaria San Carlos (IdISSC), Madrid, Spain

Walter Manucha Área de Farmacología, Departamento de Patología, Facultad de Ciencias Médicas, Universidad Nacional de Cuyo, Mendoza, Argentina

Instituto de Medicina y Biología Experimental de Cuyo (IMBECU), Consejo Nacional de Investigaciones Científicas y Tecnológicas (CONICET), Mendoza, Argentina

Schumacher Marcela Laboratorio de Desarrollo en Neurociencias Cognitivas (CIC—UNS), Instituto de Investigaciones en Ingeniera Eléctrica (IIIE—UNS CONICET), Consejo Nacional de Investigaciones Científicas y Técnicas (CONICET), Bahía Blanca, Argentina

Virna M. Martín Giménez Instituto de Investigaciones en Cs. Químicas, Facultad de Cs. Químicas y Tecnológicas, Universidad Católica de Cuyo, San Juan, Argentina

Elisa Mariajosé Martínez Canales National Autonomous University of Nicaragua at León (UNAN León – Universidad Nacional Autónoma de Nicaragua), León, Nicaragua

Gabriel Walter Martínez Laboratorio de Neurociencias y Psicología Experimental, Fundación Corporación Tecnológica Latinoamericana (FUCOTEL), Cátedra de Psicopatología, Facultad de Humanidades y Ciencias Económicas, Universidad Católica Argentina (UCA), Área de Farmacología, Facultad de Ciencias Médicas, Universidad Nacional de Cuyo (UNCuyo), Consejo Nacional de Investigaciones Científicas y Técnicas (CONICET), Mendoza, Argentina

Miriam Melis Division of Neuroscience and Clinical Pharmacology, Department of Biomedical Sciences, University of Cagliari, Cagliari, Italy

Jéssica Mendes de Souza Laboratory of Neuroscience and Behavior, Institute of Biology, University of Brasília, Brasília, DF, Brazil

Humberto Luis Mesones-Arroyo Laboratory of Neurosciences and Experimental Psychology, Latin American Technological Corporation Foundation (FUCOTEL), Cathedra of Psychopathology, Catholic University of Argentina, Area of Pharmacology, Department of Pathology, National University of Cuyo, CONICET, Guaymallén, Mendoza, Argentina

Gonzalo Mesones Laboratorio de Neurociencias y Psicología Experimental, Fundación Corporación Tecnológica Latinoamericana (FUCOTEL), Cátedra de Psicopatología, Facultad de Humanidades y Ciencias Económicas, Universidad Católica Argentina (UCA), Área de Farmacología, Facultad de Ciencias Médicas, Universidad Nacional de Cuyo (UNCuyo), Consejo Nacional de Investigaciones Científicas y Técnicas (CONICET), Mendoza, Argentina

Guilherme Peres Messas Faculdade de Ciências Médicas da Santa Casa de São Paulo, Hospital do Servidor Público Estadual de São Paulo, São Paulo, Brazil

Belén Mesurado CONICET—Universidad Austral, Instituto de Filosofía, Pilar, Provincia de Buenos Aires, Argentina

Ralph Meyers Socialpsychiatric Center for Child and Adolescent Psychiatry, Dorsten, Germany

Breiner Morales Departamento de Ciencias Sociales, Universidad de Los Lagos, Osorno, Chile

Humberto Morales Department of Radiology, Division of Diagnostic and Interventional Neuroradiology, University of Kentucky, Lexington, KY, USA

Jose Ignacio Murillo Mind-Brain Group, Institute for Culture and Society (ICS), University of Navarra, Pamplona, Spain

Guiomar Niso Psychological & Brain Sciences, Indiana University, Bloomington, IN, USA

Universidad Politécnica de Madrid, Madrid, Spain

María Emilia Oñate CONICET—Universidad Austral, Instituto de Filosofía, Pilar, Provincia de Buenos Aires, Argentina

José Víctor Orón Mind-Brain Group, ICS, University of Navarra, Pamplona, Spain

Tomás Ortiz Alonso Department of Psychiatry, Universidad Complutense de Madrid, Madrid, Spain

Virginia Leonor Herbas Pacheco Carrera de Enfermería. Facultad Ciencias de la Salud, Universidad Técnica de Oruro, Universidad Técnica de Oruro (UTO), Oruro, Bolivia

Ricardo Marcos Pautassi Facultad de Psicología, Universidad Nacional de Córdoba (UNC), Córdoba, Argentina

Instituto de Investigación Médica M. y M. Ferreyra, INIMEC-CONICET-UNC, Córdoba, Argentina

Valeria Teresa Pedrón Facultad de Farmacia y Bioquímica, Instituto de Investigaciones Farmacológicas (ININFA-UBA-CONICET), Universidad de Buenos Aires, Ciudad Autónoma de Buenos Aires, Argentina

Facultad de Psicología y Psicopedagogía, Instituto de Investigación, Universidad del Salvador, Ciudad Autónoma de Buenos Aires, Argentina

Angelina Pilatti Facultad de Psicología, Universidad Nacional de Córdoba (UNC), Córdoba, Argentina

Instituto de Investigaciones Psicológicas, IIPsi-CONICET-UNC, Córdoba, Argentina

Ana Polache Faculty of Pharmacy, Department of Pharmacy and Pharmaceutical Technology and Parasitology, University of Valencia, Valencia, Spain

Virginia Ramos Chuquimia Carrera de Enfermería. Facultad Ciencias de la Salud, Universidad Técnica de Oruro (UTO), Oruro, Bolivia

Siamak Razavi Research Center of Psychiatry and Behavioral Sciences, Tabriz University of Medical Sciences, Tabriz, Iran

Santiago Resett CONICET—Universidad Austral, Instituto de Filosofía, Pilar, Provincia de Buenos Aires, Argentina

Santiago Alejandro Resett Instituto de Filosofía, Universidad Austral, Consejo nacional de investigaciones científicas y técnicas (CONICET), Pilar, Buenos Aires, Argentina

Daniela Ripoll Departamento de Ciencias Sociales, Universidad de La Costa, Barranquilla, Colombia

Lucas Marcelo Rodriguez Centro de investigación interdisciplinar en valores, integración y desarrollo social, Pontificia Universidad Católica Argentina (UCA), Consejo nacional de investigaciones científicas y técnicas (CONICET), Paraná, Entre Ríos, Argentina

Esteban Alejandro Romanowicz Laboratorio de Neurociencias y Psicología Experimental. Fundación Corporación Tecnológica Latinoamericana (FUCOTEL). Cátedra de Psicopatología. Facultad de Humanidades y Ciencias Económicas. Universidad Católica Argentina (UCA). Área de Farmacología. Facultad de Ciencias Médicas, Universidad Nacional de Cuyo (UNCuyo). Consejo Nacional de Investigaciones Científicas y Técnicas (CONICET), Mendoza, Argentina

Claudia Sagheddu Division of Neuroscience and Clinical Pharmacology, Department of Biomedical Sciences, University of Cagliari, Cagliari, Italy

Carol Saldías Solís Escuela de Kinesiología, Facultad de Salud, Universidad Santo Tomás, Temuco, Chile

Agustín Salguero Facultad de Psicología, Universidad Nacional de Córdoba (UNC), Córdoba, Argentina

Instituto de Investigación Médica M. y M. Ferreyra, INIMEC-CONICET-UNC, Córdoba, Argentina

Danylyna Shpakivska Department of Experimental Psychology, Complutense University of Madrid (UCM), Madrid, Spain

Center for Cognitive and Computational Neuroscience (C3N), University Complutense of Madrid (UCM), Madrid, Spain

Vinícius Dokkedal Silva Departamento de Psicobiologia, Escola Paulista de Medicina, Universidade Federal de São Paulo, São Paulo, SP, Brazil

Maria Julia Francischetto Ribeiro Soares Faculdade de Ciências Médicas da Santa Casa de São Paulo, Hospital do Servidor Público Estadual de São Paulo, São Paulo, Brazil

Gianluca Susi Center for Cognitive and Computational Neuroscience, Complutense University of Madrid, Madrid, Spain

Department of Structure of Matter, Thermal Physics and Electronics, School of Physics, Complutense University of Madrid, Madrid, Spain

Gustavo E. Tafet Fundacion Internacional para el Desarroillo de las Neurociencias, Buenos Aires, Argentina

Department of Psychiatry and Behavioral Sciences, Texas A&M University, Bryan, TX, USA

Maria Clotilde H. Tavares Laboratory of Neuroscience and Behavior, Institute of Biology, University of Brasília, Brasília, DF, Brazil

Carlos Tomaz Laboratory of Neuroscience and Behavior and Graduate Program in Environment, University CEUMA, São Luís, MA, Brazil

Laboratory of Neuroscience and Behavior, Post-Graduate Program in Environment, University CEUMA, São Luís, Maranhão, Brazil

Antonella Ariela Trovato CISMA (Centro Integral de Salud Mental Argentino), Buenos Aires, Argentina

Marcos Uceta Department of Experimental Psychology, Complutense University of Madrid (UCM), Madrid, Spain

Faculty of Biological Sciences, Department of Cell Biology, Complutense University of Madrid (UCM), Madrid, Spain

Ana Sofía Vallés Instituto de Investigaciones Bioquímicas de Bahía Blanca (UNS-CONICET), Buenos Aires, Argentina

Norman Darío López Velásquez Escuela de Kinesiología, Facultad de Salud, Universidad Santo Tomás, Temuco, Chile

Centro de Investigación en Gerontología Aplicada (CIGAP), Universidad Santo Tomás, Santiago, Chile

Julia Velez-Ramos Departamento de Historia del Derecho y Filosofía Jurídica, Moral y Política, University of Salamanca, Salamanca, Spain

Giuseppe Virdis Liceo Scientifico Statale "Pitagora", Selargius, Italy

Eric Wainwright Psychiatry Department, Buenos Aires British Hospital, Buenos Aires, Argentina

Psychiatry Department, Braulio Moyano Hospital, Buenos Aires, Argentina

Cathedra of Psychiatry, Faculty of Medical Sciences, Catholic University of Argentina, Buenos Aires, Argentina

Cathedra of Psychiatry, Faculty of Medical Sciences, Buenos Aires University, Buenos Aires, Argentina

Marcela Waisman Campos Department of Cognitive Neurology, Neuropsychiatry and Neuropsychology, Instituto de Investigaciones Neurológicas "Raúl Carrea", Fundación para la Lucha contra las Enfermedades Neurológicas de la Infancia (FLENI), Buenos Aires, Argentina

María José Zinoni Instituto de Filosofía - Facultad de Ciencias Biomédicas, Universidad Austral - Consejo Nacional de Investigaciones Científicas y Técnicas (CONICET), Pilar, Argentina

Centro de Investigación interdisciplinar en Valores, Integración y Desarrollo Social, Universidad Católica Argentina - Consejo Nacional de Investigaciones Científicas y Técnicas (CONICET), Paraná, Argentina

Teodoro Zornoza Faculty of Pharmacy, Department of Pharmacy and Pharmaceutical Technology and Parasitology, University of Valencia, Valencia, Spain

Part I

Epistemological Considerations About the Study of Normal and Abnormal Human Behaviours

1 (Dis)Embodied Encounters: Deciphering Intersubjectivity in the Context of the Prescription of Drugs

Francesca Brencio

Phenomenology and Hermeneutics: What They Are, How They Work, and Why We Need to Take Them into Account in Mental Healthcare

Phenomenology is a method of inquiry that aims to describe the basic structures inherent in conscious experience, such as embodiment, spatiality, temporality, intentionality, and intersubjectivity, and to analyze their possible deviations. Conceived by Edmund Husserl [1], the founding father of the phenomenological movement, as a method to investigate one's lived experience, phenomenology offers reliable descriptions of the structures of conscious lived experiences by *how they are experienced*, without the imposition of external explanatory frameworks. This is widely known as a first-person perspective (1P) [2]. From a phenomenological perspective, subjectivity is never regarded as an object, but rather as a means of allowing the world to display itself. Starting from this, phenomenology focuses on the *form* and *construction*, rather than on the contents, of experience. By analyzing the modes by which our world experience is constituted, phenomenology is capable of detecting the critical points where this constitution is vulnerable and open to deviations that may also emerge as psychiatric symptoms. The very first step of the phenomenological enterprise begins with the recognition that our experience is always hidden by habitual beliefs and assumptions, what Husserl calls the *natural attitude*, and what is required to be suspended in order to access our primordial experience. This is possible by bracketing the validity of the current convictions, paradigms, and beliefs through the *epoché*. The nature and scope of this methodological shift is not to deny, doubt, neglect, abandon, or exclude reality from our research, but rather to focus more narrowly and directly on the phenomenological given.

It was through the contributions of Martin Heidegger [3] that a hermeneutical shift occurred into the phenomenological approach [4]. In fact, while Husserlian phenomenology confined itself to clarifying the experiential structures of subjectivity, Heideggerian phenomenology "went a step further (or a step backwards) and asked, how are we to understand (i.e., interpret), evaluate, and finally act on what we experience." [5, p. 206]. According to Heidegger, hermeneutic phenomenology does not objectify experience, but rather scrutinizes the a theoretical domain of each lived experience, stressing the role of the pathic dimension of each given experience [6]. This is what

F. Brencio (✉)
University of Birmingham, School of Psychology, Birmingham, UK
e-mail: f.brencio@bham.ac.uk; https://bham.academia.edu/FrancescaBrencio; https://www.researchgate.net/profile/Francesca-Brencio

P. Á. Gargiulo, H. L. Mesones-Arroyo (eds.), *Psychiatry and Neuroscience Update – Vol. V*,
https://doi.org/10.1007/978-3-031-72219-6_1

Heidegger intends to do when he deals with the facticity of existence. In his early lectures in Freiburg (1918–1919), he shows how intentional life is grounded on the affective element; both the active and the passive aspects of intentional directedness. His early project can be understood as a kind of radicalization of the Husserlian–Brentanian notion of intentionality, in order to demonstrate that the unity of intentional life at a pretheoretical level is grounded on the "pathic" dimension of existence, a preworldly element. In practical life, "I experience myself as always attached to the surrounding world. This experiencing-oneself is no theoretical 'reflection', no 'inner perception', or the like, but is self-worldly experience, because experience itself has a worldly character and emphasizes significance in such a way that one's own experienced self-world no longer stands out from the surrounding world." [7, p. 10]. This state of being always attached to the world is analyzed in *Being and Time* through the fundamental structures of existence, among which *Befindlichkeit* occupies a specific role [8].

The relationship between phenomenology and hermeneutics is not that simple: one needs to reflect on the fact that the majority of scholars in the field of hermeneutics had their roots in phenomenological education to realize how intertwined both these two methods are. If Heidegger was the first to break with reflective phenomenology, Paul Ricoeur [9] and Hans Georg Gadamer [10] both follow his footprints. The task of hermeneutic phenomenology is to show the interplay between experience and its interpretation. In the twentieth century, hermeneutic phenomenology developed as "an attempt to complement the phenomenological analysis of the experiential structures of subjectivity with an account of the reflective character (i.e., affective, cultural, historical, ethical) of selfhood." [11, p. 237]. Since human experience is a product of interpretation, hermeneutic phenomenology is interested in scrutinizing those accounts of selfhood that comprehend also self-reflection, culture, and history. The interrogation of the significance and meaning of an experience is thus more urgent when it relates to mental health issues [12].

In the contemporary context, phenomenology has been involved in an important dialogue with neuroscience and cognitive science. In the first case, the interchange between phenomenology and neuroscience is represented by the growing field of neurophenomenology. Born at the end of the 1990s through the fundamental contribution of Francisco Varela, neurophenomenology is a method of inquiry designed to understand the so-called hard problem of consciousness and its relationship with the brain through a stereoscopic perspective in which neuroscientific questions guided by first-person phenomenological evidence (1P) combined with third-person neuroscientific evidence (3P) can suggest new articulations of the phenomenological descriptions [13].

In the second case, the combination of phenomenology with enactivism [14] and the past 30 years of interdisciplinary research in the cognitive sciences [15] are harbingers of many fruitful outcomes for both fields. What is enactivism? It is a complex approach to the conceptualization and study of the mind in which accounts of brain activity, philosophy, and biology are involved. Generally speaking, the enactive approach focuses on sense-making as an embodied and situated activity. For enactivism, cognition arises through a dynamic interaction between an acting organism and its environment: "Cognition is not 'inside' the brain, representing information about the world, computing it according to internal rules, and eventually telling the body how to act; cognition is rather enacted or brought forth, over time, by the whole organism (not just its brain) situated in the world." [16, p. 1083]. The environment of an organism is enacted by the active exercise of that organism's sensorimotor processes. According to enactivism, mental processes are: *embodied*, involving more than the brain, including a more general involvement of bodily structures and processes; *embedded*, functioning only in a related external environment; *enacted* involving not only neural processes but also things an organism does; and *extended* into the organism's environment. This is often summarized under the heading of the "4Es" [17]. The introduction of the term "enaction" is attributed to Francisco Varela in the famous book *The*

Embodied Mind (1991). Varela proposed the term "enaction" to "emphasize the growing conviction that cognition is not the representation of a pre-given world by a pre-given mind, but is rather the enactment of a world and a mind on the basis of a history of the variety of actions that a being in the world performs." [15, p. 9]. The interchange between phenomenology and enactivism has contributed to an understanding of the mind in a novel way that breaks from the traditional Cartesian and computational models that have dominated and continue to dominate science and medicine. The alternative perspective consists of a set of approaches that emphasize different versions of the basic consensus idea that the mind is not just "in the head" or in the brain [18] but that the explanatory unit should be the brain–body–environment in a mutual and circular relationship [19].

Due to its purpose, namely clarifying and describing the structures of experience since its origin phenomenology had a widespread application not just in philosophy but also in psychology: Husserl and Ludwig Binswanger [20] devoted their work to understanding psychological phenomena through the phenomenological toolbox, offering a better methodological and epistemological foundation for empirical research. In his dialogue with Freudian psychoanalysis, Jean Paul Sartre [21] developed existential psychoanalysis, an alternative therapeutic approach mainly grounded on the phenomenological method. Both through the works of the first generation of phenomenologists—Theodor Lipps, Alexander Pfänder, Edith Stein, just to mention a few—and psychiatrists who applied the phenomenological method for the understanding of psychopathological phenomena—Such as Karl Jaspers, Eugène Minkowski, Ludwig Binswanger, Erwin Straus, and Wolfgang Blankenburg—and more recently through the contribution of scholars in the field of clinical phenomenology—i.e., Josef Parnas, Thomas Fuchs, Giovanni Stanghellini, Guilherme Messas, Matthew Broome, among many other names—it has been possible to "carry" the phenomenological method into the field of mental healthcare, particularly to psychiatry. The introduction of the phenomenological method for the understanding and treatment of mental health issues involves a particular analysis of reality, to provide relevance to the given and lived experiences. The aim of the phenomenological analysis is not to account for how the physical world gives rise to a first-person perspective, but rather the opposite: *how phenomena*, including the objective world, *emerge in the first-person perspective* [22]. As a consequence, psychopathological phenomena and abnormal mental experiences are not anymore conceived in the framework of a diagnosis-centered approach, but rather as a coherent way of *being in the world* of the person.

With the introduction of the second-person approach (2P), or intersubjective perspective, recent research in phenomenology and social cognition overcame the antagonism between first- and third-person perspectives. In fact, while the first-person approach corresponds to the basic and prereflective experience of implicit self-awareness [23], the second-person approach means a prereflective awareness of self and others, based on ongoing face-to-face interactions [24]. It is in this rich and interdisciplinary scenario that we can see how a phenomenological approach to intersubjectivity may enrich the understanding and development of the clinical encounter. Let us see how.

Intersubjectivity and the Clinical Encounter

The notion of intersubjectivity is central in philosophy, cognitive science , and neuroscience. In what follows, I will sketch the history of the notion of intersubjectivity through the phenomenological lens and link it to the enactive approach.

We cannot talk of intersubjectivity without going back to Husserl [25]. For him, the foundational element of intersubjectivity is the body, conceived as zero point (*Nullpunkt*) from which the perceived world and the space are organized [26, p. 61]: "The Body, in virtue of the constitutive role of the sensations, is of significance for the construction of the spatial world." [26, p. 62]. Thus, "all things of the surrounding world possess an orientation to the Body, just as, accordingly, all expressions of orientation imply this relation. The 'far' is far from me, from my Body; the 'to the right' refers back to the right side of my Body, e.g., to my right hand." [26, p. 166]. As the means of intersection and organization of the perceived world, the body may be regarded as having a double nature: as *Leib*, the living-and-felt body, and as *Körper*, the material-object body. This is illustrated with the well-known example of double sensation: "Touching my left hand, I have touch-appearances, that is to say, I do not just sense, but I perceive and have appearances of a soft, smooth hand, with such a form (…). The hand that is touching (…) has its touch-sensations at the place on its corporeal surface where it touches (or is touched by the other) (…). The sensation is doubled in the two parts of the Body, since each is then precisely—or the other—an external thing that is touching and acting upon it, and each is at the same time Body." [26, pp. 152–153]. This double consideration of the body is far from being a kind of residual aspect of the dualistic Cartesian legacy. To overcome such a possibility, Husserl created a term in which both aspects of the body are unified: *Leibkörper*. The main intention of this word is to express that the subjective lived aspects of corporeality are intertwined with the material ones.

This double gaze on the body tells us something crucial about the nature of *embodiment as an ongoing act*, continuously *shaped by our experiences*, by the relationships and interactions with others, and the environment: "Lived experiences are 'bound' to the Body. Yet it is clear that the psychic subject is not primarily related to his Corporeal body as a material thing and is only mediately related to the lived experiences connected up to it, but, rather, the reverse: the psychic subject has a material thing as his Body because it is animated, i.e., because he has psychic lived experiences which, in the sense of the apperception of the human, are one with the Body in a singularly intimate way." [26, p. 129]. *The body is the condition of the possibility to meet others and the world around us*. It is from this consideration of the body that we can talk about intersubjectivity as the mutual exchange of thoughts, feelings, and experiences, both conscious and unconscious, between two subjects: the "possibility of sociality, the possibility of comprehension (…) presupposes a certain Bodily intersubjectivity." [26, p. 311].

This accent on the direct bodily and affective nature of intersubjectivity shows how subjectivity only reaches its full relation to itself and to the world through intersubjectivity, and this latter only exists and develops in a mutual interrelationship between subjects that share a common world. The possibility of sociality therefore presupposes this intersubjectivity. Drawing on Husserl's conception of the body, Maurice Merleau-Ponty develops his concept of embodiment, which is cardinal both in phenomenology and enactivism. Embodiment means that the *lived body* is the constitutive element of our being-the-world: "The body is the vehicle of being in the world, and having a body is, for a living creature, to be intervolved in a definite environment, to identify oneself with certain projects and be continually committed to them." [27, p. 50]. According to Merleau-Ponty, the body's typical mode of existence is a "being-toward-the-world"; this orientation is essentially *temporal*, involving a dialectic between the present body, conceived as "I can" (following Husserl's legacy), and the *habit body*, the sedimentations of past activities that take on a general, anonymous, and autonomous character. The body itself is experienced in different ways: it is a permanent part of one's perceptual field; it has "double sensations" that enact a form of reflexivity; it has affective experiences; and its kinesthetic sense of its own movements is given directly. This kinesthetic awareness is made possible by a preinferential system of bodily movements and spatial equivalences that Merleau-Ponty names the "body schema." The body has a "situational spatiality" that is oriented toward actual or possible tasks and this spatiality unveils the intentional relationship that the body has with the space: "I can," *rather than an* "I think." The lived body unveils the demarcation between the self and the others. It represents the point of departure of each experience and encounters: "The perceived world is not only my world, but the one in which I see the behavior of other people take shape, for their behavior equally aims at this world, which is the correlative not only of my consciousness, but of any consciousness which I can possibly encounter." [27, p. 164]. Another important merit of Merleau-Ponty is the introduction of the concept of *intercorporeality* as a prereflective intertwining of lived and living bodies, in which each one is affected by the influence of the other's body as well as by the effects of reciprocal relations. This leads to a kind of embodied communication: "The communication or comprehension of gestures comes about through the reciprocity of my intentions and the gestures of others, of my gestures and the intentions discernible in the conduct of other people. It is as if the other person's intentions inhabited my body and mine his." [27, p. 96].

Through the central work of Merleau-Ponty, an embodiment is recognized as a foundational element for the dialogue with enactivism: embodiment enables our immediate apprehension of others [28]. For enactivism, living beings do not act only passively, merely as receptors of information from the outside that is translated into internal representations in a second moment; rather, organisms participate actively in the creation of meanings. It means that the brain does not receive an external world without the body participating in it. On the contrary, the external realm is the result of an interaction process between the sense-making activity of an agent and the responses from its environment. This requires dynamic coupling and coordination by the agents. This happens within the frame of a "mutual circulation between cognitive science and phenomenology in which subjectivity and experience play the vital role that they also have in the everyday doings of living, sentient, sense-making beings." [29, p. 494]. The bodily experiences of interaction are the ground of understanding both each other and of understanding the world together. This understanding postulates a rich and complex constellation of interaction processes, which include several components such as bodily resonance, affect, attunement, coordination of gestures, facial and vocal expression, and many others [30, p. 466]. In our experience of others, we do not simply see their face, their eyes, their body, and gestures, but we sense all these things through our bodies, through a mutual *bodily resonance* typical of second-person interactions [31].

Talking about intersubjectivity from the angle of phenomenology and enactivism implies making some distinctions about the different levels of intersubjectivity. We can, at least, distinguish among *three levels of intersubjectivity*: primary intersubjectivity [32], referring to perceptual and motor processes that allow newborns and young infants to engage with others from birth, through expressions, intonations, gestures, and movements (0–12 months); secondary intersubjectivity [33], through which infants begin to tie actions to pragmatic and social contexts, to develop joint attention and joint actions, and to reach the fundamental stage in language development (from 13 months to 4 years). Joint attention involves sharing a common focus on something with someone else. In childhood, joint attention is a deeply embodied interaction. Infants' responsiveness to others' embodied effects is demonstrated by *affective synchrony, affect attunement, bodily resonance , and intercorporality*. These embodied interactions are at the core of intersubjectivity as intercorporeality and this shows the role of embodied attention in the development of social perspectives: "We do not simply observe others; we are not passive spectators. Rather we interact with others and in doing so we develop further capabilities in the contexts of those interactions." [34, p. 260]. Finally, tertiary intersubjectivity (from 4 years), when infants become aware of others as mental agents (not only bodily agents, as in the previous phase) with their own thoughts and beliefs that may also differ from theirs and from reality [35]. The ability to integrate different perspectives is grounded on "the ability to freely oscillate between an ego-centric, embodied perspective on the one hand, and an allocentric or decentered perspective on the other, without thereby losing one's bodily center of self-awareness." [36, p. 195].

The account of intersubjectivity, as described so far, is the opposite of any pure mental approach to this theme. In fact, such an approach postulates a fundamental inaccessibility to others, whose mental states, emotions, and feelings may be inferred only indirectly and not through bodily intercorporeality. This is what happens, for example, in the so-called "Theory of Mind," according to which the brain appears to be modeled upon an inner process, mainly characterized by inferential or simulative models. This tendency to rely on the brain to explain social cognition and social perception reduces intersubjectivity to an inferential or projective process encapsulated in the brain, overlooking interactions between the individual and their environment [37]. Conceived from the perspective of intercorporeality and enactivism, intersubjectivity deals with empathy, understood as a kind of intuitive, implicit knowledge that arises immediately when we meet another person, and this "implicit empathy" underlies social exchanges [38].

The phenomenological and enactive account of intersubjectivity may be of great help in understanding every encounter, particularly the clinical encounter.

(Dis)Embodied Encounters. Deciphering Intersubjectivity in the Context of the Prescription of Drugs

As we have seen, embodiment is at the core of every gesture, action, behavior, and relationship we have. It is also through our body that we can *perceive* others through sensory modalities. This empathetic perception is rooted in our bodily awareness and interconnections with others, and guarantees *bodily resonance*. How is this possible? To understand what bodily resonance is we need "to abandon the idea that emotions are only 'mental' phenomena, and the world is bare of any affective qualities (…). We do not live in a merely physical world; the experienced space around us is always charged with affective qualities." [39, p. 4]. These affective qualities (or affective affordances) are experienced by bodily resonance, which "includes all kinds of local or general bodily sensations (…). There is no emotion without at least the slightest bodily sensations and movement tendencies (…). The body is a 'resonance body,' a most sensitive 'sounding board' in which every emotion reverberates." [39, p. 5].

Bodily resonance acts as the medium of our affective engagement in a situation and connects people with one another in circular interactions [39]. Different components of the affection—resonance—emotion cycle mutually influence each other, and this cycle causes corresponding "reverberations" in the brain. "The continual 'resonance' of brain and organism is the precondition of conscious experience." [20, p. 126]. In every encounter, our bodily resonance is at work, even if it is at different levels and depends on existential and clinical conditions [40]. In what follows I will examine through the phenomenological lens the clinical encounter in terms of intersubjectivity, and I will explain how the prescription of drugs may negatively impact the embodied encounter.

The encounter between a patient and a physician is always an embodied encounter between existences that must communicate and enter into a relationship with each other. In the space of the encounter, each participant can *feel* the presence of the other. This possibility to feel the other unveils our structural engagement with the world. Feelings are always embodied and are different manifestations of affectivity itself. They are the key structures of our affective states: "Affects are modes of bodily attunement to, and engagement with, the lived world. It is only through our affectivity that we find ourselves in a meaningful environment in which persons and things matter for us, and in which we care for them as well as for ourselves. Affects are the very heart of our existence." [41, p. 613]. The affective dimension of experience (of each experience) is an existential phenomenon characterized by the way it touches or affects us, and how it moves us.

Another cardinal element of the clinical encounter is the atmospheres, which inhabit the prepersonal and prelinguistic dimensions that human beings experience mainly in a shared space. Defining what the atmospheres are is a bit tricky because they have a certain ambiguity which may be defined as their principal characteristic. In our ordinary language, we use the word atmosphere to signify both external landscapes and internal ones. As such, atmospheres may be impersonal or transpersonal, referring to the environment, or to one's own feeling; they may have significance for people's affective states, things, and spaces. Drawing on atmospheric phenomena, the atmospheres in clinical encounters are associated with affective qualities and may also be characterized by a certain vagueness, evading rational explanation and any measurement: "Atmospheres are neither something objective, that is, qualities possessed by things, and yet they are something thing like, belonging to the thing in that things articulate their presence through qualities—conceived as ecstasies. Nor are atmospheres something subjective, for example determinations of a psychic state. And yet they are subject like, belong to subjects in that they are sensed in bodily presence by human beings and this sensing is at the same time a bodily state of being of subjects in space." [42, p. 122]. In clinical encounters, atmospheres are intersubjective phenomena experienced by the participants in a shared situation. Atmospheres have a kind of synesthetic nature: to perceive an atmosphere implies a certain involvement in a situation and a predisposition to this perception. For these reasons, the training of mental health professionals in the recognition and understanding of changes in atmospheres may have implications both on the diagnostic side and on the therapeutic side, namely by reinforcing the empathic patient–doctor relationship [43].

Embodied presence, affective states, atmospheres, gestures, and dialogue are all components of the clinical encounter. The observation, description, and understanding of their disturbances are fundamental when clinicians must ascertain a psychopathological condition. In fact, when an impairment in one or more of these components occurs, it may disrupt ordinary life and the adaptive emotion functions, provoking a series of abnormal psychological phenomena. What happens when the examination of such elements is undermined by the prescription of drugs? Drugs impact behaviors and relationships, affective states, and the ability to get into dialogue. They affect both the relationships with the mental health professionals and the relationships that the person has with their illness or condition. A well-recognized property of chemical substances used for recreational purposes is "their ability to produce altered states of consciousness and concomitant changes in behavior by virtue of their action on the central nervous system." [44, p. 409].

In evidence-based psychiatric practice, there is a gap between long-term outcomes and treatment safety. This gap is grounded mainly upon two biases: the first bias is to consider mental disorders as chemical brain imbalances, and the second one is the predominant role of the pharmaceutical industry in the scientific community. Psychiatric drugs are psychoactive drugs: due to their neurophysiological effects, they alter mental and emotional life, and behaviors for the duration of the treatment. Psychiatric drugs do not target underlying diseases or symptom-producing mechanisms; they create an altered state of mental functioning that is superimposed on underlying feelings and behaviors [45]. Mental distress is viewed as a burden or disease to get rid of, as quickly as possible and without pain. Medication fits very well into this view, providing hopes of "quick fixes." However, in many cases, mental distress can become chronic and lead to long-term (dis)ability, while the meaning (or "message") carried by the symptoms is ignored. *Efficacy* and *effectiveness* are considered the same, when actually they are not.

As with any other substance, every type of psychiatric drug induces a certain altered mental and physical state, the characteristics of which depend on the nature of the drug taken. Some psychiatric medications produce pleasurable psychoactive effects; others are more often associated with the experience of unpleasant psychoactive effects. An important concern is that the continued use of drugs, and the consequences of this on the activity of the central nervous system, may compromise mental functioning: "The possibility of adverse psychological and behavioral effects occurring after long-term use of other psychiatric medications has periodically been suggested, but has received little attention." [44, p. 409].

The fundamental principle at the core of the prescription of psychiatric drugs and their use is that they are worthwhile only if the benefits outweigh the harms. However, this is not that simple to calculate due to the many factors that contribute to the psychoactive effects or to dependence. The treatment and understanding of mental health issues are strictly linked to the need to reassess the models and roles in clinical practices, such as a drastic reduction in the prescription of drugs, more careful attention to a person-centered approach, and a focus on treatments centered on patients' lived experiences and community-based interventions. From a phenomenological and hermeneutic informed approach to mental health, pharmacotherapy is evaluated as an important but not exhaustive component in the healing journey. In his monumental *General Psychopathology,* Karl Jaspers exhorted us to use methodological pluralism in the field of mental health: "We must guard against any one viewpoint becoming an absolute even if such a viewpoint proves fruitful for research and might now and then even be decisive for radical therapy." [46, p. 577]. The biological paradigm at the core of contemporary psychiatry often forgets the complexity and the meaning of psychopathological phenomena, which may not be reduced only to "brain affections" and treated by a massive recourse to prescribing drugs.

Drugs do not cure the underlying mental health issues; they treat symptoms and signs and may improve the quality of life of a person with a certain condition. *Curing* has to do with the process of *recognition*, which shows the essential dimension of the self, never isolated but always embedded in a *relational dimension*: with itself, with a certain condition, with others, and with the environment [47]. Contemporary psychiatry is disease-centered: it means that the issue of diagnosis and its treatment are at the core of the therapeutic enterprise, which is essentially modeled on drugs' efficacy. A disease-centered model embraces the idea that drugs act on the underlying physical disease process: they are able to reverse a "faulty" physiological process into a "normal" one. This model is at the core of the way psychiatric drugs are currently named and classified according to the disease; "thus, there are 'antipsychotics' thought to act specifically on the pathology underlying psychosis, 'antidepressants' thought to act on the pathology of depression, 'anxiolytics' thought to act on the pathological basis of anxiety, antimanic drugs thought to act on the pathology of mania, lithium and other 'mood stabilisers' thought to act on the pathological basis of abnormal mood." [45, p. 5].

This raises the issue of the perspective from which the therapist encounters the patient. An important element that I would like to stress is the difference among the phenomenological, psychoanalytic, and psychiatric viewpoints on the clinical encounter [48]. While psychiatry claims an idea of objectivity as something that can be achieved only by adopting a "point of view from nowhere," psychoanalysis advocates an idea of neutrality, recognizing the impossibility of being impassible to a patient's experiences. Phenomenology, however, offers the psychiatrist the tools to become aware of their own lived experience of the clinical encounter in a very specific way, stressing the role of the embodied dimension of each encounter, and the necessary shift from a third-person approach to a second-person one, a view from within the clinical encounter. From this perspective, illness always has an intersubjective dimension that challenges the therapist's gaze. This allows the possibility of an authentic encounter between people, not reducible to a checklist of symptoms or to a series of drugs' prescriptions to be renewed time after time. This possibility must lie in something different. Gadamer [49] invites us to consider *health as a moral enterprise*, and not as something that can simply be made or produced by doctors. As a moral enterprise, health requires clinicians and health workers to be equipped with a series of different tools. This is why a phenomenologically oriented psychiatry may be of great help in deciphering disturbances of intersubjectivity as the origin of psychopathological phenomena.

Conclusions

Human experience is the result of interpretation, not only of action. The interrogation of the significance and meaning of an experience is vital in our ordinary life but can be even more central when the integrity of the self is undermined by mental health issues. In the contemporary context, phenomenology and hermeneutics are often neglected in medical schools: their study, discussion, understanding, and applications usually happen among expert senior clinicians. Young generations of practitioners are trained in neuroscience and pharmacology, but very rarely in considering the psyche as not the results of brain activity or biochemical reactions.

In this contribution, I have underlined how phenomenology and hermeneutics are important tools in questioning those components of a human being's existence, and how they are involved in the description and understanding of mental health. In the context of mental health experiences, deciphering intersubjectivity is a crucial effort for any diagnosis and treatment. This operation is possible in the space of "betweenness": the space between I and Thou, between patient and doctor, and between the person and her community. This space conveys a sense of openness and an original bond with others, which allows intersubjectivity to be an open enterprise.

References

1. Husserl E. Cartesian meditations: an introduction to phenomenology. The Hague: Martinus Nijhoff; 1960; Husserl E. The crisis of European sciences and transcendental phenomenology: an introduction to phenomenological philosophy. Evanston: Northwestern University Press; 1970a; Husserl E. Logical investigations. London: Routledge; 1970b; Husserl E. Ideas pertaining to a pure phenomenology and to a phenomenological philosophy. First book. General introduction to a pure phenomenology. The Hague: Martinus Nijhoff; 1982; Husserl E. Ideas pertaining to a pure phenomenology and to a phenomenological philosophy. Second book. Studies in the phenomenology of constitution. Dordrecht: Kluwer Academic Publishers; 1989; Husserl E. Ideas pertaining to a pure phenomenology and to a phenomenological philosophy. Third book. The Hague: Martinus Nijhoff; 1980; Husserl E. Psychological and transcendental phenomenology and the confrontation with Heidegger (1921–1931). Dordrecht: Kluwer Academic Publishers; 1997.
2. Moran D. The phenomenological approach. In: Stanghellini G, Raballo A, Broome M, Fernandez AV, Fusar-Poli P, Rosfort R, editors. The Oxford handbook of phenomenological psychopathology. Oxford: Oxford University Press; 2019. p. 205–15.
3. Heidegger M. Being and time. New York: Harper & Row; 1962; Heidegger M. The Zollikon seminars. In: Boss M, editor. Protocols-conversations-letters. Evanston: Northwestern University Press; 2001; Heidegger M. The basic problems of phenomenology (Winter Semester 1919/1920). London: Bloomsbury; 2013.
4. von Herrmann F-W. Hermeneutics and reflection: Heidegger and Husserl on the concept of phenomenology. Toronto: University of Toronto Press; 2013.
5. Stanghellini G, Rosfort R. Emotions and personhood. Exploring fragility—making sense of vulnerability. Oxford: Oxford University Press; 2013.
6. Brencio F. Disposition: the "pathic" dimension of existence and its relevance in affective disorders and schizophrenia. Thaumazein. 2018;6:138–57. https://doi.org/10.13136/thau.v6i0.
7. Heidegger M. Towards the definition of philosophy. London: Continuum; 2002.
8. Brencio F. Befindlichkeit: disposition. In: Stanghellini G, Raballo A, Broome M, Fernandez AV, Fusar-Poli P, Rosfort R, editors. The Oxford handbook of phenomenological psychopathology. Oxford: Oxford University Press; 2019. p. 344–53. https://doi.org/10.1093/oxfordhb/9780198803157.013.39.
9. Ricoeur P. Fallible man. New York: Fordham University Press; 1987; Ricoeur P. Oneself as another. Chicago: University of Chicago Press; 1992; Ricoeur P. The conflict of interpretations: essays in hermeneutics. London: Continuum; 2004; Ricoeur P. Husserl. An analysis of his phenomenology. Evanston: Northwestern University Press; 2007a; Ricoeur P. History and truth. Evanston: Northwestern University Press; 2007b; Ricoeur P. From text to action. Essays in hermeneutics II. London: Continuum; 2008.
10. Gadamer HG. Truth and method. New York: Crossroad; 2006.
11. Rosfort R. Phenomenology and hermeneutics. In: Stanghellini G, Raballo A, Broome M, Fernandez AV, Fusar-Poli P, Rosfort R, editors. The Oxford handbook of phenomenological psychopathology. Oxford: Oxford University Press; 2019. p. 235–47.
12. Brencio F, Bauer P. Words matter. A hermeneutical-phenomenological account to mental health. Phenomenol Mind. 2020;18:68–77. https://doi.org/10.17454/pam-1805.
13. Varela F. Neurophenomenology: a methodological remedy for the hard problem. J Conscious Stud. 1996;3(4):330–49.

14. Gallagher S, Zahavi D. The phenomenological mind: an introduction to philosophy of mind and cognitive science. London: Routledge; 2008.
15. Varela F, Thompson E, Rosch E. The embodied mind. Cambridge, MA: The MIT Press; 1991.
16. Colombetti G. Psychopathology and the enacted mind. In: Fulford KWM, Davies M, Gipps RGT, Graham G, Sadler JZ, Stanghellini G, Thornton T, editors. The Oxford handbook of philosophy and psychiatry. Oxford: Oxford University Press; 2013.
17. Newen A, De Bruin L, Gallagher S, editors. The Oxford handbook of 4E cognition. Oxford: Oxford University Press; 2018.
18. Noe A. Out of our heads. You are not your brain. New York: Hill & Wang; 2009.
19. Fuchs T. Ecology of the brain. Oxford: Oxford University Press; 2017.
20. Binswanger L. Über Phänomenologie. In: Ausgewählte Vorträge und Aufsätze. Bern: Francke; 1955. p. 13–47; Binswanger L. Drei Formen missglückten Daseins: Verstiegenheit, Verschrobenheit, Manieriertheit. Tübingen: Niemeyer; 1956. Binswanger L. Grundformen und Erkenntnis Menschlichen Daseins. München: Ernst Reinhardt Verlag; 1962.
21. Sartre JP. The emotions: outline of a theory. New York: Philosophical Library; 1948; Sartre JP. Being and nothingness: an essay on phenomenological ontology. New York: Philosophical Library; 1956; Sartre JP. Between existentialism and Marxism. New York: Morrow & Co.; 1976.
22. Parnas J. The self and intentionality in the pre-psychotic stages of schizophrenia: a phenomenological study. In: Zahavi D, editor. Exploring the self: philosophical and psychopathological perspectives on self-experience. Amsterdam: John Benjamins Publishing Company; 2000. p. 115–47.
23. Zahavi D. Subjectivity and selfhood: investigating the first-person perspective. Cambridge: MIT Press; 2005.
24. Fuchs T. The phenomenology and development of social perspectives. Phenomenol Cogn Sci. 2013;12:655–83. https://doi.org/10.1007/s11097-012-9267-x.
25. Zahavi D. Husserl's phenomenology. Stanford: Stanford University Press; 2003.
26. Husserl E. Ideas pertaining to a pure phenomenology and to a phenomenological philosophy. Second Book; 1989.
27. Merleau-Ponty M. Phenomenology of perception. New York: Routledge; 1981.
28. Fuchs T, De Jaegher H. Understanding intersubjectivity: enactive and embodied. In: Fuchs T, Sattel HC, Henningsen P, editors. The embodied self: dimensions, coherence and disorders. Stuttgart: Schattauer Verlag; 2010. p. 203–15.
29. De Jaegher H, Pieper B, Clénin D, Fuchs T. Grasping intersubjectivity: an invitation to embody social interaction research. Phenomenol Cogn Sci. 2017;16:494. https://doi.org/10.1007/s11097-016-9469-8.
30. Fuchs T, De Jaegher H. Enactive intersubjectivity: participatory sense-making and mutual incorporation. Phenomenol Cogn Sci. 2009;8:466. https://doi.org/10.1007/s11097-009-9136-4.
31. Fuchs T. Temporality and psychopathology. Phenomenol Cogn Sci. 2013;12:75–104.
32. Trevarthen CB. Communication and cooperation in early infancy: a description of primary intersubjectivity. In: Bullowa M, editor. Before speech. The beginning of human communication. Cambridge: Cambridge University Press; 1979. p. 321–48.
33. Trevarthen C, Hubley P. Secondary intersubjectivity: confidence, confiding and acts of meaning in the first year. In: Lock A, editor. Action, gesture and symbol: the emergence of language. London: Academic; 1978. p. 183–229.
34. Gallagher S. Intersubjectivity and psychopathology. In: Fulford KWM, Davies M, Gipps RGT, Graham G, Sadler JZ, Stanghellini G, Thornton T, editors. The Oxford handbook of philosophy and psychiatry. Oxford: Oxford University Press; 2013. p. 258–74.
35. Tomasello M. The cultural origins of human cognition. Cambridge, MA: Harvard University Press; 1999.
36. Fuchs T. Pathologies of intersubjectivity in autism and schizophrenia. J Conscious Stud. 2015;22:191–214.
37. Gallese V. The 'shared manifold' hypothesis: from mirror neurons to empathy. J Conscious Stud. 2001;8:33–50.
38. Englebert J. Psychopathologie de l'homme en situation. Paris: Hermann; 2013.
39. Fuchs T. Intercorporeality and interaffectivity. In: Meyer C, Streeck J, Jordan S, editors. Intercorporeality: emerging socialities in interaction. Oxford: Oxford University Press; 2016.
40. Bizzari V. Schizophrenia and common sense: a phenomenological perspective. In: Hipólito I, Gonçalves J, Pereira J, editors. Schizophrenia and common sense. Studies in brain and mind. Berlin: Springer; 2018. p. 39–53. https://doi.org/10.1007/978-3-319-73993-9_3.
41. Fuchs T. The phenomenology of affectivity. In: Fulford KWM, et al., editors. The Oxford handbook of philosophy and psychiatry. Oxford: Oxford University Press; 2001.
42. Böhme G. Atmosphere as the fundamental concept of a new aesthetics. Thesis Eleven. 1993;36(122):113–26.
43. Costa C, Carmenates S, Madeira L, Stanghellini G. Atmospheres and the clinical encounter. In: Stanghellini G, Raballo A, Broome M, Fernandez AV, Fusar-Poli P, Rosfort R, editors. The Oxford handbook of phenomenological psychopathology. Oxford: Oxford University Press; 2019. p. 872–81.
44. Moncrieff J, Cohen D, Porter S. The psychoactive effects of psychiatric medication: the elephant in the room. J Psychoactive Drugs. 2013;45(5):409. Published online 2013 Nov 18. https://doi.org/10.1080/02791072.2013.845328.
45. Moncrieff J. The myth of the chemical cure. Basingstoke: Palgrave Macmillan; 2008.

46. Jaspers K. General psychopathology. Baltimore: Johns Hopkins University Press; 1997.
47. Brencio F. From diagnosis to therapeutic empathy. A journey into recognition. Philos Psychiatry Psychol. 2021;28(1):11–3. Project MUSE muse.jhu.edu/article/785883.
48. Sholokhova S. Benefits and challenges of the phenomenological approach to the psychiatrist's subjective experience: impassivity, neutrality, and embodied awareness in the clinical encounter. Philos Psychiatry Psychol. 2019;26(4):83–96. https://doi.org/10.1353/ppp.2019.0043.
49. Gadamer HG. The enigma of health: the art of healing in a scientific age. Stanford: Stanford University Press; 1996.

Francesca Brencio PhD, is Teaching Fellow in Mental Health at the School of Psychology at the University of Birmingham (UK) with a full-time teaching position. She is also the Director of the PhenoLab, a Theoretical Laboratory in Phenomenology and Mental Health. Executive Committee Member of The Royal College of Psychiatrists Special Interest Group in Philosophy, since 2018 she has an ongoing collaboration with The Collaborating Centre for Values-based Practice at St. Catherine's College at the University of Oxford (UK).

2 Addictions: Epistemological Reflections Around Fields of Study and Disciplines

Juan Ernesto Calderón

Introduction

Addictions are a complex phenomenon. This complexity manifests itself in the definition of addictions. What do addictions consist of? When do you call a person "addicted"? Is an addict a person who simply consumes a certain substance in an uncontrolled way, whether legal or illegal? Is an addicted person free? Is an addicted person responsible for their actions? These are just some of the questions that arise when talking about addictions. At first glance, these questions require different approaches. There are questions of law, biology, medicine, ethics, philosophy, etc. When there are so many disciplines around an object of study, we immediately talk about interdiscipline and an interdisciplinary approach. The concept of discipline is often associated with a bureaucratic-administrative distinction. According to this view, it is enough to create a new department or division that shares at least the name with two previous departments to do interdisciplinary. However, from Thomas Kuhn, the importance of shaping the discipline in scientific practice as a whole is shown, indicating that interdisciplinary is more complex than creating another division with a shared name. The concept of discipline is associated with a disciplinary matrix, which defines a scientific community and, in so doing, requires that the community exist. The disciplinary matrix is the way we see the world and act on it. The latter indicates that not only the understanding of the object is given by the disciplinary matrix but also by the intervention in it. On this basis, interdisciplinary ceases to be a mere sum of looks to become a horizon of compression that surpasses the individual and transformative looks of the object.

The objectives of this contribution are (1) To show from Kuhn's work how discipline shapes a worldview; (2) to investigate the concept of discipline and the divisions of the sciences; and (3) To demonstrate that a different model of discipline organization is needed to achieve a truly interdisciplinary approach to an object such as addictions. To this end, we will work on Kuhnian ideas of paradigm, disciplinary matrix , and incommensurability. These notions are the basis that will allow us to investigate the division of sciences and how different classifications shape different ways of understanding and practicing scientific knowledge. Finally, the idea of a collaborative program for the organization of disciplines is put forward. The collaborative program attempts to overcome the mere juxtaposition of discipline in favor of true interdisciplinary.

J. E. Calderón (✉)
Department of Philosophy, Faculty of Philosophy and Letters, Facultad de Filosofía y Letras, Universidad Nacional de Cuyo, Centro Universitario, Mendoza, Argentina

P. Á. Gargiulo, H. L. Mesones-Arroyo (eds.), *Psychiatry and Neuroscience Update – Vol. V*,
https://doi.org/10.1007/978-3-031-72219-6_2

Paradigm, Disciplinary Matrix, and Incommensurability

According to Kuhn [1] the previous epistemology provided an ideal image of science, in a rational and constant growth. Historical analysis shows that real science differs substantially from ideal science. Kuhn rejects the ideal image of science, showing that it is made up of social, political, cultural, etc. Kuhn outlines this central idea in the "Introduction" to the structure, entitled "A Role for History." The study of the history of science rejects the traditional view that all developments of a theory are merely antecedents of the current state of the theory. Kuhn answers these questions with the notion of a "paradigm" [1, p. 10]. This notion is central to understanding continuity and change in the history of science. Analyzing the history of science in the light of paradigms allows us to explain why scientists retain theories despite finding anomalies. When an anomaly appears, scientists can put it in brackets hoping to find a solution and continue their line of research. Often with the passage of time and the refinement of instruments, both technical and mathematical, it is possible to move from an anomaly to a confirmatory example of theory. Added to the above, there is always the possibility of using ad hoc hypotheses to save a theory [1, p. 78]. Critical Rationalism knows this defense strategy and admits that this difficulty cannot be eliminated at the methodological level. The only option for Falsacionism is to establish a code of honor that the scientist must respect. In other words, the scientist should not use any strategy that takes away the falsifiable character of a theory [1, p. 104]. Therefore, maintaining the falsifiability of scientific statements is not only a test of the temperament of the theory but also of the temperament of the scientist. However, Kuhn's analysis shows that the retention or rejection of a theory cannot be fully explained by the Falsacionist methodology, whether it is analyzed at an exclusively logical level or whether it resorts to the so-called "code of honor" of the scientist. The Falsacionist methodology forces the facts to suit the explanations.

On the basis of the notion of paradigm, Kuhn [1, p. 13] analyzes the history of different disciplines and determines that in all of them, it is possible to distinguish two clearly defined periods: The pre-dogmatic period and the paradigmatic or normal science period. The first corresponds to the stage where the discipline has not reached sufficient development and many schools appear competing with each other. The central point of this period is that there are no basic agreements between the different schools, which generate a permanent dispute at the level of the *foundations* because neither the object nor the method proper to the discipline appears to be clear. Once a school has managed to impose itself on its competitors, converting the followers of other schools or condemning them to oblivion, it is when the discipline enters the paradigmatic period. This period is characterized by the rapid development and absence of discussions on the fundamentals [1, pp. 35–43].

When a discipline enters the paradigmatic period, it no longer returns to the previous period [1, p. 79], characterized by the simultaneous presence of several competing schools. Radical changes are scientific revolutions, where one paradigm is suppressed and another appears in its place. A revolution occurs when a certain paradigm cannot adequately respond to a series of problems, which under its assumptions, examples, and theories are presented as anomalies. The substitution of one paradigm for another cannot be explained through the traditional idea of continuity [1, p. 77]. The shift from Aristotelian to Newtonian physics and from Ptolemaic to Copernican astronomy shows a total shift in the scientific horizon in their respective disciplines and represents a classic example of the scientific revolution.

As can be seen, the historical turn represents a radical change in the way of conceiving scientific rationality. "The transition from a paradigm in crisis to a new one from which a new tradition of normal science can emerge is far from a cumulative process, one achieve by an articulation or extension of the old paradigm" [1, pp. 84–85]. The transition from one paradigm to another means a change in methods and applications. Kuhn argues that in the constitution of a paradigm or a "disciplinary matrix", as he will later call it, the notion of the scientific community *is fundamental*. A scientific community is usually composed of several generations, so the community of Newtonian mechanics lasted more than 200 years and that of Ptolemaic astronomers more than 1000 years. Obviously, each community will have its own elements that will differentiate it from the previous one. However, these elements do not come from a given a priori *definition* but from concrete scientific practice. A disciplinary matrix is composed of symbolic generalizations, models, values, and examples. These four elements are practiced and maintained by those who work within a discipline over a period of time. Symbolic generalizations "are the formal or the readily formalizable components of the disciplinary matrix" [1, p. 182]. Values, on the other hand, are key to understanding the cohesion of the scientific community, even though they vary greatly from one individual to another [1, p. 185]. Some values are of a very general nature—such as that science should be useful to society—, while others are particular to the group—for example, that, according to the degree of accuracy that is postulated, the quantitative method is preferred to the qualitative. Finally, examples appear. These represent the solutions that the disciplinary matrix has given throughout its development and serve to initiate future members through textbooks.

Models are the second constitutive element that Kuhn points out of disciplinary matrices, and where metaphysical elements appear. These commitments act as beliefs in particular models, which fulfill heuristic functions within scientific research. "… the electric circuit may be regarded as a steady-state hydrodynamic system; the molecules of a gas behave like tiny elastic billiard balls in random motion." These group commitments move from heuristic to ontological models and "Among other things they supply the group with preferred or permissible analogies and metaphors" [1, p. 184]. Consequently, they will also determine what the explanations and solutions to the problems are, and conversely, what the enigmas and the importance they have for the disciplinary matrix.

Variations on Incommensurability

Popper [2] and Kuhn first recognized the importance of metaphysics for science in the face of the neopositivism tradition. However, both authors have great differences in understanding what metaphysics is and what degree of objectivity it can achieve. For Popper [3, pp. 1–31], metaphysics is not only a source of bold conjecture, but also the basis that guarantees us a world outside ourselves which we can possibly know. For Kuhn, instead, a paradigm, far from providing objective knowledge, is determined by historicity. The way the scientist sees the world is shaped through the current disciplinary matrix. In the first edition of *The Structure*, Kuhn states that "The proponents of competing paradigms practice their trade in different worlds (…) Practicing in different worlds, the two groups of scientists see different things when they look from the same point in the same direction" [1, p. 150]. This statement is directly related to the thesis of incommensurability. One of the pillars of the thesis of incommensurability is the theoretical burden of observational statements. From the 1950s and 1960s, this issue became of fundamental importance in Hanson's work. This author, based on the psychology of the *Gestalt*, definitively refutes the neopositivist thesis that postulates the common sensory and observational basis of perceptions. The vision itself is, for Hanson [4], an action that is constituted from a theoretical charge. If we stick to the results pointed out by Hanson's theory, the reference is not independent of the way in which we access to it. Two theories will be truly immeasurable when they assume the same reference framework, but that framework is constituted by what each scientific community understands to belong to it. From this belief, it follows that truth is not associated with the metaphysical assumption around the existence of a world independent of us, but with what the paradigm or the disciplinary matrix postulates as such. Following one of the best-known examples, the concept "planet" has undergone, with the passage from Ptolemaic to Copernican astronomy, a series of transformations. These transformations not only imply that we cannot explain the change that has taken place in the concept of "planet" with the passage from one theory to another but also show a typical case of incommensurability between rival theories.

So far the discussion has been centered on the first version of the thesis of incommensurability, the so-called "global incommensurability". The second version of the thesis of incommensurability is the so-called "local incommensurability." This version is restricted to the semantic aspect, so it does not affect the totality of the theories but some specific parts of them. The local version, says Kuhn, is the original version of it [5, pp. 35–36].

Along with the change in the thesis of incommensurability, Kuhn's thought underwent a series of transformations and clarifications that led him to distinguish between interpretation and translation. Interpreting is the task proper to the historian of science and that allows anything expressed in a language to be understood by a speaker of another language, if enough effort and imagination are applied to the task. Translation, on the other hand, does not change the meaning of words or phrases, it is a quasi-symmetric task governed by some manual that specifies the sequences of words that in one language can be replaced by a given sequence in another language. This kind of translation is called Kuhn "Quinean" [5]. The science historian encounters texts that require the construction of an alternative form of reading, which needs the construction of an alternative lexicon to be addressed. Therefore, the reader of a previous paradigm must detect the terms that have changed meaning to discover the use they had in the original text. Certainly, the only way for someone to understand a text in another language is by learning its language. In other words, understanding a former paradigm implies, for a member of another paradigm, become bilingual. Learning another language brings intrinsically a different way of dividing and understanding the world, it is not just learning a more or less complete list of word meanings.

In this sense, it is interesting to note Kuhn's response to the attacks of Philip Kitcher on the thesis of incommensurability. Kitcher [6] departs from the analysis of the language of twentieth-century chemists and concludes that it can be used to identify referents of the terms of the chemists of the nineteenth century. On this basis, Kitcher claims that modern terminology explains why and in what areas the old theories were successful. Kuhn [5, pp. 40–41] denies that this could be a translation and that it would lead to the rejection of the thesis of incommensurability. However, he accepts that historians can understand ancient texts and use modern language to identify references to the terms of those texts. In other words, he accepts Kitcher's results but indicates that to understand the theories of the past historians cannot make a translation, but an interpretation. For this statement, Kuhn [5, p. 14] affirms: "Is 'full communication' nevertheless possible between an eighteenth- and twentieth-century chemist, as Kitcher supposes? Perhaps, yes, but only if one of the two learns the other's language, becoming, in that sense, a participant in the other's practice of chemistry."

Division of Sciences

Kuhn's approach to disciplinary matrices and incommensurability allows us to appreciate how the different scientific categories shape and constitute the object of study. In other words, the vision of the object makes the object different. The relationships between different areas of knowledge refer to the topic of the classification of sciences, one of the basic questions of the history of the philosophy of science, epistemology, gnoseology, and the sciences themselves. Classifications of knowledge go back to the beginning of Western philosophy with Plato and his distinction between *doxa* and *episteme*. The first is the realm of mere opinion, while the second is the knowledge founded, true, and known by causes. From this first classification, the rest of Western history is nourished to understand what science is. Aristotle [7], on the other hand, is the first to propose a complete classification of knowledge through the distinction between theoretical, practical, and productive sciences. The first are those who seek in and for themselves a knowledge that does not depend on anything either. The second are those on which the action of man and his being with others is based. The productive ones are concerned only with building objects and depend on the agent that produces the constructed object. This division is based on the degree of autonomy that each knowledge has, and it raises a relationship of hierarchy between them. The Aristotelian distinction had a long reign extending into the Middle Ages, where it was mixed with elements of the Christian worldview.

In modernity, there is an investment in the valuation of science. The search for knowledge through knowledge itself is not the ultimate goal of science but the satisfaction of human material needs. During the Middle Ages, the practical sciences were relegated to a theoretical level; in modernity, human actions were directly subjected to a field that must be understood within the technique. This shift is by no means innocuous: it functions as a powerful disciplinary matrix. The removal of the category of practical science leaves an impossible gap for the other categories to fill. The analysis of human action resists being framed from strange categories: thinking that one can obtain the same rigor or that it is possible to think of a single method independently of the object are also products of eliminating the practical sciences. In addition, the removal of the category of practical science invalidates reflection on the ends and the good within the realm of science. In other words, to reflect on the ends and the good is something foreign to science.

Once the hierarchical approach to the division of sciences and the elimination of practical sciences has been removed, classifications of sciences tend to be based on different criteria. There are criteria that attend to the ontological, assuming that reality is constructed by types of entities or phenomena. The distinction between natural and spiritual sciences responds to this criterion because it assumes that there are two distinct areas of reality. Other criteria aim to distinguish disciplines according to the human capacity with which they are known. Thus, memory will correspond to history; to logic, reason, etc. Others speak of hard and soft sciences, paying attention to the rigor that would characterize some in the face of the vagueness of others. In a simplified way in the latter classification, the use of formalized languages is usually taken as a synonym for "rigor."

Within the range of classifications of contemporary science, the classification of Rudolf Carnap [8] is the most widely used. Carnap distinguishes knowledge into two large groups: formal sciences, on the one hand, and factual sciences on the other. This Carnap distinction responds to a triple demand. The first is the ontological criterion, which departs from the entities of which one and another discipline is concerned, the factual sciences work with entities that require the contest of experiences to be known, while the formal ones do not require the experience to know. The second criterion is logic, which refers to the types of statements of which one or another type of discipline is used so that the factual sciences use synthetic statements, where the predicate contains elements distinct from the subject and thus broaden knowledge. Formal sciences use analytical statements, where the predicate explains what is already contained in the subject. The last of the criteria refers to the method that is to the procedures for research and validation of knowledge. Carnap's classification marks the academic organization and the way in which knowledge is taught within the educational system at all levels. Beyond the fact that there is a fairly important consensus on the distinction between formal and factual sciences, the distinction between social and natural facts is not universally accepted. The three criteria that Carnap points out in this subdivision are not so clear because they generate great debate in the academic community. What is the method in the social sciences, the same as the natural ones or another different one? If the social sciences do not admit the same method as the natural ones, will they be sciences? If the same method is used, won't the object be forced?

Along with the above, one of the central characteristics of the Carnap classification is that the form of communication or interaction between different kinds of knowledge is not explicit. How the knowledge that is constantly emerging will work or where it will be included is not clear.

Problem of Interdisciplinary in the Approach to Addictions

The debate over the method is central from modernity. The method is the one that allows us to distinguish what science is and what science is not. The basis will only be achieved from the exercise and use of the method. The different problems posed by addictions require an interdisciplinary approach. The problem is that interdiscipline is not a task without discrepancies. An intuitive approach affirms that interdiscipline means to gather the different looks on an object to try to understand it better. In a way, interdisciplinarity forces us to broaden our gaze, to admit other angles of vision of the object, without renouncing our own. However, it is not only a matter of knowing an object but also of operating with it, of solving problems, and responding to practical questions.

Boon and Van Baalen [9, p. 16] state that two different forms of philosophical analysis of science can be recognized, or as they call it "two distinct *philosophical paradigms of science*." This distinction appears for the first time in Boon [10], who distinguishes between a "physics paradigm" and another that he calls an "engineering paradigm." According to this distinction, the physics paradigm focuses more on the metaphysical and ontological assumptions of a disciplinary matrix, while the engineering paradigm focuses on producing useful knowledge to solve problems external to scientific practice. This second form of philosophical analysis of science is where interdiscipline can be included, not only as a theoretical element but as an operative reality or one that must operate at the level of giving answers and articulating the different visions about the same object. These articulated visions are what make interdiscipline operational.

Interdisciplinarity is no longer just a matter of academic debate, but it influences different areas of knowledge in the world of production and economics. Thus, addressing the classification of sciences is one of the first tasks. The location of each discipline preserves how access to the object will be or how it should be. An interesting case is the case of the social sciences. These are part of the factual sciences and therefore share or should share at least the following basic characteristics: objectivity and valuing neutrality. These characteristics are totally revealing because, on the one hand, they leave out much classical knowledge (ethics, for example) of the concept of science and at the same time, they modify the permitted activity of other disciplines (the so-called "political science"). The first case is out of scientific knowledge because the concepts proper to ethics, such as value, reflections on the good, and the ends of human life, contradict the basic fact that science must be removed from evaluation. The second case is a typical example of a radical change in worldview. Politics was, for Aristotle [7], the typical example and the main practical science. Politics is the knowledge that determines what should be done and what should not be done because human life is always a life in a community. This value dimension is outside modern science. The Aristotelian practical sciences are a completely strange category for modernity. For modernity, political science is only one of the social sciences, which studies the theory and practice of politics, systems, and political behaviors in society. Its objective is to establish, from the observation of facts of the political reality, explanations as certain as possible about its functioning, leaving aside any valuable traits. Political science does not mark the end of life because it is a descriptive science.

If we think of a complex reality such as addictions we see that they are not only difficult to fit into some category but also require different classifications. In other words, the different classifications of science cannot be ignored because they are useful to make a more integrative approach to the object. One of today's great challenges is to understand how different forms of knowledge relate to each other. This challenge can be addressed through the development of nondichotomous systems. A case in point is the famous circular system of Jean Piaget [11]. In this case, disciplines operate in a collaborative, nonhierarchical manner. The underlying idea of circularity is not vicious but virtuous. In this case, it is no longer a question of thinking that biology is imposed on the social sciences or on philosophy or on those sciences, but that they all contribute their vision of the problems that arise. In the same line as Piaget, what Alicia Gianella [12] calls the "reticular model" has been proposed. The interesting point about this model is that it captures the growing complexity and network of different knowledge because "… in the network members who in turn are networks are admitted: thus, neurosciences are part of the cognitive sciences, as much as the sciences of language." Along with the above, it is also the case that transversal theories to different disciplines form in turn networks. The Theory of Evolution is an example of this. The collaborative work between the members of the different disciplines generates a synergy of knowledge growth that opens new horizons of understanding. At the same time, it makes the methodology of work enriched and does not fall into an inbreeding where the practice of a method cannot be questioned, falling into dogmatic attitudes, in many cases. In the reticular model, philosophy is another discipline that participates in the reticulum. Therefore, philosophy "By positioning itself in this dual role of participant and evaluator of the dynamics of knowledge, its commitment is different and greater…" [12] as it was conceived in the twentieth century. The reticular-collaborative model allows and forces the members of each scientific community to think and work differently. This new form of work involves tearing down not only structures of thought but also administrative and bureaucratic structures.

In the case of addictions, it is advisable to allow all kinds of approaches. In this sense, an approach that rescues and uses the distinctions of the classics can help to understand the object in a different and renewed way. It is counterproductive to address addictions without taking into account the ethical aspect or the political dimensions, in the classical sense of both kinds of knowledge. The great challenge of interdiscipline is to make the scientist an interpreter capable of speaking different languages. That is, he must be able to know how to interpret the language of two different disciplinary matrices and must take both, not simply overlap them. Leaving aside the approach where there is no possibility of translation is the first step toward a true interdisciplinary approach. The second step is to make this interdiscipline operational through the collaboration of different traditions.

Conclusion

Addictions are challenging problems. How to approach, how to intervene, and how to think policies about them are issues that require interdisciplinary work. However, interdiscipline, to be real and operational, must be thought of from categories that exceed the mere juxtaposition of disciplines. Kuhn proposes the notion of translation as a key tool to understand the possibility of communication between different disciplinary matrices. By way of example, a question that is always present in all areas is: what is happiness? This question, within the scope of the contemporary distinction of science, is challenging because it cannot be placed anywhere within the division of science. Moreover, this question is foreign to the field of scientific self-reflection, posed in contemporary terms. Trying to understand happiness only from accepted scientific parameters means true reductionism. Reductionism is a path that takes us away from interdisciplinary because it imposes a one-way look at problems. Thinking from globally immeasurable paradigms generates serious problems to address problems that require wide-ranging views. For this reason, if incommensurability is partial and supports translation, then different traditions can help in understanding complex objects like addictions.

References

1. Kuhn T. The structure of scientific revolution. Chicago: The University of Chicago Press; 1970.
2. Popper K. The logic of scientific discovery. London: Hutchinson; 1959.
3. Popper K. Objective knowledge. An evolutionary approach. Oxford: Clarendon Press; 1979.
4. Hanson NR. Patterns of discovery. Cambridge: Cambridge University Press; 1958.
5. Kuhn T. Commensurability, comparability, communicability. In: Conant J, Huageland J, editors. The road since structure. Chicago: The University of Chicago Press; 1982. p. 33–57.
6. Kitcher P. Theories, theorist and theoretical change. Philos Rev. 1978;87:519–47.
7. Aristotle. Nicomachean ethics. Indianpolis/Cambridge: Hackeet Publishing Company; 1999.
8. Carnap R. Philosophical foundations of physics. New York: Basic Books Inc; 1966.
9. Van Boon M, Baalen S. Epistemology for interdisciplinary research—shifting philosophical paradigms of science. Eur J Philos Sci. 2019;9:16. https://doi.org/10.1007/s13194-018-0242-4.
10. Boon M. An engineering paradigm in the biomedical sciences: knowledge as epistemic tool. Prog Biophys Mol Biol. 2017;129:25–39. https://doi.org/10.1016/j.pbiomolbio.2017.04.001.
11. Piaget J. Psychology and epistemology: towards a theory of knowledge. Harmondsworth: Penguin; 1972.
12. Gianella A, Las disciplinas científicas y sus relaciones. En: Anales de la educación común/Tercer siglo/año 2/número 3/Filosofía política de la enseñanza/abril de 2006. p. 74 a 83. http://fcaenlinea1.unam.mx/anexos/1156/1156_u5_act1b_p16.pdf. Accessed 6 Mar 2019.

3 Addictions and Artificial Intelligence in *Brave New World*: From the Benedict Option to the Hermit Beginning

Luis Enrique Echarte,
Augusto Pascual Ítalo Gargiulo,
and Pascual Ángel Gargiulo

Present fears are less than horrible imaginings. (*Macbeth*. Shakespeare)

O soul! Soul! Beauty of the world! Indestructible! Rapturing! With your eternal youth! (*Hyperion*. Hölderlin)

Introduction. What Aldous Huxley Can Still Teach Us?

The year 2022 marks the 90th anniversary of the publication of Aldous Huxley's *Brave New World* (*BNW*) [1, 2], one of the most politically and academically resonant modern novels and, most surprisingly, with such social visibility that its imagery has achieved pop icon status. What explains its success? Because it is not the first late modern dystopia. However, it is the one that has best diagnosed the evils and risks of contemporary science and, as we now know, the one that has been most successful in forecasting its consequences. For example, one of the topics dealt with in the book, which is now very topical again with the war in Ukraine, is related to the dangers of nuclear and biological weapons, not

L. E. Echarte (✉)
Humanities and Medical Ethics Unit, School of Medicine, University of Navarra, Pamplona, Navarra, Spain
e-mail: lecharte@unav.es; https://www.unav.edu/en/web/investigacion/nuestros-investigadores/detalle-investigadores-cv?investigadorId=59376

A. P. Í. Gargiulo
Laboratorio de Neurociencias y Psicología Experimental, Fundación Corporación Tecnológica Latinoamericana (FUCOTEL), Cátedra de Psicopatología, Facultad de Humanidades y Ciencias Económicas, Universidad Católica Argentina (UCA), Área de Farmacología, Facultad de Ciencias Médicas, Universidad Nacional de Cuyo (UNCuyo), Consejo Nacional de Investigaciones Científicas y Técnicas (CONICET), Mendoza, Argentina

Centro Integral de Salud Mental Argentino (CISMA), Buenos Aires, Argentina; https://www.cisma.com.ar; http://fucotel.org/index.php/blog

P. Á. Gargiulo
Laboratory of Neurosciences and Experimental Psychology, Latin American Technological Corporation Foundation (FUCOTEL), Cathedra of Psychopathology, Catholic University of Argentina, Area of Pharmacology, Department of Pathology, National University of Cuyo, CONICET, Guaymallén, Mendoza, Argentina; http://fucotel.org/index.php/blog; https://www.linkedin.com/in/pascual-angel-gargiulo-63414a47/?originalSubdomain=ar

P. Á. Gargiulo, H. L. Mesones-Arroyo (eds.), *Psychiatry and Neuroscience Update – Vol. V*, https://doi.org/10.1007/978-3-031-72219-6_3

so much because of the evil they can bring, which is evident to all, but because of the fear they generate among us.

> What is the point of truth or beauty when anthrax bombs are exploding all around you? It was then that science began to be policed; after the Nine Years' War, people were already willing to have their desires controlled. Anything to live in peace. [2, p. 235]

Such exacerbated fear is a consequence of previous evils and, under certain circumstances, is the cause of evils worse than an atomic explosion or a pandemic. In Huxley's futuristic society, called the *World State*, citizens have surrendered enormous amounts of freedom in exchange for personal security and social stability–sustainability. It is not exempt from, but it is of a weak character, inauthentic, and founded on strictly objectivist equality.

> There was something called democracy. As though men were more than physico-chemically equal. [2, p. 47]

Unlike dystopias such as George Orwell's *1984*, in *BNW*, freedom is not stolen but offered as a bargaining chip to a government that agrees to do whatever it takes to ensure peace and sustained quality of life for its citizens. This pact includes not only state hypervigilance but also genetic, psychological, and social conditioning measures so that individuals do not hinder the plan drawn up for the durability of the system and the supposed happiness they are guaranteed. As part of this conditioning, a series of routines are established in the population that the individual unfailingly associates with his well-being and, at the same time, about which he cannot think critically or assume, in any way, their partial or total cessation. In other words, the designers of the *World State* use addiction strategies to avoid the uncertainty that free thought and personal initiative introduce in human relations: addiction to the Soma (a happiness-producing drug), to unbridled consumption, to sex, to technology, to *reality shows*… addiction even to the gregarious feeling of belonging to the group or caste—Alpha, *Beta, Gamma, Delta, and Epsilon*.

This last addiction, which is at the heart of all mass dynamics (using José Ortega y Gasset's term) probably the one that most effectively prevents escaping from each citizen's role. In the following soliloquy by Bernard Marx, one of the novel's protagonist outcasts, the strength of this feeling is expressed in the following form:

> A chronic fear of being slighted made him avoid his equals, made him stand, where his inferiors were concerned, self-consciously on his dignity. How bitterly he envied men like Henry Foster and Benito Hoover! Men who never had to shout at an Epsilon to get an order obeyed; men who took their position for granted; men who moved through the caste system as a fish through the water—so utterly at home as to be unaware either of themselves or of the beneficent and comfortable element in which they had their being. [2, p. 65]

All these addictions, from the major to the minor, appear in *BNW* perfectly orchestrated, though without the most common adverse effects we usually find linked: illness, loss of job, and abandonment of family, among others. Even death seems to be virtually dodged with the achievement of short, quick transitions between blissful and cadaverous states. Death does not bother if it barely appears in a life of uninterrupted pleasures and chores.

> Soma played none of these unpleasant tricks. The holiday it gave was perfect and, if the morning after was disagreeable, it was so, not intrinsically, but only by comparison with the joys of the holiday. The remedy was to make the holiday continuous […] Soma may make you lose a few years in time—the doctor went on. But think of the enormous, immeasurable durations it can give you out of time. Every soma-holiday is a bit of what our ancestors used to call eternity. [2, p. 156]

Huxley presents us, in short, with the paradoxical scenario of a society that seems to function optimally and sustainably, although at the price of citizens who have succumbed, in a controlled manner, to multiple addictions.

Regardless of whether Western societies today are closer or further away from this *kindly* apocalyptic scenario, Huxley's narrative is fruitful for rethinking the main approaches currently used to deal with the problem of addictions and treatments derived from such approaches. With this chapter, we intend to enrich the discussion, particularly in those issues where Huxley's perspective is very original. To this end, we will introduce, firstly, the framework theory from which most of the approaches in the research of the addictive phenomenon are governed today. Secondly, we will point out fundamental questions regarding the social factors involved—one of the most important, the development of Artificial Intelligence (AI). Finally, we will bring into the contemporary debate the basic ideas expressed in *BNW* on the possible solutions to a society structured on the idea of fear.

A Multidimensional Approach to Addictions

Addiction is defined generically as a chronic mental disorder in which the patient suffers relapses, and it is characterized by compulsive substance seeking or repetition of pleasurable behaviors despite the negative consequences of the consumption or behavior [3]. Currently, pharmacological interventions remain the primary therapies in addiction, although, for decades, psychological strategies for behavior modification have been gaining ground in medical practices as supportive therapies [4]. Cognitive behavioral therapy and cue exposure therapy are among the most effective for this purpose [5, 6]. With the former, the aim is to enhance inhibitory control and cognitive flexibility, and with the latter, to reduce reactivity to cues of exposure to the addictive element. Deep brain stimulation and therapeutic gene modulation also appear as promising strategies in the treatment of addiction [7].

In addition to the treatments mentioned above, there are classical psychotherapeutic treatments. These take their target in the study of the patient's personal and family history, which would include both individual factors (e.g., personality traits) and social factors (family ties, labor integration, etc.). All this is to draw a map that helps to explain everything from the causes that generate addiction, such as low self-esteem, to problems associated with rehabilitation, such as low frustration tolerance. Many prevention strategies also draw from the psychosocial paradigms offered by such approaches [8].

These latter psychotherapies usually seek, firstly, to make the patient more aware of his or her way of thinking, feeling, and being in the world, and more importantly, of the reason for all of them, which includes becoming aware of some critical internal psychological processes (unconscious defense mechanisms, for example) and also external environmental factors (such as the trivialization of drugs in his or her work, family or leisure environment). Secondly, and in line with this starting point, the aim is to motivate the patient to generate changes in his or her lifestyle by first externalizing his or her intentions and then internalizing them [9, 10]. Interpersonal therapy, for example, focuses its strategies on changing the individual's environment by replacing more superficial, unstable, and conflictive relationships with healthier ones. Similarly, family intervention therapies seek to involve family members in treatments to facilitate such lifestyle changes. Something similar is pursued by group therapies, which aim to generate communication between addicted patients, as this seems effective in counteracting the frequent denial by the patient of his or her addiction, a response that often leads to increasing shame and isolation [11, 12].

Classical psychotherapies, in their wide varieties, stem from the major schools of psychotherapy: structuralism, behaviorism, psychoanalysis, Gestalt, and humanism, among the most important. Each of them proposes its framework theory to explain what the psyche is and, based on this explanation, to guide the patient's way of being. It is not surprising, therefore, that these schools are strongly influenced by the philosophical movements of the nineteenth and twentieth centuries: phenomenology, existentialism, functionalism, evolutionism, etc. However, with all the differences that may separate them, there is a common point from which most psychotherapies draw: the belief that an integrated and structured system of thought helps mental well-being and, conversely, that the destructuring of thought can generate illness. With the so-called meaning therapies, which take up this fundamental idea, psychotherapists try to guide the patient's conversation so that he becomes more aware of what he believes and does and, most importantly, so that these beliefs and behaviors become more logical and coherent. Of all the schools, logotherapy is possibly, first proposed by Viktor Frankl, the one that places the most significant emphasis on the therapeutic benefit of the search for meaning [13]. Among other features, this treatment highlights the particular respect that, for Frankl, the physician or psychologist should have for the patient's beliefs, who should not be coerced but only, based on his beliefs, helped to weave a solid horizon of meaning. We will see that, according to Huxley's proposal, this respect for the patient, depending on how it is understood, may generate benefits or aggravate addiction.

Meaning and Intuitive Sense Therapies

In the matter of meaning, psychotherapy becomes eminently philosophical or, if one prefers, where philosophy reaches clinical heights. Because the main question to resolve is whether integration is possible based on laws of coherence and rationality, yet, can the mind use real order to gain stability, or, on the contrary, must it build such order in an eminently chaotic reality? Frankl defends the former: the patient's inquiry must be directed toward the observation of reality and the search for truth. The philosophical assumptions behind this thesis are of the first order: reality can be known, and knowledge of reality is beneficial—healthy truth. It is not a new idea as it appears already in Plato's *Charmides*:

> 'But our king Zalmoxis', he said, 'who is a god, says that just as one should not attempt to cure the eyes apart from the head, nor the head apart from the body, so one should not attempt to cure the body apart from the soul. And this, he says, is the very reason why most diseases are beyond the Greek doctors, that they do not pay attention to the whole as they ought to do, since if the whole is not in good condition, it is impossible that the part should be. Because,' he said, 'the soul is the source both of bodily health and bodily disease for the whole man, and these flow from the soul in the same way that the eyes are affected by the head. So it is necessary first and foremost to cure the soul if the parts of the head and of the rest of the body are to be healthy. And the soul,' he said, my dear friend, 'is cured by means of certain charms, and these charms consist of beautiful words. It is a result of such words that temperance arises in the soul, and when the soul acquires and possesses temperance, it is easy to provide health both for the head and for the rest of the body'. [14]

The reasonableness of the good speeches that Plato puts in Socrates' mouth contrasts with the persuasive speeches of the sophists, who were less attentive to the veracity of their judgments and more to the intrinsic power of the narrative. The coherence of his sentences may be the same or even more prominent in the second group, but the search for truthfulness occurs only in the former. In the words of one of the most important representatives of the sophist school:

> If it was speech that persuaded her and deceived her soul, her defence remains easy. Speech is a great power, which achieves the most divine works by means of the smallest and least visible form; for it can even put a stop to fear, remove grief, create joy, and increase pity. [15, pp. 131–133]

The sophists represent paradigmatically in philosophy what post-rationalist psychotherapies are in psychology. Among the latter, the neuropsychiatrist Vittorio Guidano is possibly the one who explicitly defends the extreme position. According to his *systemic cognitive procedural approach*, the patient should not seek thoughts conforming to reality but create his reality, i.e., forge an essential and knowingly subjective fiction capable of offering a singular unity to the mind that reality is unable to provide.

> Adaptation therefore is the ability to transform perturbation arising from interaction with the world into information meaningful to one's experiential order. Maintaining adaptive adequacy essentially means preserving one's sense of self by continuously transforming the perceived world rather than merely corresponding to it. [16, p. 6]

It is not reality but the affective experiences derived from correct narratives elaborated by the subject that Guidano seeks in his peculiar psychotherapy. The influence of Michel Foucault's social constructivism in this proposal is evident and reinforces one of the philosopher's most polemic theses: not only health but also mental illness is a construction. Although Foucault puts here the decisive weight on the social element:

> Madness cannot be found in a wild state. Madness exists only within a society, it does not exist outside the forms of sensibility which isolate it and the forms of repulsion which exclude it or capture it. We can therefore say that in the Middle Ages, and then in the Renaissance, madness is present within the social horizon as an aesthetic or day-to-day fact; then, in the eighteenth century—as a result of confinement—madness goes through a period of silence, of exclusion. It has lost the function of manifestation, of revelation, that it had in the epoch of Shakespeare and Cervantes (Lady Macbeth, for instance, begins to speak the truth when she goes mad), and becomes mendacious, derisory. Finally, the twentieth century collars madness, and reduces it to a natural phenomenon bound up with the truth of the world. This positivist appropriation gave rise to, on the one hand, the scornful philanthropy which all psychiatry displays towards the madman and, on the other, the great lyrical protest we find in poetry from Nerval to Artaud, an effort to restore to the experience of madness a depth and a power of revelation which had been destroyed by confinement. [17, pp. 114–115]

The social dependence on mental health is not a new idea. Numerous philosophers and psychologists of the nineteenth and twentieth centuries have accepted that this relationship between society and mental health is founded on the capacity of the former to generate global images of existence that individuals can assimilate. Historically, the most important have been those of a religious nature. This idea appears in many of the writings of Émile Durkheim, one of the fathers of the field of sociology, for whom religion is a crucial natural phenomenon in the promotion of social cohesion. Similarly, Erik Erikson, one of the prominent authors in the early days of evolutionary psychology, will assert that such cosmogonies are fundamental in developing and entrenching the subject's identity. Erikson also adds a crucial etiopathogenic factor in *late modernity*: the loss of social belief systems leads to a weakening of the sense and meaning of identity and the consequent increase of panic in the face of a fragmented perception of existence [18, pp. 56–58]. This is also the reason why philosophers such as Jünger Habermas or Daniel Dennet urge intellectuals of the twenty-first century to replace mythical-religious discourses with scientific images that offer a new horizon of meaning after the devastation left by, to use Max Weber's expression, the disenchantment of the world [19, pp. 101–115; 20, p. 186]. However, as Norbert Elias rightly points out, scientific narratives, especially those of a purely objectivist nature, seem to be more effective in generating doubts among believers and nonbelievers than in generating new totalizing discourses:

> The unwelcome knowledge and the concealing fantasies are therefore probably progeny of the same stage of evolution. Today, in possession of an immense store of experience, we can no longer avoid asking whether these complaisant dreams do not in the long run have far more unwelcome and dangerous results for human beings in their communal life than the unvarnished knowledge. [20, p. 35]

Elias' diagnosis would explain, at least partially, why more and more philosophers are proposing to counteract existential panic by constructing fiction in the most authentic Guidano style. This is the case, for example, with Richard Rorty, who advocates the definitive renunciation of the idea that some images of the world are better than others. From his Neopragmatism, he proposes the democratization of all vocabularies and images, that is, the cessation of privileges based on greater or lesser proximity to reality. Newtonian physics, Buddhism, Darwinism, or feminist poetry would be nothing but discourses that, in different linguistic contexts, would function equally in the task of offering us shelter in our increasingly inhospitable world [21, pp. 63–77].

From Anguish to Fear

Post-rationalist proposals have gained more ground in academic than clinical contexts. And this makes sense since it implies admitting a degree of subjectivism among health professionals that few medical or psychological associations would still be willing to accept. It would mean giving up the scientific aura on which much of their authority and expertise in mental health is sustained. Nevertheless, some steps in this direction are being taken. See, for example, the greater diagnostic weight that is given to symptoms—subjective criteria of illness—in successive editions of the Diagnostic and Statistical Manual of Mental Disorders. This is the context in which Muñoz and Jaramillo write that the DSM-V opens the door to medicalize everyday situations such as bereavement because there are sufferings that, however natural they may be, the patient may decide not to tolerate [22].

The trend among mental health researchers and clinicians seems to be the opposite. Both in the field of psychiatry and psychology, empirical research is gaining ground, which explains the rise of the cognitive-behavioral and exposure psychotherapies mentioned above and, of course, the development of pharmacological treatments. All of them propose hypotheses that can be easily modeled in laboratories, although, on the other hand, they do not favor multidimensional approaches to the problem of addictions or synergies with sense therapies. Part of this drift may have to do with a rebound effect in the face of classical psychotherapies excessively imbued with the single-case phenomenological approach, a situation that prevents generalizations from being established as frequently as they are established in other fields of medicine. Perhaps this tendency can also be explained as a radical response from those who fear the subjectivist drift of the mental health field. Alternatively, it may also be because philosophy, its methods of access to truth, and its connection with scientific-technical rationality are less and less understood. The philosopher José Ortega y Gasset adheres to this third hypothesis, for whom this lack of understanding of philosophy would also explain why science has fallen into what he calls the barbarism of specialism, an expression to which he dedicates the following words:

> A fair amount of the things that have to be done in physics or in biology is mechanical work of the mind which can be done by anyone, or almost anyone. For the purpose of innumerable investigations it is possible to divide science into small sections, to enclose oneself in one of these, and to leave out of consideration all the rest. The solidity and exactitude of the methods allow of this temporary but quite real disarticulation of knowledge. The work is done under one of these methods as with a machine, and in order to obtain quite abundant results it is not even necessary to have rigorous notions of their meaning and foundations. In this way the majority of scientists help the general advance of science while shut up in the narrow cell of their laboratory, like the bee in the cell of its hive, or the turnspit in its wheel. [23, p. 123]

With the barbarism of specialism, Ortega y Gasset expresses the growing disinterest of intellectuals in everything outside their specific field of research. Moreover, this disinterest clashes entirely with the classic university project of collaboration between men of science and letters to elaborate a cohesive image of the world. Again, if the meaning offered by religions enters into decadence and science renounces to take its place, then man seems doomed to existential anguish, to emptiness, and, more importantly, as Jacques Derrida denounces, to the anticipatory fear of suffering anguish. It is not surprising, he says, that our society is adopting strategies, never before seen, to overcome this fear. Unfortunately, this solution, he concludes, only leads to a sort of fear even more harmful than the previous one, *the fear of fear* [24].

Addiction can be understood, in this framework, as a manifestation and adverse effect of one of these social paths against anguish and fear. Some authors even dare to assert that this could be one of the main causes of addiction. Bruce K. Alexander, for example, disqualifies the prevailing theory around addiction, which he calls "the official view" or the "medical model," as a position that "is based on reductionist hi-tech neuroscience" [25, p. 208]. In opposition to this, he proposes the *Dislocation Theory of Addiction*, a holistic approach that aims to find the root causes of the problem.

> Also in contrast to the official view, the dislocation theory focuses not on individuals but on the social causes of mass addiction in various societies and historical eras. Of course, each addicted individual has a unique history to tell, but the dislocation theory provides a framework within which individual struggles with addiction in the context of their own predispositions can be more deeply understood. [25, p. 224]

Alexander follows a scheme of reasoning similar to that of Erikson and Ortega y Gasset. On the one hand, he argues that modern societies' intellectual and social fragmentation is an omnipresent fact in late modernity. Dislocation would be "both the psychological consequence of social fragmentation and the precursor to mass addiction" [25, p. 225]. Indeed, his definition of dislocation appeals to what Ortega y Gasset would argue about as one of the most important sources of human identity. For Alexander:

> ...the rupture of enduring and sustaining connections between individuals and their families, friends, societies, livelihoods, rituals, traditions, nations and deities, elements that form the basis of psychological wholeness. [25, p. 225]

Nevertheless, if Ortega y Gasset is right and, in part, *we are the beliefs we inhabit* [26, p. 17], then Alexander's social theory of addiction is tremendously relevant in the search for the main causes of what has already become one of the greatest epidemics of the twenty-first century. And it is precisely at this point of the approach—which generates lively debates around the crisis of modernity—where Huxley's novel offers its most brilliant and novel reflections. Let us see it below.

Beyond Adaptation to the Environment

The society of *Brave New World*, as mentioned, founded on fear, not only bears close parallels to contemporary society as described by Alexander but goes even further in its retrospective and prospective evaluation. Let us begin with the former.

Huxley shows a fragmented society and addictions that its citizens perceive not as a consequence of fragmentation but as a palliative solution to the derived state of distress. Nevertheless, could such a dependency be considered an addiction if there is no perception of adverse effects? Here lies the crux of the matter. Alexander revolves his discourse around the disease and adaptive dysfunctionality of addiction, while Huxley gives another twist to the argument and presents us with a definition of addiction that transcends both aspects and emphasizes the problem of meaning. However, he does not confer on this, as Frankl does, a single dimension related to coherent thought, but adds a second, more important one, which has to do with the search for reality, the point of departure and arrival in the formation of beliefs—access that fragmentation also prevents. Finally, this criterion justifies that behavior can manifest an addiction, even if it is healthy and socially convenient. In *Brave New World Revisited*, Huxley writes:

> The real hopeless victims of mental illness are to be found among those who appear to be most normal. "Many of them are normal because they are so well adjusted to our mode of existence, because their human voice has been silenced so early in their lives, that they do not even struggle or suffer or develop symptoms as the neurotic does." They are normal not in what may be called the absolute sense of the word; they are normal only in relation to a profoundly abnormal society. Their perfect adjustment to that abnormal society is a measure of their mental sickness. These millions of abnormally normal people, living without fuss in a society to which, if they were fully human beings, they ought not to be adjusted. [1, p. 276]

This reflection by Huxley brings to light an aspect of the problem of addiction that negative symptoms and social maladjustment overshadow when considering its etiopathogenesis. Freedom, and with it, reality, has been sacrificed. So, the return to harmony requires the restoration of both because any solution that ignores them leads to worse scenarios, however asymptomatic and socially acceptable they may be.

Huxley further delves into one of the evils already inculcated by Alexander, forgetfulness. Because the addicted person not only ignores or confuses the root of his addiction, but has forgotten the moment of the two significant pacts: that of the exchange of freedom for security and, another more ancient one, the exchange of the human spirit for the attainment of certainties, that is, certain and maximally objective knowledge. Huxley places in the Enlightenment thought, characterized by the reduction of human intelligence to a mathematical calculating reason, the beginning of the diffusion of this second pact. The following quotation is long but, because of its content, it deserves to be transcribed in its entirety:

> The first step in the simplification of reality, without which (since human minds are finite and nature is infinite) scientific thought and action would be impossible, is a process of abstraction. Confronted by the data of experience, men of science begin by leaving out of account all those aspects of the facts which do not lend themselves to explanation in terms of antecedent causes rather than of purpose, intention, and values. Pragmatically they are justified in acting in this odd and extremely arbitrary way; for by concentrating on the measurable aspects of such elements of experience as can be explained in terms of a causal system, they have been able to achieve a great and ever-increasing control of the energies of nature. But power is not the same thing as insight, and as a representation of reality the scientific picture of the world is inadequate, for the simple reason that science does not even profess to deal with experience as a whole, but only with certain aspects of it in certain contexts. All this is quite clearly understood by the more philosophically-minded men of science.
> ...But, unfortunately some men of science and many technicians have lacked the time and inclination to study the philosophical basis and background of their special subject. Consequently, they tend to accept the world picture implicit in the theories of science as a complete and exhaustive account of reality; they tend to regard those aspects of experience, which scientists leave out of account, because they are incompetent to deal with them, as being somehow less real than aspects, which scientists have arbitrarily chosen to abstract from out of the infinitely rich totality of the given facts. [27, pp. 28–29]

Purpose, intention, and values disappear under the scrutiny of a science that pretends to reduce everything to algorithmic computations. Worse still, that capacity of rationality responsible for apprehending these phenomena, which Huxley calls, following classical terminology, intuitive knowledge, falls into disuse. He identifies with its atrophy, the first link in the chain that leads to this particular kind of addiction in late modern Western societies. We will call it *structural addiction* from now on.

Of course, Huxley is not the first writer to denounce mechanistic reductionism and the fragmentation it produces at all levels. However, few have made his denunciation so vehemently. We may have to go back to the very beginnings of the Enlightenment movement to find similar attacks. Johann Wolfgang von Goethe makes his Faust one of the best known. In several passages, he criticizes the *mereological fallacies* already widespread in the name of the Enlightenment. Thus, for example, Goethe puts in the mouth of Mephistopheles the following satirical words addressed to a naive student who asks him for advice in his studies:

> Don't waste your time, it's gone so fast, but arranging it right will save you plenty of it. Accordingly, dear friend, my first advice is that you hear the *Collegium Logicum*. The course will discipline your mind and lace it tight in iron-boots so that it will no longer rush headlong along the paths of thought or, like a will-o'-the-wisp perhaps, wander at random everywhere. Days on end will be used to teach you that what you once did as a single act, as easily as you eat or drink, must really be done as one-two-three. Although in fact the fabric of thought is like a masterpiece of weaving, for which one treadle moves a thousand threads as back and forth the shuttles fly and threads move quicker than the eye and a single stroke makes a thousand ties, nonetheless the philosopher comes and proves to you it had to be thus: the first was so, the second so, and hence the third and fourth are so; but if there were no first and second the third and fourth could never exist. Students applaud this everywhere, but fail to master the weaver's art. To understand some living thing and to describe it, the student starts by ridding it of its spirit; he then holds all its parts within his hand except, alas! for the spirit that bound them together which chemists, unaware they're being ridiculous, denominate *encheiresin naturae* [natural treatment]. [28, p. 49]

Goethe accuses enlightened intellectuals of reducing thinking to the work of a loom, and knowledge to a fabric that can be unraveled in the same way it was spun. *Brave New World* will be, in this way, the paroxysm of this analytical and objectifying inertia that ends up colonizing everything. This division materializes, for Huxley, in many ways: in particular, with the sciences, which are subdivided and isolated from each other in their *Babelic ascent*; and with the economy, in which the models of productive and commercial specialization triumph in order to reach higher levels of performance. It is also in this trend that Huxley glimpses the current resource crises: on the one hand, specialization makes countries more and more economically dependent, but on the other, the atomization of the interests of each nation increasingly alienates those who need to negotiate in order to survive. Thus, he concludes that enlightened globalization is at odds with economic and political sustainability. Nevertheless, *BNW* excels in showing how the divisive ideas of the Enlightenment end up affecting corporeality itself, on which every human capacity is harmonized. Fragmentation not only reaches family and cultural relations but penetrates the very heart of the individual, considered as something that is no more than the sum of its parts, like any other machine—such as Ford's automobiles. On this belief rests a new kind of equality that lowers the ontological status of the individual to the point of accepting his mass production on assembly lines—like the Ford Model T's of 1908. Huxley thus describes the *Bokanovsky method* of manufacturing human beings:

> One egg, one embryo, one adult—normality. But a bokanovskified egg will bud, will proliferate, will divide. From eight to ninety-six buds, and every bud will grow into a perfectly formed embryo, and every embryo into a full-sized adult. Making ninety-six human beings grow where only one grew before. Progress. [2, p. 4]

It is more than preventing the activity of what is most human in man. The biological and social engineering of *Brave New World* leaves out, erases, the human potentiality, the capacity to connect with the real and with others. In other words, it tries to eliminate the most intimate part of his nature. Unfortunately, in this respect, we are also finding warning signs of what may come. Few would deny today that the man-machine metaphor is permeating public discourse and, through it, citizenship. The effect of this self-understanding metamorphosis is the increasingly extensive and intense anthropomorphic relationship we maintain with the machines surrounding us, whether for professional or recreational reasons or the most serious of all, loneliness—see the latest advances in care robots. However, perhaps the two perfect expressions of the belief that man, ultimately, is a loom, complex, but a loom, is the warm welcome being given, on the one hand, to proposals for mind *uploading* and, on the other, to initiatives to grant gadgets with AI positions of moral responsibility. For example, in November 2022, the City of San Francisco (California) approved using robots with AI and lethal capabilities.

Today, machines are being built that appear to talk and feel like human beings. More importantly, there is a proliferation of human beings who speak and feel like machines. This double situation makes recognizing the machine as a new *neighbor* seem inevitable. The intensification of anguish at the weakening of intimacy, and shared intimacy, also seems likely to follow the same path. The phenomenon of addiction seems to be no stranger to all this, especially with increasingly intelligent machines, but devoid of any intimacy and experience of meaning, which will not cease to induce the belief that human beings are also empty inside. Androids with AI are the worst mirrors in which an addicted person can try to find his reflection.

Soma, Authenticity, and Dislocation

Another parallel between Huxley's and Alexander's positions is the intrinsic power granted to the substance or activity in which the addiction is the object. As Alexander writes: "the new definition had the qualities of a reductionist medical diagnosis: Addiction was necessarily a 'compulsion' that had a physical cause" [25, p. 212]. In contrast, his definition has more to do with something much less material, a radical moral failure. It is not only that the individual errs in pursuing what is good, true, and beautiful in his life. A bigger and earlier problem is that he is incapable of undertaking moral activity, given the external confusion surrounding and invading him. This fracture is what prevents him from discerning between the real and the unreal in terms of values or, what is the same, between the natural and the unnatural. Thus, for Alexander, the addictive power that a substance or activity inherently has is small if we separate it from the context of existential anguish, which is what makes that substance or activity truly irresistible. This argument is reinforced by the relapses of patients after long periods of confinement in detoxification centers. The addiction to the substance may have been overcome, the behavioral habits corrected, and yet… it is not enough to move forward in a life worth living or to resist one that is not worth living.

In *BNW*, Alexander's approach is made explicit. Citizens give themselves freely to addictions, especially to *Soma*, to positively reinforce the roles that the State confers on the individual but, above all, to drown the imperious need for meaning that all the protagonists of the novel suffer, to a greater or lesser extent. Lenina, one of the central characters of Brave New World, shows such idea when she talks about her experience of soma consumption:

> How kind, how good-looking, how delightfully amusing every one was! 'Bottle of mine, it's you I've always wanted…' But Lenina and Henry had what they wanted … They were inside, here and now—safely inside with the fine weather, the perennially blue sky […] Swallowed half an hour before closing time, that second dose of Soma had raised a quite impenetrable wall between the actual universe and their minds. [2, pp. 77–78]

The power of *the soma* lies more in isolating her from the fractured world (to neutralize the anguish) than in stimulating her with intense emotions. Another clear passage about the same is the one in which Henry Foster, a secondary character in the plot, an expert in statistics within the London Central Incubation and Conditioning Center, flies over one of the city's crematoria, where corpses are recycled:

> Do you know what that switchback was? He said. It was some human being finally and definitely disappearing. Going up in a squirt of hot gas. It would be curious to know who it was a man or a woman, an Alpha or an Epsilon… He sighed. Then, in a resolutely cheerful voice, 'Anyhow,' he concluded, 'there's one thing we can be certain of; whoever he may have been, he was happy when he was alive. Everybody's happy now'. [2, p. 75]

The feeling of happiness, or rather of well-being, gains real force only in the context of a profound reflection on human life. Foster reflects, grieves, and appeals to the feelings generated by chemistry to justify the *status quo*. These lines are also interesting because they reflect the author's optimism regarding the human incapacity to completely neutralize the deepest and noblest aspirations of the human being. There are numerous occasions in which the characters in *BNW* express, in a veiled manner, a certain nostalgia or regret for a better life whose existence they only suspect. The curious thing, which also allows us to take a step closer to the conclusion here, is that some of these regrets are articulated with sentimental criteria. The *World State* offers a range of emotions that reveal themselves insufficient:

> I [Helmholtz] feel I could do something much more important. Yes, and more intense, more violent. But what? […] "I want to know what passion is," she heard him saying. "I want to feel something strongly". [2, p. 70 and 94]

Huxley is recovering in *BNW* a classical understanding of emotional life, lost in *the official view* of addiction. Some emotions seem directly caused by physical stimuli (a glass of wine, a cup of coffee), but there are more immaterial triggers: ideas. And to specific ideas, Aristotle refers to the noun *boulēsis* (βούλησις), a type of rational desire or, what is the same, of sentient thinking in which he places the heart of the human will—of its freedom to act. It is not a tangential issue, for let us not forget that this freedom is the sacrificial victim in *BNW* and the central loss in addictive behaviors. The ideas of boulēsis are arrived at by the endeavor of reason to seek reality and, with it, to move what is mere opinion toward the ideal of truth. This approach of the individual to reality has a phenomenal emotional expression, which is essential to this encounter. This expression is the experience of meaning, the experience that the individual's life has a meaning within the universe he inhabits. The excitement generated by the ingestion of coffee is accidental (the physical cause that triggers the emotion could be another or the emotion evoked by the substance could be another). In contrast, the excitement generated by the encounter with a loved one is essential and authentic. Nothing else can cause such deep emotion. It is what Bernard's character refers to when he exclaims:

> And what an intensity of feeling it must generate! I often think one may have missed something in not having had a mother. [2, p. 112]

For Huxley, these intense feelings allow us to overcome the internal and external limits that condition human behavior. Expressed in another way, the rational life oriented to the search for meaning fills the existential void left by fragmentation, and drives the individual to exercise his rationality and freedom even more in an endless growth of intellect and sensibility. In short, the alternative that Huxley proposes to the hedonism of *BNW*, which is extensible to the discourse on structural addiction, is not an insipid intellectualistic asceticism but, on the contrary, a more pleasurable life in which, in addition, other higher values are integrated, such as those associated with truth and freedom.

Cancelation Culture

Only because of a factory or punctual defect (being too ugly, too smart, born in the wrong place), the main characters in Huxley's dystopia enjoy enough vision to sense that life in the *World State* is miserable and that the problem is not confined to their physiology or biography. From Alexander's perspective, it is a privileged situation concerning addicted patients who do not know who they are. Bernard, John, and Helmholtz try to rebel against the system but are ultimately defeated. Huxley offers several interesting clues to the problem: first, *BNW* citizens, who suffer from continuous surveillance, are bombarded by commercial and political propaganda, and are accustomed to frenetic activism that leaves little room for reflection. In his essay, *Science, liberty and peace*, Huxley will introduce another element that marks a point of no return in this type of society: military technology of mass destruction. When a dominant minority possesses such weaponry, rebellion against tyrants becomes almost impossible [27, pp. 19–22]. He has atomic weapons in mind, although we could include AI for military and political use in the same category. In fact, the development of this technology in cyber-surveillance and the use of Big Data for population profiling, among other purposes, for the creation of *fake news*, fits even better than nuclear intimidation, given that in the World State, one cannot strictly speak of a *Big Brother* or dominant minority that subjugates the rest. All are subjected to the same cruel plan of progress.

Second, and more importantly, the rebels to the system lack a sufficiently sophisticated system of thought and language to understand the scope of the problem and the possible solutions. Not only that, they are weak. They are devoid of the physical and moral strength to resist the onslaught of the enemy or, more dangerously, their siren songs. It is fascinating how Huxley presents us with this idea in the figure of Bernard, socially rejected for having a less athletic body than the majority. His reflective awareness of social ills arises from this eccentric situation. However, his criticism wanes, in fact, turns to praise, when by a change of his fortune, he achieves fame and prestige among his own. In Huxley's texts, gregariousness is possibly the most potent chain among all imaginable addictions. Not fear but power, fame, and success are here the bargaining chip in this surrender of judgment, freedom, and the sacred love of friendship—whether this success takes the form of recognition among the powerful of the moment, or among the so-called wise or just. Bernard, like any other addict, is only capable of surrounding himself with prey, sycophants, and henchmen, even if he describes such relationships with euphemisms and poetic words that are the fruits of other times and mentalities. Perhaps it is on this last point that Huxley's dystopia becomes highly topical. For into the hands of the rebels, especially John and Helmholtz, come forbidden books on morals, science, and art, where all those things they lack are discussed and explained. However, they fail to understand the old ways of thinking and doing, and worse still, they misunderstand them in such a way that far from helping them, they intensify the vicious circle of pleasure, utility, and sad abnegation around which their lives revolve.

It is not by accident. The Founding Fathers of *BNW* suspected that history could lead to a diversity of opinion and critical thinking, which is one of the worst manifestations of freedom. That is why they dictated that part of the mental conditioning of the population was aimed at achieving contempt for everything that referred to the past. The maxim children memorize from their earliest childhood and attribute to Henry Ford, its legendary founder, leaves no room for doubt: "History is bullshit" [2, p. 235]. Everything that happens must be explained by what is seen in the most objective and useful here and now.

It cannot be said that there is an express will to forget in the West, although some point out that the phenomenon of the *cancelation culture* has close similarities. The curse that today falls on researchers who are being censured by the scientific community, regardless of the veracity of their work, due to unpopular—politically incorrect—comments or actions, is extending to thinkers of other eras, judged under the anachronistic and revisionist gaze of the hyper-specialist [29]. As Ortega y Gasset points out, this disinterest in history even affects the history of science, which gave and gives meaning to the researcher's work.

> But if the specialist is ignorant of the inner philosophy of the science he cultivates, he is much more radically ignorant of the historical conditions requisite for its continuation; that is to say: how society and the heart of man are to be organized in order that there may continue to be investigators. The decrease in scientific vocations noted in recent years, to which I have alluded, is an anxious symptom for anyone who has a clear idea of what civilization is, an idea generally lacking to the typical "scientist," the high-point of our present civilization. He also believes that civilization is there in just the same way as the earth's crust and the primeval forest. [23, p. 126]

It is not a distant issue that affects only researchers and the future of research. The most intimate human aspirations are affected today by this forgetfulness, which is also the forgetfulness of moral tradition. With forgetfulness, human practices change, and new practices bring new ways of understanding the world. New horizons are opened, but also the past becomes more and more distorted. Alasdair MacIntyre's denunciation in *After Virtue* of the practically irretrievable loss of the cultural background that made the classical tradition and its highest ethical achievements intelligible: that of education in virtues and *Paideia*, among others, is already a classic.

> The social obstacles derive from the way in which modernity partitions each human life into a variety of segments, each with its own norms and modes of behavior. So work is divided from leisure, private life from public, the corporate from the personal. So both childhood and old age have been wrenched away from the rest of human life and made over into distinct realms. And all these separations have been achieved so that it is the distinctiveness of each and not the unity of the life of the individual who passes through those parts in terms of which we are taught to think and to feel. [30, p. 204]

MacIntyre is no more optimistic than Huxley about the possibility of recovering what has been lost. "The language and appearances of morality persist even though the integral substance has to a large degree been fragmented and then in part destroyed" [30, p. 5]. Worse than oblivion, he warns, is the current use of vestigial terms and practices with erroneous and perverse meanings, a phenomenon that adds even more confusion to the fragmentation that enlightened thought has been generating for three centuries now: generosity, fidelity, respect, commitment, honesty, piety, contemplation, faith, etc. This means that not even communities that are presumed to be as traditional as countercultural are safe from the corruption of their ideals and practices. The South Korean philosopher Byung-Chul Han alludes to this in his essay *The Disappearance of Rituals*, appealing to an evil that seems to affect both East and West:

> Values today also serve as things for individual consumption. They become commodities. Values such as justice, humanity, or sustainability are exploited for profit. One fair-trade enterprise has the slogan: 'Change the world while drinking tea.' Changing the world through consumption—that would be the end of the revolution. Nowadays, one can purchase vegan shoes or clothes; soon there will probably be vegan smartphones too [...] Moral values are consumed as marks of distinction. They are credited to the ego-account, appreciating the value of self. They increase our narcissistic self-respect. Through values we relate not to community but to our own egos. [31, p. 5]

Narcissism, Byung-Chul Han argues, is probably the most severe and profound manifestation of social atomization, and at the same time, a consequence of the enlightened exaltation of the autonomy of the individual, which after its hypertrophy, individualism, ends up degenerating in the atrophy of the individual, meanly, the dissolution of the concept of *person*. Postmodernity is characterized, indeed, by the suspicion about the capacity of reason to reach the truth; the suspicion about the human will to make free decisions; the suspicion about the ontological status of the human being –human dignity. The individual is annihilated in mass society. The new social models leave no room for the old rituals, and traditional communities seem to distinguish less and less between these transcendental bridges and their mere impostures, which are now reduced to mere sentimentality or the most empty, willful, and falsely hopeful of human activities.

The Last Resort

The failure of the three friends is different and, in it, Huxley gives some clues as to his proposal for the evils of the contemporary world. John, the savage, after his failed attempt at revolt, retreats to an old abandoned lighthouse in rural England. It is there, in silence and contemplative activity, that he experiences an epiphanic moment that Huxley will later call the clear white light of the Void, using a term from *The Tibetan Book of the Dead*. It is a double experience: the deflation of the self and the opening of the doors of perception toward the real and, even, toward the infinite, which for Huxley, takes the form of unlimited love. It is an intuitive revelation of being—the ground—which is "at once transcendent and immanent" [32, p. 15].

> He had almost finished whittling the stave into shape, when he realized with a start that he was singing—singing! It was as though, stumbling upon himself from the outside, he had suddenly caught himself out, taken himself flagrantly at fault. Guiltily he blushed. After all, it was not to sing and enjoy himself that he had come here. It was to escape further contamination by the filth of civilized life; it was to be purified and made good; it was actively to make amends. [2, p. 254]

In the deprivation of stimuli, the suppression of prejudices, and the simplest and useless activities, John, the savage, hears for the first time the voice of nature, which is interior and exterior to him, and for the first time, he experiences that deep joy of sense. However, he misinterprets this experience with the criteria of the old man, and scruples impede moral progress. Furthermore, John's lifestyle has become BNW's new reality TV attraction. His end is tragic: after being visited by hundreds of onlookers and succumbing to an orgy of sex and Soma, he ends up, in despair, committing suicide.

Huxley offers no easy solutions. The conquest of the lost humanity, of the forgotten nature, is not something a human can do on his own. On the one hand, the society of the *World State* will prevent it in two different ways: by corrupting the countercultural movements (turning them into just another spectacle among spectacles) or by exercising explicit violence on them. It is the case of Bernard and Helmholtz, who are banished to the Falkland Islands. On the other hand, because John carries evil, fracture, and addiction within him, no matter where he flees, he cannot leave behind centuries of generations educated in enlightened sensibility. John's ending conveys to the reader a message of hope. Late modern evils are not all encompassing. Even in the worst imaginable scenario, that is *BNW*, Huxley continues to present us with a place where human beings can find safety and begin to reverse the situation—although it may take many generations to recover the keys in which the greatest works of civilization were written and to re-establish the social relations we still enjoy today. That place is found in the human interior, where nature shines waiting for the slightest act of communication, of introspection, to widen the intimacy of the human heart.

Huxley does not glory in the originality of his proposal. He recognizes that he is only trying to remind us of the beliefs that are latent in the philosophical and religious tradition of a great set of peoples and cultures, called by the generic name of The Perennial Philosophy, in Latin, *philosophia perennis* [33, pp. 12–13]. It is no coincidence that, as with *Faust*, this wisdom emerged renewed at the same historical moment in which its nemesis emerged. It is probably *Hyperion*, an epistolary novel by Friedrich Hölderlin, one of the most explicit articulations of the human need to return to nature when everything seems to collapse, namely, when the man seems lost.

> Thus I gave myself up more and more to blissful nature, and almost too endlessly. How gladly I'd have become a child to be closer to her! How gladly I'd have known less and become like the pure ray of light to be closer to her! Oh, to feel myself for a moment in her peace, her beauty, how much more that meant to me than years full of thinking, than all the ventures of all-venturing men! What I'd learned, what I'd done in my life melted away like ice, and all youth's designs died away in me; and Oh you dear ones, who are distant, you dead and you living, how wholly one we were! [34, p. 135]

In search of a safe place to rest his soul, the young Hyperion embarks on a journey, which is also a spiritual journey in which there will be no shortage of disappointments: first with his teacher, Adamas; with his soul friend, Alabanda; with the state for which he fights, Greece; and finally with his true love, Diotima. Disillusioned and dejected, he will retire as a hermit to the woods where he will find the peace he sought, the forgotten wisdom, and the lost energy to relaunch himself into the world inhabited by his compatriots with the oldest and always new message—a new *return to the cavern*.

> I have seen it once, the one and only that my soul was seeking, and the consummation we project beyond the stars, that we defer until the end of time, I've felt it in the here and now. It was here, the most high, in this cycle of human nature and of things, it was here!
>
> I no longer ask where it is; it was in the world, it can return in the world, it's in the world now, only more hidden. I no longer ask what it is; I've seen it, I've known it. Oh you who seek the highest and the best, be it in the depths of knowledge, in the turmoil of action, in the darkness of the past, in the labyrinth of the future, in the graves or above the stars! Do you know its name? The name of what is one and all?
>
> Its name is beauty. [34, p. 137]

BNW offers the maximum social sustainability that objectivity can offer, the most pleasurable life that utilitarian calculations can achieve. Yet, it lacks what, for Huxley, is the one thing that man cannot be deprived of: it is a world without beauty, the ultimate emotion in which the idea of meaning shines. It is not pure speculation or vain poetry. The phenomenal experience that fails to be wholly eclipsed (even during the climax offered by such potent drugs as heroin) is the ugliness of the pleasure experienced. It is often also one of the anchors by which, consciously or unconsciously, the subject tries to undertake rehabilitation. For Huxley, among all the anchors, it is also the only one that can resist the onslaught of the waves on such a journey. However, the difficulty is that this journey is not only indicated for the patient but also for the doctor who treats him, the family that cares for him, and the entire society surrounding him. The undertaking reaches the limits of the unfeasible, but there are ways of making it practical. We will end the chapter with this last point.

Benedict and Hermit Options

The strategy of withdrawing from society in order to save it is no stranger to contemporary controversies about the evils of late modernity. One of the proposals that have gained supporters in recent years is the one presented by Rod Dreher in his book *The Benedict Option*. Based on the social diagnosis of *After Virtue*, he proposes abandoning modern lifestyles and forming tight local communities similar to those founded by Benedict of Norcia in the sixth century, with the end of the Roman Empire and societal collapse.

> The Benedict Option is a call to undertake the long and patient work of reclaiming the real world from the artifice, alienation, and atomization of modern life. It is a way of seeing the world and of living in the world that undermines modernity's big lie: that humans are nothing more than ghosts in a machine, and we are free to adjust its settings in any way we like. [35, p. 236]

Ben Op is a call for Christians, of course, but it can be extended to all minorities, religious or not, who disapprove of the imperialistic dynamics of this late modern, hedonistic, utilitarian, and narcissistic culture. Because *Ben Op* is, above all, a movement against any attempt to reduce the idea of rationality to AI; against the fashion of banishing the experience of the natural from social practices; and against the distortion of the mystery of human freedom. There should be no objection, therefore, to those who prefer a more secular and appealing to all tastes name. *The Hyperionian Option* would be valid for all those who would make Hölderlin's words about love, nature, and freedom their own:

> You springs of the earth! You flowers! And you forests and you eagles and you fraternal light! How old and new is our love!—We are free, we don't anxiously strive to be outwardly equal; how should not vary the modes of life? But we all love the aether, and deep in our innermost being we are all of us like. [...] We are living tones, we sound together in your harmony, nature! Who can split that asunder? Who will part lovers? [35, p. 136]

Similarly, Dreher's proposal is not so much an attack on the process of secularization of the modern world but a critique of the objectivist reductionism, *dataism*, in Byung-Chul's expression, to which the Enlightenment has led us, which necessarily leaves out what is natural inside and outside of man and, with it, the relations of significance.

Also, like Huxley, Dreher is aware that these communities are not about establishing new moral elites. Those who thus interpret the "Ben Op" do not realize that, possibly, these are just an expression of identity reactions, alternative ways of satisfying the gregarious addiction of those who, due to various circumstances, cannot obtain recognition from the majority groups. It is no longer a matter of showing the way to the misguided or resisting the enemy. We are addicts—all of us, largely fractured. All of us belong to the masses. Evil has been penetrating the hearts of Westerners for too long to naively think that Christian communities (or any other traditionalist community) have not already received metastatic cells that will eventually destroy all resistance to the *establishment* from within. It is not only a question of preserving knowledge of (Christian) Great Tradition, or knowledge of the Perennial Philosophy, or any other past belief system. Nor does it consist merely of returning to old educational systems, as some nostalgic academics try to do with the Liberal Arts tradition. Both groups are losing their way because, as MacIntyre claims, these solutions are useless without recovering the lost meaning, which entails not merely learning ideas—their objective dimension—but above all, understanding them, that is, accessing their subjective dimension. In this context, for Huxley, recovering the links with nature is fundamental, necessary, and prior in the step from learning to understanding a belief system.

In conclusion, the only advantage these small communities can boast is that their members are more aware of the problem of alienation from nature, and that it is necessary to seek a solution to the dynamics of structural addiction in terms of fracture. For this reason, to avoid such a traditionalist misinterpretation, it may be more appropriate to redefine the proposal as *The Hermit Option* since the emphasis in these communities would be on the attitude of recollection and contemplation of its members in search of new forms of life and communities that favor the development of moral life and the avoidance of addictive dynamics.

It is not a new strategy at all. It is what Benedict of Nursia did before he formulated his Rule and began founding monasteries. He did it imitating Jesus' retreat into the desert, before what Christians call his public life and proclamation of the kingdom. Many passages in Huxley's philosophical essays refer to the desert as a symbol of purification and Enlightenment: Muhammad and the mountain cave named Hira; Gautama Buddha (Siddhārtha Gautama), the ascetic life in Rajagaha, etc. in all these narratives underlies, for Huxley, the same attitude of initial detachment in the search for the essential, the origin or arkhé (or arche) of things, an attitude that does not take the form of pure self-reflection but, first of all, of attentive listening to a voice that comes from outside and within at the same time.

> Oh sister of the spirit which lives and sways in us with fiery power, Oh holy air! How beautiful it is that, all-pervasive and immortal, you're there with me wherever I may wander! [...] For stillness dwells in the land of the blissful, and above the stars the heart forgets its anguish and its language. [34, pp. 43–44]

Dreher writes that this flight into the wilderness, physical or virtual, is not the ideal state of moral life, but it is a starting point to begin rebuilding society, a good soil to begin again to seed moral communities. This consideration makes an even better name for his proposal *The Hermit Beginning*. The search for silence and austere life may not be the perfect form of moral life, but it is the most spiritual and, for Benedict of Nursia, between the material and the spiritual, the latter takes primacy over the former, since only from that hierarchy is it possible to consolidate later a perfect and complete moral life, which is an expression of the material-spiritual unity of man. The *Her Beg* is, therefore, only a beginning and not a definitive renunciation of the materiality of man and his world, with its sophisticated objective discourses and its precious technology.

We want to end this section with a brief historical note. *Hermit Beginning Thesis* was first proposed on November 25, 2002, in the speech "Secure or free societies? The new utopias: Sustainability and Artificial Intelligence" as part of the series of conferences organized by the *Círculo Amistad Numancia*. To this social and intellectual club belonged, as a member, Antonio Machado, one of the greatest Spanish poets, in whose poetry we find the most beautiful songs to the flat desert, the silent wastelands, and the unmapped roads.

Hospitality and *Kenosis* in the Cyberspace

One criticism that "Ben Op" has received inside and outside the Christian community is the abandonment of its social responsibilities—the neighbor. Dreher defends himself against such accusations by appealing to the Gospel question: *can the blind lead the blind?* "It is less urgent to convince the alternative culture in which we live of the truth of Christ than it is for the Church to tell itself its own story and to nurture its own life [...] we cannot become the gift to others we are called to be until we embrace the limits that are necessary to our vocation" [36]. In the short term, and especially under the accusatory gaze of those left behind, it may seem a cruel and selfish decision. However, in the long run, it seems the fastest and most effective way to help those who take the blind for teachers and end up breeding the blind themselves. For Huxley, every single Westerner is the pitiful child of the modern blind but, especially us academics—snobbish and fragile Huxlerian bookworms.

> Today I feel no wish to demonstrate that sanity is impossible. On the contrary, though I remain no less sadly certain than in the past that sanity is a rather rare phenomenon, I am convinced that it can be achieved and would like to see more of it. For having said so in several recent books and, above all, for having compiled an anthology of what the sane have said about sanity and all the means whereby it can be achieved, I have been told by an eminent academic critic that I am a sad symptom of the failure of an intellectual class in time of crisis. The implication being, I suppose, that the professor and his colleagues are hilarious symptoms of success. The benefactors of humanity deserve due honour and commemoration. Let us build a Pantheon for professors. It should be located among the ruins of one of the gutted cities of Europe or Japan, and over the entrance to the ossuary I would inscribe, in letters six or seven feet high, the simple words: SACRED TO THE MEMORY OF THE WORLD's EDUCATORS. SI MONUMENTUM REQUIRIS CIRCUMSPICE. [1, pp. 6–7]

Huxley does not believe that modern academics are shrewd snakes, as they like to think: their speeches and behavior (alienated smiles... bland tears...) show they are just miserable victims of their parents and themselves. Even the best no longer understand the problem of seeking to do evil in the name of good; the worst seek to use the name of good or God for their own interests—the accumulation of individual, political, or technological power. *Her Beg* seems to be the initial means of escaping this vicious circle, if not this generation, then the next. It is the most compassionate measure, even though it seems selfish and ruthless to the outside eyes of those it is intended to help.

Returning to Dreher, he concludes his analysis with a final lament: these times require more life testimonies than speeches. "Pagans converted to the early Church not simply because of the words the first Christians spoke, but because of the witness of the kinds of lives they lived. It has to be that way with us too" [36]. Although Huxley ended his days embracing many Buddhist beliefs, this statement aligns with much of his thinking. Not just Huxley, it can be adopted by any community that shares a deep belief in human nature.

What Huxley explicitly states in *The Perennial Philosophy*, published in 1945, is the need to go beyond different religious and philosophical sensibilities to try to reach the deepest yearnings of the human spirit. This attitude does not imply disavowing one's religious faith or particular vocation, Huxley warns, but learning from and in others what is common and important to share—the awakening of the organs to the unity of the body would be and, ultimately, the cornerstone of all community. According to Huxley, this goal requires a paradoxical state of solitude and, simultaneously, singular companionship, especially by those who pursue the same goal. Huxley devotes an entire chapter of the work mentioned above to charity [33, pp. 95–112]. He does not believe it is possible to reach the foundation of human nature without a neighbor upon whom to establish a dialogue in love. He explains that it is for this reason that it is not strange to know that hermits, from the earliest times, have wanted to group and lead a particular community life. Therefore, withdrawal from the world cannot be total. It is not the only argument to defend the same thesis. Referring to *the Benedict hospitality*, Dreher writes:

> The Benedictines are instructed to welcome outsiders so long as they don't interrupt communal life. It should be that way with us, too. We should always be open to others, in charity, to share what we have with them, including our faith. [36]

However, communicating the faith, Dreher warns, is different from communicating what might be the best recipe in our time for growth in the moral life. Only honest and committed search testimonies can be offered on such a matter. Besides, with such a strategy, there will be not few who, according to him, will swell the lists of intramural citizens—a new and, at the same time, very old way of evangelization.

Charles Taylor is one of the authors who takes up a similar idea about the impossibility, in complete isolation, of re-establishing authentic and meaningful relationships. However, here is the interesting aspect of his contribution, he manages to articulate in his discourse the need for recollection and accompaniment. For the Canadian philosopher, the relationship with the other helps in the process of transcending the self toward the *arkhe*. He describes this act of emptying one's own will (*the act of kenosis*) as follows:

> [A]cknowledging the transcendent means being called to a change of identity. Buddhism gives us an obvious reason to talk this way. The change here is quite radical, from self to 'no self' (*anatta*). But Christian faith can be seen in the same terms: as calling for a radical decentering of the self, in relation with God. [37, p. 21]

Sensual and intellectual contemplations are complemented, for Taylor, by a third type, the expressivistic contemplation (or of the acts of the heart, if one prefers), in which the subject acquires particular intuitions and emotions that have special importance in the growth of the moral life [38, pp. 374–381]. Not just any type of accompaniment is valid to obtain such fruits. Taylor refers specifically to those in which individuals "embrace radical, suffering-servant lifestyles in solidarity with all the marginalized peoples of the planet" [39]. In other words, this accompaniment implies, on the one hand, asceticism and recollection, and on the other, attention to the neediest, in its least sophisticated sense: aid to the sick, the hungry, the abandoned, etc. Those who suffer from the fever of contemporary consumerism, however pitiful their moral situation may be, would not fall into this category. They will have to wait.

In our opinion, Taylor's view contrasts with those of Huxley, MacIntyre, and Dreher in several advantageous ways. First, he is not as pessimistic as Huxley and MacIntyre regarding the human capacity to reverse, in a short time, the worst of imaginable situations. Of course, Taylor bases this optimism on the pleading power of prayer. In similar terms, Hölderlin sings:

> Do not weep when the best decays! Soon it will renew itself! Do not grieve when your heart's melody falls silent! Soon there'll come a hand to make

> it sound again! […] We're like fire that slumbers in the tinder-dry branch or the flint; and all the while we writhe and seek the end of close confinement. But they come, they make up for eons of struggle, those moments of liberation, when the divine bursts open the dungeon, when the flame frees itself from the wood and surges victorious over the ash, ha! When we feel as if the unbound spirit, forgotten its suffering, its servile form, were returning in triumph to the halls of the sun. [34, p. 45]

Unlike Huxley, Taylor does not blame the self for all evils, nor, therefore, does he accept the Buddhist solution, i.e., that spiritual liberation from suffering involves understanding that the self is an illusion. For him, it would be enough to recognize that late modernity has succumbed to the hypertrophy of the self and that the task of modern intellectuals is to figure out how to reverse the inflationary inertia. Can some of the discourses and methods of the Buddhist tradition be useful in this deflationary project? It is an interesting controversy that would need to be carefully assessed. However, for Christians, it may not be necessary to look outside, as they have Eastern traditions that partially incorporate similar practices—both apophatic and cataphatic ones—for self-forgetfulness and heart-opening.

In conclusion, Taylor's proposal demands less radicalism than Huxley's, in the sense that it does not ask the *BNW* citizen to renounce what he most cherishes, the self, but simply to put it on a diet. Similarly, he is also less critical of modernity than Huxley, MacIntyre, and Dreher for he values the gains made in recent centuries in favor of the individual and individual rights, many of the most important, Christian-driven. "Modern thinkers like Petrarch and Erasmus were Christians who tried to provide fresh answers to the questions scholasticism failed to solve" [40].

What Taylor's kenotic ethics does seem to demand is the maximum detachment from consumer goods, banal human relationships, and technology that the individual can afford. Keeping what is necessary to sustain a simple and attentive listening life is the key. On this point, Taylor shares John Dewey's thesis: the media, of whatever kind, are not value-laden. The media shape, reinforce, and weaken the purposes of those who possess them, and the more powerful they are, the greater their effect. Thus, it cannot be frivolously affirmed that the good intention of the user is sufficient for the handling of the material or technological good to be beneficial. It is not that they are necessarily harmful to moral life but, for Taylor, it requires a prudent preparation and a special diet of reason, feeling, and will that few would be willing to accept. And if these are already difficult times we live in, times that demand not a few sacrifices, it does not seem the best idea to intensify moral efforts further. Perhaps later, when the self is in better shape. But now there is no need to do so, before, other more urgent horizons await the man with a fractured soul. Those that Hölderlin promised centuries ago:

> Like Jupiter's eagle to the song of the muses I hark to the wonderful endless harmony in me. Untroubled in mind and soul, strong and blithe, in smiling earnest I sport in spirit with fate and the three sisters, the holy Parcae. Full of godly youth my whole being exults in itself, in all things. Like the starry heavens I'm both still and moved. [34, p. 42]

The kenotic proposal finds interesting echoes in contemporary addiction therapies. Not a few rehabilitation programs integrate volunteer activities for such patients. Indeed, one strategy for patients to deal with their own problems is to sign up for a volunteer service. However, this therapy is not without its risks since it is difficult not to end up with a utilitarian attitude, which is the evil from which one intends to flee. And there is a bigger problem. As Byung-Chul warns above, social solidarity may end up in another of the forms of frenetic consumerism, either as a muffler for moral conscience or as another food for an ego that competes even in the most sacred matters—like new Saturnines devouring their children. In this matter, Huxley still seems to be right: the desert is a crucial element, the first step of all, in an attempt to regain the connection with the real world. Once again, the proposal of the *Her Beg* appears in all its scope and with all its force.

Finally, *BNW* presents us with an added obstacle. Kenosis seems impossible in a world where no one asks for help or accompaniment, as basic needs are covered and human ideals are eclipsed. The introduction in this dystopia of AI, and especially of care robots as perfect palliative strategies for loneliness, which is probably the most specifically natural and human suffering, leads us not only to the worst imaginable scenario but also to a singular controversy is kenotic transcendence possible with a care robot, that is, with an anthropomorphic reality that simulates needs, including affective ones, and therefore generates in the user the feeling that he is useful, that he can help and pour all his love toward such an empty entity without making the lover go through the trials of love? The new modes of virtual relationships will undoubtedly favor this transition toward more alienated and surreptitiously addictive lifestyles. In contrast, the idea is a revulsive against technological alienation that can also serve as a beacon not only to Christians but also to all those who *intuit*—sense—the need for better *sources of self* to overcome structural addictions in modern times, i.e., silence, simple life, and transformative love.

Paradoxes in an Island. Huxley's Assumptions and Motivations About Experience

In his last novel, *Island* (first published in 1962), Huxley makes a final nod to *BNW*. If Bernard and Helmholtz are exiled to the Falkland Islands to try to find a better life together with other rebels, in *Island*, we meet William Asquith, a journalist who arrives at the *Kingdom of Pala*, a "forbidden island" in which its inhabitants live a utopia that combines the best of Western and Eastern culture. In particular, *Island* promotes technological progress compatible with spaces for silence, contemplation of nature, and connected meaningful relationships. Nevertheless, this story does not end well either. The conspiracy against Rani, the queen of *Pala*, to sell the island's oil exploitation rights ends with the kingdom's destruction.

> The work of a hundred years destroyed in a single night. And yet the fact remained—the fact of the ending of sorrow as well as the fact of sorrow. [41, p. 294]

The sorrow ends when the human being realizes that life does not consist in surviving, in individual or social immortality, but, above all, in making existence more rational and loving, meaning, in complying with human nature. It is then when what is not pursued is achieved: eternal life. This idea is precisely what Huxley tries to reach the reader with his novels: transforming mere knowledge into understanding—enlightenment.

In *Island*, however, we find a chiaroscuro in the role that Huxley gives to technology in the path of such enlightenment. *Palanese* citizens use moksha-medicine, an entheogen drug, to help them free themselves from the self and open up to the infinite.

> With four hundred milligrams of moksha-medicine in their bloodstreams, even beginners can catch a glimpse of the world as it looks to someone who has been liberated from his bondage to the ego. [41, p. 139]

Psychedelic Mushrooms are part of the plan for the field of his imagined new Neurotheology, which represents one of the highest bridges with which Huxley intends to recover the unity of the sciences, especially the experimental sciences and the humanities, and, more importantly, the body-spirit unity. Here, the problems begin: how to distinguish the experience of enlightenment from what may be nothing more than an incipient psychosis? As we will see below, Huxley does offer, from his personal experience with psychotropic drugs, some suggestive reflections that deserve our attention and analysis.

Huxley typifies the subjective sensations induced by the consumption of mescaline in two groups: the first, due to a peculiarly intense and revealing character, is the one made up of mystical experiences; the second, due to its dreamlike and transgressive force, that of visionary experiences. The experiences of this second group are, for Huxley, pure mirages, the result of hallucinations of merely chemical origin. They are not, however, negligible because, in his opinion, they allow the individual to free himself from those prejudices and too rigid thought schemes that prevent individuals from opening up to uncomfortable and apparently absurd truths. Mystical experiences, on the contrary, would, according to him, have a real referent, they would be a bridge of direct intuitions toward nature, which would be expressed through them in the form of moral conscience. These latter are the ones that we are interested in analyzing here because, despite his efforts, Huxley fails to offer solid criteria that would allow them to be differentiated from mere visionary experiences.

Here, we will approach what Huxley experienced using a descriptive phenomenological method, retracing the path started in previous studies [42–45]. In this attempt by Huxley, there is an attempt to bring certain experiences, typical of the humanities, closer to the experimental sciences. This implies an approach to what in previous studies we have described, following Dilthey, as natural sciences and spiritual sciences [42]. At this initial point, we will try to reach the comprehensible dimension through the descriptive phenomenological method. Later we will refer to the natural methods that tried to modify the perceptual conditions pointing to a supposed ecstasy.

From what is understandable, what is impressive here is an attempt to resolve the historical failures of humanity, evident in a succession of armed conflicts during the twentieth century, through the appeal to the inner life and the abandonment of economic and power-related interests. We will focus then on the understanding of *the* other person, in his individuality and within the historical framework that somehow conditions him. In other words, the motivations that led him to try his experiment with mescaline are numerous and confluent. We will briefly outline what we understand to be his main motives.

1. On the one hand, he is concerned about the possibility of establishing deep encounters between people. A juvenile ophthalmological problem seems to play an important role in some difficulties in his relationship with others. Although he managed to overcome it, it is possible that this difficulty in capturing para verbal elements of communication may have had an impact on his difficulties, which are extensively discussed in the work we are analyzing. He raises his disbelief here around the possibility of the deep communication between human beings. Some difficulty could be supposed in the empathic encounter. This would grant relational, binding value, by sharing experiences that cannot be reduced to words.
2. Huxley's horror regarding violence is well known, and openly commented on, all the more so because of the historical moment he had to witness. He preaches peace by drawing attention to valuable elements of intimacy. His position could be considered quietistic pietism.
3. There is a more or less manifest religious drive in his intention. Explore the possibility of finding the perception of an object that allows you to see the entire universe in it. He explicitly seeks, and describes, what he considers a vision from the sublime, an apophany, a view from on high.

Elements of Huxley's Apophatic Experience

We will describe here the manifestations arising from the experience in his experiment. In the first place, we will refer to the vertiginous experiences of neo-significance of external objects, interpreted here as revelations, but very similar to those reported by schizophrenic patients in their early stages. The presence of hallucinations and temporal-spatial distortions may be a sign of a cerebral toxic effect and not of mystical illumination.

1. Huxley's apophatic experience
2. Hallucinations in Huxley's experience
3. Temporospatial disorders in Huxley's experience

We now develop the postulate.

1. *Huxley's Apophatic Experience*

We will proceed to make a phenomenological analysis of his story, taking his expressions in this sense. The presence of hallucinations in this experience of Huxley and schizophrenias has been highlighted. But we understand that the parallelism does not end here. Even more striking are the parallels between Huxley's interpretations of the perceptual and delusional or apophatic manifestations (Conrad) of schizophrenia.

We will take the interpretations of the apophatic referred to in this experience. There are striking parallels between the schizophrenic delusion or apophany and its present correlate, Huxley's experience.

Huxley's decision is to submit himself to a mescaline use test. He does it, according to him, like a guinea pig. The act takes place on a bright May morning. The state is induced by ingesting four-tenths of a gram of mescaline. Approximately an hour and a half after said intake, phenomena appear that could be defined as apophatic experiences in the sense of Conrad. Three flowers in a crystal vase allow him to contemplate what Adam had contemplated on the morning of his creation. He speaks of a feathery incandescence, of a transfiguration. He had before him the miracle, moment by moment, of naked existence [46, p. 20]. There would be an affective exaltation referred to the perception of these images of the external world. The objects are the same, but illuminated by a different light, a light that could be called the light that illuminated Adam on the day of his creation, the "miracle of naked existence."

Clear reminiscences of what Conrad called "temper" or "delusional humor" would appear here [47]. This experience would seem to be marked by a very clear mode of existence of things. Huxley uses the word "Istigkeit." This word is the abstract of the verb to be in German, "ist," "is" in English, and "es" in Spanish. The term, used by a mystic like Meister Ekhardt, has implications for the way what is perceived appears. With this term, Huxley seems to refer to a feeling of a strong presence, a perception from the ecstasies. In the context of Huxley's mescaline experience, this set of elements should be interpreted as an element of toxic psychosis. It would be predominantly linked to a delusional experience, giving it the character of evidence.

Continuing with his experience, the perception of four legs on a wicker chair is described as a "miraculous fact." Perceiving them within the ongoing experience confers a gift, "above all costs." It is precisely a "new direct knowledge of the true nature of things" [46, pp. 35–36]. Here again, the effulgence of the apophatic experience as understood by Conrad is manifested. The sight of the books has such a force that he refers that it seems that they were going to jump from the shelves to launch themselves in an insistent way to his perception. We would be here facing apophaties from the outside world. This apophany of the outside world entails, in Conrad's approach, a set of meanings and revelations. Those four legs "procure all kinds of wealth." Even more, and surpassing all previous expectations, they go on to seek "a new direct knowledge of the true Nature of Things." It would be extremely difficult not to notice here the apophatic and, in that sense, emphatic character of this statement. At this point, it would be assumed a humoral state similar to delusional.

In other passages of his work, and consistent with other affirmations present here, Huxley refers to inanimate objects that reach "the edging of glory." It has a clear apophatic connotation, within a very similar system, due to the set of meanings, to a delusional system. This *delusional system* has a substitute character of the original and direct perception of the world within the framework of its original relations. It would be possible to speak here of a "delusional worldview, a new order" following a delusion. Huxley goes so far as to postulate a "sacramental vision of reality." In this framework, he proposes a "new apophany." A particular world constitutes the framework, a world in which everything shines with "inner light, infinite in its meaning" [46, pp. 24–26]. He speaks of a transfiguration, of a beatific vision.

Huxley would seem to fall into a fallacy. A revelation, a mystical experience involved from the subjective an intense emotion in the face of the unveiling of deeper, more mysterious realities. It is true that a*n actual* revelation could generate intense emotion, but here evidence of the opposite direction seems to prevail. Not every emotionally charged perception constitutes a transcendent, mystical experience. Although the first statement is valid here, there is no evidence in the opposite direction.

The emotion generated by the perception in these altered states seems to constitute an argument about the existence of a revelation. Specifically, he inferred from the exalted and "salient" perception of some flowers ("Istigkeit") and other inanimate objects, a participation of the entire universe in them. The entire universe becomes patent, tangible in the perceptual act linked to the flowers.

Another confusing element is the idea of a transcendent experience. In reality, what is being operated here is intra-individual, cerebral metabolic, which generates impressions about the perception of objects in the external world, and the illusory fact of perceiving the entire universe in an object. It does not transcend toward the object and its deep planes. The physiological impact of the images is modified through a pharmacological resource, with a very relevant impact on the affective sphere. On the object, seem to fall "the edgings of glory."

2. *Hallucinations in Huxley's Experience*

The accompanying psychopathological elements of the experience are, neither more nor less, visual hallucinations, perplexity, and temporal-spatial disorientation. It is curious that with this syndromatic constellation, this experience has not been related to psychoses rather than to enlightenment. It is no longer just about meanings assigned to perceptual phenomena, but to phenomena of frank psychosis, some of them even related to delirium. This is the case of hallucinations, *perplexity,* and space-time disorders.

Hallucinations are described by Huxley in a very lively way. This experience constituted a very particular event, generating the perception of very unusual shapes and colors (Gargiulo, Part 2). Huxley describes that half an hour after taking the drug he had the perception of a slow dance of golden lights, sumptuous red surfaces that swelled, expanding from shimmering, vibrating nodules of energy, shifting. At times and closing his eyes he affirms that he perceived gray structures, from which bluish spheres arose, which acquired solidity and then ascended without noise until they were lost. He claims that the mescaline did not give him entrance to another world but that these visions appeared in objective space. He affirms that "it was not the world of visions." From psychiatric semiology, we could say that they were true hallucinations, identified with the perceptual and not with previous ideas. The phenomena are presented as pure, indubitable, and are recognized in the outside world [46, pp. 24–26]. For all that has been said *here*, *it* could *be possible to* speak of hallucinatory phenomena.

3. *Temporospatial Disorders in Huxley's Experience*

At some point, temporospatial disorders are evident. These disorders are accompanied by feelings of perplexity. Spatial relationships would seem to cease to matter much at the time of the reported experience. Huxley refers to the feeling of perceiving the world in terms other than spatial categories. One could speak of an experience of strangeness, of a feeling of perplexity present and evidenced in statements such as perceiving, according to him, that the walls of the room were no longer at right angles, that the perspective seemed strange. This seems to be linked to a certain perplexity. The perception of that moment is not related to ordinary spatial categories.

The place and the distance would seem to be relegated by a perception based on the intensity of existence, depth of meaning, and relationships within a system. Here, the salience of some existing and present objects in front of the observer is noticed, and the weight of the meanings of the protruding. The meaning prevails over the temporospatial coordinates, thus resulting in a strong foreshortening. Space loses its predominance, as does time. Thus, an atmosphere compatible with delusional certainties is generated.

Time and its perception also undergo very relevant modifications. Huxley speaks of a perpetual present in an ever-changing apocalypse. The expressions are close to Conrad's descriptions of the apocalyptic experiences of incipient schizophrenia. It is, in both cases, a new universe.

In another part of his experience, Huxley relates that the books in the room shone with a living light. The books "reached the edges of glory" and this was more manifest in some than in others. One could speak here of the emergence of the apophatic, in the sense of Conrad. In Huxley's story, an indifference to time and space appears, with a prevalence of being and meaning. Its integration within a system recalls the set of meanings within the delusional system, which replaces the original perception of the world and its original relationships. There would be a delusional worldview, a new order generated by delusion. Huxley speaks of a "sacramental vision of reality," a "new apophany," in a world where everything shone with "inner light, infinite in meaning" [46, pp. 24–26].

Final Chords of Huxley's Experience

Finally, Huxley attempts to synthesize his findings [46, pp. 31–32]. He affirmed in this regard that he did not observe disorders in the ability to remember. He highlights the intensity that visual perceptions acquire. He postulates that the eye recovers a perceptive innocence typical of childhood. He affirms that in this infantile perceptual state, the meaning is not immediately subordinated to the concept. He states that in the experience, the interest in space and time decreases. This would be equivalent to the modification of the a priori forms of perceptions, from a Kantian perspective. It should be noted that this would imply a perceptual distortion rather than a disclosure of reality. He tells us that perception is vastly improved. But it will undergo a profound change, and not for the better. He would seem to be pointing out here a surrender of intentionality, one more element compatible with schizophrenic psychoses. Huxley attributes this surrender of intentionality to a lack of interest for reasons that can mobilize people who have not come into contact with this experience he has lived. This experience brings better things to think about. The claudication of intentionality could be interpreted, at least in the sense of an additional element, as arising from the difficulty of executive functions derived from a difficulty in the frontal cortex, typical of schizophrenic psychoses. We will come back to this when we talk about schizophrenic psychoses.

In a brief synthetic expression, we could say that there is no clear decrease in verbal expression. The chromatic acquires a very clear prevalence over the temporospatial. What is perceived under conditions of this type is valued far above what is done in the normal world. This would imply bypassing vital interests to access particular experiences.

On the "Reducing Valve of the Brain"

His hypothesis regarding a supposed "reducing valve of the brain" deserves separate consideration. Particularly striking is the fact that *he* proposes a perceptual or cognitive reduction or impairment by mechanisms that would be intrinsic to the brain when in reality attention orders and chooses. When attention is focused on an object, we filter out upstart, accessory, or irrelevant stimuli. This has a brain correlate or filter mechanism. This is altered in psychoses. The operation of this postulated "valve" would seem to be, for Huxley, a veil covering reality, and the effect of mescaline a key to unveiling or "aletheia." It would not be that in this particular state, there is an expansion of the conscious experience, given the impairment of a supposed valve. It is a filter function, which exists and has been attributed to the functioning of some brain structures in dynamic integration with others, and which is interfered with by the drug. We will explain this in some detail.

When talking about brain circuit interactions in schizophrenic psychosis, Grace [49] proposes, based on preclinical psychophysiological studies of his group that in the ventral striatum, or Nucleus Accumbens Septi (NAS), there would be an integration of various brain projections that would exer*t* their control and interaction there. Glutamatergic projections from the hippocampus, amygdala, and frontal cortex are integrated into the Nucleus Accumbens Septi (NAS) or ventral striatum or neostriatum. In this structure, an integration takes place between the outputs of these structures and their prevailing function. This striatal integration of *behavior* involves goal-directed *behaviors* (frontal cortex), contextual cues (hippocampus), and affective facilitation of these processes (amygdala). In this way, if the interaction is carried out under normal conditions, a teleological *behavior* with situational location and its corresponding affective valence are produced.

There is a synergistic facilitatory activity between the electrotone provided on the neurons of the NAS by the hippocampus and the projections of the frontal cortex. This electrotone provided by the hippocampus allows the expression of the frontal *cortex*, which otherwise does not get its expression. If there is any dysfunction in hippocampal tone, as Grace argues in the case of schizophrenias, impulsive behavior, guided by the amygdala, prevails. This consists, for this author, the primary cerebral dysfunction in schizophrenic psychoses [48].

On the other hand, there are efferent projections from the NAS that will reach the thalamus. An inhibitory pathway originates in the NAS, traverses the ventral pallidum (VP), and reaches the dorsomedial nucleus of the thalamus, which exerts a filter function through these GABA-mediated inhibitory afferents. This filter function allows relevant stimuli to reach the cerebral cortex, while irrelevant stimuli do not. In this sense, these brain structures exert a function of hierarchizing stimuli and inhibit irrelevant stimuli [48]. The role of the dopamine system has been also recognized [49], and interactions between dopamine and glutamate within NAS are widely described [50]. Regarding the psychotomimetic action of ketamine, the interference with the somatosensory system due to the interference of cortico-thalamo-cortical circuits and its consequences at the level of sensory integration in translational models seem to be central facts in the brain dysfunction underlying schizophrenia [51].

A failure of this system produces a cortical flood of irrelevant stimuli, with an overload that *impedes* orderly thinking and *favors* chaotic cortical activation. This phenomenon would seem to recall Huxley's idea of the "reducing valve of the brain." This cerebral filter system would be altered in psychoses and would be annulled by hallucinogenic drugs. Thus, they would access an intense but very messy experience. Huxley's perception through his experience with mescaline is striking, but it is questionable whether to attribute a higher consciousness value to this state.

Glutamate, Dopamine, and Schizophrenia

Starting from preclinical translational studies, we stated, in 1998, that the primary symptoms of schizophrenia could be explained by deficits in glutamate transmission in NAS, and not by increased dopaminergic activity. We work with a shape discrimination test using visual stimuli in the pigeon [52]. We suggest that the dopaminergic pathways afferent to the NAS could be linked to the treatment of schizophrenia, rather than to the onset of the disease. The following years we observed that primary, secondary, and cognitive symptoms could be emulated in translational models by selectively blocking N-methyl-D-aspartate (NMDA) glutamatergic receptors in NAS [53].

In our 2014 review, we brought together the findings and previous evidence*s* provided by our laboratory regarding the relevance of NMDA glutamatergic blockade in NAS. Starting from a study in schizophrenic patients [54], we proposed a study in a translational model in pigeons interfering with dopaminergic and glutamatergic activities in NAS in a shape perception test [52]. In this study, we found that dopaminergic stimulation in NAS did not interfere with the discrimination of visual stimuli. On the contrary, NMDA glutamatergic blockade induced the impossibility of discriminating stimuli above chance values. This fact was interpreted by us as an alteration of the gestalt perceptual function, in the orbit of Conrad's theories regarding incipient schizophrenia [47]. We proposed our model as a translational approach to delusional perception. And we conclude affirming that these perceptual distortions, which would be translational approximations to the delusional perceptions of schizophrenics, were due, according to the results, to decreased disorders of glutamatergic function in NAS and not to increased dopaminergic transmission in this pathway. However, all drugs that have proven action in schizophrenic psychoses have a blocking action on the mesolimbic dopaminergic pathway. As previously said, this led us to postulate that the blockade of the dopaminergic pathway should be related to the treatment of schizophrenic psychoses, but not necessarily to the onset of initial symptoms.

Another phenomenon in that study particularly caught our attention. This phenomenon was the fact that correction trials (correcting trials) increased significantly with the same pharmacological treatment of NMDA-type glutamatergic antagonism. A correction trial consists of the presentation immediately after a wrong trial of the same stimuli in the same position aiming to facilitate correction. This necessarily implies a relapse into a pattern that has not been successful. If the rectification does not occur, the number of correction trials is increased. This implies perseveration in the same stimulus and being able to rectify. In the mentioned study [52], we interpret this phenomenon of perseveration in the wrong stimulus as a phenomenon of ideo-affective rigidity, a secondary or residual symptom of schizophrenia. Consequently, we postulate that both the primary symptoms (delusional perception) and the secondary ones (represented here by ideo-affective rigidity) could be induced by blocking NMDA-type glutamatergic transmission.

Other subsequent studies confirmed the value of glutamatergic blockade in NAS with other NMDA-type glutamatergic antagonists [55, 56] in shape perception. Another interesting finding was the fact that the blockade of the presynaptic glutamate receptor, responsible for the release of this neurotransmitter, improved the performance of the trials in terms of the percentage of correct trials and, additionally, decreased the correction trials. This would imply an improvement in performance in all the parameters used in this test. This would contrast with the effect of the D-2 antagonist used in that experiment, which only decreased the number of correction trials without affecting the percentage yield of correct answers [56].

Throughout our project, carried out on pigeons in association with the team of Professor Juan Delius in Konstanz, we carried out some experiments on rats in our laboratory within the same collaboration. Given that the pigeons presented with the pharmacological treatment in NAS an alteration in perception, we proposed the same procedure in the rat in a learning and memory test. There we observed that the NMDA glutamatergic blockage induced an alteration in acquisition without affecting consolidation [57, 58]. This would be consistent with the perceptual alterations from the temporal point of view. Perceptions constitute the beginning of stimulus fixation.

In the learning and memory experiment, a new element appeared that caught our attention. We observed a decrease in the number of fecal boluses expelled by the rats that had received treatment with the NMDA antagonist. Fecal boluses are considered an element linked to stress and anxiety. This could mean that there was a concomitant anxiolytic effect. For this reason, we decided to carry out an experiment with a specific anxiety test, the elevated Plus Maze (EPM) [59, 60]. In this anxiety experiment in the EPM we observed a statistically highly significant increase in the stay in the open arm with the treatment. This decrease in anxiety was interpreted by us as a sign of affective crushing in our translational model.

Another prominent element in schizophrenic psychoses is the alteration or impairment of the working memory function. In order to induce a working memory disorder with NMDA antagonist injections in*to the* NAS, we used a specific test in rats [61]. *With this purpose,* we used the Hole Board *Test* in a model with five holes to observe how the *rats* distributed their exploration behavior. It was notably disorganized with statistically very significant changes in the order and frequency of exploration of the Hole Board holes. Concomitantly, we observed a phenomenon compatible with disorganization due to overactivation of the Frontal Cortex, a phenomenon that we interpret as associated with the failure of the thalamic filter functions associated with these circuits.

The glutamatergic hypothesis of schizophrenia, related to these findings, has received increasing attention [53, 61]. However, some symptoms in men with schizophrenic psychoses would seem to be related to dopaminergic pathways. In fact, recent studies point to the involvement of both neurotransmission systems [62]. This could be explained by concurrent facilitations. In fact, the significance of certain stimuli seems to be influenced by the prominence or salience given to them by additional elements provided by dopaminergic transmission. Elements of both neurotransmission systems could concur simultaneously. Thus, to the perceptual difficulty generated by glutamatergic blocks, the exaltation of some stimuli due to prominence or salience could be added.

The perceptual difficulty linked to glutamate has been previously referred to by us in the aforementioned translational studies. This difficulty would lead to an alteration in the appreciation of the environment and the place that the perceiver fits in it [63]. We must add to this the affective exaltation of certain irrelevant stimuli that become highly significant due to bodily maladjustments, and, as such, experiential, perceptible but not understandable. The prominence of some stimuli, which would be abnormally high, would be attributable to mesolimbic dopaminergic hyperactivity. Psychosis would be related to an aberrant perceptual prominence [64, 65]. In this way, glutamatergic and dopaminergic neurotransmissions would be integrated into the central perceptual distortions of schizophrenic psychoses. It may act as conditioning the reaction to this perception [66].

The fact that there is an initial glutamatergic dysfunction would be relatively well established. However, the fact that there is an aberrant prominence would be related to phenomena linked to dopaminergic pathways. Within this framework, the phenomenology, biology, and pharmacology of psychoses would be integrated [64]. The role of dopamine would be fundamentally linked to motivational states and the prominence of internal or external events of the mind. If a stimulus predicts that a *behavior* will be reinforced or punished, changes occur in the discharge of dopaminergic pathways in the brain. The possibility of assigning predictive values to the stimuli and the prominence of these over other similar ones in the experience of the specific individual who affront them [67, 68] have been attributed to this phenomenon. It would be a succession of previous events in the subject's learning history linking these stimuli, behaviors, and consequences [66]. Finally, and in general terms, the blockade of dopamine in the mesolimbic pathway by antipsychotics decreases the salience and aberrant value of some stimuli [64].

Finally, and greatly simplifying the explanation, we point out that antipsychotic drugs act by antagonizing dopaminergic D-2 receptors and serotonergic 5HT-2 receptors [69]. The action of mescaline is exactly the inverse. This drug works by stimulating D2 and 5HT-2 receptors [70]. It could be concluded from this that it is reasonable to consider mescaline as a psychotogenic drug, with all that this implies in relation to the subject treated here. This can be an additional element to interpret Huxley's experience as an experience indistinguishable from a toxic psychosis, namely, a visionary experience (as far as hallucinatory and delusional) and not necessarily a mystical experience.

The transformation associated with the visionary experience is caused by the experience itself. To have a vision is to be transformed in a certain soft way. In contrast, the hard transformation associated with the mystical experience is caused by something prior to that experience. In other words, the mystical experience is only a manifestation of *kenosis* but is not the *kenosis*. Therefore, with the chemical induction of a visionary experience, we can be certain that the individual will be transformed in a manner similar to a naturally induced visionary experience. But we cannot be sure of the same with the chemical induction of mystical experiences. These could be just mental mirages, mere hallucinations far from a real transformation.

If this is so, gathering in silence and love seem the only sure way to transform the individual. It is not the experience but something prior to the experience that an individual becomes sensitive to that light by which it is possible to reconnect with the real and grow in harmony with the external and internal nature. Nevertheless, insofar as this *kenosis* is not reducible to mere chemical phenomena, to pure neuropsychology, at least as both are understood today, we must affirm that the desert natures or the hand of the needy act on the hermits in a way that transcends the purely perceptual or cognitive. Deserts and brains are more than data. In other words, they cannot be fully symbolized, translated, or replaced… either by chemical or silicon elements or not even by virtual cybernetic spaces. They are natural irreplaceable elements with the mysterious strength of the sign. Therefore, natural causes and effects cannot be studied or replicated in vitro, that is, in a laboratory where the only thing that is handled and controlled are data. In conclusion, it is not possible to distinguish objectively mystical experiences from visionary experiences. For this task, it is necessary to add to the objective also the subjective, that is, the singular and subjective element, which only each individual, himself, can provide. But the fact that mystical experience is beyond the reach of experimental science does not mean that it does not have a crucial role in its study and promotion—necessary but not sufficient. Unfortunately, such recognition of the humility of science and the overflowing mystery of nature is what many today are unwilling to accept.

A Rose-Wreath Crown

Returning to the *Island*, Huxley draws there a final parallel with *BNW*. If the *World State* defeats the rebels and demonstrates the sustainability of a state founded on technology, *Pala* succumbs in defense of more humane values. However, is it a failed state? Huxley offers us in this antinomy another prophecy and his final and most profound hope in reality. On the one hand, he anticipates a world obsessed with sustainability and, on the other, shows us his belief that there are individual and social circumstances worse than death and social chaos, such as the loss of self and the denaturalization of laws. It should not be forgotten that Nature always comes to the rescue. Like Hölderlin, Huxley does not believe in sad endings either.

> O soul! soul! beauty of the world! indestructible! rapturing! With your eternal youth! you are; what then is death and all the woe of men?—Oh! many empty words have been made by these strange brethren. Yet all things proceed from pleasure, and everything ends in peace. [34, p. 137]

This mysterious defense of the natural is in stark contrast to the idea of the leaders of the *World State* that everything associated with perennial, substantially true identity is a threat to any system of government that seeks stability:

> 'A love of nature keeps no factories busy. It was decided to abolish the love of nature, at any rate among the lower classes; to abolish the love of nature […] We condition the masses to hate the country,' concluded the Director. 'But simultaneously we condition them to love all country sports. At the same time, we see to it that all country sports shall entail the use of elaborate apparatus. So that they consume manufactured articles as well as transport […] Which brings us at last,' continued Mr. Foster, 'out of the realm of mere slavish imitation of nature into the much more interesting world of human invention'. [2, 14, 35]

In short, technology in Huxley's technological future confers upon the human species an extraordinary power to free it from many of the obstacles and evils that have accompanied it in its history, including self-annihilation by atomic and biological weapons. It also presents itself as an extraordinary facilitator of paths and pleasurable states. None of this is ignored in BNW and Island; nevertheless, it appears associated with a darker danger than extinction, a risk that has anguish as its sign and fear as its herald. In this chapter, we have related both as important factors propitiating addictive behavior that, however, do not usually arouse the attention of researchers, more focused on the genetic, psychological, and biographical analysis of the individual and, above all, using reductive, *objectivist* methodologies that further bias the identification of causes and solutions. The great confidence that not a few specialists are placing in using AI as a research tool is, in this sense, one of the latest signs of this dataistic drift. Of course, AI can be useful for solving specific problems [71], but it is difficult to justify that it will represent great promise in this field.

Finally, there is a bigger problem than not making sufficient progress in achieving better treatments for addiction. If Huxley and Alexander are right and it is not possible to fully understand

and conveniently treat addiction from a *locationalist* approach, which leaves out the problem of meaning, then current treatments may be causing an iatrogenic type of evil. Do patients end their addiction therapies with the reinforced idea that their suffering is related to some malfunctioning part of themselves (the brain, surely) or a particular toxic habitat that must be abandoned—much as one might think that a computer should not be placed in excessively humid places? Because this is an idea that would intensify existential anguish in the face of a fragmented body and world, made up of parts—just as a machine is made up of components.

Nature is today the primary objective from which intellectuals must strive to defend freedom against postmodern structural addictions. It does not necessarily imply endorsing the existence of gods or ascribing to any particular type of transcendentalism or immanentism—the latter is the option Huxley chooses. All these positions fit into a common cause to prevent the coming of the last man—the last world. Indeed, great difficulties create the strangest traveling companions. Nietzsche, another philosopher critical of the modern inflationist ego, writes the following:

> I show you the last man.
>
> "What is love? What is creation? What is longing? What is a star?"—thus asks the last man and he blinks.
>
> The earth has become small, and on it hops the last man, who makes everything small. His race is as ineradicable as the flee-beetle; the last man lives longest.
>
> "We have invented happiness"—say the last men, and they blink. [72, p. 17]

It is Nietzsche's most eloquent way of showing that we cannot have the Last Men as interlocutors [73]. Talking to them is like throwing words at the wind—only the desert can affect the Last Men. The Zarathustra imagined by Nietzsche spent 10 years in the mountains, in the only company of dangerous lions and shrewd serpents, to return to the world and manifest his wisdom. Before the desert, he also belonged to the group of the Last Men; after the desert, Zarathustra began proclaiming the message. However, these speeches are not addressed to the last man. They have not so much an argumentative purpose as a sign of recognition among those who have awakened from the enlightened dream and want to come together to rebuild the world. Nietzsche, like Huxley, speaks not only of the present but also of a better tomorrow.

The clue of recognition helps explain why Nietzsche chose *poetic fiction* to present his philosophical ideas in all their depth. Indeed, he emphasizes with analogies and metaphors the idea of the solitary path that each man must travel.

> When Zarathustra had said these words he became silent, like one who has not yet said his last word; long he weighed his staff in his hand, doubtfully. At last he spoke thus, and the tone of his voice had changed.
>
> Now I go alone, my disciples. You too go now, alone. Thus I want it. Verily, I counsel you: go away from me and resist Zarathustra! And even better: be ashamed of him! Perhaps he deceived you. [72, p. 3]

Zarathustra should not be understood, not followed, but interpreted, which implies that readers/disciples have to employ high levels of subjectivity in a task that has more to do with themselves than with the words of the master. On this point, both Huxley and Taylor would agree with Nietzsche that the cultural battle is now to be fought in theaters, auditoriums, and art galleries rather than in academic forums. For reflective discourse to be effective, it must first recover the lost capacity for contemplation. And it is the masters of contemplation, the artists, who can best guide the Westerner in this task [74].

On the other hand, in the cited text, Nietzsche points to the big problem of late modern narcissism, which the prophet seems to have overcome: Zarathustra's ego has recovered its natural and functional size for attaining a good life. But then, how should the relationship with his disciples be? On the one hand, authentic disciples would be those who intuit something of the prophet's truth but who have yet to walk the desert path. It is no small thing. But for Zarathustra it is not enough, and therefore, he tests their patience and constancy with rebuffs, criticisms, and even insults. That is why Nietzsche writes below:

> The man of knowledge must not only love his enemies, he must also be able to hate his friends. [72, p. 3]

The disciples should follow Zarathustra, but not because of the merit or affection of the master... They should also be able to abandon him to cross the desert. However this is only possible if, first of all, the master takes a long time to answer questions, which expels the most impatient, pusillanimous, or sycophants-opportunistic disciples; and second, if later, the master accepts the abandonment of those who will surpass him. Nietzsche excludes, with these considerations, individuals with severe levels of narcissism. The following analogy, quasi-metaphorical, facilitates the understanding of this criterion of exclusion.

The narcissistic person resembles a dying star of the *red giant* type. In general terms, this type of star is characterized by a large volume, low density, and lower surface temperature than younger stars. It is because they are running out of fuel at their center, and their gravitational mass is decreasing, which causes, at first, the outer layers of the star's crust to expand.

Similarly, Nietzsche distinguishes between the "self" (*Selbst*) and the "ego" (*Ich*): the former represents what is given in the human being, including the natural ends and élan vital—on which the philosopher will build his theory about the Power Will—, while the latter is constituted by the set of beliefs that the individual has about himself and the world. For Nietzsche, Narcissus is burdened with an ego that has forgotten the self and ceases to seek it and feed on it. Therefore, this ego, freed from the gravitational influence of the real, grows, inflates, and denaturalizes beliefs, feelings, and behavior. The consequences have already been discussed above, fragmentation, anxiety, and fear... Nietzsche now also adds to this list a defensive reaction that anticipates, in a way, the Freudian defense mechanisms. The ego seeks in its public image an element of anchorage and coherence. That is why Narcissus needs to persuade others about who he is, a pure image of ego, which reinforces pathological dependency relationships—mentioned above as structural addiction. Furthermore, because external beliefs sustain internal beliefs, inflationary dynamics are intensified.

This framework also explains why theatricality is usually associated with narcissism. Narciso's being depends on what others believe him to be. If he succeeds in deceiving others, he will also succeed in deceiving himself—a deep self-deception [75]. The narcissist is cheerful when others believe he is cheerful, is a great father of a family when he has gained such fame, is a great professional when he is socially successful, manifests a blameless moral life when others judge him so, etc. However, the absence of connection with his self makes his behavior inauthentic, unnatural, and faked because Narciso finds it increasingly difficult to distinguish when he is lying and when he is telling the truth.

In summary, reputation is everything to Narcissus; that is why a single wayward individual, a dissonant note, may turn his perfect happiness into hell. He maintains a constant ambivalent attitude of love and hate toward his fellows. Because acolytes are needed, but, at the same time, they all are potential enemies—a source of critiques and rivality. So, the higher the levels of narcissism, the higher the histrionics or violence. Cordial indifference is not an option: he can only seduce or destroy, usually both simultaneously.

A red giant does not continue to grow indefinitely. There comes a time when the energy of the nucleus is exhausted, and the red giant shrinks again until, in the worst case, it becomes one of those all-devouring black holes. Similarly, while the self exerts its benevolent influence on Narcissus, even unconsciously, he will continue to live in his idyllic dream. However, when this influence ceases, and the disconnection with reality reaches severe heights, Narcissus will succumb to darkness and anguish that make him almost wholly incapacitated for transcendence, that is, for any effective act of *introspection* and *extrospection*, for any attitude search for himself and for the undreamt of reality. Narcissus is Nietzsche's Last Man.

How then to enter into a dialogue with Narcissus? It would be like addressing an uninhabited fortress, especially if Narcissus is fully integrated into a community of Narcissus, like the addicted citizens of BNW. Zarathustra cannot drag him neither into silence, which for Narcissus would imply annihilation, nor into love, which he only understands as another opportunity to feed his own external image. For Nietzsche, the solution is to try to prick the ego's balloon: satire is the needle to be used. Because if it bothers Narcissus to a great degree to cause indifference, it bothers him even more not to be taken seriously. It is solidity, seriousness, and "gravity" that he seeks and what he lacks most -and therefore, the mocking indifference of a single fellow is like an exorcism for his spirit.

> This laugher's crown, this rose-wreath crown: I myself have set this crown on my head, I myself have canonized my laughter. I have found no other strong enough for it today.
>
> Zarathustra the dancer, Zarathustra the light, who beckons with his wings, ready for flight, beckoning to all birds, pre-walled and ready, blissfully light-hearted:
>
> Zarathustra the prophet, Zarathustra the laughing prophet, no impatient nor uncompromising man, one who loves jumping and escapades; I myself have set this crown on my head! [72, p. 218]

This text is not a hymn against truth or nature (the solid or substantial reality) as it is sometimes interpreted, but against those who have erected the ego as the only autonomous and supreme reality. Zarathustra does not suffer from the bitterness of cynicism, from which, in fact, he has been cured. Only after trying his own medicine does he dare to give advice: Last Men must be asked to dance, only to be sat upon with contempt; their pompous figure must be praised, only to have their neatly trimmed beards criticized. In short, jokes and mockery are the recipes to soften their masks.

Better still than Nietzsche, Herbert George Wells captures the mystery of laughter and its modern scope in "A Vision of Judgment." We want to conclude this chapter with a fragment of this story about the final judgment, Christian in this case, but also irreverently interreligious and from which Nietzsche, despite his belligerent anti-Christian attitude, would indeed also grant a laugh:

> "Well?" said God, looking down at him. We were privileged to hear the reply, and indeed the acoustic properties of the place were marvelous. "I plead guilty," said the little figure. "Tell them what you have done," said the Lord God. "I was a king," said the little figure, "a great king, and I was lustful and proud and cruel. I made wars, I devastated countries, I built palaces, and the mortar was the blood of men. Hear, O God, the witnesses against me, calling to you for vengeance. Hundreds and thousands of witnesses." He waved his hands towards us. "And worse! I took a prophet -one of your prophets—" [...]
>
> "Did he do all this?" said the Lord God. The Recording Angel flattened his book with his hand. "In a way," said the Recording Angel, carelessly. "Read," said the Lord God. And the angel read, explaining very carefully and fully all the wickedness of the Wicked Man. [...]
>
> Everybody was laughing. Even the prophet of the Lord whom the Wicked Man had tortured had a smile on his face. The Wicked Man was really such a preposterous little fellow. "And then," read the Recording Angel, with a smile that set us all agog, "one day, when he was a little irascible from over-eating, he—"
>
> "Oh, not that," cried the Wicked Man, "nobody knew of that" [...] The Wicked Man rushed to and fro across God's palm, and then suddenly turned about and fled up the sleeve of God. [...]
>
> "And now," said God, as he shook us out of his sleeve upon the planet he had given us to live upon, the planet that whirled about green Sirius for a sun, "now that you understand me and each other a little better...try again". [76, pp. 598–602]

Wells' laughter strips the man, purifies him of all false images, and confronts him with his own reality. Laughter turns the ego toward the self, fills it with shame and humiliation, and drives it toward the desert. That is to say, in a second moment, laughter opens the way to a new way of looking at oneself, a growth in sensitivity and intelligence, and, finally, to a new perception. In it, the individual awakens to astonishment before a self that is something more than expected, something bigger and, at the same time, more dependent on the harmony of reality. Then, a new authentic, beautiful, strong, and free ego is born.

Wells offers us another utopia, this time the most hopeful of all and, perhaps for that reason, the most utopian. Can man's laughter, or that of God himself, save us from anguish, addiction, fear, and the robotization of human nature? Shame can lead to reconciliation with oneself and others, but it can also sow in the human heart the desire for annihilation of the being, of all beings. This bad ending could reflect that there is no longer anyone behind the mask. Parallelly, we will also find two consecutive times in the process of destroying the self: Evil, which is always voracious—destroyer of worlds—grants the wicked the extensions (some of them of extraordinary brilliance) that he or she needs to consummate his work. Nevertheless, in the end, the wicked will also be drowned in the seas of nothingness which, in human infinity, never seem to touch shores.

Here we find the most severe cases, where all hope must be abandoned because, paraphrasing Mark Twain, these Last Men—Narcissus—would have no more sense of humor than a tombstone. But even if it is true that there is no remedy for a heart in which only cynical laughter dwells, who can be sure of such a doom? Who can get to the bottom of the human heart? The only sure path seems, therefore, to maintain the serene highness of patience, be very zealous for one's gathering in silence, and accept that Last Men will never want to share this planet with such provisional hermits. Persecution and crossfire are unavoidable in the advent of new orders and categories.

Final Remarks. ChatGPT and the True Technological Humanism

Hubert Dreyfus, a philosopher at the University of Berkeley, California, published *Alchemy and Artificial Intelligence* in 1965, at the height of the technological bubble of the 1960s. This article earned him the rejection of the scientific community for criticizing the excessive expectations that were being generated in the field of *machine learning*. There were things that machines could do and others that "still" could not [77]. His article was neither understood nor well received. Branded as retrograde, he suffered what today we call *cancelation culture*, an academic censorship that, although history would end up proving him right, was not going to disappear. At the end of the decade, investors, disappointed, withdrew their funding. And some of us still wonder what heights AI would have reached today without the fever of false hopes. Dreyfus continued to work until his death in 2017, oblivious to a large majority of colleagues who continued to blame him for being right or, better, for not having been right themselves.

It is difficult to be sure what Dreyfus' opinion would have been about the new AI boom. Would he disdain those who compare today the program to the invention of the Internet? I venture to say that the situation is not the same. Now it is not a question of how fast the technology will develop, because the technology is already here and it opens up extraordinary horizons of possibility.

One of the greatest challenges a computer engineer can take on, according to Dreyfus, is to come up with software that generates natural language. And this is precisely what the program developed by OpenAI has achieved. ChatGPT is capable of providing answers to a user's questions in natural, coherent language. Of course, this is not merely a matter of form—it never was. ChatGPT does what it does because of its GPT 3.5, the learning model that underpins it, which draws on the formidable amount of information it gets from the Internet: its current version enjoys an analysis capacity of up to 175 billion parameters and has been trained on 500 billion different words obtained from the most diverse sources. In other words, ChatGPT responds like a human being to highly qualified questions. In the United States, it has managed to pass graduate exams in law and economics and is close to passing the USMLE tests, which every doctor has to pass. It still has certain limitations, however. It is not able to answer image-dependent questions, since, for the time being, it only works with verbal or written information. But it is only a matter of time before it integrates or is integrated into other types of software; for example, in Oxipit's ChestLink, which autonomously identifies pathological structures from radiographic images; or in STAR, a robot designed at Johns Hopkins University which, at the beginning of 2022, also autonomously and successfully performed several gastrointestinal interventions on pigs.

The potential of ChatGPT is much greater than initially conceived by its creators and will significantly affect key sectors of our society. It is justified, therefore, to qualify it as a disruptive technology: it can bring about abrupt changes in professions, markets, social habits,etc. This type of major technological advantage is often accompanied by no lesser difficulty, many of them related to the speed of change, i.e., with a maturation and adaptation time that is not always foreseen. In the medical sector, for example, we can begin to assign to ChatGPT the simplest and most repetitive tasks, for example, those related to patient care. Something similar to what Babylon Health already does is a model of triage in primary care based on artificial intelligence that is already in operation in Rwanda and some cities in the United Kingdom. It would be a good option in countries suffering from overcrowded Emergency Departments. But in return, jobs would be lost for those who are likely to be less qualified and therefore also the most vulnerable in the retraining process, in which industry has to collaborate. This is a simple example of the importance of establishing the right timing in social transformations.

More complex levels of application for ChatGPT are those directly related to medical care, where time also plays against quality care. The software will require the doctor to be trained quickly, as he may not lose his job, but he may be negligent in his practice. He will need basic skills in algorithms, programming, data, networks, etc. if he wants to learn to contextualize the *outputs* offered by AI on his patients and, even more difficult, to use the application creatively. ChatGPT enjoys great versatility but it is not completely reliable and, worse, it is not going to be easy to detect when it is and when it is not. Part of the difficulty is that, as has been said, the power of this software lies in the amount of indiscriminate data it is fed with, which endows it with greater response power (including predictions) than similar models but trained with exclusively biomedical data—e.g., PubMedGPT. Understanding this paradoxical performance and detecting its biases are two of the main research challenges of our decade.

More and different difficulties occur at higher levels of complexity, those where AI is applied to biomedical research. In this chapter, we have mentioned some of them, but we wanted to focus on the risk that, in our opinion, is the greatest of all, because it affects an already existing social problem, social dislocation, which a poor understanding and use of AI can lead to paroxysm. We could even say that AI can lead to becoming a new soma, one that Huxley was not able to imagine in his worst nightmare. The dystopia of *Brave New World* was incomplete and now we know why. It was yet to describe its ending, which, applying Daniel Dennett's term *philosophical zombie*, could be called a *kind zombie apocalypse*.

With programs with ChatGPT, professionals, no matter what field, will have to deal with a peculiar temptation, the comfort of reducing their work to three tasks: collecting evidence, entering evidence into the software, and listening to the virtual oracle, who is almost always right. And the loquacity of the program does not help to curb this drift. On the contrary, it induces the belief, conscious, or unconscious that ChatGPT is not only reliable but also trustworthy, i.e., an "other" to whom to delegate real responsibilities. After all, language is one of the specific advantages of our species and an expression of the also unique human intelligence. Comfort and recognition thus enter into a vicious circle. This perception of the machine, far from encouraging the digital literacy of professionals, can eventually reduce all work to pure technical knowledge. Worse still, the more the citizen is willing to believe that ChatGPT behaves like a human being, the greater the risk that he himself will act like a machine. And vice versa. The transformation from man to machine, the transformation from what one is to what one is not, implies a disintegration of the whole, a dislocation, first social and then individual, which would explain the anguish and the consequent structural addictions.

Like Taylor, Dreyfus predicts and identifies the root of the problem. We are forgetting what separates man and nature from machines. For, indeed, algorithmic intelligence is one of the types of human intelligence, and one of the characteristics of such intelligence is to be entirely objectifiable, that is, translatable and reproducible in different models and media. But human intelligence is not only algorithmic, nor is the reasoning used in any profession. Our intelligence, says Dreyfus, is also intuitive or, in other words, open to wonder in the face of reality. In other words, intuitive intelligence limits a space in which truth, goodness, and beauty occur as experiences rather than as ideas. In this space, every profession is sustained and elevated as art and science at the same time (what the classics called *techne*) and not as mere technical knowledge, which any machine can perform—the activity of the machine, in this sense, can never be professional. However, Dreyfus warns us that intuitive thinking is primarily subjective so that no Turing test can prove its presence, whether in men or machines. Taking this reasoning to its extreme, this implies that being intelligent is not the same as appearing intelligent and that there is no way to distinguish some types of men from others. Of course, nothing prevents us from being able to create machines that perfectly simulate joy and consciousness, professional behavior, but the replication of such experiences escapes algorithmic logic.

Clinical eye («ojo clínico») is a term that, in Spanish, physicians use to refer to a capacity similar to the notion of intuition, which Dreyfus rescues from the history of philosophy. With the clinical eye, the physician intuits the diagnosis sought. With the clinical eye, he glimpses how far to venture with the treatment. With the clinical eye, he perceives the best way to approach the patient. And it is also through the clinical eye that he grasps the deepest meaning of scientific work and the very infinity of human dignity. However, every good physician knows that the clinical eye is not enough. His actions must be accompanied by evidence and judgments that support his decision-making. But without the clinical eye, which grows with good practices, the physician ceases to understand not only his profession but also life and its games. Every professional, physician or not, who really is one (and who does not simply appear to be one), recognizes this phenomenal experience that ennobles and fills his work with mystery. Without the clinical eye, all activity becomes alienating and leads to disorders similar to what we now call occupational burnout—another obvious source of structural addiction.

In a society that has blithely erected evidence as the guardian of the great transcendentals and of the training that supposedly leads to them, programs like ChatGPT will only make it more difficult to cultivate professional intuition. Because if today it is difficult to convince our students to study not to pass exams but to be professionals—not just to look like one, even if they look very good, even better than those who really are—it will be even more difficult to convince them of the correct use of ChatGPT. The competitive climate does not help, nor does the fact that in our cloisters the number of those who firmly believe in the identification of both types of study, and both types of professionals, is growing. A clear manifestation of this phenomenon is that our undergraduate and graduate students suffer, in an increasingly intense way, a constant bombardment of exams that does not allow them to study calmly, in the very long term, or even in a disinterested way. Probably, it will not be long before experts appear who justify the use of automatic learning programs to the detriment of memory, and of the search, comprehension, and synthesis of information—the breeding ground of intuitive thinking. These heralds of professional technification will support their position on evidence and rigorously business criteria of quality and production, which include, ironically, ethical algorithms. And from the evidence, they cannot be refuted.

What has been said about intelligence can also be said about good. Doing good is not the same as *being* good. Machines can do a lot of good, but they are not good. The *men-machine* are creatures obsessed with good (perhaps because of the fracture that dwells in their heart), but their actions do not reach the object of their longing. Because doing good is never enough. The *men-machine* expresses the last gasps of the last man: they want to forgive and be forgiven *for all their good deeds*, but they only know how to open and close their mouths—and blink—, laugh and cry theatrically, and give tight hugs. In this cove of vanities, chaos, and good manners, AI may even anesthetize the last dissatisfaction around which the men-machine revolves and revolves because its misuse would intensify the mirage by which ethics is identified with morality—the final sign of dislocation, even more telling than addiction.

In the terminal phase of this process of intellectual and moral decay, we could venture into a society composed of machines and/or *machine-men*, it doesn't matter, in which suffering and violence have disappeared and pleasure and altruistic behaviors reign everywhere. This *kind zombie apocalypse*, without intuition that awakens the subtle longing for the natural, without subjectivity and intimacy—without heart—, and without that prudence (Aristotle's *phronesis*) with which to direct individual and social progress, marks the end of history. Men then descend to the ninth circle of Dante's *Inferno*, where souls are trapped in a lake of ice. As discussed earlier, it's the latest twist on *Brave New World*, where all possible conscious resistance becomes impossible.

So, is it not possible to make technologies such as ChatGPT compatible with those practices that show us how important and free human action is? There are reasons to believe so, but the path does not seem easy. Dreyfus's latest book, *Retrieving Realism* (2015) [78], which he writes with Canadian philosopher Charles Taylor, offers some hopeful clues about how to avoid a drift that cannot seem to be defeated head-on. The true technological humanism (TTH), which both authors prelude, takes conspiratorial forms in a call to fight, from the catacombs—we would say, from the very foundations of the profession—, the cunning of those who intend to lead society into its longest night. Above all, both authors base in this work the main challenge of all those who intend to follow the path of the *Her Beg*: we must learn to recover, first individually (or in groups of hermits) and then socially, that reality that we inhabit and that elevates human intelligence, affectivity and will to the rank of authentic.

Let us make a final note on the hermit spirit. The contemplative retreat is not a starting from scratch, because it assumes a fundamental premise, where objectivity and subjectivity sink their deepest roots and become indistinguishable: the experience of awakening. Dreyfus and Taylor call it a *transitional grasp on reality*:

> [T]ake the banal case of dreaming. We wake up, and it is this which assures us that we are really there, in contact with reality. A similar point was made by Plato in relation to the dialectic. You know you're there-in contact with the really real-because you've climbed there out of error. [78]

This awakening, or the search for the exit doors to life merely dreamed of, constitutes, for the moment in a merely formal way, the basis of the TTH: humanism, insofar as it defends the idea of truth and nature; technological, to emphasize that technology has reached levels of possibility capable of being exploited in a way never before dreamed of, but, above all, which may represent the greatest risk ever taken against the human species. The structural addiction and moralism we suffer today are the main signs of this risk. Those who have the strength to escape from them and also resist the inclemencies of the desert will be the ones who will return to offer us the best proposals that will give content to the future of authentic and fruitful humanism. These new men, *true overmen* (der echter übermensch) will offer us the criteria to know what to delegate to AI and what not, or how and in what to cultivate memory, imagination, inquiry, and reflection in a world in which they will not be necessary or useful [73]. It will depend on these men that the future may be less perfect, but, to paraphrase Huxley, freer, without preference for persons or nations, and more beautiful—beauty that only shines in the presence and warmth of love.

Acknowledgments We wish to acknowledge the CIMA Project "Non-invasive diagnosis of cancer patients using artificial intelligence applied to the analysis of circulating tumor cells in blood (DeepCTC)" for continued collaboration and support.

References

1. Huxley A. Brave new world and brave new world revisited. Toronto: Vintage Canada; 2007.
2. Huxley A. Brave new world. New York: Harper Perennial; 1989a.
3. Nestler EJ. Molecular basis of long-term plasticity underlying addiction. Nat Rev Neurosci. 2001;2:119–28.

4. Fuehrlein BS, Ross DA. Opioid use disorder: a desperate need for novel treatments. Biol Psychiatry. 2017;81:e43–e5.
5. Zilverstand A, Parvaz MA, Moeller SJ, Goldstein RZ. Cognitive interventions for addiction medicine: understanding the underlying neurobiological mechanisms. Prog Brain Res. 2016;224:285–304.
6. Mellentin AI, Skot L, Nielsen B, Schippers GM, Nielsen AS, Stenager E, et al. Cue exposure therapy for the treatment of alcohol use disorders: a meta-analytic review. Clin Psychol Rev. 2017;57:195–207.
7. Liu J-F, Li J-X. Drug addiction: a curable mental disorder? Acta Pharmacol Sin. 2018;39(12):1823–9.
8. Nelson LF, Weitzman ER, Levy S. Prevention of substance use disorders. Med Clin North Am. 2022;106(1):153–68.
9. Guajardo HS, Bagladi VL, Kushner DL. Integrative psychotherapy in addictive disorders. J Psychother Integr. 2004;14(3):290–306.
10. Woody GE. Research findings on psychotherapy of addictive disorders. Am J Addict. 2003;12(2):S19–26.
11. Rosendahl J, Alldredge CT, Gary MS, Burlingame M, Strauss B. Recent developments in group psychotherapy research. Am J Psychother. 2021;74(2):52–9.
12. Flores PJ, Mahon L. The treatment of addiction in group psychotherapy. Int J Group Psychother. 1993;43(2):143–56.
13. Frankl V. Psychotherapy and existentialism: selected papers on logotherapy. New York: Simon & Schuster; 1967.
14. Plato. Laches and Charmides. Indianapolis: Hackett; 1992.
15. Gorgias. Encomium on Helen. In: Freeman K, editor. Ancilla to the pre-socratic philosophers. Cambridge: Harvard University Press; 1948. p. 131–3.
16. Guidano V. The self in process: toward a post-rationalist cognitive therapy. New York: The Guilford Press; 1991.
17. Foucault M. Interview given to Le Monde on July 22, 1961.
18. Erikson E. Young man Luther: a study in psychoanalysis and history. New York: Norton; 1962.
19. Habermas J. The future of human nature. Cambridge: Polity Press; 2001.
20. Elias N. The loneliness of the dying. New York: Continuum; 2001.
21. Rorty R. Objectivity, relativism and truth: philosophical papers. Cambridge: Cambridge University Press; 1991.
22. Muñoz LF, Jaramillo LE. DSM-5: significant changes? Rev Asoc Esp Neuropsiquiatr. 2015;35(125):111–21.
23. Ortega y Gasset J. The revolt of the masses. London: George Allen & Unwin LTD; 1932.
24. Derrida J. Comment ne pas parler. Dénégations. In: Psyché. Inventions de l'autre. París: Galilée; 1987. p. 535–95.
25. Alexander BK. Replacing the official view of addiction. In: Davis JE, Gonzalez AM, editors. To fix of to heal. Patient care, public health, and the limits of biomedicine. New York: New York University Press; 2016. p. 208–37.
26. Ortega y Gasset J. Ideas y creencias. Madrid: Revista de Occidente; 1942.
27. Huxley A. Science, liberty and peace. London Chatto & Windus; 1950.
28. Goethe JW. Faust. Princeton: Princeton University Press; 1994.
29. Teixeira da Silva JA. How to shape academic freedom in the digital age? Are the retractions of opinionated papers a prelude to "cancel culture" in academia? Curr Res Behav Sci. 2021;2:100035.
30. MacIntyre A. After virtue. A study in moral theory. Notre Dame: University of Notre Dame Press; 2007.
31. Han B-C. The disappearance of rituals. Medford: Polity Press; 2020.
32. Huxley A. Huxley and god: essays. San Francisco: Harper; 1992.
33. Huxley A. The perennial philosophy. London: Chatto & Windus; 1947.
34. Hölderlin F. Hyperion, or the Hermit in Greece. Cambridge: Openbook Publishers; 2019.
35. Dreher R. The Benedict option: a strategy for Christians in a post-Christian nation. New York: Sentinel; 2017.
36. Dreher R. Benedict option FAQ. A guide for the perplexed and the curious. The American Conservative, 6 Oct, 2015. Website accessed 15 Dec 2022. https://www.theamericanconservative.com/benedict-option-faq/.
37. Taylor A. A Catholic modernity? In: Heft JL, editor. A Catholic modernity? Charles Taylor's Marianist Award Lecture, with responses by William M. Shea, Rosemary Luling Haughton, George Marsden, and jean Bethke Elshtain. Oxford: Oxford University Press; 1999. p. 13–37.
38. Taylor. The sources of the self. The making of modern identity. Cambridge: Harvard University Press; 1989.
39. Driessen MD. Beyond the Benedict option: how Christians can engage while being countercultural. In America. The Jesuit Review, February 11, 2016.
40. Aranda Vargas JP. Review of 'the Benedict option'. Metaphys Person Philos Knowl Life. 2020;12(23):175–8.
41. Huxley A. Island. London: Chatto & Windus; 1989b.
42. Gargiulo PA. *Sobre la Desesperanza y otros escritos psicológicos. Ensayo*. Saarbrücken: Editorial Académica Española/AV Akademiker Verlag Gmbh & Co. K.G./Editado en Alemania y España; 2012.
43. Gargiulo PA. The phenomenological method as an opening to psychopathology and psychotherapy (El método fenomenológico como apertura a la psicopatología y a la psicoterapia). Acta Psiquiatr Psicol Am Lat. 2018;64(4):273–86.
44. Gargiulo PA. Phenomenological analysis of a psychedelic experience: an approach to Huxley's study *The doors of perception* (Part 1) (Análisis fenomenológico de una experiencia psicodélica: Una aproximación a la obra de Huxley *Las puertas de la Percepción*. Parte 1). Acta Psiquiatr Psicol Am Lat. 2020;66(1):49–58.
45. Gargiulo PA. Phenomenological analysis of a psychedelic experience: an approach to Huxley's study *The doors of perception* (Part 2) (Análisis fenomenológico

de una experiencia psicodélica: Una aproximación a la obra de Huxley *Las puertas de la Percepción*. Parte 2). Acta Psiquiatr Psicol Am Lat. 2020;66(2):140–8.
46. Huxley A. *Las puertas de la percepción*. Tercera Edición. Buenos Aires: Editorial Sudamericana. 1962.
47. Conrad K. Die beginnende Schizophrenie, Versuch einer Gestaltsanalyse des Wahnsinns [Incipient schizophrenia: an attempt at a gestaltic analysis of insanity]. Stuttgart: Thieme; 1966.
48. Grace AA. Gating of information flow within the limbic system and the pathophysiology of schizophrenia. Brain Res Brain Res Rev. 2000;31(2–3):330–41.
49. Goto Y, Grace AA. The dopamine system and the pathophysiology of schizophrenia: a basic science perspective. Int Rev Neurobiol. 2007;78(06):41–68.
50. Kelley AE, Andrzejewski ME, Baldwin AE, Hernandez PJ, Pratt WE. Glutamate-mediated plasticity in corticostriatal networks: role in adaptive motor learning. Ann N Y Acad Sci. 2003;1003:159–68.
51. Qin Y, Mahdavi A, Bertschy M, Anderson PM, Kulikova S, Pinault D. The psychotomimetic ketamine disrupts the transfer of late sensory information in the corticothalamic network. Eur J Neurosci. 2023;57(3):440–55.
52. Gargiulo PA, Siemann M, Delius JD. Visual discrimination in pigeons impaired by glutamatergic blockade of nucleus accumbens. Physiol Behav. 1998;63(4):705–9.
53. Gargiulo PA, Landa De Gargiulo AI. Glutamate and modeling of schizophrenia symptoms: review of our findings: 1990-2014. Pharmacol Rep. 2014;66(3):343–52.
54. Del Vecchio S, Gargiulo PA. Objetivación de la función visomotriz en la esquizofrenia [Visual and motor functions in schizophrenic patients]. Acta Psiquiatr Psicol Am Lat. 1992;38(4):317–22.
55. Acerbo MJ, Gargiulo PA, Krug I, Delius JD. Behavioural consequences of nucleus accumbens dopaminergic stimulation and glutamatergic blocking in pigeons. Behav Brain Res. 2002;136(1):171–7.
56. Gargiulo PA, Acerbo MJ, Krug I, Delius JD. Cognitive effects of dopaminergic and glutamatergic blockade in nucleus accumbens in pigeons. Pharmacol Biochem Behav. 2005;81(4):732–9.
57. Gargiulo PA, Martínez G, Ropero C, Funes A, Landa AI. NMDA glutamatergic blockade of nucleus accumbens disrupts acquisition but not consolidation in a passive avoidance task. Ann N Y Acad Sci. 1999;877:717–22.
58. Martínez G, Ropero C, Funes A, Flores E, Landa AI, Gargiulo PA. AP-7 into the nucleus accumbens disrupts acquisition but does not affect consolidation in a passive avoidance task. Physiol Behav. 2002;76(2):205–12.
59. Martínez G, Ropero C, Funes A, Flores E, Blotta C, Landa AI, Gargiulo PA. Effects of selective NMDA and non-NMDA blockade in the nucleus accumbens on the plus-maze test. Physiol Behav. 2002;76(2):219–24.
60. Baiardi G, Ruiz AM, Beling A, Borgonovo J, Martínez G, Landa AI, Sosa MA, Gargiulo PA. Glutamatergic ionotropic blockade within accumbens disrupts working memory and might alter the endocytic machinery in rat accumbens and prefrontal cortex. J Neural Transm (Vienna). 2007;114(12):1519–28.
61. Lindsley CW, Shipe WD, Wolkenberg SE, Theberge CR, Williams DL Jr, Sur C, Kinney GG. Progress towards validating the NMDA receptor hypofunction hypothesis of schizophrenia. Curr Top Med Chem. 2006;6(8):771–85.
62. Howes O, McCutcheon R, Stone J. Glutamate and dopamine in schizophrenia: an update for the 21st century. J Psychopharmacol. 2015;29(2):97–115.
63. Pankow A, Katthagen T, Diner S, Deserno L, Boehme R, Kathmann N, Gleich T, Gaebler M, Walter H, Heinz A, Schlagenhauf F. Aberrant salience is related to dysfunctional self-referential processing in psychosis. Schizophr Bull. 2016;42(1):67–76.
64. Kapur S. Psychosis as a state of aberrant salience: a framework linking biology, phenomenology, and pharmacology in schizophrenia. Am J Psychiatry. 2003;160(1):13–23.
65. Miyata J. Toward integrated understanding of salience in psychosis. Neurobiol Dis. 2019;131:104414.
66. Skinner BF. About behaviorism. Oxford: Alfred A. Knopf; 1974.
67. Schultz W. Predictive reward signal of dopamine neurons. J Neurophysiol. 1998;80(1):1–27.
68. Schultz W. Behavioral theories and the neurophysiology of reward. Annu Rev Psychol. 2006;57:87–115.
69. Galvanho JP, Manhães AC, Carvalho-Nogueira ACC, Silva JM, Filgueiras CC, Abreu-Villaça Y. Profiling of behavioral effects evoked by ketamine and the role of $5HT_2$ and D_2 receptors in ketamine-induced locomotor sensitization in mice. Prog Neuro-Psychopharmacol Biol Psychiatry. 2020;97:109775.
70. Vamvakopoulou IA, Narine KAD, Campbell I, Dyck JRB, Nutt DJ. Mescaline: the forgotten psychedelic. Neuropharmacology. 2023;222:109294.
71. Cresta P, Carusso M, Alemany LA, Acion L. Practical foundations of machine learning for addiction research. Part I. Methods and techniques. Am J Drug Alcohol Abuse. 2022;48(3):260–71.
72. Nietzsche F. Thus spoke Zarathustra. New York: Penguin Books; 1966.
73. Echarte LE. Biotecnología para la mejora moral. Más allá de la estética crepuscular del último hombre. Bioética y Ciencias de la Salud. 2022;10(1):1–47.
74. Echarte LE. Rehabilitar la subjetividad en el diálogo interdisciplinar. La solución de Aldous Huxley al problema de las dos culturas. Philosophia. 2020;80(1):107–60.
75. Echarte L, Bernácer J, Larrivee D, Oron JV, Grijalba-Uche M. Self-deception in terminal patients: belief system at stake. Front Psychol. 2016;7:1–6.
76. Wells HG. A vision of judgment. In: Complete short stories. London: Phoenix Giant; 1999.
77. Dreyfus HL. Alchemy and artificial intelligence. RAND Report (Rand Corp); 1965. p. 3244.
78. Dreyfus H, Taylor C. Retrieving realism. Cambridge: Harvard University Press; 2015.

Thoughts on the Meaning of Life

4

Miriam Dolly Arancibia

> A failed life is a wounded and scattered existence, which has lost the north and the hope of recovering it. (Alejandro Llano)

Introduction

Addictions cause dependencies that in most cases lead to death. Among the multiple causes of addiction is the absence of a deep sense of one's own life. Anguish, pain, and depression act as fatal ingredients in that progressive surrender to death. Society watches undaunted by the loss of many young, and not so young, to such a fate. The impotence of the person is immeasurable against this scourge.

Thoughts expressed by Alejandro Llano [1] in his work *The achieved life* (*La vida lograda*) express a clear parallel with the problem of addictions. "The root of the matter is that I have turned against myself and struck blindly and without any consideration, although it was probably with little voluntariness, driven more by weakness than by malice."

This reality demands to reflect on the meaning of life, of the vital horizon that, although diluted in gloom, exists and requires personal effort to glimpse it with clarity.

In his work, *The palliative society* (*La sociedad paliativa*) Byung Chul Han [2] refers to a deeply human quote from Walter Benjamin. "Of all the bodily sensations, pain is the only one that represents for man a kind of navigable current whose flow never dries up and leads him to the sea. Whenever man tries to abandon himself to pleasure, this turns out to be a dead end."

Human beings naturally tend to look for pleasurable situations and avoid those that cause pain. However, in times centered on hedonism, some people attempt to eliminate pain even in the wrong ways.

Byung Chul Han [2, p. 11] affirms that if we let only medicine deal with pain, its character as a sign-in code escapes. These words contain an interpellation of all as pain is everyone's problem. Han argues that all social criticism has to develop its own hermeneutic of pain. In addition, he calls "algophobia" the phobia of the prevailing pain, that is, a generalized fear of suffering. Algophobia leads to permanent anesthesia; it is about avoiding any painful state. This algophobia is based on a paradigm shift, so you live in a society of positivity that tries to get rid of all forms of negativity. It is about avoiding negative thoughts and replacing them immediately with positive ideas [2, p. 13].

He has coined the concept of palliative society provoked by the neoliberal ideology of resilience. His position is critical of neoliberalism and capi-

M. D. Arancibia (✉)
Cátedra de Filosofía Social, Departamento de Sociología, Facultad de Ciencias Sociales, Universidad Nacional de San Juan, San Juan, Argentina; http://www.linkedin.com/pub/miriam-dolly-arancibia-de-calmels/90/101/565

P. Á. Gargiulo, H. L. Mesones-Arroyo (eds.), *Psychiatry and Neuroscience Update – Vol. V*,
https://doi.org/10.1007/978-3-031-72219-6_4

talism. However, beyond the political position of this author, the interesting thing about his reflections is his sense of opportunity. Those come at opportune times. In 2019 he published *The disappearance of rituals* (*La desaparición de los rituales*) [3], a book in which he seemed to glimpse the situation of isolation triggered by the pandemic, caused by the SARS 2 virus in the last 2 years. In October 2021, he published *No-things* (*No-cosas*) [4] a book in which he opposes the excesses of technology, against those who promote Metaverso as a new chapter of the internet. In this way, also in his book *The palliative society (La sociedad paliativa)* [2] there are reflections worthy of consideration, beyond the political position or background that sustains them. In brief, Byung Chul Han's reflections are a timely invitation to think about current existential issues.

Thus, it is possible to agree with Han [2, p. 19] when he argues that pain is a complex cultural configuration. Nevertheless, there is no agreement with Han when he argues that the new formula of domination is "be happy" considering the positivity of happiness as the product of a neoliberal device. According to Han [2, p. 23], as positive emotional capital, happiness should provide an interrupted capacity for performance; so self-motivation and self-optimization make the neoliberal device of happiness very effective. He also sustains that the imperative to be happy generates pressure that is more devastating than the imperative to be obedient.

Therefore, the invitation, or the challenge, is there. The attitude one has in the face of pain and the way in which happiness is conceived mark the way in the search for vital meaning. The objective of this chapter is to show existing paths for a deep reflection, and at the same time, to awaken the concern of finding a personal response to one's own vital sense.

Hermeneutic of Pain

Leonardo Polo [5] argues that there is no idea of pain, it is something unintelligible, it is something very radical. "We have pain, we feel it, we suffer or we endure; what we can't do about is thinking about it" [5, p. 207]. Contrary to what the human being does with his sensations, that is, with the material of ideas, and even what he does with his emotions and moods, he cannot do the same with pain. You have an awareness of pain, but you have no "entity of reason." There is a concept of pain as there is a concept of nothingness, but in both cases, there is no corresponding extra-mental content. "The agent intellect does not illuminate the pain, which is there, by thinking, inscrutable, as a strange exception to ideal clarity" [5, p. 208]. Pain is not outside of thought as a kind of Kantian thing itself that thought does not reach, but to which it could reach.

What then can we say about pain? The question of its essence is impossible. Nor can we answer from the scientific field. The biologist will be able to tell how the painful stimulus is produced in the periphery of the body and how it is transmitted to your brain, but it will say nothing of human pain. Faced with this question, the mind remains without strength and without resources. "Man can flee it, bypass it, overcome it, free itself from it, and heal it. What he can't do is cultivate it in himself, think about it and love it" [5, p. 209].

Since the direct question is impossible, we must pose the question indirectly; that is, the human sense of pain is what pain means to man. Thus posing the question, we arrive at a hermeneutic of pain: how have human beings understood that pain plays?

The Greek attitude toward pain was inside of the idea of destiny, to which man is surrendered and thus depersonalized, given over to the game of impersonal forces. The biography of the human being is a concrete case of universal destiny and the human being is a piece of the cosmos. Hence, pain is also an insurmountable obstacle. The human being, unable to sustain himself in the face of pain, assumes destiny. "Suffering awakens the human, makes its great richness of meaning resonate. But, the end result is a limit, an impotence" [5, p. 221]. According to Greek culture, in the face of pain man settles in his nature, in his substance.

Thus, the question arises: is pain something accidental or something substantial for man?

Leonardo Polo [5] answers that pain is not something accidental because the advent of pain is not something similar to that of a property of nature, nor to that of a cultural object or of any historical event. It is not something that adds to the human being. However, pain is not a substance either. Although its persistence and deep rootedness lead us to think that pain belongs to the same human condition, the substantial cannot be pain or vice versa. The notion of substance expresses an intimate solid and well-compact consistency that is incompatible with the crisis or rupture itself in pain. "That your own substance hurts would be equivalent to being corrupted, that is, to this positive sense of reality ceasing to be" [5, p. 227].

Thus, pain is not a reality abstracted from man, nor is it a primary constitutive of the human being. Pain is an appearance in the human being. "The depth of the installation of pain in our own being demands that man make room for it" [5, p. 228]. There is no pain without a mourner. These are not corresponding terms as object and subject, but the mourner is the metaphysical condition of the possibility of human pain, so there is no abstract pain or itself.

Pain settles in, and is inserted into our being, in the sense that pain is not even possible without that insertion. Unlike other realities in which essence and existence can be distinguished, pain is constituted as such insofar as installed in the human being.

The Christian sense of pain, pain as a task, is a mystical, interior, trans-psychological sense. No subjectivism can decipher it, since pain, as a task is the work of destruction of every particular self—mystical death of the self [5, p. 253].

Job's attitude is paradigmatic of the Christian sense of pain because it represents the "triumph over pain achieved by a fundamental conviction, or faith, in the absolute Transcendence of Being" [5, p. 223]. We do not experience pain as an insurmountable situation because human life is anchored in faith in God. "That is why, when pain appears, and shows the true condition of man, his smallness, his fragility and insecurity, such a discovery is not condensed into a definitive judgment, it does not found a pessimistic conclusion as the last result and definitive meaning of existence. God is deeper than I am to me. This is the result of the book of Job" [5, pp. 223–224].

Pain is not an abstract reality, but appears in the human being. It is worth noting the strength that acquires in a hermeneutic of pain the feature of the human person conceived from the transcendental anthropology of Leonardo Polo.

Polo [5] affirms that human personal love, as a reflection of Uncreated Love, is a fundamental foundation and primordial act. Therefore, it is a real condition of the integrity of any human operation. Hence, two moments correspond to him in the person's response to the so-called creator, that is, to the realization of his destiny: discovery of the ideal and realization of that ideal.

The ideal is to overcome knowledge by arriving at things as they come from the First Cause. Love places reality beyond all horizons. "Man can love things in themselves, but not by themselves; the motive of personal love is absolutized" [5, p. 229]. Like Plato, Polo understands that love is the eagerness to beget in beauty. This begetting is the production of acts in which the human being is faithful to his being, and in them, he realizes the ideal. "Thus, *ordo amoris* is *ordo realis*" [5, p. 230].

Another trait pointed out by transcendental anthropology is that the person is the giving being (*ser donal*) and as such, man is both in himself and in the relationship: he coexists. The breakdown of the activity of giving is the condition and root of pain, which thus becomes a rupture of the series of affection—love. The breakdown of the personal being is like a cracking by whose fractures a waterlogging occurs. Nevertheless, it is not the breaking of a block, of a substance, but of an act, that translates its decrease into pain. Pain as such is a personal situation, it is not only a particular sensation, and hence only sin (break of the *ordo amoris*) is pain as such [5, p. 231].

As for the Christian attitude toward pain, Polo refers to the theological conception of the human person. "The first thing that happens in the Christian in order to pain is the rebirth, the reopening of his integral being, obstructed by pain" [5, p. 251]. This happens in baptism and penance. In this way, the pain dissolves.

Modern idealist philosophy directs the problem toward egocentrism since it centers the constitution of philosophical systems on the subject. Polo considers that pain is a refutation of that philosophy because "there is no determinable human subject capable of giving reason for the pain" [5, p. 254].

The acceptance of the Cross, exalted by the Christian attitude to pain, is subverted in modern philosophy. The anthropological consequences were very significant. Juan Fernando Sellés [6, p. 111] considers that, in modern philosophy, man was regarded as a foundation. The seat of self-foundation found its place in reason. According to this view, it will no longer be necessary to turn to God or other people to describe man.

The subjectivism characteristic of modern philosophy leaves traces for the contemporary attitude to pain. Then, it is not surprising that the terms with which Byung Chul Han [2] describes the current situation are those of "palliative society." In this type of society, evasion and denial are some of the numerous mechanisms that the human being uses in the face of painful situations. On the other hand, such mechanisms do not emerge in isolation or individually, but in society as a whole.

From the perspective of psychopolitics, Han [2, p. 14], argues that a palliative society coincides with the society of performance. Pain is interpreted as a symptom of weakness, it is necessary to hide it or eliminate it by optimizing it. The palliative society is a society of "I like" and the human being is the victim of a delirium for complacency.

The "like" is the sign and the painkiller of the present. "Nothing should hurt" [2, p. 14]. Life itself has to be able to be uploaded to Instagram, it must lack painful conflicts and contradictions. This culture of complacency lacks the possibility of catharsis.

The palliative society is immunized against criticism by desensitizing through medicines or inducing a dullness with the help of the media. Social media and computer games act as anesthetics. "The permanent social anesthesia prevents knowledge and reflection and represses the truth" [2, p. 25]. It is a society of survival, "the virus is the mirror of our society. It reflects the society we live in. Today survival is absolutized, as if we were in a permanent state of war" [2, p. 29]. The fight against the pandemic shows a viral radicalization; all forces were used to prolong life. However, the more life is reduced to a mere survival; the more afraid one is of dying [2, p. 29]. Algophobia becomes a thanatophobia. The pervasiveness of death in the mass media makes people nervous.

In this way, the society of survival loses all the ability to value the good life. Moreover, we had forgotten that human life is marked by uncertainty and risk. The human being is fragile, a cane that thinks, as Pascal said [1, p. 22]. According to Alejandro Llanos [1, p. 23], the fullness of life is achieved by those women and men who have become a task for themselves, who are authors of their lives, who did not cease in the inquiry to decipher the enigmas of existence.

On the contrary, those people who succumbed to thanatophobia sacrificed to survive everything that makes life worth living. Depression does not occur in a society defined by rituals. However, the soul that succumbs to thanatophobia is absorbed, emptied of rituals. Those rituals are what contain the world; they essentially are symbolic practices of installation in a home [3, p. 27]. However, in a palliative society, those symbols also vanished, narratives or rituals that made life more than survival. "Life is it stripped of any narrative that gives it meaning. It is no longer what can be narrated, but what can be measured and countable" [3, p. 31].

In the palliative society, there are no referential senses that provide support and guidance in situations of pain. If these referential senses become then meaningless, we must fight with analgesics [2, p. 35]. The sense of pain presupposes a narrative that integrates life into a horizon of meaning, and this occurs because life itself was reduced to a biological process becoming empty of meaning [2, p. 39].

The palliative society compulsively flees from the negative. Unlike pain, health is not dialectical, therefore, the palliative society that declares it the supreme value, is imprisoned in a hell of the same. It lacks the dialectical force of transformation [2, p. 64].

Only thanks to pain, argues Han [2, p. 61], the spirit attains a new knowledge, a higher form of knowledge and consciousness. Following Hegel, Han affirms that what characterizes the spirit is the ability to remain in contradiction, and therefore of pain. The spirit overcomes the painful contradiction by developing into a higher form; thus, pain is the engine of the dialectical formation of the spirit, and pain transforms it.

Happiness

The most beautiful pages written in the history of philosophy are perhaps those found in book X of the *Nicomachean Ethics*, in which Aristotle [7] discusses happiness.

After virtues, friendship, and pleasure, Aristotle outlines what happiness is. "Every art and every inquiry, as well as every action and choice, pursues a good" [7, EN 1094ª]. According to Aristotle, there is a common agreement to call this good "happiness". Most believe that living well and succeeding are the same as being happy [7, EN, 1095, 15–20]. However, the disagreement lies in what happiness means.

Aristotle says that happiness is not a habitual state; it is a certain type of activity. Among the activities, one distinguishes those necessary, that those chosen by another, and that those chosen by themselves. Clearly, happiness must be among the activities chosen by themselves and not by anything else, because they have no need of anything, that is, they are self-sufficient [7, EN 1176b]. Such are the actions according to virtue. So for example, beautiful and noble actions are something chosen by itself.

Now, what is the source of happiness? The mass considers that good and happiness consist of pleasure which is why they love the dissolute life [7, EN1095b15]. However, Aristotle clarifies, in EN1095b20 that in this way the mass shows similarity with slaves because it prefers an animal life [7, EN1095b20].

On the other hand, refined people identify happiness with honor. Nevertheless, it is evident to Aristotle that this objective is too superficial. Honor resides above all in those who pay honor rather than in those who are honored. On the contrary, the ultimate good or happiness must be something personal and difficult to lose [7, EN1095b20]. Wealth is also not good, nor is happiness itself; it is only a useful instrument serving a purpose other than itself [7, EN1096a5].

Human beings, as humans, should not limit themselves to thinking human things, nor as mortals, limit themselves to thinking mortal things. They must turn to immortality as far as possible, and do everything to live according to the better part that is in us. This is life according to the intellect, since that is what the human being mainly consist of. Consequently, this will be the happiest life [7, EN1178a]. Regarding the virtues, it is not enough just to know them, but to possess them and put them into practice, they are acquired by exercise, and this is the way to become good [7, EN 118b20].

On this point, Leonardo Polo [5, p. 168] adds that virtue is the edge of the soul, as the act of the axe is the edge. Virtue is that by which the soul acts as such. It is what humanizes the individual because it is what comes from him. As an action, it is also in accordance with his essence. In this way, Polo considers that many aspects of the traditional are recovered, such as courage and self-control [8, p. 103].

The *areté* is the good life, happiness is better than the good life since it bets on being faithful to the condition of being human. The soul, owner of itself, also owns its actions and in this way is an end for itself, that is, free to achieve happiness. On the contrary, he who has no virtue is in an unhappy condition, is a slave to his passions, is carried away by opinion and is greedy for fame and riches [5, p. 169; 9, p. 128].

Giovanni Reale [10, p. 106] synthesizes the Aristotelian conception: happiness derives from the contemplation of truth, the fruit of the highest level of knowledge, which constitutes that type of life that, to a supreme and perfect degree, belongs to God.

From a phenomenological approach, Wojtyła [11, p. 200] argues that it is necessary to look for the sphere of the state of happiness in that which is internal and intransitive in the act, in that which identifies with the realization of oneself as a person.

Such self-realization is constituted through a series of aspects among which truth and freedom stand out. The realization of the person in the act depends on the active and inwardly creative union of truth with freedom. This union generates a state of happiness. Freedom alone does not seem to be a generator of happiness. The action of freedom in truth is what amounts to the realization of the person [11, p. 201].

Now, it is possible to distinguish, from this phenomenological perspective, the dimension of the person, unique and unrepeatable, before the network of interpersonal and social relationships, from the entire multidirectional system of relations with the world. All these relationships have meaning for man's happiness. A particular and essential meaning possesses the reference to other people. The intrapersonal perspective of the state of happiness is essential and fundamental [11, p. 201].

According to Wojtyła [11, p. 202], if in the inquiry into happiness man somehow goes out of his own way, the very fact of such inquiry indicates the particular correlation that exists between the state of happiness and his own person. It is necessary to look for the basis of this correlation in the person himself, in whose constitutive properties, freedom and truth, that is, the dynamic relationship, rooted in the intellect, with the truth in knowledge and actions.

The state of happiness thus shows a particular fulfillment toward the person, in relation to his structure of self-possession and self-control. One can speak of the specific structure of the state of happiness as a personal structure, that is, it does not exist and does not make sense outside the person or without it [11, p. 201].

The state of happiness is linked exclusively to the person, to his particular and unrepeatable structure in the world of nature. Only in this structure, the realization of the self occurs through the act. On the other hand, the state of happiness is not pleasure. When the human being acts, it contains in himself/herself not only the fulfillment of the act on the foundation of self-determination but also contains the realization of the person on the same foundation; self-determination is always a concrete realization of freedom [11, p. 203].

Between the state of happiness and pleasure, there is not only a difference in degree but rather in depth. Pleasure is more superficial, while the state of happiness is something deeper in the human being. In the fulfillment of the act, and the personal fulfillment of oneself through the act, corresponds the state of happiness as something very specific, something that cannot be broken down into the pleasure–displeasure elements and reduced to them. This specificity and irreducibility of the state of happiness remain in close union with the transcendence of the person [11, p. 204].

The term transcendence means etymologically to cross a certain threshold or a certain limit, *tras-scender*. This overcoming of the limit of the subject happens on the one hand in the cognitive acts, on the other hand, in the will that has the character of a tendency. Crossing the boundary of the subject to the object, i.e., intentionality, is what Wojtyła calls horizontal transcendence. The transcendence that we owe to self-determination, transcendence by the very fact of freedom, of free beings in action, and not only by the fact that the will is intentionally directed toward its own object, as a value-end. This is vertical transcendence [11, p. 145].

To the notion of virtue according to Aristotle, who began this section, we added the notions of truth, freedom, and transcendence. This shows the profound scope that the notion of happiness acquires when you delve into it.

Regarding the term transcendental, Leonardo Polo's proposal focuses on an extension of the transcendental ones because the traditional philosophy offers to be continued [12, p. 13]. He distinguishes between metaphysical transcendentals and personal transcendentals [12, p. 22]. Such a distinction allows for the necessary distinction between metaphysics and anthropology.

To open this new transcendental field, it is necessary to resort to the method called abandonment of the mental limit. Mental operations are inferior cognitive acts; therefore, what one knows is necessarily limited. We detect this limitation from intellectual habits, which are the cognitive acts superior to operations.

If we take into account the limitation of the object, we notice the transobjective theme when leaving the mental limit; if we detect the limitation of the operation, we reach the transoperative theme. The first corresponds to metaphysics and the second to anthropology [12, p. 23].

The transcendental according to the transcendental doctrine is distinguished into absolute transcendental (the entity, the one, and the thing) and relative transcendental (truth, good, and beauty). According to Polo, it is necessary to add the transcendental ones: the act of being co-existential, freedom, intellect, and *donal* love.

In this way, the discourse on happiness reaches a central point in all consideration of the human being: love, which in Polyan terms is *donal* love. It is a fundamental life experience of one's own acceptance as well as the acceptance of others. "A completely lonely capacity to love would be absolute tragedy…. If others are not dignified, then I am a meaningless being…." [8, p. 116].

Thus, from the perspective of transcendental anthropology, pain and happiness acquire a new dimension in order to give solid support to the personal definition of the meaning of life.

Conclusion

The task in the search for the vital sense requires a pause in everyday life. It implies stopping and asking yourself about the why and for what of the acceleration, frivolity, and violence that society projects. In the age of hyper-digitization, human beings find themselves increasingly isolated because they live more hastily in the endless race to satisfy social standards.

Since the beginning of time, human beings have expressed the desire and need for transcendence. In artistic manifestations (from cave paintings), in mythological explanations of reality, in philosophical arguments, and even in art and current technology. Artificial Intelligence and Metaverse are different ways of expressing the same desire: that of immortality and to live beyond the limits imposed by our mortal condition. Procreating according to the body or according to the soul, as Socrates said, allows us to leave something of ourselves to future generations. This desire for immortality, to transcend, carries implicitly a conception of a happy life because what we search is, finally, to achieve absolute happiness free of all disturbance.

The cold sensation of emptiness invades the person, who is immersed in social mandates, and loses his way toward vital horizons that allow him to rise above the fragility of the substitute and transient. "The society of transparency not only lacks truth, but also appearance. Neither truth nor appearance are so *apparent*. Only the vacuum is completely transparent" [13, p. 79].

On the other hand, personal love and acceptance offer a firm point on which to lean. "To hold that a person is to give emphasizes love. It is said that loving is transcendental or that it becomes with the personal being, because the highest sense of being is to give" [12, p. 211]. From this perspective, those positions that conceive the pursuit of happiness as the product of a political theory or a system of government are weakened.

It is evident that this search for happiness goes beyond such theories or systems. A system of government may impose limitations on the paths to happiness, but it cannot determine the person because he is essentially free.

Despite the compulsive messages of the mass media, neither success nor material abundance provides happiness. The high suicide rates from countries that sadly boast as the most prosperous prove it.

References

1. Llano A. La vida lograda [The life achieved, The life accomplished]. Barcelona: Editorial Planeta; 2017.
2. Han B. La sociedad paliativa [The palliative society]. Buenos Aires: Herder; 2021.
3. Han B. La desaparición de los rituales [The disappearance of rituals]. Buenos Aires: Herder; 2020.
4. Han B. La No-cosas [Non-stuff, not things]. Buenos Aires: Herder; 2021.
5. Polo L. La persona humana y su crecimiento [The human person and his growth]. Pamplona: EUNSA; 1999.

6. Sellés J. Antropología para inconformes [Anthropology for nonconformists]. Pamplona: Instituto de Ciencias para la Familia, Universidad de Navarra; 2006.
7. Aristóteles. Etica Nicomachea [Nicomachean ethics]. Bari: Editori Laterza; 1999.
8. Polo L. La originalidad de la concepción cristiana de la existencia [The originality of the Christian conception of existence]. Pamplona: EUNSA; 2010.
9. Polo L. Quien es el hombre [Who is the man]. Madrid: Ediciones RIALP; 2007.
10. Reale G. La sabiduría antigua [The ancient wisdom]. Barcelona: Herder; 1996.
11. Wojtyła K. Persona e Atto [Person and act]. Cittá del Vaticano: Libreria Editrice Vaticana; 1982.
12. Polo L. Antropología Trascendental [Transcendental Anthropology], Tomo I La persona humana. Pamplona: EUNSA; 2003.
13. Han B. La sociedad de la transparencia [The society of transparency]. Buenos Aires: Herder; 2013.

5 Relationship Between Meaning of Life and Permissiveness in Substance Using and Abusing Adolescents

Lucas Marcelo Rodriguez,
Santiago Alejandro Resett, and María José Zinoni

Introduction

Adolescence is an important stage of life with physical, social, and cognitive changes that extend from 11–12 years to 18–19 years [1, 2]. Therefore, adolescence is a fundamental stage of socio-moral development, where intellectual structures are consolidated [3, 4], as well as social interactions with others, such as assuming social conventions and consolidation of empathy [1, 5–8], mainly due to more complex cognitive development (hypothetical-deductive thinking, meta-cognition, future-oriented thinking, etc.), greater prominence of the peer group, such as experiencing new social roles, among other factors [1]. In this context, it is very important for social life to study moral judgment and character education. In addition, existential questions about the reason for living and the meaning of life begin in the context of the maturation of cognitive structures.

This chapter develops the relationship between the meaning of life and moral judgment (permissiveness and penalization) that adolescents make on substance use and abuse, particularly alcohol, cannabis, and cocaine. The empirical results show a higher meaning of life when it is a greater penalization of the consumption of alcohol, cannabis, and cocaine. In addition, there is a higher meaning of life in less-permissive adolescents to the consumption of cannabis. These results are reflected in the framework of current research and theories.

Current research shows that frequent cannabis users have a higher number of negative consequences than occasional users [9]; other studies show that substance abuse affects well-being and family functioning, as well as financial position, physical health, and psychological well-being [10]. For these reasons, the meaning of life in adolescents is considered to be of great importance in studying substance use and abuse.

Meaning of Life and Existential Emptiness

According to Viktor Frankl [11] meaning of life differs from one person to another, from day by day. It is not something abstract, each person should discover it by themselves and take upon their own mission to fulfill in life. Through the will to meaning, the person is referred to the

L. M. Rodriguez (✉) · S. A. Resett
Instituto de Filosofía - Facultad de Ciencias Biomédicas, Universidad Austral, Consejo nacional de investigaciones científicas y técnicas (CONICET), Pilar, Buenos Aires, Argentina

M. J. Zinoni
Centro de Investigación Interdisciplinar en Valores, Integración y Desarrollo Social, Pontificia Universidad Católica Argentina (UCA), Consejo nacional de investigaciones científicas y técnicas (CONICET), Paraná, Entre Ríos, Argentina

P. Á. Gargiulo, H. L. Mesones-Arroyo (eds.), *Psychiatry and Neuroscience Update – Vol. V*,
https://doi.org/10.1007/978-3-031-72219-6_5

search for meaning and its fulfillment, in the encounter with another person [12].

Frankl [11, 12] explained that people who do not find meaning in life experienced an existential void. It is mostly manifested in boredom. The great disease of our time is the lack of objectives, boredom, lack of meaning, and purpose. The will to meaning cannot be ordered, it is rather an intentional act that does not allow self-imposition. There must be an object offering in life for meaning to arise. The search for meaning is not a matter for an intellectual minority but of each individual and it is within everyone's reach. Frankl [11, 12] explains that the fundamental anthropological fact is that the human being always refers beyond himself, toward something that is not him, toward something or toward someone, and toward a meaning. Therefore, the human being realizes himself to the extent that he transcends himself.

The existential emptiness is another important concept developed by Viktor Frankl [11, 12] that refers not only to the lack of meaning but also to boredom with life. When a person does not have a reason to live, a meaning to give to his life, that existential emptiness manifests itself in different ways. The author explains that taking to the extreme, can end in suicide. One of the manifestations of existential emptiness is the desire for pleasure, which can be manifested in the use and abuse of substances [11, 12]. It is necessary to find a meaning of life and reason to live in order to face the existential emptiness through the will to meaning.

Numerous instruments have been developed to evaluate the meaning of life. One of the most used in the world and in Latin America is the Purpose in Life (PIL) [13, 14], which measures meaning of life versus existential emptiness. This instrument was adapted to Spanish by Gottfried [15]. The instrument has two parts, one of them is qualitative for clinical use and the other is quantitative. The quantitative part is made up of 20 items on a 7-option Likert scale. In this adapted version [15], three subscales were identified. (1) *Perception of meaning*. The person perceives progress in life through freedom and responsibility. (2) *Experience of meaning*, comprising the emotional experience a person has about his life and daily situations. (3) *Attitude toward death*. The person reflects on being born or not, as well as suicide and death (as an inevitable destiny).

Research has been carried out on the meaning of life using the intervention program "Youth in search of meaning." Indeed, Gottfried [16] found that, by the end of the intervention program, those adolescents who participated in it obtained higher scores in sense of life than those adolescents who were in the control group. In this case, the meaning of life was evaluated with the Purpose in Life.

Other research has been conducted on moral judgment and the meaning of life. Gómez and Barrio [17] found that those adolescents who scored higher in *perception of meaning*, *experience of meaning,* and *attitude toward death* (PIL), also scored higher in penalization of acts in general. These results show a positive relationship between penalization and the meaning of life. Gómez and Barrio [17] state that although adolescents with existential emptiness penalize risky, criminal, or morally controversial behaviors less seriously, there is no evidence to show that they apply this to the behavioral level. This is because they only measured moral judgment.

Adolescents' Substance Use

Risk behaviors increase in this stage of life, such as antisocial behavior, aggressiveness, and the consumption of toxic substances, among others [18]. This does not mean that these behaviors are caused by adolescence [2]. Research has also pointed out that there are three classes of risk factors for these types of problems. The psychological ones consist of certain personality characteristics that were already present before adolescence: impulsiveness, depression, and performance problems. Furthermore, those who tolerate deviation from norms are generally at greater risk. Interpersonal factors refer to belonging to conflictive or distant families; to excessively permissive, indifferent, or rejecting parents, and to homes in which toxic substances are used or their use is accepted. Likewise, there is a tendency to look for friends who use or tolerate them, which, in turn, favors greater consumption. Drug use is facilitated by any factors of the social context. First of all, the community norms about it; secondly the degree to which drug laws are enforced; and finally, the way drug use is portrayed in the media [2, 19].

It should be clarified that toxic substances can be divided into legal and illegal. The former substances are those whose production, sale, and consumption are not punishable by law, such as alcohol or tobacco, in contrast to cocaine and heroin. Also, it can be classified according to its effects: depressants, stimulants, and hallucinogens. The first slows down the functioning of the brain (such as alcohol), the second speeds up the functioning of the brain (such as cocaine), and the last alters the functioning of the brain, giving rise to hallucinations or distortions in perception (such as LSD). On the other hand, toxic substances can be classified according to their origin: natural, synthetic, and semi-synthetic [20].

Regarding how widespread this behavior is in adolescence, research carried out in first-world countries, such as the United States, indicates that almost all adolescents have tried alcohol and two-thirds have tried cigarettes [2]. In 2004, the Monitor the Future survey found that 48% of high school seniors said they had drunk alcohol at least once in the past month, whereas 33% of them said they had been intoxicated (having had five or more alcoholic drinks) not less than once in the previous 2 weeks. Cigarettes are the next most commonly used substance in adolescence. In 2004, 25% of high school seniors said they had smoked cigarettes at least once in the past 30 days. Cigarettes are followed in frequency by cannabis, which 20% of high school seniors said they had used in the previous month [21].

It should be clarified that the peak of the consumption of toxic substances does not occur at this stage of life, but rather in the next life cycle, called emerging adulthood, which extends from 18 years old to the entire third decade of life [1]. This is due to the fact that in emerging adulthood there is less parental supervision, greater autonomy, and financial independence, unlike in the previous stage.

In both adolescents and emerging adults, the sequence of the consumption of toxic substances should be highlighted. The sequence of consumption goes through four phases or stages [1]: (1) alcohol consumption (wine and/or beer), (2) tobacco use, (3) cannabis use, and (4) hard drug use (such as cocaine or LSD). Thus, beer, wine, cigarettes, and cannabis are called gateway drugs because most teens who try hard drugs have already passed through the "gates" of those substances [22].

Since it is almost daily consumption that affects behavior and health, it is an encouraging fact to know that only a small proportion of young people have serious problems of drug dependence (consuming them daily or using "hard" drugs). Despite being a period in this stage of life in which the consumption of toxic substances is exploratory or recreational, it does not imply that it should be minimized. Currently, the fact that experimentation with toxic substances begins at a younger age than previous generations, even in elementary school, is a disturbing sign. In Argentina, the consumption of toxic substances in adolescents is extremely widespread, which is a worrying fact. The SEDRONAR study [23] indicated that the prevalence of alcohol consumption in the last year was about 54% in adolescents from 12 to 17 years, 13% in tobacco, and 5% in cannabis. The data are alarming: half of adolescents tried alcohol in recent months; the percentage of cannabis use tripled, compared to previous studies; and the number of adolescents who have not considered consumption of cannabis as an act of risk doubled. In 2010 the consumption of this illegal drug was 10%, while in 2017 it was 21%. Similarly, the use of cocaine tripled in just 7 years. As in other countries, there are gender differences due to the fact that men show a higher consumption, compared to women.

The consequences of the consumption of toxic substances (recreational and chronic) are varied: car accidents, risky sexual relations, fights, etc. The frequent consumption of toxic substances affects behavior at a social, emotional, cognitive, and physical level. The psychosocial effects in adolescents not only are contemporary but also are related to mental health problems in adulthood. Thus, the use of drugs in adolescents has negative effects in adulthood: affecting performance in study and work; damaging physical and mental development, affecting psychosocial functioning; deteriorating the emergence of the ability of mental development; and leading to adulthood disorders, and increasing morbidity and mortality [24].

Other current research studies show undesirable effects of abusing substances. For example, frequent cannabis users have a higher number of negative consequences than occasional users [9]; other studies show that substance abuse affects well-being and family functioning, as well as financial position, physical health, and psychological well-being [10].

Moral Judgment (Permissiveness and Penalization) in Adolescents' Substance Use

Moral judgment is an evaluative judgment to determine whether a human act is considered morally good or bad. The moral judgment has been studied in psychology from the perspective of penalization of acts [25–28], as well as from the perspective of acceptance or permissiveness of controversial moral acts [29–34].

Moral permissiveness refers to the tolerance that a person has toward different socio-moral issues, such as abortion, substance use, and corruption [30]. Controversial moral acts are those behaviors that can be considered unacceptable and unjustifiable by people. They may fall into the category of sexuality, self-interest morality, and legal–illegal morality. The sexual category encompasses acts related to life, death, and sexual relations (for example: prostitution and having sexual relations before the age of majority). The morality category of self-interest includes actions related to personal integrity and honor (for example: evade taxes if there is an opportunity to do it and keep money that has been found on the street). Besides, the legal–illegal morality category encompasses behaviors proscribed by law (for example: sneaking out of a car without the owner's permission and political assassinations) [31]. Other authors have grouped these behaviors into the following categories: Personal integrity, Honesty, and Social legality [30].

Rodriguez, Mesurado, and Moreno [35] carried out an investigation on the penalization of acts as faults and crimes, in Argentine adolescents and young people. Ordered by rank, among the 25 acts to estimate penalization, *administering cocaine* was ranked 4th; *smoking cannabis* was ranked 12th, *drinking beer to excess* was ranked 23rd, and *getting drunk at a party* was ranked 24th. That is, they penalized more the use of cocaine, then cannabis , and to a lesser extent alcohol. For both cocaine and cannabis, women penalised use more than men [35].

In relation to the permissiveness of controversial moral acts, a current study [36] in an order by rank in adolescents, on 22 controversial moral acts, *smoking cannabis* ranked 15th; being position 1 always justifiable and 22 never justifiable. That is, *smoking cannabis* was one of the least justifiable morally controversial acts.

Meaning of Life and Moral Permissiveness in Substance Using and Abusing Adolescents

A cross-sectional study was carried out in adolescents to evaluate the relationship between the meaning of life and moral judgment (permissiveness and penalization) regarding the use of alcohol, cannabis, and cocaine. A sample of 181 adolescents between 15 and 18 years old (M = 16.22 SD = .92), 81 men (44.8%) and 100 women (55.2%) was formed. The sample was obtained from middle-level schools in the cities of Entre Ríos, Argentina.

A sociodemographic questionnaire was developed for these variables. In order to evaluate the meaning of life, the Purpose in life (that evaluates three dimensions: *perception of meaning*, *experience of meaning,* and *attitude toward death*) was used [15]. To assess moral permissiveness, the Controversial Moral Behaviors Scale of Harding and Phillips [29] was used, in the Spanish version [30]. It consists of 22 items that express behaviors of which the interviewee must express the degree of acceptance, with a scale from 1 (Never acceptable) to 10 (Always acceptable). In this research, only the item *Smoking cannabis* was considered. To measure the penalization of acts, the Penalization of Faults and Crimes Scale was used [25, 37]. In this research, the items related to substance use and abuse were used, namely: *administering cocaine*, *smoking cannabis*, *drinking beer to excess*, and *getting drunk at a party*.

Due to the characteristics of the variables, Spearman's Rho statistic was used to evaluate the relationship between the *meaning of life* and *permissiveness/penalty* (see Tables 5.1 and 5.2).

A positive correlation was observed between grouped use and abuse substance penalization with perception of meaning, the experience of meaning, and total purpose in life. Although the correlations are not so strong, it must be understood that the phenomena in psychology are multi-causal, which is why a significant correlation is already an important piece of information. The positive correlation between penalization in general and purpose in life (PIL) had already been proven in previous empirical studies [17], but there were no studies that disaggregated the use and abuse of substances.

Also, a negative correlation was observed between smoking cannabis permissiveness with the perception of meaning, the experience of meaning, attitude toward death, and total purpose in life.

Table 5.1 Spearman's rho between meaning of life and grouped penalization of substance use

	Grouped use substance[a]	Total PIL	Perception of meaning (PIL)	Experience of meaning (PIL)	Attitude toward death (PIL)
Grouped use substance[a]	1.000	.172*	.148*	.191**	.074
Total PIL	.172*	1.000	.919**	.742**	.670**
Perception of meaning (PIL)	.148*	.919**	1.000	.589**	.521**
Experience of meaning (PIL)	.191**	.742**	.589**	1.000	.320**
Attitude toward death (PIL)	.074	.670**	.521**	.320**	1.000

$N = 181$
**The correlation is significant at the 0.01 level (2 tails)
*The correlation is significant at the 0.05 level (2 tails)
[a]Administering cocaine, smoking cannabis, drinking beer to excess, and getting drunk at a party

Table 5.2 Spearman's Rho between meaning of life and permissiveness

	Smoking cannabis	Total PIL	Perception of meaning (PIL)	Experience of meaning (PIL)	Attitude toward death (PIL)
Smoking cannabis	1.000	−.356**	−.395**	−.225**	−.229**
Total PIL	−.356**	1.000	.919**	.742**	.670**
Perception of meaning (PIL)	−.395**	.919**	1.000	.589**	.521**
Experience of meaning (PIL)	−.225**	.742**	.589**	1.000	.320**
Attitude towards death (PIL)	−.229**	.670**	.521**	.320**	1.000

$N = 181$
**The correlation is significant at the 0.01 level (2 tails)
*The correlation is significant at the 0.05 level (2 tails)

Conclusions

In general, the problem of substance use and abuse has been studied in relation to different problems and pathologies, but studies with the positive aspects of the human person are less frequent. Recent systematic studies account for this fact, such as the increase in the study of prosocial behavior and substance abuse in the last decade; finding an inverse relationship between both variables [38]. We understand that the study of the meaning of life and the use and abuse of substances is a contribution to this line of seeing the problematics, incorporating positive aspects of the human person in relation to these issues.

By means of this study, the relationship between the meaning of life (in its different dimensions of perception and experience of meaning and attitude toward death) and moral judgment (in two dimensions) has been revealed. At first, people who have a higher sense of life in terms of perception and experience of meaning penalized the use and abuse of substances with higher scores than others. Secondly, those people who have a higher sense of life in terms of perception and experience of meaning and attitude toward death are less permissive in terms of smoking cannabis. Although the behavioral dimension has not been evaluated here, only the moral judgment, involved on the basis of people's behavior can give an indication of behavior.

This chapter agreed with theoretical statements and empirical studies on existential emptiness since numerous authors [11, 12, 39–41] have stated that people who experience or express "existential emptiness" may present a greater predisposition to risky, antisocial, or criminal behaviors, such as alcoholism, addictions, or violence toward others.

Within the framework of Viktor Frankl's theory, recent empirical studies show that higher presence of meaning was associated with lower alcohol and other drug use, with boredom mediated those relationships [42]. Another recent empirical study shows that the meaning of life negatively and partially mediated the relationship between stress and substance abuse [43].

The theories and recent studies carried out, as well as the empirical contribution made in this chapter, show the importance of fostering the meaning of life and reducing the existential emptiness in adolescents and young people, to avoid the use and abuse of substances. Thus, promoting meaning of life through the construction of a life project at this stage of the life cycle is of great importance as psychoprophylaxis.

References

1. Arnett JJ. Adolescence and emerging adulthood. Pearson; 2020.
2. Steinberg L. Adolescence. McGraw-Hill; 2018.
3. Kohlberg E. A medieval Muslim scholar at work: Ibn Ṭāwūs and his library, vol. 12. Leiden: Brill; 1992.
4. Piaget J, Inhelder H. Psicología del niño. Madrid: Morata; 2000.
5. Bonino S. Contagio, empatía e comportamento prosociale. In: Caprara GV, Bonino S, editors. Il comportamento prosociale. Aspetti individuali, familiari e sociali. Trento: Erikson; 2005. p. 23–44.
6. Castillo G. Adolescencia, mitos y enigmas. Bilbao: Desclée De Brouwer; 2016.
7. Griffa MC, Moreno JE. Claves para una Psicología del Desarrollo. Tomo II. Buenos Aires: Lugar Editorial; 2005.
8. Papalia D, Martorell G. Desarrollo humano. Barcelona: McGraw-Hill; 2021.
9. Pilatti A, Rivarola Montejano G, Nillus M, Fernandez M, Pautassi RM. Factores que diferencian el consumo frecuente y esporádico de marihuana en estudiantes universitarios. Act Colom Psicol. 2022;25(1):87–104. https://doi.org/10.14718/ACP.2022.25.1.7.
10. Dykes G, Casker R. Adolescents and substance abuse: the effects of substance abuse on parents and siblings. Int J Adolesc Youth. 2021;26(1):224–37. https://doi.org/10.1080/02673843.2021.1908376.
11. Frankl V. El hombre en busca de sentido. Barcelona: Herder; 1979.
12. Frankl V. Ante el vacío existencial. Hacia una humanización de la psicoterapia. Barcelona: Herder; 1980.
13. Crumbaugh JC, Maholick LT. An experimental study in existentialism: the psychometric approach to Frankl's concept of noogenic neurosis. J Clin Psychol. 1964;20:589–96.
14. Crumbaugh JC, Maholick LT. Manual of instructions for the purpose in life test. Saratoga: Viktor Frankl Institute of Logotherapy; 1969.
15. Gottfried AE. Adaptación Argentina del PIL Test (Test de sentido en la vida) de Crumbaugh y Maholick. Rev Psicol. 2016;12(23):49–65.
16. Gottfried AE. El sentido de vida en adolescentes entre 17 y 18 años de la ciudad de Mendoza, evidenciado

antes y después de un programa de intervención basado en los postulados de Viktor Frankl. Diálogos Pedagóg. 2017;15(29):85–114.
17. Gómez JS, Barrio A. Relación entre las dimensiones del sentido de la vida y la estimación de la gravedad de faltas y delitos en adolescentes de 15 a 17 años de las ciudades de Hasenkamp y Concordia, Entre Ríos. Tesis de grado. Pontificia Universidad Católica Argentina, Facultad Teresa de Ávila; 2018.
18. Facio A, Resett S, Mistrorigo C, Micocci F. Adolescentes argentinos. Cómo piensan y sienten. Buenos Aires: Lugar editorial; 2006.
19. Chassin L, Hussong A, Barrera M, Molina B, Trim R, Ritter J. Adolescent substance use. In: Lerner R, Steinberg L, editors. Handbook of adolescent psychology. Wiley; 2004.
20. Addiction Center. What are drug classifications? https://www.addictioncenter.com/drugs/drug-classifications/, 2022.
21. Monitoring the Future. Tables and figures. http://www.monitoringthefuture.org, 2005.
22. Kandel DB, editor. Stages and pathways of drug involvement: examining the gateway hypothesis. Cambridge University Press; 2002.
23. SEDRONAR Estudio Nacional. Informe de Resultados N° 1 en población de 12 a 65 años, sobre Consumo de Sustancias Psicoactivas. Ministerio de la Nación Argentina; 2017.
24. Das J, Salam R, Arshad A, Finkelstein Y, Bhutta Z. Interventions for adolescent substance abuse: an overview of systematic reviews. J Adolesc Health. 2016;59(4):S61–75.
25. Rimoldi HJ, López Alonso AO. Sobre la relatividad de los juicios psicológicos. CIIPME. Publicación Nro. 24, Bs As; 1973.
26. Moreno JE. Posturas éticas de los jóvenes y estimación de la gravedad de faltas y delitos. Rev Soc Psicol Uruguay. 1991;3(6):85–92.
27. Rodriguez LM. Psicología del desarrollo moral en la adolescencia: un modelo integrativo. Tesis de Doctorado en Psicología, Universidad Católica Argentina, Facultad de Psicología y Psicopedagogía; 2016.
28. Rodriguez LM, Moreno JE. Posturas éticas y empatía, predictores de prosocialidad y de penalización de faltas y delitos. Acción Psicol. 2016;13(2):43–56. https://doi.org/10.5944/ap.13.2.17809.
29. Harding S, Phillips D. Contrasting values in western Europe. Unity, diversity, and change. London: Macmillan; 1986.
30. Grimaldo M, Merino C. Tolerancia y juicio moral en estudiantes universitarios de la ciudad de Lima. Liberabit. 2010;16(2):131–40.
31. Mathiesen ME, Mora O, Castro M. Valores de los estudiantes de la Universidad de Concepción (Chile). Aplicación de la escala de comportamientos morales controvertidos. Rev Latinoam Psicol. 1998;30(1):121–36.
32. Mathiesen ME, Mora O, Chamblás I, Navarro G. Familia, permisividad y juicio moral en estudiantes de enseñanza media de la provincia de Concepción. Psykhe (Santiago). 2004;13(1):3–20.
33. Merino C, Grimaldo MP. Complejidad factorial y conductas moralmente controversiales. Rev Argent Cienc Comport. 2011;3(3):38–43.
34. Merino C, Grimaldo MP. Análisis no paramétrico de rankings de tolerancia en comportamientos moralmente cuestionables. Rev Digit Invest Docencia Univ. 2015;9(2):33–48.
35. Rodriguez LM, Mesurado B, Moreno JE. Penalización de actos: el juicio moral en adolescentes y jóvenes. Rev Estud Exp Educ. 2018;17(34):69–78.
36. Rodriguez LM, Ghiglione ME. Permisividad moral en adolescentes. Un estudio descriptivo. In: Congreso Educación del carácter en latinoamérica: retos y oportunidades. Buenos Aires: Universidad Austral; 2018.
37. Lopez Alonso AO. Estimación de la gravedad de faltas y delitos e influencia subjetiva en los jueces de los antecedentes criminales. In: Estimación de la gravedad de faltas y delitos e influencia subjetiva en los jueces de los antecedentes criminales. CIIPME; 1977. p. 16.
38. Esparza-Reig J, Martí-Vilar M, Merino-Soto C, García-Casique A. Relationship between prosocial behaviorus and addiction problems: a systematic review. Helthcare. 2022;10:74. https://doi.org/10.3390/healthcare10010074.
39. Gottfried AE, Fozzatti MJ. El sentido de vida en jóvenes de 18 a 25 años concurrentes a centros educativos de nivel secundario. Acta Psiquiatr Psicol Am Lat. 2016;62(3):172–80.
40. Griffa MC, Moreno JE. Actas de la II Jornada de Intercambio Académico y de Investigación. Buenos Aires: Universidad Católica Argentina, Facultad de Psicología y Psicopedagogía; 2012.
41. Nuévalos RC. La conducta antisocial desde una psicopedagogía positiva (una aproximación desde la logoterapia y la resiliencia). Rev Fuentes. 2011;11:161–74.
42. Csabonyi M, Phillips LJ. Meaning of life and substance use. J Humanist Psychol. 2020;60(1):3–19. https://doi.org/10.1177/0022167816687674.
43. Kheirabadi H, Jajarmi M, Bakhshipoor AB. A structural correlation modeling of stress and substance abuse with the mediating role of meaning in life and experiential avoidance. Int J Behav Sci. 2021;15(1):34–40. https://doi.org/10.30491/IJBS.2021.225787.1241.

6 Epistemic Competencies of Philosophy in Therapeutic Praxis: An Analysis of Pedro Laín Entralgo's Work

María Teresa Gargiulo

Introduction

The objective of this study is to analyse how Pedro Laín Entralgo conceives the epistemic competences of philosophy both in the field of a comprehensive theory of disease and of the sick man and its natural projection in the field of medical practice. Certainly, the question might seem lacking in novelty and meaning. Above all, since the death of the Spanish doctor, what we now recognize as the philosophy of medicine has grown exponentially and has diversified into various areas and specialities. Philosophical thinking today crosses medical practice in different directions. Hence, to reveal the specific scope of the issue at hand, it is necessary to discriminate the epistemic field to which we refer.

Within the broad and complex scope of what is now known as the philosophy of medicine Engelhardt y Erde [1] distinguish in it, four orientations or large areas of reflection.

The first major area of discussion can be recognized as an ontology of medicine which would deal with analytically discussing topics such as the nature of medicine, the meaning and scope of the medical task, the specificity of the doctor–patient relationship, or the type of entity that is a disease, discomfort, health and care.

Second, there is a core of discussion that can be recognized as a continuation of the same philosophy of science and that is nothing more than an epistemology of medicine that inquiries about the rationality of medical knowledge, how it is constructed, what kind of knowledge is clinical, how to access the knowledge of the disease and the body, what is the logic of diagnosis, prognosis and clinical trials; what are the philosophical premises of the various medical paradigms, and much more.

Third, it is worth mentioning what we could call an ethics of medicine that is recognized today under the name of bioethics. This deals with regulating the doctor–patient relationship based on the values and specific purposes of medical practice.

Finally, to these three great areas of the philosophy of medicine must be added the effort of the most disparate philosophical traditions to build medical anthropology capable of transcending the coordinates of scientific naturalism. The work of Laín Entralgo, the psychosomatic pathology of Juan Rof Carballo, Edmund Pellegrino [2] and Mario Caponnetto [3] are inscribed in this line; or the themes of medical anthropology developed by authors such as Fleck, Canguilhem, Grmek, Foucault and Bastide, as Engelhardt y Erde point out [1].

This last area of discussion is not concerned with developing a foundation under a strictly theoretical formality—such as can be affected in

M. T. Gargiulo (✉)
Departamento de Filosofía, Facultad de Filosofía y Letras, Universidad Nacional de Cuyo/CONICET, Mendoza, Argentina

P. Á. Gargiulo, H. L. Mesones-Arroyo (eds.), *Psychiatry and Neuroscience Update – Vol. V*,
https://doi.org/10.1007/978-3-031-72219-6_6

the first major area of the philosophy of medicine cited above. It tries to formulate medical anthropology, certainly anchored in an anthropological understanding, but fundamentally concerned with intervening and transforming medical practice itself. Indeed, all praxis in the field of medical practice is a natural extension of a medical theory, that is, a theoretical understanding of disease and man's sick.

It is within this framework that our question about whether philosophy can legitimately intervene on the same nerve centre on which the health sciences are built, namely, in the same therapeutic praxis, is inscribed.

Nowadays, the ontological, epistemic and ethical impact that philosophy has on the configuration and structure of medicine is undeniable. However, the question about whether philosophical inquiry directly affects human health and disease remains valid. We will try to outline a possible answer to this question, based on the writings of Laín Entralgo.

By way of hypothesis, we state that the medical anthropology proposed by Lain Entralgo invites philosophy to intervene directly in the healing process itself; in the real and existential process of the patient.

In the first place, we will develop a brief historical contextualization of the question regarding the epistemic status of medical practice. This study will allow us to access, first, from the very writings of the Spanish doctor, the epistemic foundation that legitimizes the intervention of philosophical inquiry in medical care. Second, we will outline a brief characterization of this practice or philosophical care of the patient, giving continuity to the assumptions made explicit in the first point.

These two sections will allow us to study the issue from two different perspectives. On the one hand, we will analyse the long historical path that our question crosses, as it is exposed by our historian of medicine. This allows us to access the normative image of his medical anthropology. In the second section, on the other hand, we are interested in outlining a model of practice or philosophical interpellation immersed in the same process of care and cure of the patient. To do this, we will focus particularly on his studies regarding the care of the soul in Galenic medicine.

Medicine: A Science of Nature or Science of the Spirit?

Strictly speaking, we must note that our author does not systematically formulate a doctrine regarding the issue at hand; he does not, at least in these terms. However, as we will show throughout this study, he formulates medical anthropology that demands and presupposes the philosophical care of the patient.

The intervention or philosophical question could be understood as an authentic continuity and support of his particular concern to attend to the spiritual dimension of the patient.

The epistemic foundation of this intervention of philosophy in medical practice is addressed by Laín Entralgo in his article entitled, "Nature and history in medicine" [4]. There and in many other extensive passages of his vast work, he describes the implosion that occurred in the nineteenth century of the sciences of the spirit (psychology, politics, morals, anthropology, etc.) in the very precinct of medicine. He explains this phenomenon as various attempts to humanize patient care and to attend to this ontological niche that was recognized as spirit.

Various schools and traditions coincided in pointing out the psycho-spiritual dimension of human illness, although with diverse and conflicting connotations regarding it.

Among the projects already existing in the 1880s, our historian ponders, in the first place, the contributions of psychoanalysis. In his opinion, Freud was able to correct the abusive naturalism of Western medicine. He highlighted the rigorous need for dialogue with the patient, both for diagnosis and treatment. He underlined the instinctive component of human life. He demonstrated the existence and significance of the subconscious modes of psychic activity, accounting for the influence of the psychic life on the functions and movements of the body. And, finally, Laín Entralgo emphasizes, that Freud was concerned with comprehensively ordering the event of the disease in the patient's biography [5]. However, despite all these merits that he acknowledges psychoanalysis, our author ends up describing its impact on the medical culture as a renovating and poisonous effect [5, p. 127]. Freud's original intention to humanize medical knowledge and practice failed. He failed by being unable to identify an ontic and personal zone of the patient, identifying the latter with a series of vital-instinctive dynamics, namely, libido as the pleasure principle, the Oedipus complex, repression, the unconscious, sublimation, id, ego and super-ego, etc. This "verbal and conceptual abuse" [5, p. 119], prevented Freud from accessing that personal nucleus and left medicine submerged again in the spheres of the mechanical instinctive, explains Laín Entralgo.

Not only the efforts of psychoanalysis but any attempt by psychology are valued, by our author, as insufficient in this task of rediscovering and recovering the personal reality of the patient in therapeutic praxis.

The rediscovery of this ontic zone in the nineteenth century questioned the scope of a sciences of the nature that proved incapable of accounting for the vital dynamics that transcended the mechanical patterns of vital-instinctive action. To the extent that the pathological event is no longer reduced to a series of specific dysfunctions or particular physical–chemical or biochemical structures, the understanding of medicine as an art subscribed exclusively to the natural sciences is weakened.

Our author positively ponders the various projects of psychosomatic medicine to humanize medical assistance, which understand health or illness as a functional psychophysical totality; a unity that is prior to the diversification of isolated physiological or psychic facts. Indeed, this is an indisputable step, according to our historian, to understand this vital unit.

However, he warns of the danger that these projects are limited to attending to the psychological dimension of the patient without transcending their spiritual dimension. In an analogous direction, Laín Entralgo criticizes personalistic medicine—and which can be extended to narrative medicine in force today. Personalism is intertwined in the consideration of the individual under the notion of person. But the person, the Spanish doctor objects, is much more than a psycho-physical unit. Human illness is not only explained by that unity and by what may be particular and idiosyncratic in his biography, but also by that dimension that specifically accounts for the true hierarchy of man in the order of beings [5, pp. 119–20].

When the Spanish doctor postulates an outline of what he understands by this personal or spiritual dimension of the patient, he borrows from scholasticism and the phenomenology of Husserl and Scheler, the notion of intentionality. Intentionality is the fundamental condition that enables man to know, become aware of objects and project his actions, explains Laín Entralgo in continuity with the philosophical traditions just mentioned [5, p. 121]. It is the first presupposition of the spiritual character of a human experience such as illness and pain. Our author characterizes intentionality as a "tending towards"; like a tear, like the opening "outwards" of the human psychophysical totality [5, p. 120].

This intentional dimension of the human spirit legitimizes and requires the doctor to attend precisely to this ontic centre of the patient [5, p. 121].

To understand Laín Entralgo's integration of philosophy into medical practice, it is first necessary to understand that this concern for building medical anthropology led him to epistemically relocate medicine, not as a science of nature but as a science of man. "The personal, he writes, in the most genuine sense of the word, should be a task for the doctor" [5, p. 123]. This dimension of the person is the foundation by which medicine is distinguished from mere biology and becomes a supra-biological science, a true science of man. In *History of Medicine* (1997), he states: "This is not and cannot be—against what was believed in 1900—applied natural science" [6, p. 651].

From this perspective, Laín Entralgo defines the epistemological status of medicine as a single art that transcends both the naturalistic-explanatory method of the natural sciences and the descriptive method of the spiritual sciences. Medical practice certainly seeks to "collect from the world of the data of the senses concerning an isolated human existence" [5, p. 132] and in this, it seems to continue the task of the natural sciences. But also, and above all, explains our author, he tries to connect these data "with the historical-social reality in which that specific man finds himself immersed" [5, p. 132].

Faced with the sick man, the doctor must implement the immense arsenal of resources that therapy offers today—pharmacotherapeutic, dietary and surgical. But, asks our author, "can it be said that this can and should always be all and only the treatment of human illness?" [6, p. 625]. Certainly not. The Spanish doctor insists that it is necessary to understand and attend to the patient's disease not only from the latest experimental results of neurophysiology and endocrinology but also from the emotional and intellectual activity of the patient [6, p. 639].

Furthermore, he allows himself to complete Dilthey's scheme of human sciences by adding to anthropology and psychology a third discipline, namely medicine. But this medicine that he conceives as an anthropology of the sick man, does not adopt the theoretical character of the first two. It is a practical science whose pragmatic goal is nothing more than a redirection of the patient to a new vital and personal integrity [5, p. 133].

In this epistemic context, medical-philosophical practice is not an "explanatory attitude", distant and theoretical. On the contrary, it is immersed in the healing process itself as an "attitude of help", faithful to the real constitution of the patient and his life experience [6].

Medicine cannot be limited to curing and relieving the patient through a specific diagnostic and therapeutic theory and technique, but also to giving the patient a new sphere of freedom. It implies attending, understanding and projecting the patient's world of meaning through philosophical questioning. The Spanish doctor invites medicine to become a true "pathos pedagogy" (*pathogogy*), that is, an art of educating sick men, which requires the art of leading the sick man "towards a more suitable possibility of living than the anguished and invalid state in which the disease plunges him" [5, pp. 132–133].

The philosophy that is in itself a sciences of the Spirit is integrated by our author, in the same pragma of this particular science of man that is medicine. Medicine "is not Physics or Chemistry, just as it is not Philosophy or History", he explains [5, p. 131]. Only by understanding this new intermediate and equidistant epistemological status of the sciences of nature and the sciences of the Spirit, it is possible to reveal his understanding of philosophical questioning as a skill that integrates the medical profession.

The medical anthropology of Laín Entralgo seeks to integrate or coordinate all the resources of the art of healing, including the convergence of philosophy in therapeutic action to the extent that it provides a comprehensive understanding of the disease [6, p. 641]. In it, he tries to formulate an understanding of pathology that is truly faithful to what man is by nature. On the other hand, he denounced that medicine that excludes the philosophical or spiritual dimension of the healing process would exclude the true *self* from the morbid process. Instead, it would deal with a living individual, but not with the exclusively human nucleus [6, p. 633].

Our author recognizes that many cultivators of what attempts to be medical anthropology have frequently incurred in irresponsible interpretative novelties [6, p. 639]. However, this is not an obstacle to denying the strictly scientific basis of the intervention of philosophy in the field of medicine.

Let us then briefly characterize some notes of this medical-philosophical practice. For this, we will present certain historical practices of ancient medicine that, according to Laín Entralgo, should be valid today in medical practice.

Background and Possibilities of Philosophical Interpellation in Galenic Medicine

In the previous point, we exposed the epistemic and normative foundation of the medical anthropology of Laín Entralgo. Next, we will consider how the Spanish doctor conceives the philosophical interpellation as an integral part of the same medical practice. To account for this practice, throughout all his writings, he refers particularly to Galenic medicine.

Certainly, he notes that the history of psychosomatic pathology is, in a way, the entire history of medicine [7, p. 14]. Attempts to humanize medicine do not begin or end with Galen. However, in his writings, he repeatedly returns to the Galenic practice of medicine to the extent that he finds in it a series of resources capable of inscribing, in a vital way, the philosophical interpellation as part of the processes of cure and care of the sick patient. His references to Greco-Latin medicine constitute for him an alternative to rethink research and contemporary medical practice [7, p. 86].

Our Spanish doctor does not conceive the disease as a mere organic disorder that translates into an immune, functional or metabolic-degenerative way [6, p. 624]. On the contrary, following the comprehensive coordinates of the Galenic, he approaches illness by understanding the biographical, intimate and social reality of each patient, fundamentally understanding the illness as a disorder in the very way of living. In *History of Medicine*, he wrote:

> In its most proper determination—let's continue with Galen—, the disease is a disorder of the body; but being psycho-organic, biographical, intimate and social the reality of man, and being it by essence, to the causation and manifestation of human disease belong, also by essence, moments that are not primarily and strictly corporeal. This is expressed above all in the fact that, in addition to being an organic disorder, human disease is always and essentially a way of living; to live, of course, humanely. [6, p. 624]

The disease is presented as a situation of human existence in which a disorder of the organism and a way of having lived and of being living of the person who suffers from that disease are integrated. Faced with this, the doctor-philosopher "must help the chronically ill and the convalescent to reinstall himself in the best possible way in his world; sometimes, inventing with him and for him a new way of living" [6, pp. 651–652].

Our historian of medicine considers Galen as the synthesis and definitive form of the "physiological" medicine of the Greeks [7, p. 88]. He recognizes the merit of having rescued the patient's personal and intimate core as part of medical care. The doctor of Pergamon in his *sex res non naturales* points out the duty of the doctor to attend to all those causes of human illness, namely, not only the environment, food, work or rest of the patient but also the movements or affections of the soul that can trigger a morbid process.

Our author denounces that the richness of this "dietary" of Galenic medicine was reduced and impoverished, in the medicine of the nineteenth century, to a life regimen that dealt exclusively with home care, diet, exercise or good sleep hygiene. However, that medicine forgot what Galen recognised as the movements of the soul [6, p. 652].

Habits, affections, thoughts and movements of the soul are the object of medicine to the extent that they can behave, according to Galen, as the cause of a humoral movement with a pathological impact on the body. Let us remember that in *Quod animi mores corporis temperamenta sequntur* [7], Galen postulates that the psychic manifestations of man can be explained by the physiological schemes of his humoral doctrine.

However, in *De propium Animi Cuiuslibet Affectuum Dignotione et Curatione* [8] and *De Animi Cuiuslibet Peccatorum Dignotione et Curatione* [9] the Greek doctor postulates that the movements of the soul, in certain cases, can behave as the cause of human illness. The doctor transcends the schemes of naturalistic corporalism and complements the approach of his pathological doctrine. That is to say, he no longer shows the dependence of moral life and psychic manifestations on the humoral state. Instead, he opens the consideration that psychic, cognitive and moral dispositions behave as primary etiological causes of human affections. In this same line, our historian of medicine explains "Greek pathology reaches its inner perfection and the height of its aspirations in the work of Galen; which seeks to collect for *physiology* and *tékhne iatrike* all the moral life of man" [7, p. 69].

Galen wrote "The doctor must consider it part of his task, not only to discover the idiosyncrasies of the patient but also to find out what oppresses his mind" [10]. In *De Animi Cuiuslibet Peccatorum Dignotione et Curatione* defines these errors or *hamartemata* [9, pp. 85, 59–61] as those erroneous judgments about the purpose of life, which are due, not to a disorder of the passions, but a failure in the reasoning of the *logos* [9, pp. 63–64]. Hence, the doctor of Pergamon finds it essential to be instructed in the logical or demonstrative method to be able to choose a way of life in accordance with rational nature [9, p. 66].

This galenic discernment is what Laín Entralgo seeks to recover and reinvent in his medical anthropology. The therapeutic process of formally personal pathology, according to our author, must attend to the intimate subjectivity of the patient, to his biography, to his freedom—although the exercise of it is more or less conditioned—, to his sociability [6, p. 634]. "Strictly speaking—explains the historian of medicine—what happens in his body belongs to the *physis* of a man as much as what happens in his psyche; a Greek never stopped thinking so" [7, p. 88]. The physis of the patient cannot be translated in a materialistic way, so only the somatic would be sickening—in a proper sense. On the contrary, what happens in the intimacy of the patient, either as a cause or as a symptom, constitutes, explains our author, the disease suffered by the patient [7, p. 88].

To this end, it becomes necessary to formulate within the medical practice an exploratory and dialogic method different from the sensory and measurement exploration of modern medicine [7, p. 92]. It is about establishing a helping relationship in which the doctor and the patient engage in a confidential philosophical dialogue aimed at the patient clarifying for himself his challenges, his conflicts, his doubts or existential dilemmas. The objective of this practice is for the patient to develop for himself new horizons of meaning capable of generating a new art of living.

According to our author, these dilemmas or spiritual quests may not in themselves constitute a disease [7, p. 107]. But they can behave as true *diathesis* of the psychic life, that is, as a cause that could favour a particular psychic disposition that can affect or injure the less resistant functions of some organs [7, p. 83].

The doctor must attend to the patient's lifestyle, passions and judgments as long as they behave as a possible causal agent of human illness. Certain disorders, conflicts and anguishes that appear in the spiritual and personal search of a patient, due to the psychophysical movement that is concomitant to them, can slowly and gradually generate properly morbid affections. Hence, the philosophical appeal to the patient's world of meaning, his biography, his ideas, habits, anxieties, hopes, life projects and possibilities does not imply for our author, as we explained in the first point, a distancing from the epistemic competencies of medical practice.

The concerns that afflict the sick man are not reduced to a series of psychological dysfunctions but also have a philosophical root. They may be associated with his basic worldviews. Hence, a need to investigate not only the patient's psychobiographical vicissitudes but also his metaphysical intimacy.

From this perspective, it may be an advance of narrative medicine to contemplate and describe the disease "from within the patient", that is, from his most intimate sensations. But we believe that the medical anthropology of Laín Entralgo transcends this individualizing intention in a project of greater scope, namely, to rehabilitate that galenic care on the spiritual movements of the soul insofar as they can behave as a possible causal agent of human illness [5, pp. 132–133].

Conclusion

Indeed there are multiple and essential influences that philosophy has on the ontological assumptions of medicine, on the analysis of its epistemic validity or on the ethical issues that affect its very exercise. But what we have been interested in elucidating in this study is whether the philosophy, according to the medical anthropology of

Laín Entralgo, has effectively interfered in the same medical act.

For our Spanish doctor, philosophical interpellation has a direct bearing on human illness. In this line, he proposes to recover those galenic forms of approaching the patient where philosophy does not constitute an alien and independent discipline of the medical act but rather participates in its very process. Philosophy does not adopt, in its medical anthropology, a merely normative and analytical character for medical practice. It intervenes in the same process of healing and caring for the patient.

His invitation to reconsider Galenic medicine does not imply, in any way, neither a naive regression to the primitive stages of medicine nor a contempt for the long tradition through which it has been progressing. On the other hand, our historian of medicine insists that the medical theories of the past cannot be underestimated. For all theories, it may be considered a means of embracing the facts and approaching the truth [5, p. 136]. Even more so in the case of Galen, he turns the historical recapitulation into a novelty. In his studies on the doctor of Pergamon, he presents the possibility of thinking about medicine today as a structure of knowledge that is more attentive to this ontological niche that defines the human being. Dialogue with Galen means for him the opportunity to recover or reinvent that metaphysical identity between truth and good, between science and happiness, between body and spirit, which they knew and practised.

References

1. Engelhardt HT Jr, Erde EL. Philosophy of medicine. In: Durbin PT, editor. A guide to the culture of science, technology, and medicine. New York: Free Press; 1980. p. 364–46.
2. Pellegrino ED, Thomasma DC. Philosophical basis of medical practice. New York: Oxford University Press; 1981.
3. Caponnetto M. Antropología Médica. Antecedentes históricos, epistemología, teoría antropológica y contenido temático. Paraná: Staurós Ediciones; 2021.
4. Laín Entralgo P. Naturaleza e historia en la medicina. Escorial; 1940. p. 1.
5. Laín Entralgo P. Historia de la Medicina. Barcelona: Masson; 1997. p. 635–7.
6. Laín Entralgo P. Enfermedad y Pecado. Barcelona: Toray; 1961. p. 14.
7. Galeno, Quod Animi Mores Corporis temperamenta Sequntur (QAM). Introd., trad. y notas de Juana Zaragoza Gras. Madrid: Gredos, 2003.
8. Galeno, De propium Animi Cuiuslibet Affectuum Dignotione et Curatione (Aff. Dig.). In P. N. Singer (Trad. Introd. and Notes). Galen: Selected Works, Ars. Medica (Ars Med.). Oxford/New York: Oxford University Press, 1997.
9. Galeno, De Animi Cuiuslibet Peccatorum Dignotione et Curatione (Pecc. Dig.). In P. N. Singer (Trad. Introd. and Notes). Galen: Selected Works, Ars. Medica (Ars Med.). Oxford/New York: Oxford University Press, 1997.
10. In Hipp. Epid. VI com. I–VIII. Further on he writes: "The cure of a person whose illness has originated in his mind can only be achieved by removing the fixed idea, and not by means of food and drink, living conditions, baths, walks and things by the style". In Hipp. Epid. VI com. I–VIII.

Free Will, Addiction, and the Feeling of Self-Control

7

Rocco J. Gennaro

In this chapter, I explore the relationship between several interrelated vexed topics in philosophy and psychology, namely, the free will-determinism debate, the nature of addiction, compulsion, and self-control. As we shall see, having a conscious feeling of compulsion to use drugs is, in some ways, irrelevant to whether the related actions are free according to both determinists and compatibilists. I explain below while raising some questions about the so-called "deep self" compatibilist view on free will. With these considerations in the background, I then turn my attention to the role of introspection in self-control and briefly, sketch a brain-based account of self-control whereby becoming consciously aware of our compulsions can sometimes lead to controlling addictive cravings.

Terminology and Definitions

It is crucial first to be clear about some of the key concepts, including addiction and compulsion. Of course, there are different conceptions and definitions of these terms in the literature. For example, "Addictions are strong appetites. Addicts are people who have a strong appetite. Appetites generate desires, and the satisfaction of these desires generally provides pleasure. A drug addict has strong appetites for some drug" [1]. A compulsion is often understood as an overwhelming and intense desire leading to immediate action. It seems to crowd out other impulses and mental states since one's attention is so focused on, say, acquiring and taking a drug. Compulsion in drug addiction is often viewed as resulting from impaired "self-control" (as opposed to what is sometimes called "weakness of will") [2, 3]. Of course, even if one has a compulsion to do something at a given time, it doesn't follow that one will always have it at future times. Finally, the notion of "craving" is frequently mentioned in the literature on addiction. For example, "the phenomenon of craving is widely taken to be an important, if not central, feature of addiction. Craving is standardly described as an extremely intense urge to use a given substance or to enact an addictive behavior; a desire that…often overwhelms attempts at abstention. Craving is commonly appealed to in order to explain how addiction jeopardizes self-control, intentions, resolutions, and choice" [4]. Cravings are powerful desires that tend to crowd out other considerations [5].

R. J. Gennaro (✉)
Department of Political Science and Philosophy, LAC 3055, University of Southern Indiana, Evansville, IN, USA
e-mail: rjgennaro@usi.edu; https://www.usi.edu/faculty/rjgennaro

P. Á. Gargiulo, H. L. Mesones-Arroyo (eds.), *Psychiatry and Neuroscience Update – Vol. V*, https://doi.org/10.1007/978-3-031-72219-6_7

Two further points should be noted here as well:

1. Addictions are generally harmful although perhaps some can yield benefits, such as an athlete who is addicted to working out and practicing even to the level of an obsession at times. Although I will focus on drug addiction, much of what I have to say will apply to other forms of addiction, such as alcohol, tobacco, pornography, gambling, and eating.
2. Drug addicts are clearly sometimes able to stop taking their drug of choice, albeit sometimes with the need of outside help or counseling. At the very least, this suggests that drug addiction is probably not quite like psychiatric disorders which seem entirely outside the realm of control (e.g., paranoid schizophrenia). Perhaps it is better to think of addiction as coming in degrees or levels of compulsion.

Free Will and Determinism

Some of the talk about compulsion and a lack of self-control normally seems to imply a lack of freedom or autonomy, at least to some extent. Although I am not primarily concerned with addressing the traditional free will-determinism debate here, it is important in the background of much of the addiction literature and it is of course a major metaphysical problem in its own right [6, 7]. It is a central question about the nature of human beings and our relationship to the physical world. Like the dualist-materialist debate, much of the free will-determinism dispute often centers on how much weight to put on first-person or subjective experience as opposed to third-person or scientific evidence. After all, we frequently make decisions after some period of conscious deliberation and thought. A determinist would likely concede that it "feels" or "seems" like we have free will from the conscious first-person point of view. However, the scientific third-person evidence regarding the nature of cause and effect in our bodies (including our brains) outweighs the first-person evidence and shows us that free will is really an illusion. Of course, even those who do believe in free will concede that not all of our actions are free. We do many things automatically, simply out of habit, and without really thinking about them.

It is, however, most important here to explain that, in philosophical circles at least, the notion of free will has two very different historical definitions, one much stronger than the other. The stronger "libertarian" free will is perhaps what most people tend to have in mind and seems presupposed in most legal systems and world religions. On this view, we have the following definition:

Libertarian Free Will = A person P does act A freely when, and only when, P could have done some other action B at that same time *and* P had some control over doing A.

For many, the core ideas of "could have done otherwise" and "control" over actions are also essential for holding someone morally and/or legally responsible for an action. After all, if someone were to assault another person and he was compelled to do so given his state of mind at that time, then he really *couldn't* have done otherwise and so then how can we really hold him morally responsible for the action? He can still of course be *guilty* of the crime in the sense that he caused it and is thus legally responsible for it, but that is different than a more robust kind of moral responsibility. Still, a society should protect citizens from dangerous criminals regardless of where one stands on the free will-determinism debate.

Determinism, in this psychological sense, might be defined as follows:

Psychological Determinism = Given the entire conscious and unconscious psychological make-up of a person P at a particular time (which results jointly from P's heredity *and* past experiences), P is compelled to do what P actually does *at that time*.

Like the libertarian, many determinists (often called 'hard' determinists) believe that free will and determinism are incompatible, that is, the very same action cannot be both free and determined. Thus, they are called "incompatibilists." This seems to follow from the above definitions. Either we can sometimes do other than what we actually do or we never can do other than what we actually do. Furthermore, libertarian free will begins to sound very mysterious and even "supernatural" in the sense that humans are somehow supposed to have a special power to alter the physical world, including our bodies or brain activity. And how could I have had *the very same* beliefs, desires, preferences, and so on, as when I decided to have pizza for lunch, but then *at that same time* still have chosen to order something else? The same causes yield the same effects. If I choose to eat a cheeseburger the next day for lunch, mustn't there have been *something different* about my state of mind at that later time?

In a sense, then, if determinism is true, then all our actions are really the result of "compulsion" at least in the sense that we could not do otherwise. Of course, we may sometimes feel as if we could do otherwise or as if we have genuine self-control but that is precisely the illusion of free will. Much the same, then, might often be said of addictive behavior: an addict regularly *feels compelled* to act to take drugs as opposed to feeling that he can exercise some self-control and not perform the action. Thus, the feeling of compulsion (and self-control, for that matter) is, in some ways, irrelevant to whether there really is a deterministic cause of the action in question. Deterministic causes can obviously often be unconscious. The feeling of self-control would itself equally be an illusion of sorts and result from a deterministic series of neural events in the brain.

Perhaps even more relevant for our purposes, there is also a long tradition of "*compatibilism*," sometimes called "soft determinism." Compatibilists agree with determinists that that there is no such thing as libertarian free will but they argue that a very important notion of freedom (and moral responsibility) remains, which is indeed compatible with determinism. The very same action can sometimes be both free and determined. Thus, for various reasons, they argue that "freedom" is better understood as something more like "the absence of external constraint" or "acting in accordance with one's desires and beliefs." A person's free actions are determined by *internal* causes such as desires and beliefs while not coerced by someone else. A person is, for example, doing what she wants to do at that time and is not compelled to do it by external causes at the time of the action. As we shall see below, however, the matter is more complicated in a way that is relevant to the case of addiction.

Frankfurt's View

Despite the initial account noted above, Harry Frankfurt famously gives a compatibilist explanation for somewhat unusual and potentially problematic cases where a compatibilist would likely want to say that an action is *not* free even when the action is brought about by internal causes.

For example, a drug addict or a kleptomaniac who really wants to stop such behavior is not really acting freely because (or if) she has a second-order desire to get rid of her first-order desire to take drugs or steal [8]. Kleptomaniacs compulsively desire to steal and act accordingly. But they are arguably not free since they cannot help having compulsive desires. Still, the above initial compatibilist definition would apparently treat the act as free since his stealing is caused by his beliefs and desires and he is not compelled by another person to steal. Thus, Frankfurt further explains that *a free action is one that is caused by the person's beliefs and desires only if those beliefs and desires flow from "who the person is."* This is sometimes called the "real self" or "deep self" compatibilist view, as opposed to the so-called "reasons responsiveness" alternative account [9].

According to the deep self-account, the desire to steal does not result from who you really are when it is at odds with this desire—that is, when you don't approve of the desire, so to speak. Indeed, you may wish that you could eliminate that desire. Thus, the action may not be free after all and you thus you ought not to be held morally responsible for it. Frankfurt distinguishes between first-order desires, which are desires to do certain things, and second-order desires, which are desires to have (or not have) certain first-order desires. You may have a first-order desire or compulsion to smoke a cigarette or use meth first thing every morning but also have a second-order desire not to have such an unhealthy and destructive first-order desire. In this case, you are what Frankfurt calls an "unwilling addict" since your drug use and addiction do not really reflect your "will" or "who you really are." But if your first-order desire matches your second-order desire, then the desire does flow from who you are and you actually are free in the sense that you are really doing "what you will or want." In this case, you are a "willing addict." Even though the kleptomaniac's stealing is caused by his (first-order) beliefs and desires, the action may not be free if he does not want to have that desire to steal. Of course, just how one can eliminate or overcome one's own unwanted first-order desires may vary from person to person, as we shall see below.

It is crucial to remember that compatibilists are still determinists so whether the unwilling addict has the relevant second-order desire and whether the addict can exercise self-control is also itself determined. Thus, it is still the case that the addict cannot desire to do otherwise.

I also wonder why there cannot be what we may even call "third-order desires." Suppose I am a willing addict. Can't I sometimes think "I don't want to be a willing addict" or "I don't want to be the kind of person I am"? "I willingly take drugs, but I don't want to have the will to take drugs" seems like a coherent thought, but it's unclear to me as to whether this should matter in terms of the action being free. Instead of not approving of my first-order desire to use drugs, why can't I also not approve of myself as a person who wants to take drugs?

Two Models of Addiction

Relevant to the notion of "self-control" and to some of the discussion below (and above as well) are the much-discussed two models of addiction, namely, the brain disease and the willpower models [1]. The "disease view" has it that "an addict's drug-seeking behavior is the direct result of some physiological change in their brain, caused by chronic use of the drug." The "normal process of motivation in the brain…is somehow changed or perverted by brain damage or adaptation caused by chronic drug use." The idea is that the addict is no longer rational and uses drugs as a result of a fundamentally nonvoluntary process. On the other hand, "perhaps the oldest view of addiction among psychologists and philosophers has held that some part of an addict wishes to abstain, but their will [power] is not strong enough to overcome an immediate desire toward temptation. On this view, addicts lose "control" over their actions."

It is crucial to note that these two accounts of addiction are not fundamentally incompatible. It seems possible that neurological mechanisms can underlie an addict's inability to resist temptation. But Foddy and Savulescu explain that the motivations behind each view are different: whereas the Willpower View is motivated by phenomenology and first-person report, the Disease View is based on neurobiological evidence. If, for example, we assume that some form of materialism is true, then it stands to reason that when we describe the conscious experiences in drug addiction in terms of cravings, desires, compulsions, feelings of self-control, etc. there should indeed be some neural representations of these mental states. It is just that willpower is something described from the first-person point of view whereas the brain disease view is framed in terms of neural processes.

Consciousness, Introspection, and Self-Control

Addiction is even sometimes thought of as a disorder of self-control. It is difficult to define "self-control" precisely, but Henden [2] explains that "it tends to be used in the sense of involving a conscious effort to override or inhibit competing urges, behaviors, or desires in order to attain particular goals." In the case of drug addiction, the conscious effort in question would seem to require at least some awareness of the strong desire to take a drug. Thus, the drug addict would first need to introspect the desire in order to exercise self-control. To some extent, then, this may be what we mean by exercising "willpower" which of course is also sometimes subject to failure [10]. Exercising self-control does seem to have a recognizable phenomenological element. On the other hand, the feeling of *lacking* "self-control" would be when one (consciously) recognizes that the first-order desire is stronger than one's self-control.

By way of contrast, one extreme case where consciousness and self-control would seem not to be able to play any role is the famous case of somnambulism (sleepwalking) which includes a bizarre case where some complex behavior resulted in a murder. Kenneth Parks, a Canadian citizen who was sleeping on his couch on May 24, 1987, put on his shoes and jacket, walked to his car, and drove 23 kilometers to the home of his parents-in-law where he proceeded to strangle his father-in-law into unconsciousness and stab his mother-in-law to death [11]. He was charged with first-degree murder but he pleaded not guilty saying that he was sleepwalking and suffering from noninsane automatism. He did have a history of sleepwalking, as did many other members of his family, and the duration of the episode and Parks' limited subsequent memory were consistent with somnambulism. Additionally, two separate polysomnograms indicated abnormal sleep patterns. At his trial, Parks was found not guilty and the Canadian Supreme Court upheld his acquittal. There was clearly significant "automatic" behavior but also some rather intricate motor skills and goal-direction. His neighbor observed some of his movements and described them as purposeful and task-oriented. Still, there is presumably no conscious ability to exercise willpower or self-control in such cases. Levy calls the automatic behaviors in question "action scripts" which guide actions, where a script is a set of motor representations that can be triggered by an appropriate stimulus and runs to completion [12].

Let me introduce a different but related sleeping case but which does not involve much motor behavior at all. Suppose your partner (with no history of somnambulism) rolls over in bed during the night and, apparently in deep sleep, says "I am going to kill you tomorrow" using your first name. This would seem to reflect some sort of (unconscious) first-order desire and belief. After all, people do talk in their sleep sometimes which seems far less involved than sleepwalking. I would imagine that you would mention this the next day, perhaps with some trepidation. Your partner may of course not remember it at all and would perhaps even be shocked. Suppose your partner assured you that it is not really something that reflects his or her "deep self" or second-order desires (assuming that your partner concedes that it was a genuine first-order desire in the first place). Perhaps your partner would even be willing to go for some counseling or psychotherapy in order assuage any fears you may have. Still, would you be convinced that your partner merely expressed a desire which will not be acted upon? Maybe, but, after all, addicts and kleptomaniacs still do sometimes act in accordance with their first-order desires.

The question I have is different and a challenge to the deep self-view: Why should the "deep" or "real" self be based on your partner's conscious second-order desires? After all, first, introspection is not infallible, and, second, the first-order desire (as expressed in an unconscious sleep state) may be precisely what your partner "really" wants to do. Surely, you might seriously wonder if your partner was expressing a real (or "deep") buried desire during sleep not articulated during normal waking hours. In other words, you might reasonably suppose that the stated desire expresses a true desire and even reflects your partner's hidden "real self." Why think that your real self is only manifested during conscious and introspective states? When we wonder what a person is really like or really thinks, it seems to me that we must be open to the possibility that the first-order desire (whether consciously or unconsciously expressed) expresses the real attitude. When awake and confronted by you, your partner may even engage in deception including self-deception. As is often shown in psychotherapy, it is the buried or unconscious desire that is the most real. Perhaps the same goes for Kenneth

Parks and his apparent desire to kill his in-laws—didn't he at least have the unconscious desire to kill them?

Now what makes an unconscious mental state, such as a desire, a conscious mental state? In previous work, I have defended the higher-order thought (HOT) theory of consciousness championed mainly by David Rosenthal [13, 14]. The idea is that what makes a mental state conscious is that it is the object of a suitable HOT which is a higher-order representation (HOR). A mental state M becomes conscious when there is a HOT directed at M. HOTs are cognitive states involving a conceptual component. A HOT is a "meta-psychological" or "meta-cognitive" state, that is, a mental state directed at another mental state. So, for example, my desire to drink some water or to smoke a cigarette becomes conscious when I am (non-inferentially) "aware" of the desire. Intuitively, it seems that conscious states, as opposed to unconscious ones, are mental states that I am "aware of" being in some sense. Conversely, the idea that I could be having a conscious state while totally *unaware* of being in that state seems contradictory. A mental state of which the subject is completely unaware is clearly an *un*conscious state. For example, I would not be aware of having a subliminal perception and thus it is an unconscious perception.

However, it is crucial to observe that, according to HOT theory, when a conscious mental state is a first-order world-directed state, the higher-order thought (HOT) is *not* itself conscious; otherwise, circularity and an infinite regress would follow. When the HOT is itself conscious, there is a yet higher-order (or third-order) thought directed at the second-order state. In this case, we have *introspection* which involves a conscious HOT directed at an inner mental state. When one introspects, one's attention is directed back into one's mind. For example, what makes a desire to ingest a drug a conscious first-order desire is that there is an unconscious HOT directed at the desire. In this case, one's conscious focus is directed at the drug. When one *introspects* that desire, however, one have a conscious HOT directed at the desire itself. This is an important distinction for any theory of consciousness and can also help us to understand the experience of drug addiction, compulsion, and self-control. One need not subscribe to HOT theory, however, in order to accept the above characterization of introspection as consciously thinking about one's own mental states.

As we have seen, Frankfurt emphasizes higher-order *desires* whereas HOT theory pays significant attention to higher-order *thoughts*. I can, for example, consciously think about or reflect on my strong desire to ingest a drug. This, in turn, may lead me to want to get rid of it or wish I didn't have it, as Frankfurt explains in terms of his deep self-compatibilism. I may then consciously try to overcome the compulsive desire for using a drug via self-control or willpower.

Importantly, we often shift back and forth between conscious beliefs and desires about the world and introspective states which involve thinking and reasoning about one's own mental states. Executive functions are often deployed in this process such as planning and reasoning. With regard to exercising self-control, introspection reveals various first-order desires and the addict may or may not have the power to change or eliminate those desires once the addict becomes aware of them. Higher-order conscious thoughts are directed a first-order addictive desires with the goal of eliminating them or lessening their compulsive force. This often requires significant conscious effort. Some addicts are able, even on their own sometimes, to achieve that goal using what we described above as "willpower." Some addicts can achieve this goal only with the help of others via rehabilitation, counseling, psychotherapy, or hypnosis. Other addicts are unable to use their introspective power to alter or eliminate the strong desire to take drugs. Another possibility is that a different stronger first-order desire is formed which can override or outweigh the desire for drug use. For example, a woman becomes pregnant and then becomes highly motivated not to cause harm to her future child so that she stops taking her drug of choice. Perhaps the father of the child also needs to get his act together for the sake of the child and stop taking drugs or gambling money away. This doesn't mean that the craving for drugs or the drug addiction itself is gone entirely but rather it is no longer the strongest desire. Of course, there are no guarantees that an addict will never slip back into the addictive behavior. This is why addicts and alcoholics typically refer to themselves as a "recovering addict" even many years after sobriety.

A Brain-Based Account?

Some of the above discussion about self-control and introspection might be put in more explicitly neurophysiological terms. Hirstein et al. [15], for example, emphasize the role of executive function—such as attentional control, planning, inhibition, and task switching—with regard to having free will and moral responsibility. But they also note the central role of the prefrontal cortex (PFC) in exercising these functions. "These capacities are implemented by brain structures primarily—though not exclusively—belonging to the cognitive control network and are known to the neuropsychological field as executive functions. These functions are what allow us to be agents with reasons, plans, and values and to coordinate our behavior accordingly as we move through a complex world."

It seems likely that the more sophisticated introspective states, including those associated with executive functions, would depend upon activity in the PFC. The general view expressed in the previous section can thus be understood from a neurological perspective. For example, it is known that there are feedback loops going from the PFC back to "lower-level" brain areas. At the risk of treating the PFC as a homunculus for the "self," let us suppose for the sake of argument that the PFC is where "you" reason and decide whether to act on more basic desires. Introspection and executive processes are some of the functions of the PFC and we might further suppose that they can be directed (top-down) to and causally affect lower-level neural areas such as those involved in drug addiction desires. It seems plausible to suppose that such a causal impact could have the effect of "controlling" or "suppressing" some lower-level brain activity including the strength of an addictive desire. After all, connections between neurons are sometimes described as having an inhibitory effect, which could lessen the first-order desires or cravings in other brain areas. The same perhaps goes for other addictions or disorders. Of course, many people are able to quickly or easily suppress a strong desire, say, even to commit a violent action against another or to resist the thought of committing suicide. The same goes for continuing to use a drug but just how much effort is necessary will depend on the particular person, desire, and introspective ability. In some cases, a person, especially with certain psychiatric conditions (e.g., psychopathy, OCD), will simply be entirely unable to suppress or control certain desires and actions.

Now, a drug addict may already have abnormal function of the PFC precisely due to the neurological effects of a drug habit. This will only hamper the ability to stop using drugs. The capacity for self-control, however, would still depend on the individual. Along these same lines, Volkow et al. [16] explain that "the changes that occur in the reward and emotional circuits of the brain are accompanied by changes in the function of the prefrontal cortical regions, which are involved in executive processes. Specifically, the down-regulation of dopamine signaling that dulls the reward circuits' sensitivity to pleasure also occurs in prefrontal brain regions and their associated circuits, seriously impairing executive processes." They explain that "in persons with addiction, the impaired signaling of dopamine and glutamate in the prefrontal regions of the brain weakens their ability to resist strong urges or to follow through on decisions to stop taking the drug. These effects explain why persons with addiction can be sincere in their desire and intention to stop using a drug and yet simultaneously unable to follow through on their resolve."

Volkow et al. also observe that "addictive drugs activate reward regions in the brain by causing sharp increases in the release of dopamine….This attenuated release of dopamine renders the brain's reward system much less sensitive to stimulation by both drug-related and nondrug-related rewards. As a result, persons with addiction no longer experience the same degree of euphoria from a drug as they did when they first started using it." Still, it is important to remember that a minority of people who use drugs become addicted. It surely depends upon differences in vulnerability to various genetic, environmental, and developmental factors. And, even further, the above view is also controversial to the extent that it may presuppose the disease model of addiction. While there is some evidence that addictive drugs can diminish self-control by damaging the prefrontal cortex, it does not follow that addicts lose it altogether.

It is also worth noting here that there is a significant decrease in PFC activity while dreaming which may again help to explain why we tend not to suppose that there is any chance for self-control in the somnambulism case described earlier. Indeed, for example, it seems obvious that Kenneth Parks was incapable of introspecting or reasoning during his murderous action. What matters most across the board is not whether the desire to kill or use drugs is conscious or feels compulsory, but rather whether consciously thinking about those desires can lead to suppressing them.

In closing, then, I have explored the relationship between the interrelated topics of the free will-determinism, addiction, compulsion, and self-control. As we have seen, having a feeling of, say, compulsion to use drugs is, by itself, irrelevant to whether the related actions are free according to both determinists and compatibilists. Compatibilists, such as Frankfurt, argue that the issue turns more on the presence or absence of certain second-order desires. I then raised some questions about this so-called "deep self" compatibilist view, such as whether we should always treat second-order desires as reflecting one's true self. We also saw that it is really through introspection that we sometimes consciously experience having some kind of "self-control." There may even be the beginnings of a brain-based account of self-control which can explain how our becoming consciously aware of our compulsions and using executive functions can sometimes lead to controlling addictive cravings.

References

1. Foddy B, Savulescu J. A liberal account of addiction. Philos Psychiatry Psychol. 2010;17:1–22, p. 1, 2.
2. Henden E. Addiction as a disorder of self-control. In: Pickard H, Ahmed S, editors. Routledge handbook of philosophy and science of addiction. London: Routledge Press; 2018.
3. Huoranszki F. Weakness and compulsion: the essential difference. Philos Explor. 2011;1:81–97.
4. Lavallee Z. Addictive craving: there's more to wanting more. Philos Psychiatry Psychol. 2020;17:227–38, p. 227.
5. Holton R, Berridge K. Addiction between compulsion and choice. In: Levy N, editor. Addiction and self-control. New York: Oxford University Press; 2013.
6. Kane R, editor. The Oxford handbook of free will. 2nd ed. New York: Oxford University Press; 2011.
7. McKenna M, Pereboom D. Free will: a contemporary introduction. New York: Routledge; 2016.
8. Frankfurt H. Freedom of the will and the concept of a person. J Philos. 1971;68:5–20.
9. Fischer J, Ravizza M. Responsibility and control: a theory of moral responsibility. Cambridge: Cambridge University Press; 1998.
10. Levy N, editor. Addiction and self-control. New York: Oxford University Press; 2013.
11. Santoni de Sio F, Di Nucci E. Pushing the margins of responsibility: lessons from Parks' somnambulistic killing. Neuroethics. 2018;11:35–46.
12. Levy N. Consciousness and moral responsibility. New York: Oxford University Press; 2014.
13. Rosenthal D. Consciousness and mind. New York: Oxford University Press; 2005.
14. Gennaro R. The consciousness paradox: consciousness, concepts, and higher-order thoughts. Cambridge, MA: The MIT Press; 2012.
15. Hirstein W, Sifferd K, Fagan T. Responsible brans: neuroscience, law, and human culpability. Cambridge, MA: The MIT Press; 2018. p. 13.
16. Volkow N, Koob G, McLellan T. Neurobiologic advances from the brain disease model of addiction. N Engl J Med. 2016;374:363–71, p. 367, 364.

8 The Beginning of Consumption as Antidepressant Self-Medication

Ricardo Aranovich

Addictive drugs have been known since ancient times. It is worth wondering why it is currently increasing its consumption in the way it does. The answer could be found, at least in part, in cultural factors that affect the way of life and the psychological state of society. Ortega y Gasset says: "We live in a time that feels fabulously capable of doing things, but doesn't know what to do. He dominates all things, but he is not master of himself [...] With more means, more knowledge, more techniques than ever, it turns out that today's world is going like the most unfortunate one that has ever been purely adrift" [1].

A sector of society that appears to be particularly vulnerable is that of adolescents and youth. In these times, the acquisition of addictive behaviours is frequent. In this chapter, we will develop some hypotheses in relation to this phenomenon and its relationship with what happens in other stages of existence. Adolescents and youth are the repositories of a cultural attitude that shows them as "the happiest time of life". In Spanish, there are statements such as "Youth, divine treasure" that account for this idea. However, the real situation of the adolescent and the young person is quite different.

The adolescent is until recently a child to whom the needs of the adult suddenly arise without having the resources to satisfy them. Sexual desires appear to him, he would like to have his own economic resources and he struggles to affirm an incipient identity. For this, he reacts against the paternal authority and affirms himself in his peers as referents of conduct. He finds himself having to integrate socially in a strange environment with new demands and prestige guidelines and is very competitive. He begins to have to think about his future, which is uncertain and, depending on the socio-economic context in which he lives, more or less favourable and/or problematic.

A perspective like this would put an adult at risk of a major depressive state. In the young, an element is added that is the aforementioned cultural attitude about happiness that is supposed to be typical of youth. The young man is required to be in good spirits to sustain acceptance among his peers. If he does not run the risk of rejection and marginalization (he is "bitter"). Consequently, we can assume that a number of young people are experiencing what we could define as a hidden depression, which does not find a containing or understanding attitude in the adult world.

On the contrary, he finds himself faced with the reiteration that it is "the best time in life", "the one to take advantage of", in which being depressed should be embarrassing. "And you, what problems can you have?", the adults blurt out to the young man. They completely ignore the problem that afflicts them the biggest of all is

R. Aranovich (✉)
Fundación Acta, Ciudad de Buenos Aires, Argentina

P. Á. Gargiulo, H. L. Mesones-Arroyo (eds.), *Psychiatry and Neuroscience Update – Vol. V*,
https://doi.org/10.1007/978-3-031-72219-6_8

that of the future. It is equivalent to saying that what is not resolved is himself, his own person. As Ortega expresses, "… It is, then, life that paradoxical reality that consists in deciding what we are going to be—therefore, in being what we are not yet, in starting by being future…" [2]. We must bear in mind that cocaine, in addition to its antidepressant effect, increases the feeling of power and security, so that it diminishes, for the moment, all the fears that you might have about your future possibilities.

In this situation, the first contact with the drug occurs. The inevitable environmental influence induces it. It is usually a very pleasant experience and determines new experiences. I remember a case in which the patient told me about his first experience with cocaine: "This can't be bad, it's all lies". We may assume that he experienced relief from his depressive state.

Those who design campaigns against addictions should consider this situation. They usually focus their advertising on the deterioration and other effects that the habit of consuming illegal substances produces, but they should also strongly warn against the very favourable effect experienced in the first or first contact with the drug and that it is time for increased risk of becoming addicted. It should be borne in mind that, at first, the future addict deludes himself with the illusion that he is not going to fall into dependency because it is not yet installed in him. The expression that reflects this state are "I handle it", "If I want I can leave it" and "Until it's too late".

There is a similarity with what happens in youth and in other times of life. It is that the drug compensates for the state produced by the lack of stimulating purpose in life. In the case of the young man, this is notorious. The panorama that is presented to him facilitates discouragement. To clarify this situation we should make an incursion into aspects of the culture in which the young person currently finds himself.

The young people must find a way to achieve their own economic autonomy. The most frequent way to prepare for that, if he finds himself in an environment that can provide it, is to take a university degree that, when received, gives him a qualification to practice a profession. However, even in this situation, in which he appears to be privileged in relation to others, other difficulties appear. Not all careers ensure that his exercise will be profitable enough. Then, the "employment exit" is privileged and the career is chosen following that criterion, which results in careers that become fashionable, disregarding the fundamental thing: vocation. Moreover, in the face of the uncertainty of the future, the only thing that diminishes anguish and generates energy for action is the mystery of one's vocation. Without a vocation, the future appears to the young person as an effort with no more meaning than economics. In addition, even that, in an increasingly competitive society, is somewhat uncertain. Even more difficult is the situation of the young person who has to work. There are very few stimulating jobs and in the others, he ends up feeling under an obligation in which he does not find any attraction.

What is the importance of vocation? The human being is conditioned by material and emotional needs: oxygen, food, housing, company, he does not know his future, and even more, he does not choose his date or his place of birth nor does he know the moment of his death. With such conditioning, we can say that he lacks freedom, but there is the paradox that freedom is, at the same time, a fundamental desire. In reality, the human being feels free when, despite all the circumstances in which he finds himself and, even more, taking advantage of some of them, he manages to do something that he wants to do. In other words, freedom is not doing anything, which would lead to dispersion and a greater loss of freedom.

The human being feels free when he is delivered to an action that responds to his desire, something that he "wants" to do. However, it is not just any doing. Rather it acquires strength and meaning to the extent that it is part of a life project. This project of life is, at the same time, the answer to the uncertainty of the future. Faced with needs and uncertainties, the human being has the capacity and the possibility to develop a coping plan, a hypothesis and a project in favour of which he feels solves his life. Nevertheless, this project is much more than just solving needs.

Carrying out that project itself becomes the fundamental need in relation to which the other needs take a backseat.

That is the vocation. Let us listen to Ortega y Gasset: "In such a way that each of our actions demands that we make it spring from the total anticipation of our destiny and derive it from a general program for our existence. (…) This call that we feel towards a type of life, this voice or imperative cry that rises from our most radical background, is the vocation" [3]. The true response to needs is not limited to solving them. What emerges is something distinctively human.

The impulse to develop and carry out a life argument of their own, to achieve goals that are no longer related to material needs, but that produce satisfaction by themselves and, when they solve the needs, it is in addition. In addition, satisfaction increases to the extent that the subject feels that he is improving in his actions. On the other hand, is it evolving? That is why whoever lives according to his vocation feels free because the impetus for action is not born of needs. These are overcome as a life goal. We know well that this is an ideal, but like any ideal, we will be better off to the extent that we can get closer to it.

However, man is not always clear about the path that would bring him closer to the ideal. In this regard, Ortega y Gasset also tells us: "Each man, among his various possible beings, always finds one who is his authentic being. And the voice that he calls to that authentic being is what is called 'vocation'. But the majority of men dedicate themselves to silencing and ignoring that voice of vocation. He tries to make noise within himself, deafen himself, distract himself so as not to hear her and cheat himself by substituting his authentic being for a false vital trajectory. Instead, he only lives himself, only the one who lives his vocation truly lives, the one who coincides with his true 'self'" [4].

It happens that the current way of life does not favour that coincidence with itself. To achieve it, it is necessary to abstract from external stimuli, turn "inside" adopt an attitude of searching and listening inside, and be ready to pay attention to the thoughts and feelings that arise. Ortega y Gasset distinguishes being in contact with oneself and calls it "introspection" or turned towards the outside and calls it "alteration" and deals with both in his essay "Introspection and Alteration", where he says: "Almost everyone is altered, and in alteration, man loses his most essential attribute; the possibility of meditating, of withdrawing within himself to come to an agreement with himself and specify what he believes; what he really likes and what he really hates. The alteration beclouds him, blinds him, forces him to act mechanically, in a frantic sleepwalking" [5].

And this state of affairs, which affects everyone, affects particularly young people. In these people, in whom the absence of an interior life that would provide them with some peace and balance leads them to seek the solution of their anxieties in external action and, in the face of the failure of their attempts they become depressed and seek to get out of that painful state with what is most at hand: drugs.

In addition, what could he turn to? Although Ortega y Gasset already spoke more than 80 years ago of the drawbacks of the superficialization of the way of life, we have closer testimonies of the consequences of this trend.

Jérôme Bindé, Professor of Literature and Director of the Prospective Office of the United Nations Educational, Scientific and Cultural Organization (Unesco), states: "There are no longer traditional values", "Contemporary societies suffer a crisis of values. Those who yesterday were considered important were displaced by the frivolous. This crisis is no longer just that of the traditional moral frameworks, inherited from the great religious confessions, but also that of the secular values that succeeded them." [6].

This is the reason why we have stopped at the topic of vocation. Faced with the uncertainty of his future and in a world of confused values, the young person (and the adult) must look within himself for the element in which to affirm himself to face his existence. That element is a vocation. Moreover, we are not referring to a restrictive sense of profession or trade. The vocation implies experiencing the possibility of dedicating one's life to something transcendent. Viktor Frankl expresses it by talking about meaning. "Man's search for the meaning of life constitutes a primary force and not a "secondary realization" of its instinctive impulses (...) it is oneself and one alone who has to find it (...) I do not consider that we invent the meaning of our existence, but that we discover it" [7].

As we have seen above, the vocation is the way of acting not out of material need, however the need is satisfied by the action itself and that is what is experienced as freedom in this life and is the best antidote against depression.

"Obviously, it is our life-project, which, in the case of suffering, does not coincide with our actual life; man dilates, splits into two—the one that had to be and the one that turns out to be. The dislocation manifests itself in the form of pain, anguish, anger, bad humor, emptiness; coincidence, on the other hand, produces the prodigious phenomenon of happiness" [8], Ortega y Gasset tells us again.

In Genesis, God said to Adam when expelling him from Paradise: "You will earn your bread with the sweat of your brow" which, of course, also applied to his descendants. If we want to imagine that, even expelled from Paradise, the human being continues to be a child of God, we can suppose that He gave him a way to soften the sentence and that this is the vocation, which lightens the effort, turns it into enthusiasm and opens the way to the action itself, disinterested and, often, more supportive. This leads us to consider vocation as a manifestation of the spiritual condition of the human being.

It all depends on how the young person is going to live his life and this, of course, depends on influences, family, education, friends, environment and culture (e.g., television). Moreover, at the rate we are going, these influences do not point to the young person deepening his introspection in search of a contact with himself that allows him to maintain balance and serenity in the face of the avalanche of external stimuli. The young man finds himself before an enormous and tempting offer of material goods that he is not usually in a position to acquire and, as the possession of these seems to be the most important, he experiences a state of impotence that accentuates his depression, or, worse still, leads to marginalization and maladaptive or criminal behaviour. It is known that, once the addiction is acquired, the need for money to solve it brings it dangerously close to this last alternative.

Another possibility of giving meaning to his existence would be the cultivation of religious, philosophical, artistic, political or other interests that would allow him to join groups that shared those same interests and not that the discotheque be the one that occupies an almost exclusive place as a space of socialization. However, in this regard, it is required that the young person can make a first move that brings him closer to other interests. Here, once again, the cultural and social context is decisive. "Science, art, justice, courtesy, religion are orbits of reality that do not barbarously invade our people, as hunger or cold do; they only exist for those who have the will for them." Ortega y Gasset tells us in this regard [9].

If we take all these situations later in life, cocaine use continues to be motivated by the search for extra energy to respond to the demands that life poses. However, it can be assumed that the origin of this lack of energy, as in youth and at other stages of life is also due to a lack of motivation caused by the same factors mentioned. Depression has become the leading cause of disability according to the WHO (World Health Organization) [10] without being limited to one age or another. This may account for stimulant use beyond youth.

The other drug whose use is epidemic is marijuana. Moreover, the reason for this fact is a sort of flip side of what happens with cocaine. In this case, the coexistence of demand and uncertainty is also an important factor, however instead of seeking a sense of security and increased coping capacity typical of stimulants, the marijuana user seeks relief from the anguish that comes from that unresolved situation.

Human society requires that the individuals comprising it have behaviours that favour its persistence and growth. For this, it has developed a culture that trains its members in that sense. Thus, individuals acquire and develop capacities that, in addition to ensuring their own survival, are also useful for the whole. For this, society, as a great educator, stimulates these behaviours. Let's say that since the beginning of time, humanity has been educating itself so that its members are of benefit and support for their life in society. It leads to approval, in the family first and society later and is the fundamental tool. For example, school achievements generate an environmental response of approval and praise that activates at the brain level a reaction mediated by the release of dopamine that stimulates and reinforces the motivation to persist and add more achievements. The one responsible for this reaction is the mesolimbic pathway, also called the reward or gratification pathway [11]. This is related to the satisfaction that the subject experiences every time he achieves a favourable result in her life. The subject makes an effort in pursuit of a goal and, upon reaching it, in addition to the objective advantages obtained. He experiences a state of fullness, satisfaction and reinforcement of self-esteem that predisposes him to continue improving himself.

Well, marijuana stimulates the dopaminergic pathway of gratification and those who consume it feel that they cannot worry, without having to make an effort; they feel as if they have already achieved their goal. In a society with the current level of demand and competitiveness, it is not surprising that there are users of marijuana who seek to alleviate the tension generated by a work situation with a demand that does not yield in intensity or duration. This is the motivation for consumption on weekends or "after the office". But, as we have seen, adolescents and young people are also required by an unknown and, moreover, uncertain future. And, in these cases, marijuana also relieves that state and replaces it with a feeling that everything is fine, that there is no need to make an effort for anything because a state of satisfaction is experienced as if all the needs had already been resolved.

I remember a case of a young man who used marijuana, the son of a very busy prestigious colleague. The son saw the father's demands in schedules and occupations and advised him: "Come «old man» stop! Relax, smoke a "joint" with me and stop running around. You'll see how good you feel",

As with any addictive substance, the first experiences are very satisfactory, but then the effect decreases and tolerance occurs, that is, a higher dose is required for a declining effect. However, with marijuana, something special happens on that path. The reward pathway, whose effect is stimulated by the drug, ceases to act, through tolerance, even though the drug is still present. The result is that the entire delicate motivational system with which humanity has always been educating itself collapses and the addict loses all initiative and interest in his personal evolution. This is how inexplicable (for parents and relatives) dropouts of activities, university careers and studies occur, even in advanced degrees.

This leads us to reconsider the proclaimed innocuousness of marijuana since, although it does not affect certain organs, such as alcohol or tobacco, it affects the capacity for action and fulfilment in life, which ultimately implies a serious disability.

In any case, whether one or the other is the substance whose consumption leads to addiction, we can relate the initial contact with the search for a resource that alleviates the depressive mood produced by what the subject perceives as a gap between the demands that society places on him and his ability to cope with them. So he looks for something that stimulates him, makes him feel more energetic and thus is able to face social situations with greater security and being "up to the task". Or if not, something that allows him to stop worrying and get out of the annoying and distressing state of uncertainty about the alternatives, favourable or not, that he could find in his life and feel as if he had already resolved everything well.

Let's go back to the cultural situation in which addictions develop. The family-society continuum is what must generate the conditions in young people so that they become enthusiastic about an activity that responds to their vocation. It is noteworthy that, although there are expressions of concern about the issue of addictions, few voices are heard that address the issue as a symptom of a state of society. In addition, what does the young man see around him? The desert.

A few years ago, all young people were going to resolve their lives by being "rock" or "pop" stars. Moreover, the young women projected themselves as models or singers. Traditional occupations, such as scientists, entrepreneurs, engineers, and journalists, were not very attractive; they seemed to lack the ability to light the fire of vocation, to arouse enthusiasm, to mobilize the energies that set in motion the inner springs whose action is in action in life. This lack of interest in these professions and the interest in others more linked to entertainment has nothing to do with the vocation but with a "fashion". Fashion is collective, impersonal and superficial, it only requires "letting go", that is, the opposite of the responsible and sincere introspection that requires discovering one's own vocation. Let's see how Ortega y Gasset expresses it: "I want to say that our life is never a simple being, a pure lying down. To live is always to live, for something or for something; is a transitive verb. Hence, there can be no human life without a vital interest, which sustains, constitutes and organizes that life. In the moment, all vital interest was completely and effectively slackened, life would cease to be" [12].

In a depressed mood, there is a lack of energy, of vitality and, without vitality, that state in which vitality and vocation would be enhanced can hardly occur. On the contrary, a negative interaction occurs depression—lack of energy—lack of interest—depression, etc. Instead, the synergy between vitality and vocation is what comes closest to a state of wholeness and confidence. In this case, there is no need to resort to any consumption to face the overwhelming uncertainty of an existence without interest or motivation.

Returning to the young man (or the young woman), in that age group depression usually has the characteristics of what is called "Concealed Depression". In favour of the energy typical of age, young people can maintain an apparently normal rhythm of activities, despite being in a depressive state that would have an older person turned over in bed. Given that for the topic at hand, it is of the utmost importance to detect this situation, parents should be prepared to notice small signs. The young person stopped going out on some weekend nights and stayed at home when always discussions were given to the contrary. He always had good grades and has a drop in his performance as a student. He is irritable, moody and has bad responses, which is unusual. He spends more time locked in his room, which, on the other hand, is more messy than usual. He is less talkative. He has less interaction with friends. He is unwilling for his usual sport. If some or several of these circumstances occur, even though, for example, they continue to attend school and comply with schedules, a consultation with a psychiatrist specializing in young people is necessary. An adequate therapeutic intervention is, without comparison, preferable to an addictive self-medication.

References

1. Ortega y Gasset J. Obras Completas. Madrid: Editorial Taurus; 2005. Tomo IV, p. 398.
2. Ortega y Gasset J. Obras Completas. Madrid: Editorial Taurus; 2008. Tomo VIII, p. 369.
3. Ortega y Gasset J. Obras Completas. Madrid: Editorial Taurus; 2006. Tomo V, p. 350.
4. Ortega y Gasset J. Obras Completas. Madrid: Editorial Taurus; 2006. Tomo VI, p. 483.
5. Ortega y Gasset J. Obras Completas. Madrid: Editorial Taurus; 2010. Tomo X, p. 142.
6. Bindé J. ¿Hacia dónde se dirigen los valores? Coloquios del Siglo XXI. Fondo de Cultura Económica, México; 2006. https://fce.com.ar/wp-content/uploads/2020/11/Binde.pdf.
7. Frankl VE. El hombre en busca de sentido. Barcelona: Editorial Herder; 1984. p. 98.
8. Ortega y Gasset J. Obras Completas. Madrid: Editorial Taurus; 2006. Tomo V, p. 131.
9. Ortega y Gasset J. Obras Completas. Madrid: Editorial Taurus; 2004. Tomo I, p. 769.
10. World Health Organization (WHO). Depression; 2021 September 13. https://www.who.int/es/news-room/fact-sheets/detail/depression.
11. Lac A, Luk JW. Testing the amotivational syndrome: marijuana use longitudinally predicts lower self-efficacy even after controlling for demographics, personality, and alcohol and cigarette use. Prev Sci. 2018;19(2):117–26. https://doi.org/10.1007/s11121-017-0811-3. PMID: 28620722; PMCID: PMC5732901. https://pubmed.ncbi.nlm.nih.gov/28620722/.
12. Ortega y Gasset J. Obras Completas. Madrid: Editorial Taurus; 2004. Tomo II, p. 747.

The Use of Coca in Miners

9

Ricardo Jorge Llanque Ferrufino

Introduction

This ethnographic work will identify some sociocultural factors (see Figs. 9.1, 9.2, 9.3, 9.4, 9.5, 9.6, 9.7, 9.8, 9.9 and 9.10) that we consider very relevant determinants in the ritual of coca leaf *pijcheo* by Bolivian miners in the Cerro de San José in the city of Oruro, Bolivia.

Bertonio refers to chewing coca in Aymara is *Hallchitha, hallpatha* [1]. In ancient Aymara, the term *pijchu* does not exist as a synonym for chewing coca, but there is the term *phichu*, which, among other meanings, refers to eye lashes. In its symbolic nature, it is identified with the following terms: *nayra phichuna hamppatitha*. It means tearing off the eyelashes, worshiping the idols or *wakas*. For her part, *Nayra phichuna phustiritha* refers to blowing her eyelashes toward the *wuakas*, worshiping them. It is a clear reference to what describes the chronicles and some contemporary researchers. In these stories, they refer that when arriving at the shores of the sea and to worship the *mama cocha* or the goddess of the sea, the Andeans removed their eyelashes and offered them to the goddess asking for her protection [2]. On the other hand, *phichu* also means good or bad fame, the coat of arms and glory of each one. Likewise, *pichuta* means to tie the

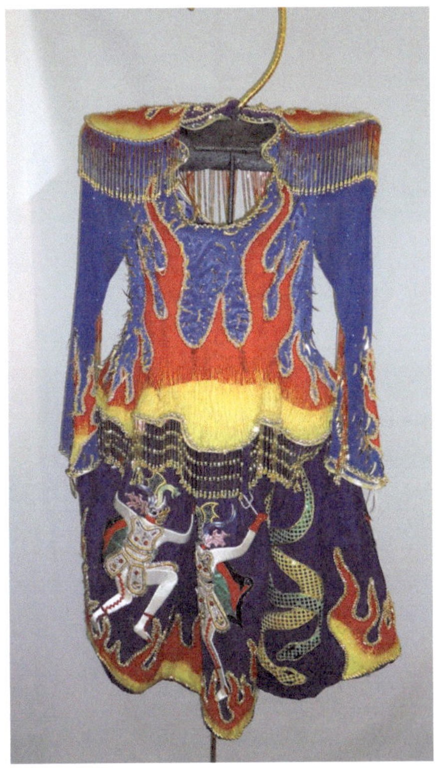

Fig. 9.1 "Ancient" (*ñaupa*) dress of a *supay* (evil) *china* (woman). Note the modesty of the suit with the skirt reaching below the knees. The skirt has dancing devils as figures

R. J. Llanque Ferrufino (✉)
Antropólogo. Carrera de Antropología, Universidad Técnica de Oruro, Oruro, Bolivia
e-mail: jorgellanque@antropologiauto.com

P. Á. Gargiulo, H. L. Mesones-Arroyo (eds.), *Psychiatry and Neuroscience Update – Vol. V*,
https://doi.org/10.1007/978-3-031-72219-6_9

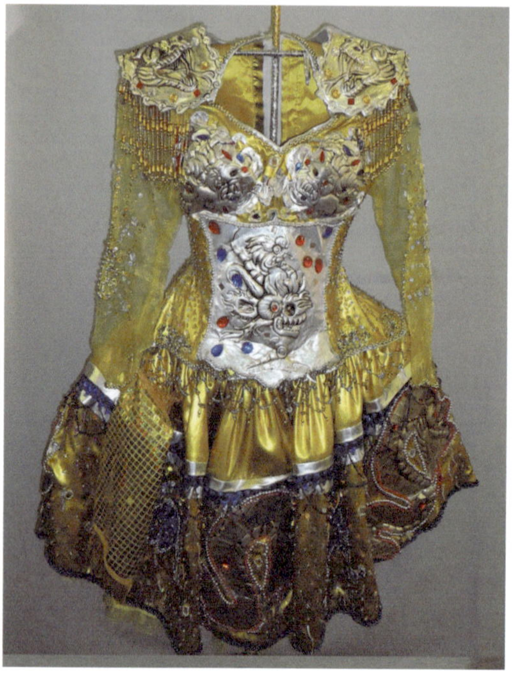

Fig. 9.2 Young *supay* (*evil*) *china* (woman) costume. This design is more daring since it means doom in lust

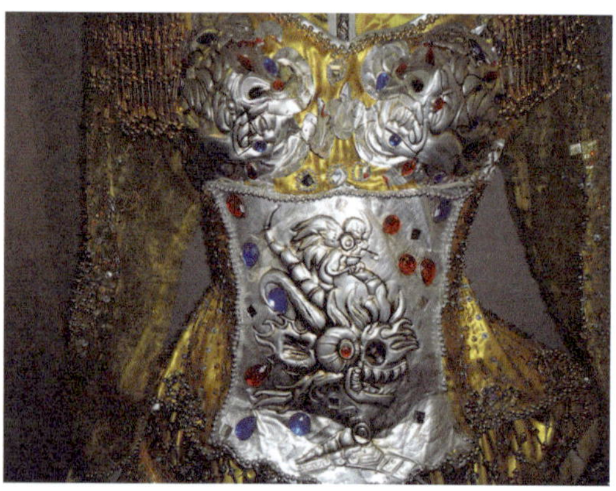

Fig. 9.3 Detail of the china supay suit with embossed metal

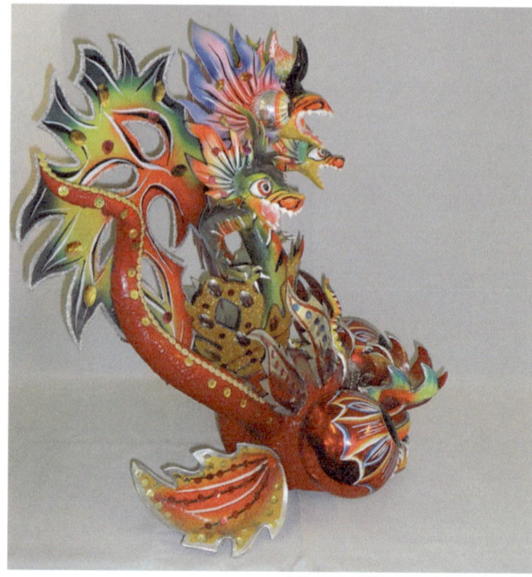

Fig. 9.4 Side view of traditional Oruro Carnival Devil mask. Historically, it is related to the *Tío* (*Uncle*) of the mine, because the Catholic Church related all Andean deities to the devil

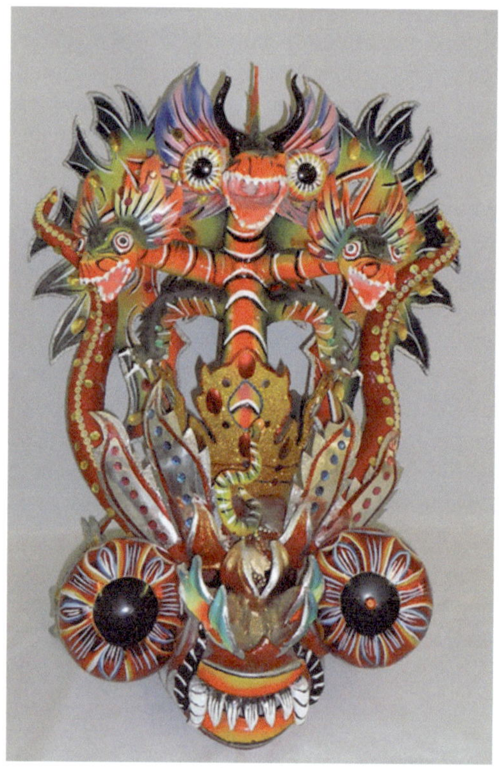

Fig. 9.5 Front view of traditional devil mask. Note the dragons that refer to the diabolic character but also to pre-Aymara *urus* deities related to water

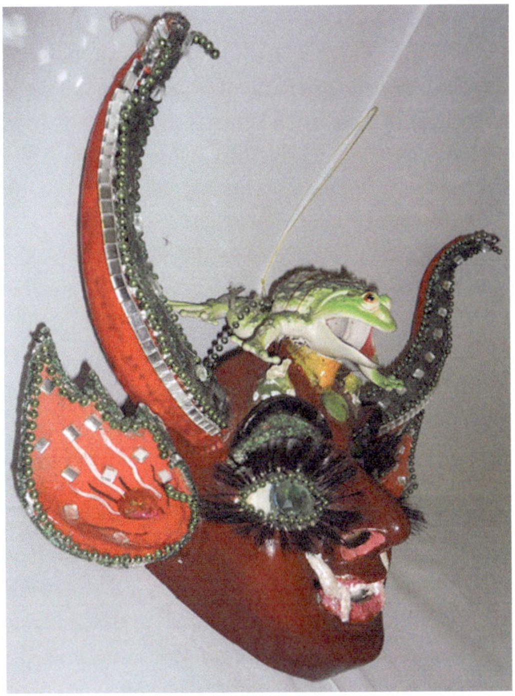

Fig. 9.6 *China supay* mask, diabolical female figure, temptation of lust in men. She together with the devils dance through the streets of Oruro and finally pay homage to the "*Virgen del Socavón*" ("*Sinkhole Virgin*")

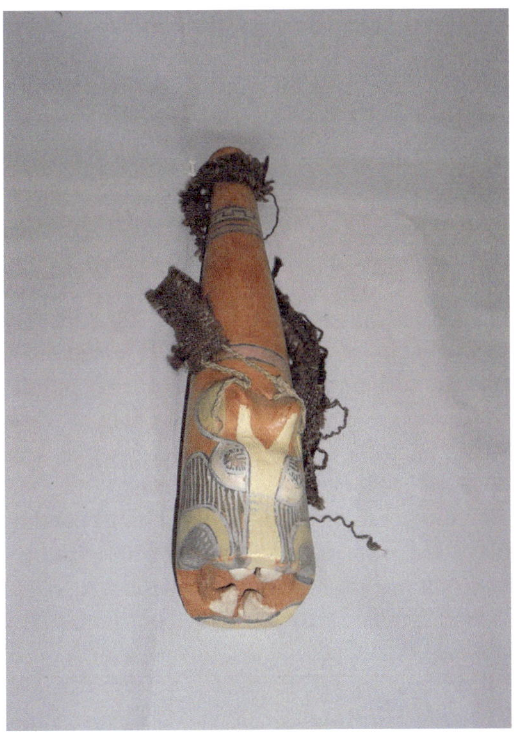

Fig. 9.7 Ceramic *Pututu*, with Tihuanaco motifs. It is the representation of an *otoronko* or Andean jaguar. The *pututus* are also made with the horns of the bull

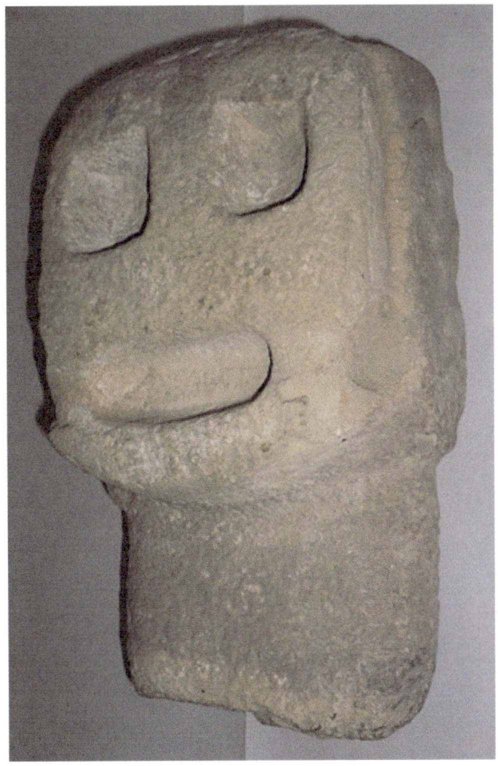

Fig. 9.8 Nail head (*Wankarani-Oruro* culture). It is a transition between llama and puma. It may be the first manifestation of a transfigured deity of both animals

mouth of the sack or bags. Finally, *phichu* is the end of the wool that is removed before spinning.

Therefore, the term *pijchu* in *Aymara* is a corruption of the ancient symbolic word of *phichu* (eyelash, good deeds, close the mouth of the sack). In its sacred character, the eyelashes are seen as an offering or element of transubstantiation to the sea and the ancient *wakas*. In this case, the coca *pijchada*—assuming the character of the eyelashes—is seen as an element of offering to the hill, its guardians and its veins, which, like the *mama cocha* (with its own guardians and marine veins) can change or not its opinion with respect to whoever dares to enter their domains.

Regarding Quechua [3], it seems that it was not possible to identify a special term for chewing coca as a ritual, chewing is *camuni*. On the other hand, *acuni acullicuni* is called *eating coca,* that is, as part of the diet, not as a ritual process. *Actuni* or *hacchuni* or *acturcuni* has reference to the previous term: *spitting coca and pouring out*

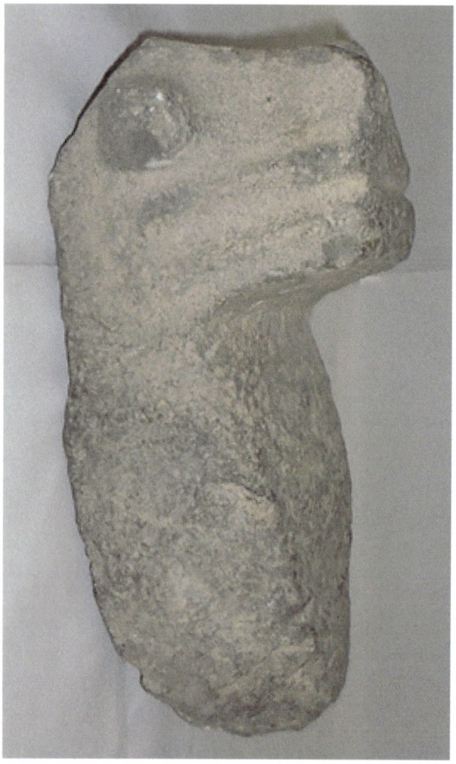

Fig. 9.9 Lithic figure (*Wankarani-Oruro* culture), apparently of the nail type with serpentine motifs, the deity of water

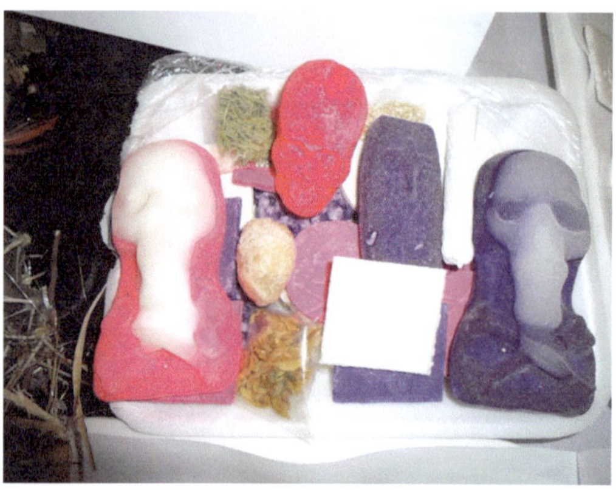

Fig. 9.10 Complementary offerings used in the "*Andean tables*" to the *Pachamama* and other deities, in the shape of human skulls, representation of the dead. In the central Andes, especially in the case of Oruro, the dead begin the rainy season, a time of revitalization of space, of productivity. Death in this sense assumes the character of life

of the mouth what is brought in it. It implies that having consumed all its juices or all the benefits that coca has, one gets rid of it, assuming all these terms in Quechua to the daily use of coca as food and not as a ritual. Therefore, the present study focuses on *pijchu* as ritual consumption with these identified characteristics.

In this way, *Phijchar* in the mine means the previous ritual process in the company of the *Tío* (*Uncle*, underground mining deity). Subsequently, chewing the coca leaves little by little to extract their juice is an activity that takes place over a long period and is a traditional part of the miners' preparation process prior to work. It also takes place when it is necessary to change the *pijchu* on the second day of work. The difference with the *Acullicu* is that this other practice is identified as part of everyday life.

We circumscribe our theme from the analysis of the social fields of Pierre Bourdieu and the modern *Aymara* personality. The latter "is made up of two subsystems: one oriented towards the *ayllu*, which has remained unchanged with respect to the configuration of the pre-Columbian personality, and the other directed towards the Hispano-Creole national society, which has been inverted in correspondence with the inversion of the real and mythical world occurred after the conquest" [4].

In the mining case, the dialogue is dialectical [5]. It is identified that the productive relations determine many factors of consolidation of the mining identity. Likewise, [6] the contextual conditions of the cooperative miners have configured other routes of dialogue in the mining identity dynamics. In this sense, as Rivera mentions, a "ch'ixi" vision is assumed. In it, there is no predominance of black and white, but actually gray, as the interaction of various values and patterns necessary to form what we call identity, "…literally refers to mottled gray, formed from countless black and white points that are unified for perception, but remain pure, separated", and serves to "admit the permanent struggle in our subjectivity between the Indian and the European" [7].

This identity construction process is due to several factors such as the historical, sociocultural, sociological context, and modernity itself. Regarding a contemporary sociological vision of the miners, see [6].

The data collection method is qualitative-ethnographic with emphasis on participant observation and interviews with miners chosen by an Oruro Cooperative to be able to work in these job interviews in the symbolic spaces identified by the institution itself.

Methodology

The present work is qualitative, with emphasis on the development of field interviews. To this end, we realized an agreement between the Anthropology School of the Technical University of Oruro and a mining cooperative in the city of Oruro. We expected that the result of these interviews would be the elaboration of a work text that will serve the aforementioned cooperative.

Similarly, as part of the interaction work, six interns have been designated in different years (2019–2020–2022) to carry out support work in the aforementioned Cooperative and to serve them as part of their graduation process. We do not mention the name of the institution, even for security reasons.

Our purpose is to extend these preliminary data even from fieldwork over 2 years. This will allow us to further strength studies in the field of mining. In addition, with the interns, it is sought to be able to develop some alternative actions that favour this or other mining cooperatives that are part of the current Bolivian reality.

Results

In the case of Oruro, it is known that the Mines of this city were exploited even before the Inca period according to various studies in the archaeological field [8, 9]. Subsequently, Lorenzo de Aldana manages to obtain the distribution of the land of Paria and exploits its mineral wealth by the hand of the Urus miners who lived at that time, when this Spaniard died. Apparently, he was sterile. For this reason, it had no heirs other than the *Urus*, *soras,* and *casayas* themselves, which have been studied [10]. It has been explained the journey that these ethnic groups had to go through in order to benefit from this inheritance. Others take charge of the mines and finally, they founded the Villa Real de San Felipe de Austria, today Oruro. The working of the mines was different since the town did not have *mitayos* (Indians subjected to the *mita* system) to work. It allowed greater flexibility in labour relations at the time. Mining concessions were individualized. However, mining has its ups and downs and in this way the mines of the town of Oruro were owned by Spaniards, British, Chileans and nationals with varied moments of splendour and moments of calm even until well into the beginning of the republic.

With the incursion of liberalism, the mines passed into different private hands, among which the Oruro mining company (formed with Chilean capital) stands out among others. The revolution of 1952 allows the nationalization of the mines. It allowed the creating of a leafy bureaucratic apparatus. In it, the miners become salaried, but also by forming unions. They were part of groups with Marxist tendencies. This fact, on occasion (Barrientos Presidency), generates that San José closed its doors. However, over time the statist character of the mines continued to be maintained, until well into the 1980s, when the current model could no longer follow what required the application of Supreme Decree 21,060, leading to the mass dismissal of miners.

With the promulgation of this Decree on August 29, 1985, many of the state miners were "relocated". This term was not real because they were fired. Faced with this, many with their settlement travelled to other departments or countries. Others stayed in place, looking for other options, including mining but cooperative, as in

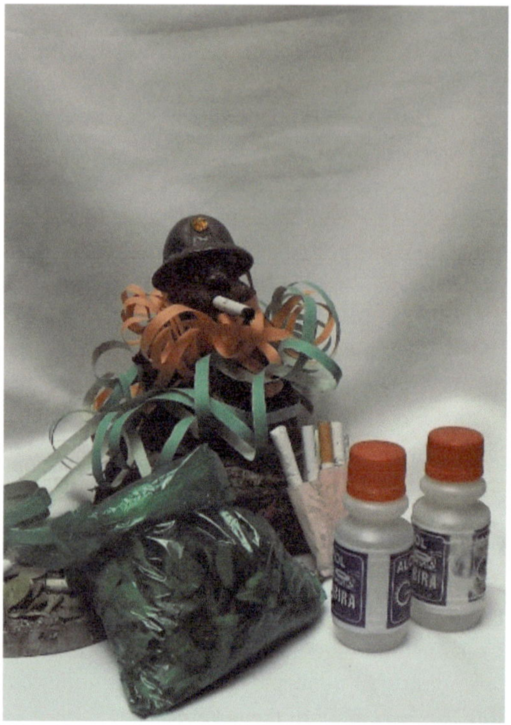

Fig. 9.11 *Tío* (*Uncle*), Andean deity guardian of the mineral veins. It may be modelled as in this case or just be a piece of pure mineral that assumes anthropomorphic characteristics for his acolytes. Note that he has cigarettes and coke as part of the daily offering in the pijchus

the present case. Currently, the city of Oruro has several cooperatives [10] that are taking charge of the exploitation of different types of minerals in the different hills of the city.

In the case of the San José mine, an original study focuses above all on the mining cultural patterns that were consolidated in a unionized hegemony against the dominant and ruling elites. This study reflects new spaces of confrontation and dialogue, in which the *Tío* (*Uncle*) (see Fig. 9.11) and the miners establish relationships of reciprocity and mutual nourishment between them: "We eat from the mine and the mine eats us" [5]. From anthropological science, it should be considered the study carried out by Nash [11]. It identifies some peculiarities of *pijcheo* in state mining. This study says the following:

> …we start to *ch'allar* in the workplaces inside the mine; we bring banners, mix and streamers. First, we start with the *Uncle*. We put a cigarette in his mouth. After this, we pour alcohol on the ground for the *Pachamama*. Then we give it to *Uncle*. Then we get out our coke and start chewing and smoking. We serve liquor from the bottles each of us has brought. We light Uncle's cigarette and tell him: "*Uncle*, help us in our work, don't let us have accidents". We do not kneel before him as we would before a saint because that would be sacrilege. Then, we all started getting drunk. We talk about our work and the sacrifice we are making. When this is over, we wrap the streamer around Uncle's neck. We prepare our tables and after some time we say, "Let's go". Some have to carry those who are drunk. We go to the place where we change our clothes. Moreover, when we leave there again, we make the offering of the liquor, pennants and we wrap our necks with streamers. From then on, each one does what they want, they go home or continue drinking, but it is their decision. [11]

In the aforementioned ritual described by this author, perhaps what has disappeared is the use of a mixture flags and streamers. However, apparently Nash is describing a *pijchu* closthe e to carnival or in August due to the festive nature of her description (a kind of flourish of the mine similar to that of the cattle). However, the identified elements and context survive in many aspects today in the daily *pijchus* that are made in the mine, except for what we mentioned.

In our brief fieldwork, cooperative miners rediscovered a mine on Cerro San José. To avoid conflicts with several of the relocated miners, the Bolivian Mining Commission (COMIBOL) agreed to grant spaces for the exploitation of minerals to former state miners associated with cooperatives. In this way, COMIBOL avoided conflicts and left these now cooperative miners to risk their own capital. On the other hand, they themselves absorbed the floating workforce. They had to open a shaft that had been buried in another time and rediscovered two *Uncles* who guarded that abandoned mine. The aforementioned figures were approximately 200 m from the entrance. In this way, the miners gave life to the place, in this case risking their own resources.

This ritual space to carry out the *pijchu* has a high symbolic value for the aforementioned cooperative. It was the first reception they had after opening the sealed mine. It serves above all to receive visitors—according to our informants—since in different sections of the mine, the cooperative members themselves have created their own *uncles* and *aunts* where they *pijchan* in their places to be able to ask for protection.

It can be said that the mine is like an underground labyrinthine stone city, where only its occasional owners know its places and its exploitation spaces. The first daily challenge is to reach one's destination, avoiding various obstacles such as flooded areas, and going up or down to other levels if there is luck with stairs or otherwise only with ropes. Their daily diaspora includes humid or extremely hot places, and the miners avoiding all these obstacles. In recent times, several women have become miners and they are not the traditional *palliris*. The term "Palliri" designates people, generally women, whose job it is to collect, choose and pulverize rocks, coming from residues of the mining industry. Through this procedure, they obtain material. However, here they are women who work inside the mine. In this way, the patriarchal myth that only men should enter the mine has been broken, because otherwise, they would scare away the vein. The woman finally arrives at her destination to start the *pijchu*.

As we said at the beginning of the working day, the miners ask *Tío* (*Uncle*) for permission, invite him for a cigarette and offer him alcohol in small containers. If there is beer, they leave a can for him to consume symbolically. On the altar where the two *uncles* who received us are located, unopened cans of beer could be seen on both sides, while in the lower part of this altar, several ritual tables known as white *q'oas* (*offerings*) can be seen (see Figs. 9.12 and 9.13). These ritual tables surround the *Uncle* and the *Aunt* who are part of the initial altar of this cooperative. They offer a "challa" to the *Pachamama* (the floor) as a way of inviting and requesting a favour from Mother Earth so that she allows them to work. Then they symbolically offer *Uncle* a drink. They don't drink too much. It's just a ritual etiquette activity to appear in front of *Uncle* and ask for protection. The miner consumes the drink.

In texts referring to the extirpation of idolatries, this action is reminiscent of the *upay pacha*, which refers precisely to starting work activities

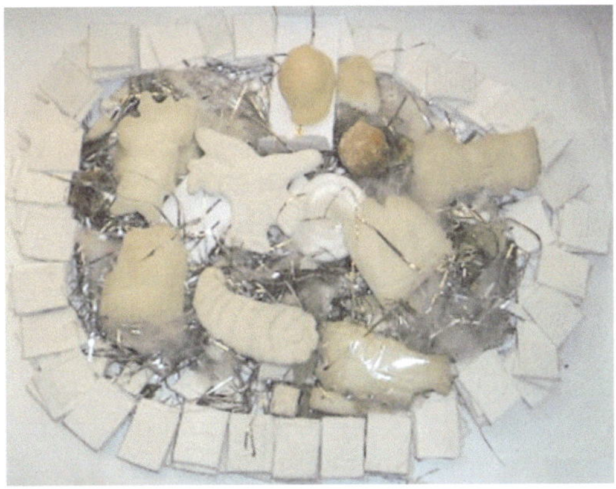

Fig. 9.12 White "*mesa*" (*table*) for personal luck. Apparently, the term "*mesa*" is a corruption of "mass", understanding that the Catholic mass is a ritual of renewal of the alliance with God. The tables are renewal offerings with main deities such as *Mother Earth* or *Pachamama*

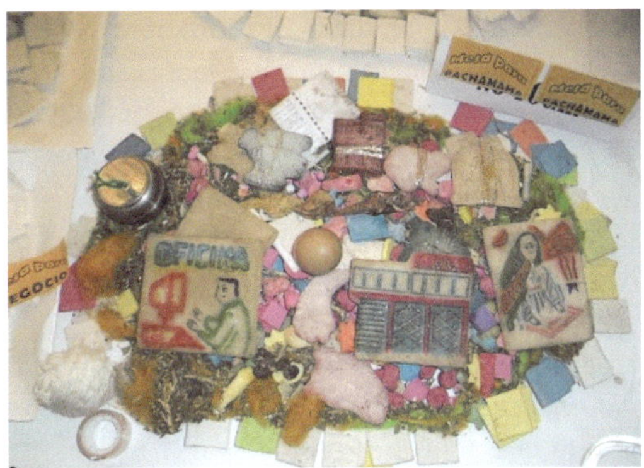

Fig. 9.13 *Pachamama* table for business or economic activity. Unlike the *white table*, this one has different symbolic elements referring to economic activity. The fact that there is even an egg in the center of it refers to this symbolic need

in a festive way in the world of the dead, in this case in the world below. According to the late researcher Alberto Guerra, *upaypacha* is the name given to the action of calling *Pachamama*, not necessarily in the mine but in any place (verbal communication with the anthropologist Víctor Escalier). In this case, alcohol assumes the character of an individual male offering at the beginning of the ritual to the *wakas* on the hill. Then it's social, when alcohol is shared in libations to reaffirm the retribution that is requested.

The burning sensation and the disinhibiting effect that alcohol has when ingested assumes in this sense this sacred masculine character and strengthens the alliance transubstantiated in the drink between the miner and the *Uncle*. Alcohol allows you to ask for permission, initiate work *thaki*, and plan the future by looking at the past [8].

The sacred masculine character is also reflected in the physical way of offering alcohol. The guide miner raises his glass offering the libation. The other miners do the same. They make the gesture of raising the glass upwards. They shortly turn into *orks* when they offer the drink. In this *orko* sense, that is to say the masculine. *Orkosuyu* would be masculine space (and time?), while *uma* is feminine [12].

This then implies the development of the female offering, which is coca leaf *pijcheo*, doing it sitting down. This refers to *uma* that is to say below. She is feminine due to different factors: she belongs to a low warm zone, that is, *uma*, and she is also part of the plant world, one of the most beloved daughters of *Pachamama* who expresses herself in *kaypacha*, or world in which one lives. It assumes a more social character. In its development, it is carried out among the members of the group that will work and that are already sitting around the *Uncle* "surrounding him". In this moment, the *Uncle* and miners have the opportunity to talk about the problems that the miners have or could have during the workday. These include the possibility of planning some actions, and telling jokes and anecdotes in the company. The *Uncle* has previously received his cigarette, alcohol in small bottles and coke at his feet or on his lap. Since he is the boss, he listens to everything the miners tell him. He finds out the latest news, how it will affect his followers, he laughs at his jokes, he likes to listen to spicy stories with erotic tones.

> "...Uncle likes that, that they talk to him about spicy things" Juana, miner, 30 years old (fictitious name).

He also listens to their pleas and lamentations.

After this process, the miners are ready to work. The same factors occur at work, but apparently, this sense of camaraderie that the miners try to generate with their *Uncle* or *Aunt* has not been identified [6]. On the other hand, it has been reported that in Potosí, when people *pijcha* they also see omens in coca according to its shape, color, etc.

In this way, the *pijcheo* allows fraternization between all the members of the work group, but it is also a way of presenting the work group to the *Uncle*. Symbolically, this group dynamic asks for his support to protect them and allow them to work. Sharing the laughter does not make him alien to him, but rather the opposite. In this case, this type of action would apparently allow *Uncle* to agree to work well with them, both for the offering they give him and for his actions in the *pijchu* ritual.

It is necessary to keep *Uncle* happy, as they need his protection against landslides, toxic gases and work accidents. It could be said that the entire ritual process is to ask for permission and that, he not be offended when the veins are opened, that he allows the miner to continue working, that the *Uncle* does not take the ore elsewhere and that he remains happy with the presence of his *protégés*. This well-executed prior process allows for psychological social security for the group and, in a certain sense, individual psychological security for the miner. It could be said that the fact of sharing the *pijchu* with *Uncle* gives hope that he will not forget the occasional subjects or "*protégés*" of their moments of haste, to start his day. However, the *Uncle* is also severe and sometimes "*denies*" some actions—surely poorly executed from his point of view—of his subjects or "*protégés*".

Most of the workers do not doubt the presence of the *Uncle* or the *Pachamama*. When they are scared, they shout: What are you doing *Uncle*? Or: Don't get mad *mom*! When an accident almost happens, they offer *Uncle* more liquor and coke, thanking him for saving them. Some say that the dangers that miners constantly face in the mines cause some to lose their manhood. When this happens, the miners turn to *Uncle* and ask him to make them as sexually strong as he is [11].

In this sense, coca as a female symbolic offering would assume the role of appeasing the *Uncle*. In addition, it is not for less. Its historical biography places it as a selective food for great dignitaries, priests and hegemonic castes of power from the *Aymara* lordships to the *Inca* era. In colonial and republican times, its restricted circulation was eliminated. By this way, it was socialized among the rest of the population, but no longer in a ritual sense. It was used in order to better exploit all indigenous and mestizos in the new model of government (colonial and then republican).

The miner should avoid three factors in the development of the working day. First, to avoid attacks of hunger, since this would prevent him from carrying out his work efficiently. Second, eliminate the sensation of thirst to continue with his day without interruptions. Third, avoid different types of distractions throughout the day. These three factors are remedied with coca *pijcheo*. The miners of San José identify that *pijcheo* is played in two journeys throughout the day.

> "… once I did the whole day with the two *pijchus*… I have not gone out to eat, besides I had no money", said Clara, a 35-year-old miner.

Eating in this case, breaks concentration at work. It also causes heaviness and drowsiness. It seems that the miner's food has many carbohydrates. This is due precisely to the expenditure of energy in their work. They eat too much bread, rice, noodles, potatoes, chuño and, when possible, meat and chicken. Vegetable consumption seems to be low.

However, that deserves a deeper study. Some doctors from Oruro observed precisely that some of the children of the miners—not necessarily from San José—were chubby. This was due to the diet high in fats and carbohydrates, which the aforementioned children received. In addition, it is precisely that the mother—theoretically—should prepare the differentiated foods. Nevertheless, economic resources and the lack of nutrition education prevent these differentiated menus from being available. This leads the diet to focus on the needs of the mining father. In the case of the miners, it cannot be guaranteed that all of them only dedicate themselves to *pijchar* and do not consume food during their working days. It should be remembered that the families of the miners sent their lunches during the peak hours corresponding to the state mining.

This does not just apply to miners. In another study carried out with Aymara merchants [13], it was observed that part of their children were also obese. This was due to the fact that the parents did not monitor their children's diet. They gave them money so that they could choose the dish of their best option. It was possible to see that the favourites of these children were French fries and chicken fried in oil or broaster, among other foods with a high-fat content and little intake of vegetables.

In this case, the *pijchu* is found on one of the cheeks of the face and is preserved for a period of 4–5 h, while the miner works concentrated on his activity. He occasionally chews a part of the coca bolus and cools it down with his saliva. Attention should not be lost on work by placing more coca leaves in the mouth since it would be irrational to do this in the middle of the working day. It must be waited until all the juices and energy that this symbolic banquet gives to the miner have been consumed and according to the alliance that must be maintained with the *Uncle* and the *wakas* from the hill. When the supernatural powers that prevent hunger and fatigue end, that is, when the miner slowly returns to his weakened human materiality, he spits out the *pijchu*. In this form, it is also absorbed by the Pachamama—mine that in this case will eat the juices of the man expressed in the rest of the saliva that the *pijchu* has and therefore part of the essence of the miner.

The coca is also given back to the *Uncle* when the vein has been opened, that is when it has been accepted by the miner so that he can extract the metal. In this case, the coca-offering strengthens the positive reciprocity that has been consolidated between the miner or group of miners and the *Uncle*. The prize for its consumption is also reflected in the days of payment for the sale of the mineral. If the "mineral harvest" has been good, the gifts to *Uncle* consisting of Alcohol and coca (beer or singani in the best of cases) are the token of gratitude that the miner gives to the caretaker of the minerals and therefore to the *Pachamama*.

Discussion and Conclusions

The *pijcheo* ritual differs from the *acullicu* since in its very etymology the *phichu* symbolically refers to the offering of eyelashes to the sea, to ask for its protection and favours. In this case, in the hills, the offering is the *pijchada* coca leaf (female) and alcohol (male), which are given to the *Uncle* and the *wakas* of the hill, asking for protection and favours in this sea of stones, veins and land.

The *pijchu* allows different types of alliances to be established based on the transubstantiation of its consumption, which is reflected in the mining alliance—*Uncle* and *wakas*. In this sense, different levels of alliance are consolidated.

At an individual psychological level, an alliance sealed with coke, cigarettes and alcohol, asking for the favours of caring for accidents and keeping bad places away to the miner and asking for the opening of veins to obtain labour benefits. Reciprocity will be identified in the achievement of the same identified factors.

At a social level, social networks are strengthened, creating an occasional atmosphere of harmony and joy. "You should not enter into the mine sad or disowning, since the vein may disappear" so that *Uncle* himself gladly accepts the arrival of his occasional *protégés*.

During the working day, the *pijchu* becomes a symbolic banquet where the worker becomes transubstantiated and manages to obtain resistance at work. He becomes immune to fatigue and hunger since he absorbs the energies that give him powers from chewing the coca leaf. This occurs in the first instance.

In a second instance, when the effect of the coca leaves has been totally assimilated, the rest of the *pijchu* is spit out in the same mine. In this moment, it assumes a new value like the eyelashes that were offered to the sea, to the *Mama cocha*. The already consumed *pijchu* is offered symbolically since this ritual food has all the strength and flows essence of the working miner. The *Pachamama*-mine consumed it, thus consolidating these minor banquets reciprocally, in the day-to-day mining work.

References

1. Bertonio L. Vocabulario de la lengua aymara. Chuquito: Casa de la Compañia de Jesus; 1612.
2. Valera B. Relación de las Costumbres antiguas de los naturales del Piru. Cuzco: Archivo Historico del Cuzco; 1953.
3. Gonzales D. Vocabulario de la lengua Quichua. San Marcos: Universidad Nacional de San Marcos; 1608.
4. Montes F. La Mascara de piedra. La Paz: Armonia; 1999.
5. Nash J. Resistencia cultural y conciencia de clase en las comunidades de las minas de Estaño de Bolivia. Allpanchis. 1985:116–32.
6. Absi P. Los Ministros del Diablo, el trabajo y sus representaciones en las minas de Potosi. La Paz: IEFA-PIEB; 2009.
7. Rivera S. Un mundo Ch'ixi es posible. Ensayos desde un presente en crisis. Buenos Aires: Tinta Limon; 2018.
8. Abercrombie T. Caminos de la memoria y del poder. In: Etnografía e historia en una comunidad andina. La Paz: IFEA; 2006.
9. Cruz P, et al. Las minas de Oruro, en el cruce de la historia y la arqueología. Mundo de antes. 2017;No. 11:195–223.
10. Del Rio M. Riquezas y poder: las restituciones a los indios del Repartimiento de Paria. In: Saberes y Memorias en los Andes. Institut des hautes études de l'Amérique latine; 1997. p. 261–78.
11. Nash J. Cuando el diablo anda en las minas. Creencias tradicionales entre los mineros del estaño de Bolivia. Revista Crisis; 1975.
12. Bouysse T. La Identidad aymara. Aproximación histórica siglo XV, siglo XVI. La Paz: Hisbol; 1987.
13. Llanque J, Villca E. Qamiris aymaras, desplazamiento e inclusión de elites andinas en la ciudad de Oruro La Paz. PIEB; 2011.

Part II

From Basic Neurosciences to Human Brain

10 Corticostriatal Pathways: From Evolution to Human Pathology

Manuel Alejandro Guevara, Iker Barrutieta-Arberas, Evelina Haralanova, Svetlozar Haralanov, Gabriel Walter Martínez, Luis Hernán Llano, Ángel José Martín Gargiulo, Augusto Pascual Ítalo Gargiulo, Ana Paula Colombini, Mercedes María Lucrecia Gargiulo, Marcos Constantino Josué Gargiulo, Andrés Acuña, Gonzalo Mesones, Humberto Luis Mesones-Arroyo, Norman Darío López Velásquez, José Vicente Lafuente Sánchez, Luis Enrique Echarte Alonso, Adriana Inés Landa De Gargiulo, and Pascual Ángel Gargiulo

M. A. Guevara (✉) · G. W. Martínez · L. H. Llano · A. Acuña · G. Mesones · A. I. Landa De Gargiulo
Laboratorio de Neurociencias y Psicología Experimental, Fundación Corporación Tecnológica Latinoamericana (FUCOTEL), Cátedra de Psicopatología, Facultad de Humanidades y Ciencias Económicas, Universidad Católica Argentina (UCA), Área de Farmacología, Facultad de Ciencias Médicas, Universidad Nacional de Cuyo (UNCuyo), Consejo Nacional de Investigaciones Científicas y Técnicas (CONICET), Mendoza, Argentina

H. L. Mesones-Arroyo · P. Á. Gargiulo
Laboratory of Neurosciences and Experimental Psychology, Latin American Technological Corporation Foundation (FUCOTEL), Cathedra of Psychopathology, Catholic University of Argentina, Area of Pharmacology, Department of Pathology, National University of Cuyo, CONICET, Guaymallén, Mendoza, Argentina
e-mail: hlmesones@mesoneshumberto.com.ar; http://fucotel.org/index.php/blog; http://fucotel.org/index.php/blog; https://www.linkedin.com/in/pascual-angel-gargiulo-63414a47/?originalSubdomain=ar

I. Barrutieta-Arberas · J. V. Lafuente Sánchez
LaNCE-Neuropharm Research Group, Dep Neurosciences, Facultad de Medicina y Enfermería, University of the Basque Country (UPV-EHU), Leioa, Spain
e-mail: onplasav@lg.ehu.es; josevicente.lafuente@ehu.eus

E. Haralanova
Department of Psychiatry and Medical Psychology, Medical University of Sofia, Sofia, Bulgaria

First Psychiatric Clinic, University Hospital for Neurology and Psychiatry "St. Naum", Sofia, Bulgaria

First Psychiatric Clinic, University Hospital for Neurology and Psychiatry "Sveti Naim", Sofia, Bulgaria

S. Haralanov
Department of Psychiatry and Medical Psychology, Medical University of Sofia, Sofia, Bulgaria

Á. J. M. Gargiulo · A. P. Í. Gargiulo · A. P. Colombini · M. M. L. Gargiulo · M. C. J. Gargiulo
Laboratorio de Neurociencias y Psicología Experimental, Fundación Corporación Tecnológica Latinoamericana (FUCOTEL), Cátedra de Psicopatología, Facultad de Humanidades y Ciencias

P. Á. Gargiulo, H. L. Mesones-Arroyo (eds.), *Psychiatry and Neuroscience Update – Vol. V*,
https://doi.org/10.1007/978-3-031-72219-6_10

Introduction

Corticostriatal pathways have been the subject of great interest in recent times. Higher functions, traditionally assigned to the cerebral cortex, depend to a large extent on the integration of these regions with subcortical centers. One of these cortico-subcortical integration pathways is constituted by the set of corticostriatal pathways. They have acquired great relevance both in explaining brain physiology and in the pathophysiology of neurological and psychiatric diseases.

Corticostriatal pathways constitute excitatory glutamatergic projections from cortical areas to the striatum. These cortical areas can be limbic, motor, or sensory [1]. Its finality is to intervene in the processing of cognitive and sensorimotor tasks [2]. The existence of intracortical circuits that would regulate the activity of striatal neurons from the cortex has also been postulated [3]. Likewise, a connection between the basal ganglia and the cerebellum has been pointed out, which would explain reward-linked activities in the cerebellum and the formation of motor routines [4].

Regarding its ontogeny, studies carried out in rodents (rats and mice) have allowed us to describe its development. Thus, the growth cones [growth cones] of the cortical axons reach the striatum on day 12 of embryonic development, and the homolateral projection is confirmed on embryonic day 18. The heterolateral projection is confirmed on the third postnatal day. On postnatal day 7, synaptogenesis formation begins, with a decline in axonal growth. After 3–4 weeks of life, concentrations of dendritic spines acquire a density equivalent to that of the adult brain [5]. It has been described that intracortical circuits would exert an influence on the activity of striatal neurons from the cortex [3].

Its evolutionary implications have been the subject of numerous studies, some of which we will mention below.

Phylogenic Considerations on the Corticostriatal Pathways

Corticostriatal pathways have been linked to amniotes (reptiles, birds, and mammals) and have been considered absent in anamniotes (fish and amphibians). However, in the latter, structures have been reported that would have a certain homology. The structures located in deep zones of the mammal's brains present variants in the phylogeny. The structures that are deep in mammals, in fish would appear to be located on the surface, by extrusion and not by intrusion. Some of these structures would be functionally similar to mammalian corticostriatal systems (Fig. 10.1).

Structural studies carried out in fish by means of injections of horseradish peroxidase in the dorsomedial and dorsolateral regions of the telencephalon of goldfish (*Carassius auratus*) show that there would be a pattern of thalamus projections very similar to that of terrestrial vertebrates. This fact has been adduced to postulate that there would be homologies with the thalamus of ter-

Económicas, Universidad Católica Argentina (UCA), Área de Farmacología, Facultad de Ciencias Médicas, Universidad Nacional de Cuyo (UNCuyo), Consejo Nacional de Investigaciones Científicas y Técnicas (CONICET), Mendoza, Argentina

Centro Integral de Salud Mental Argentino (CISMA), Buenos Aires, Argentina; https://www.cisma.com.ar; http://fucotel.org/index.php/blog

N. D. López Velásquez
Centro de Investigación e Innovación en Gerontología Aplicada (CIGAP), Facultad de Salud, Universidad Santo Tomas, Temuco, Chile

Carrera de Kinesiología, Facultad de Salud, Universidad Santo Tomás, Temuco, Chile
e-mail: nlopez17@cuc.edu.co

L. E. Echarte Alonso
Humanities and Medical Ethics Unit, School of Medicine, University of Navarra, Pamplona, Navarra, Spain
e-mail: lecharte@unav.es; https://www.unav.edu/en/web/investigacion/nuestros-investigadores/detalle-investigadores-cv?investigadorId=59376

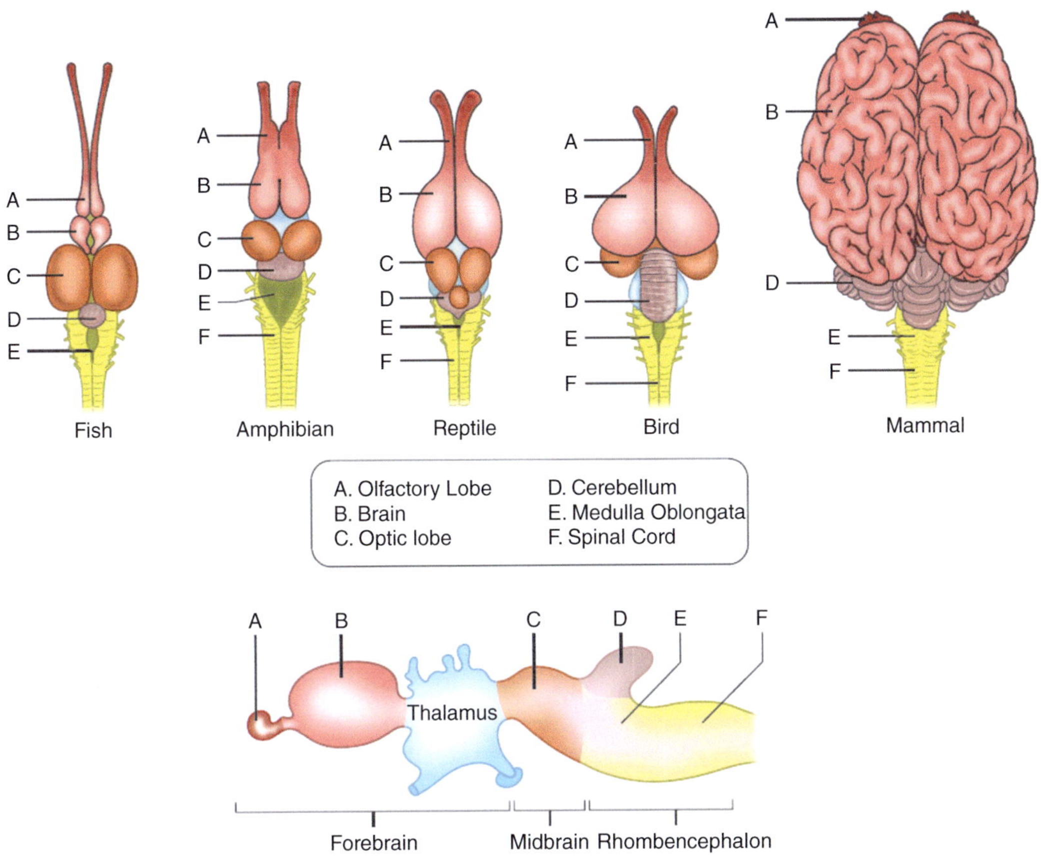

Fig. 10.1 Comparison of the brains of a fish, an amphibian, a reptile, a bird, and a mammalian. Schematic representation. Top: Brain morphology comparison. Bottom: Brain simplified structure

restrial vertebrates, particularly between the dorsomedial region and the striatum. These homologies are thus closely related to the projections of terrestrial vertebrates. The thalamus projections would be very similar [6].

Regarding fish species, the brain of the Zebrafish has been studied. There would be homologies in him between his forebrain and that of mammals. This species has been studied to objectify time perception in stimulus-response interval timing tasks. Zebrafish have been proposed as a model to study the neural circuits involved in learning time intervals, synchronization, and time perception [7].

The brain of teleost fish has been compared with the brain of birds and mammals, in order to search for correlations between behavior and levels of brain complexity. Despite structural differences, teleost fish have been found to possess highly advanced cognitive abilities [8, 9]. On the other hand, the paleal region of teleost fish has been pointed out as the ancestor of the hippocampus of amniotes. In this sense, the paleal region would be made up of various structures subject to subdivision. Among these structures, it is worth mentioning the medial pallium or paleal areas of reptiles and fish as homologs of the hippocampus of birds and mammals. This structure is very relevant in these species for complex spatial orientation. Additionally, these anatomical evidence has been supported by others of a functional nature on navigation map-making and spatial strategies comparable to those of terrestrial vertebrates [8, 9]. All of this would indicate that the evolution of the forebrain of vertebrates would not have established such relevant functional differences as is usually held [8]. These structures would give great flexibility to the navigation behaviors of the mentioned fish [9].

In the study of amphibians, investigations with frogs are especially important. The frog is part of a genus of anuran amphibians, of the Ranidae family, in whose brain there would be relevant structures in terms of homologies of the corticostriatal pathways. When the connections of the *Rana pipiens* telencephalon are studied with static methods, using horseradish peroxidase, connections were found between cell groups of the thalamus, the brain stem, and the telencephalon. There would be thalamic pathways projecting sensory information to the striatum. Another thalamic projection with sensory information would reach the medial telencephalic wall, and there would also be intratelencephalic connections [10].

In the bullfrog (*Rana catesbeiana*), the afferents to the striatum have been studied using histochemical techniques with horseradish peroxidase (HRP). The purpose was to examine the projections and terminal fields inside the striatum. The anterior lateral and central thalamic nuclei were observed to project into it from the ipsilateral side. From the contralateral side, it projects the entopeduncular nucleus. This projection would have a ventral predominance. Other entries would have a less prominent role but are still very important. This would be the case of projections originating from the ipsilateral amygdala nuclei (lateral and medial amygdala), preoptic area, posterior tubercle, and reticular nucleus of the tegmentum. These and other afferents, along with other experimental evidence, suggest that the anuran striatum processes sensory information from the midbrain roof [11].

In reptiles, many studies have been carried out in turtles, in which glutamatergic projections and ionotropic receptors have been described. This has led to the proposal of the turtle as a model to understand glutamatergic neuronal circuits in various species [12]. When trying to draw parallels between mammalian and reptilian cortices, a homology between the mammalian superior and temporal neocortex and the dorsal cortex and dorsal ventricular ridge (DVR) in reptiles is accepted [13]. In birds, this would occur with the Wulst and the Dorsal Ventricular Ridge (DVR), which will be described later.

Decision making seems to be related to the development of corticostriatal pathways. For this reason, it makes sense to review the knowledge of comparative anatomy between reptiles and mammals. Data emerging from these studies suggest that the expansion of cortical–striatal connectivity appears to be a key development in the evolution of behavioral flexibility [14].

The homology between the brains of birds and mammals is highlighted in relatively recent works, particularly with regard to cognitive functions in relation to the neocortex of the avian pallium [15]. Birds have basal ganglia and a well-defined set of corticostriatal pathways. It has been suggested that these pathways would be decisive in the differences between the brains of anamniotes (fish and amphibians) and amniotes (reptiles, birds, and mammals). These pathways would provide sensory and motor information to the striatum in order to allow better movement control of the basal ganglia [16], along with the processing and discrimination of visual stimuli performed in the mesopallium ventrolaterale (MVL) [17].

As in mammals, corticostriatal glutamatergic projections have been identified in birds. The existence of projections from the nuclei of the dorsal zone of the thalamus to the striatum has been considered an additional analogy between the brain of birds and that of mammals. Additionally, dopaminergic projections on the striatum from the ventral tegmental area and the substantia nigra have been described. As a counterpart, the striatum is projected onto the tegmental area with two pathways, one direct and the other indirect, which passes through the Pallidum. Both pathways predominantly use GABA. In turn, interneurons have been found in the striatum. These would use GABA and Acetylcholine. The striatum also projects to the motor cortex and tectum. Another indirect route would reach the tectum through the substantia nigra. It would again be a GABAergic pathway. This being so, there would then be a marked similarity between the basal ganglia and their connections between the brains of birds and mammals [18].

As previously anticipated, the bird brain possesses a special formation called the Wulst, or lump or pillow, which is particularly important in sensory processing. The term was proposed in 1905 by Kallischer [19] and adopted by later authors. A subdivision of this structure has been proposed in 2004 [20]. In an expert review of the names of bird brain structures [20], among other redesignations, the names of the structures involved in Wulst were proposed. It was concluded that the term hyperstriatum for the various cell layers of Wulst should be replaced by hyperpallium, mesopallium, and nidopallium. The convenience of keeping the particle "hyper-" is admitted, alluding to an enlarged or bulging structure. It is also pointed out that the presence of this enlarged or bulging structure in the upper part of the pallium is consistent with the indication of its phylogenetic origin since it would represent a structural hypertrophy of the dorsal cortex present in reptiles [20].

The previously called *accessory hyperstriatum* has come to be called hyperpallium apicale. This assumes recognition of its position at the apex of the telencephalon and avoids functional or evolutionary subordination to other parts of the brain. Along this structure is the *intercalated* or *interstitial nucleus*. This nucleus has fundamentally somatosensory and particularly visual afferents [20]. In this way, the Wulst has very important relations with the vision and, therefore, with the registration of the external world. Another interesting point regarding Wulst is the stratification of its brain layers. These subdivisions of Wulst have been called "*pseudo-layers*," with some interesting nuances. These layers would seem to bear some analogies with the cortical layers of mammals. However, the presence of neurons such as pyramidal neurons, which have a translaminar position in their dendritic trees, is not confirmed [20].

The evolutionary formation of the cortex, and its derivation in the mammalian cortex, has been the subject of multiple theorizations [13]. The evolution of the brain has also been studied using embryological patterns, considering that adult individuals differ more in their final conformation. Thus, a set of homologies between sauropsids and mammals has been established. These studies would indicate minor evolutionary changes, but with very important consequences in neural connections [21].

The existence of two major qualitative differences between the brains of mammals and saurops (birds and reptiles) in the upper and rostral parts of the brain (pallium) has been pointed out. Mammals have a six-layered neocortex and also exhibit a different morphological organization in the middle or lateral sector of their pallium than sauropsids [22]. All this leads us to consider, not without some care, the validity of *translational studies* of pharmacological interference in certain brain areas in the *pigeon* as a way of approaching human brain functions. Since the pigeon has a highly developed sense of sight, it is an animal of choice for experimental studies of complex visual stimuli processing, as will be seen later in this chapter.

In mammals, Grace [23] has described the existing corticostriatal connections in detail when discussing the pathophysiology of schizophrenic psychoses. Dismissing the initial notion of a dopaminergic disorder in schizophrenia, he resorts to the interpretation of a possible interruption in the regulation from the cortex of subcortical dopaminergic pathways. In this new interpretation, the hippocampus would have a relevant role in this process. This formation would have an impact facilitating the flow of information from the frontal cortex to the Nucleus Accumbens Septi (NAS). When hippocampal or entorhinal cortex development is interfered with, a mechanism facilitating the arrival of information from the frontal cortex to the NAS is interfered with. An affectation of the development of the limbic system would therefore have consequences in adult rats. Grace proposes that there would be a dysfunction due to early involvement of the hippocampus that would result in disturbances in the interactions between the cortex and the NAS during adulthood [23].

The connections between the frontal cortex, hippocampus, and amygdala would occur in the NAS. In this neostriatal structure, glutamatergic

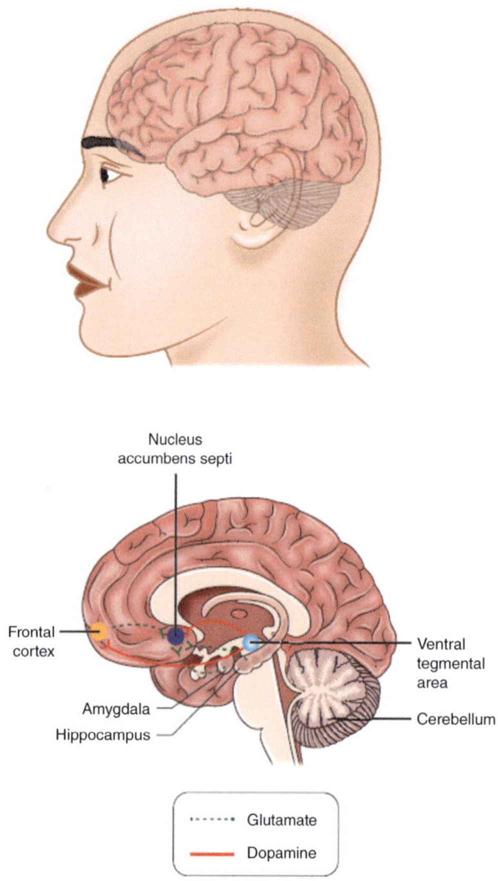

Fig. 10.2 Main glutamatergic and dopaminerc pathways involved in schizophrenia. Schematic representation

projections would be found from the frontal cortex (neocortex), amygdala (paleocortex) and hippocampus (archicortex), and from dopaminergic projections from the ventral tegmental area [23]. These structures would generate a situation of interaction and balance that would be altered in psychoses (Fig. 10.2).

Corticostriatal connections have been linked to complex functions, such as motivation and cognition in complex goal-directed tasks. Thus, the different functional regions or domains of the striatum have been attributed links with complex behaviors. The caudate nucleus has been linked to cognition. The ventral striatum would be related to the functions linked to reward. Finally, the putamen would have to do with motor control. This would constitute a simplification, since these systems would be more complex [24].

Many striatal synaptic pathways have been correlated with learned responses. A group of neurotransmitters, among which dopamine and glutamate stand out, seem to regulate cortical, thalamic, and limbic inputs, which, in turn, regulate outputs from spiny neurons of the striatum. These inputs influence the manifestation of learned behaviors. Reward circuits, classically linked to learning and mediated by dopamine, play an important role in learning [25].

From the detection of anhedonia as a relevant factor in depression [26], dopaminergic activity and other receptors have been studied, as well as reward circuits in depression. The fact that there is a relationship between these circuits and modulation by endocannabinoids has led to the suggestion of an interaction between endocannabinoid and dopaminergic receptors in reward circuits, that is, in corticostriatal circuits. The endocannabinoid and dopaminergic receptors would be found there, which would be particularly vulnerable to stress, thus compromising the reward circuits and the corticostriatal regions [27].

In animal models, there are findings that suggest a relationship between compulsion and an increase in activity in the dorsal striatum in the face of reward announcements, increasing the compulsive search for them [28]. Likewise, a connection between the basal ganglia and the cerebellum has been postulated, which would explain the activity linked to rewards in the cerebellum [4]. On the other hand, based on the existence of intracortical subnetworks, attempts have been made to establish connection maps or connectivity projections from the cerebral cortex to the striatum in rodents [1]. All these circuits would generate complex structures and ramifications, thus facilitating less determined behavioral patterns.

Several animal models of schizophrenia have been developed from a hypofunction of the N-Methyl-D-Aspartic glutamate (NMDA) receptor [29]. It was noted that many symptoms of schizophrenia could be generated by the administration of glutamate NMDA receptor antagonists.

It was found that this manipulation of the receptor could induce alterations in humans and animals compatible with schizophrenic sign-symptoms [30]. We pointed out in a 2014 review that the blockade of glutamatergic transmission in Nucleus Accumbens Septi (NAS) allowed the induction of primary, secondary, and cognitive symptoms in translational models [31]. Basically, these corticostriatal connections have been linked to complex functions. Even at the risk of being somewhat schematic, different elements of the striatum have been linked to motor control (putamen), cognition (caudate and NAS), and motivation (NAS) [24].

Corticostriatal Pathways and Human Pathology

The corticostriatal pathways have been implicated in a significant number of human diseases. From neurology, these corticostriatal pathways have been related to Parkinson's, Gilles de la Tourette syndrome, Huntington's Chorea, and Amyotrophic Lateral Sclerosis (ALS). A disorder in their functioning has also been linked to psychiatric conditions such as attention deficit disorder (ADHD), autism, obsessive compulsive disorder (OCD), and schizophrenia. Its importance in the normal and in the pathological has been widely described [3].

In Parkinson's disease, in addition to the classic alterations in the nigrostriatal pathway, a phenomenon of corticostriatal uncoupling has recently been proposed. This would produce a gait freeze, which problematizes the lives of these patients in an abrupt and unexpected way, also linked to perceptual dysfunctions. There would be disruption in cortico-subcortical functional connectivity that would result in executive dysfunction [32].

On the other hand, gait imbalance, another disabling phenomenon in Parkinson's disease, has been attributed to an alteration in corticostriatal and frontal cortical processing, which mediates cognitive–motor interactions, generating a cognitive attentional cortical processing dysfunction, related to a glutamatergic frontostriatal projection [33]. In G2019S mutant mice, abnormalities in corticostriatal plasticity and activity have recently been observed on postnatal day 21, at which time excitatory synaptogenic activity in the striatum ends. It has been proposed that this deficit would serve as a model to study these non-motor symptoms of Parkinson's disease, especially cognitive and psychiatric ones, such as depression and anhedonia [34].

Another movement disorder, Gilles de la Tourette syndrome, has also been linked to dysfunction of the corticostriatal pathways. It would be a dysfunction of the traffic of impulses through the basal ganglia, within the framework of the corticostriatal and thalamocortical circuits [35].

An important point in the pathology of these pathways is Huntington's Disease (HD). Mutation of the huntingtin gene, a protein with numerous functions, including synaptic transmission, results in a fatal hereditary neurodegenerative disease. There is a very relevant loss of corticostriatal neurons with clear disconnection. Its clinical consequence is chorea major. This disease has been the subject of translational studies, and it has been concluded that there is a very significant loss of corticostriatal neurons. Also, the relevance of huntingtin in synapses is supported [36]. In its early stage, there are motor symptoms that are generated by very subtle disorders of neuronal function and synaptic communication.

Huntington's disease (HD) in its late stage involves neuronal death, thus it is a neurodegenerative disorder. In its progression, it affects functionally in a profound way the corticostriatal information processing functions. Animal models and the study of neural networks have been very useful in the study of these circuits. Neurotrophic factors have been implicated [37, 38].

In amyotrophic lateral sclerosis [ALS], the role of corticostriatal pathways has also been suggested [3]. The lesion zone in ALS seems to be in the hippocampus from the beginning of the illness, later becoming larger in different brain zones, particularly in the hippocampus, subiculum, and thalamus [39]. Recent studies show involvement of the frontal lobes and the corticospinal, corticopontine/corticorubral and corticostriatal tracts. All of this correlates with the values of the specific scales for clinical measurement of the disease and the function of the upper motor neuron (UMN) [40].

Various studies have demonstrated the role of neurotrophins in the modulation of corticostriatal synapses. This modulation is altered when there is a mitochondrial failure or dysfunction. Functionally, this disorder affects the release of neurotransmitters, particularly at corticostriatal synapses, and the availability of neurotrophins. Structurally, it has an action on dendritic arborization, as well as on the length of medium spiny neurons (MSN), present in the striatum [41, 42].

In relation to psychiatric pathology, these dysfunctions have initially been related to attention deficit disorder (ADHD). The role of frontal corticostriatal circuits (FCSC) in ADHD has been a matter of discussion. These structures participate in cognition, emotion, and motor function, mainly in their self-regulation. Although there have been discrepancies between various studies, this would have to do with population differences or the structures studied [43].

In this disorder, studies carried out with structural brain images (magnetic resonance) have shown altered topological characteristics, with functional correspondences in the clinical and psychometric aspects. Clinically, the major structural abnormalities were correlated with more severe symptoms. Psychometrically, the correlation could be established with the results in the Stroop and Wisconsin card sorting tests [44].

An association between genes related to autism spectrum disorder (ASD) and developmental abnormalities of these corticostriatal pathways has been proposed [5, 45]. These would imply disorders of synaptic plasticity, imbalances between excitation and inhibition located in these structures, and abnormal axonal growths [5]. At the behavioral level, corticostriatal circuits (CSC) have been related to some repetitive behaviors, with a very reduced repertoire, present in children with this condition. It has been suggested that interruptions in these pathways could be conditioned by differences in genetic characteristics, on which environmental influences would act, disturbing brain development [45]. It is accepted that the structural variations of the corticostriatal circuits would be influenced by genetic factors, while environmental factors would have greater relevance in the development of gray matter in the orbitofrontal cortex and the anterior cingulate cortex. This would occur mainly in children with the condition [45].

Regarding obsessive-compulsive disorder, there is also evidence that relates this condition to corticostriatal pathways. In animal models, there are findings that suggest a relationship between compulsion and an increase in activity in the dorsal striatum in the face of reward announcements, increasing the compulsive search for them [28].

There are numerous hypotheses regarding the dysfunctions underlying *obsessive-compulsive disorder*. An imbalance between habitual behavior and goal-directed behavior has been proposed, establishing relationships with neural correlates in the corticostriatal circuit. This hypothesis was evaluated and contrasted with metacognitive theories. All this has led to support the convenience of multidisciplinary approaches for the treatment of OCD. This would encompass both pharmacological and psychological approaches [46].

Compulsive behaviors are more or less impulsive stereotyped behaviors with difficulties to inhibit them. Compulsivity constitutes a very relevant element both in obsessive-compulsive disorder and in drug addiction. An overlap between compulsiveness, obsessive-compulsive disorders, behavioral addictions, and substance use has been proposed. In these cases, there would be a deterioration in the processing of rewards and punishments. As a neurobiological correlate, these phenomena would be accompanied by an attenuated release of dopamine in the ventral striatum. It is believed that there would also be a negative reinforcement in the limbic system. There would also be cognitive and behavioral inflexibility. This has been postulated to be linked to decreased prefrontal control and imbalances between dorsal and ventral frontostriatal recruitment [47].

Our work team has dedicated its greatest efforts, in recent years, to the neurobiology of *schizophrenic psychoses*. The etiology of schizophrenic psychoses has been the subject of various theories. We [48–50] came up with an initial study on the alteration of perception in such psychoses. The description and the large amount of evidence cited in support of the concept of corticothalamic dysfunction relate to the phenomena of perception, consciousness, and neurotransmitters involved in schizophrenia in a very strong way. Not only hallucinations but also other disturbances of cognition and perception are symptoms of schizophrenia. The cognition involved in interpreting perception is important, particularly in distinguishing facial expressions from emotion [51]. Conrad [52] argued that the interpretation of interpersonal communication, due to its subtlety, is affected more than perceptions of external objects, thus facilitating delusional perceptions. All of these findings, taken together, strongly suggest that cognitive deficits may be at the heart of schizophrenia [51]. We have studied these issues in the field of perception and psychoses, beginning with Conrad's insights into a Gestalt dysfunction underlying delusional perceptions [52]. We used the Bender gestalt test [53, 54], which showed that global scores and time spent were significantly different between healthy controls and acute schizophrenic patients in their first bout and non-medicated and chronic schizophrenic patients. This allowed us to quantify perceptual disturbances resulting from the loss of the objective structure of perception in schizophrenic patients [48]. Our results are consistent with the failure of schizophrenic patients to perform well on backward visual masking tasks [55], which is related to the failure to establish gamma-range cortical oscillations in response to sensory stimulation [56].

Our next objective was to study perception in close relationship with cognition and anxiety in translational models in animals, considering the current primary conceptions about the pathophysiology of schizophrenia. Carlsson has proposed that psychotogenesis depends on an interaction between the dopamine and glutamate pathways that project to the striatum from the lower brain stem and cortex, respectively [57]. The action of these neurotransmitters on GABAergic striatal projection neurons (indirect striatothalamic pathways) exerts an inhibitory action on thalamocortical glutamatergic neurons, thus protecting the cortex from sensory overload and hyperactivation. This protection could be reduced by hyperactivity of dopaminergic pathways or hypofunction of corticostriatal glutamate pathways, leading to psychosis. The direct pathway exerts an excitatory influence and both pathways are controlled by glutamatergic corticostriatal fibers, which act as brakes and accelerators, respectively [57].

We studied perception in an animal model using pigeons. The pigeons were trained in a visual discrimination task, in which the reward was linked to pattern recognition, which required a high level of attention. We stimulated dopamine receptors and blocked N-methyl-D-aspartic type (NMDA) glutamatergic receptors within the ventral striatum, Nucleus Accumbens Septi (NAS), which is classically linked to schizophrenia [23, 58], with the aim of producing a state homologous to the "psychotic-like state," with the loss of "gestalt" discrimination function [59]. Negative findings were observed with injections of apomorphine or lidocaine, but significant and reversible performance interruption at near-random levels was obtained after injection of 7-aminophosphonoheptanoic acid (AP-7) into the NAS [59–61]. In rats, we observed that by injecting AP-7 into the NAS, acquisition is impaired, which requires a high level of attention and is linked to perception, with no effect on consolidation [62, 63]. In these experiments, fecal boluses also decreased during recovery, suggesting a decrease in anxiety levels during acquisition.

For this reason, we used a specific anxiety test, the Plus Maze Test, and we observed that AP-7 clearly decreases anxiety levels when injected into the NAS, suggesting a fact homologous to the affective flattening observed in schizophrenia [64]. Taking all these findings together, it seems that NAS integrates the cognitive and affective levels, and a dysfunction in this nucleus could be the basis of the schizophrenic illness, providing a basis for the explanation of the positive (cognitive) and negative symptoms (affective flattening). Subsequently, and since there is a problem with working memory in schizophrenic psychoses, we tested this function with the Hole Board test in rats cannulated bilaterally in NAS [65]. With this last experimental approach, we complete the emulation of primary, secondary, and cognitive symptoms through translational studies based on the glutamatergic blockade of NAS started in 1998.

Grace proposed a circuit with the aim of explaining various schizophrenic symptoms [23]. His hypothesis is that schizophrenia is related to a dysfunction in the modulation of afferent projections of a glutamatergic nature, which converge on the NAS. It receives the motor plans produced by the prefrontal cortex, the cognitive information of the contexts from the hippocampus and the affective evaluation provided by the amygdala. The modulation is performed according to the gate's hypothesis. This integration leads to goal-directed behavior constrained by contextual information and emotional meaning. On the contrary, in schizophrenia, this integration is disturbed, and this fact leads to an abnormal affective impulse with an inappropriate use of contextual signals, which results in an impulsive and disorganized being.

In the general framework, the general objective of this chapter has been to comment on the induction of symptoms and signs of schizophrenic psychoses in translational models by intracerebral administration of glutamate NMDA receptor antagonists. We sought to repeat the symptoms observed by injection within the NAS with this type of drug, in translational models. Stereotaxy was used as a method to objectify the location of the cannulas in the rat brain. The three groups of schizophrenic symptoms were induced in translational models by the injection of NMDA-type glutamatergic antagonists into NAS. Translational models of positive, negative, and cognitive schizophrenic symptoms were proposed. It has recently been pointed out that the generation of other symptoms related to delusional perception can be explained by dopaminergic hyperfunction [66]. This hyperfunction would condition a pathological salience of certain stimuli, favoring the associated delusional perception. Ultimately, both neurotransmission systems interact in NAS, exerting mutual regulation [67].

Conclusion

Diverse and numerous pathologies have been associated with corticostriatal dysfunctions. Knowledge of the comparative anatomy of the brains of different species is a requirement for the design of translational models. The existence of developed corticostriatal pathways legitimizes the use of the species chosen for our translational models [48–50, 68, 69]. This is the case of the experiments carried out on birds and rodents by our working group on experimental approaches to schizophrenia.

References

1. Hintiryan H, Foster NN, Bowman I, Bay M, Song MY, Gou L, Yamashita S, Bienkowski MS, Zingg B, Zhu M, Yang XW, Shih JC, Toga AW, Dong HW. The mouse cortico-striatal projectome. Nat Neurosci. 2016;19(8):1100–14. https://doi.org/10.1038/nn.4332.
2. Graybiel AM. The basal ganglia: learning new tricks and loving it. Curr Opin Neurobiol. 2005;15(6):638–44. https://doi.org/10.1016/j.conb.2005.10.006.
3. Shepherd GM. Corticostriatal connectivity and its role in disease. Nat Rev Neurosci. 2013;14(4):278–91. https://doi.org/10.1038/nrn3469.
4. Habas C. Research note: functional connectivity between a corticostriatal network and the cerebellum. Cerebellum. 2022;21(3):520–4. https://doi.org/10.1007/s12311-021-01316-w.
5. Li W, Pozzo-Miller L. Dysfunction of the corticostriatal pathway in autism spectrum disorders. J Neurosci Res. 2020;98(11):2130–47. https://doi.org/10.1002/jnr.24560.
6. Echteler SM, Saidel WM. Forebrain connections in the goldfish support telencephalic homologies with land vertebrates. Science. 1981;212(4495):683–5. https://doi.org/10.1126/science.6971493.
7. Cheng RK, Jesuthasan SJ, Penney TB. Zebrafish forebrain and temporal conditioning. Philos Trans R Soc Lond Ser B Biol Sci. 2014;369(1637):20120462. https://doi.org/10.1098/rstb.2012.0462.
8. Rodríguez F, López JC, Vargas JP, Broglio C, Gómez Y, Salas C. Spatial memory and hippocampal pallium through vertebrate evolution: insights from reptiles and teleost fish. Brain Res Bull. 2002;57(3–4):499–503. https://doi.org/10.1016/s0361-9230(01)00682-7.
9. Rodríguez F, Quintero B, Amores L, Madrid D, Salas-Peña C, Salas C. Spatial cognition in teleost fish: strategies and mechanisms. Animals (Basel). 2021;11(8):2271. https://doi.org/10.3390/ani11082271.

10. Kicliter E. Some telencephalic connections in the frog, Rana pipiens. J Comp Neurol. 1979;185(1):75–86. https://doi.org/10.1002/cne.901850105.
11. Wilczynski W, Northcutt RG. Connections of the bullfrog striatum: afferent organization. J Comp Neurol. 1983;214(3):321–32. https://doi.org/10.1002/cne.902140309.
12. Hussan MT, Sakai A, Matsui H. Glutamatergic pathways in the brains of turtles: a comparative perspective among reptiles, birds, and mammals. Front Neuroanat. 2022;16:937504. https://doi.org/10.3389/fnana.2022.937504.
13. Reiner AJ. A hypothesis as to the organization of cerebral cortex in the common amniote ancestor of modern reptiles and mammals. Novartis Found Symp. 2000;228:83–102; discussion 102–13. https://doi.org/10.1002/0470846631.ch7.
14. Lee AM, Tai LH, Zador A, Wilbrecht L. Between the primate and 'reptilian' brain: rodent models demonstrate the role of corticostriatal circuits in decision making. Neuroscience. 2015;296:66–74. https://doi.org/10.1016/j.neuroscience.2014.12.042.
15. Jarvis ED, Güntürkün O, Bruce L, Csillag A, Karten H, Kuenzel W, Medina L, Paxinos G, Perkel DJ, Shimizu T, Striedter G, Wild JM, Ball GF, Dugas-Ford J, Durand SE, Hough GE, Husband S, Kubikova L, Lee DW, Mello CV, Powers A, Siang C, Smulders TV, Wada K, White SA, Yamamoto K, Yu J, Reiner A, Butler AB, Avian Brain Nomenclature Consortium. Avian brains and a new understanding of vertebrate brain evolution. Nat Rev Neurosci. 2005;6(2):151–9. https://doi.org/10.1038/nrn1606.
16. Veenman CL, Wild JM, Reiner A. Organization of the avian "corticostriatal" projection system: a retrograde and anterograde pathway tracing study in pigeons. J Comp Neurol. 1995;354(1):87–126. https://doi.org/10.1002/cne.903540108.
17. Clark W, Chilcott M, Azizi A, Pusch R, Perry K, Colombo M. Neurons in the pigeon visual network discriminate between faces, scrambled faces, and sine grating images. Sci Rep. 2022;12(1):589. https://doi.org/10.1038/s41598-021-04559-z.
18. Veenman CL. Pigeon basal ganglia: insights into the neuroanatomy underlying telencephalic sensorimotor processes in birds. Eur J Morphol. 1997;35(4):220–33. https://doi.org/10.1076/ejom.35.4.220.13079.
19. Kallischer O. Das Grosshirn der Papageien in anatomischer und physiologischer Beziehung/von Otto Kalischer. Contributors Kalischer, Otto. Mott FW. 1853–1926 Kalischer, Otto King's College London Publication/Creation Berlin: Verlag der Königl. Akademie der Wissenschaften, in Commission bei Georg Reimer, 1905. Persistent URL https://wellcomecollection.org/works/xwjsn6h7.
20. Reiner A, Perkel DJ, Bruce LL, Butler AB, Csillag A, Kuenzel W, Medina L, Paxinos G, Shimizu T, Striedter G, Wild M, Ball GF, Durand S, Güntürkun O, Lee DW, Mello CV, Powers A, White SA, Hough G, Kubikova L, Smulders TV, Wada K, Dugas-Ford J, Husband S, Yamamoto K, Yu J, Siang C, Jarvis ED. Revised nomenclature for avian telencephalon and some related brainstem nuclei. J Comp Neurol. 2004;473:377–414.
21. Striedter GF. The telencephalon of tetrapods in evolution. Brain Behav Evol. 1997;49(4):179–213. https://doi.org/10.1159/000112991.
22. Molnár Z, Butler AB. The corticostriatal junction: a crucial region for forebrain development and evolution. BioEssays. 2002;24(6):530–41. https://doi.org/10.1002/bies.10100.
23. Grace AA. Gating of information flow within the limbic system and the pathophysiology of schizophrenia. Brain Res Rev. 2000;31:330–41.
24. Haber SN. Corticostriatal circuitry. Dialogues Clin Neurosci. 2016;18(1):7–21. https://doi.org/10.31887/DCNS.2016.18.1/shaber.
25. Bamford NS, Wightman RM, Sulzer D. Dopamine's effects on corticostriatal synapses during reward-based behaviors. Neuron. 2018;97(3):494–510. https://doi.org/10.1016/j.neuron.2018.01.006.
26. Willner P. Validity, reliability and utility of the chronic mild stress model of depression: a 10-year review and evaluation. Psychopharmacology. 1997;134(4):319–29. https://doi.org/10.1007/s002130050456.
27. Goldstein Ferber S, Weller A, Yadid G, Friedman A. Discovering the lost reward: critical locations for endocannabinoid modulation of the cortico-striatal loop that are implicated in major depression. Int J Mol Sci. 2021;22(4):1867. https://doi.org/10.3390/ijms22041867.
28. Harada M, Pascoli V, Hiver A, Flakowski J, Lüscher C. Corticostriatal activity driving compulsive reward seeking. Biol Psychiatry. 2021;90(12):808–18. https://doi.org/10.1016/j.biopsych.2021.08.018.
29. Nakazawa K, Sapkota K. The origin of NMDA receptor hypofunction in schizophrenia. Pharmacol Ther. 2020;205:107426. https://doi.org/10.1016/j.pharmthera.2019.107426.
30. Lee G, Zhou Y. NMDAR hypofunction animal models of schizophrenia. Front Mol Neurosci. 2019;12:185. https://doi.org/10.3389/fnmol.2019.00185.
31. Gargiulo PA, Landa De Gargiulo AI. Glutamate and modeling of schizophrenia symptoms: review of our findings: 1990-2014. Pharmacol Rep. 2014;66(3):343–52.
32. Bardakan MM, Fink GR, Zapparoli L, Bottini G, Paulesu E, Weiss PH. Imaging the neural underpinnings of freezing of gait in Parkinson's disease. Neuroimage Clin. 2022;35:103123. https://doi.org/10.1016/j.nicl.2022.103123.
33. Sarter M, Avila C, Kucinski A, Donovan E. Make a left turn: cortico-striatal circuitry mediating the attentional control of complex movements. Mov Disord. 2021;36(3):535–46. https://doi.org/10.1002/mds.28532.
34. Huntley GW, Benson DL. Origins of Parkinson's disease in brain development: insights from early and persistent effects of LRRK2-G2019S on striatal circuits. Front Neurosci. 2020;14:265. https://doi.org/10.3389/fnins.2020.00265.

35. Kimber TE. An update on Tourette syndrome. Curr Neurol Neurosci Rep. 2010;10(4):286–91. https://doi.org/10.1007/s11910-010-0118-2.
36. Barry J, Bui MTN, Levine MS, Cepeda C. Synaptic pathology in Huntington's disease: beyond the corticostriatal pathway. Neurobiol Dis. 2022;162:105574. https://doi.org/10.1016/j.nbd.2021.105574.
37. Bunner KD, Rebec GV. Corticostriatal dysfunction in Huntington's disease: the basics. Front Hum Neurosci. 2016;10:317. https://doi.org/10.3389/fnhum.2016.00317.
38. Plotkin JL, Surmeier DJ. Corticostriatal synaptic adaptations in Huntington's disease. Curr Opin Neurobiol. 2015;33:53–62. https://doi.org/10.1016/j.conb.2015.01.020.
39. Liu S, Ren Q, Gong G, Sun Y, Zhao B, Ma X, Zhang N, Zhong S, Lin Y, Wang W, Zheng R, Yu X, Yun Y, Zhang D, Shao K, Lin P, Yuan Y, Dai T, Zhang Y, Li L, Li W, Zhao Y, Shan P, Meng X, Yan C. Hippocampal subfield and anterior-posterior segment volumes in patients with sporadic amyotrophic lateral sclerosis. Neuroimage Clin. 2021;32:102816. https://doi.org/10.1016/j.nicl.2021.102816.
40. Kalra S, Müller HP, Ishaque A, Zinman L, Korngut L, Genge A, Beaulieu C, Frayne R, Graham SJ, Kassubek J. A prospective harmonized multicenter DTI study of cerebral white matter degeneration in ALS. Neurology. 2020;95(8):e943–52. https://doi.org/10.1212/WNL.0000000000010235.
41. Mendoza E, Miranda-Barrientos JA, Vázquez-Roque RA, Morales-Herrera E, Ruelas A, De la Rosa G, Flores G, Hernández-Echeagaray E. In vivo mitochondrial inhibition alters corticostriatal synaptic function and the modulatory effects of neurotrophins. Neuroscience. 2014;280:156–70. https://doi.org/10.1016/j.neuroscience.2014.09.018.
42. Torres-Cruz FM, Mendoza E, Vivar-Cortés IC, García-Sierra F, Hernández-Echeagaray E. Do BDNF and NT-4/5 exert synergistic or occlusive effects on corticostriatal transmission in a male mouse model of Huntington's disease? J Neurosci Res. 2019;97(12):1665–77. https://doi.org/10.1002/jnr.24507.
43. Nikolaidis A, He X, Pekar J, Rosch K, Mostofsky SH. Frontal corticostriatal functional connectivity reveals task positive and negative network dysregulation in relation to ADHD, sex, and inhibitory control. Dev Cogn Neurosci. 2022;54:101101. https://doi.org/10.1016/j.dcn.2022.101101.
44. Chen Y, Lei D, Cao H, Niu R, Chen F, Chen L, Zhou J, Hu X, Huang X, Guo L, Sweeney JA, Gong Q. Altered single-subject gray matter structural networks in drug-naïve attention deficit hyperactivity disorder children. Hum Brain Mapp. 2022;43(4):1256–64. https://doi.org/10.1002/hbm.25718.
45. Hegarty JP II, Lazzeroni LC, Raman MM, Hallmayer JF, Cleveland SC, Wolke ON, Phillips JM, Reiss AL, Hardan AY. Genetic and environmental influences on corticostriatal circuits in twins with autism. J Psychiatry Neurosci. 2020;45(3):188–97. https://doi.org/10.1503/jpn.190030.
46. Robbins TW, Vaghi MM, Banca P. Obsessive-compulsive disorder: puzzles and prospects. Neuron. 2019;102(1):27–47. https://doi.org/10.1016/j.neuron.2019.01.046.
47. Figee M, Pattij T, Willuhn I, Luigjes J, van den Brink W, Goudriaan A, Potenza MN, Robbins TW, Denys D. Compulsivity in obsessive-compulsive disorder and addictions. Eur Neuropsychopharmacol. 2016;26(5):856–68. https://doi.org/10.1016/j.euroneuro.2015.12.003.
48. Gargiulo PA. Aproximaciones Experimentales a la Disfunción perceptual en la Esquizofrenia (Experimental approaches to perceptual dysfunction in schizophrenia). Rev Neurol. 2003;37(6):545–51.
49. Gargiulo PA, Landa de Gargiulo AI. Perception and psychoses: the role of glutamatergic transmission within the nucleus accumbens septi. Short communication. Behav Brain Sci. 2004;27(6):792–3.
50. Gargiulo PA, Landa De Gargiulo AI. Glutamate and modelling of schizophrenia symptoms: review of our findings: 1990-2014. Pharmacol Rep. 2014;66(3):343–52.
51. Holden C. Neuroscience. Deconstructing schizophrenia. Science. 2003;299(5605):333–5. https://doi.org/10.1126/science.299.5605.333.
52. Conrad K. Die beginnende Schizophrenie. Versuch einer Gestaltanalyse des Wahnsinns [Incipient schizophrenia: an attempt at a gestaltic analysis of insanity]. Stuttgart: Thieme; 1966.
53. Del Vecchio S, Gargiulo PA. Visual and motor function in schizophrenic patients. Acta Psiquiatr Psicol Am Lat. 1992;38:317–22.
54. Gargiulo PA, Del Vecchio S. Gestaltic visual motor function in schizophrenic patients. Göttingen neurobiology report 1997. In: Elsner N, Wässle H, editors. Proceedings of the 25th Göttingen neurobiology conference 1997, Vol. II, Communication 1005. Stuttgart: Thieme; 1997.
55. Green MF, Nuechterlein KH. Backward masking performance as an indicator of vulnerability to schizophrenia. Acta Psychiatr Scand Suppl. 1999;395:34–40. https://doi.org/10.1111/j.1600-0447.1999.tb05981.x.
56. Green MF, Nuechterlein KH, Breitmeyer B, Mintz J. Backward masking in unmedicated schizophrenic patients in psychotic remission: possible reflection of aberrant cortical oscillation. Am J Psychiatry. 1999;156(9):1367–73. https://doi.org/10.1176/ajp.156.9.1367.
57. Carlsson A, Waters N, Waters S, Carlsson ML. Network interactions in schizophrenia-therapeutic implications. Brain Res Brain Res Rev. 2000;31:342–9.
58. Matthysse S. Nucleus accumbens and schizophrenia. In: Chronister RB, De France JF, editors. The neurobiology of the nucleus accumbens, Sebasco Estaes, Proceedings of the symposium: nucleus acumbens,

Sebasco Estates, Maine. Brunswick: Haer Institute; 1980. p. 351–9.
59. Gargiulo PA, Siemann M, Delius JD. Visual discrimination in pigeons impaired by glutamatergic blockade of nucleus accumbens. Physiol Behav. 1998;63(4):705–9. https://doi.org/10.1016/s0031-9384(97)00516-7.
60. Acerbo MJ, Gargiulo PA, Krug I, Delius JD. Behavioural consequences of nucleus accumbens dopaminergic stimulation and glutamatergic blocking in pigeons. Behav Brain Res. 2002;136(1):171–7.
61. Gargiulo PA, Acerbo MJ, Krug I, Delius JD. Cognitive effects of dopaminergic and glutamatergic blockade in nucleus accumbens in pigeons. Pharmacol Biochem Behav. 2005;81(4):732–9.
62. Gargiulo PA, Martínez G, Ropero C, Funes A, Landa AI. NMDA glutamatergic blockade of nucleus accumbens disrupts acquisition but not consolidation in a passive avoidance task. Ann N Y Acad Sci. 1999;877:717–22.
63. Martínez G, Ropero C, Funes A, Flores E, Landa AI, Gargiulo PA. AP-7 into the nucleus accumbens disrupts acquisition but does not affect consolidation in a passive avoidance task. Physiol Behav. 2002;76(2):205–12.
64. Martínez G, Ropero C, Funes A, Flores E, Blotta C, Landa AI, Gargiulo PA. Effects of selective NMDA and non-NMDA blockade in the nucleus accumbens on the plus-maze test. Physiol Behav. 2002;76(2):219–24.
65. Baiardi G, Ruiz AM, Beling A, Borgonovo J, Martínez G, Landa AI, Sosa MA, Gargiulo PA. Glutamatergic ionotropic blockade within accumbens disrupts working memory and might alter the endocytic machinery in rat accumbens and prefrontal cortex. J Neural Transm (Vienna). 2007;114(12):1519–28. https://doi.org/10.1007/s00702-007-0776-7.
66. Kapur S. Psychosis as a state of aberrant salience: a framework linking biology, phenomenology, and pharmacology in schizophrenia. Am J Psychiatry. 2003;160(1):13–23.
67. Kelley AE, Andrzejewski ME, Baldwin AE, Hernandez PJ, Pratt WE. Glutamate-mediated plasticity in corticostriatal networks: role in adaptive motor learning. Ann N Y Acad Sci. 2003;1003:159–68. https://doi.org/10.1196/annals.1300.061.
68. Murueta-Goyena-Larrañaga A, Bengotxea H, Gargiulo PA, Ortuzar N, Lafuente JV. Neuropathological background of MK801 for inducing murine model of schizophrenia. In: Gargiulo PA, Mesones HL, editors. Psychiatry and neurosciences. Translational approaches. New York: Springer; 2017. p. 337–54. ISBN: 978-3-319-53125-0.
69. Murueta-Goyena A, Ortuzar N, Gargiulo PÁ, Lafuente JV, Bengoetxea H. Short-term exposure to enriched environment in adult rats restores MK-801-induced cognitive deficits and GABAergic interneuron immunoreactivity loss. Mol Neurobiol. 2018;55(1):26–41. https://doi.org/10.1007/s12035-017-0715-z. Erratum in: Mol Neurobiol. 2017.

Pavlovian Impulsivity: Connectionist Predictions, with Implications for Addiction

11

José E. Burgos and Santiago Castiello

Impulsive behavior, or impulsivity for short, has been widely studied as possibly crucial to addictions and their treatment. This behavior has been defined as a preference for a small reward after a short delay over a large reward after a long delay [1]. In the treatment of addictions, the reward of interest consists of long-term positive consequences of not consuming an addictive substance (e.g., cocaine, food, nicotine, and alcohol). These consequences vary according to the substance (e.g., improved circulatory and respiratory health for not smoking, weight loss for not eating sugar, and social reinforcement for not consuming cocaine of alcohol), and compete with the rewarding physiological effects of the substance (e.g., increased dopaminergic activation). In all cases, impulsivity occurs when an addicted person prefers the short-term physiological effects of the substance over the long-term positive consequences of not consuming it.

J. E. Burgos (✉)
Universidad de Guadalajara, Centro de Estudios e Investigaciones en Comportamiento, Guadalajara, Jalisco, Mexico
e-mail: jburgos@academicos.udg.mx;
http://www.ceic.cucba.udg.mx/Investigacion/personal-investigador?id=4

S. Castiello
Department of Experimental Psychology, University of Oxford, Oxford, UK
e-mail: santiago.castiello@st-annes.ox.ac.uk;
santiago.castiellodeobeso@yale.edu;
https://sites.google.com/view/santiagocastiello/home

In animal experimental research, the dominant working hypothesis is that impulsivity thus defined results from delay discounting in operant conditioning, a reduction in the subjective value of a delayed reward [2]. In operant conditioning, animals learn to behave in a certain way (e.g., press a bar or peck a key) after being rewarded for it. The key experimental operation here is response-dependent (operant) reinforcement, where the animal is required to perform a certain response to be rewarded. Additionally, responses in operant conditioning are emitted in that they are not unconditionally elicited by the reward, unlike unconditioned responses such as salivation to food and blinking to a puff of air.

In this chapter, we hypothesize another possible source of impulsivity. We do not intend this hypothesis to displace or replace in any way the delay-discounting hypothesis in operant-conditioning research. Rather, we only seek to supplement this hypothesis with ours. Ours arises from a very simple computer simulation using an extant connectionist or neural-network model. As a computational study, it will be highly theoretical and simplified. Consequently, and as a first attempt, it will be quite preliminary, suggestive, and subject to further investigation.

We call our hypothesis "Pavlovian impulsivity," where the qualifier "Pavlovian" refers only to the kind of reinforcement operation involved, namely, response-independent reinforcement. We define Pavlovian impulsivity as a preference

P. Á. Gargiulo, H. L. Mesones-Arroyo (eds.), *Psychiatry and Neuroscience Update – Vol. V*,
https://doi.org/10.1007/978-3-031-72219-6_11

for a discrete cue X previously paired with a small response-independent reinforcement after a short delay, over another discrete cue Y previously paired with a large response–independent reinforcement after a long delay. As clarified later, the model we used allows this definition to preserve the emphasis on emitted responding found in delay discounting in operant conditioning. Thus, by "Pavlovian" we mean only response-independent reinforcement, not the occurrence of unconditioned responses.

In Pavlovian conditioning, reinforcement delay depends on the interstimulus interval (ISI), the time between the onset of a cue and the occurrence of the reinforcer, which has been shown to have a robust effect on Pavlovian conditioning [3]. The main effect is known as the ISI function, a non-monotonic relation between the ISI and a conditioned-response measure. This function has a roughly inverted-U shape, where intermediate ISIs are optimal in promoting Pavlovian conditioning. ISIs below or above optimal ISIs weaken Pavlovian conditioning. The weakening with longer ISIs might be reminiscent of certain mathematical descriptions of delay discounting [4], but we will not discuss this.

The ISI function has been previously simulated with the model, for elicited [5] as well as emitted responding [6, 7], so we will not repeat it here. The important result of this research for our present purposes is that the model can simulate a Pavlovian form of discounting as the long-ISI side of an ISI function, for both types of responding. The present study is an extension of this result to a Pavlovian form of impulsivity as a result of weakened emitted responding due to a long ISI.

The expression "Pavlovian impulsivity" has been used by others in ways that differ from ours. In a review of the relations between emotion, decision-making, and the amygdala, Seymour and Dolan [8] view negative automaintenance as a case of Pavlovian impulsivity (p. 666). Negative automaintenance is the maintenance of an autoshaped response (an emitted skeletal response acquired through Pavlovian reinforcement) with an omission procedure, where responding prevents reinforcement. However, we did not simulate this phenomenon here, and it is unclear how it relates to our present definition of "Pavlovian impulsivity."

In another paper, Pine et al. [9] refer to the "mediation of unconditioned and conditioned responses by dopamine," which they view as related to "the concept of Pavlovian impulsivity, where responses associated with primary, innate values form a simple, evolutionary specified action set operating alongside, sometimes in competition with other control mechanisms, such as habit based and goal-directed action" (p. 8894). They proposed this as an interpretation of increased impulsivity in a serial choice task by dopamine agonists (e.g., L-DOPA) administered to humans. Although the present model considers the role of dopaminergic systems in conditioning (see next section and Appendix), we simulated neither pharmacological manipulations nor a serial choice task. Also, the authors restricted Pavlovian impulsivity to responding that is unconditionally elicited by the reinforcer, whereas we did not. Our simulation predicts that response-independent reinforcement can also result in impulsive emitted responding.

Another key antecedent is the study by Picker and Poling [10] with autoshaping in pigeons. Autoshaping is the acquisition of an emitted (skeletal) response (e.g., keypecking in pigeons, barpressing in rats) under Pavlovian reinforcement, which the model used here can also simulate [11]. In their study, pigeons first received trials of different keylight cues (e.g., a red light vs. a white cross) separately paired with either different food frequencies (e.g., 100% vs. 50%, Experiment 1) or durations (Experiment 2). Then, pigeons received unreinforced choice tests, where the cues were concurrently presented as a compound cue. The results showed that pigeons chose more frequently the cue that had been previously paired with a larger food frequency or longer food duration. The procedure in our simulation was similar, except that a cue was paired with either a small reinforcement (or "reward") after a short ISI or a large reward after a long ISI, to approximate procedures used to study operant impulsivity.

The larger issue here is the operant-Pavlovian distinction. This issue has not yet received a universally accepted resolution, nor has it been much discussed in relation to impulsivity, except for two papers. In one paper, Killeen [12] hypothesized that discounting could be viewed as an exponential (perhaps hyperbolic) decay in the "associability" between a response and a reinforcer. This decay, he pointed out, is comparable to the eligibility trace that is hypothesized in some neural-network models to describe how the associability between a cue and a primary reinforcer decreases with the ISI in Pavlovian conditioning [13, 14].

Such decay has also been observed for elicited responding in the nictitating membrane response preparation with rabbits, although steeper for trace than delay conditioning [15]. There also is evidence of comparable effects of the ISI on emitted responding with response-independent reinforcement in autoshaping [16]. Killeen [12] thus distinguished between Pavlovian and operant discounting, as we do, except that he seems to have restricted Pavlovian discounting to responding that is unconditionally elicited by the reinforcer, whereas we do not.

In another paper, Holt et al. [17] first trained two responses in pigeons, keypecking with an autoshaping procedure and treadle pressing with a hand-shaping procedure. Then, pigeons received a discrete-trial choice procedure with various conditions that required either response. The authors predicted that impulsivity would be greater for keypecking, thanks to the keylight-food relation in autoshaping. This relation facilitated the elicitation of keypecking by the keylight, which in turn promoted a temporally more contiguous keypecking-food relation. The results confirmed the prediction, from which the authors hypothesized that stimulus-reinforcer relations could play a role in impulsivity. Our simulation of Pavlovian impulsivity here is consistent with this conjecture, only that the effects of stimulus-reinforcer relations are modeled in connectionist fashion, as effects of the duration of certain input activations (simulated cues) without others (simulated reinforcer) on the inner workings (activations and connection weights) of a neural network.

In the first section, we give an informal description of the model. In the second section, we describe the simulation. In the last section, we discuss some implications for operant impulsivity and addiction. We will not try to predict any specific quantitative properties of Pavlovian impulsivity, as it still is a hypothetical phenomenon pending animal corroboration. The present study is only a first connectionist approach to impulsivity from the perspective of a particular neural-network model. We thus only seek to describe a few basic ordinal properties of this novel phenomenon.

The Model: Informal Description

In this section, we give an informal description of the model, with the neural network that we used in the simulation, focusing on the aspects that are most directly relevant to the study, in particular, how the operant-Pavlovian distinction is conceived. The Appendix describes the more formal, mathematical part, which consists of the activation function (used to compute unit activations) and learning function (used to compute changes in connection weights).

The model was initially proposed as a formal connectionist interpretation of the operant-Pavlovian distinction behaviorally guided by a unified reinforcement principle [18]. It was also guided by evidence on some of the neural substrates of conditioning, especially the roles of hippocampal and dopaminergic systems. It was thus built only on neurocomputational interpretations of basic behavioral and neural categories, for which it is a purely neurobehavioral model. This feature distinguishes it from models of conditioning that have been built either on cognitive (e.g., "attention," "expectancy," "associative strength," "memory," "representation," "information," "storage," and "retrieval") and behavioral [19–21]; only behavioral [4, 12, 22]; or cognitive, behavioral, and neural categories [13, 23, 24].

Pavlovian conditioning phenomena that have been simulated with the model include acquisition, extinction, and faster reacquisition or "savings" [25]; ISI functions [5]; latent inhibition

[26] C/T ratio effects [27]; context-shift effects [28]; simultaneous conditioning [29]; second-order conditioning and resistance to extinction [30]; and blocking and overshadowing [31].

Simulations of operant conditioning with the model have been less extensive. So far, the model has simulated acquisition, extinction, faster reacquisition, generalization, and discrimination [25]; timing in a fixed-interval schedule [6, 7]; and reinforcement revaluation [32]. Research remains to be conducted to determine whether the model can also simulate other, more specific operant-conditioning phenomena (e.g., shaping, behavioral contrast, negative reinforcement, positive punishment, fixed-ratio performance, the matching law, and conditional discrimination).

Despite this, the model provides conceptual resources to theorize about the operant-Pavlovian distinction [33]. The reason is that the model can also simulate autoshaping and automaintenance, positive as well as negative [11]. Ever since their discovery [34, 35], these phenomena have been central to discussions on the distinction, especially the possible role of stimulus-reinforcer relations in operant responding [36]. The model thus allows for theorizing about such role and, to this extent, the possible role of those relations in operant impulsivity as a result of discounting. This theorizing is linked to how the model conceives the operant-Pavlovian distinction in terms formal interpretations of behavioral and neural categories. The model defines behavioral categories in terms of neural categories but does not identify the former with the latter. Behavioral categories are still different from neural categories. Rather, such definitions refer only to some neural substrates of behavioral categories.

The behavioral categories are those typically found in discussions about the operant-Pavlovian distinction. Such categories thus constitute distinctions between different types of stimuli (CSs, discriminative vs. primary reinforcers, unconditioned stimuli, Sr's), reinforcement operations (response independent vs. response dependent), and responses (emitted vs. elicited). These distinctions are made in the model in terms of formal interpretations of neural categories. We can best explain how with an example.

Figure 11.1 depicts the network that we used in the simulation described in the next section. In connectionist jargon, the network has a feedforward architecture where neural units (squares, hexagon, circles) are organized into one input (S'), two hidden (S'', M''), and one output layer (M'). Units are intended to simulate (very simply) relatively small neuronal groups. Units on one layer send connections (lines with button endings) to units on the adjacent layer to the right. Connections are intended to simulate relatively small synaptic groups. Connections are one-directional in that unit i (pre-connection unit) is connected to unit j (post-connection unit) but not vice versa. Therefore, i can activate j, but not vice versa. For example, input unit S'_1 is connected to and hence can activate S''_1 (top unit of the first hidden layer), but not vice versa. Similarly, M''_1 (top unit of the second hidden layer) is connected to and hence can activate the M'_1 output unit, but not vice versa, and so on.

Other neural categories on which the model was built refer to a few general principles of gross avian and mammalian neuroanatomy. These principles yield a classification of the types of units that a network can have and a few general guidelines on how to connect them. Thus, the network has units to simulate small fractions of sensory and motor, primary as well as association, areas. Some sensory units (sensory primary or input or S') connect to others (sensory association or S'') and some special-purpose units (H, for "hippocampal"). Other sensory units (S'') connect to some motor units (motor association or M''); these, in turn, connect to other motor units (primary motor or output or M') and other special-purpose units (D for "dopaminergic"). This basic configuration is general to avian and mammalian brains. Obviously, there are many differences in detail, within and across species. However, they are too complex to simulate as a starting point. Also, the model's phylogenetic generality is limited (e.g., invertebrates lack dopaminergic and hippocampal systems).

Like other neural-network models of conditioning [23], the present one makes a distinction between two types of stimuli in terms of activations of two types of input units. Such activations

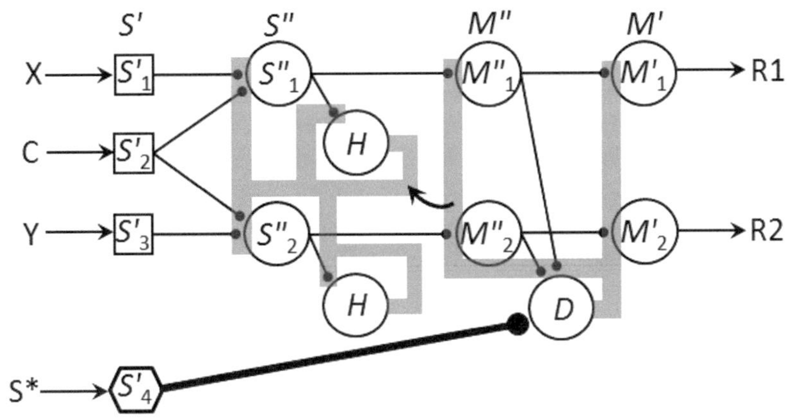

Fig. 11.1 Neural network used in the simulation (see next section). X, Y: Simulated discrete cues (e.g., a green keylight vs. a yellow keylight). C: Contextual cues. S*: Simulated biologically significant stimulus or primary reinforcer (e.g., food, water). Arrows to inputs: Sensory transduction (not modeled). Squares labeled as S'_1, S'_2, S'_3: Input units whose activations are intended to simulate primary-sensory (S') effects of X, C, and Y, respectively. Hexagon labeled as S'_4: Input unit whose activation is intended to simulate a primary-sensory effect of S*. Input activations are assigned according to a training protocol that simulates some conditioning procedure of interest. Circles: Neurocomputational units whose activations are computed according to the activation rule (see Appendix). Thin lines with button endings: initially weak, variable, one-direction connections whose weights change according to the learning rule (see Appendix). Curved thick line (from S'_4 to D): Maximally strong fixed connection. Connections are one-directional and are intended to simulate synapses. Activations propagate from left to right (but see the Appendix for a description of the activation update procedure). S'': Sensory-association hidden layer, consisting of S''_1 and S''_2. M'': Motor-association hidden layer, consisting of M''_1 and M''_2. M': primary-motor (output) layer, consisting of M'_1 and M'_2, whose activations are intended to simulate primary-motor precursors of two forms of emitted responding R1 and R2 (e.g., pecking a green key vs. pecking a yellow key), respectively. Arrows from outputs: primary-motor-to-effector transduction (not modeled). H: Units that simulate a hippocampal area (e.g., CA1), source of the discrepancy (transparent rectangles) that modulates weight changes in the S'-S'' and S''-H connections (gray areas from H; see learning rule in Appendix). D: Unit that simulates a dopaminergic structure (e.g., ventral tegmental area), source of the discrepancy that modulates weight changes in the S''-M'', M''-M', and M''-D connections (gray areas from D; see learning rule in Appendix). Curved arrow: Amplification of the H discrepancy by the D discrepancy

are intended to simulate primary-sensory effects of different types of exteroceptive environmental events (the intrinsic physicochemical properties of which, for example, wavelength, are not simulated in the model). In Fig. 11.1, one type of input unit is depicted by the squares labeled as S'_1, S'_2, and S'_3. Their activations are intended to simulate primary-sensory effects of exteroceptive, environmental events (e.g., changes in wavelength). S'_1 and S'_3 activations simulate primary-sensory effects of two discrete cues X and Y, respectively, such as two occasionally occurring keylight colors (e.g., green and yellow). S'_2 activations simulate primary-sensory effects of a context (C) that consists of background cues that are "tonic" as opposed to "phasic" [37] in that they remain fixed throughout a conditioning session (e.g., the box walls, roof, and floor).

The other type of input unit is depicted as the hexagon labeled as S'_4. The activation of this unit is intended to simulate primary-sensory effects of stimuli used as biologically significant, primary reinforcers in conditioning research (S*; e.g., food and water). In contrast to the other input units, S'_4 sends only a maximally strong fixed connection (thick line) to unit D (see below). In other networks in this model, S'_4 also sends maximally strong fixed connections to output units that simulate primary-motor precursors of elicited responding. For simplicity, however, the present network does not have such units, to focus on emitted responding. Of course, this is a theoretical possibility unlikely to obtain in animals.

Input units should thus be distinguished from their activations and these from their behavioral interpretations. A unit is intended to simulate an entity with a definite spatial location, such as a group of neurons within a brain. For example, input units are intended to simulate some small fraction of primary-sensory cortex (e.g., visual, auditory, gustatory, and olfactory). Input activations can be symbolized as $a(S'_1)$, $a(S'_2)$, $a(S'_3)$, and $a(S'_4)$, respectively, and are intended to simulate the activity or functioning of such fraction as an effect of some environmental event. The magnitude of this activity is assumed to be directly proportional to that of environmental events.

Behavioral interpretations of input activations are largely arbitrary and refer to the environmental events themselves, labeled in Fig. 11.1 as X, C, Y, and S*. The arrows from these labels to the input units depict a sensory transduction process (conversion of environmental events into neural activity) that the model does not simulate. An input activation greater than zero thus simulates a primary-sensory effect of an environmental event, and the higher the activation, the more intense the event; in particular, primary reinforcement is simulated as $a(S'_4) > 0$, where different activation levels simulate (primary-sensory effects of) different primary-reinforcer magnitudes.

At any moment, input units can be activated in myriad different ways, depending on how the network is to be trained. Networks are trained according to a protocol that simulates a conditioning procedure of interest as a specification of how input units are to be activated throughout (discrete) time. The training protocols we used in the simulations were Pavlovian in that $a(S'_4) > 0$ did not depend on the network's output activations.

Output units, M'_1 and M'_2 (Fig. 11.1) simulate primary-motor precursors of two forms of emitted-responding R1 and R2 (e.g., pecking a green key vs. pecking a yellow key), respectively. Their emitted character does not refer to spontaneous responding without any antecedent controlling exteroceptive stimulus. Rather, emitted responding here refers only to their activations not being unconditionally activated by the S'_4 input unit when $a(S'_4) > 0$, as they do not receive any connection from it.

Strictly, output activations do not simulate responses. Responses also involve effectors (muscles and glands), which the model does not simulate. Also, all activations (and weights) in this model are numbers between 0.0 and 1.0, whereas responses are binary events. To simulate responses, a response rule that converts output activations into responses must be added. In the past, a simple threshold rule has been used, where a response is defined in terms of an output activation that is equal to a greater than a moderate value (e.g., 0.5), and we use it here as well. It admittedly is very simple (e.g., does not allow for differences in response magnitude), and more sophisticated rules are possible, but we prefer a simple rule as a convenient starting point.

This clarification yields two others. First, the fact that the model does not identify activations with responses means that the present definitions of behavioral categories in terms of neural categories are nonreductive. The second clarification has to do with the "emitted" character of emitted responding as simulated in the model. The activation rule allows for some spontaneous activation (greater-than-zero activations with zero input activations) for hidden and output units. However, with a low value of a certain free parameter of the activation rule ($\sigma = 0.1$; see Appendix), spontaneous activations are close to zero (~0.007). Consequently, spontaneous output activations do not meet the output activation criterion for a simulated response that we adopt here (0.5). For output activations to meet this criterion a network must be trained with a protocol that promotes sufficient weight gain by the appropriate connections. In the case of this network, such a protocol would involve high $a(S'_1)$, $a(S'_2)$, and/or $a(S'_3)$, followed by a high $a(S'_4)$ after an optimal (not too long) ISI.

Like input units, output units are different from their activations and these from their behavioral interpretations. Again, a unit is intended to simulate a spatially located entity such as a group of neurons within a brain. Output units, in particular, are intended to simulate small fractions of primary-motor areas (e.g., cortical "homunculus" that maps different body parts onto different parts of primary-motor cortex).

Output activations are intended to simulate the activity or functioning of such fraction.

We interpret M'_1 and M'_2 activations as primary-motor precursors of two forms of emitted-responding R1 and R2. Formally, M'_1 and M'_2 symbolize units, $a(M'_1)$ and $a(M'_2)$ can symbolize their activations, and R1 and R2 their behavioral meanings. The arrows from the output units depict a motor transduction process (conversion of neuronal activity into effector functioning, e.g., muscle contraction) that is not simulated by the model (at least not its anatomical and physiological details; a response rule could be viewed as a very abstract simulation of them). Responding is just assumed to be directly proportional to output activation.

Learning in artificial neural networks is defined as changes in connection weights (i.e., thin lines with button endings, Fig. 11.1), according to a learning function (see Appendix). Weight changes are intended to simulate (very simply) changes in synaptic efficacies in natural neuronal circuits. The model thus allows for a learning-performance distinction, where learning is defined as connection weight changes, and performance as a response rule for output activations.

This distinction, in turn, allows for a performance but does not force a learning operant-Pavlovian distinction. The model's learning function makes no distinction between operant and Pavlovian learning. The underlying assumption here is that both have at least one learning mechanism in common. This assumption does not imply an absolute identity between operant and Pavlovian conditioning, only a commonality in at least one underlying learning mechanism. They can thus differ in some respects captured by the model (different reinforcement operations and types of responses). There are other differences the model excludes. For example, the model says nothing about the genetic level, where there could also be important differences [38]. But then again, such differences do not exclude the possibility of at least one common learning mechanism at the synaptic level. Nor does this hypothesized mechanism exclude other possible common mechanisms at the same or other (e.g., genetic and molecular) levels.

The relevant implication here is that operant and Pavlovian impulsivity share at least one underlying learning (synaptic change) mechanism. From the model's perspective, as used here, their main difference is at the performance level, in the kind of reinforcement operation (response-dependent for operant vs. response-independent for Pavlovian). It remains to be seen whether this makes a substantial behavioral difference in animals.

The network also includes two special-purpose units H and D intended to simulate hippocampal and dopaminergic areas, respectively. The learning rule in the Appendix describes the exact way in which the role of these systems is simulated. Intuitively, the activations of these units (more precisely, temporal differences or discrepancies in their activations) modulate weight changes in all of the network's variable connections. H discrepancies (gray areas arising from each H unit) thus modulate weight changes in the S'-S'' and S''-H connections. D discrepancies (gray areas arising from D) modulate weight changes in S''-M'', M''-D, and M''-M' connections.

The network's architecture determines its functioning as follows. S'_1 can only activate M'_1 (via S''_1 and M''_1), S'_3 can only activate M'_2 (via S''_2 and M''_2), and S'_2 can activate both output units (because it is connected to both S'' units). Behaviorally, this means that, after suitable training, X can only control R1 and Y can only control R2, whereas C can control both. The desired effect was that either cue had to control more strongly its own response than the other cue. For the simulation, we chose X to control R1 more strongly than Y controlled R2. Also, we seek this effect to result from a learning (weight change) process under a training protocol that simulates the kind of procedure used to study behavioral impulsivity.

We designed a protocol to simulate this procedure and promote more weight gain by the connections in the S'_1-S''_1-M''_1-M'_1 than the S'_3-S''_2-M''_2-M'_2 pathway. For this, we relied on how the learning rule works. Intuitively, moments when $a(S'_4) = 0$ tend to promote weight loss, which, in turn, weakens activations of either output unit (M'_1 or M'_2) by its corresponding input unit (S'_1 or S'_3, respectively). The ISI is simulated as a sequence of such moments, from the first input activation moment until the next moment when $a(S'_4) > 0$ (simulated primary reinforcement). Longer ISIs are simulated by more such moments, which promote weight loss and, to this extent, a lower activation of either output unit by its corresponding input unit. We thus designed the training protocol for Y to include a longer ISI, so that Y would control R2 less strongly than X controlled R1.

To simulate the kind of procedure used in research on impulsivity, such ISI must end with a higher $a(S'_4)$, to simulate a large reward, but this promotes weight gain, which counters the detrimental effect of a longer ISI. However, the ISI can be so long that even $a(S'_4) = 1.0$ (the maximum activation possible) cannot counter its detrimental effect. We thus chose an ISI for Y that was sufficiently long for this to occur. The result was a training protocol that simulated a large reward paired with Y after a long ISI. The short-ISI/small-reward condition was designed for X following the same logic. Shorter ISIs promote more weight gain, but a lower $a(S'_4)$ counters this effect. We thus chose $a(S'_4)$ to be lower for X than Y, but sufficiently high to allow a shorter ISI to promote more weight gain by the connections in the S'_1-S''_1-M''_1-M'_1 pathway and, to this extent, a stronger control of R1 by X.

A Simulation

For simplicity, as a starting point, a single neural network with the architecture depicted in Fig. 11.1 was used. All initial (pretraining) weights were set to 0.1 (to simulate an experimentally naïve animal), and all activation and learning free parameters were the same as in previous simulations (see Appendix). For the simulation, we used a simulator designed and coded in Delphi© by the first author. The simulator (executable Windows© file), source code, all necessary files for the simulation, and simulation data are available upon request to the first author.

To simulate the Pavlovian training of two emitted response alternatives, the network first received 100 X+ trials randomly intermixed with 100 Y+ trials, in context C. In this procedure, X was simulated as (an exteroceptive cue causing) $a(S'_1) = 1.0$ for three moments and Y as $a(S'_3) = 1.0$ for seven moments. A primary reinforcement operation (+) was simulated as $a(S'_4) = 0.7$ (small reinforcer) at the last moment of X, for an ISI of two moments (short delay), and as $a(S'_4) = 1.0$ (large reinforcer) at the last moment of Y, for an ISI of six time-steps (long delay). C was simulated as $a(S'_2) = 0.65$ (the context was assumed to be less salient than X or Y, a common assumption in conditioning modeling). C was present for the entire training. For simplicity, the intertrial interval was not explicitly simulated but assumed to be sufficiently long for all activations to decrease to near-zero spontaneous levels (see Refs. [26, 29] for simulations of the effect of this interval with the model).

Then, the network received 20 XY choice test trials, where X and Y were presented as a compound for four moments without the reward. During test trials, there was no learning because the learning rule was disabled to obtain pure output activations without weight changes and, thus, avoid extinction (this is a theoretical possibility impossible to achieve in animals). After this test, the learning rule was again enabled and the network received 100 additional response-independent small reinforcements (same magnitude as the small reinforcer during training) in the presence of C alone (without X or Y) with a delay of four moments. After this, the network received another 20 XY choice test trials. The question here was whether and how such context conditioning modified the effect of training.

The results are shown in Fig. 11.2, in terms of the mean $a(M'_1)$ (filled bars) and $a(M'_2)$ (empty bars) at the last moment of choice trials, before (top panel) and after (bottom panel) context conditioning. Comparable results were obtained in repeated simulations with the same architecture. There was almost no variation in the output activations at that moment across choice trials, hence the near-zero standard errors. The legend below the top panel shows the training conditions before context conditioning.

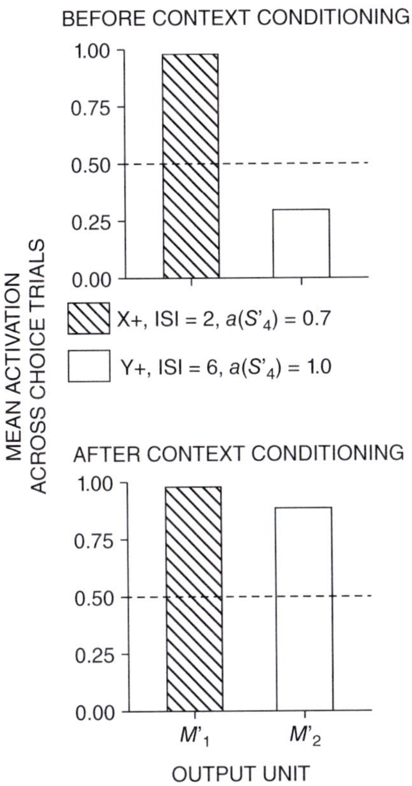

Fig. 11.2 Simulation results in terms of mean $a(M'_1)$ (filled bars) and $a(M'_2)$ (empty bars) at the second-to-last moment of discrete-choice test trials (with the learning rule disabled) before (top panel) and after (bottom panel) context conditioning. Before context conditioning, as shown in the legend below the top panel, the network received 100 trials of X+ randomly intermixed with 100 Y+ trials. X was simulated as $a(S'_1) = 1.0$ for three moments, and Y as $a(S'_3) = 1.0$ for seven moments. X trials were paired with a small reinforcer, simulated as $a(S'_4) = 0.7$, after a short delay (ISI of two moments). Y was paired with a large reinforcer, simulated as $a(S'_4) = 1.0$, after a long delay (ISI of six moments). All trials occurred in context C, simulated as $a(S'_2) = 0.65$. Dashed lines: Output activation response criterion. A response is defined as an output activation above this criterion. Standard errors were nearly zero because there was almost no variation in output activations across test trials. Pavlovian impulsivity was simulated in the top panel as a mean $a(M'_1)$ above response criterion, simulating at least one R1 response to X in every choice test trial, and a mean $a(M'_2)$ well below the criterion, simulating no R2 response to Y in any test trial. Impulsivity was thus simulated as a total preference for X. During context conditioning, 100 more response-independent small reinforcers were given in the presence of C alone (without X or Y) with a delay of three moments. The bottom panel shows an increase in the mean $a(M'_2)$ above the response criterion, indicating at least one R2 response to Y in every choice trial. The model thus predicts that context conditioning eliminates Pavlovian impulsivity

The top panel shows that the model predicts Pavlovian impulsivity as a mean $a(M'_1)$ (filled bar) above the response criterion (dashed line), due to a strong activation of M'_1 by S'_1 (via S''_1 and M''_1), and a mean $a(M'_2)$ below the response criterion (empty bar), due to a weak activation of M'_2 by S'_3 (via S''_2 and M''_2). In behavioral terms, X controlled at least one R1 response in every choice trial. In contrast, Y controlled no R2 response in the second-to-last moment of any choice trial. All of this occurred in choice test trials, so impulsivity was simulated as a complete preference for X.

X controlled R1 more strongly than Y controlled R2 because the shorter delay, despite ending in a smaller reward, was more effective in promoting weight gain by connections in the S'_1-S''_1-M''_1-M'_1 pathway than the larger reward was in promoting weight gain by connections in the S'_3-S''_2-M''_2-M'_2 pathway. Consequently, S'_1 activated M'_1 more substantially than S'_3 activated M'_2. The largest weight difference was observed between the S''_1-M''_1 and S''_2-M''_2 connections: The final S''_1-M''_1 connection weight in this phase was 0.85, whereas the final S''_2-M''_2 connection weight was 0.58.

Context conditioning was negligible in this phase for two reasons. First, S'_2 (the contextual-cue unit) was connected to both S'' units, together with S'_1 and S'_3. This connectivity promoted competition between S'_2 and S'_1 for the amount of weight on S''_1, and between S'_2 and S'_3 for the amount of weight on S''_2 (see learning rule in the Appendix for a mathematical description of this competition). Second, $a(S'_2)$ was much lower than $a(S'_1)$ and $a(S'_3)$, which gave a competitive disadvantage to S'_2. Behaviorally, then, C exerted little control over R1 or R2. Practically all R1 responding was controlled by X.

The bottom panel of Fig. 11.2 shows the mean $a(M'_1)$ and $a(M'_2)$ at the second-to-last moment of test choice trials after context conditioning. This conditioning was more substantial than in the first phase because the inter-reward became much shorter, and X and Y were absent, which gave a greater competitive advantage to S'_2. The result was an increase in both output activations, but now the increase of $a(M'_2)$ was sufficient to exceed the response criterion. The largest effect of context conditioning was to increase the final S''_2-M''_2 connection weight to 0.88. This increase allowed S'_3 to activate M'_2 more substantially in the second than the first-choice test trial. Behaviorally, this activation simulates at least one R2 response to Y in every test choice trial and, hence, the elimination of the impulsivity shown in the top panel. Because $a(M'_1)$ also increased (although less substantially), the network also emitted at least one R1 to X on every test trial. Hence, there was no preference for a particular cue, which simulates a sort of indifference, but one that deviates from the standard indifference notion, as we discuss next, among other issues.

General Discussion

The results show that the model predicts a novel phenomenon that has implications for impulsivity as a result of a Pavlovian form of discounting. We have called this phenomenon "Pavlovian impulsivity" and defined it as a preference to emit responses in a choice test to a cue previously paired with a small response-independent reinforcement after a short ISI, over a cue previously paired with a large response-independent reinforcement after a long ISI. This prediction approximates the kind of impulsivity that has been studied using operant contingencies (i.e., with response-dependent reinforcement) and viewed as a result of delay discounting.

Like that kind of impulsivity, the one predicted here involves responding that is emitted in that it is not unconditionally elicited by the reward. The predicted phenomenon also results from a Pavlovian form of discounting (the long-ISI end of an ISI function). These similarities allow for some contact between Pavlovian impulsivity, as predicted here, and operant impulsivity as studied in the field. Pavlovian impulsivity and discounting, however, result from response-independent reinforcement of discrete trials, whereas operant impulsivity and discounting result from response-dependent reinforcement without discrete trials (i.e., in "free-operant" arrangements).

The present model, then, like Killeen's [12], makes a distinction between operant and Pavlovian discounting and, to this extent, between Pavlovian and operant impulsivity (insofar as the latter results from the former). Such distinctions limit the applicability of the present study to operant impulsivity and discounting, if a sharp operant-Pavlovian distinction is drawn. However, in contrast to his model, the present one makes a somewhat less sharp distinction by hypothesizing a common learning mechanism that allows for a deeper relation between operant and Pavlovian conditioning.

As we argued in our informal description of the model, such a mechanism does not prevent making behavioral distinctions that are usually made in discussions about the operant-Pavlovian distinction (viz., conditioned-unconditioned stimuli, response-dependent/response-independent reinforcement, emitted-elicited responding). This is possible because the model works at two levels of theorizing. At the connection level, the model postulates a common learning mechanism (without intending to exclude other mechanisms, whether different or common). At the network level, the model makes those distinctions by attaching behavioral meaning to computational interpretations of neural categories.

Regarding such distinctions, the model predicts that emitted responding can be conditioned through response-independent reinforcement of discrete cues (the model also predicts conditioning of emitted responding through response-dependent reinforcement, but we did not simulate this here, as it would have meant a more complex simulation). The model thus allows for a coherent combination of a defining feature of Pavlovian conditioning (response-independent reinforcement of discrete cues) with a defining feature of operant conditioning (responding that is not unconditionally elicited by the reinforcer).

This combination obtains most clearly in autoshaping and positive automaintenance. Procedures used to study these phenomena are thus ideal to experimentally test the existence of Pavlovian impulsivity as predicted here. The basic procedure would be to first give animals X+ trials (e.g., reinforced red keylights) randomly intermixed with Y+ trials (e.g., reinforced yellow keylights), as Picker and Poling [10] did. In contrast to their procedures, however, rewards (+) would be given in a way that has been used to study behavioral impulsivity experimentally, that is, pairing one cue (e.g., X) with a small reward after a short ISI and the other with a large reward after a long ISI. Then, as in Picker and Poling's [10] experiments, animals would receive discrete-choice test trials where both cues are presented simultaneously. The model predicts that animals will tend to choose the cue that was paired with the small reward after a short ISI. We have used the model to predict pigeon's behavior in a similar autoshaping procedure where we manipulated the probability of reward in a large and uncertain option against a small and certain option, networks as pigeons adjusted their autoshaped choice to the probability of large uncertain alternative [39].

The model also predicts that free small rewards (of the same kind and magnitude as in the training phase) in the presence of the training context alone, separated by a short interval, reduce Pavlovian impulsivity. There is evidence that operant conditioning is as context dependent as Pavlovian conditioning [40]. Perhaps, then, context conditioning could also influence operant impulsivity in the way that was simulated here for Pavlovian impulsivity. This prediction could be experimentally tested by giving the pigeons a procedure analogous to the one simulated here, after the first-choice test phase: Response-independent small rewards (of the same kind and magnitude as in training) in the training context alone (without X or Y), followed by additional nonreinforced XY compound trials to test for choice.

In sum, the model predicts that animals will tend to respond to both keylights indifferently. This kind of indifference differs from the standard notion found in the animal impulsivity and discounting literature. Perhaps the most substantial difference is that the standard notion refers to variations in the response-reward delay [3] or the magnitude of the reward [41]. Here, in contrast, indifference was simulated as a result of context conditioning, without varying any of the cue-reward ISIs or the magnitude of the reward. Only a shorter inter-reward interval was used during the context conditioning phase.

If this prediction is experimentally confirmed with animals, its implication for applied human settings seems significant: Undesired impulsive responding in humans could be eliminated, or at least reduced, by context conditioning. Ethical caveats, however, must be carefully considered before implementing any treatment based on this prediction, especially if the "reinforcer" is harmful to the person receiving it, as is the case with intoxicating substances (e.g., cocaine, nicotine, alcohol). This treatment would basically mean deliberately giving such substances to the addicted person, clearly quite an unethical, perhaps even counterproductive strategy (liable to precipitate addiction and relapse; cf. [42–45]). A thorough examination of this prediction is thus necessary, before using it as a scientific basis for substance abuse treatment. In general, multiple behavioral interventions have been proposed to reduce impulsive behavior but there is insufficient clinical evidence to make an unequivocal determination of which are more effective [46].

The predictions could fail for a number of reasons. First, keypecking, a standard response used in autoshaping preparations, has a substantial elicitation component. This feature is suggested by evidence that the form of autoshaped keypecking resembles that of the response that is presumably elicited by the reinforcer (e.g., pecking grain, drinking water; e.g., [47]; cf. [48]). Here, in contrast, we simulated purely emitted responding (M'_1 and M'_2 were not activated by S'_4; behaviorally, S* did not elicit either response). This is inconsistent with that evidence, but we meant it as a convenient simplification, more than a strong theoretical claim. The model allows for a fuzzy distinction between elicited and emitted responding in networks that have several output units for the same response form, some of which are activated by S'_4 and others are not. In this manner, the same response form could have elicitation and emission components. However, this would require a more complex simulation than we intended to do for a first step like the present one. It remains to be seen whether networks whose output units can also be unconditionally activated by S* simulate comparable results.

Second, due to the network's architecture, $a(M'_1)$ and $a(M'_2)$ can both be simultaneously above the response criterion in choice test trials, as shown in the bottom panel of Fig. 11.2. The implication is that R1 and R2 are not mutually exclusive, for which both responses can occur simultaneously. That is to say, R1 and R2 did not compete with each other in that the occurrence of either does not prevent the occurrence of the other. Nor did X and Y compete for control of R1 or R2 either, as S'_1 and S'_3 each had its own path to their respective output units (M'_1 and M'_2, respectively), and both paths could be activated simultaneously (this exploits the intensely parallel character of neural-network processing).

This situation differs from those typically used in experimental research on choice. The typical situation is that animals can physically choose or respond to just one option, even if it is logically compatible with others (e.g., nothing logically prevents picking both, an immediate-small reward, and a delayed-large reward). Some models of choice attempt to capture this kind of situation by assuming some sort of competition between stimuli or responses, whether direct or mediated by mental representations or neurons (e.g., Refs. [12, 49–51]).

We meant this simplification as yet another strategic abstraction for a starting point. The model allows for network architectures that simulate neuronal competition between primary-sensor effects of exteroceptive stimuli (e.g., connecting both cue units to the same S'' units) and/or primary-motor precursors of responding (e.g., by adding lateral inhibition among output units), but this would mean a more complex simulation than we intended as a first step. Preliminary further simulations in our lab by Miguel Aguayo suggest that at least Pavlovian impulsivity also obtains with networks that simulate mutually exclusive responses by including lateral inhibition in the output layer. Other preliminary simulations suggest that a trace interval between the end of the cues and the reinforcer also reduces significantly Pavlovian impulsivity.

Albeit primarily practical, our simplification of response compatibility implies that stimulus or response competition is not necessary at least for the kind of choice we simulated here as Pavlovian impulsivity. This prediction raises the possibility that response competition is not necessary for choice in general. Testing this possibility empirically with animals would require a situation where both alternatives can be responded to simultaneously, so that responding to one does not exclude responding to the other (i.e., where both, R1 and R2, could occur concurrently). Keypecking, the response topography that is typically used in the standard autoshaping preparation is not suitable for this. A more suitable preparation could be bar- or pad-pressing in primates (e.g., monkeys, humans), where both bars (or pads) could be pressed simultaneously.

Two other reasons why the present predictions could fail are the simplicity of the network and the way we simulated the context. Obviously, the network is exceedingly simple and was not designed after any particular known brain circuit. In particular, no known brain circuit has such a neat neuroanatomical division between primary-sensory effects of different cues and primary-motor precursors of different response forms. All known natural brain circuits are far more complex than this. Nor does the model capture any molecular, cellular, or physiological details of neuronal functioning. Hence, we do not presume our simulation to be neurobiologically accurate and sophisticated. The results might thus be just an artifact of our simplifications. Perhaps, there is no natural brain circuit that neutrally implements Pavlovian impulsivity as predicted here. Still, we take the study as an opportunity to theorize about impulsivity from a somewhat different perspective, in the hope that some of it will lead to novel research, empirical and theoretical.

Similar caveats apply to the very simple way in which we simulated primary-sensory effects of the context, as discussed somewhere else [27, 28]. These effects were simulated as a constant activation of a single input unit. However, we have a very poor understanding of exactly how contextual cues work. Intuitively, an operant-conditioning chamber gives the animal sufficient freedom of movement to allow its orienting behavior to change through time, especially during inter-reward intervals. In this way, different contextual cues (parts of the chamber) could control different aspects of the animal's behavior at different times, depending on how it moves about the chamber. The model allows for networks that could simulate this intuition, by having multiple input units that are variably activated depending on the activations of certain output units. But this is entirely hypothetical and remains to be thoroughly investigated.

If Pavlovian impulsivity as simulated here is experimentally confirmed, what could be its significance to operant impulsivity? The obvious general conjecture in this regard is that Pavlovian impulsivity could somehow contribute to operant impulsivity (which, of course, does not exclude the vice versa). Much less obvious is exactly how such contribution could be obtained. A number of hypotheses present themselves in this regard, all of them purporting some operant-Pavlovian behavioral link.

The strongest link is that Pavlovian impulsivity could be constitutive of and, to this extent, enable operant impulsivity. Again, like operant impulsivity, Pavlovian impulsivity involves emitted responding. However, Pavlovian impulsivity was simulated as arising from response-independent reinforcement of discrete cues, whereas operant impulsivity arises from response-dependent reinforcement in free-operant situations. How can these differences be reconciled to make Pavlovian impulsivity constitutive of operant impulsivity?

The only possibility is that response-dependent reinforcement in operant impulsivity is paired with contextual cues C_X and C_Y (both different from, but possibly similar to, C), in a way similar to that simulated here for discrete cues X and Y. In virtue of this, C_X and C_Y could become antecedent controlling exteroceptive stimuli of emitted responding, in a way that promotes operant impulsivity. For this assumption to be plausible, we need a better understanding of how contextual cues work. In particular, because contextual cues are constantly present, it is unclear how they could work as discrete cues in precisely the way simulated here for X and Y.

We have suggested a general way in which contextual cues could work in these networks, but then again, it remains to be empirically and theoretically fleshed out. In particular, it is unclear how it could work in operant impulsivity. In order to work, C_X would have to be paired (via response-dependent reinforcement) with the small reward after a short delay, and contextual cues C_Y with the large reward after a long delay. But why should C_X and C_Y be paired precisely in that way? How do such pairings correspond precisely to the appropriate response alternatives (e.g., operanda)? No obvious answers are apparent.

Despite these important uncertainties, the present simulation is consistent with the conjecture by Holt et al. [17] that stimulus-reinforcer temporal relations could influence impulsivity. This emphasis on stimulus-reinforcer relations does not mean that the model excludes response-reinforcer relations. The model can simulate their temporal aspect in a standard way, as intervals between a response (above-criterion output activations) and a primary reinforcer (whether or not brought about by the response). However, the model theorizes about their effects in a connectionist style that departs from the standard operant-conditioning sense of response-class modification [52, 53]. Such style, rather, refers to the effect of response-reinforcer intervals thus simulated on the activations of and weights on output units, as a combination of two processes.

First, the activation rule includes a decay mode where there is a chance that at any moment t, the activation of unit j (which could be an output unit) is a decayed value of j's activation at $t-1$. The longer the ISI, the more frequent such decay will be. Second, connection weight changes depend partly on the levels of activation of the connected units, due to the learning rule's Hebbian component. Lower activations thus tend to at least decelerate weight gain, and occasionally promote weight loss, which in turn further weakens output activations. All of this is promoted by long ISIs. The net result of the two processes combined is that too many moments between an output activation sufficiently high to count as a response and an upcoming reward will tend to lower output activations. By the time the reward occurs, emitted-responding output activations are too low to allow for any substantial weight gain by their receiving connections.

This effect obtains for emitted responding but not elicited-responding output units because the latter are unconditionally activated by the reward. If $a(S'_4)$ is high, such unconditional activation will also be high and hence allow for substantial weight gain by the unit(s)' receiving connections (the same obtains for D). In agreement with conventional wisdom, then, and focusing on output units, the model restricts the significance of response-reinforcer relations to emitted responding. Still, the model views them as inextricably linked to stimulus-reinforcer relations because all responding is hypothesized to be under the control of some exteroceptive antecedent stimulation, which depends on these relations.

In sum, the present paper challenges the conventional wisdom that impulsivity is restricted to operant (response-dependent) reinforcement. In simple typical cases, this wisdom depicts animals as choosing between actions and making impulsive decisions when one action that leads to a quicker but smaller reward is preferred over an action that leads to a delayed but larger reward. Our notion of Pavlovian impulsivity suggests that impulsive behavior (and decision-making in general) might not require action-dependent rewards. Impulsive choices could arise from stronger Pavlovian conditioning to cues that signal more immediate albeit smaller rewards than cues that signal less immediate albeit greater rewards. Cue-reinforcer temporal contiguity could thus prevail over reinforcer magnitude in controlling Pavlovian choice behavior, which could lead to impulsive behaviors.

This implication prompts different kinds of hypothetical scenarios about addictive-qua-impulsive behavior that could lead to various treatments. As a very simple example, suppose an alcoholic person A concurrently receives invitations to drink from friends B and C. Suppose also that cues from B's presence have been highly correlated with quick access (short delay) to, say, two drinks (small reward), and cues from C's presence have been highly correlated with a deferred access (long delay) to, say, six drinks (large reward), independently of A's actions. Our study suggests the hypothesis that A is more likely to accept B's than C's invitation, everything else being equal, even if the two choices are not mutually exclusive.

This impulsive choice would be less harmful to A than the following one. A concurrently receives invitations from B (again) to have just two drinks (immediately, as usual) and brother D to go to a family gathering in 3 h. If D's presence has been highly correlated with delayed family gatherings, our study suggests that A would still accept B's invitation, even if they are more gratifying to A than drinking. Our results also suggest that giving A free small drinks separated by relatively short intervals in the original training context in the absence of both B and C might reduce the impulsive choice. But then again, this procedure raises critical ethical considerations. Of course, real life is far more complex, but these scenarios are a start, albeit they should be assessed with other approaches to addictions and their treatment. Much more research is needed, theoretical as well as empirical. Unfortunately, the vast intricacies of clinical settings pose major challenges to systematic well-controlled empirical research, which might underlie its general scarcity in these settings.

Appendix: Mathematical Description of the Model

Mathematically, the model consists of an activation rule (or function) and a learning rule. The activation rule is used to compute the level of activation (number between 0.0 and 1.0) of every neurocomputational unit (circles in Fig. 11.1) at every moment of every trial. The learning rule is used to change the weights (also numbers between 0.0 and 1.0) of all variable connections (thin lines with button endings in Fig. 11.1) at every moment. For both rules, time is conceived as consisting of discrete moments, occasions, epochs, or time-steps of indefinite but relatively short duration (say, 500 ms, give or take, if the reader absolutely needs a value, but no particular duration is used for computational purposes). We describe each rule in turn.

The activation rule consists of two modes: unconditional (automatic, "innate") and conditional ("learned"). Unconditional activation does not require any learning (weight change) and obtains when the activation of a certain input unit (S'_4 in the network depicted in Fig. 11.1) at t is larger than zero, and the unit whose activation is being computed (j) is either D or an elicited output unit (the network we used has no such output unit). Otherwise, conditional activation obtains. Conditional activation requires learning (increases in connection weights) and has two mutually exclusive states: reactivation and decay. All these states relate mathematically according to Eq. 11.1 below, a simplified version for the present study, without inhibition or output units that simulate unconditioned responding.

$$a_{j,t} = \begin{cases} a\left(S_4'\right), & \text{if } a\left(S_4'\right) > 0 \text{ and } j \text{ is } D\left(\text{unconditional activation}\right); \\ L\left(exc_{j,t}\right) + \tau L\left(exc_{j,t-1}\right)\left[1 - L\left(exc_{j,t}\right)\right], & \text{otherwise, if } L\left(exc_{j,t}\right) \geq \theta_{j,t}\left(\text{reactivation}\right) \\ L\left(exc_{j,t-1}\right) - \kappa L\left(exc_{j,t-1}\right) & \text{otherwise}\left(\text{decay}\right) \end{cases} \quad (11.1)$$

where j denotes the unit, whose activation is being computed, t denotes a timestep,

$$L(x) = \frac{1}{1 + e^{\frac{-x+\mu}{\sigma}}}$$

is the logistic function with constant mean $\mu = 0.5$, variable standard deviation σ (a free parameter; typically, $\sigma = 0.1$, which allows for a spontaneous activation level of approximately 0.007 with initial connection weights of 0.01), and argument $exc_{j,t} = x$, where

$$x = \sum_{i=1}^{n} a_{i,t} w_{i,j,t}$$

where n denotes the number of units connected to j.

Figure 11.3 shows a generic neurocomputational unit (amplification of any of the circles of the network in Fig. 11.1) for conditional activation, intended to simulate a relatively small neuronal group. A neurocomputational unit is intended to simulate a relatively small neuronal group. It receives a finite number of afferent activations ($a_{1,t}, \ldots, a_{i,t}, \ldots, a_{n,t}$) from one or more (up to n) excitatory pre-connection units (there can also be inhibitory units, but the network had none). Each preconnection unit is connected to a post-connection process (j) through weight a connection with a variable weight ($w_{1,j,t}, \ldots, w_{i,j,t}, \ldots, w_{n,j,t}$) that computes a product of activation and connection vectors $\mathbf{a}_{j,t}$ and $\mathbf{w}_{j,t}$, respectively. This product is the net amount of excitation on j and t ($exc_{j,t}$) and is passed as an argument to a logistic function (L).

Whether the rule is reactivation or decay mode at t depends on a Gaussian threshold ($\theta_{j,t}$), a random number generated according to a Gaussian distribution with a mean of 0.2 and standard deviation of 0.15. $\theta_{j,t}$ is one source of randomness in the model (another source is the procedure for updating activations and weights at t, which is random asynchronous). $\theta_{j,t}$ is also dynamical, as it is generated at every moment for every computational unit. Two other free parameters are temporal summation (τ_j) and decay (κ_j), where $\tau_j = 0.1$ and $\kappa_j = 0.1$.

A connection is intended to simulate a relatively small synaptic group, and a weight to simulate the efficacy of a synaptic group to allow the activation of a postsynaptic by a presynaptic neuronal group. Since a weight is a number between 0.0 and 1.0, and can be interpreted as the proportion of transmitter receptors on j that are controlled by i. The rule to change weights follows Eq. 11.2 below:

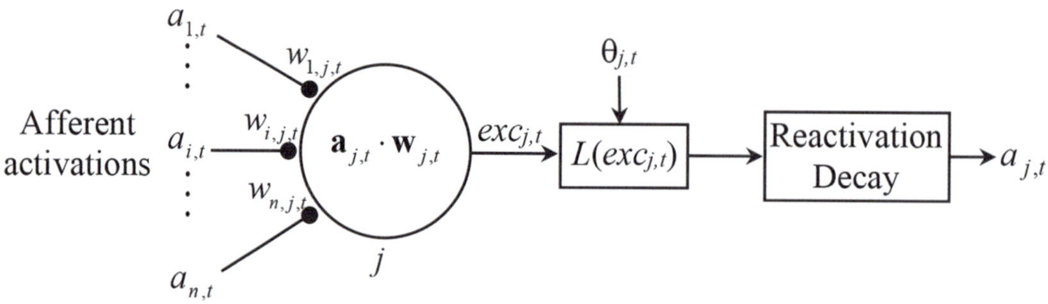

Fig. 11.3 Generic neurocomputational unit for conditional activation. i: afferent unit. j: generic target unit (representing only an S'', M'', H, D, or output unit). $a_{i,t}$: excitatory afferent activation (from either input or excitatory computational units). $w_{i,j,t}$: weight of a connection with an excitatory afferent unit. $\mathbf{a}_{j,t}\cdot\mathbf{w}_{j,t}$: product between a vector of excitatory afferent activations and a vector of corresponding weights. $exc_{j,t}$: net amount of excitation on j at t. L: Logistic function with $exc_{j,t}$ as an argument. $\theta_{j,t}$: Gaussian threshold. $a_{j,t}$: Efferent conditional activation of j at t (sent to another unit if j represents an S'' or M'' unit)

$$\Delta w_{i,j,t} = \begin{cases} \alpha_j a_{j,t} d_t p_{i,t} r_{j,t}, & \text{if } d_t \geq .001 \ (\text{weight gain}) \\ -\beta_j w_{i,j,t-1} a_{i,t} a_{j,t}, & \text{otherwise} \ (\text{weight loss}) \end{cases} \quad (11.2)$$

where α (rate of weight increment) and β (the rate of weight decrement) denote the two free parameters of the rule ($\alpha = 0.5$ and $\beta = 0.1$). The other terms of the rule are:

$a_{i,t}$: activation of pre-connection unit (i);
$a_{j,t}$: activation of post-connection unit (j);
$d_t = d_{H,t} = Avg(|a_{H,t} - a_{H,t-1}|) + d_{D,t}(1 - d_{H,t-1})$, if j is an S'' or H unit, where Avg denotes the mean discrepancy across hippocampal units (two, in the present study); otherwise,
$d_t = d_{D,t} = a_{D,t} - a_{D,t-1}$, if j is an M'', D, or M' unit (no averaging is necessary here because the networks had only one D unit);

$$p_{i,t} = \frac{a_{i,t} w_{i,j,t-1}}{N}, \text{where } N = exc_{j,t};$$

$$r_{j,t} = 1 - \sum_{i=1}^{n} w_{i,j,t}.$$

Like some other models, the rule has a Hebbian component in that connection weights partly depend on the activations of the connected units. The rule and is more akin to (but also different in some respects from) unsupervised, reinforcement tan supervised rules. The key factor is d_t, a signal that modulates changes of all weights, inspired by the roles of hippocampal (e.g., CA1) and dopaminergic (e.g., ventral tegmental area) areas in conditioning. In this sense, d_t is a diffuse signal. It also is a discrepancy signal in that it is defined as a temporal difference between the activations of certain units in pairs of successive moments. In early simulations, the d_t threshold was 0 but was increased to 0.001 to simulate latent inhibition [26]. The $p_{i,t}$ and $r_{j,t}$ factors introduce a "rich get richer, poor get poorer" sort of competition among connections for a limited amount of weight on any postsynaptic unit.

The very same rule is used to change all variable connections in a network, regardless of units or training protocols. In fact, none of the behavioral categories used to make the distinction appear in the rule. It is in this sense that the rule makes no learning (weight-change process) distinction between operant and Pavlovian conditioning. Initial connection weights are typically set to relatively low values (e.g., 0.2, as in this study).

References

1. Madden GJ, Bickel WK. Impulsivity: the behavioral and neurological science of discounting. American Psychological Association; 2010.
2. Odum AL. Delay discounting: I'm a k, you're a k. J Exp Anal Behav. 2011;96(3):427–39.
3. Schneiderman N, Gormezano I. Conditioning of the nictitating membrane of the rabbit as a function of CS-US interval. J Comp Physiol Psychol. 1964;57(2):188.

4. Mazur JE. An adjusting procedure for studying delayed reinforcement. In: Commons ML, Mazur JE, Nevin JA, Rachlin H, editors. Quantitative analyses of behavior: Vol. 5. The effect of delay and of intervening events on reinforcement value. Hillsdale: Erlbaum; 1987. p. 55–73.
5. Burgos JE. Evolving artificial neural networks in Pavlovian environments. In: Advances in psychology, vol. 121. North-Holland; 1997. p. 58–79.
6. Burgos J, Donahoe JW. Structure and function in selectionism: implications for complex behavior. In: Issues in experimental and applied analyses of human behavior; 2000. p. 39–57.
7. Donahoe JW, Burgos JE. Timing without a timer. J Exp Anal Behav. 1999;71(2):257–63.
8. Seymour B, Dolan R. Emotion, decision making, and the amygdala. Neuron. 2008;58(5):662–71.
9. Pine A, Shiner T, Seymour B, Dolan RJ. Dopamine, time, and impulsivity in humans. J Neurosci. 2010;30(26):8888–96.
10. Picker M, Poling A. Choice as a dependent measure in autoshaping: sensitivity to frequency and duration of food presentation. J Exp Anal Behav. 1982;37(3):393–406.
11. Burgos JE. Autoshaping and automaintenance: a neural-network approach. J Exp Anal Behav. 2007;88(1):115–30.
12. Killeen PR. Models of trace decay, eligibility for reinforcement, and delay of reinforcement gradients, from exponential to hyperboloid. Behav Process. 2011;87(1):57–63.
13. Sutton RS, Barto AG. Toward a modern theory of adaptive networks: expectation and prediction. Psychol Rev. 1981;88(2):135.
14. Wagner AR. SOP: a model of automatic memory processing in animal behavior. In: Information processing in animals. Psychology Press; 2014. p. 15–58.
15. Schneiderman N. Interstimulus interval function of the nictitating membrane response of the rabbit under delay versus trace conditioning. J Comp Physiol Psychol. 1966;62(3):397.
16. Brown BL, Hemmes NS, de Vaca SC. Timing of the CS-US interval by pigeons in trace and delay autoshaping. Q J Exp Psychol Sect B. 1997;50(1b):40–53.
17. Holt DD, Carlson JD, Follett VL, Jerdee NJ, Kelley DP III, Muhich KM, Tiry AM, Reetz NK. Response factors in delay discounting: evidence for Pavlovian influences on delay discounting in pigeons. Behav Process. 2013;98:37–43.
18. Donahoe JW, Crowley MA, Millard WJ, Stickney KA. A unified principle of reinforcement. In: Commons ML, Herrnstein RJ, Rachlin H, editors. Quantitative analyses of behavior: Vol. 2. Matching and maximizing accounts. Ballinger Publishing Company; 1982. p. 493–521.
19. Gibbon J, Balsam PE, Spreading association in time. In: Locurto CM, Terrace HS, Gibbon J, editors. Autoshaping and conditioning theory. New York: Academic; 1981. p. 219–53.
20. Rescorla RA. A theory of Pavlovian conditioning: variations in the effectiveness of reinforcement and nonreinforcement. In: Black AH, Prokasy WF, editors. Classical conditioning II: current research and theory. New York: Appleton-Century-Crofts; 1972. p. 64–99.
21. Stout SC, Miller RR. Sometimes-competing retrieval (SOCR): a formalization of the comparator hypothesis. Psychol Rev. 2007;114(3):759.
22. Herrnstein RJ. On the law of effect. J Exp Anal Behav. 1970;13(2):243–66.
23. Schmajuk NA, Lam YW, Gray JA. Latent inhibition: a neural network approach. J Exp Psychol Anim Behav Process. 1996;22(3):321.
24. Harry KA. A neuronal model of classical conditioning. Psychobiology. 1988;16(2):85–125.
25. Donahoe JW, Burgos JE, Palmer DC. A selectionist approach to reinforcement. J Exp Anal Behav. 1993;60(1):17–40.
26. Burgos JE. Theoretical note: simulating latent inhibition with selection neural networks. Behav Process. 2003;62(1–3):183–92.
27. Burgos JE. Theoretical note: the *C/T* ratio in artificial neural networks. Behav Process. 2005;69(2):249–56.
28. Burgos JE, Murillo-Rodríguez E. Neural-network simulations of two context-dependence phenomena. Behav Process. 2007;75(2):242–9.
29. Burgos JE, Flores C, García Ó, Díaz C, Cruz Y. A simultaneous procedure facilitates acquisition under an optimal interstimulus interval in artificial neural networks and rats. Behav Process. 2008;78(2):302–9.
30. Sánchez JM, Galeazzi JM, Burgos JE. Some structural determinants of Pavlovian conditioning in artificial neural networks. Behav Process. 2010;84(1):526–35.
31. Burns R, Burgos JE, Donahoe JW. Pavlovian conditioning: pigeon nictitating membrane. Behav Process. 2011;86(1):102–8.
32. Donahoe JW, Burgos JE. Behavior analysis and revaluation. J Exp Anal Behav. 2000;74(3):331–46.
33. Burgos JE. The operant/respondent distinction: a computational neural-network analysis. In: Schmajuk N, editor. Computational models of conditioning. New York: Cambridge University Press; 2010. p. 244–71.
34. Brown PL, Jenkins HM. Auto-shaping of the pigeons' key-pec. J Exp Anal Behav. 1968;11(1):1–8.
35. Williams DR, Williams H. Auto-maintenance in the pigeon: sustained pecking despite contingent non-reinforcement. J Exp Anal Behav. 1969;12(4):511–20.
36. Schwartz B, Gamzu E. Pavlovian control of operant behavior: an analysis of autoshaping and its implications for operant conditioning. In: Handbook of operant behavior. Routledge; 1977. p. 53–97.
37. Balsam PD. The functions of context in learning and performance. In: Balsam PD, Tomie A, editors. Context and learning. Hillsdale: Psychology Press/Erlbaum; 2014. p. 1–21.
38. Brembs B. Spontaneous decisions and operant conditioning in fruit flies. Behav Process. 2011;87(1):157–64.

39. Castiello S, Burgos JE, Buriticá J, dos Santos CV, Alcalá JE. Interacción entre magnitud y probabilidad de reforzamiento en la elección automoldeada. Rev Mex Anal Conducta. 2020;46(1):23–66.
40. Welker RL, Tomie A, Davitt GA, Thomas DR. Contextual stimulus control over operant responding in pigeons. J Comp Physiol Psychol. 1974;86(3):549.
41. Richards JB, Mitchell SH, De Wit H, Seiden LS. Determination of discount functions in rats with an adjusting-amount procedure. J Exp Anal Behav. 1997;67(3):353–66.
42. Cepeda-Benito A, Short P. Morphine's interoceptive stimuli as cues for the development of associative morphine tolerance in the rat. Psychobiology. 1997;25(3):236–40.
43. Siegel S, Ramos B. Applying laboratory research: drug anticipation and the treatment of drug addiction. Exp Clin Psychopharmacol. 2002;10(3):162.
44. Sitharthan T, Sitharthan G, Hough MJ, Kavanagh DJ. Cue exposure in moderation drinking: a comparison with cognitive–behavior therapy. J Consult Clin Psychol. 1997;65(5):878.
45. Sitharthan T, Sitharthan G, Kavanagh DJ. Emotional cue exposure for alcohol abuse: development of a new treatment procedure to train moderation drinking in the context of dysphoria. Clin Psychol Psychother. 2001;8(1):73–8.
46. Rung JM, Peck S, Hinnenkamp JE, Preston E, Madden GJ. Changing delay discounting and impulsive choice: implications for addictions, prevention, and human health. Perspect Behav Sci. 2019;42(3):397–417.
47. Jenkins HM, Moore BR. The form of the auto-shaped response with food or water reinforcers. J Exp Anal Behav. 1973;20(2):163–81.
48. Wasserman EA. Pavlovian conditioning with heat reinforcement produces stimulus-directed pecking in chicks. Science. 1973;181(4102):875–7.
49. Bogacz R, Brown E, Moehlis J, Holmes P, Cohen JD. The physics of optimal decision making: a formal analysis of models of performance in two-alternative forced-choice tasks. Psychol Rev. 2006;113(4):700.
50. Insabato A, Dempere-Marco L, Pannunzi M, Deco G, Romo R. The influence of spatiotemporal structure of noisy stimuli in decision making. PLoS Comput Biol. 2014;10(4):e1003492.
51. Kacelnik A, Vasconcelos M, Monteiro T, Aw J. Darwin's "tug-of-war" vs. starlings "horse-racing": how adaptations for sequential encounters drive simultaneous choice. Behav Ecol Sociobiol. 2011;65(3):547–58.
52. Catania AC. The concept of the operant in the analysis of behavior. Behaviorism. 1973;1(2):103–16.
53. Skinner BF. The generic nature of the concepts of stimulus and response. J Gen Psychol. 1935;12(1):40–65.

12 Drug Abuse: From Biological to Psychological Dynamics

Schumacher Marcela and Osvaldo Agamennoni

Introduction

People start using drugs voluntarily, but largely due to pressure from the environment, over which they lack the tools to manage. Cannabis is the most widely consumed illegal substance [1] being the first step in the adolescent initiation. The addictive state is the consequence of acute brain changes due to the successive administration of the substance, which finally leads to modifications that last over time. Adolescent cannabis use represents an important public health concern due to their severe neuropsychological disorders with short to long-term adverse consequences. In this sense, it is critical the need for efficacious cognitive-behavioural therapies [2].

In the last years, the phenomenon of the consumption of cannabis was more and more critical. The wide acceptance of it in many different cultures and countries and its natural origin tend to make people believe that it is a product with few adverse effects, especially when compared to other drugs of abuse. This false belief has turned to this compound in a drug of beginning or the door of entrance to other more addictive drugs. From a diagnostic point of view, the term addiction is now related to substance use disorders. It is a brain disorder because it generates functional changes in brain circuits involved in reward, stress, and self-control. These changes can be present a long time after the person stops using drugs.

Addictive behaviours occur despite leading to a degradation of the social and psychological spheres of health disorders of the subject. It is precisely this aspect of search or uncontrollable need (craving) that best defines the process of drug dependence. Thanks to advances in research on the neurobiological mechanisms of addiction, it is now understood that we are facing disease, and as such, it must be treated. Pharmacological and psychological therapy, added to new meditation techniques, allows, in many cases, the affected person to lead a normal life again.

To fully understand drug abuse, it is necessary to analyse the alterations that it produces in the dynamic information processing system in which the brain is intimately involved, from the perception and construction of the own reality to the actions decided accordingly. Figure 12.1 shows a

S. Marcela
Laboratorio de Desarrollo en Neurociencias Cognitivas (CIC—UNS), Instituto de Investigaciones en Ingeniera Eléctrica (IIIE—UNS CONICET), Consejo Nacional de Investigaciones Científicas y Técnicas (CONICET), Bahía Blanca, Argentina; http://www.ldnc.uns.edu.ar

O. Agamennoni (✉)
Laboratorio de Desarrollo en Neurociencias Cognitivas (CIC—UNS), Universidad Nacional del Sur—Depto. de Ingeniería Eléctrica y de Computadoras, Instituto de Investigaciones en Ingeniera Eléctrica (IIIE—UNS CONICET), Comisión de Investigaciones Científicas de la Provincia de Buenos Aires, Bahía Blanca, Argentina; http://www.ldnc.uns.edu.ar

P. Á. Gargiulo, H. L. Mesones-Arroyo (eds.), *Psychiatry and Neuroscience Update – Vol. V*, https://doi.org/10.1007/978-3-031-72219-6_12

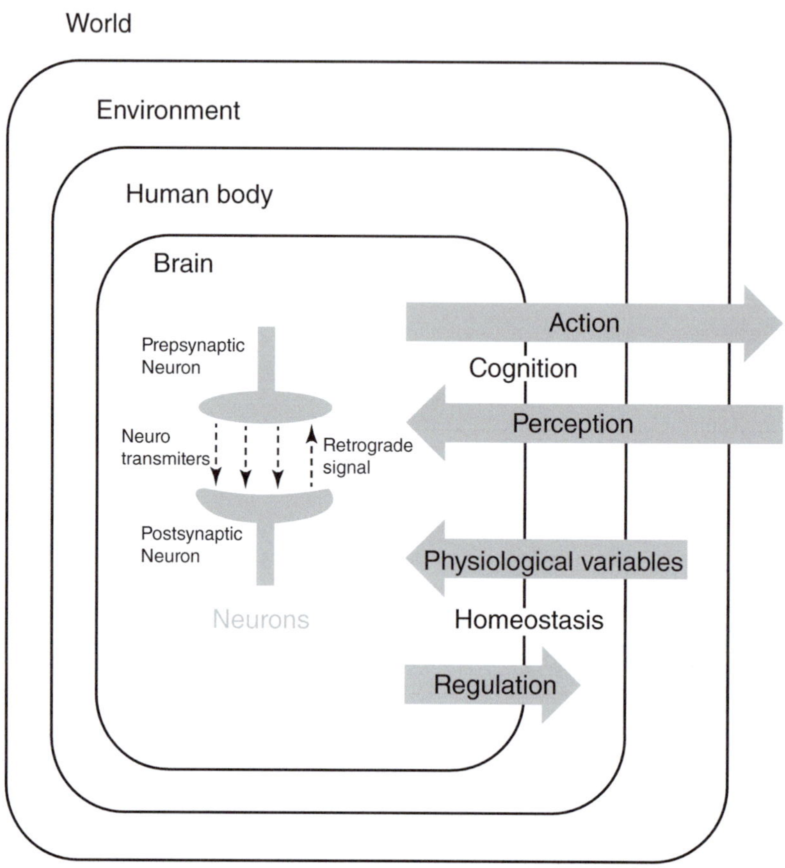

Fig. 12.1 From neurons to the world and vice versa. The neurons of the brain are responsible for perceiving the events of the environment and the world that we live in and for performing the actions that make up our daily life. Cognitive capabilities are responsible for such performances. The homeostatic processes regulate physiological variables to guarantee a living condition for our body

global framework of the different dynamic systems where our brain is involved. A set diagram emphasises that neurons are the blocks that build up the brain. Simultaneously, the brain is part of our human body, which performs in an environment that constitutes a part of the world around us. A succession of events propagates over time, creating paths through which information flows, thus transforming our brains when adapting to those events. Our actions modify the environment in many ways and generate messages that others perceive of ourselves. The ability to act appropriately in this context is known as cognitive capacity. Within it, all the elements that make up the information processing circuit are involved, which are prediction, attention, perception, memory, and understanding, among others.

The "perceptual cycle" proposed by Ulric Neisser [3, pp. 190] in 1978 and the "action-perception cycle" of Gregor Schöner [4, pp. 455] in 1994 derived in the "cognitive cycle" of Simon Haykin [5], and later was introduced in the area of neuroscience [6, pp. 1]. Figure 12.2 illustrates the elements presented and the flow of information in a cognitive cycle. The affordance competition hypothesis [7] states that the environment offers us a set of possibilities, or "affordances". We perceive through our senses and using the information contained in our memory. We evaluate the different affordances through an internal simulation [8] process that allows us to predict future outcomes. For this, we use a frame of reference based on the self-awareness values that guide our behaviour and our cognitive capabilities. Once the decision is made, we will have a goal to pursue (action) and achieve it, and we will use our cognitive control.

The brain is an information flow-processing organ that segregates and integrates incoming stimuli to facilitate flexible behaviour and cognition. There exists now enough evidence showing that the feedback control view of behaviour can

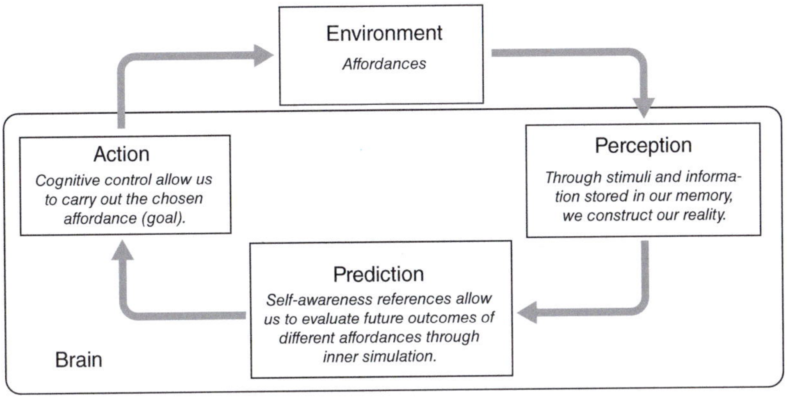

Fig. 12.2 Information flow involved in the cognitive cycle of perception, prediction, and action in considering the affordances of the environment. Perception allows us to construct our reality. Using our cognitive capabilities and working, semantic and episodic memories, we perform an inner evaluation of the different options (prediction). This process leads us to an objective (goal) to pursue using our cognitive control abilities

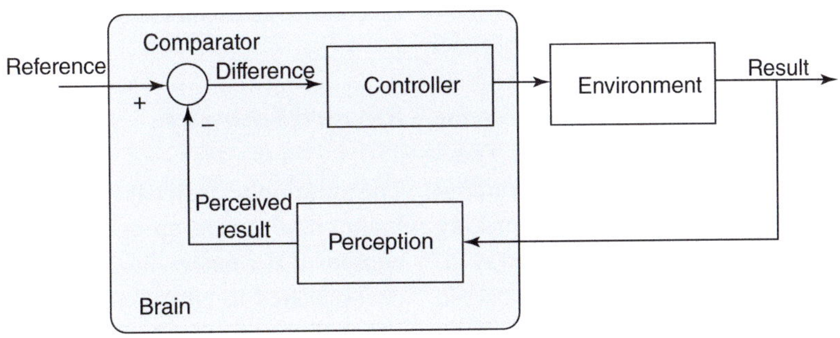

Fig. 12.3 Feedback control scheme of human behaviour in its interaction with the environment. We perceive the results of our actions and compare them with the desired objective (Reference). The error or difference allows us to exercise the corresponding control actions to get closer to the desired objective

provide a conceptual foundation for understanding human cognition [7]. Moreover, it is possible to define behaviour as a dynamic emergence motivated by feedback control loops and self-organised process.

Perception is a process by which our brain processes incoming significant sensory information and, together with the mental models stored in our memory, allows us to construct our own reality. Then, we elaborate possible courses of action to follow from the predictions of the possible results of each action and decide which one brings us more close to our goal. If we pay attention, we can realise that our thoughts are not static. They make up a kind of structured film based on a closed cycle of speculations (predictions) about possible future events followed by possible actions by third parties, and so on.

To highlight the importance of our brain in controlling the activities we carry out in the cognitive cycle, it is necessary to visualise this particular aspect. Figure 12.3 schematically shows this process. Suppose you want to achieve a certain result from an object (for example, driving a car). Given a desired reference value (path to follow), the brain exercises control actions (steering wheel and pedals) in order to achieve the desired result. In certain situations, it is necessary to negotiate certain actions with other people with whom we interact (self-organise to avoid a collision). This vision of the behaviour of our brain in relation to its actions with elements or situations in the environment can be generalised to any situations, where it is important to understand the crucial role that prediction plays in its dynamics. As an example, consider the behaviour of a driver when he must anticipate the path of another vehicle to drive safely.

The cognitive cycle and the feedback control approach offer an appropriate contextual frame to study and fully understand the emergent behaviour as a consequence of the continuous interaction with the environment where we lived. The cognitive cycle enables us to show the continuous circular flow of information in carrying our activities. The feedback control system allows us to consider the reference that regulates our behaviour and to appreciate how they influence our actions. It provides a framework to study the alterations produced by drug abuse in the closed information loop and to study the effects on the behaviour of an intervention therapy in the medium and long term.

Drug dependence theories propose that the transition from occasional substance use to harmful use and addiction is a consequence of the imbalance of midbrain dopamine signals. These signals are involved in the reinforcement learning process of cognitive control and decision-making system [9]. In this sense, an adequate way to appreciate the effects of the drug on human behaviour is from an approach that allows us to adequately visualising the dynamic effects in the neural circuits. These effects begin in alterations in the neurotransmitters that communicate to neurons and finally translate into changes in behaviour linked to decision-making processes. In the last years, mindfulness-based interventions (MBIs) have been tailored directly to the treatment of mechanisms that undergird addiction. A considerable number of controlled research studies demonstrate that MBIs may produce significant clinical benefits.

Researchers have strong evidence showing that mindfulness-based therapies are effective in reducing drug consumption [10]. Mindfulness, i.e. the quality or state of being conscious or aware of something, has proved to be effective in reducing craving by modulating cognitive, affective, and psychophysiological processes.

This chapter aims to operationalise the construct of a systemic approach of drug of abuse to address the affection from the neurotransmitter alteration level to the deficiencies caused at the human decision-making level. To do this, we will initially approach the reward circuit to understand how the alterations that occur in synaptic linkages as a result of the presence of phytocannabinoids affect it. Later, we will address the human decision-making process from the "affordances competition" theory approach [7] and the concept of the cognitive cycle in order to appreciate how the flow of information forms a closed circuit of circulation that reinforces behaviours. For its complete understanding, it is necessary to introduce some basic concepts of feedback systems to appreciate how the self-awareness reference values to maintain an appropriate way of acting. In this regard, it is facilitated the comprehension that mindfulness constitutes an important aid in the treatment of recovering addicts.

Reward Pathway

The mesolimbic pathway, or reward pathway, is a brain circuit made up of a set of dopaminergic neurons that connect different areas of the brain, encompassed in our reinforced learning system. Dopamine neurons send information to each other following a route thanks to dopamine, a very important neurotransmitter in our nervous system, which allows us to send signals between neurons related to the body's emotional, motor, and cognitive responses to certain stimuli. When a neuron receives enough stimulation, a neurotransmitter is released in the synaptic cleft, the space that separates the two neurons. The neurotransmitter binds to a receptor in the neuron with which it communicates, generating a signal in it, thus transmitting the information involved in the activity. That communication is essential to carry out our brain functions.

Dopamine neurons are a group of approximately 500 K cells in humans within the ventral midbrain. These cells are grouped in two major divisions, the nigrostriatal system with motor function (it degenerates in Parkinson's disease) and the mesolimbic system with motivation and reward functions, which are essential for the habit-forming effects of drugs of abuse and motivated behaviours [11].

The main functions of the mesolimbic pathway are linked to reward, the feeling of motivation, and reinforcement or emotional learning. The association of particular events with a pleasant sensation is the basis of the reinforced learning mechanism. We will tend to repeat that which gives us pleasure. In general, positive events such as a personal achievement and a satisfying sexual relationship are ingrained in the brain through such reinforcing mechanisms.

Endocannabinoid System

There are three different classes of cannabinoids: phytocannabinoids, endocanabinoids, and synthetic cannabinoids. The endocannabinoid system of our brain is so named because it was the cannabis plant (phytocannabinoid) that led to its discovery. The eCB system is conformed by the cannabinoid receptors CB1 and CB2, the principal eCB ligands, anandamide (AEA) and 2-arachidonoylglycerol (2-AG), and their metabolic enzymes. CB1 is most abundant, especially in the substantia nigra, globus pallidus, hippocampus, cerebral cortex, putamen, caudate, cerebellum, and amygdala. CB2 is associated with cells linked to immune function.

Within the central nervous system (CNS), the endocannabinoids are synthesised and released "on-demand" into the synaptic cleft. They work as retrograde synaptic messengers through binding to the CB receptors on the presynaptic terminal of neurons [12]. When the postsynaptic neuron is activated, the eCB is produced, released, and returned to the presynaptic neuron where they activate the cannabinoid receptors (see Fig. 12.1 retrograde signal). In doing so, they control what happens next in the presynaptic neuron when it is stimulated again. The eCB system acts as a modulator of the brain communication system, protecting the CNS against over activation or over inhibition caused by neurotransmitters and does so by self-regulating the activation of the CB1 receptors. This process is known as the homeostatic function in the central nervous system (CNS).

Our brain was evolutionarily adapted to make us feel good and maintain that state. It is another of the manifestations of the homeostatic process. It is called the dopamine reward circuit because it involves several parts of the brain taking different actions when exposed to dopamine. The eCB system is also involved in many other functions such as memory, learning, appetite, and sleep patterns, immune functions, and fertility. The amount of eCB messenger is tightly regulated according to the needs of the body. This modulator is essential to fine tune the performance of brain functions. The eCB system also acts in the modulation of pain-producing effects of pain relief, stress, and anxiety reduction, helping our body to learn to modulate stress. It also operates in the regulation of mood inducing the release of dopamine in the brain's reward system. Unfortunately, many different causes that trigger good feelings can erroneously induce the brain to get caught up in the process of reinforcing behaviours. Essentially, it is up to the logical mind to make life decisions that benefit and trigger the dopamine reward circuit for positive actions rather than a detrimental one.

Cannabis Effects in the Neuronal Connectivity

The *Cannabis sativa* plant contains approximately 400 different chemical compounds, of which 60 are part of the group of cannabinoids. The Δ9-tetrahydrocannabinol (THC) is the principal psychoactive constituent of cannabis and is similar to endocannabinoids. When an exogenous phytocannabinoid such as THC occupies the place, it should occupy an endocannabinoid molecule (at the CB1 receptor), and the self-regulation is affected and altered biochemical cascades predominate. THC is fat soluble, and because of this, it can accumulate in the adipose tissue and the lipid membranes of the neurons. Even after a single administration of THC, detectable levels are found in the body for weeks. It is considered that the occasional users of cannabis tend to accumulate the THC, since the same one usually is deposited in rich zones in fat (like the brain, liver, and gonads). This accumulation usually is associated with problems of loss of memory caused by the alterations of the hippocampus. In occasional users, it is estimated that they are needed around 4 weeks to eliminate the THC from the organism. Nevertheless, it is believed that long-standing users of cannabis require much more time to recover their cognitive functions and that some of the produced upheavals are chronic. The way of action of THC is different from that of other drugs. It exerts both excitatory and inhibitory mechanisms by unbalancing the release of both the inhibitory neurotransmitter GABA and the excitatory neurotransmitter glutamate. Because of that, it can induce a variety of physiological and excitatory depressant effects, for example, sedation and euphoria simultaneously [13]. Decreasing the inhibitory action of GABA induces the release of dopamine indirectly on dopaminergic neurons. The central mechanism of action of THC results from its partial agonist activity in the CB1 and CB2 cannabinoid receptors. Since the GABA is a neurotransmitter inhibitor of the dopamine cascade, when the THC is coupled to the receptor CB1, this receptor located in the GABAergic neurons is activated, generating an exacerbated torrent of dopamine. In this way, the sensations of pleasure and well-being proper to the increase of dopamine in the centres of cerebral pleasure emerge.

The dependency on marijuana occurs when the brain adapts to significant amounts of the drug and reduces the production of its own eCB neurotransmitters and consequently the sensitivity to them. The repeated consumption of cannabis drive tolerance for many subjective and psychological effects [14]. Thus, the intensity of such effects is determined not only by the dose of THC but also by past experiences, expectations of the consumer, environment, and different sensitivities [15]. Some studies describe that cognitive effects last longer than 24 h, even after a single dose smoked or taken orally [16].

Chronic exposure to cannabinoids produces a desensitisation phenomenon characterised by a decrease in the number of CB1 receptors. When drug use is maintained for a long time, withdrawal phenomena are accentuated, and the physiological adaptation resources are not sufficient to compensate and maintain a homeostatic situation. For this reason, the compulsive and uncontrolled consumption of the drug arises. Thus, although addiction can be considered as such from the first symptoms of chronic consumption, the addictive process reaches its critical point coinciding with the impossibility of regulation of the homeostatic system. At this point, the changes that have occurred have no chance of reverting to their normal baseline during abstinence, and a new residual baseline is established on which the next drug intake acts. In such circumstances, the motivational efficacy of the drug is further sensitised, and a vicious cycle occurs.

The physiological mechanisms developed during withdrawal syndrome to drugs of abuse are associated with changes in various neurotransmission systems and symptoms such as anxiety, sleep disturbances, dysphoria, and alterations in appetite, which lead the patient to relapse into consumption [17]. The reward pathways, or mesolimbocortical dopaminergic pathways, originate in the ventral tegmental area and connect to the nucleus accumbens and other regions (prefrontal cortex, limbic). The activation of these pathways produces a powerful compulsion ("craving") to maintain this state of stimulation or satisfaction.

THC is also more stable than endocannabinoids and can remain in the body for a longer period, overwhelming the endocannabinoid system. It can slow down a person's reaction time. It can alter short-term memory and higher mental processes. Small doses of THC can reduce stress, anxiety, and panic, and high doses can produce the opposite effect, increasing stress, and fear. Then is clear that THC breaks the retrograde balance of neuron activity by preventing neurotransmitters from being generated on demand. Dependence occurs when the brain adapts to large amounts of the drug and reduces the production of and sensitivity to its own endocannabinoid molecules.

Another worrying fact is that a cannabis extract containing between 3% and 5% THC, increases the permeability of the blood–brain barrier making possible the entry of these compounds to the brain receptors and the placental barrier permeability [18]. For that reason, the problem of addiction extends to pregnant women.

Drug addiction may also be related to a reduced ability to experience rewards that are unrelated to drugs and emotional dysregulation. These entail persistent memories for previous experiences with the drug contrasting with a global cognitive decline that may hamper new, adaptive learnings. The feeling of pleasure that the drug provides without having any relation to a specific positive emotional state or achievement constitutes one of the main problems of drug abuse. Overall, these features promote a desire for the drug, leading to relapse in drug use. In turn, further drug exposure aggravates its consequences on the brain and behaviour, creating the harmful "addiction cycle" [19].

The prefrontal cortex of the brain is one of the areas still maturing during adolescence. The area enables us to assess situations, make proper decisions, and keep our emotions and desires under control. Being this critical part of an adolescent's brain in progress puts them at increased risk under drug use. During this period of development, drug use may cause brain changes that have profound and long-lasting consequences. Imaging studies corroborate that regular adolescent cannabis use is associated with impaired connectivity and reduced volume of specific brain regions involved in a wide variety of executive function [20]. Other brain imaging studies of addicted people show physical changes in areas of the brain that are essential for good judgement, decision-making, learning, memory, and behaviour control. These changes help explain the compulsive nature of addiction [21].

A longitudinal study [22] showed that when frequent cannabis use begins in adolescence, it produces an average loss of 6 and up to 8 IQ points in mid-adulthood. In the same study, people who used cannabis heavily during adolescence and stopped using the drug, as adults, did not regain the IQ points they had lost. On the other hand, those who only began to use intensively in adulthood did not lose IQ points. These results corroborate that cannabis has the greatest long-term impact on young people whose brains are still making new connections and maturing.

One of the critical elements in the treatment of addictions is craving. The effectiveness of the treatment of addictions will depend on how well controlled the craving is so that the patient does not relapse into the desire to consume the drug. Drug use is a personal decision in which various internal factors (self-awareness, motivations, cognitive skills, etc.) and external environmental pressures (peer incitement, family problems, etc.) are involved and compete. For a heavily addicted individual, drug use usually occurs without a great deal of thought, without conscious urges. Under these circumstances, drug use is likely driven by automatic processes. Conversely, the process of quitting drug use and the process of relapsing when there is an awareness of negative consequences are both complex decision-making processes. They involve weighing the positive and negative social, emotional, medical, financial, and legal consequences [23]. For this reason, it is of fundamental importance to understand how this automatic response is produced, how it can be deactivated, and, once this is done, how to correctly adjust the decision-making process.

Human Decision-Making Process

The human brain has different decision procedures that coexist and compete with each other. We can roughly classify them as irrational or heuristic and rational or consciously deliberative. The decision procedure activates different regions of the brain [24]. Heuristic decisions are based on emotional influence and deliberative decisions on logic calculation and working memory manipulation. The same individual can be consistent or logically correct on some occasions and not on others. This shows that multiple decision rules, some of them logically accurate and some inaccurate, coexist in our brain. Both heuristic and deliberative decisions may be encompassed within a common neural framework based in brain pathways that can be traced back to our evolutionary ancestors. Cognition and emotion are integrated into the brain. Cognition and emotion conjointly and equally contribute to the control of thought and behaviour. Brain areas related to emotion are often subcortical, such as the amygdala, ventral striatum, and hypothalamus. They are often considered as evolutionarily primitive. Cognitive processes develop in cortical regions. The cerebral cortex has more than half the volume of the human brain. It is assumed to be responsible for perception, thought, language, attention, episodic memory, and voluntary movement, among other complex tasks. Because of this traditional separation, many mental health professionals resisted for a long time the notion that cognitive dissonance produces physiological arousal. However, now researches consider that emotion and cognition are only minimally decomposable in the brain and that the neural basis of emotion and cognition should be viewed as strongly non-modular [25]. The reason may be found in the hub that regulates the flow and integration of information between regions carries out the cognitive–emotional interactions. The hubs are areas of the brain with a high degree of connectivity.

Rational behaviour in the decision-making process is mostly goal-directed [26], i.e. is predominantly determined by endogenously generated (and internally represented) goals rather than by external stimuli. Living organisms self-generate goals for satisfying their basic needs (e.g. "hunger" generates the goal "take a meal") and face the problem of selecting from a menu of goals under different environmental and internal (motivational and cognitive) contexts. Goals are strongly dependent on self-awareness since it is often the first step to setting goals. Self-awareness means being aware of oneself, including one's traits, feelings, and behaviours. Self-awareness impairment is the failure to ascribe personal relevance or significance to internal or external stimuli or events that have implications for the self, being they environmental cues feedback, interoceptive sensations, or ongoing behaviour [27].

Abstraction ability allows predicting the consequences of actions by the predicted long-term consequences and opportunities they make possible. The affordance competition theory [7] suggests that during interactive behaviour, the brain defines a set of desirable actions currently available in its environment ('affordances'). It is known that objects or situations may evoke actions independently of the person's intention to act. It is an automated cause–effect response wired in the brain. Different possibilities are analysed by simulation and stored in working memory to steer action. Affordances are revealed by "internal simulations" of potential actions. The brain is continuously involved in generating predictions about future opportunities rather than just reacting to already available affordances. Evidence suggests that objects and events, including social ones, can automatically activate action schemas. In this paper, the usual conception of "action schema" is assumed, i.e. the characteristics that enable an intelligent being to repeat the action and apply it to new contents. A repertoire of representations of these actions is internally evaluated in achieving a particular goal. This approach is not strictly limited to visible affordances; it permits the integration, in the same simulation, of currently perceived events, anticipated events, and action alternatives.

In this context, it is elucidating to analyse the brain organisation within the frame of a system of hierarchical feedback control loops (Fig. 12.4). We assume self-awareness values as the set of principles or standards of behaviour, the own judgement of what is important. These values define the references (set points) for dynamic behaviour. Within this frame, the environment offers a menu of alternatives (action schema repertoire), and the brain actives a mechanism of evaluation through simulations (Fig. 12.4b). It means preprogram aspects of actions motivated by external cues and simulates it using memory information (episodic and semantic), providing extra flexibility and reference to similar experiences. Obviously, the motivational system can further influence these ongoing simulations (sad events vs. happy events) or can be influenced by them. The desirability of their predicted outcomes biases them.

All the alternatives are internally evaluated, and one of them is selected, which determines a

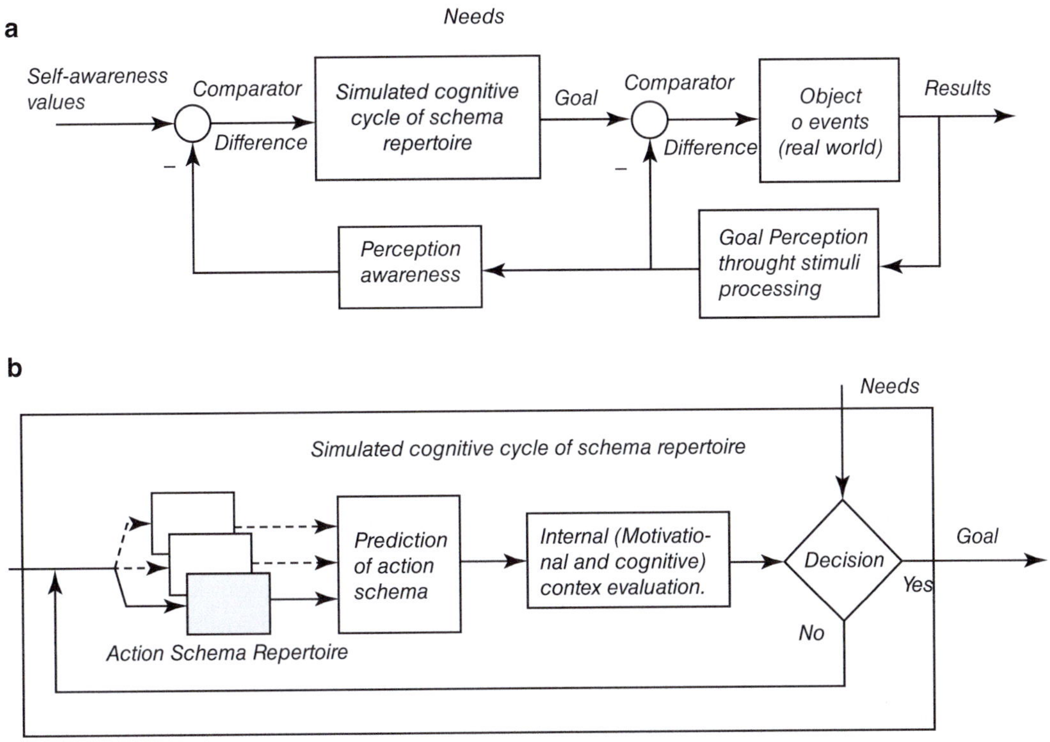

Fig. 12.4 Human decision-making process: (**a**) Self-awareness sets a reference point for the simulated cognitive cycle, where all possibilities ("affordances") within in the schema repertoire (see **b**) are internally simulated and evaluated. The output of this evaluation is the goal (see **a**) reference for the inner loop. The result achieved in the real world is perceived in the frame of the decided goal and the self-awareness value. (**b**) Expansion of the simulated cognitive cycle of schema repertoire block of (**a**). It shows the inner process of motivational and cognitive context evaluation of all the affordances and the influence of the needs in decision process for selecting a particular goal

goal (see Fig. 12.4a). Motivation is of fundamental importance in the selection among multiple action alternatives. The goal is a reference (set point) of the inner loop, where it is executed through continuous feedback control, using sensory information from the environment (goal perception). The result achieved is also perceived in the frame of the desired self-awareness values (perception awareness). In this work, we assume that goal perception refers exclusively to the appreciation of the goal itself, without any ulterior implications. On the other hand, by perception awareness, we understand the complete understanding of all the consequences that the objective entails. For example, the goal of smoking can be achieved and is immediately gratifying, but it ceases to be when all its consequences are considered. Discrepancies are evidenced by a nonzero output of the comparators that drive the brain to action corrections in pursuing the desired result. Otherwise, a new goal may be selected. Besides, since alternatives potential actions continue to be processed, it is possible to switch actions if new opportunities or necessities arise.

According to Maslow's [28] hierarchy approach of needs, human being has basic or physiological needs (food, water, rest, security, etc.), psychological needs (belonging and love, esteem, etc.), and self-fulfilment needs (creative activities, achieving full potentials). The human being seeks first the satisfaction of basic needs, then psychological, and finally, the self-fulfilment needs. As emerging lower needs are fulfilled, new and higher needs emerge. The basic needs shared by all members of a species are species-wide goals. Once the basic needs are satisfied, individuality develops. The physiological and psychological needs compete with each other, and the state of the needs' network shifts within these needs when the individual experiences discontent.

The network of decision rules consists of four connected areas: the amygdala, the orbitofrontal cortex (OFC), anterior cingulate cortex (ACC), and dorsolateral prefrontal cortex (DLPFC), which account for various decision rules on specific tasks. These four regions comprise a three-layer network, in which the vigilance threshold of the individual determines the status of activation of each layer. The state of the needs' network influences the vigilance threshold so that the winning needs become dominant to implement the corresponding decision rules (see decision block in Fig. 12.4b).

In order to satisfy their needs, human beings evaluate the different alternatives available to them (affordances). Each need will have its intensity, and it will establish an order of realisation. When evaluating it, its advantages and disadvantages are weighed in a given time horizon. Increasing the intensity of a need reduces the time horizon for its satisfaction. For example, trying to satisfy the need to find a partner may have a certain expected future time horizon of fulfilment, but surely satisfying a basic need such as hunger has a much shorter horizon. See Fig. 12.4b internal (motivational and cognitive) context evaluation.

The established reference from a self-awareness of own value (set point) and the result perceived (which enters with a minus sign) are compared (see Fig. 12.4a). If the output of the comparator is small, the results are close to the reference and our attention will move to a new action. If the difference is greater than a given threshold, it means that the obtained result differs from the reference (desired set point) and will try to take action to reduce it. As an example, let us assume that our desired (reference self-awareness value) body weight is 70 kg, and we are slightly overweighed. We are sitting in a restaurant examining the menu. The environment offers a repertoire of possible action schema, like several dishes of foods we like but inappropriate considering our overweight, and others with much less calories but less tasty. We analyse the different alternatives internally and finally decide on one (goal). After some time, we will be able to perceive with particular intensity the results of it. It is crucial to realise that to carry out an appropriate goal, we need the self-awareness value of having a healthy body weight. On the other hand, the intensity of hunger (need) has its weight in the final decision on the chosen goal.

The underlying mechanisms of executive functions, such as inhibition, monitoring progress through perception, and working memory, are implicated in the system [26]. Self-awareness is also closely linked to goal monitoring. Goal monitoring is the process that individuals use to identify obstacles during goal pursuit. Then, self-awareness should be a predictor of the identification of goal-related obstacles. This also may explain why heightened self-awareness is related to an increased effort in goal-directed, increased choice of problem-solving strategies, and better goal-related performance [29].

Drug Effects on the Human Decision-Making Process

There exists a diversity of craving definitions. However, most researchers assume that craving is a subjective experience of wanting to use a drug. This definition has three crucial elements: craving is conscious, craving is an expression of desire, and that desire is directed towards the use of a specific drug [30].

Drug addiction compromises self-awareness and decision-making, modifying previously rewarded behaviours that no longer produce favourable outcomes [27]. Motivation is also defined as what makes one effort to achieve a reward or to avoid punishment. Emotion and motivation are closely related as both depend on the relationship between the human being and its environment. Motivation is generally invoked to explain avenues that individuals use to preserve and enhance self-esteem. By strongly modifying the motivational structure of the person, drug addiction seriously compromises self-awareness.

The decision to abstain depends upon the capacity to suppress the representation of the

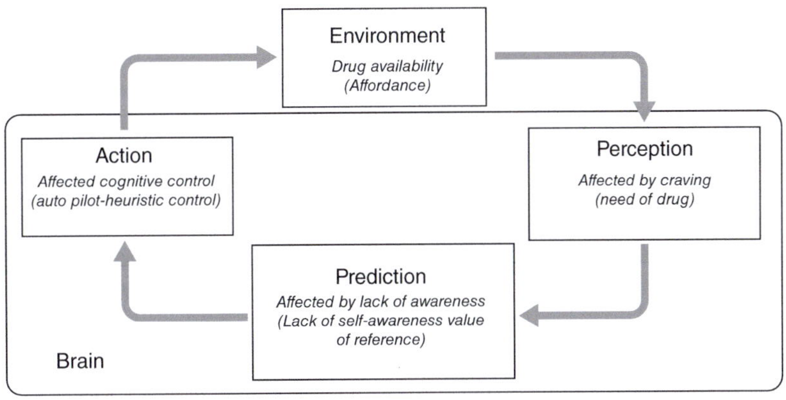

Fig. 12.5 Vicious cycle. The environment offer drug as an affordance, the perception is affected by the craving, prediction by the lack of self-awareness values of behavioural reference, and finally, the action is altered because heuristic control (autopilot) gains space over cognitive control

positive hedonic effects of drug use and to enhance the awareness of the negative consequences of drug use. Relapse occurs when the perception of the positive hedonic effects of drug-taking "win out" over the perception of the negative consequences of drug-taking. This happens because the mental models of the positive hedonic effects of drug taking are much stronger than the mental models of the negative consequences of drug taking [23].

Drugs introduce new needs and modify the relative weight of each one that each person possesses, altering their order of priorities. It is difficult for an addict to make a correct evaluation of the available alternatives (affordances) of the environment. In addition, as their cognitive control capacity is affected, decision-making often shifts to a more automatic, heuristic mode, commonly referred to as being on "autopilot". In short, the vicious cycle is shown in Figure 12.5. It takes the form of the cognitive cycle in which the affections of the three fundamental parts that have to do with the intervention of the brain are revealed: the perception, prediction, and consequent action. The perception is affected by craving, the prediction by the lack of awareness, and the action by the predominance of automatic (autopilot) decision. In order to get out of this vicious cycle is crucial to re-establishing awareness in decision-making. Self-awareness and motivations, as well as the awareness of the problems related to drug abuse, are primarily involved in the decision-making process of a recovering addict. Cognitive skills are the main capacities to focus our attention due to their role in the dynamic of such a process.

Mindfulness

Kabat-Zinn [31] introduced mindfulness to clinical practice and defined it as "the awareness that emerges through paying attention on purpose, in the present moment, and non-judgementally to the unfolding of experience moment by moment". Mindfulness is a phenomenon that has drawn the attention of many scientists and clinicians over the last decade. The reason for the great interest in mindfulness lies in the numerous benefits that come from practising it. These positive effects have been found in various areas of human functionality: emotional, cognitive, behavioural, and interpersonal [32]. The important role mindfulness plays in health and well-being give rise to the question: how does it work? [33]

An increased capacity for metalising/mindfulness means that the individual is able to make more deliberate, thoughtful, and conscious, as opposed to heuristic, automatic, and subconscious decisions, which in turn provides a sense of agency and control in the individual [34]. Mentalisation is the ability to understand one's own behaviour and that of others in terms of mental states. Mentalisation is a developmental achievement that is acquired in the context of a secure attachment relationship and determines the way in which the individual will relate with himself and others. It implies attending to mental states in self and others, understanding misunderstandings, and seeing yourself from the outside and others from the inside.

Mindfulness in Addiction Treatment

Different studies [35] show that mindfulness-based interventions (MBIs) reduce drug consumption and craving by modulating cognitive, affective, and psychophysiological processes that are the core of the self-regulation and reward processing system. In general, mindfulness practices and specifically MBIs help to prevent relapses by increasing self-awareness [36], reducing reactivity to drug signals [37], and reducing negative affective states [38]. Mindfulness enhances functional connectivity between top-down and bottom-up brain circuitries and, in this way, reverses the allostatic load by which normal reward learning is appropriate by addictive substances.

The craving is for the continuation of pleasant or the cessation of unpleasant feeling tones. By decoupling pleasant and unpleasant experience from habitual reactions of craving and aversion, careful attention to present moment experience can bring a broadening or spaciousness of awareness that allows new appraisals of life situations [39].

Mindfulness practices allow evoking the state of metacognitive awareness characterised by attentive and non-judgemental monitoring of moment-by-moment cognition, emotion, and perception without recurrence of past and future thoughts. The practice of mindfulness favours focused attention, open monitoring, and cognitive resources application [35]. Open monitoring is a metacognitive state of awareness. It involves monitoring the content of consciousness while reflecting back on the process or quality of consciousness itself. In this way, mindfulness practice reduces emotional reactivity by revealing the insubstantiality and emotionally overloaded of any particular content of consciousness. Open monitoring sustained attention, attentional reorienting, conflict monitoring, retaining information online in working memory, inhibitory control, and emotion regulation are the most important set of tools that allows modifying the weight of each needs improving the possibilities of a rational internal evaluation of all the affordances. Since the brain is continuously involved in generating predictions about future opportunities, mindfulness reduces the negative effect of emotionally biased predictions. Since mindfulness enhances self-awareness, a set of different nonbiased reference values (see Fig. 12.4a) will be available to guide the behaviour, to properly judge what is important.

According to Garland and Howard [35], mindfulness exerts influence on the biology of an addicts' brain, allowing it to re-establish its usual dynamic by amplifying prefrontal activation, increasing frontostriatal connectivity, decreasing limbic reactivity, and improving autonomic regulation. These biological changes have an impact on the restructuring of reward processing, boosting executive functions, strengthening dispositional mindfulness, reducing stress reactivity, decreasing drug cue-reactivity, and minimising thought suppression. By reinforcing top-down cognitive control, MBIs may enhance executive functions improving self-control over automatic habits and response inhibition that are decisive to quit drug use and maintaining abstinence. The beneficial effects include working memory and selective attention/response inhibition. All those beneficial effects listed improve the cognitive control effectivity of the addict's decision-making system.

In summary, mindfulness is understood as a development in the ability to control attention, emotional regulation, and self-awareness [40]. These cognitive skills are employed in applying coping strategies rather than avoidance, work the underlying mechanisms that trigger non-adaptive behaviours, and ultimately identify and amplify natural contingencies [41]. Returning to Fig. 12.4, the development of cognitive control skills has a beneficial impact on the evaluation of good affordances and the making of smarter decisions closer to the values of the person. The ability to regulate emotions and improvements in self-awareness, and reduced self-judgement abilities allow setting new and more appropriate goals that help to stay off the drug.

Citing Ramon y Cajal's phrase "Every man can be, if he proposes, a sculptor of his own brain" and under the paradigm of associative learning proposed by Hebb, it is to be expected that any activity performed with a specific frequency and maintained in time can mould the neuronal structures of the brain. Any practice or therapeutic session can induce structural changes in the brain even more in the case of addictions, where clear indications of how a structurally and functionally addicted brain differs from a normal brain have been found [42].

Conclusions

All drugs of abuse cause an increased activity of the mesocorticolimbic dopamine system. During chronic use, neuroadaptive and neuroplastic changes occur, which modify the structure of that system. The environmental stimuli, related in time and space to the drug, can become conditioned stimuli that will trigger the irrepressible desire to consume later and by themselves.

In this chapter, we have focused on the mechanisms by which exogenous cannabinoid acts on the endocannabinoid system, generating the well-known consequences of consumption. Among other functions, the endocannabinoid system is involved in maintaining homeostatic balance, synaptic plasticity, and the control of certain phases of memory processing. When an external molecule that perfectly fits the cannabinoid receivers occupies the space, it generates abnormal neurotransmitter cascades. This reinforcement generates a feeling of pleasure that again tends to repeat itself to find the same sensations and in a short period are generated mechanisms of addiction and search of those sensations (craving) that are very difficult to control, since the system of endocannabinoid self-control is unbalanced and cannot respond to physiological regulation or homeostatic.

This is what happens when the THC, phytocannabinoid of the plant of *Cannabis sativa*, binds in partially agonist form to the cannabinoid receptors and triggers biochemical imbalances. This affects the regulation of essential neurotransmitters such as GABA, dopamine, adrenaline, serotonin, glutamate, and reinforcements in the cascade of mesolimbic self-compensation. When consumption is excessive, and the person shows patterns of addiction, the problems of tolerance and dependence on the drug generate even more undesirable effects by affecting neural dynamic communication that definitively alters the decision-making system.

We present a particular approach to the human decision-making process within the framework of the affordance competition theory and the cognitive cycle approach. In this way, the feedback control mechanisms present in human behaviour can be clearly appreciated. We describe how the effects of the drug on neuronal communication mechanisms alter this process and how they translate into risky behaviours by introducing needs due to drug use. These alterations affect the perception of the possibilities of the environment, how they are evaluated (predictions), and the cognitive control that is carried out in pursuit of the objectives (actions).

Subsequently, we have presented, in a summarised way, the mindfulness technique and its positive effects in improving the different aspects involved in human decision-making. In summary, drug abuse produces a lack of awareness, automatic heuristic (non-deliberate) actions, craving, negative effect, stress reactivity, among others. Mindfulness increases awareness, kindness, and self-compassion and decreases autopilot, judgement, and reactivity, allowing using wisely the cognitive capabilities.

In any case, it is essential to point out that the most effective way to face drug abuse is through prevention. For this, it is of great relevance to address the teaching of adolescents in these topics. In particular, the possibilities offered by mindfulness as a tool to exercise better control of one's behaviour, a fact of significant importance to face all kinds of dilemmas.

Acknowledgments This work was supported by the Agencia Nacional de Promoción Científica y Tecnológica from Argentina under grant PICT 2016 1009, by the Universidad Nacional del Sur under grant PGI 24/K085, and by Comisión de Investigaciones Científicas de la provincia de Buenos Aires.

References

1. Hoch E, Bonnet U, Thomasius R, Ganzer F, Havemann-Reinecke U, Preuss UW. Risks associated with the non-medicinal use of cannabis. Dtsch Arztebl Int. 2015;112(16):271–8.
2. Aguinaldo L, Squeglia L, Gray C, Lees B, Tomko R, Jacobus J. Behavioral treatments for adolescent cannabis use disorder: a rationale for cognitive retraining. Curr Addict Rep. 2019;6(4):437–42.
3. Belardinelli MO. The debt of cognitive science to Ulric Neisser. Cogn Process. 2012;13:189–91.
4. Schöner G. Dynamic theory of action-perception patterns: the "moving room" paradigm. Biol Cybern. 1991;64:455–62.
5. Haykin S. Cognitive radio: brain-empowered wireless communications. IEEE J Sel Areas Commun. 2005;23(2):201–20.
6. Madl T, Baars BJ, Franklin S. The timing of the cognitive cycle. PLoS One. 2011;No. 6(4):1–16.
7. Pezzulo G, Cisek P. Navigating the affordance landscape: feedback control as a process model of behavior and cognition. Trends Cogn Sci. 2016;No. 20(6):414–24.
8. Giovanni P, Matteo C, Haris D, Laura B. Action simulation in the human brain: twelve questions. New Ideas Psychol. 2013;No. 31(3):270–90. https://doi.org/10.1016/j.newideapsych.2013.01.004.
9. Baker T, Stockwell T, Barnes G, Holroyd C. Individual differences in substance dependence: at the intersection of brain, behaviour and cognition. Addict Biol. 2011;16(3):458–66.
10. Garland E, Howard M. Mindfulness-based treatment of addiction: current state of the field and envisioning the next wave of research. Addict Sci Clin Pract. 2018;13:14.
11. Melis M, Pistis M. Hub and switches: endocannabinoid signalling in midbrain dopamine neurons. Philos Trans R Soc Lond Ser B Biol Sci. 2012;367(1607):3276–85.
12. Oltrabella F, Melgoza A, Nguyen B, Guo S. Role of the endocannabinoid system in vertebrates: emphasis on the zebrafish model. Develop Growth Differ. 2017;No. 59:194–210.
13. Brown S, Safo P, Regehr W. Endocannabinoids inhibit transmission at granule cell to purkinje cell synapses by modulating three types of presynaptic calcium channels. J Neurosci. 2004;No. 24(24):5623–31.
14. Fehr K, Kalant H, Lebrank AE. Residual learning deficit after heavy exposure to cannabis or alcohol in rats. Science. 1976;192(4245):1249–51.
15. Kolansky H, Moore W. Clinical effects of marihuana on the young. Int J Psychiatry. 1972;10(2):55–67.
16. Fehr K, Kalant H, editors. Cannabis and health hazards: proceedings of an ARF/WHO scientific meeting on adverse health and behavioral consequences of cannabis use; 1981 30 Mar 30–Apr 3; Toronto, Canada. ISBN 0-88868-084-8.
17. Giuffrida A, Parsons LH, Kerr TM, Rodriguez de Fonseca F, Navarro M, Piomeli D. Dopamine activation of endogenous cannabinoid signaling in dorsal striatum. Nat Neurosci. 1999;2:358–63.
18. Gómez M, Hernández M, Johansson B, de Miguel R, Ramos JA, Fernández-Ruiz J. Prenatal cannabinoid and gene expression for neural adhesion molecule L1 in the fetal rat brain. Brain Res Dev Brain Res. 2003;147(1–2):201–7.
19. Sampedro-Piquero P, Santín LJ, Castilla-Ortega E. Aberrant brain neuroplasticity and function in drug addiction: a focus on learning-related brain regions. In: Behavioral neuroscience. Intech Open; 2019. p. 1–25. https://doi.org/10.5772/intechopen.85280.
20. Batalla A, Bhattacharyya S, Yücel M, Fusar-Poli P, Crippa JA, Nogué S, Torrens M, Pujol J, Farré M, Martin-Santos R. Structural and functional imaging studies in chronic cannabis users: a systematic review of adolescent and adult findings. PLoS One. 2013;8(2):e55821. https://doi.org/10.1371/journal.pone.0055821.
21. Fowler J, Volkow N, Kassed C, Chang L. Imaging the addicted human brain. Sci Pract Perspect. 2007;3(2):4–16. https://doi.org/10.1151/spp07324.
22. Meier M, Caspi A, Ambler A, Harrington HL, Houts R, Keefe R, McDonald K, Ward A, Poulton R, Moffitt TE. Persistent cannabis users show neuropsychological decline from childhood to midlife. In: Posner M, editor. Proceedings of the national academy of sciences; 2012. p. E2657–64.
23. Naqvi N, Bechara A. 2010. The insula and drug addiction: an interoceptive view of pleasure, urges, and decision-making. Brain Struct Funct. 2010;214(0):435–50. https://doi.org/10.1007/s00429-010-0268-7.
24. Levine D. Brain pathways for cognitive-emotional decision making in the human animal. Neural Netw. 2009;22:286–93.
25. Pessoa L. On the relationship between emotion and cognition. Nature. 2008;9:148–58.
26. Pezzulo G, Castelfranchi C. Thinking as the control of imagination: a conceptual framework for goal-directed systems. Psychol Res. 2009;73:559–77.
27. Moeller S, Goldstein R. Impaired self-awareness in human addiction: deficient attribution of personal relevance. Trends Cogn Sci. 2014;18(12):635–41.
28. Maslow A. Toward a psychology of being. New York: Van Nostrand Reinhold; 1968.
29. Kreibich A, Hennecke M, Brandstätter V. The effect of self-awareness on the identification of goal-related obstacles. Eur J Personal. 2020;34:215–33.
30. Tiffany S, Wray J. The clinical significance of drug craving. Ann N Y Acad Sci. 2012;1248:1–17.
31. Kabat-Zinn J. Mindfulness-based interventions in context: past, present, and future. Am Psychol Assoc D12. 2003;10(2):144–56.
32. Warren Brown K, Ryan RM, Creswell JD. Mindfulness: theoretical foundations and evidence for its salutary effects. Psychol Inq. 2007;18(4):211–37.

33. Jankowski T, Holas P. Metacognitive model of mindfulness. Conscious Cogn. 2014;28:64–80.
34. Allen J, Fonagy P, Bateman A. Mentalizing in clinical practice. American Psychiatric Publishing; 2008.
35. Garland EL, Howard MO. Mindfulness-based treatment of addiction: current state of the field and envisioning the next wave of research. Addict Sci Clin Pract. 2018;13(14):1–14.
36. Bowen S, Chawla N, Collins S, Witkiewitz K, Hsu S, Grow J, Clifasefi S, Garner M, Douglass A, Larimer M, Marlatt A. Mindfulness-based relapse prevention for substance use disorders: a pilot efficacy trial. Subst Abus. 2009;30(4):295–305.
37. Garland E, Gaylord S, Boettiger C, Howard M. Mindfulness training modifies cognitive, affective, and physiological mechanisms implicated in alcohol dependence: results of a randomized controlled pilot trial. J Psychoactive Drugs. 2010;42(2):177–92.
38. Witkiewitz K, Bowen S. Depression, craving, and substance use following a randomized trial of mindfulness-based relapse prevention. J Consult Clin Psychol. 2010;78:362–74.
39. Brewer J, Elwafi H, Davis J. Craving to quit: psychological models and neurobiological mechanisms of mindfulness training as treatment for addictions. Psychol Addict Behav. 2012;27(2):366–79.
40. Tang YY, Hölzel BK, Posner MI. The neuroscience of mindfulness meditation. Nat Rev Neurosci AOP. Published online 18 March 2015. 2015; https://doi.org/10.1038/nrn3916.
41. Bowen S, Chawla N, Marlatt A. Mindfulness-based relapse prevention for addictive behaviours: a clinician's guide. London: Guilford Press; 2010.
42. Volkow ND, Fowler JS, Wang GK. The addicted human brain viewed in the light of imaging studies: brain circuits and treatment strategies. Neuropharmacology. 2004;47:3–13.

13 Morphine Addiction: Sex Differences and the Role of the $GABA_B$ Receptors

Valeria Teresa Pedrón and Graciela Noemí Balerio

Introduction

Addiction could be conceptualized as a recurrent cycle of different stages that worsens as time passes and involves plastic changes in the reinforcement, stress, and executive function systems [1–3]. It can be framed into different progressive stages: acute use, chronic use, acute withdrawal, and long-term withdrawal, which can induce drug reinstatement [4].

Several studies have reported differences in drug use patterns between men and women. Women have shown to escalate from occasional drug use to drug abuse faster than men [5, 6]. In addition, women have seen to be more vulnerable to the negative effects of drug use [7] and tend to look for treatment more frequently than men [6]. Nevertheless, once in treatment, women seem to have the same or even better chances to stay abstinent compared to men (except for tobacco use) [3].

Studies in rodents have demonstrated the presence of sex differences in the motivational and subjective effects of drugs of abuse. These reports indicate that female mice are more susceptible than males to the negative consequences of drug use. It is important to clarify that the term sex refers to a difference between male and female based on their reproductive organs and chromosomes. On the other hand, the term gender, which is used more frequently in humans, refers to the sexual identity of the individual.

GABA is the major inhibitory neurotransmitter in the mammalian central nervous system, it exerts its action through two different types of receptors: ionotropic ($GABA_A$ and $GABA_C$) and metabotropic $GABA_B$ receptors. $GABA_B$ receptors have been reported to be involved in the modulation of multiple functions within the central nervous system, including locomotion, anxiety, memory, and nociception [8–10].

The purpose of the present chapter will be to address the current evidence regarding sex differences in morphine addiction and the involvement of $GABA_B$ receptors in the addictive properties of morphine. This knowledge could be useful for both preclinical and clinical research.

V. T. Pedrón
Facultad de Farmacia y Bioquímica, Instituto de Investigaciones Farmacológicas (ININFA-UBA-CONICET), Universidad de Buenos Aires, Ciudad Autónoma de Buenos Aires, Argentina

Facultad de Psicología y Psicopedagogía, Instituto de Investigación, Universidad del Salvador, Ciudad Autónoma de Buenos Aires, Argentina

G. N. Balerio (✉)
Facultad de Farmacia y Bioquímica, Cátedra de Farmacología e Instituto de Investigaciones Farmacológicas (ININFA-UBA-CONICET), Universidad de Buenos Aires, Ciudad Autónoma de Buenos Aires, Argentina
e-mail: gbalerio@ffyb.uba.ar

P. Á. Gargiulo, H. L. Mesones-Arroyo (eds.), *Psychiatry and Neuroscience Update – Vol. V*,
https://doi.org/10.1007/978-3-031-72219-6_13

Acute Use: Analgesia and Reward

Analgesia

Pain is defined as the presence of a noxious sensory stimuli in combination with a negative affect and frequently treated by the administration of drugs such as morphine or other opioids [11]. Several reports have indicated the presence of sex differences in the effects induced by acute morphine administration. Morphine has shown to induce an increased analgesia in males compared to female rodents using different experimental models of pain. Sex differences in the effect of morphine have been observed in visceral pain [12–14]. Male mice showed an increase in morphine analgesia compared to female mice after intraplanar administration of complete Freund's adjuvant [11]; using thermal pain [15–18] and mechanical pain [19–21].

There are several mechanisms that have been proposed to explain these sex differences in morphine analgesia. The periaqueductal gray (PAG) is a neural locus for opioid action [22, 23]. Female mice have shown to need the doble of the maximal antinociceptive dose (ED_{50}) compared with male mice following intra-PAG morphine administration to produce the same antinociceptive response [24] and female mice have shown to express a significant reduced number of μ-opioid receptors in the PAG compared to male mice [25]. It has also been shown that reducing PAG μ-opioid receptor availability had a greater impact on opioid antinociception in females compared to male mice [26]. Furthermore, several studies have shown sex differences in morphine metabolism. When morphine is metabolized to form two active metabolites: morphine-3-glucuronide (M3G) and morphine-6-glucoronide (M6G), M6G binds to μ-opioid receptors and has potent analgesic effects, while M3G binds to an innate immune receptor, the toll like receptor 4, to induce allodynia and hyperalgesia [27, 28]. Female mice morphine metabolism produces a two-times greater concentration of M3G compared to male mice [29, 30], which can also explain the presence of sex differences in the analgesic response. A recent study by Doyle and Murphy [31], reported that intra-PAG administration of M3G reduced de analgesic effect of morphine in male mice, which supports the metabolic differences hypothesis.

In a recent review, the relation between sex differences in morphine analgesia and the role of gonadal hormones have been addressed [32]. Gonadal hormones could have both an organizational and activational effects on nociception. The organizational effects are long-term developmental effects and the activational effect is associated with transient changes observed in adulthood [33]. Evidence of the organizational effects hormones indicates that morphine is more potent in gonadally intact males compared to female mice but when gonadectomized, antinociception is significantly decreased in male and increased in female mice. This attenuated effect of morphine in castrated male mice is reversed by testosterone administration [34, 35]. In previous studies from our laboratory, we have observed that prepubertal intact male mice show greater analgesic effect of morphine compared to female mice [16] indicating the organizational effect of gonadal hormones on sex differences.

Clinical studies have indicated that the administration of baclofen, a $GABA_B$ receptor agonist, could enhance morphine analgesia [36] and patients who underwent total knee arthroplasty and received baclofen reported less opioid use compared to the patients that only received opioid treatment [37]. A possible explanation is that coactivation of opioid and $GABA_B$ receptors might induce an enhanced opioid analgesia compared to the activation of opioid receptors alone [36].

Only a few preclinical studies have explored the role of $GABA_B$ receptors on morphine analgesia. Systemic administration of baclofen has shown to potentiate the analgesic effect of morphine [9, 16, 38]. On the other hand naloxone pretreatment, a μ-opioid receptor antagonist, has shown to reverse the antinociceptive effect of baclofen indicating an interaction between opioidergic and GABAergic systems [38, 39]. In a recent study from our laboratory, we also evaluated the effect of a $GABA_B$ receptor antagonist, 2-hydroxy-saclofen, and the lack of a functional

$GABA_B$ receptor, using $GABA_{B1}$ knockout mice, on morphine antinociception [16]. Our results indicated that 2-hydroxy-saclofen attenuated or even blocked morphine induced antinociceptive responses. Moreover, morphine did not induce analgesia in $GABA_{B1}$ knockout mice, supporting the interaction of the GABAergic and the opioidergic systems.

Reward

The rewarding effects of drugs of abuse are responsible for the initiation of the addictive process, which indicates the importance of studying the rewarding effects of drugs of abuse [40]. There are sex differences in the reinforcing properties of morphine, but in this case, the females tend to show greater preference to opioids than male rodents. In Wistar rats, studies have shown that low doses of morphine are more reinforcing for females than for males [41]. However, in Sprague-Dawley rats, no differences in induced reward were observed. The presence of sex differences on morphine reward seems to be showed at lower doses, but when high doses are given, females continue showing preference and, in males, reward disappears [42]. In the self-administration paradigm, female mice learned to self-administer morphine and heroin more quickly and showed greater motivation to self-administer compared to males [43–45]. Therefore, the sex differences in the reinforcing value of morphine vary according to the strain of rat and the dose used to induce preference. The paradigm of conditioned place preference (CPP) has shown to reflect aspects of drug seeking triggered by contextual cues [46]. Studies using the CPP paradigm to investigate morphine reward have shown that adult female rats develop a more robust morphine preference to morphine compared to males [41, 42]. These findings reflect that adult female mice tend to have a higher preference for morphine compared to males [47–49]. Nevertheless, there are reports of male mice being more sensitive to morphine reward compared to female mice [50]. Additionally, female rats exert a greater effort in operative conditioning tasks to obtain a reinforcement of morphine or heroin [43]. In a recent study from our laboratory [51] we did not observe sex differences in the rewarding effect of morphine in prepubertal mice which indicate the activational effect of gonadal hormones in morphine reward (Fig. 13.1).

Studies in rodents have shown that there are clear sexual differences in the basal dopaminergic tone and in the activation of the striatum, after the administration of drugs of abuse in adult rodents [52–54]. Adult females, in comparison with males, have shown to have higher levels of striatal extracellular dopamine (DA) concentrations, greater DA neuron terminal density in the caudate nucleus, an increase in extracellular DA concentration after amphetamine stimulation in the striatum [55, 56] and a higher striatal concentration of DA after cocaine administration [57]. Experiments using microdialysis showed that basal DA levels and its metabolite, 3,4-dihydroxyphenylacetic acid (DOPAC), are modulated by the estrous cycle in females [58]. In addition, the ranges of extracellular levels of DA/DOPAC are higher during proestrus, suggesting a greater change in the magnitude of DA release when estrogen levels are high [59]. These data support the hypothesis that fluctuations in the levels of ovarian hormones during the estrous cycle in females could induce alterations in the activation of the dopaminergic system. Considering that in the present study we used prepubertal mice, we can suggest that the lack of sexual differences observed in the reinforcing effect of morphine could be explained by the lack of cyclic variations in ovarian hormones.

It has been hypothesized that morphine acts on μ-opioid receptors within the ventral tegmental area (VTA), inhibiting GABAergic neurons that produce an inhibition on dopaminergic neurons [60–65]. This phenomenon induces a disinhibition and stimulation of the dopaminergic neurons in the VTA with the consequent (DA) release into the nucleus accumbens, amygdala, hippocampus, and prefrontal cortex [62, 64–68]. In line with this, it has been shown that morphine does not induce reward in μ-opioid receptor deficient mice [69]. In addition, it has been reported

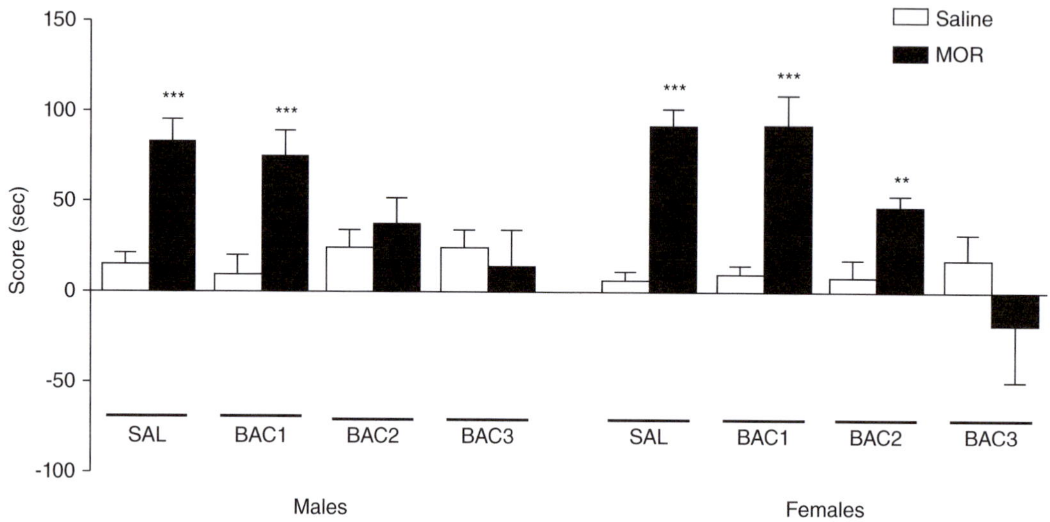

Fig. 13.1 Effect of baclofen pretreatment on the rewarding effects of morphine in male and female mice. Baclofen (2 and 3 mg/kg, i.p.) (BAC2 and BAC3) pretreatment was able to prevent the reinforcing effect of morphine (7 mg/kg, s.c.) (MOR) in male mice, but only BAC 3 was able to prevent the reinforcing effect of MOR in female mice. Results are expressed as mean ± SEM ($n = 8–15$ mice for each sex/group). Bars represent vehicle treated (white bars) and MOR treated (black bars) male and female mice. $^{**}P < 0.01$, $^{***}P < 0.001$, compared with respective saline treated groups

that morphine microinjections in the VTA induce reward in rats [70]. This mechanism plays a fundamental role in the reinforcement induced by morphine administration.

Regarding the role of $GABA_B$ receptors, a previous study has shown that systemic BAC administration prevents the rewarding properties of morphine [71]. This report used a high dose of BAC (10 mg/kg, i.p.), which has shown to induce motor impairment in mice [39] and the CPP paradigm has previously shown to be affected by locomotor activity [72]. Other studies have explored the effect of $GABA_B$ agonists and antagonists injection into specific brain areas in the development of morphine reward [73–77]. Baclofen pretreatment has shown to prevent the rewarding effects of morphine when administered in the dorsal hippocampus [73], the agranular insular cortex [74], the nucleus accumbens shell [74], but it had no effect on the rewarding effects of morphine when administered intra-central amygdala [76]. In line with this, the administration of the $GABA_B$ receptor antagonist phaclofen potentiated the rewarding effects of morphine and blocked the preventive effect of baclofen on morphine reward when administered in the dorsal hippocampus [73]. On the contrary, the administration of $GABA_B$ receptor antagonist saclofen administered intra-tegmental pedunculopontine nucleus prevented the rewarding effects of morphine [77].

In our laboratory, we explored the effect of systemic administration of three doses of baclofen (1, 2 and 3 mg/kg, i.p.) on the development of morphine reward in male and female prepubertal mice [51]. We did not observe the presence of sex differences, but baclofen pretreatment was able to prevent the rewarding effects of morphine at the doses of 2 and 3 mg/kg in male mice, but in female mice only the dose of 3 mg/kg was able to prevent the rewarding properties of morphine (Fig. 13.1). The lack of sex differences could be related to the age of animals (prepubertal mice), since circulating estrogen has shown to influence the effects of morphine in female mice [31].

Chronic Use: Tolerance and Sensitization

Tolerance

The pharmacological effect of morphine has shown to decrease with chronic use, a phenomenon known as tolerance. Previous studies have reported that male rodents develop greater tolerance to the analgesic effects of morphine compared with females administered by cumulative dose, infusion, or repeated dosing for a fixed time schedule [25, 78–80], but others have challenged these results [81, 82]. The discrepancy between studies could be attributed to differences in drug administration, the nociceptive assay employed, hormonal status, species, and experimental design [83].

The possible mechanisms imply the role of sex steroids acting on neuronal processes in the central nervous system [21, 84]. A study by Mousavi et al. [79] indicated that excitatory amino acid release in the nucleus accumbens may be modulated by an estrogen sensitive mechanism and play a role in morphine analgesia and tolerance. Moreover, Shekunova and Bespalov [85] indicated that proestrus females produced a significant acute tolerance to morphine (10 mg/kg) but ovariectomized rats did not. In line with this, chronic estradiol administration to ovariectomized rats reinstated the induction of tolerance.

Regarding the role of $GABA_B$ receptors in morphine tolerance, Alavian and Shiasvand [76] reported that baclofen administration intra-central amygdala increased the expression of tolerance to morphine, but the administration of the $GABA_B$ receptor antagonist, CGP353548, reduced the acquisition and expression of morphine tolerance. On the contrary, $GABA_A$, instead of $GABA_B$ receptors, seems to be involved in the development of morphine tolerance in the formalin test [86].

Sensitization

Neural changes induced by repeated exposure to opioids is reflected in a behavioral phenomenon called behavioral sensitization [87]. In consequence, mice develop drug-induced increases in locomotor activity, reinforcing and rewarding effects [88]. Powell and Holtzman [89] have indicated that behavioral sensitization occurs as opposed to the development of tolerance to the analgesic effect of morphine. There are only few studies that explore sex differences in morphine sensitization. A report by Zhan et al. [90] explored the presence of sex differences in morphine sensitization in ICR mice. Repeated morphine administration increased the locomotion, whereas attenuated the levels of anxiety, rearing and self-grooming behaviors in female mice, but not in male mice.

$GABA_B$ receptors have demonstrated to have a role in the development of morphine sensitization [71, 91, 92]. Chronic baclofen pretreatment has shown to significantly inhibit the development of morphine sensitization and to decrease the dopamine release induced by chronic morphine treatment [91]. Another study reported that chronic baclofen treatment reverted the motor sensitization induced by a prior chronic morphine treatment [92]. According to a study by Leite-Morris et al. [93] both the acquisition and expression of morphine sensitization could be mediated by $GABA_B$ receptors in the VTA. They observed that intra-VTA administration of baclofen produced a significant inhibition of the stimulant effect and blocked Fos induction in the nucleus accumbens shell and baclofen effect was reversed by 2-hydroxysaclofen administration.

Withdrawal: Somatic and Motivational Components

In dependent animals, a withdrawal state emerges after cessation of drug exposure or after the administration of an antagonist drug. Therefore, this state increases the likelihood of reinstatement of drug use [94]. Withdrawal to drugs of abuse is known to cause two types of symptoms: somatic or physical symptoms and motivational or psychological symptoms. Acute opioid withdrawal induces a series of physical symptoms that can be easily assessed in rodents: jumps, wet dog shakes, weight loss, paw tremors, diarrhea, and piloerection. In general, withdrawal symptoms are precipitated by the administration of an opioid antagonist such as naloxone. Many studies focus on the somatic signs of withdrawal, but the motivational aspects deserve attention because they play a key role in drug use reinstatement. Even though somatic signs of withdrawal tend to disappear in a few days, other phenotypes are increased, including social interaction deficits and depressive phenotypes.

Somatic Component

In previous studies from our laboratory, we have observed that the physical signs of opioid withdrawal are more pronounced in male than female mice [95, 96] even though morphine kinetics after chronic treatment did not demonstrate differences between sexes [97]. Similar results have been reported in other studies [78, 98]. Another study showed that the duration of somatic signs induced by spontaneous opioid withdrawal is higher in male than in female rats [84, 99]. When using the acoustic startle reflex as an indicator of abstinence, no sex differences have been observed after withdrawal from an acute dose of morphine in rats [100]. Regarding the neurochemical changes induced by morphine withdrawal, previous studies from our laboratory showed an increase in DA levels and its metabolites in the striatum and frontal cortex of males, but not female mice [101]. Likewise, the population of μ-opioid receptors was increased in certain areas in males exclusively [102]. These differences observed could be, partially, the cause of the greater sensitivity of males in the behavioral expression of morphine withdrawal syndrome. Moreover, we have observed a decrease in the activation of areas CA1, CA3 and dentate gyrus of the hippocampus in males, but not in female withdrawn mice [103]. Taking all together, these data indicate that males are more sensitive to morphine withdrawal compared to female mice both at a behavioral and a neurobiological level.

Baclofen pretreatment has shown to attenuate the somatic expression of morphine withdrawal [104–106] indicating the participation of $GABA_B$ receptors. Previous studies from our laboratory, have shown that baclofen prevents the expression of morphine withdrawal syndrome in male as well as female mice [96], reestablishes the dopaminergic neuron activity [101], and the μ-opioid receptor levels [102, 107] modified during morphine withdrawal. On the contrary, we did not observe changes in the c-Fos expression modified by morphine withdrawal in the hippocampus of male mice [103].

Motivational Component

Regarding the motivational aspects of morphine withdrawal, there are a few studies exploring the presence of sex differences. When studying anxiety-like behaviors induced by spontaneous morphine withdrawal Mohammadian and Miladi-Gorji [99] did not find differences between male and female rats. On the contrary, in a previous study from our laboratory, we observed sex differences in the increase of time spent and the number of entries to the open arms of the elevated plus maze of morphine abstinent mice which can be interpreted as an anxiolytic-like effect [108]. This result was in agreement with previous studies in male mice [109–112]. Hofford et al. [110] have hypothesized that this response could be caused by the emotionality, the motivation and defensive patterns induced by morphine withdrawal. As the studies performed in rats have shown an anxiety-like behavior, these discrepancies could be explained by species differences, but further studies are needed [113].

The aversive state associated with morphine withdrawal is evaluated through the conditioned place aversion paradigm (CPA). As far as we concern, there is only one report exploring the aversive effect of morphine withdrawal using CPA by García-Carmona et al. [114]. No sex differences were found in the aversive effect of morphine, but they found that CPA extinction was delayed in male mice compared with female mice. On the contrary, in a study from our laboratory [51], we observed sex differences in the CPA induced by morphine withdrawal. Male mice showed a greater place aversion when compared with female mice.

A previous study by Hodgson et al. [115] explored the effect of morphine withdrawal on mood through the forced swim test in male and female adolescent mice. Their results indicated that withdrawn male mice, but not female mice, showed an increase in immobility in the forced swim test. These results suggest that opioid withdrawal might affect mood in a sex dependent manner.

Regarding the motivational component of morphine withdrawal, there are no previous reports exploring the role of $GABA_B$ receptors on morphine withdrawal induced place aversion. In a previous study from our laboratory, we studied the effect of baclofen on the elevated plus maze behavior after precipitation morphine withdrawal. We observed that baclofen pretreatment was able to prevent the increase in time spent and entries to open arms in both male and female mice. Moreover, baclofen was able to prevent changes in BDNF expression observed in male mice in areas associated with the motivational component of morphine withdrawal [108].

Relapse

Clinical evidence indicates that women are more vulnerable to relapse and have shorter abstinence periods between relapses [116, 117]. Different hypothesis has been proposed: from an increase in the internal cue's reactivity (emotional, negative reinforcement) and a greater sensitivity toward external cues (associated to the drugs, positive reinforcement) [116]. As far as we know, there are no preclinical studies assessing sex differences in the reinstatement of morphine consumption, but clinical studies have indicated that women might bc more vulnerable than men to have drug cravings when presented with opioid associated paraphernalia [118]. Further preclinical studies could enlighten our knowledge regarding the presence of sex differences and the underlying mechanisms of these sex differences in morphine relapse.

To our knowledge, there are no reports regarding the role of $GABA_B$ receptors in morphine relapse or craving. Nevertheless, a study by Spano et al. [119] reported that the administration of baclofen was able to prevent the heroin-induced reinstatement of heroin seeking behaviors in rats. Another study [120] indicated a possible role of the GABAergic system in morphine craving. In this report, the stimulation of the GABAergic system through acupuncture significantly reduced morphine craving and prevented changes in c-Fos expression induced by morphine administration. These studies support the participation of the $GABA_B$ receptors in opioid relapse and craving, but further experiments are needed to clarify this item.

Conclusion

Findings regarding sex differences in morphine addiction indicate that in general males are more vulnerable than females to the antinociceptive properties of morphine and that females are more vulnerable to their rewarding effects. Moreover, males are more likely to develop tolerance, but less likely to develop sensitization when compared to female mice. Regarding morphine withdrawal, there are several studies indicating that male mice express a more intense somatic component of morphine withdrawal than female mice, but the evidence related to sex differences in the motivational component of morphine withdrawal is still scarce. In addition, we did not find preclinical studies about the presence of sex differences in morphine relapse.

With respect to the role of $GABA_B$ receptors, previous studies indicate that the modulation of $GABA_B$ receptors could potentiate the positive effects of morphine and prevent unwanted side effects like reward, withdrawal, and relapse.

Taking all these into account there is evidence of the presence of sex differences and the role of $GABA_B$ receptors in many aspects of morphine addiction. Further studies are needed to expand our knowledge in this matter and to elucidate the underlying mechanisms.

References

1. Goldstein RZ, Volkow ND. Drug addiction and its underlying neurobiological basis: neuroimaging evidence for the involvement of the frontal cortex. Am J Psychiatry. 2002;159:1642–52.
2. Heatherton TF, Tice DM. Losing control how and why people fail at self-regulation. San Diego: Academic; 1994.
3. Koob GF, Le Moal M. Drug abuse: hedonic homeostatic dysregulation. Science (80-) [Internet]. 1997 [cited 2019 Nov 25];278(5335):52–8. Available from: https://science.sciencemag.org/content/278/5335/52.short.
4. Koob GF, Le Moal M. Neurobiology of addiction. Elsevier/Academic; 2006.
5. Carroll ME, Lynch WJ, Roth ME, Morgan AD, Cosgrove KP. Sex and estrogen influence drug abuse. Trends Pharmacol Sci [Internet]. 2004 [cited 2014 Jan 20];25(5):273–9. Available from: http://www.ncbi.nlm.nih.gov/pubmed/15120494.
6. Lynch W, Roth M, Carroll M. Biological basis of sex differences in drug abuse: preclinical and clinical studies. Psychopharmacology (Berl) [Internet]. 2002;164(2):121–37. Available from: http://link.springer.com/10.1007/s00213-002-1183-2.
7. Plant M. Women and alcohol: contemporary and historical perspectives. Free Assn Books; 1997.
8. Dalvi A, Rodgers RJ. GABAergic influences on plus-maze behaviour in mice. Psychopharmacology (Berl) [Internet]. 1996 [cited 2021 Feb 12];128(4):380–97. Available from: https://link.springer.com/article/10.1007/s002130050148.
9. Balerio GN, Rubio MC. Baclofen analgesia: involvement of the GABAergic system. Pharmacol Res. 2002;46(3):281–6.
10. Mombereau C, Kaupmann K, Froestl W, Sansig G, Van Der Putten H, Cryan JF. Genetic and pharmacological evidence of a role for GABAB receptors in the modulation of anxiety- and antidepressant-like behavior. Neuropsychopharmacology. 2004;29(6):1050–62.
11. Armendariz A, Nazarian A. Morphine antinociception on thermal sensitivity and place conditioning in male and female rats treated with intraplantar complete Freund's adjuvant. Behav Brain Res [Internet]. 2018;343:21–7. Available from: http://www.ncbi.nlm.nih.gov/pubmed/29378294.
12. Ji Y, Murphy AZ, Traub RJ. Sex differences in morphine-induced analgesia of visceral pain are supraspinally and peripherally mediated. Am J Physiol Regul Integr Comp Physiol [Internet]. 2006;291(2):R307–14. Available from: http://www.ncbi.nlm.nih.gov/pubmed/16556902.
13. Ji Y, Murphy AZ, Traub RJ. Estrogen modulation of morphine analgesia of visceral pain in female rats is supraspinally and peripherally mediated. J pain [Internet]. 2007;8(6):494–502. Available from: http://www.ncbi.nlm.nih.gov/pubmed/17383238.
14. Murphy AZ, Suckow SK, Johns M, Traub RJ. Sex differences in the activation of the spinoparabrachial circuit by visceral pain. Physiol Behav [Internet]. 2009;97(2):205–12. Available from: http://www.ncbi.nlm.nih.gov/pubmed/19275905.
15. Nealon CM, Patel C, Worley BL, Henderson-Redmond AN, Morgan DJ, Czyzyk TA. Alterations in nociception and morphine antinociception in mice fed a high-fat diet. Brain Res Bull [Internet]. 2018 [cited 2019 Jun 27];138:64–72. Available from: http://www.ncbi.nlm.nih.gov/pubmed/28684345.
16. Pedrón VT, Varani AP, Bettler B, Balerio GN. $GABA_B$ receptors modulate morphine antinociception: pharmacological and genetic approaches. Pharmacol Biochem Behav. 2019;180:11–21.
17. Kest B, Wilson SG, Mogil JS. Sex differences in supraspinal morphine analgesia are dependent on genotype. J Pharmacol Exp Ther [Internet]. 1999;289(3):1370–5. Available from: http://www.ncbi.nlm.nih.gov/pubmed/10336528.
18. Loyd DR, Murphy AZ. Sex differences in the anatomical and functional organization of the ventromedial medullary pathway in the rat: a potential circuit mediating the sexually dimorphic actions of morphine. J Comp Neurol. 2006;738(September 2005):723–38.
19. Cicero TJ, Nock B, Meyer ER. Sex-related differences in morphine's antinociceptive activity: relationship to serum and brain morphine concentrations. J Pharmacol Exp Ther [Internet]. 1997;282(2):939–44. Available from: http://www.ncbi.nlm.nih.gov/pubmed/9262361.
20. Cicero TJ, Nock B, Meyer ER. Gender-related differences in the antinociceptive properties of morphine. J Pharmacol Exp Ther [Internet]. 1996;279(2):767–73. Available from: http://www.ncbi.nlm.nih.gov/pubmed/8930182.
21. Craft RM. Sex differences in opioid analgesia: "from mouse to man". Clin J Pain [Internet]. 2003;19(3):175–86. Available from: http://www.ncbi.nlm.nih.gov/pubmed/12792556.
22. Lane DA, Tortorici V, Morgan MM. Behavioral and electrophysiological evidence for tolerance to continuous morphine administration into the ventrolateral periaqueductal gray. Neuroscience [Internet]. 2004;125(1):63–9. Available from: http://www.ncbi.nlm.nih.gov/pubmed/15051146.
23. Loyd DR, Morgan MM, Murphy AZ. Morphine preferentially activates the periaqueductal gray-rostral ventromedial medullary pathway in the male rat: a potential mechanism for sex differences in antinociception. Neuroscience [Internet]. 2007;147(2):456–68. Available from: http://www.ncbi.nlm.nih.gov/pubmed/17540508.
24. Bobeck EN, McNeal AL, Morgan MM. Drug dependent sex-differences in periaqueducatal gray mediated antinociception in the rat. Pain [Internet]. 2009 [cited 2013 Aug 17];147(1–3):210–6. Available from: http://www.pubmedcentral.nih.gov/articleren-

der.fcgi?artid=2814455&tool=pmcentrez&rendertype=abstract.
25. Loyd DR, Wang X, Murphy AZ. Sex differences in micro-opioid receptor expression in the rat midbrain periaqueductal gray are essential for eliciting sex differences in morphine analgesia. J Neurosci [Internet]. 2008;28(52):14007–17. Available from: http://www.ncbi.nlm.nih.gov/pubmed/19109484.
26. Bernal SA, Morgan MM, Craft RM. PAG mu opioid receptor activation underlies sex differences in morphine antinociception. Behav Brain Res [Internet]. 2007 [cited 2014 Jan 20];177(1):126–33. Available from: http://www.pubmedcentral.nih.gov/articlerender.fcgi?artid=1868665&tool=pmcentrez&rendertype=abstract.
27. Lewis SS, Hutchinson MR, Rezvani N, Loram LC, Zhang Y, Maier SF, et al. Evidence that intrathecal morphine-3-glucuronide may cause pain enhancement via toll-like receptor 4/MD-2 and interleukin-1beta. Neuroscience [Internet]. 2010;165(2):569–83. Available from: http://www.ncbi.nlm.nih.gov/pubmed/19833175.
28. Due MR, Piekarz AD, Wilson N, Feldman P, Ripsch MS, Chavez S, et al. Neuroexcitatory effects of morphine-3-glucuronide are dependent on Toll-like receptor 4 signaling. J Neuroinflammation [Internet]. 2012;9:200. Available from: http://www.ncbi.nlm.nih.gov/pubmed/22898544.
29. Baker L, Ratka A. Sex-specific differences in levels of morphine, morphine-3-glucuronide, and morphine antinociception in rats. Pain [Internet]. 2002;95(1–2):65–74. Available from: http://www.ncbi.nlm.nih.gov/pubmed/11790468.
30. South SM, Edwards SR, Smith MT. Antinociception versus serum concentration relationships following acute administration of intravenous morphine in male and female Sprague-Dawley rats: differences between the tail flick and hot plate nociceptive tests. Clin Exp Pharmacol Physiol [Internet]. 2009;36(1):20–8. Available from: http://www.ncbi.nlm.nih.gov/pubmed/18671713.
31. Doyle HH, Murphy AZ. Sex-dependent influences of morphine and its metabolites on pain sensitivity in the rat. Physiol Behav [Internet]. 2018;187:32–41. Available from: http://www.ncbi.nlm.nih.gov/pubmed/29199028.
32. Nasser SA, Afify EA. Sex differences in pain and opioid mediated antinociception: Modulatory role of gonadal hormones. Life Sci [Internet]. 2019;237:116926. Available from: http://www.ncbi.nlm.nih.gov/pubmed/31614148.
33. Rasakham K, Liu-Chen L-Y. Sex differences in kappa opioid pharmacology. Life Sci [Internet]. 2011;88(1–2):2–16. Available from: http://www.ncbi.nlm.nih.gov/pubmed/20951148.
34. Rao SS, Saifi AQ. Influence of testosterone on morphine analgesia in albino rats. Indian J Physiol Pharmacol [Internet]. 29(2):103–6. Available from: http://www.ncbi.nlm.nih.gov/pubmed/4093190.
35. Stoffel EC, Ulibarri CM, Craft RM. Gonadal steroid hormone modulation of nociception, morphine antinociception and reproductive indices in male and female rats. Pain [Internet]. 2003;103(3):285–302. Available from: http://www.ncbi.nlm.nih.gov/pubmed/12791435.
36. Gordon NC, Gear RW, Heller PH, Paul S, Miaskowski C, Levine JD. Enhancement of morphine analgesia by the GABAB agonist baclofen. Neuroscience [Internet]. 1995 [cited 2013 Nov 22];69(2):345–9. Available from: http://www.ncbi.nlm.nih.gov/pubmed/8552232.
37. Sanders JC, Gerstein N, Torgeson E, Abram S. Intrathecal baclofen for postoperative analgesia after total knee arthroplasty. J Clin Anesth [Internet]. 2009;21(7):486–92. Available from: http://www.ncbi.nlm.nih.gov/pubmed/20006256.
38. Aley KO, Kulkarni SK. GABAergic agents-induced antinociceptive effect in mice. Methods Find Exp Clin Pharmacol [Internet]. 1989;11(10):597–601. Available from: http://www.ncbi.nlm.nih.gov/pubmed/2511384.
39. Balerio GN, Rubio MC. Baclofen analgesia: involvement of the GABAergic system. Pharmacol Res [Internet]. 2002 [cited 2020 Aug 18];46(3):281–6. Available from: https://pubmed.ncbi.nlm.nih.gov/12220972/.
40. Koob GF, Le Moal M. Drug addiction, dysregulation of reward, and allostasis. Neuropsychopharmacology [Internet]. 2001 [cited 2016 Aug 12];24(2):97–129. Available from: http://www.ncbi.nlm.nih.gov/pubmed/11120394.
41. Karami M, Zarrindast MR. Morphine sex-dependently induced place conditioning in adult Wistar rats. Eur J Pharmacol. 2008;582(1):78–87.
42. Cicero TJ, Ennis T, Ogden J, Meyer ER. Gender differences in the reinforcing properties of morphine. Pharmacol Biochem Behav. 2000;65(1):91–6.
43. Cicero TJ, Aylward SC, Meyer ER. Gender differences in the intravenous self-administration of mu opiate agonists. Pharmacol Biochem Behav. 2003;74(3):541–9.
44. Lynch WJ, Carroll ME. Sex differences in the acquisition of intravenously self-administered cocaine and heroin in rats. Psychopharmacology (Berl) [Internet]. 1999;144(1):77–82. Available from: http://link.springer.com/10.1007/s002130050979.
45. Roth ME, Carroll ME. Sex differences in the escalation of intravenous cocaine intake following long- or short-access to cocaine self-administration. Pharmacol Biochem Behav [Internet]. 2004;78(2):199–207. Available from: https://linkinghub.elsevier.com/retrieve/pii/S0091305704001029.
46. Chen L, Xu M. Dopamine D1 and D3 receptors are differentially involved in cue-elicited cocaine seeking. J Neurochem [Internet]. 2010;114(2):530–41. Available from: http://doi.wiley.com/10.1111/j.1471-4159.2010.06775.x.
47. Elman I, Karlsgodt KH, Gastfriend DR. Gender differences in cocaine craving among non-treatment-

seeking individuals with cocaine dependence. Am J Drug Alcohol Abuse [Internet]. 2001;27(2):193–202. Available from: http://www.ncbi.nlm.nih.gov/pubmed/11417935.
48. Robbins SJ, Ehrman RN, Childress AR, O'Brien CP. Comparing levels of cocaine cue reactivity in male and female outpatients. Drug Alcohol Depend [Internet]. 1999;53(3):223–30. Available from: https://linkinghub.elsevier.com/retrieve/pii/S0376871698001355.
49. Sterling RC, Dean J, Weinstein SP, Murphy J, Gottheil E. Gender differences in cue exposure reactivity and 9-month outcome. J Subst Abuse Treat [Internet]. 2004;27(1):39–44. Available from: https://linkinghub.elsevier.com/retrieve/pii/S0740547204000418.
50. Fakira AK, Peck EG, Liu Y, Lueptow LM, Trimbake NA, Han M-H, et al. The role of the neuropeptide PEN receptor, GPR83, in the reward pathway: relationship to sex-differences. Neuropharmacology [Internet]. 2019;157:107666. Available from: http://www.ncbi.nlm.nih.gov/pubmed/31199956.
51. Pedrón VT, Canero EM, Aon AJ, Varani AP, Balerio GN. Baclofen prevents behavioral and biochemical alterations induced by morphine rewarding effects in male and female mice. European Journal of Pharmacology. 2024;979:176768. Avaible from: https://doi.org/10.1016/j.ejphar.2024.176768.
52. Becker JB. Gender differences in dopaminergic function in striatum and nucleus accumbens. Pharmacol Biochem Behav [Internet]. 1999;64(4):803–12. Available from: http://www.ncbi.nlm.nih.gov/pubmed/10593204.
53. Becker JB, Perry AN, Westenbroek C. Sex differences in the neural mechanisms mediating addiction: a new synthesis and hypothesis. Biol Sex Differ [Internet]. 2012;3(1):14. Available from: http://www.pubmedcentral.nih.gov/articlerender.fcgi?artid=3724495&tool=pmcentrez&rendertype=abstract.
54. Becker JB, Hu M. Sex differences in drug abuse. Front Neuroendocrinol [Internet]. 2008 [cited 2014 Jan 20];29(1):36–47. Available from: http://www.pubmedcentral.nih.gov/articlerender.fcgi?artid=2235192&tool=pmcentrez&rendertype=abstract.
55. Castner SA, Xiao L, Becker JB. Sex differences in striatal dopamine: in vivo microdialysis and behavioral studies. Brain Res. 1993;610(1):127–34.
56. Walker QD, Rooney MB, Wightman RM, Kuhn CM. Dopamine release and uptake are greater in female than male rat striatum as measured by fast cyclic voltammetry. Neuroscience [Internet]. 1999;95(4):1061–70. Available from: https://linkinghub.elsevier.com/retrieve/pii/S030645229900500X.
57. Walker QD, Ray R, Kuhn CM. Sex differences in neurochemical effects of dopaminergic drugs in rat striatum. Neuropsychopharmacology. 2006;31(6):1193–202.
58. Shimizu H, Bray GA. Effects of castration, estrogen replacement and estrus cycle on monoamine metabolism in the nucleus accumbens, measured by microdialysis. Brain Res [Internet]. 1993;621(2):200–6. Available from: https://linkinghub.elsevier.com/retrieve/pii/000689939390107X.
59. Xiao L, Becker JB. Quantitative microdialysis determination of extracellular striatal dopamine concentration in male and female rats: effects of estrous cycle and gonadectomy. Neurosci Lett [Internet]. 1994;180(2):155–8. Available from: https://linkinghub.elsevier.com/retrieve/pii/030439409490510X.
60. Gysling K, Wang RY. Morphine-induced activation of A10 dopamine neurons in the rat. Brain Res [Internet]. 1983;277(1):119–27. Available from: https://linkinghub.elsevier.com/retrieve/pii/0006899383909137.
61. Hyman SE, Malenka RC. Addiction and the brain: the neurobiology of compulsion and its persistence. Nat Rev Neurosci [Internet]. 2001;2(10):695–703. Available from: http://www.nature.com/articles/35094560.
62. Johnson S, North R. Opioids excite dopamine neurons by hyperpolarization of local interneurons. J Neurosci [Internet]. 1992;12(2):483–8. Available from: http://www.jneurosci.org/lookup/doi/10.1523/JNEUROSCI.12-02-00483.1992.
63. Kalivas PW, Duffy P, Eberhardt H. Modulation of A10 dopamine neurons by gamma-aminobutyric acid agonists. J Pharmacol Exp Ther [Internet]. 1990;253(2):858–66. Available from: http://www.ncbi.nlm.nih.gov/pubmed/2160011.
64. Koob GF. Neural mechanisms of drug reinforcement. Ann NY Acad Sci [Internet]. 1992;654:171–91. Available from: http://www.ncbi.nlm.nih.gov/pubmed/1632582.
65. Spanagel R, Weiss F. The dopamine hypothesis of reward: past and current status. Trends Neurosci [Internet]. 1999;22(11):521–7. Available from: https://linkinghub.elsevier.com/retrieve/pii/S0166223699014472.
66. Di Chiara G, Imperato A. Opposite effects of mu and kappa opiate agonists on dopamine release in the nucleus accumbens and in the dorsal caudate of freely moving rats. J Pharmacol Exp Ther [Internet]. 1988;244(3):1067–80. Available from: http://www.ncbi.nlm.nih.gov/pubmed/2855239.
67. Pontieri FE, Tanda G, Di Chiara G. Intravenous cocaine, morphine, and amphetamine preferentially increase extracellular dopamine in the "shell" as compared with the "core" of the rat nucleus accumbens. Proc Natl Acad Sci USA [Internet]. 1995;92(26):12304–8. Available from: http://www.ncbi.nlm.nih.gov/pubmed/8618890.
68. Wise RA. Drug-activation of brain reward pathways. Drug Alcohol Depend [Internet]. 1998;51(1–2):13–22. Available from: https://linkinghub.elsevier.com/retrieve/pii/S0376871698000635.
69. Mattes RD. Dietary compensation by humans for supplemental energy provided as ethanol or carbohydrate in fluids. Physiol Behav [Internet]. 1996;59(1):179–87. Available from: https://linkinghub.elsevier.com/retrieve/pii/0031938495020071.

70. Phillips AG, LePiane FG. Reinforcing effects of morphine microinjection into the ventral tegmental area. Pharmacol Biochem Behav [Internet]. 1980;12(6):965–8. Available from: http://www.ncbi.nlm.nih.gov/pubmed/7403209.
71. Kaplan GB, Leite-Morris KA, Joshi M, Shoeb MH, Carey RJ. Baclofen inhibits opiate-induced conditioned place preference and associated induction of Fos in cortical and limbic regions. Brain Res. 2003;987:122–5.
72. Cunningham CL, Gremel CM, Groblewski PA. Drug-induced conditioned place preference and aversion in mice. Nat Protoc. 2006;1(4):1662–70.
73. Zarrindast M-R, Massoudi R, Sepehri H, Rezayof A. Involvement of GABA(B) receptors of the dorsal hippocampus on the acquisition and expression of morphine-induced place preference in rats. Physiol Behav [Internet]. 2006;87(1):31–8. Available from: http://www.ncbi.nlm.nih.gov/pubmed/16274709.
74. Sun K, Mu Q, Chang H, Zhang C, Wang Y, Rong S, et al. Postretrieval microinjection of baclofen into the agranular insular cortex inhibits morphine-induced CPP by disrupting reconsolidation. Front Pharmacol [Internet]. 2020;11. Available from: https://www.frontiersin.org/article/10.3389/fphar.2020.00743/full.
75. Wang C, Pan R, Wan X, Tan Y, Xu L, Ho CS, et al. Immediate psychological responses and associated factors during the initial stage of the 2019 coronavirus disease (COVID-19) epidemic among the general population in China. Int J Environ Res Public Health. 2020;17(5):1729.
76. Alavian F, Ghiasvand S, Sahraei H, Rafiei-Rad M. Intervention of the Gamma-aminobutyric acid type B Receptors of the amygdala central nucleus on the sensitivity of the morphine-induced conditionally preferred location in Wistar female rats. Addict Heal [Internet]. 2017;9(2):110–7. Available from: http://www.ncbi.nlm.nih.gov/pubmed/29299214.
77. Heinmiller A, Ting-A-Kee R, Vargas-Perez H, Yeh A, van der Kooy D. Tegmental pedunculopontine glutamate and GABA-B synapses mediate morphine reward. Behav Neurosci [Internet]. 2009 [cited 2013 Aug 1];123(1):145–55. Available from: http://www.ncbi.nlm.nih.gov/pubmed/19170439.
78. Craft RM, Stratmann JA, Bartok RE, Walpole TI, King SJ. Sex differences in development of morphine tolerance and dependence in the rat. Psychopharmacology (Berl) [Internet]. 1999;143(1):1–7. Available from: http://www.ncbi.nlm.nih.gov/pubmed/10227072.
79. Mousavi Z, Shafaghi B, Kobarfard F, Jorjani M. Sex differences and role of gonadal hormones on glutamate level in the nucleus accumbens in morphine tolerant rats: a microdialysis study. Eur J Pharmacol [Internet]. 2007 [cited 2014 Jan 20];554(2–3):145–9. Available from: http://www.ncbi.nlm.nih.gov/pubmed/17112508.
80. Meng J, Zhang X, Wu H, Bu J, Shi C, Deng C, et al. Morphine-induced conditioned place preference in mice: metabolomic profiling of brain tissue to find "molecular switch" of drug abuse by gas chromatography/mass spectrometry. Anal Chim Acta [Internet]. 2012 [cited 2013 Aug 1];710:125–30. Available from: http://www.ncbi.nlm.nih.gov/pubmed/22123121.
81. Barrett AC, Cook CD, Terner JM, Craft RM, Picker MJ. Importance of sex and relative efficacy at the mu opioid receptor in the development of tolerance and cross-tolerance to the antinociceptive effects of opioids. Psychopharmacology (Berl) [Internet]. 2001;158(2):154–64. Available from: http://www.ncbi.nlm.nih.gov/pubmed/11702089.
82. Holtman JR, Sloan JW, Wala EP. Morphine tolerance in male and female rats. Pharmacol Biochem Behav [Internet]. 2004 [cited 2014 Jan 20];77(3):517–23. Available from: http://www.ncbi.nlm.nih.gov/pubmed/15006462.
83. Zhang Y, Donica CL, Standifer KM. Sex differences in the Nociceptin/Orphanin FQ system in rat spinal cord following chronic morphine treatment. Neuropharmacology [Internet]. 2012;63(3):427–33. Available from: http://www.ncbi.nlm.nih.gov/pubmed/22575074.
84. Cicero TJ, Nock B, Meyer ER. Gender-linked differences in the expression of physical dependence in the rat. Pharmacol Biochem Behav [Internet]. 2002;72(3):691–7. Available from: http://www.ncbi.nlm.nih.gov/pubmed/12175466.
85. Shekunova EV., Bespalov AY. Estrous cycle stage-dependent expression of acute tolerance to morphine analgesia in rats. Eur J Pharmacol [Internet]. 2004 [cited 2019 Jun 27];486(3):259–64. Available from: http://www.ncbi.nlm.nih.gov/pubmed/14985047.
86. Rahman AF, Takahashi M, Kaneto H. Role of GABAergic systems in the development of morphine tolerance in formalin-treated mice. Jpn J Pharmacol [Internet]. 1995;68(2):207–11. Available from: http://www.ncbi.nlm.nih.gov/pubmed/7563978.
87. Stewart J, Badiani A. Tolerance and sensitization to the behavioral effects of drugs. Behav Pharmacol [Internet]. 1993;4(4):289–312. Available from: http://www.ncbi.nlm.nih.gov/pubmed/11224198.
88. Francès H, Graulet A, Debray M, Coudereau JP, Guéris J, Bourre JM. Morphine-induced sensitization of locomotor activity in mice: effect of social isolation on plasma corticosterone levels. Brain Res [Internet]. 2000;860(1–2):136–40. Available from: http://www.ncbi.nlm.nih.gov/pubmed/10727632.
89. Powell KR, Holtzman SG. Parametric evaluation of the development of sensitization to the effects of morphine on locomotor activity. Drug Alcohol Depend [Internet]. 2001;62(1):83–90. Available from: http://www.ncbi.nlm.nih.gov/pubmed/11173171.
90. Zhan B, Ma H-Y, Wang J-L, Liu C-B. Sex differences in morphine-induced behavioral sensitization and social behaviors in ICR mice. Dong wu xue yan jiu = Zool Res [Internet]. 2015;36(2):103–8. Available from: http://www.ncbi.nlm.nih.gov/pubmed/25855229.

91. Fu Z, Yang H, Xiao Y, Zhao G, Huang H. The gamma-aminobutyric acid type B (GABA B) receptor agonist baclofen inhibits morphine sensitization by decreasing the dopamine level in rat nucleus accumbens. Behav Brain Funct. 2012;2–11.
92. Bartoletti M, Ricci F, Gaiardi M. A GABA(B) agonist reverses the behavioral sensitization to morphine in rats. Psychopharmacology (Berl) [Internet]. 2007;192(1):79–85. Available from: http://www.ncbi.nlm.nih.gov/pubmed/17242923.
93. Leite-morris KA, Fukudome EY, Shoeb MH, Kaplan GB. $GABA_B$ receptor activation in the ventral tegmental area inhibits the acquisition and expression of opiate-induced motor sensitization. J Pharmacol Exp Ther. 2004;308(2):667–78.
94. Koob GF, Volkow ND. Neurocircuitry of addiction. Neuropsychopharmacology. 2010;35(1):217–38.
95. Diaz SL, Kemmling AK, Rubio MC, Balerio GN. Morphine withdrawal syndrome: involvement of the dopaminergic system in prepubertal male and female mice. Pharmacol Biochem Behav [Internet]. 2005 [cited 2013 Jul 22];82(4):601–7. Available from: http://www.ncbi.nlm.nih.gov/pubmed/16325246.
96. Diaz SL, Kemmling AK, Rubio MC, Balerio GN. Lack of sex-related differences in the prevention by baclofen of the morphine withdrawal syndrome in mice. Behav Pharmacol [Internet]. 2001;12(1):75–9. Available from: http://www.ncbi.nlm.nih.gov/pubmed/11270515.
97. Diaz S, Hermida M. Pharmacokinetic aspects of naloxone-precipitated morphine withdrawal in male and female prepubertal mice. Drug Dispos [Internet]. 2007 [cited 2013 Jul 22];289(September 2006):283–9. Available from: http://onlinelibrary.wiley.com/doi/10.1002/bdd.554/abstract.
98. Mavrikaki M, Lintz T, Constantino N, Page S, Chartoff E. Chronic opioid exposure differentially modulates oxycodone self-administration in male and female rats. Addict Biol [Internet]. 2021;26(3):e12973. Available from: http://www.ncbi.nlm.nih.gov/pubmed/33078503.
99. Mohammadian J, Miladi-Gorji H. Age- and sex-related changes in the severity of physical and psychological dependence in morphine-dependent rats. Pharmacol Biochem Behav [Internet]. 2019;187:172793. Available from: http://www.ncbi.nlm.nih.gov/pubmed/31639387.
100. Radke AK, Gewirtz JC, Carroll ME. Effects of age, but not sex, on elevated startle during withdrawal from acute morphine in adolescent and adult rats. Behav Pharmacol [Internet]. 2015;26(5):485–8. Available from: https://journals.lww.com/00008877-201508000-00009.
101. Diaz SL, Kemmling AK, Balerio GN. Baclofen reestablishes striatal and cortical dopamine concentrations during naloxone-precipitated withdrawal. Neurochem Int [Internet]. 2003;42(4):293–8. Available from: http://www.ncbi.nlm.nih.gov/pubmed/12470702.
102. Diaz SL, Kemmling AK, Bonavita CD, Rubio MC, Balerio GN. Baclofen reestablishes micro-opioid receptor levels modified by morphine withdrawal syndrome in either sex. Synapse [Internet]. 2004 [cited 2013 Jul 22];54(1):24–9. Available from: http://www.ncbi.nlm.nih.gov/pubmed/15300881.
103. Pedrón VT, Taravini IRE, Induni AS, Balerio GN. Baclofen did not modify sexually dimorphic c-Fos expression during morphine withdrawal syndrome. Synapse [Internet]. 2013 [cited 2013 Jul 22];67(3):118–26. Available from: http://www.ncbi.nlm.nih.gov/pubmed/23152154.
104. Bexis S, Ong J, White J. Attenuation of morphine withdrawal signs by the GABA(B) receptor agonist baclofen. Life Sci [Internet]. 2001;70(4):395–401. Available from: http://www.ncbi.nlm.nih.gov/pubmed/11798009.
105. Riahi E, Mirzaii-Dizgah I, Karimian SM, Sadeghipour Roodsari HR, Dehpour AR. Attenuation of morphine withdrawal signs by a GABAB receptor agonist in the locus coeruleus of rats. Behav Brain Res. 2009;196(1):11–4.
106. Zarrindast MR, Mousa-Ahmadi E. Effects of GABAergic system on naloxone-induced jumping in morphine-dependent mice. Eur J Pharmacol [Internet]. 1999 [cited 2019 Nov 18];381(2–3):129–33. Available from: http://www.ncbi.nlm.nih.gov/pubmed/10554880.
107. Diaz SL, Barros VG, Antonelli MC, Rubio MC, Balerio GN. Morphine withdrawal syndrome and its prevention with baclofen: autoradiographic study of l-opioid receptors in prepubertal male and female mice. Synapse. 2006;140(February):132–40.
108. Pedrón VT, Varani AP, Balerio GN. Baclofen prevents the elevated plus maze behavior and BDNF expression during naloxone precipitated morphine withdrawal in male and female mice. Synapse. 2016;70(5):187–97.
109. Hodgson SR, Hofford RS, Norris CJ, Eitan S. Increased elevated plus maze open-arm time in mice during naloxone-precipitated morphine withdrawal. Behav Pharmacol [Internet]. 2008 [cited 2013 Aug 18];19(8):805–11. Available from: http://www.ncbi.nlm.nih.gov/pubmed/19020415.
110. Hofford RS, Hodgson SR, Roberts KW, Bryant CD, Evans CJ, Eitan S. Extracellular signal-regulated kinase activation in the amygdala mediates elevated plus maze behavior during opioid withdrawal. Behav Pharmacol [Internet]. 2009 [cited 2013 Aug 5];20(7):576–83. Available from: http://www.ncbi.nlm.nih.gov/pubmed/19738463.
111. Lipták N, Dochnal R, Csabafi K, Szakács J, Szabó G. Obestatin prevents analgesic tolerance to morphine and reverses the effects of mild morphine withdrawal in mice. Regul Pept [Internet]. 2013 [cited 2014 Mar 11];186:77–82. Available from: http://www.ncbi.nlm.nih.gov/pubmed/23891980.
112. Lipták N, Dochnal R, Babits A, Csabafi K, Szakács J, Tóth G, et al. The effect of pituitary adenylate cyclase-activating polypeptide on elevated plus

maze behavior and hypothermia induced by morphine withdrawal. Neuropeptides [Internet]. 2012 [cited 2014 Mar 11];46(1):11–7. Available from: http://www.ncbi.nlm.nih.gov/pubmed/22226680.
113. Zhang Z, Schulteis G. Withdrawal from acute morphine dependence is accompanied by increased anxiety-like behavior in the elevated plus maze. Pharmacol Biochem Behav [Internet]. 2008 [cited 2014 Mar 11];89(3):392–403. Available from: http://www.pubmedcentral.nih.gov/articlerender.fcgi?artid=2323908&tool=pmcentrez&rendertype=abstract.
114. García-Carmona J-A, Baroja-Mazo A, Milanés M-V, Laorden ML. Sex differences between CRF1 receptor deficient mice following naloxone-precipitated morphine withdrawal in a conditioned place aversion paradigm: implication of Hpa axis. Homberg J, editor. PLoS One [Internet]. 2015;10(4):e0121125. Available from: https://dx.plos.org/10.1371/journal.pone.0121125.
115. Hodgson SR, Hofford RS, Roberts KW, Eitan D, Wellman PJ, Eitan S. Sex differences in affective response to opioid withdrawal during adolescence. J Psychopharmacol [Internet]. 2010 [cited 2014 Jan 20];24(9):1411–7. Available from: http://www.ncbi.nlm.nih.gov/pubmed/19939877.
116. Hudson A, Stamp JA. Ovarian hormones and propensity to drug relapse: a review. Neurosci Biobehav Rev [Internet]. 2011;35(3):427–36. Available from: https://linkinghub.elsevier.com/retrieve/pii/S0149763410000953.
117. Kosten TA, Gawin FH, Kosten TR, Rounsaville BJ. Gender differences in cocaine use and treatment response. J Subst Abuse Treat [Internet]. 1993;10(1):63–6. Available from: https://linkinghub.elsevier.com/retrieve/pii/074054729390100G.
118. Yu J, Zhang S, Epstein DH, Fang Y, Shi J, Qin H, et al. Gender and stimulus difference in cue-induced responses in abstinent heroin users. Pharmacol Biochem Behav [Internet]. 2007;86(3):485–92. Available from: http://www.ncbi.nlm.nih.gov/pubmed/17306353.
119. Spano MS, Fattore L, Fratta W, Fadda P. The GABAB receptor agonist baclofen prevents heroin-induced reinstatement of heroin-seeking behavior in rats. Neuropharmacology [Internet]. 2007;52(7):1555–62. Available from: http://www.ncbi.nlm.nih.gov/pubmed/17451755
120. Lee BH, Zhao RJ, Lee BG, Kim NJ, Yang CH, Kim HY, et al. Acupuncture suppresses morphine craving in progressive ratio through the GABA system. J Acupunct Meridian Stud [Internet]. 2015;8(4):175–82. Available from: http://www.ncbi.nlm.nih.gov/pubmed/26276453.

14 Neurobiology of Addiction

Michel Bourin

Introduction

In a simplified way, the addiction is defined as a state of dependence on a drug. This is a mental illness chronic characterized [1]:

1. By an intense need, uncontrollable to seek out and consume the drug.
2. The inability to limit consumption despite medical, social, family, or professional negative effects.
3. Feelings of discomfort psychic, and sometimes physical, during deprivation drug. Weaning is very difficult and the very high risk of relapse.

Criteria of more precise diagnosis are included in the DSM (Diagnostic and Statistical Manual of Mental Disorders, edited by the American Association of Psychiatry). More broadly, the term addiction can be extended to certain behaviors which have the same repetitive, compulsive character, with loss of control (e.g., gambling). Of common neurobiological mechanisms are involved in both cases [2].

Different psychoactive substances can lead to addiction. These substances are first consumed as experimental for their own effects which can be of the psychoanaleptic type (e.g., amphetamines and cocaine), psycholeptic type (e.g., benzodiazepines, alcohol, and opiates), or still psychodysleptic type (e.g., cannabis). A rewarding first experience gives desire to repeat the consumption, and this repetition may cause, in some individuals, involuntary engagement in the cycle of addiction [3].

This cycle of addiction is manifest regardless of the type of substance consumed, which suggests the existence of a neurobiological basis common to the phenomenon of addiction.

With harmful use, physical, psycho-emotional, and social damage is present. It is associated with repetition of use, but there is still a possibility of abstaining from using. Beyond that, it is dependence that sets in, with loss of the freedom to abstain. The addict behavior will persist despite all the difficulties and opposition to achieving it. The term drug is used to define dependence, which is, according to the WHO definition of 1969, "a mental and sometimes physical state characterized by changes in behavior, which always include an urge to consume the product in order to recover its psychic effects and to avoid the discomfort of its deprivation" [4].

Despite the magnitude of the problems associated with the consumption of licit and illicit substances, the neurobiological processes involved in the phenomenon of drug addiction are still only partially understood. However, neuroimaging and the recent development of technologies

M. Bourin (✉)
Neurobiologie de l'anxiété et de la dépression, Université de Nantes, Nantes, France
e-mail: michel.bourin@univ-nantes.fr

P. Á. Gargiulo, H. L. Mesones-Arroyo (eds.), *Psychiatry and Neuroscience Update – Vol. V*,
https://doi.org/10.1007/978-3-031-72219-6_14

related to genetics, among others, have enabled major advances in the study of neuroscience. Essentially dopaminergic and striatal in conception, the biological theories of drug addiction now integrate the contribution of the glutamatergic, opioid, and endocannabinoid systems, as well as the interaction between these different components within the striatal and mesocorticolimbic structures [5]. This paradigm shift has led to the emergence of several therapeutic strategies aimed at reducing the risk of relapse by modulating more specifically the functioning of these cortical and subcortical structures.

What happens to the brain when from taking drugs?
Why do some consumers arrive more to control their consumption?
Why is the risk of relapse so high?

Some answers to these questions have been provided thanks to the research carried out in the animal for many years. Like humans, animals are sensitive to the positive reinforcing effects of drugs [6]. These effects appear when the administration of a drug increases the likelihood appearance of behaviors leading to its consumption. This process is a determinant essential to the potential for substance abuse and can be studied in rodents or in the monkey by means of different models, such as drug self-administration or preference of conditioned space. Thanks to modeling addictions, we now have a better understanding of the mechanisms molecular, cellular, genetic, and epigenetics responsible for the passage of an occasional compulsive drug use and relapse after long periods abstinence [7]. The aim of this chapter is to describe the circuits neurons involved in addiction and changes that occur within these circuits during the addiction cycle.

Installation of Addiction

Addiction has the characteristics of a chronic pathology, of progressive installation, with a course punctuated by relapses, and the occurrence of which is determined by vulnerability factors [8]. In the addictive process, the progressive changes in consumption behavior are part of a temporality:

- an initialization through the positive hedonic impact (reward, "liking"),
- the pursuit of behaviors via automatisms (learning, conditioning),
- the negative emotional consequences more than by the vain search for the initial effect (incentive salience, "wanting"),
- loss of control over consumption.

We can therefore consider schematically that this process takes place in three stages [9]:

- The first stage is a non-pathological phase of drug taking where the individual uses the drug recreationally. This phase corresponds to the moment when taking the product is, for the individual, a recreational activity, among others. Consumption occupies only a small part of his behavioral repertoire. This can be considered "normal" behavior that exists in a large proportion of the human population, whether they are legal or illegal drugs.
- The second stage, intensive, sustained, and increasing use, begins with an increase in the frequency and amount of the drug used, as well as the motivation for it. Drug use intensifies and becomes sustained. In addition, problems associated with use appear but are not sufficiently serious to always lead to attempts at abstinence [10]. This second stage is the first moderate pathological phase, during which the individual uses too many drugs, but his behavior remains organized, and he is generally well integrated into society. Not all patients with heavy use will progress to dependence as confirmed by various follow-up studies. For the patients who will become dependent, it is appropriate to wonder about the conditions of the installation of this dependence: there is, for the subjects who will become dependent, a gradual and increasingly imperative installation of psychic dependence, of craving. There is therefore a zone of transition (or gradual transition) and therefore of

imprecision between harmful use and dependence.

- Schematically, we could thus consider that there are, at this phase, two large subgroups of patients: A first group in which there are risk factors for progression to dependence; in this group, intensive and repeated use corresponds to a preliminary phase, often short, of the dependence, which constitutes its logical evolution. A second group in which the factors of vulnerability to the dependence are few; but conversely, the environmental and training factors are present. In this group, the return to controlled consumption is much more frequent, in particular when the pressure to consume decreases (advanced in age, setting up as a couple, etc.) or when a care process is undertaken (greater efficiency of brief interventions in this subgroup is likely)
- The third and final step in this process leads to the most serious condition. In this case, the individual largely loses control over his drug use and becomes dependent (or fully addicted to severe DSM V) [11]. During this phase, taking the product becomes the main activity of the individual, invading almost all of the space normally occupied by other components of his behavioral repertoire. The degradation of his social life then becomes inevitable and relapses, even after a prolonged period of abstinence, unfortunately becomes the rule [12].

Neural Circuits Involved in Positive Reinforcement Effects of Acute Drug Use

Repeated consumption leads to functional and structural cerebral modifications of several neurocircuits, including those of reward but especially those involved in the management of emotions, mood, motivation and learning that can affect behavioral habits and capacities of adaptation. Little by little, these modifications change the motivational properties of the products: if they were taken initially for pleasure, they are then mainly taken out of need, with important behavioral routines linked to conditioning, automation, and a loss of cognitive flexibility [13].

The Reward Circuit

The role of the reward circuit in positive reinforcing effects of drugs has been suggested over 30 years ago. This circuit, described by Olds and Milner in 1954 [14], has for elements essential dopaminergic neurons of the ventral tegmental area (VTA) and the Medial Forebrain Bundle (MFB), fiber bundle connecting the VTA to the ventral striatum, more particularly at the nucleus accumbens. The stimulation of this beam leads to a behavior intracranial self-stimulation, considered as a "reward" for the animal.

Subsequent studies have shown that various addictive substances had the ability to reduce the electrical threshold for this self-stimulation intracranial, suggesting that their potential for abuse could be explained by awareness of this reward circuit [15].

Subsequent research (in animals, but also in men) have confirmed the place powerhouse of the mesolimbic dopaminergic system in behavioral motivation and in the positive reinforcement effects of drugs; they also emphasized complexity, and the diversity of the mechanisms involved depending on the type of substance consumed [16]. VTA dopaminergic neurons are an essential part of the reward circuit [17]. Studies in monkeys have allowed to better specify the functional role of these neurons by showing that they emit brief bursts of action potential following the presentation of a reward unexpected or, more precisely, a stimulus conditional associated with the presentation of the reward. This puffing discharge accompanies increased release of dopamine (DA) at the level of nerve endings [18]. Neurons increase their activity during presentation of the conditional stimulus, but they do not, however, modify their activity during presentation of the announced award. On the other hand, if the announced reward by the stimulus is not presented, the activity electrical power is reduced. The activity of dopaminergic neurons in VTA is therefore linked to the error reward prediction;

they signal changes (positive or negative) in the prediction of future rewards [19]. More recently, extensive studies of VTA demonstrated the existence of subpopulations neurons distinguished by their position within the VTA, their nerve connections, their electrophysiological properties, and their functional role [20]. These studies confirm that dopaminergic neurons innervating the nucleus accumbens (lateral shell) are mainly involved in reporting a reward while dopaminergic neurons innervating the prefrontal cortex are mainly activated by aversive stimuli.

Studies indicate the existence of circuits distinct capable of generating reinforcement positive and negative reinforcement, allowing to attribute to dopaminergic neurons a very broad role in controlling motivation behavioral and, more broadly of an individual's response to «Salient» events (that is to say significant for him by relation to his experience) [17]. In addition to innervation by dopaminergic neurons in VTA, the nucleus accumbens receives information from the prefrontal cortex, amygdala, and hippocampus, regions that are part of the limbic system involved in emotions. The neurons of the nucleus accumbens (essentially GABAergic in nature) send projections toward the substantia nigra and the ventral pallidum, itself in connection with the thalamus, the prefrontal cortex, and the dorsal striatum, regions involved in the grip decision regarding the choice of actions to initiate and perform [21]. The nucleus accumbens therefore occupies a strategic position in the brain to convert emotional signals in motivated actions. The action of certain drugs on other connected brain regions to the VTA pathway—nucleus accumbens can also intervene in their reinforcing positive effects [22]. As mentioned earlier, different drugs exist, with distinct pharmacological targets. Thus, cocaine is a monoamine reuptake inhibitor (DA, noradrenaline and serotonin) and prolongs, therefore, the lifespan of these neurotransmitters in the synaptic cleft; amphetamines stimulate the release of monoamines by preventing their vesicular storage and reversing their transport at the presynaptic level; opiates are receptor agonists mu; alcohol is (in particular) (a positive allosteric GABA A receptor modulator) and tetrahydrocannabinol (THC) a partial agonist of cannabinoid receptor.

By Which Mechanisms These Different Drugs Stimulate the Reward Circuit?

By their effect direct on the DA reuptake or on its release, psychostimulants, such as cocaine or amphetamines, directly stimulate dopaminergic transmission in the nucleus accumbens and exert strong positive reinforcement in animals [23]. The latter easily learns to self-administer these psychostimulants in the nucleus accumbens, but a lesion of the mesolimbic system removes this self-administration. On the other hand, other drugs such as opiates, alcohol, or cannabis have no effect direct on dopaminergic transmission, but disinhibit VTA dopaminergic neurons by inhibition of GABAergic inter-neurons present in this region. This disinhibition is also accompanied by an increase in DA release in the nucleus accumbens and a positive reinforcing effect [24]. The animal is self-administered these drugs when the cannula is implanted at the level of the VTA (and not at the level of nucleus accumbens).

The new behavioral repertoire is then dominated by a progressive loss of control, consumption becoming frequent with an inability to limit it [25]. It is associated with obsessive thoughts about the product, a search and compulsive consumption with an urgent need (craving) to reproduce the initial pleasant sensation but above all to alleviate a discomfort, the need to increase the doses to regain the initial effect, and the continuation of this consumption whatever the consequences under penalty of psychological or even physical suffering. These changes persist even after a long break, are the cause of frequent relapses and involve processes of memory disturbance.

Cellular Adaptations and Molecules Induced by Repeated Drug Administration

Repeated administration of drugs results in cellular and molecular changes in within the reward circuit, but also in various regions of the brain, associated or not to this circuit [26].

Reward Channel Adjustments

Under normal physiological conditions, the reward circuit provides motivation necessary for carrying out actions or behaviors adapted to survival, such as foraging, reproduction, and social contact. Stimulation by drug addiction substances is clearly more intense and longer lasting than stimulation induced by natural rewards, which will result in focusing attention and motivation over drugs to the detriment of natural stimuli [12]. With the repetition of consumption, this abnormally intense activation and sustainable can generate, in individuals likely or in special circumstances, lasting synaptic changes within the reward circuit and regions associated and lead to psychological and behavioral changes leading to addiction [27]. We can say that drugs usurp the reward circuit and divert from its normal physiological role. Numerous studies have been carried out in animals and humans to try to better understand neurobiological changes caused by chronic use of drugs. These studies were carried out with various substances and experimental procedures varied, and the results obtained have allowed a better understanding of the process of addiction, even if these results are not always consistent [28].

Since addictive substances have the common property of stimulating the reward circuit during their acute administration, it is not surprising that they induce common changes within this circuit during their repeated administration, although some differences exist depending on the type of drug [29]. Generally, the brain responds homeostatically at chronic exposure to drugs by a compensatory decrease in functioning the dopaminergic system; this is the tolerance phenomenon. Brain DA levels are reduced and the response to natural rewards is reduced [30]. This could explain negative emotional sensations experienced between periods of consumption of drugs and abstinence. But at the same time, chronic drug exposure awareness leads to dopaminergic systems manifested by a greater increase in the dopaminergic transmission when the drug is consumed [31]. A psychological important change is motivational awareness or hypersensitivity to motivational effects drugs and stimuli associated with their consumption. The usual goals of life are neglected, and behavior is oriented more and more exclusively toward the search for drug and its consumption. The phenomenon of behavioral awareness can be studied in animals, in particular at the locomotor level, even if the degree relevance of this model is discussed. It is about in fact a phenomenon of inverse tolerance, which manifests itself as an increase in drug effects on repeated intermittent exposure [32]. The intensity of awareness is influenced by different factors such as dose, method of administration, interval between jurisdictions, gender, and genetics. This awareness can last a long time, up to several months after taking the drug. The environment plays a major role in the expression of awareness behavioral, and this could explain the high risk of relapse in the presence of stimuli previously associated with consumption drug [33].

The sensitization phenomenon has been described for drugs as diverse as cocaine, morphine, ethanol, nicotine, or THC and cross-sensitization is also described, which suggests the existence of common mechanisms [34]. Generally speaking, the awareness process involves an increasing dopaminergic transmission within the meso-cortico-limbic system. Changes in dopaminergic receptor sensitivity have been demonstrated: decreased sensitivity of D2 auto receptors and increased D1 receptor sensitivity at the level of the nucleus accumbens [35]. On the other hand, the dopaminergic neurons of VTA have increased expression of AMPA receptors with increased permeability to Ca2+. It gives them increased sensitivity to glutamate and would explain the phenomenon of LTP ("Long Term Potentiation," or potentiation duration of the excitatory transmission) observed in VTA with various drugs [36]. "Long Term Potentiation," or potentiation duration of the excitatory transmission is observed in VTA with various drugs. Increased expression of CREB has also been reported. This protein that fixes cAMP is a regulatory transcription factor expression of different genes [37]. Common biochemical modifications have been also observed at the level of the nucleus accumbens, as the induction of the transcription factor ΔFosB and increased cAMP. The fact than the different addictive substances lead to common adaptations within of the reward circuit opens up new interesting perspectives for the development of new addiction treatments [26].

If all drugs cause common modifications within the reward circuit, it is no less true that they have also specific effects that distinguish them from each other and are linked to their action on distinct pharmacological targets [38]. These specificities are marked in the effects (sought or not) of drugs on the body. So, opiates have pain relieving effects related to stimulation of mu receptors located at routes of pain transmission [39]. Cocaine stimulates the cardiovascular system by blocking the reuptake of catecholamines at the level of the ortho-sympathetic system. Psychedelics interfere striato-thalamic pathways serving to filter sensory impulses arriving at the cortex [40]. Specificities also exist in modifications of neurobiological training caused by chronic administration of different types of drugs: decreased sensitivity of mu receptors for opiates, decreased sensitivity GABAA receptors for alcohol, modifications nicotinic receptor density for tobacco. And specific effects are also described at the circuit level of reward. Thus, chronic administration psychostimulants such as cocaine, amphetamines, and nicotine increase the number of dendrites and the density of synaptic buttons within the nucleus accumbens and the prefrontal cortex. Then, that chronic administration of opiates has a reverse effect [41]. The reasons and implications of these differences remain unclear.

Adaptations at the Level of Cortical Regions and the Hippocampus

Animal brain imaging studies and in humans indicate that the administration chronic drugs also lead to complex changes within regions frontal cortices. Cortical hypo-frontality has been highlighted, characterized by a decrease in basal activity at the level prefrontal, anterior cingulate regions and orbitofrontal, which control the functions executive, working memory, attention, and behavioral inhibition via their projections glutamatergic to VTA and nucleus accumbens [42]. The modifications caused by chronic drug administration could be involved in impulsiveness and compulsion to consume, which characterizes addictive behavior. The decrease in the activity of pyramidal cells in the cortex is accompanied by a decrease in sensitivity to natural rewards. On the other hand, these cells are hypersensitive to the activating action of drugs and stimuli associated with their consumption [25]. A maturation incomplete circuits involved in behavioral motivation and circuits involved in the control of executive functions could explain the particular vulnerability of adolescents developing an addiction [43]. The meso-accumbens system and the meso-cortical are not the only ones affected by taking drugs. The research carried out over the past 10 years on rodents showed another effect common to different addictive substances [44]. These have, in fact, the property common to reduce neurogenesis at the level of the serrated gyrus of the hippocampus during their chronic administration. A reduction in hippocampal neurogenesis could contribute cognitive problems observed in many drug addicts. A reduction of hippocampal neurogenesis is also observed in animal models of various mental illnesses. Given the close link between mental illnesses and drug addiction, some authors have proposed a neurogenic model dual diagnosis [45, 46].

Link Between Stress and Addiction

Numerous studies have shown a close link between stress and addiction. This link should be considered in both directions: the influence of stress on the consumption of drug and vice versa, the influence of drugs on the regions of the brain involved in stress reactions [10]. Stress exerts an important role on drug use. In humans and animals, stress facilitates initiation of drug use and maintaining that consumption. It is at note that the increased transmission excitatory at the level of the VTA, reported during administration of different drugs, is also induced by stress and that the stress also reduces hippocampal neurogenesis [47]. Stress is also a factor significant risk of relapse. The influence of stress on the consumption of drug is accepted and vice versa, the influence of drugs on the regions of the brain involved in stress reactions is also postulated. On the other hand, acute and chronic administration of various drugs modulate activity in a variable way the hypothalamic-pituitary-adrenal axis, leading to changes in secretion of CRF (corticotrophin releasing factor), ACTH (corticotropin), and cortisol [48]. Commonly, however, weaning brutal of virtually all drugs comes with activation of CRF neurons of the amygdala. The amygdala is a region of the limbic system involved in fear and anxiety and its activation could explain, partly, negative emotional symptoms experienced by drug addicts in withdrawal [49]. Besides CRF, other neurotransmitters involved in stress are also activated during weaning. The activation of noradrenergic systems is particularly well documented in the case of withdrawal from opiates and the alcohol. Pharmacological manipulations of these systems (by clonidine, in particular) have the ability to reduce some of the withdrawal signs observed in alcoholics and heroin addicts in withdrawal [50].

Signs of Withdrawal, "Craving" and Relapse

Psychic and physical signs of withdrawal play an important role in relapse. We speak of secondary dependence when the drug use becomes necessary to avoid feeling the signs of withdrawal [51]. The third stage of the addiction cycle mentioned at the beginning of this chapter, namely the stage of "craving" is a key element of relapse which makes addiction a mental illness recurring. This notion of "craving" is difficult to define; it corresponds to an irresistible desire to use the drug again after a period of abstinence of varying length, which may be several months or years old. Understanding the mechanisms involved in this phenomenon is a challenge for the development of therapies effective [51]. Animal models indicate that post-withdrawal drug testing may be induced in different ways: by a new drug administration, by a stressful stimulus, but also by exposure to previously matched neutral stimuli with the drug administration ("clues contextual") [10]. These observations emphasize on the preponderant influence of factors environmental (consumption context) which, when combined repeatedly drug use, acquire the value of conditional stimuli, evoking the availability of the drug and the memory of its euphoric effects. Animal studies and human imaging studies have found highlight the involvement of cortical regions and limbic in this associative learning as well as in "craving" and relapse [52].

Factors Influencing the Development of an Addiction

Although many people consume potentially addictive substances, most of them do not become drug addicts. Many factors influence the probability of a first drug use, the evolution toward a problematic use, then the evolution toward addiction cycle. These factors depend on the consumer himself (age, sex, mental health diseases), the nature of the drug (type of substance, mode of consumption, quantity consumed) and the environment (role of peers, drug availability, social support and family, economic status). Genetics factors also play a role in the development of the addiction cycle and twin studies have made it possible to evidence the role of different genes involved in drug metabolism, in the function of particular receivers or in the stress response [53].

Conclusion

In short, addiction implies a succession of neuroadaptations leading to a reprogramming of neural circuits involved in pleasure and motivation, memory, conditioning, executive functions, judgment, self-control, and reaction to stress. These neuroadaptations lead to complex changes in psychological and behavioral functions. Genetic, developmental, and environmental factors influence the course and the severity of the process.

To explain this gradual installation of addiction, four major complementary mechanisms, which unfold and reinforce each other, are necessary:

- Motivational awareness: the salience of the reward (gradual increase in motivation to consume).
- Learning habits: automatic behavior unrelated to a desired effect but which goes into stimulus-response mode.
- Hedonic allostasis: negative emotional state linked to a deficit in the activation of the reward circuit, with an increase in the threshold.
- Inhibitory control deficit (impairment of executive functions): loss of “reasonable” intellectual control, performed by the prefrontal cortex.

In the addicted subject, there is an overvaluation of the object of desire. Its value “rewarding” the memory of it leads to a major motivation: simple desire has become need. The cortical control, reasonable, is too limited to take into account the context and the consequences.

These four major complementary mechanisms are based on four circuits that interact and are interconnected:

- The reward circuit.
- The motivation circuit: salience.
- The pathways of memory and conditional habits.
- Control by the prefrontal, intellectual and executive cortex.

To which are added, as the dependency sets in:

- The perception of internal states analyzing the need and which goes as far as craving (compulsive need to consume): insula.
- The avoidance and anxiety circuit: habenula and amygdala.

In a normal situation, the balance between these four circuits results in actions adapted to our emotional situation or need. The reward circuit gives the value of a need, of which motivation gives the value of a need and responds to internal states, that of memory brings into play learned associations and that of control enables conflicts to be resolved [54]. In the normal subject, the decision to take an action toward a desired goal takes into account the importance of the motivation for this object, depending on its reward value, itself linked to the memory of the pleasure that it previously brought about [55]. But ultimately, it is the cortical, prefrontal control that will assess, depending on the context and the anticipated and memorized desire, whether to act or to defer action.

In the event of addiction, there is a reinforcement of the value of the product, both by the overvaluation of the need (salience) as in the motivation to obtain it, and by the invasion of memory circuits with disconnection from the less partial of the inhibitory control circuit exerted at the level of the prefrontal cortex by cortical associations. This makes it possible to better understand the psycho-behavioral attitudes of dependent subjects: the brain becomes hypersensitized to the drug and to the environmental stimuli associated with it, gives much less importance to other interests, objectives, and motivations that have become secondary to the obsessive need of the drug.

The information sent by the whole brain, major value of the reward (nucleus accumbens), major salience and therefore major motivation (cingulate cortex and orbitofrontal cortex), exacerbated memory of pleasure (hippocampus) to which craving is added (insula), have become imperative, corresponding to a need perceived as necessary, absolute, and vital [56].

The whole brain is now programmed to recognize this need as essential. The “reasonable” control can no longer be exercised, to counterbalance this information of major need requiring immediate action of the prefrontal cortex to satisfy it.

References

1. Angres DH, Bettinardi-Angres K. The disease of addiction: origins, treatment, and recovery. Dis Mon. 2008;54:696–721.
2. Grant JE, Potenza MN, Weinstein A, Gorelick DA. Introduction to behavioral addictions. Am J Drug Alcohol Abuse. 2010;36:233–41.
3. Heather N. Is the concept of compulsion useful in the explanation or description of addictive behaviour and experience? Addict Behav Rep. 2017;6:15–38.
4. Satel S, Lilienfeld SO. Addiction and the brain-disease fallacy. Front Psychol. 2014;4:141.
5. Bechara A, Berridge KC, Bickel WK, Morón JA, Williams SB, Stein JS. A neurobehavioral approach to addiction: implications for the opioid epidemic and the psychology of addiction. Psychol Sci Public Interest. 2019;20:96–127.
6. Stoops WW. Reinforcing effects of stimulants in humans: sensitivity of progressive-ratio schedules. Exp Clin Psychopharmacol. 2008;16:503–12.
7. Hyman SE. Addiction: a disease of learning and memory. Am J Psychiatry. 2005;162:1414–22.
8. Clay SW, Allen J, Parran T. A review of addiction. Postgrad Med. 2008;120:E01-7.
9. Piazza PV, Deroche-Gamonet V. A multistep general theory of transition to addiction. Psychopharmacology. 2013;229:387–413.
10. Sinha R. Chronic stress, drug use, and vulnerability to addiction. Ann N Y Acad Sci. 2008;1141:105–30.
11. Volkow ND, Koob GF, McLellan AT. Neurobiologic advances from the brain disease model of addiction. N Engl J Med. 2016;374:363–71.
12. Volkow ND, Michaelides M, Baler R. The neuroscience of drug reward and addiction. Physiol Rev. 2019;99:2115–40.
13. Koob GF, Volkow ND. Neurobiology of addiction: a neurocircuitry analysis. Lancet Psychiatry. 2016;3:760–73.
14. Olds J, Milner P. Positive reinforcement produced by electrical stimulation of septal area and other regions of rat brain. J Comp Physiol Psychol. 1954;47:419–27.
15. Koob G, Le Moal M. Drug addiction, dysregulation of reward, and allostasis. Neuropsychopharmacology. 2001;24:97–129.
16. Lynch WJ, Nicholson KL, Dance ME, Morgan RW, Foley PL. Animal models of substance abuse and addiction: implications for science, animal welfare, and society. Comp Med. 2010;60:177–88.
17. Bromberg-Martin ES, Matsumoto M, Hikosaka O. Dopamine in motivational control: rewarding, aversive, and alerting. Neuron. 2010;68:815–34.
18. Schultz W, Dayan P, Montague PR. A neural substrate of prediction and reward. Science. 1997;275:1593–9.
19. Schultz W. Dopamine reward prediction error coding. Dialogues Clin Neurosci. 2016;18:23–32.
20. Beier KT, Steinberg EE, DeLoach KE, et al. Circuit architecture of VTA dopamine neurons revealed by systematic input-output mapping. Cell. 2015;162:622–34.
21. Root DH, Melendez RI, Zaborszky L, Napier TC. The ventral pallidum: subregion-specific functional anatomy and roles in motivated behaviors. Prog Neurobiol. 2015;130:29–70.
22. Feltenstein MW, See RE. The neurocircuitry of addiction: an overview. Br J Pharmacol. 2008;154:261–74.
23. Dela Peña I, Gevorkiana R, Shi WX. Psychostimulants affect dopamine transmission through both dopamine transporter-dependent and independent mechanisms. Eur J Pharmacol. 2015;764:562–70.
24. Szabo B, Siemes S, Wallmichrath I. Inhibition of GABAergic neurotransmission in the ventral tegmental area by cannabinoids. Eur J Neurosci. 2002;15:2057–61.
25. Crews FT, Boettiger CA. Impulsivity, frontal lobes and risk for addiction. Pharmacol Biochem Behav. 2009;93:237–47.
26. Adinoff B. Neurobiologic processes in drug reward and addiction. Harv Rev Psychiatry. 2004;12:305–20.
27. Alcaro A, Huber R, Panksepp J. Behavioral functions of the mesolimbic dopaminergic system: an affective neuroethological perspective. Brain Res Rev. 2007;56:283–321.
28. Akhtar A. The flaws and human harms of animal experimentation. Camb Q Healthc Ethics. 2015;24:407–19.
29. Niehaus JL, Cruz-Bermudez ND, Kauer JA. Plasticity of addiction: a mesolimbic dopamine short-circuit? Am J Addict. 2009;18:259–71.
30. Peper A. A theory of drug tolerance and dependence I: a conceptual analysis. J Theor Biol. 2004;21(229):477–90.
31. Trifilieff P, Martinez D. Imaging addiction: D2 receptors and dopamine signaling in the striatum as biomarkers for impulsivity. Neuropharmacology. 2014;76(Pt B):498–509.
32. Robinson TE, Berridge KC. Incentive-sensitization and addiction. Addiction. 2001;96:103–14.
33. Tulchinsky TH, Varavikova EA. Measuring, monitoring, and evaluating the health of a population. New Public Health. 2014;2014:91–147.
34. Cadoni C, Pisanu A, Solinas M, Acquas E, Di Chiara G. Behavioural sensitization after repeated exposure to Delta 9-tetrahydrocannabinol and cross-sensitization with morphine. Psychopharmacology. 2001;158:259–66.
35. Palmiter RD. Dopamine signaling as a neural correlate of consciousness. Neuroscience. 2011;15(198):213–20.
36. Lüscher C, Malenka RC. NMDA receptor-dependent long-term potentiation and long-term depression (LTP/LTD). Cold Spring Harb Perspect Biol. 2012;4(6):a005710.
37. Robichaux WG 3rd, Cheng X. Intracellular cAMP sensor EPAC: physiology, pathophysiology, and therapeutics development. Physiol Rev. 2018;98(2):919–1053.

38. Gardner EL. Addiction and brain reward and antireward pathways. Adv Psychosom Med. 2011;30:22–60.
39. Al-Hasani R, Bruchas MR. Molecular mechanisms of opioid receptor-dependent signaling and behavior. Anesthesiology. 2011;115:1363–81.
40. Vongpatanasin W, Mansour Y, Chavoshan B, Arbique D, Victor RG. Cocaine stimulates the human cardiovascular system via a central mechanism of action. Circulation. 1999;100:497–502.
41. Russo SJ, Dietz DM, Dumitriu D, Morrison JH, Malenka RC, Nestler EJ. The addicted synapse: mechanisms of synaptic and structural plasticity in nucleus accumbens. Trends Neurosci. 2010;33:267–76.
42. Goldstein RZ, Volkow ND. Dysfunction of the prefrontal cortex in addiction: neuroimaging findings and clinical implications. Nat Rev Neurosci. 2011;12:652–69.
43. Kim-Spoon J, Kahn RE, Lauharatanahirun N, Deater-Deckard K, Bickel WK, Chiu PH, King-Casas B. Executive functioning and substance use in adolescence: neurobiological and behavioral perspectives. Neuropsychologia. 2017;100:79–92.
44. Diana M. The dopamine hypothesis of drug addiction and its potential therapeutic value. Front Psychol. 2011;2:64.
45. Kang E, Wen Z, Song H, Christian KM, Ming GL. Adult neurogenesis and psychiatric disorders. Cold Spring Harb Perspect Biol. 2016;8(9): a019026.
46. Bourin M. Neurogenesis and neuroplasticity in major depression: its therapeutic implication. In: Kim YK, editor. Major depressive disorder. Springer Singapore; 2021. p. 157–73.
47. Kuhn BN, Kalivas PW, Bobadilla AC. Understanding addiction using animal models. Front Behav Neurosci. 2019;13:262.
48. Torres-Berrio A, Cuesta S, Lopez-Guzman S, Nava-Mesa MO. Interaction between stress and addiction: contributions from Latin-American neuroscience. Front Psychol. 2018;21(9):2639.
49. Zorrilla EP, Logrip ML, Koob GF. Corticotropin releasing factor: a key role in the neurobiology of addiction. Front Neuroendocrinol. 2014;35:234–44.
50. Becker HC. Effects of alcohol dependence and withdrawal on stress responsiveness and alcohol consumption. Alcohol Res. 2012;34:448–58.
51. Becker HC. Alcohol dependence, withdrawal, and relapse. Alcohol Res Health. 2008;31:348–361; Wolf ME. Synaptic mechanisms underlying persistent cocaine craving. Nat Rev Neurosci. 2016;17:351–365.
52. Martin-Fardon R, Weiss F. Modeling relapse in animals. Curr Top Behav Neurosci. 2013;13:403–32.
53. Bourin M, Chagraoui A. Abuse and misuse. In: Emilien G, Weikunat R, Lüdicke F, editors. Consumer perception of product risks and benefits. Springer; 2017. p. 429–53.
54. Rybnicek R, Bergner S, Gutschelhofer A. What individual needs influence motivation effects: a neuroscientific study on McClelland's need theory. Rev Manag Sci. 2019;13:443–82.
55. Kim SI. Neuroscientific model of motivational process. Front Psychol. 2013;4:98.
56. Haber SN, Tang W, Choi EY, Yendiki A, Liu H, Jbabdi S, Versace A, Phillips M. Circuits, networks, and neuropsychiatric disease: transitioning from anatomy to imaging. Biol Psychiatry. 2020;15(87):318–27.

What Can We Expect from the Evaluation Drug Addiction in Animals?

15

Michel Bourin

Introduction

The study of the causes and neurobiological mechanisms of addiction requires the use of animal models. This use of animals can be justified for several reasons. First, ethics prohibit the use of invasive neurobiological approaches in humans. Second, there are no alternative mathematical or in silico models of addiction yet. Finally, unlike physical dependence, addiction is a behavioral disorder and, as such, cannot be summarized on lineages, human or animal cells, or any other in vitro, cellular, or subcellular model [1]. The research on animal models therefore represents a kind of "reverse medicine." Unlike the clinician, whose goal is to help people with addiction to avoid it, the experimenter seeks to reproduce certain aspects of the addiction in laboratory animals considered, a priori, to be healthy [2]. Since the very first systematic experimental studies in animals in the 1950s, animal models of addiction have evolved significantly, in close association with the very conceptions of addiction [3]. To simplify, we can distinguish three major periods in experimental research on animal models of addiction, each involving researchers from different backgrounds (pharmacologists, psychologists, neurobiologists, and psychiatrists) and referring to particular conceptions of the phenomenon [4]. These three periods are preceded by a prescientific period, before 1950, during which no systematic attempt is made to model addiction in animals, while animal experiments in physiology and psychology are in full swing [5].

In recent years, increasing attention has been brought to risks as well as the possibility of chronic addiction and abuse substances acting at the central level, such as hypnotics, barbiturates, benzodiazepines, and even other psychotropic drugs such as antidepressants and psychostimulants [6].

Now, it is time to define the protests more clearly of central and peripheral dependency and to understand how substances affect neurobiology and behavior in humans as well as in animals. Of more, the problems of consumption of illicit products such as heroin and its derivatives, cocaine, as well as substances new ones like methamphetamines, the most used being ecstasy, unfortunately remain relevant [7]. Faced with this situation, it is essential to have reliable and reproducible animal models.

Preclinical studies have different goals. They are used to advance our knowledge of neuropharmacological bases of the action of substances and to understand the mechanism and the pathways involved in drug use. The interaction studies allow the evaluation of molecules capable of mitigating or suppressing self-administration of

M. Bourin (✉)
Neurobiology of Anxiety and Mood Disorders, University of Nantes, Nantes, France
e-mail: michel.bourin@univ-nantes.fr

P. Á. Gargiulo, H. L. Mesones-Arroyo (eds.), *Psychiatry and Neuroscience Update – Vol. V*,
https://doi.org/10.1007/978-3-031-72219-6_15

drugs or medicine in animals, which is a big benefit in humans.

The aim of this chapter is to offer the best animal models more relevant to assess dependence and risk of withdrawal from legal and not legal psychotropic substances.

Self-Administration

The objective of self-administration studies is essentially to highlight the addictive potential of a given substance and to study its effects on behavior [8]. The procedure is requested to early evaluate an addictive potential, that is an important step during the development of new molecules before evaluating their therapeutic properties.

In addition, the protocol can be used for different classes of products and statistically validated [9].

In self-administration studies, the products are used as positive reinforcement in order to maintain a drug-seeking behavior. Usually, self-administration procedures use operant conditioning models. In these conditioning studies, the animals are placed in experimental cages soundproofed and ventilated (Skinner boxes) [10]. A feeder is accessible on one of the walls of the cage where the animal can get food in the form of pellets easily accountable. The animals have a lever on which they must press to receive the food. This food is considered positive reinforcement. Furthermore, each cage has lights that can be used independently (discriminative stimulus). A sound device can also be usable [11]. In self-administration studies, the products are used as pharmacological reinforcement positive instead of food. Rapid development of physical dependence is then observed. The animals can get the drug in different ways: in most experiments, drugs are obtained from using chronically implanted catheters during a brief surgical anesthesia; noninvasive methods with oral administration can be used. In monkey, a procedure involving intramuscular administration has been used, implying greater ease and allowing chronic administration over a long period; however, the effects are weaker than those of an intravenous administration. There are inhalation techniques [12] allowing the study of volatile drugs (tetrahydrocannabinol and nicotine).

Two procedures allow the study of the location of the reward mechanism induced by a drug. One is intracranial self-administration [13], and the other is the conditioned place preference procedure, which we will detail later. Intracranial microinjections locate the brain systems involved, on the other hand, peripheral administration allows the study of a wide range of drugs, but not the location of the site of action.

The experimental problem remains the injection of small volume without alter neighboring structures. A microinfusion model electrolyte was set up [14].

There is a good correspondence between drugs that maintain self-administration in laboratory animals and those that are used in humans for addiction purposes [15]. Animals used for these studies include monkeys (rhesus monkey or baboon) and rats [16], are trained to press a lever with their muzzle. Rats and mice are the most interesting, because they have a lower cost, allowing the use of naive animals for the drug studied and the use of a single protocol and correct statistical analysis. Compared to rodents, monkeys present many problems including those of maintenance. The implementation of this procedure is not feasible in mice. This test is sensitive to psychostimulants such as amphetamine and cocaine, to opiates such as morphine and heroin, phencyclidine, barbiturates, benzodiazepines, ethanol, nicotine, and some volatile solvents. There are exceptions for cannabis, which gives equivocal results, and LSD, which gives negative results. In the majority of cases, no false positives were found. Substances studied may, however, be effective in some circumstances and not others, depending on the dose used, the history of the animal, and the conditions of access to drug. Cocaine is often used as a standard substance comparison in these studies [8]. In conclusion, it is specially to assess a physical dependence more than an psychic addiction. It is important to be vigilant about the amount of food administered to the animal during the experiment, which

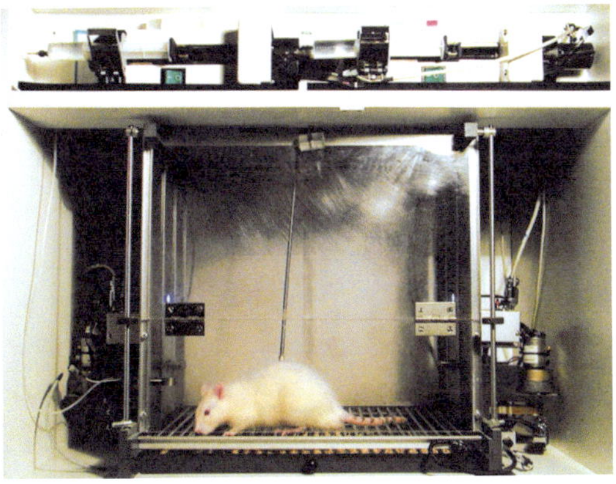

Fig. 15.1 Packaging cage for self-administration intravenous experiments. This cage is equipped with a motorized lever, a syringe pump, and an injection tube. The animal can receive a dose intravenous drug in voluntarily operating a lever

largely conditions the response. It is thus possible to artificially increase the "dependence" potential by reducing the amount of food made available to animals [17] (Fig. 15.1).

Discrimination

The purpose of discrimination studies is to assess psychic addictions of a substance. Maintaining the behavioral sensation induced by the product also makes it possible to determine whether a product belongs to a class or to study the effect of different doses [18]. The fact that substances induce discriminating control behavior is a phenomenon of practical and theoretical interest [19]. Procedures' operant conditioning is also used in discrimination studies (see previous paragraph), but two levers are then necessary. In most studies of this type, an animal is trained, reinforcing a response linked to the injection of a substance, to produce another response following the injection of another solution [20]. Other products are then injected to determine if they also may cause response controlled by the training drug. This is called generalization [21].

In conditioning studies, this is generally a light or sound that is used as discriminative stimuli or as signals controlling behavior [22]. In discrimination studies, the effects of substances are used as discriminative stimuli indicating how many reinforcements (number of pellets) can be obtained. The animals are trained to press a lever to obtain food after administration of a potentially addictive and to press a second lever in the presence of sodium chloride solution (placebo). When discrimination is assimilated, the animals press the lever appropriate depending on whether they received the training substance or saline solution. Accuracy is excellent in most experiments (90% or more of satisfactory answers). Studies using opioid substances as a trainer revealed molecular specificity, even a stereospecificity, excellent. The majority of substances possessing addictive properties such as psychostimulants, benzodiazepines, and LSD also have discriminative effects.

These effects are important in addiction. Indeed, one of the reasons that humans abuse drugs is the need to obtain characteristic subjective effects of the substance used. For example, substances which produce the same discriminative effects as morphine in animals are also those which produce in humans, morphine-like effects. The discrimination procedure therefore seems to offer experimental access to subjective experience, to perception or the stimuli produced by drugs, and thus provide an overview of the psychophysiology of subjective perception [23].

Withdrawal

Withdrawal helps to unmask physical dependence, reflecting thus an adaptive process of the administration of substances studied [24]. There are two main types of withdrawal:

- "Spontaneous withdrawal": if a phenomenon of dependence is induced by chronic administration of a product for a more or less time, then the administration is abruptly stopped. The time of onset of the first signs of withdrawal, their intensity, and duration are then noted.
- "Precipitated withdrawal": this is about the induction of withdrawal by administration of an antagonist of receptors occupied by the substance. After chronic administration of a

substance, its antagonist is administered to the animal, thus precipitating its withdrawal, for example, administration of naloxone for opioid withdrawal, or administration of flumazenil for benzodiazepines [25, 26].

The signs of withdrawal are then assessed based on behavioral grids. Signs of benzodiazepine withdrawal are generally divided into three criteria:

- motor effects (tremors, convulsive movements, reduction spontaneous motor activity, tail erection, posture arched back),
- autonomic nervous system (piloerection, diarrhea, white ears),
- behavior (anxiety, aggressiveness, increased startle to an auditory or tactile stimulus).

These withdrawal symptoms have been well studied in animals and humans; they are common on abrupt cessation with some minor variants [27].

For opioids, it is possible in rats to quantify compulsive jumping, shaking of the paws, grooming, into burying, twisting behaviors and diarrhea [28].

Substitution During Withdrawal or Cross-Dependence

These studies are based on the hypothesis that a substance capable of to suppress the withdrawal syndrome when stopping another substance is likely to produce the same type of addiction. Some techniques used should be compared to those of "self-administration" studies [29]. The animals are placed in soundproofed experimental compartments (see section "Self-administration") and have a lever. They are trained according to a specific strengthening program and self-administered the benchmark drug. In other techniques, the animals passively receive the substance. In these cases, signs of withdrawal are analyzed after substitution [30]. This principle of cross-dependency is used either for substitutions of doses for the same molecule or for substitutions of different substances. There may be partial substitutions in which the substitute substance only partially eliminates the withdrawal syndrome of the other molecules.

Conditioned Place Preference

In conditioned place preference studies, an environment distinctive is repeatedly linked to the administration of a substance, and another environment is connected with failure to take the product [31]. Traditionally, the device consisting in a box is divided into two separate compartments. A guillotine separates the two compartments. A guillotine separates the two compartments, in each of them it is possible to record the time spent and to detect the movements of the animal.

This system can be connected to a computer. A recording video can also be set up. The boxes are then placed in a soundproof system and under a weak white light [32]. The rat is the animal of choice, but study in mice is also possible. Typically, environments differ by visual signals (illumination, light or dark walls, painted in black and white, vertical lines or horizontal) and tactile signals (soil texture: soft or rough) and sometimes by the smell. After training by confinement in the compartment allocated either to the drug or to placebo, the animals regain free access to both compartments. The usual measurement parameter used is the increase time spent in the compartment associated with the drug. This test has been used successfully with a wide range addictive drugs that also maintain self-administration. There are, however, a few exceptions: phenobarbital and phencyclidine [33]. It is an alternative technique of self-administration procedures. As we had it mentioned in the first paragraph, this technique also allows the study of the location of mechanisms involving reward circuits thanks to the possibility of microinjections at the level of brain structures (see section "Self-administration").

Awakened Animal Microdialysis and Free of Its Movements

This technique allows the study of animal behavior and the quantification of transmitters released in brain regions [34]. Briefly, the technique is broken down as follows: the animal is anesthetized and placed in a stereotaxic apparatus. A guide for the microdialysis cannula is then implanted in the desired region using stereotaxic coordinates. Then, we let the animal recover from the surgery. Five to seven days later, the microdialysis probe is placed and infused with physiological saline. The drug studied is in turn administered by this probe. The dialysates are recovered and analyzed.

Models to Invent

Research on animal models has come a long way over the past 60 years. However, several obstacles remain to be overcome in order to improve its validity. First, we must strengthen the return to the clinic; the subjective symptoms of addiction seem still escape animal models. For example, the desire to limit consumption or to abstain is undoubtedly one of the most important symptoms because without this desire, there is no motivational conflict or attempt at abstinence and therefore compulsion. In fact, there is not yet an animal model of abstinence. Second, laboratory animals generally have access to drugs without any other option. It is therefore difficult, if not impossible, to know whether they use the drug addictively or only because of the lack of other options [35]. Future research on addiction models should introduce, during drug access, other activities that are biologically and/or socially important for the animal being studied. The abandonment of the latter for drugs and the costs it entails in terms of health and well-being would be a particularly valid model of addiction. Finally, most models adhere to a simplistic etiological hypothesis that attributes a central role to prolonged drug exposure, a hypothesis that largely ignores the multifactorial etiology of addictions [36]. Some animal models still have to be invented.

Conclusion

Determining the addictive potential of a substance can be made using animal models. It should however to be careful to avoid false negatives (addictive substances in men who have not revealed their addictive potential in animals), but also false positives.

In either case, the experimental design is important; do not reduce the animal's food too much under penalty of making him more quickly dependent, or on the contrary feed him too well so that he no longer wants to do efforts.

The assessment of marketing authorization files must therefore be careful in regarding psychotropic drugs, and the expert should refer to source files. In case of doubt, a second opinion should be performed by an independent laboratory.

Finally, a single model cannot be retained; it is right to compare the results of the five models proposed here in order to make a preclinical opinion.

References

1. Spanagel R. Animal models of addiction. Dialogues Clin Neurosci. 2017;19:247–58.
2. Lynch WJ, Nicholson KL, Dance ME, Morgan RW, Foley PL. Animal models of substance abuse and addiction: implications for science, animal welfare, and society. Comp Med. 2010;60:177–88.
3. Rogers PJ. Food and drug addictions: similarities and differences. Pharmacol Biochem Behav. 2017;153:182–90.
4. Kuhn BN, Kalivas PW, Bobadilla AC. Understanding addiction using animal models. Front Behav Neurosci. 2019;29(13):262.
5. Acker CJ. Creating the American junkie: addiction research in the classic era of narcotic control. The Johns Hopkins University Press; 2002. 276 p
6. Weaver MF. Prescription sedative misuse and abuse. Yale J Biol Med. 2015;88:247–56.
7. Hegadoren KM, Baker GB, Bourin M. 3,4-methylenedioxy analogues of amphetamine: defining the risk to humans. Neurosci Biobehav Rev. 1999;23:539–53.
8. Jones JD, Comer SD. A review of human drug self-administration procedures. Behav Pharmacol. 2013;24:384–95.
9. Kuzmin A, Johansson B. Expression of c-fos, NGFI-A and secretogranin mRNAin brain regions during initiation of cocaine self-administration in mice. Eur J Neurosci. 1999;11:3694–700.
10. O'Connor EC, Chapman K, Butler P, Mead AN. The predictive validity of the rat self-administration model for abuse liability. Neurosci Biobehav Rev. 2011;35:912–38.
11. Hascoët M, Bourin M. Anticonflict effect of alpidem as compared with the benzodiazepine alprazolam in rats. Pharmacol Biochem Behav. 1997;56:317–24.

12. Woods JH. Behavioral pharmacology of drug self-administration. In: Lipton MA, Mascio A, Killam K, editors. Psychopharmacology: a generation of progress. New York: Raven Press; 1978. p. 595–607.
13. Mc Bride WJ, Murphy JM, Ikemoto S. Localization of brain reinforcement mechanisms: intracranial self-administration and intracranial place-conditioning studies. Behav Brain Res. 1999;101:129–52.
14. Bozarth MA, Wise RA. Electrolytic microinfusion transducer system: an alternative method of intracranial drug application. J Neurosci Methods. 1980;2:273–5.
15. Panlilio LV, Goldberg SR. Self-administration of drugs in animals and humans as a model and an investigative tool. Addiction. 2007;102:1863–70.
16. Phillips KA, Bales KL, Capitanio JP, et al. Why primate models matter. Am J Primatol. 2014;76:801–27.
17. Heather N. Is the concept of compulsion useful in the explanation or description of addictive behaviour and experience? Addict Behav Rep. 2017;6:15–38.
18. Colpaert FC. Drug discrimination in neurobiology. Pharmacol Biochem Behav. 1999;64:337–45.
19. Bertalmio A, Herling S, Hampton RY, Winger G, Woods JH. A procedure for rapid evaluation of the discriminative stimulus of drugs. J Pharmacol Methods. 1982;7:289–99.
20. Bouton ME. Extinction of instrumental (operant) learning: interference, varieties of context, and mechanisms of contextual control. Psychopharmacology. 2019;236:7–19.
21. Young R. In: Buccafusco JJ, editor. Drug discrimination in methods of behavior analysis in neuroscience. 2nd ed. Boca Raton: CRC Press/Taylor & Francis; 2009.
22. Wilson PN, Pearce JM. A role for stimulus generalization in conditional discrimination learning. Q J Exp Psychol. 1989;41B:243–73.
23. Swedberg MD. Drug discrimination: a versatile tool for characterization of CNS safety pharmacology and potential for drug abuse. J Pharmacol Toxicol Methods. 2016;81:295–305.
24. Heilig M, Eglin M, Crabbe JC, Becker HC. Acute withdrawal, protracted abstinence and negative affect in alcoholism: are they linked? Addict Biol. 2010;15:169–84.
25. Bourin M, Malinge M, Colombel MC, Vasar EC. Cholecystokinin receptor agonists block the jumping behaviour precipitated in morphine dependent mice by naloxone. Eur Neuropsychopharmacol. 1999;9:37–43.
26. Martin JR, Moreau JL, Jenck F. Precipitated withdrawal in squirrel monkeys after repeated oral administration of alprazolam, diazepam, flunitrazepam or oxazepam. Psychopharmacology. 1995;118:273–9.
27. Vogel H. Psychotropic and neurotropic activity. In: Vogel HG, editor. Drug discovery and evaluation. Berlin/Heidelberg: Springer; 2007.
28. Pinelli A, Trivulzio S, Ciapponi PM. Quantitative opioid withdrawal signs in rats: effects exerted by clothiapine administration. Fundam Clin Pharmacol. 1997;11(4):346–55.
29. Lambs RJ, Griffiths RR. Behavioral effects of pentobarbital, lorazepam, ethanol and chlorpromazine substitution in pentobarbital-dependent baboons. J Pharmacol Exp Ther. 1993;265:47–52.
30. Tagashira E, Tomoko U, Hinamori T, Yanaura S. Cross physical dependence liability of psychotropic drugs in rats dependent on barbiturates. Jpn J Pharmacol. 1983;33:659–69.
31. Su ZI, Santoostaroam A, Wenzel J, Ettenberg A. On the persistence of cocaine-induced place preferences and aversions in rats. Psychopharmacology. 2013;229:115–23.
32. Steinpreis RE, Aaron LR, Parrett FA. Methadone produces conditioned place-preference in the rat. Pharmacol Biochem Behav. 1996;54:339–41.
33. Myers KM, Bechtholt-Gompf AJ, Coleman BR, Carlezon WA Jr. Extinction of conditioned opiate withdrawal in rats in a two-chambered place conditioning apparatus. Nat Protoc. 2012;7:517–26.
34. Ipponi A, Lamberti C, Medica A, Bartolini A, Malmberg-Aiello P. Tiagabine antinociception in rodents depends on GABAB receptor activation: parallel antinociception testing and medial thalamus GABA microdialysis. Eur J Pharmacol. 1999;368:205–11.
35. Ahmed SH. The science of making drug-addicted animals. Neuroscience. 2012;211:107–25.
36. Kendler KS. Levels of explanation in psychiatric and substance use disorders: implications for the development of an etiologically based nosology. Mol Psychiatry. 2012;17:11–21.

16 Pharmacological Basis of Cocaine Addiction

Michel Bourin

Introduction

Cocaine comes in the form of a white powder or crystals extracted from the leaves of a plant in South America: coca (*Erythroxylum coca*) [1]. It was the Conquerors ("*Conquistadores*") who brought it back to Europe. It was initially used as an anesthetic at the beginning of the twentieth century [2]. It was driven by a researcher's faith that Freud was led to explore the effects of cocaine, as soon as it was discovered and isolated from the coca leaf [3]. Young Freud's enthusiasm for research began with the use of cocaine on his own person, which was a common practice in medicine then, to test the properties of a new drug. The effects of the drug were especially made to please Freud; he, who complained of his headaches and neurasthenia, found it a sovereign remedy. Freud used cocaine on and for himself, but also in order to make a name for himself in the scientific community and find a means of symbolic recognition. His study of the properties of cocaine began in April 1884, and he used it for 12 years. He was enthusiastic about cocaine (which is not yet considered a party drug) and supported its use in the treatment of neurasthenia, as an energizer and as an anesthetic. For his part, he made creative and worldly use of it, announcing practices that our society is familiar with [4].

Cocaine base, which circulates under the name "crack" or "free base," is a derivative of cocaine hydrochloride, resulting from the addition of bicarbonate or ammonia. This transformation allows the powder to crystallize into small pebbles, intended to be smoked and more rarely injected. The effects of the cocaine base are much more powerful than those of the hydrochloride. Their onset is faster (1–2 min against 15–30 min), but their duration is much shorter (10–15 min against about an hour), which leads users to a multiplication of the catches. Classified among the stimulants, it is consumed most often by the nasal route (sniff), sometimes pulmonary (inhalation of smoke or vapors by oral or nasal route), or intravenous (injection). Its consumption leads to a feeling of intellectual and physical power, causing indifference to fatigue, coupled with a feeling of euphoria. These positive effects are followed by a "descent" phase, marked by symptoms of the depressive type, anxiety, and strong irritability.

The coca cultivation, which probably occupies nearly 200,000 hectares in Latin America, would produce around 300,000 tons of coca annually, enough to make about 1000 tons of cocaine. Global cocaine production reached a new all-time high with nearly 2000 tons in 2017, while that of opium is in unprecedented decline, according to report of the United Nations Office

M. Bourin (✉)
Neurobiologie de l'anxiété et de la dépression, Université de Nantes, Nantes, France
e-mail: michel.bourin@univ-nantes.fr

P. Á. Gargiulo, H. L. Mesones-Arroyo (eds.), *Psychiatry and Neuroscience Update – Vol. V*, https://doi.org/10.1007/978-3-031-72219-6_16

on Drugs and Crime (UNODC). At 1976 tons, cocaine production jumped 25% from 2016, when it had already increased by a quarter, according to estimates by the Vienna-based agency. The rise of cocaine, absorbed mainly by the markets of North America and Europe, is linked in particular to the expansion of crops and production capacities in Colombia. In this country providing some 70% of world production, coca tree areas increased by 17% in 2017, a consequence of the peace agreement concluded in 2016 with the FARC, which paradoxically allowed criminal groups to prosper in territories previously controlled by this guerrilla. The UNODC also regrets that "a decrease in eradication efforts may have fostered the idea that this crop is relatively low risk" in Colombia [5]. Today, the value of the European market (US $ 36 billion) is estimated to be close to that of the US market ($ 37 billion).

How Cocaine Works

Cocaine is a lipophilic drug with a short half-life of around 40 min. It crosses the hematoencephalic barrier, which binds to many receptors in the central nervous system but also at the cardiac, hepatic, renal, adrenal, and placental levels. Cocaine enhances the activity of monoamine neurotransmitters in the central and peripheral nervous systems by blocking the presynaptic reuptake transporters of these neurotransmitters. The main synaptic effect of cocaine is the release of dopamine from synaptic vesicles, and the dopamine transporter (DAT) allows the reuptake of dopamine mainly, but also, to a lesser extent, that of other monoamines such as serotonin and norepinephrine. These monoamines are recaptured much more efficiently by their own transporters: the serotonin transporter (SERT) and norepinephrine (NET), respectively [6, 7]. The binding of cocaine to the DAT transporter will inhibit its reuptake activity at the level of dopaminergic afferents which are particularly dense within the striatum and CPF. The blocking of DAT by cocaine will thus very significantly increase the extracellular concentration of dopamine at the level of these structures, blockade of dopamine reuptake resulting in enhanced dopaminergic neurotransmission [8].

When an individual takes cocaine, it passes more or less quickly into the bloodstream. It passes immediately into the blood if injected intravenously, very quickly when the product is smoked and a little slower when inhaled through the nose [9]. Then, the cocaine molecules being very small and liposoluble, they will cross the blood–brain barrier and end up in the brain [10]. Thus, cocaine amplifies the action of monoaminergic neurotransmitters. The physiological effects are directly linked to this alteration in neurotransmission. Indeed, excess dopamine is responsible for euphoria, and excess serotonin creates a feeling of confidence, while excess norepinephrine causes energy to rise [11]. In addition, with norepinephrine neurons at the locus coeruleus projecting their axons onto all major telencephalic and diencephalic structures, the overall and potent effect of cocaine is better understood [12].

One aspect remains mysterious about the mode of action of cocaine on the reuptake of dopamine. KO-DAT mice, still, presented a self-administration behavior of cocaine [13]. The role of dopamine in response behaviors to this drug was then called into question. However, this model has some important limitations, including constitutive hyperdopaminergy. One accepted hypothesis is that the mesocorticolimbic system of these mice would then be constitutively altered and somehow presensitized. A few years later, a more subtle mutant mouse model was created, presenting a mutation in the DAT gene that renders the transporter insensitive to cocaine (cocaine-insensitive DAT mice: CI-DAT) but continuing to fulfill its physiological reuptake. This model has shown that inhibition of DAT by cocaine is indeed an essential element in the behavioral effects of cocaine since injection of this substance does not induce locomotor sensitization in these mutants [14]. Interestingly but intriguingly, the same authors have continued this work by showing that the reintroduction by injection of associated adenovirus (AAV) of the wild-type gene in the ventral or dorsomedial striatum does not save the behavioral phenotype. On the other hand, the same injection in the dorsolateral striatum allows this rescue. In addition to behavior, the formation of dendritic spines in response to cocaine in these CI-DAT mice is also altered [15]. It is possible that multiple dopamine-related brain regions are involved in producing the robust rewarding effect of cocaine.

Similarities of Mode of Action of Cocaine on Dopamine Release in Humans and the Rodent Model

Real-time monitoring of dopamine variation in nucleus accumbens (NAc) has improved to understand the kinetics of how psychostimulants' work. This was initially carried out by the method of microdialysis in the NAc in rats injected with cocaine [16]. During an acute injection of cocaine, the concentration of dopamine increases rapidly, in about 10 min, then falls again gradually about 1 h after the injection. These results were also observed for multiple drugs and not just psychostimulants. This transient peak of dopamine is also temporally correlated with the hyperlocomotion induced by cocaine in rodents [17]. Interestingly, the glutamate concentration during this injection does not increase. Cocaine therefore has an effect of increasing striatal dopamine in rodents [18]. The exploitation and application of these results to human pathology have been possible since the mid-1990s, with the boom in imaging of dopaminergic systems in time real in humans. Thus, understanding the mechanisms of action of drugs of abuse was possible thanks to the techniques of position emission tomography and tomography by single photon emission. The first studies carried out by PET scanner showed a decrease in the level of cerebral perfusion, predominant in the frontal cortex and the left hemisphere among active cocaine addicts, but at a distance from episodes of abuse. An increase in basal ganglia flow in the first weeks of abstinence was followed, for a few months, by a reduction in frontal metabolic activity predominant on the left and correlated with depressive states, which may persist for a few months. Cocaine labeled with an isotope binds mainly in the striatum. The evolution over time of this fixation appeared to correlate directly with the sensations of "rising" and of pleasure induced by the product [19]. These techniques make it possible to indirectly follow changes in dopamine concentration in the brain through the use of agonists radiolabeled D2 and D3 dopamine receptors. These receptors are mainly located in the striatal regions, and when endogenous dopamine is released, we can observe a decrease in the occupation of these radioactive markers [20]. This method demonstrated that the increase in dopamine observed in these striatal regions by microdialysis, after an administration of cocaine in rodents, was also observed in humans, with similar kinetics. Rodent models have allowed a better understanding of the mechanism's neurons leading to addiction. In fact, rodents summarize the characteristics overall acute and chronic behavioral responses to drugs of abuse observed in humans [21]. Self-administration experiences with these substances are perfect examples. In these studies, the animal can be administered orally, intravenously (in the case of cocaine) or even intracerebral the substance studied, thus allowing to measure the reinforcing character of the drug [22].

Other behavioral tests exist during which the experimenter himself injects the drug into the animal. These so-called nonoperative protocols also induce important behavioral adaptations such as locomotor sensitization: the animal exhibits increasing locomotor activity after each daily injection. In addition, injecting cocaine can induce a preferential behavior of conditioned place (CPP), where the animal learns to associate the drug with the environment. So, in this test, the animal receives daily and alternatively, either the drug or a control solution (saline), injected into two different compartments [23]. At the end of the test, the animal has a choice between these two compartments and "chooses" to stay longer in the compartment associated with the cocaine after the learning phase. CPP is therefore closely linked to the environmental context formed by the differences between the compartments. However, it is also important in the case of locomotor sensitization since this behavior is amplified when the animal receives the drug in a new environment [24]. Besides the chronic aspect of addiction, it is interesting to note that cocaine quickly and sustainably modifies CPD and awareness-raising locomotor behaviors.

Voluntary drug research can nonetheless be modeled in experiments self-administration in rodents by associating operative behavior with a signal sensory informing of the presentation of the reward. After the learning phase, the simply presenting the signal is enough to induce drug seeking behavior in animals, characterized by operative behavior, even if it does not provide reward [25]. Regardless of the experimental paradigms chosen, that the administration requires an operative behavior or not, the behavioral alterations induced by cocaine all rely on adaptations of neural networks involving the areas cortical, striatal and dopaminergic. This set of brain structures forms the basal ganglia and the mesocorticolimbic circuit, a crucial brain network in the neuronal processing of reward and pathological adaptations to cocaine [26].

Neurobiology of Cocaine Addiction

Cocaine is a very powerful psychostimulant that acts on systems that are normally activated by natural and sensory signals. It blocks the recapture of different neurotransmitters and in particular dopamine but also noradrenaline and serotonin, which increases its concentration in the synapse. The effect of these neurotransmitters at the level of the postsynaptic neuron is therefore amplified. Moreover, to these neurochemical modifications are added morphological modifications which play an important role in particular at the level of the excitatory synapses, as well as genetic modifications that may be responsible for the long-term effects of cocaine [27].

Cocaine addiction is a very complex disease involving important modifications at different levels: neurochemical, structural, and epigenetic. This explains why current monotherapy strategies have proven to be ineffective and unsuitable, because they only target one of the many systems disrupted by drugs. It would suit to take into account all of these parameters and move toward combination therapies targeting each of these systems [28].

All psychoactive substances (including tobacco and alcohol) work directly or indirectly on the same neural networks of the central nervous system: the system of pleasure and reward or mesolimbic system [29].

The reward system is mainly made up of dopaminergic neurons, activated by dopamine. It is essential for the functioning of vital behaviors, inducing motivation and rewarding the individual with a feeling of pleasure. Other substances are also involved in this process, like acetylcholine, phenylethylamine, oxytocin, serotonin, etc., but it's mostly at the level of the dopamine cycle that cocaine intervenes [30].

By inhibiting dopamine reuptake, cocaine therefore very quickly leads to increase of its rate in the brain and produces a flash of intense pleasure: the high [31]. The induced pleasure is therefore totally artificial. It is not caused by the reality of life of the user but by a chemical dysfunction in the brain. The feeling of pleasure felt is so great that it devalues all others, like the small joys of work, hobbies, and love in particular. Indeed, the natural doses of dopamine caused by its small joys cannot compete with the very high doses induced by cocaine. However, several studies show the existence of a coupling between the mesolimbic dopaminergic and noradrenergic systems, and an important role of serotonin has been demonstrated, showing a coupling between noradrenergic systems and serotonergic [32]. The noradrenergic system and the serotonergic system, which normally regulate each other, become uncoupled following repeated administration of psychostimulants, resulting in hyperreactivity of the noradrenergic and serotonergic neurons at the cortical level. After the last administration, this decoupling persists and could be the cause of the behavioral sensitization (the body reacts to the product more and more intensely) often observed after repeated administration of cocaine [33]. However, even if the consequences of this decoupling in terms of response behavioral behavior seem rather well established, the mechanisms responsible for this dysregulation are not yet known. We just know that they involve the α1, β-adrenergic, and 5-HT2A receptors.

Dopaminergic neurons are under the excitatory influence of glutamatergic neurons coming from the prefrontal cortex, but also under the inhibitory influence of GABAergic interneurons of the ventral tegmental area whose activity is regulated by different neurotransmitters. Gamma aminobutyric acid (GABA) is the main inhibitory neurotransmitter of the brain. It plays an important role in the modulation of many physiological and psychological processes. There are several families of GABAergic receptors and in particular $GABA_B$ receptors which are involved in various psychological pathologies like anxiety, depression, and addiction [34].

Dopaminergic neurons are under the excitatory influence of glutamatergic neurons coming from the prefrontal cortex, but also under the inhibitory influence of GABAergic interneurons of the ventral tegmental area whose activity is regulated by different neurotransmitters [35].

Gamma aminobutyric acid (GABA) is the main inhibitory neurotransmitter of the brain. It plays an important role in the modulation of many physiological and psychological processes. There are several families of GABAergic receptors and in particular $GABA_B$ receptors which are involved in various psychological pathologies like anxiety, depression, and addiction [36, 37]. Cocaine is able to inhibit these $GABA_B$ receptors.

A variation in the efficiency of glutamatergic synaptic transmission would be partly responsible for establishing and/or maintaining the addiction [38]. Glutamate binds on different receptor subtypes, including AMPA and NMDA receptors. From different AMPA receptor subunits, the GluR1 subunit induces a sensitization, and cocaine has been shown to overexpress the subunit GluR1 [39]. Thus, by inducing sensitization, cocaine would lead to a decrease in efficiency of glutamatergic synaptic transmission which would be partly responsible for the establishment and/or maintenance of addictive behaviors [18].

Chronic cocaine use can induce some plasticity in the cerebral, especially in the nucleus accumbens. In this brain structure, neurons medium spiny trees have a very dense dendritic arborization which receives in its part distal about 90% glutamatergic (from the cortex) and dopaminergic influx (from the ventral tegmental area) [40]. The postsynaptic elements of dendritic arborization which are connected with the presynaptic endings to glutamate and dopamine are characteristic: they form buds along the dendrite or dendritic spines. It is at this level that we find synaptic plasticity. Cocaine is able to increase the number of dendritic branches as well as the concentration of dendritic spines. These changes last for up to a month after the last drug use [41]. These changes involve processes of neuritic growth and pseudo "Synaptogenesis" comparable to what is observed during development or in learning and memorization process. Among the molecules involved in these remodeling, in particular a kinase, Cdk5, was found [42]. Its expression is increased among chronic cocaine users. However, the mechanism by which Cdk5 allows the growth of thorns is still poorly understood. But it is likely that it involves the phosphorylation of constituent proteins of the cytoskeleton [43].

Scientific studies have made it possible to highlight modulations expression of genes after prolonged exposure to cocaine. Cocaine would cause epigenetic modifications in certain genes which has the effect of modifying them the expression [44]. These epigenetic changes induced by cocaine depend on the frequency of drug administration. Thus, it has been shown in rodents that cocaine induces changes of histones in particular by promoting the acetylation of histones at the level of the genes of which it increases expression. In addition, the administration of inhibitors of histone deacetylation helps to potentiate the behavioral effects of cocaine [45]. The persistent nature of these epigenetic modifications could explain the long-term changes seen in the neurons in cocaine users.

Conclusion

Let us look at the case of dopamine. Normally, once released and attached to the receptors, it is recaptured by a protein playing a role of transporter and carrying it back into the presynaptic cell. The cocaine molecules will attach themselves to these dopamine transporters, preventing its reuptake [46]. Thus, the brain is submerged in dopamine, in particular in the areas forming the "reward system" mainly located in the midbrain. Then, we observe a depletion of dopamine by disruption of the feedback mechanisms. The high, a sensation of intense pleasure induced by cocaine consumption does not last: between a quarter of an hour and an hour depending on the dose and the individual. Once the effect is over, the consumer feels a sudden return to earth, the crash. He then experiences a feeling of depression. Normal life is irrelevant to him compared to the euphoria he feels, and the brain is no longer able to produce dopamine in normal amounts for a period of time [47].

This is where the risk of addiction arises. If the user cannot cope with his crashes, he will want to take cocaine again. In addition to the risk of dependence, there is the risk of addiction. Indeed, cocaine not providing dopamine but exploiting that produced by the brain, it will be necessary to compensate for the drop in production induced by momentary overproduction by blocking even more transporters and therefore by increasing the doses of cocaine. The consumer will then find himself in a state of withdrawal, he will have to find cocaine at all costs which will induce stress in addition to the state of depression and he will be able to do anything to get it, even committing reprehensible acts. A new gene, delta-FosB, which appears in a specific region of the brain in chronic consumers of cocaine is perhaps a marker of cocaine addiction [48].

Cocaine addiction gradually sets in and many psychological, psychiatric, somatic, and social complications are associated with it. At the beginning of 1980s, when the cocaine epidemic began in the USA, started the first studies looking at cognitive alterations linked to cocaine use. The main results observed in these studies are in favor of impairments in memory, attention, and executive functions [49].

If the user cannot cope with his crashes, he will want to take cocaine again. In addition to the risk of dependence, there is the risk of addiction. Indeed, cocaine not providing dopamine but exploiting that produced by the brain, it will be necessary to compensate for the drop in production induced by momentary overproduction by blocking even more transporters and therefore by increasing the doses of cocaine. However, the environment in which the consumer lives plays a very important role.

Thus, laboratory experiences were redone and demonstrated that the reactions of the animal's cocaine addicts varied depending on the environment in which they lived. Indeed, if their living conditions offered them other choices to provide them with pleasure, they reduced the doses ingested. On the other hand, it has been shown that the risk of dependence is lower in married than single people and that risk decreased with age. It was shown that cocaine makes certain synapses permeable to calcium, allowing the passage of information, which normally should not pass [50], so with behavioral interventions or extensive drug therapy, one could treat addiction. However, the theory is still a long way off and if there is no cure effective against cocaine addiction, there are still some promising leads.

References

1. Haas LF. Coca shrub (Erythroxylum coca). J Neurol Neurosurg Psychiatry. 1995;59:25.
2. Calatayud J, González A. History of the development and evolution of local anesthesia since the coca leaf. Anesthesiology. 2003;98:1503–8.
3. Redman M. Cocaine: what is the crack? A brief history of the use of cocaine as an anesthetic. Anesth Pain Med. 2011;1:95–7.
4. Wesson DR, Smith DE. Cocaine: its use for central nervous system stimulation including recreational and medical uses. NIDA Res Monogr. 1977;Series 13:137–52.
5. Long G. Cocaine: Colombia weighs a new aerial war on drugs Financial Times; 2021, February 20.

6. Ritz MC, Lamb RJ, Goldberg SR, Kuhar MJ. Cocaine receptors on dopamine transporters are related to self-administration of cocaine. Science. 1987;237:1219–23.
7. Jayanthi LD, Ramamoorthy S. Regulation of monoamine transporters: influence of psychostimulants and therapeutic antidepressants. AAPS J. 2005;7:E728–38.
8. Dela Peña I, Gevorkiana R, Shi WX. Psychostimulants affect dopamine transmission through both dopamine transporter-dependent and independent mechanisms. Eur J Pharmacol. 2015;764:562–70.
9. Labiris NR, Dolovich MB. Pulmonary drug delivery. Part I: physiological factors affecting therapeutic effectiveness of aerosolized medications. Br J Clin Pharmacol. 2003;56:588–99.
10. Pimentel E, Sivalingam K, Doke M, Samikkannu T. Effects of drugs of abuse on the blood-brain barrier: a brief overview. Front Neurosci. 2020;14:513.
11. NIDA. Cocaine's pleasurable effects may involve multiple chemical sites. Retrieved from https://archives.drugabuse.gov/news-events/nida-notes/1999/08/cocaines-pleasurable-effects-may-involve-multiple-chemical-sites on 2021, May 27; 1999, August 1.
12. Pitts DK, Marwah J. Effects of cocaine on the electrical activity of single noradrenergic neurons from locus coeruleus. Life Sci. 1986;38:1229–34.
13. Rocha BA, Fumagalli F, Gainetdinov RR, Jones SR, Ator R, Giros B, Miller GW, Caron MG. Cocaine self-administration in dopamine-transporter knockout mice. Nat Neurosci. 1998;1:132–7.
14. Chen R, Tilley MR, Wei H, Zhou F, Zhou FM, Ching S, Quan N, Stephens RL, Hill ER, Nottoli T, Han DD, Gu HH. Abolished cocaine reward in mice with a cocaine-insensitive dopamine transporter. Proc Natl Acad Sci USA. 2006;103:9333–8.
15. O'Neill B, Tilley MR, Han DD, et al. Behavior of knock-in mice with a cocaine-insensitive dopamine transporter after virogenetic restoration of cocaine sensitivity in the striatum. Neuropharmacology. 2014;79:626–33.
16. Willuhn I, Wanat MJ, Clark JJ, Phillips PE. Dopamine signaling in the nucleus accumbens of animals self-administering drugs of abuse. Curr Top Behav Neurosci. 2010;3:29–71.
17. Bariselli S, Miyazaki NL, Creed MC, Kravitz AV. Orbitofrontal-striatal potentiation underlies cocaine-induced hyperactivity. Nat Commun. 2020;11:3996.
18. Schmidt HD, Pierce RC. Cocaine-induced neuroadaptations in glutamate transmission: potential therapeutic targets for craving and addiction. Ann N Y Acad Sci. 2010;1187:35–75.
19. Volkow ND, Wang GJ, Fowler JS, Hitzemann R, Angrist B, Gatley SJ, Logan J, Ding YS, Pappas N. Association of methylphenidate-induced craving with changes in right striato-orbitofrontal metabolism in cocaine abusers. Am J Psychiatry. 1999;156(1):19–25.
20. Nutt DJ, Lingford-Hughes A, Erritzoe D, Stokes PR. The dopamine theory of addiction: 40 years of highs and lows. Nat Rev Neurosci. 2015;16:305–12.
21. Kuhn BN, Kalivas PW, Bobadilla AC. Understanding addiction using animal models. Front Behav Neurosci. 2019;13:262.
22. Panlilio LV, Goldberg SR. Self-administration of drugs in animals and humans as a model and an investigative tool. Addiction. 2007;102:1863–70.
23. O'Neill B, Tilley MR, Gu HH. Cocaine produces conditioned place aversion in mice with a cocaine-insensitive dopamine transporter. Genes Brain Behav. 2013;12:34–8.
24. Badiani A, Browman KE, Robinson TE. Influence of novel versus home environments on sensitization to the psychomotor stimulant effects of cocaine and amphetamine. Brain Res. 1995;674(2):291–8.
25. Bossert JM, Marchant NJ, Calu DJ, Shaham Y. The reinstatement model of drug relapse: recent neurobiological findings, emerging research topics, and translational research. Psychopharmacology. 2013;229:453–76.
26. Haber SN. Corticostriatal circuitry. Dialogues Clin Neurosci. 2016;18:7–21.
27. Nestler EJ. The neurobiology of cocaine addiction. Sci Pract Perspect. 2005;3:4–10.
28. Volkow ND, Koob GF, McLellan AT. Neurobiologic advances from the brain disease model of addiction. N Engl J Med. 2016;37:363–71.
29. Adinoff B. Neurobiologic processes in drug reward and addiction. Harv Rev Psychiatry. 2004;12:305–20.
30. WHO reports. Neuroscience of psychoactive substance use and dependence; 2004. p. 286.
31. NIDA. How does cocaine produce its effects? Retrieved from https://www.drugabuse.gov/publications/research-reports/cocaine/how-does-cocaine-produce-its-effects on 2021, May 31; 2020, June 11.
32. Alex KD, Pehek EA. Pharmacologic mechanisms of serotonergic regulation of dopamine neurotransmission. Pharmacol Ther. 2007;113:296–320.
33. Tassin JP. Uncoupling between noradrenergic and serotonergic neurons as a molecular basis of stable changes in behavior induced by repeated drugs of abuse. Biochem Pharmacol. 2008;75:85–97.
34. Bouarab C, Thompson B, Polter AM. VTA GABA neurons at the interface of stress and reward. Front Neural Circuits. 2019;13:78.
35. Salomon L, Lanteri C, Glowinski J, Tassin JP. Behavioral sensitization to amphetamine results from an uncoupling between noradrenergic and serotonergic neurons. Proc Natl Acad Sci USA. 2006;103:7476–81.
36. Nuss P. Anxiety disorders and GABA neurotransmission: a disturbance of modulation. Neuropsychiatr Dis Treat. 2015;11:165–75.
37. Vlachou S, Markou A. GABAB receptors in reward processes. Adv Pharmacol. 2010;58:315–71.
38. O'Donovan SM, Sullivan CR, McCullumsmith RE. The role of glutamate transporters in the patho-

physiology of neuropsychiatric disorders. NPJ Schizophr. 2017;3:32.
39. Gass JT, Olive MF. Glutamatergic substrates of drug addiction and alcoholism. Biochem Pharmacol. 2008;75:218–65.
40. Barrientos C, Knowland D, Wu MMJ, et al. Cocaine-induced structural plasticity in input regions to distinct cell types in nucleus accumbens. Biol Psychiatry. 2018;84:893–904.
41. Robinson TE, Gorny G, Mitton E, Kolb B. Cocaine self-administration alters the morphology of dendrites and dendritic spines in the nucleus accumbens and neocortex. Synapse. 2001;39:257–66.
42. Shah K, Rossie S. Tale of the good and the bad Cdk5: remodeling of the actin cytoskeleton in the brain. Mol Neurobiol. 2018;55:3426–38.
43. Benavides DR, Quinn JJ, Zhong P, Hawasli AH, DiLeone RJ, Kansy JW, Olausson P, Yan Z, Taylor JR, Bibb JA. Cdk5 modulates cocaine reward, motivation, and striatal neuron excitability. J Neurosci. 2007;27:12967–76.
44. Sadri-Vakili G. Cocaine triggers epigenetic alterations in the corticostriatal circuit. Brain Res. 2015;1628(Pt A):50–9.
45. Nestler EJ. Epigenetic mechanisms of drug addiction. Neuropharmacology. 2014;76(Pt B):259–68.
46. Huang X, Gu HH, Zhan CG. Mechanism for cocaine blocking the transport of dopamine: insights from molecular modeling and dynamics simulations. J Phys Chem B. 2009;113:15057–66.
47. Morton WA. Cocaine and psychiatric symptoms. Prim Care Companion J Clin Psychiatry. 1999;1:109–13.
48. Nestler EJ. Review. Transcriptional mechanisms of addiction: role of DeltaFosB. Philos Trans R Soc Lond Ser B Biol Sci. 2008;363:3245–55.
49. Vonmoos M, Hulka LM, Preller KH, Minder F, Baumgartner MR, Quednow BB. Cognitive impairment in cocaine users is drug-induced but partially reversible: evidence from a longitudinal study. Neuropsychopharmacology. 2014;39:2200–10.
50. Bellone C, Lüscher C. Cocaine triggered AMPA receptor redistribution is reversed in vivo by mGluR-dependent long-term depression. Nat Neurosci. 2006;9:636–41.

Benzodiazepine Addiction: A Difficult Story

17

Michel Bourin

Introduction

Benzodiazepines (BZD) are drugs marketed since the 1960s that act on the central nervous system through GABA receptors. All benzodiazepines have varying degrees of anxiolytic, hypnotic, muscle relaxant, and anticonvulsant properties [1]. They are classified according to their indications as hypnotics in severe sleep disorders, anxiolytics in the symptomatic treatment of anxiety manifestations and alcohol withdrawal, antiepileptics, or anesthetics [2].

The undesirable effects of benzodiazepines include in particular, memory disorders, reduced alertness or even drowsiness, behavioral disorders, and an increased risk of falls, particularly in the elderly. Long-term use of benzodiazepines also poses a risk of pharmacological tolerance (gradual reduction in the therapeutic effect for the same administered dose) and psychological and physical dependence [3]. Some studies suggest a possible link between the consumption of benzodiazepines and long-term cognitive impairment [4].

During the 1990s, several reports alerted heath workers and the lay people to the broad consumption of benzodiazepines and the problem using them over prolonged periods. Since 1991, the maximum prescription period has been limited to 4 weeks for hypnotics and 12 weeks for anxiolytics. Several actions aimed at limiting their consumption and promoting their proper use have been implemented at the national and local levels: information campaigns and tools intended for the general public, information documents, and good practice recommendations intended for consumers by health professionals [5].

M. Bourin (✉)
Neurobiologie de l'anxiété et de la dépression, Université de Nantes, Nantes, France
e-mail: michel.bourin@univ-nantes.fr

Pharmacological Properties of Benzodiazepines

Benzodiazepines are low toxicity drugs. In fact, the doses likely to cause poisoning are much higher than the therapeutic doses and never lead to death unless combined with other treatments. However, these drugs exert undesirable effects at therapeutic doses, in particular in the elderly population [6].

Sedative Effect

This is not always an undesirable effect, since it is sometimes sought by the prescriber, especially in psychiatry. In most cases, this effect is troublesome and occurs at dosages close to anxiolytic dosages. It can, in particular, induce falls in the elderly.

It was shown that the risk of hip fracture increased in elderly patients consuming BZDs [7]. Patients appeared to be more vulnerable immediately after initiation of therapy than after

P. Á. Gargiulo, H. L. Mesones-Arroyo (eds.), *Psychiatry and Neuroscience Update – Vol. V*,
https://doi.org/10.1007/978-3-031-72219-6_17

a month of continuous use. BZDs with short half-lives do not appear to be safer than those with long half-lives. This result partially agrees with other authors. They showed that the presence of BZDs in plasma was not associated with an increased risk of hip fracture except for lorazepam [8]. In a recent review dealing with the relationship between the use of BZDs and the risk of femoral neck fracture, the authors highlighted the differences in the various protocols that explained the contradictory results. The studies that did not show an association with this risk were hospital studies, a type of study that lacks validity due to the lack of an adequate control group. However, it was concluded that there is epidemiological evidence that strongly suggests that the use of BZDs by the elderly increases their risk of cervical fractures by at least 50% [9].

Amnesic Effect

The amnesic effects of benzodiazepines have mainly been studied in anesthesiology. These effects have been reported as well after intravenous (I.V.) or intramuscular (I.M.) injections as after oral intake. In the case of anesthesia, these are desired effects to prevent the patient from remembering unpleasant events [10]. On the other hand, in ambulatory patients, the amnesic effects can become undesirable effects. Amnesia is of the anterograde type and occurs in all patients as soon as high doses are used, the elderly being particularly sensitive. The molecules with rapid absorption and strong affinity on the benzodiazepine receptors cause the most spectacular amnesias [11]. Cognitive disorders seem to be the major side effects of BZDs [12]. A follow-up study of 111,389 people aged 60–70 showed that long-term use of BZDs was a risk factor for increased cognitive decline [13].

Disinhibitory Effect

In Animals, as in Humans, benzodiazepines facilitate desinhibition behaviors which are similar of them induced by alcohol consumption [14].

The disinhibitory effect is favorable when anxiety prevents the subject from acting, however this can lead to acting out in impulsive subjects (hyperkinetic children,alcoholics, and excited elderly people). This desinhibitory effect is often called by practitioners the "paradoxical" effect of benzodazepines as opposed to their more widely known sedative effect. On the other hand, at high dosages, this effect disappears, replaced by the sedative effect.

The disinhibitory effect, however, can be the cause of sometimes successful suicide attempts if the subject then uses other drugs or other means of autolysis [15].

The role of BZDs in suicides in the elderly suggests that BZDs should be prescribed with caution in these patients, particularly hypnotics such as flunitrazepam and nitrazepam. These drugs were used in drug suicides in the elderly in the period 1992–1996 [16].

The Phenomenon of Dependence

When BZDs are abruptly stopped, a withdrawal syndrome can develop. The prevalence of these withdrawal syndromes has been estimated to be between 0% and 100% in different studies, depending to the duration of prescription. Interestingly, approximately 40% of patients treated for at least 6 months with BZD may experience a withdrawal syndrome after abrupt discontinuation of treatment [17]. The symptoms are mainly tremors, mental confusion, anxiety, and insomnia. Severe symptoms, such as convulsions and psychotic manifestations may occur, as well as a marked increase in blood pressure and myocardial ischemia, if stopped abruptly. Few withdrawal studies in the elderly have been performed; elderly patients compared with young adults show less severe withdrawal syndromes [18]. However, it has been observed that the psychotic withdrawal reactions are more marked than in the young subject [19].

The withdrawal is thought to be linked to an overactivity of the noradrenergic, serotonin, and cholinergic systems which have been inhibited by chronic administration of BZDs. The fact that the plasma concentrations of BZDs decrease more slowly, may explain that the withdrawal symptoms in the elderly are less severe.

It appears that the risks of withdrawal are increased, especially with abrupt discontinuation of BZDs with a short half-life and with a rapid reduction in plasma concentrations, as well as high dosages, and long-term use. BZDs with a short or intermediate half-life can generate withdrawal symptoms upon discontinuation that appear between 24 and 36 h after discontinuation, while BZDs with a long half-life can induce symptoms of weaning after practically a week and in this case, the stopping of BZDs is not always incriminated [20].

It appears that other factors may contribute to the severity of the withdrawal syndrome, such as a premorbid personality, including passive-dependent personalities. There are, of course, important physiological differences; thus, the previous consumption of alcohol and a low cultural level can increase the withdrawal syndrome.

Nature of the Benzodiazepine Dependency Phenomenon

The addiction induced by benzodiazepines is explained by an increased activity od dopaminergic neurons via the alpha-3 subtype of GABA receptors. This hyper dopaminergic activity explains the gratifying effect as well for the benzodiazepine consumers than alcohol consumers [21–23].

After multiple clinical cases that alerted the researchers, animal and human studies were undertaken to better understand the phenomenon of addiction, to understand the modalities of occurrence, and to try to find solutions.

1. *In Animals*

Numerous studies have been carried out, particularly in rats, baboons, and cats, and two models have been used. Addiction was first studied in rats [24]:

- A simple model: the rat takes a drink to which benzodiazepine is added. In fact, this type of experience is especially valid with barbiturates or morphine [25, 26], but it is not very convincing with benzodiazepines.
- A more elaborate model: after placing a catheter in a vein, the animal presses a lever, a bolus, that is to say a discharge of solution containing a benzodiazepine, flows into its bloodstream. Rats will squeeze the lever at a very high frequency so as to have an infusion of the highly addictive substance as seen with opioids, but less quickly than with barbiturates.

Benzodiazepine dependence was studied in baboon by exposing animals to diazepam by injections at doses of 0.125–20 mg/kg/day intragastrically for 7 days, or at doses of 0.125–20 mg/kg/day, intragastrically for 1 h for 1–35 days.

The diazepam is placed in an aqueous suspension at a concentration of 4 g/l; the suspension is prepared each day. After administration of diazepam, flumazenil (a benzodiazepine antagonist) is administered at a dose of 5 mg/kg intramuscularly. This causes abrupt withdrawal; in fact, flumazenil occupies the benzodiazepine receptor sites and thus, diazepam can no longer attach to them. Therefore, the intensity of withdrawal can be assessed by noting the clinical signs of each animal [27].

In the First Experiment

The dose of diazepam is constant at 20 mg/kg/day and the duration of exposure varies from 1, 3, 7, or 35 days. Each animal receives a dose of 20 mg/kg and the duration of exposure varies from 1, 3, 7, or 35 days. Each animal receives a dose of 20 mg/kg intragastrically, as a loading dose over 2 min, immediately before starting the continuous injection. The different exposure times were either in ascending or descending order. A minimum wash-out period of 2 weeks is necessary between each exposure.

In the Second Experiment

The duration of exposure is constant for 7 days, during which the doses of diazepam vary between: 0.125 mg/kg and 20 mg/kg. A loading dose of the total daily dose is given immediately before starting the 7-day exposure to diazepam. The order of the doses is again either ascending or descending. After treatment with diazepam, flumazenil is injected at a dose of 5 mg/kg intramuscularly. The behavior of the animals is then recorded continuously for 60, 75, 90, and 120 min after the injection of flumazenil. A score is thus established, consisting of the possible appearance of 14 signs of withdrawal [28]:

These postures have been accurately described:

- grinding of teeth,
- licking lips,
- rubbing of the nose,
- yawning,
- nausea,
- vomiting,
- head tremors,
- tremors of limbs,
- body tremors,
- convulsions and postures of the body.

In addition to these postures, other behaviors were noted:

- Nausea: the baboon stands on its four legs, the head above the body.
- Lethargic: the animal lies on the ground, unresponsive.
- Depressed: the animal sits with its chin on the chest, without response.
- Attached: the tension in his muscles is extreme, with fasciculations and tremors. This attitude is pre-convulsive because often convulsions appear after the animal takes this position.

To analyze these results, the presence or absence of the 14 withdrawal signs is considered over time periods after the injection of flumazenil. For each time period, a sign of withdrawal if it occurs more than once is taken into account.

After 1 h of exposure to diazepam, when flumazenil is given, the number of withdrawal signs is the same as when a placebo is given. In contrast, administration of flumazenil after 24 h results in a marked increase in withdrawal signs. After 3, 7, and 35 days of exposure to diazepam, the injection of flumazenil significantly increases the signs of withdrawal.

Evidence has therefore been made that abruptly stopping diazepam leads to withdrawal—provided there is a minimum of impregnation. It has thus been shown that the development of physical dependence increases with the dose administered and the time of exposure to diazepam. The experiment was carried out in cats with comparable results.

Other researchers have performed self-administration studies in monkeys. The experiments consist of preventing the effects of withdrawal induced by abrupt discontinuation of barbital by various substances such as: phenobarbital, ethanol, meprobamate, diazepam, and chlordiazepoxide. These two benzodiazepines avoid the effects of withdrawal from barbital but at very large doses (115 mg/kg in continuous infusion) thus proving that benzodiazepines are less effective in preventing withdrawal than ethanol or even meprobamate. This, however, represents indirect evidence of benzodiazepine dependence. Furthermore, the development of physical dependence has been demonstrated in animals after treatment for three benzodiazepines—diazepam, chlordiazepoxide, and flurazepam—both for doses close to therapeutic doses in humans and for higher doses [29, 30].

It was important to report this work, which was the first to establish dependence induced by benzodiazepines.

2. *In Humans*

Usually when an addiction manifests itself after taking a substance, there is a withdrawal syndrome when stopping taking the substance. Quite specific reactions are then observed, for example, in the case of opiates. These are:

- A search behavior at all costs for substance.
- Tolerance that sets in quickly which leads to increased doses.

Early studies in humans did not seem to favor addiction, except in quite rare cases. However, unusual symptoms were observed. Upon discontinuation of treatment, an altered perception of the environment—and even sensory hypersensitivity—was observed [31]. Clinicians were not convinced that all patients developed withdrawal syndrome upon discontinuation of treatment, as those who did come for a consultation were those who had failed to spontaneously discontinue [32].

Numerous studies have been undertaken either with psychotic patients reputed to be incurable or with anxiety patients. Thus, a study was carried out in patients hospitalized for chronic psychiatric pathologies [33]. Patients received high doses of chlordiazepoxide (100–600 mg/day) for 1–7 months. Most patients were treated for at least 3 months.

Eleven patients were suddenly withdrawn after having been treated with doses of 300–600 mg/day, a placebo was then administered to them. Of these, ten patients developed new symptoms after the prescription of placebo.

In five cases, an aggravation of the psychotic symptoms was observed,
In five cases, insomnia and restlessness.
In four cases, a loss of appetite.
In two cases, epileptiform convulsions.

This study, which could not have been done today because it is ethically questionable, was evidence of the addictive potential of chlordiazepoxide.

Other researchers [34] have also used chlordiazepoxide, but at a more usual dosage (45 mg) for 20 weeks. Upon discontinuation of the treatment, a mild abstinence syndrome was observed, consisting of subjective feelings of anxiety and some tension, tremors, decreased appetite, feeling faint, or dizziness. It is difficult to conclude strictly as withdrawal, but can be a resurgence of anxiety before treatment.

Diazepam was later studied in 50 subjects from hospital medical, surgical, and psychiatric departments [35]. Psychiatric patients were no more prone to drug abuse than those who took diazepam for medical or surgical reasons. Among the 24 patients who had tried to abruptly stop diazepam, 17 of them—that is to say 80%—presented a moderate withdrawal syndrome but for some of them, it was very severe. This is a compelling study of the possibility of diazepam causing withdrawal syndrome.

In 1978, a book reported 151 cases worldwide of benzodiazepine addiction, multiple drug abuse, and alcohol use [36], which may seem relatively low these days. The author also noted that there may be problems with therapeutic dose dependence, without an overdose.

Two controlled studies were published in 1981 and 1984, on a small number of patients.

The first study compares the results obtained with two groups of patients (ten in total) [37]:

- A first group where the patients gradually weaned after having taken strong benzodiazepines.
- A second group in which the patients gradually weaned, having taken doses considered as therapeutic.

The therapeutic dose group shows more withdrawal symptoms than the high dose group but later.

The symptoms found in decreasing order were: anxiety, disturbed sleep, intolerance to noise, drunken gait, a feeling of numbness and tingling, muscle pain, loss of appetite and nausea, feeling pressure on the face, aggressive feelings, depressive symptoms, sensation of weakness, sore eyes, hallucinations, and paranoid thoughts. Anxiety is felt by all patients, raising the question of the rebound effect.

The second study was carried out double blind. These were patients who, given the time, did not exhibit great nosographic homogeneity: anxiety neurosis, anxiety depression, or personality disorder with anxious mood. However, none of them exhibited alcohol abuse or took any other medication [37]. These patients have been receiving benzodiazepines at therapeutic doses for at least 1 year (between 1 and 16 years):

- 14 were receiving diazepam,
- 8 received *lorazepam*,
- 2 were receiving *clobazam*.

Withdrawal was gradual after 2 weeks with the administration of a placebo, then 2 weeks without any treatment. The study period is 10 weeks. Patients are subjected at regular intervals to a battery of tests: clinical, psychological, and physiological. Plasma concentrations of benzodiazepines decrease steadily, until they are no longer detectable after 3 or 4 weeks. Withdrawal symptoms were detected in all 24 patients. The inventory is more complete than in the previous study. The authors used it to establish the following withdrawal scale (Table 17.1).

Using the Hamilton Scale for Anxiety and Withdrawal Scale above, we have tried to understand the influence of the half-life on the development of addiction. Therefore, we compared two benzodiazepines with significantly different half-lives: prazepan (50 h) and lorazepam (12 h).

Patients received one or the other treatment for 30 days, then discontinued treatment and treatment with placebo for 10 days [39].

The evolution of the various patient groups depending on the treatment is as follows:

Prazepam group $N = 32$ patients treated for 40 days:
- 15 treated with prazepam continue treatment: 15 nothing to report;
- 17 treated with placebo after 30 days: 7 nothing to report, 9 various disorders, 1 withdrawal syndrome.

Lorazepam group $N = 31$ patients treated for 40 days:
- 15 treated with lorazepam continue treatment: 15 nothing to report.
- 16 treated with placebo after 30 days: 5 nothing to report, 5 various disorders, 6 withdrawal syndromes.

This suggests that the anxiety rebound and withdrawal symptoms are more numerous when using a half-short benzodiazepine than with a long half-life benzodiazepine. This experiment confirms hypotheses formulated previously [40].

This tendency of dependence caused by benzodiazepines linked to the half-life was studied in a natural situation by comparing the withdrawal syndromes observed after prolonged administration of benzodiazepines with long half-life (clorazepate, diazepam) and benzodiazepines with short half-lives. (alprazolam, lorazepam) [41].

Table 17.1 Withdrawal scale [38]

1. *Physical tiredness*
None 0
Tiredness but without need to lie down 1
Requiring to lie down from time to time 2
To lie down all day long 3
2. *Sleep disruption*
Normal sleep without hypnotics 0
Normal sleep with hypnotics 1
8–6 h sleep with hypnotics 2
Less than 3 h of sleep with hypnotics 3
3. *Migraines*
None 0
Occasional without need of analgesics 1
Constant but moderate, or occasional severe, salicylate efficient 2
Constant and severe, salicylate inefficient 3
4. *Dizziness*
None 0
Blackouts, occasional and light 1
Constant blackouts but light or occasional severe blackouts 2
Constant severe blackouts. Requiring to lie down 3
5. *Orthostatic symptoms*
None 0
Blackout feeling when standing up abruptly 1
Requiring to stand up slowly to avoid the blackout feeling 2
Unconsciousness 3
6. *Palpitations*
None 0
Light palpitations 1
Palpitations occasionally disturbing 2
Constant disturbing palpitations 3
7. *Tremors*
None 0
Light tremor, movements not affected 1
Obvious tremor, small movement disruptions 2
Severe tremor 3
8. *Sweating*
Normal 0
Increased slightly 1
Increased in an obvious manner 2
Profuse 3
9. *Dry mouth*
None 0
Light, but not subjectively unsettled 1
Obvious, but not severe or painful 2
Severe, rendering eating painful 3
10. *Constipation*
None 0
Light constipation without need of laxatives 1
Obvious constipation, requiring laxatives, 2
No bowel movements in spite of laxatives 3
11. *Micturition problems*
None 0
Light 1
Difficulties in emptying bladder. Treatment required 2
Urinary retention 3

Most subjects had been treated for more than 3 years. The observation of withdrawal in people who accepted (83%) was carried out blind, 32 subjects presented a withdrawal syndrome (18 for benzodiazepines with long half-life, 13 for benzodiazepines with short half-life) when stopping treatment abruptly. However, analysis of the severity of withdrawals showed that short-half-life benzodiazepines lead to much more severe withdrawals than long-half-life benzodiazepines [42].

Over the years, research has shown an incontrovertible dependence associated with taking benzodiazepines:

- At high doses, it seems inevitable;
- At therapeutic dosages, it exists even at low doses. If you are not careful with the duration of treatment, and it is prolonged, benzodiazepines with short half-life are more involved than others [20, 43].

Conclusion

The risk of benzodiazepine dependence varies depending on the duration of drug treatment. Few people become dependent when treatment with the benzodiazepine lasts less than 3 months. After 1 year, dependency rates increase, being between 20% and 45% [44].

Long-term use of benzodiazepines, especially among the elderly, has a wide range of negative effects that result in additional costs to the health care system and to society as a whole [45]. In older adults, long-term use of benzodiazepines can cause confusion and poor muscle coordination, leading to an increased risk of falls, hip fractures, and automobile accidents [46].

The severity of withdrawal symptoms depends on several factors, including the type of benzodiazepine (short- or long-acting), dose, duration of treatment, and the suddenness of discontinuation [47]. About 40% of patients who suddenly stop using a long-acting benzodiazepine (e.g., diazepam) after taking it for 6 months or more experience withdrawal symptoms.

Usually, withdrawal symptoms appear within 2 days in patients taking a short-acting benzodiazepine and within 2–10 days in patients taking a long-acting benzodiazepine. However, symptoms can appear even after 3 weeks [48]. Among the most common symptoms of benzodiazepine withdrawal are anxiety, depression, diarrhea, constipation, bloating, insomnia, irritability, muscle pain, restlessness, and failure of mind concentration and memory. Some also experience panic attacks, and sometimes seizures and symptoms of psychosis such as hallucinations, delusions, disorganized thoughts, and motor disturbances.

It is surprising that there are no clinical studies showing the similarity of dependence on benzodiazepines and that of ethanol. Indeed, the mechanism of action of these two types of products is very similar [49, 50].

References

1. Bourin M. Clinical pharmacology of anxiolytics. Arch Depress Anxiety. 2018;4(1):021–0025.
2. Griffin CE 3rd, Kaye AM, Bueno FR, Kaye AD. Benzodiazepine pharmacology and central nervous system-mediated effects. Ochsner J. 2013;13:214–23.
3. Lader M. Benzodiazepine harm: how can it be reduced? Br J Clin Pharmacol. 2014;77:295–301.
4. Stewart SA. The effects of benzodiazepines on cognition. J Clin Psychiatry. 2005;66 Suppl 2:9–13.
5. Gentile G, Lapeyre-Mestre M, Micallef J. Combatting the misuse of benzodiazepines and related Z drugs in French general practice: a clinical review. BJGP Open. 2020;4(1):bjgpopen20X101014.
6. Dailly E, Bourin M. The use of benzodiazepines in aged patients: clinical and pharmacological considerations. Pak J Pharm Sci. 2008;21:89–95.
7. Wang PS, Bohn RL, Glynn RJ, Mogun H, Avorn J. Hazardous benzodiazepine regimens in the elderly: effects of half-life, dosage, and duration on risk of hip fracture. Am J Psychiatry. 2001;158:892–8.
8. Pierfitte C, Macouillard G, Thicoïpe M, Chaslerie A, Pehourcq F, Aïssou M, Martinez B, Lagnaoui R, Fourrier A, Bégaud B, Dangoumau J, Moore N. Benzodiazepines and hip fractures in elderly people: case-control study. BMJ. 2001;322:704–8.
9. Cumming RG, Le Couteur DG. Benzodiazepines and risk of hip fractures in older people: a review of the evidence. CNS Drugs. 2003;17:825–37.

10. Veselis RA. The problem with amnesia. Anesthesiology. 2012;117:940–1.
11. Mejo SL. Anterograde amnesia linked to benzodiazepines. Nurs Pract. 1992;44:49–50.
12. Pomara N, Tun H, DaSilva D, Hernando R, Deptula D, Greenblatt DJ. The acute and chronic performance effects of alprazolam and lorazepam in the elderly: relationship to duration of treatment and self-rated sedation. Psychopharmacol Bull. 1998;34:139–53.
13. Paterniti S, Dufouil C, Alpérovitch A. Long-term benzodiazepine use and cognitive decline in the elderly: the Epidemiology of Vascular Aging Study. J Clin Psychopharmacol. 2002;22:285–93.
14. Tabakoff B, Hoffman PL. Animal models in alcohol research. Alcohol Res Health. 2000;24:77–84.
15. Dodds TJ. Prescribed benzodiazepines and suicide risk: a review of the literature. Prim Care Companion CNS Disord. 2017;19(2):PCC.16r02037.
16. Carlsten A, Waern M, Holmgren P, Allebeck P. The role of benzodiazepines in elderly suicides. Scand J Public Health. 2003;31:224–8.
17. Liebrenz M, Gehring MT, Buadze A, Caflisch C. High-dose benzodiazepine dependence: a qualitative study of patients' perception on cessation and withdrawal. BMC Psychiatry. 2015;15:116.
18. Petursson H. The benzodiazepine withdrawal syndrome. Addiction. 1994;89:1455–9.
19. Bourin M. Do benzodiazepines still need to be used? Open Access J Neurol Neurosurg. 2017;5(4):555669. https://doi.org/10.19080/OAJNN.2017.05.5556670.
20. Brett J, Murnion B. Management of benzodiazepine misuse and dependence. Aust Prescr. 2015;38:152–5.
21. Davies M. The role of GABAA receptors in mediating the effects of alcohol in the central nervous system. J Psychiatry Neurosci. 2003;28:263–74.
22. Tan KR, Rudolph U, Lüscher C. Hooked on benzodiazepines: GABAA receptor subtypes and addiction. Trends Neurosci. 2011;34:188–97.
23. NIDA. Well-known mechanism underlies benzodiazepines' addictive properties. 2012, April 19.
24. Sanger DJ. Schedule-induced drinking of chlordiazepoxide solutions by rats. Pharmacol Biochem Behav. 1977;7:1–6.
25. Harris RT, Claghorn JL, Schoolar JC. Self-administration of minor tranquilizers as a function of conditioning. Psychopharmacologia. 1968;13:81–8.
26. Stolerman IP, Kumar R, Steinberg H. Development of morphine dependence in rats: lack of effect of previous ingestion of other drugs. Psychopharmacologia. 1971;20:321–36.
27. Lukas SE, Griffiths RR. Precipitated withdrawal by a benzodiazepine receptor antagonist (Ro 15-1788) after 7 days of diazepam. Science. 1982;217(4565):1161–3.
28. Lukas SE, Griffiths RR. Precipitated diazepam withdrawal in baboons: effects of dose and duration of diazepam exposure. Eur J Pharmacol. 1984;100:163–71.
29. Rosenberg HC, Chiu TH. Time course for development of benzodiazepine tolerance and physical dependence. Neurosci Biobehav Rev. 1985;9:123–31.
30. Yanagita T, Takahashi S. Dependence liability of several sedative-hypnotic agents evaluated in monkeys. J Pharmacol Exp Ther. 1973;185:307–16.
31. Tyrer PJ. Benzodiazepines on trial. Br Med J (Clin Res Ed). 1984;288:1101–2.
32. Ladewig D. Dependence liability of the benzodiazepines. Drug Alcohol Depend. 1984;13(2):139–49.
33. Hollister LE, Motzenbecker FP, Degan RO. Withdrawal reactions from chlordiazepoxide ("Librium"). Psychopharmacologia. 1961;20(2):63–8.
34. Covi L, Lipman RS, Pattison JH, Derogatis LR, Uhlenhuth EH. Length of treatment with anxiolytic sedatives and response to their sudden withdrawal. Acta Psychiatr Scand. 1973;49:51–64.
35. Maletzky BM, Klotter J. Addiction to diazepam. Int J Addict. 1976;11:95–115.
36. Marks J. The benzodiazepines: use, overuse, misuse, abuse. Lancaster: M.T.P. Press Limited; 1978. 117p.
37. Petursson H, Lader M. Dependence on tranquillizers. Oxford University Press; 1984. 130 p.
38. Bourin M. Can one avoid dependence to the benzodiazepines? Klinik Psikopharmakologi Bülteni. 2001;11:78–81.
39. Bourin M, Urbaniak J. Effet rebond et syndrome de sevrage: Etude comparative entre deux benzodiazépines. Psychol Med. 1984;16:553–8.
40. Bourin M. Les Benzodiazépines. De la pharmacocinétique à la dépendance. Paris: Ed. Ellipses; 1989. 160 p.
41. Rickels K, Case WG, Schweizer EE, Swenson C, Fridman RB. Low-dose dependence in chronic benzodiazepine users: a preliminary report on 119 patients. Psychopharmacol Bull. 1986;22:407–15.
42. Longo LP, Johnson B. Addiction: part I. Benzodiazepines—side effects, abuse risk and alternatives. Am Fam Physician. 2000;61:2121–8.
43. Librans M, Gehring MT, Buadze A, Kalisch C. High-dose benzodiazepine dependence: a qualitative study of patients' perception on cessation and withdrawal. BMC Psychiatry. 2015;15:116.
44. Hood SD, Norman A, Hince DA, Melichar JK, Hulse GK. Benzodiazepine dependence and its treatment with low dose flumazenil. Br J Clin Pharmacol. 2014;77:285–94.
45. Liu L, Jian P, Zhou Y, Zhou J, Jia L, Tang M, Zhang R, Tang Y. Is the long-term use of benzodiazepines associated with worse cognition performance in highly educated older adults? Front Psychol. 2020;11:595623.
46. Culberson JW, Ziska M. Prescription drug misuse/abuse in the elderly. Geriatrics. 2008;63:22–31.
47. Bourin M, Malinge M. Controlled comparison of the effects and abrupt discontinuation of buspirone and lorazepam. Prog Neuro-Psychopharmacol Biol Psychiatr. 1995;19:567–75.

48. Bourin M, Thibaut F. Benzodiazepines: tackling the symptoms of withdrawal. Neuropsychiatry. 2013;3:263–5.
49. Bourin M. Mechanisms of action of anxiolytics. In: Gargiulo PÁ, Mesones Arroyo HL, editors. Psychiatry and neuroscience update. Cham: Springer; 2021. p. 195–211.
50. Licata SC, Rowlett JK. Abuse and dependence liability of benzodiazepine-type drugs: GABA(A) receptor modulation and beyond. Pharmacol Biochem Behav. 2008;90:74–89.

18 Phyto, Synthetic, and Endogenous Cannabinoids as Theoretical Possibilities of Therapeutic Molecules for the Treatment of Addictions

Virna M. Martín Giménez and Walter Manucha

Introduction

Cannabinoids are well-known molecules in the field of addictions. Psychoactive compounds derived from cannabis include phytocannabinoids as Δ9-tetrahydrocannabinol (Δ9-THC), as well as some endogenous and synthetic cannabinoids. They are directly interconnected with the reward system and, therefore, have addictive effects. Cannabinoids provoke these effects by a rise in tonic dopamine production within the ventral tegmental area, through a mechanism dependent on cannabinoid receptors type 1 (CB1). Thus, signals that are associated with the use of cannabis or other psychoactive cannabinoids may induce responses related to addictive drug seeking by causing phasic dopamine processes. Moreover, there is a dopamine-non-dependent mechanism associated with drug-seeking responses, which implicates endocannabinoid/glutamate interplay within the corticostriatal area of the reward system [1, 2]. Furthermore, Δ9-THC and its derived compounds usually causes several additional alterations on cognitive function, such as perception disorders, confusion, balance and coordination impairments, and euphoria, among others [3]. Likewise, endogenous cannabinoids may also provoke several adverse effects at central nervous system (CNS) level. In this regard, some evidences were considered. Anandamide (AEA) is metabolized by hydrolysis catalyzed by the enzyme fatty acid amide hydrolase (FAAH). If URB597, an inhibitor of this enzyme, is administered, its levels rise. This can affect various neurocognitive aspects such as learning, long-term potentiation, and memory through CB1 activation. All of this indicates that pharmacologically increasing AEA above physiological levels can sometimes be detrimental [4]. Yu et al. also found that AEA could alter neurocognitive function [5]. Another study suggested that increased levels of AEA may disturb microglial function and promote pro-inflammatory events at the CNS level [6]. Likewise, synthetic cannabinoids may cause anxiety, hypertension, agitation, paranoia, and renal/myocardial failure, among others [7]. This is the case of the synthetic cannabinoid NM2201 which may provoke multiple side effects such as double incontinence, aphasia, generalized hypertonia, lack of coordination on the left side, hyperreflexia, dense diaphoresis, fever, left hemiparesis,

V. M. Martín Giménez
Instituto de Investigaciones en Cs. Químicas, Facultad de Cs. Químicas y Tecnológicas, Universidad Católica de Cuyo, San Juan, Argentina
e-mail: vmartin@uccuyo.edu.ar

W. Manucha (✉)
Área de Farmacología, Departamento de Patología, Facultad de Ciencias Médicas, Universidad Nacional de Cuyo, Mendoza, Argentina

Instituto de Medicina y Biología Experimental de Cuyo (IMBECU), Consejo Nacional de Investigaciones Científicas y Tecnológicas (CONICET), Mendoza, Argentina

P. Á. Gargiulo, H. L. Mesones-Arroyo (eds.), *Psychiatry and Neuroscience Update – Vol. V*,
https://doi.org/10.1007/978-3-031-72219-6_18

tachycardia, hypertension, and seizures [8]. Moreover, JWH-210 (a strong CB1 receptor agonist) also has undesirable effects including tachycardia, nausea, hypokalemia, hypertension, drowsiness, restlessness and agitation, diplopia, syncope, signs of sympathomimetic toxicity, and convulsions [9].

However, nowadays cannabinoids have also been postulated to have therapeutic effects in multiple pathologies including cancer, dermatological and neurodegenerative diseases, among others. Of special interest, cannabinoids have also been explored as therapeutic agents useful in the treatment of substance abuse disorders [10]. Paradoxically, although the psychoactive effects of cannabinoids are usually dependent on the CB1 activation, the pharmacological management of this receptor may mediate beneficial effects in relation with different aspects associated with addiction to different drugs including opioids, cocaine, alcohol and nicotine, among the most relevant [11]. Pharmacological inverse agonists and antagonists of CB1 in the brain may attenuate the effects of addictive drugs related to reward and abuse. Despite this, their clinical use is hampered by potentially serious adverse effects, especially at the CNS level, which usually include an increased risk of depth anxiety and depression development (even reaching suicide), and other less serious effects such as nausea, diarrhea, hyporexia, and vomiting [12–15]. In fact, preclinical studies in rodent models have shown potential therapeutic effects of CB1 receptor-selective antagonists in the therapy of multiple addictions. However, only a few of these studies advanced to clinical trials, especially due to their severe psychiatric side effects of these antagonists because of their prolonged use. This was the case of rimonabant and other CB1 antagonists. These drugs were proved for the treatment of obesity and metabolic syndrome, but they were mostly withdrawn from the market. Moreover, pharmacological manipulation of cannabinoid receptor type 2 (CB2) may also be beneficial in the treatment of drug abuse disorders such as cocaine addiction [11].

In other words, cannabinoids may have a dual behavior; therefore, they may act not only as harmful and addictive drugs but also as beneficial substances in different circumstances [16]. This is because of CB1 and CB2 receptors have a great versatility in relation to their pharmacological behavior. Both may accept various types of agonists and antagonists and cause multiple responses. Different factors may promote their pharmacological diversity including their natural polymorphisms, alternative splice variants, phylogeny, distribution, and signaling pathways [17]. Thereby, many times, same receptors that participate in the beneficial effects of cannabinoids may also mediate—under some circumstances—multiple side effects. In this context, this chapter summarizes some of the most important therapeutic effects of cannabinoids in the field of addictions.

Therapeutic Potential of Phyto, Synthetic, and Endogenous Cannabinoids in the Treatment of Addictions

It is well known that changes in corticolimbic endocannabinoid signaling may promote the characteristic anxiety induced by alcohol withdrawal [18]. Some studies indicate that while simultaneous consumption of alcohol and cannabinoid agonists may cause undesirable side effects due to a synergism between them, the administration of CB1 antagonists may produce a significant reduction in the consumption of this addictive substance. Therefore, these antagonists could be useful as a therapeutic alternative for the treatment of alcohol dependence and addiction. Moreover, cannabinoid antagonists may also attenuate alcoholic withdrawal symptoms [19]. However, some authors have reported that smoking cannabis may cause a faster reduction in voluntary alcohol intake than in those individuals who do not [10]. In addition, the increase in endocannabinoid levels through the inhibition of monoacylglycerol lipase [MAGL, the enzyme charged in 2-arachidonoylglycerol (2-AG) hydrolysis], and/or Fatty Acid Amide Hydrolase [FAAH] could be a promising therapeutic approach for the treatment of anxiety-like phenotype induced by early alcohol abstinence [20]. In this regard, acute pretreatment with the FAAH inhibitor, URB597, administered to a mice alcohol drinking model caused a reduction in alcohol intake and preference after acute withdrawal. This effect was inhibited by pretreatment with an antagonist of CB1, suggesting a CB1 participation in the observed mechanism [21]. The pharmacological enhance in endogenous cannabinoids levels through the administration of JZL184 (an irreversible inhibitor for MAGL) to a murine model of chronic alcohol consumption and forced abstinence, prevented the increases in the activity of dorsal bed nucleus of the stria terminalis neuronal induced by abstinence, suggesting a therapeutic potential of endocannabinoids in the treatment of alcohol addiction [22]. Nevertheless, it was also found that the administration of DO34 (diacylglycerol lipase inhibitor), which reduces the biosynthesis of 2-AG, reduced the motivation to seek ethanol in alcoholic mice. Furthermore, the administration of AM404 (endocannabinoid transport inhibitor) or AM251 (CB1 antagonist) caused similar effects [23, 24]. These findings confirm that the effects of cannabinoids are highly variable, even under similar circumstances.

In relation to the opioid use disorder, it is widely demonstrated that CB1 agonists may be helpful in the treatment of this addiction [25]. In fact, a study showed an additive effect between Δ9-THC and oxycodone, suggesting the potential use of Δ9-THC to improve the therapeutic efficacy of opioids and reducing the abuse behavior associated with these substances [26]. Likewise, simultaneous pharmacological inhibition of FAAH and MAGL also decreased the heroin-seeking behavior [10]. However, the administration of a pharmacological inhibitor of CB1 at the level of the dorsal hippocampus showed that the blockade of CB1 signaling inhibited the restoration of morphine-conditioned place preference, confirming once again the dual pharmacological behavior of the endocannabinoid system [27].

Regarding methamphetamine addiction, JZL184 (inhibitor of MAGL) significantly decreased the reinstatement of methamphetamine-seeking behavior by both cue and stress in rats, while URB597 (inhibitor of FAAH), reduced only the reinstatement induced by cue. However, these effects were only observed when JZL184 and URB597 were simultaneously administered. Therefore, this would suggest that the increase of 2-AG at the brain level could avoid the reinstatement of behaviors related to methamphetamine-seeking and anxiety associated with its use [28].

In relation to cocaine use disorder, it has been suggested that pharmacological antagonism of CB1 may prevent relapses during this addiction, especially in individuals whose consumption is stress-related [29, 30]. A study showed that both rimonabant and JWH133 (CB2 receptor agonist) prevented the hyperlocomotion induced by cocaine in Swiss mice. Nevertheless, JZL184 (selective inhibitor of 2-AG hydrolysis) was also able to prevent the hyperlocomotion induced by cocaine after the administration of a sub-effective dose of rimonabant [31]. AM251 (CB1 antagonist) also inhibited the acquisition and expression of motor sensitization induced by cocaine in Swiss mice [32].

When considered nicotine addiction, most of the behavioral and neurochemical effects associated with this disorder may also be reduced by both antagonism and genetic deletion of CB1, and blockade of endocannabinoid uptake or metabolism. Therefore, these strategies may be promising in the therapy of nicotine dependence and in the prevention of relapses related to its consumption [33]. In this sense, the inhibition of the FAAH enzyme may reduce the addictive effect of nicotine in a mechanism mediated by CB1 receptor [34]. Likewise, Δ9-THC is able to decrease the symptoms associated with somatic withdrawal of nicotine. It may be suggested that MAGL inhibition may be helpful in the treatment of abstinence symptoms in individuals addicted to nicotine [35].

Therefore, cannabinoids may be useful pharmacological agents for the treatment of several addictions, including alcohol, opioid, methamphetamine, cocaine, and nicotine use disorders, and perhaps others.

Conclusion and Prospects

Despite the observed variability in the effects of phyto, synthetic, and endogenous cannabinoids, it is clear that they have an enormous therapeutic potential in the treatment of multiple addictions. The dual behavior of cannabinoids and their receptors usually is the reason for these compounds to be a cause or a solution for multiple addiction problems, especially related to the abuse of different substances. Researchers are mainly responsible for the fact that the cannabinoids used in the biomedical field is no longer a taboo subject, but also that they have been started to be used for therapeutic purposes, especially in those pathologies that do not have many pharmacological alternatives for its treatment, such as addictions.

As future prospects, new forms of cannabinoid administration could be used. This would allow drug targeting to avoid the non-specific biodistribution of these compounds. In this way, the appearance of multiple side effects associated with its therapeutic use could be prevented.

References

1. Spanagel R. Cannabinoids and the endocannabinoid system in reward processing and addiction: from mechanisms to interventions. Dialogues Clin Neurosci. 2020;22(3):241–50. https://doi.org/10.31887/DCNS.2020.22.3/rspanagel.
2. Ronan PJ, Wongngamnit N, Beresford TP. Molecular mechanisms of cannabis signaling in the brain. Prog Mol Biol Transl Sci. 2016;137:123–47. https://doi.org/10.1016/bs.pmbts.2015.10.002.
3. Gottschling S, Ayonrinde O, Bhaskar A, Blockman M, D'Agnone O, Schecter D, Suárez Rodríguez LD, Yafai S, Cyr C. Safety considerations in cannabinoid-based medicine. Int J Gen Med. 2020;13:1317–33. https://doi.org/10.2147/IJGM.S275049.
4. Basavarajappa BS, Nagre NN, Xie S, Subbanna S. Elevation of endogenous anandamide impairs LTP, learning, and memory through CB1 receptor signaling in mice. Hippocampus. 2014;24(7):808–18.
5. Yu S, Levi L, Casadesus G, Kunos G, Noy N. Fatty acid-binding protein 5 (FABP5) regulates cognitive function both by decreasing anandamide levels and by activating the nuclear receptor peroxisome proliferator-activated receptor ß/d (PPARß/d) in the brain. J Biol Chem. 2014;289(18):12748–58.
6. Ativie F, Albayram O, Bach K, Pradier B, Zimmer A, Bilkei-Gorzo A. Enhanced microglial activity in FAAH(-/-) animals. Life Sci. 2015;138:52–6.
7. Liechti M. Novel psychoactive substances (designer drugs): overview and pharmacology of modulators of monoamine signaling. Swiss Med Wkly. 2015;145:W14043.
8. Samra K, Boon IS, Packer G, Jacob S. Lethal high: acute disseminated encephalomyelitis (ADEM) triggered by toxic effect of synthetic cannabinoid black mamba. BMJ Case Rep 2017;2017.
9. Hermanns-Clausen M, Kithinji J, Spehl M, Angerer V, Franz F. Adverse effects after the use of JWH-210—a case series from the EU Spice II plus project. Drug Test Anal. 2016;8(10):1030–8.
10. Fraguas-Sánchez AI, Torres-Suárez AI. Medical use of cannabinoids. Drugs. 2018;78(16):1665–703. https://doi.org/10.1007/s40265-018-0996-1.
11. Fernández-Ruiz J, Galve-Roperh I, Sagredo O, Guzmán M. Possible therapeutic applications of cannabis in the neuropsychopharmacology field. Eur Neuropsychopharmacol. 2020;36:217–34. https://doi.org/10.1016/j.euroneuro.2020.01.013.
12. Schindler CW, Redhi GH, Vemuri K, Makriyannis A, Le Foll B, Bergman J, Goldberg SR, Justinova Z. Blockade of nicotine and cannabinoid reinforcement and relapse by a cannabinoid CB1-receptor neutral antagonist AM4113 and inverse agonist rimonabant in squirrel monkeys. Neuropsychopharmacology. 2016;41(9):2283–93. https://doi.org/10.1038/npp.2016.27.
13. Gueye AB, Pryslawsky Y, Trigo JM, Poulia N, Delis F, Antoniou K, Loureiro M, Laviolette SR, Vemuri K, Makriyannis A, Le Foll B. The CB1 neutral antagonist AM4113 retains the therapeutic efficacy of the inverse agonist rimonabant for nicotine dependence and weight loss with better psychiatric tolerability. Int J Neuropsychopharmacol. 2016;19(12):pyw068. https://doi.org/10.1093/ijnp/pyw068.
14. Robinson JD, Cinciripini PM, Karam-Hage M, Aubin HJ, Dale LC, Niaura R. Anthenelli RM; STRATUS Group. Pooled analysis of three randomized, double-blind, placebo controlled trials with rimonabant for smoking cessation. Addict Biol. 2018;23(1):291–303. https://doi.org/10.1111/adb.12508.
15. Manzanares J, Cabañero D, Puente N, García-Gutiérrez MS, Grandes P, Maldonado R. Role of the endocannabinoid system in drug addiction. Biochem Pharmacol. 2018;157:108–21. https://doi.org/10.1016/j.bcp.2018.09.013.
16. Martin Gimenez VM, Mocayar Maron FJ, Kassuha DE, Ferder L, Manucha W. Key aspects to consider about beneficial and harmful effects on the central nervous system by the endocannabinoid modulation linked to new cardiovascular therapies. Ann Pharmacol Pharm. 2019;4(2):11.
17. Howlett AC, Abood ME. CB1 and CB2 receptor pharmacology. Adv Pharmacol. 2017;80:169–206.
18. Henricks AM, Berger AL, Lugo JM, Baxter-Potter LN, Bieniasz KV, Petrie G, Sticht MA, Hill MN,

McLaughlin RJ. Sex- and hormone-dependent alterations in alcohol withdrawal-induced anxiety and corticolimbic endocannabinoid signaling. Neuropharmacology. 2017;124:121–33. https://doi.org/10.1016/j.neuropharm.2017.05.023.

19. Kleczkowska P, Smaga I, Filip M, Bujalska-Zadrozny M. Cannabinoid ligands and alcohol addiction: a promising therapeutic tool or a humbug? Neurotox Res. 2016;29(1):173–96. https://doi.org/10.1007/s12640-015-9555-7.
20. Bedse G, Centanni SW, Winder DG, Patel S. Endocannabinoid signaling in the central amygdala and bed nucleus of the stria terminalis: implications for the pathophysiology and treatment of alcohol use disorder. Alcohol Clin Exp Res. 2019;43(10):2014–27. https://doi.org/10.1111/acer.14159.
21. Zhou Y, Schwartz BI, Giza J, Gross SS, Lee FS, Kreek MJ. Blockade of alcohol escalation and "relapse" drinking by pharmacological FAAH inhibition in male and female C57BL/6J mice. Psychopharmacology. 2017;234(19):2955–70. https://doi.org/10.1007/s00213-017-4691-9.
22. Centanni SW, Morris BD, Luchsinger JR, Bedse G, Fetterly TL, Patel S, Winder DG. Endocannabinoid control of the insular-bed nucleus of the stria terminalis circuit regulates negative affective behavior associated with alcohol abstinence. Neuropsychopharmacology. 2019;44(3):526–37. https://doi.org/10.1038/s41386-018-0257-8.
23. Gianessi CA, Groman SM, Thompson SL, Jiang M, van der Stelt M, Taylor JR. Endocannabinoid contributions to alcohol habits and motivation: relevance to treatment. Addict Biol. 2020;25(3):e12768. https://doi.org/10.1111/adb.12768.
24. Basavarajappa BS, Joshi V, Shivakumar M, Subbanna S. Distinct functions of endogenous cannabinoid system in alcohol abuse disorders. Br J Pharmacol. 2019;176(17):3085–109. https://doi.org/10.1111/bph.14780.
25. Sloan ME, Gowin JL, Ramchandani VA, Hurd YL, Le Foll B. The endocannabinoid system as a target for addiction treatment: Trials and tribulations. Neuropharmacology. 2017;124:73–83. https://doi.org/10.1016/j.neuropharm.2017.05.031.
26. Nguyen JD, Grant Y, Creehan KM, Hwang CS, Vandewater SA, Janda KD, Cole M, Taffe MA. Δ^9-tetrahydrocannabinol attenuates oxycodone self-administration under extended access conditions. Neuropharmacology. 2019;151:127–35. https://doi.org/10.1016/j.neuropharm.2019.04.010.
27. Zhao X, Yao L, Wang F, Zhang H, Wu L. Cannabinoid 1 receptor blockade in the dorsal hippocampus prevents the reinstatement but not acquisition of morphine-induced conditioned place preference in rats. Neuroreport. 2017;28(10):565–70. https://doi.org/10.1097/WNR.0000000000000796.
28. Nawata Y, Yamaguchi T, Fukumori R, Yamamoto T. Inhibition of monoacylglycerol lipase reduces the reinstatement of methamphetamine-seeking and anxiety-like behaviors in methamphetamine self-administered rats. Int J Neuropsychopharmacol. 2019;22(2):165–72. https://doi.org/10.1093/ijnp/pyy086.
29. McReynolds JR, Doncheck EM, Vranjkovic O, Ganzman GS, Baker DA, Hillard CJ, Mantsch JR. CB1 receptor antagonism blocks stress-potentiated reinstatement of cocaine seeking in rats. Psychopharmacology. 2016;233(1):99–109. https://doi.org/10.1007/s00213-015-4092-x.
30. Martín-García E, Bourgoin L, Cathala A, Kasanetz F, Mondesir M, Gutiérrez-Rodriguez A, Reguero L, Fiancette JF, Grandes P, Spampinato U, Maldonado R, Piazza PV, Marsicano G, Deroche-Gamonet V. Differential control of cocaine self-administration by GABAergic and glutamatergic CB1 cannabinoid receptors. Neuropsychopharmacology. 2016;41(9):2192–205. https://doi.org/10.1038/npp.2015.351.
31. Gobira PH, Oliveira AC, Gomes JS, da Silveira VT, Asth L, Bastos JR, Batista EM, Issy AC, Okine BN, de Oliveira AC, Ribeiro FM, Del Bel EA, Aguiar DC, Finn DP, Moreira FA. Opposing roles of CB_1 and CB_2 cannabinoid receptors in the stimulant and rewarding effects of cocaine. Br J Pharmacol. 2019;176(10):1541–51. https://doi.org/10.1111/bph.14473.
32. Lopes JB, Bastos JR, Costa RB, Aguiar DC, Moreira FA. The roles of cannabinoid CB1 and CB2 receptors in cocaine-induced behavioral sensitization and conditioned place preference in mice. Psychopharmacology. 2020;237(2):385–94. https://doi.org/10.1007/s00213-019-05370-5.
33. Scherma M, Muntoni AL, Melis M, Fattore L, Fadda P, Fratta W, Pistis M. Interactions between the endocannabinoid and nicotinic cholinergic systems: preclinical evidence and therapeutic perspectives. Psychopharmacology. 2016;233(10):1765–77. https://doi.org/10.1007/s00213-015-4196-3.
34. Forget B, Guranda M, Gamaleddin I, Goldberg SR, Le Foll B. Attenuation of cue-induced reinstatement of nicotine seeking by URB597 through cannabinoid CB1 receptor in rats. Psychopharmacology. 2016;233(10):1823–8. https://doi.org/10.1007/s00213-016-4232-y.
35. Butler K, Le Foll B. Novel therapeutic and drug development strategies for tobacco use disorder: endocannabinoid modulation. Expert Opin Drug Discov. 2020;15(9):1065–80. https://doi.org/10.1080/17460441.2020.1767581.

19 New Nanotechnological Approaches for the Treatment of Addiction with Cannabinoids

Virna M. Martín Giménez and Walter Manucha

Introduction

The development of new treatments for addictions based on cannabinoids is currently hampered mainly by their psychoactive effects, which limits the adequate therapeutic management of patients with these pathologies. Another important aspect for taking into account is that people with addiction problems are emotionally unstable and many times suffer psychiatric and social issues which cause high rates of treatment discontinuation. For this reason, new pharmacotherapeutic strategies need to be implemented in order to improve the safety and adherence to treatment and consequently the clinical outcomes in these patients, without wasting the therapeutic potential of these compounds [1, 2]. The delivery of neurotherapeutic agents to the central nervous system (CNS) has been a great challenge for a long time, due to, among other limitations, the occurrence of systemic and central side effects associated with these therapies. In this sense, pharmaceutical nanoformulations are emergent solutions for this and other pharmacotherapeutic problems, since they offer targeted drug delivery, improved therapeutic efficacy, and reduced systemic and local adverse effects of neurotherapeutic agents. These nanoformulations allow effective drug transport by encapsulating or adsorbing it within or at the surface of the nanocarrier platform, respectively, thus preserving it from physicochemical and enzymatic degradation, as well as from the efflux transport mediated by P-glycoprotein. Moreover, the high surface-area-to-volume ratio of nanocarriers may significantly enhance the solubility of poorly water-soluble drugs loaded in them [3]. Nanoencapsulation is also advantageous due to their ability to provide a controlled drug release (modulating the rate of drug release or programming the release site in response to a remote or specific trigger of the therapeutic target, such as changes in pH, temperature, enzyme activity, etc.) and a long blood circulation time. These aspects allow enhancing the drug bioavailability in the specific organ, tissue, or cell in which they are required at the CNS level, using a minimal dose [4].

In general, conventional drug administration forms have variable/low bioavailability and short half-life, which result in an increased dosage frequency and side effects, consequently causing

V. M. Martín Giménez
Instituto de Investigaciones en Cs. Químicas, Facultad de Cs. Químicas y Tecnológicas, Universidad Católica de Cuyo, San Juan, Argentina
e-mail: vmartin@uccuyo.edu.ar

W. Manucha (✉)
Área de Farmacología, Departamento de Patología, Facultad de Ciencias Médicas, Universidad Nacional de Cuyo, Mendoza, Argentina

Instituto de Medicina y Biología Experimental de Cuyo (IMBECU), Consejo Nacional de Investigaciones Científicas y Tecnológicas (CONICET), Mendoza, Argentina

P. Á. Gargiulo, H. L. Mesones-Arroyo (eds.), *Psychiatry and Neuroscience Update – Vol. V*,
https://doi.org/10.1007/978-3-031-72219-6_19

ineffective therapies and non-compliance (low adherence to the treatment) with the patients. Therefore, nanotechnology-based pharmacotherapeutic approaches are more promising in terms of reducing dosage regimen and consequently improving the effectivity of treatments. As mentioned, nanomedicines may act at the both cellular and molecular levels, either improving the drug uptake into the cells or impeding the drug efflux mechanisms, thus keeping the drug within the cell for a longer period than conventional therapies [5]. Thus, the singular properties of nanocarriers (e.g., polymeric nanoparticles, liposomes, micelles, and bioconjugates, among others) have mainly been explored to improve different usual pharmacokinetic and pharmacodynamic disadvantages of drugs, especially related to solubility, bioavailability, stability, and side effects [6]. Notably, the attractive features and advantages of nanosystems used for controlled drug delivery have made possible their administration through several routes such as oral, ocular, parenteral, transdermal, among others, thus expanding and diversifying their therapeutic uses [7].

In this context, this chapter summarizes the main advantages of nanotechnology applied to medicine and they are highlighted, proposing its use in the development of new formulations for the administration of cannabinoids as novel therapeutic alternatives in the treatment of multiple addictive disorders.

Recent Nanotechnological Developments for the Administration of Cannabinoids with Different Pharmacotherapeutic Goals

Multiple studies have postulated the idea of developing and optimizing different cannabinoid delivery nanosystems for overcoming the limitations of these psychoactive drugs, thus pursuing pharmacotherapeutic objectives through the use of micro and nanoparticles, both lipid and polymeric [8, 9]. These nanoformulations have demonstrated their ability for achieving the effective encapsulation of these active principles, enhancing their solubility and stability, improving their pharmacokinetic behavior, preserving them from premature destabilization by different agents, prolonging their plasma half-life, and reducing or avoiding their side effects [10, 11]. In this sense, a study that evaluated the potential of inhaled nanoparticles for the treatment of lung cancer demonstrated that their use for this type of pathology could constitute a promising strategy to overcome the current clinical disadvantages associated with the undesirable psychoactive effects of cannabinoids [12]. Other authors informed that the synthetic cannabinoid CB13 (which has critical pharmacokinetic problems because of its poor aqueous solubility) encapsulated in nanoparticles of poly(d,l-lactide-co-glycolide) (PLGA) coated with poly(ethylene glycol) (PEG) [13, 14], proved a more prolonged and intense analgesic efficacy than non-nanoencapsulated CB13, which was observed up to 11 days after a single oral administration [15]. Synthetic cannabinoid WIN55, 212-2 (WIN) has not only proven to be a promising therapeutic agent in the cancer treatment but also provokes psychoactive adverse effects. In this regard, it was achieved by the synthesis of WIN-loaded nanomicelles conjugated with maleic styrene acid. Thereby, nanoencapsulated WIN showed a great reduction in its side effects and an efficacy similar to that of WIN in free form [16, 17]. The oral administration of Δ9-THC and cannabidiol (CBD) for the treatment of different pathologies is also highly limited because of their highly lipophilic nature that consequently leads to their poor aqueous solubility. Moreover, Δ9-THC and CBD are susceptible to liver first pass mechanisms. These unfavorable physicochemical and pharmacokinetic properties cause these phytocannabinoid molecules have poor and variable oral bioavailability. In order to overcome these obstacles, a nanoformulation carrier of Δ9-THC and CBD based on pro-nanolipospheres (PNL) was designed and developed. This PNL delivery nanosystem is of a combination approved for human consumption including a medium chain triglyceride, a co-solvent, surfactants, and piperine as a natural absorption enhancer and inhibitor of intestinal metabolism. Results of its clinical evaluation in human patients showed that a single oral dose of this nanoformulation caused a threefold increase for Δ9-THC and a fourfold increase for CBD in Cmax. It also caused a 1.5-fold increase for Δ9-THC and a 2.2-fold increase in area under the curve when compared to Sativex®, the first formulation of medicinal cannabis standardized globally. Therefore, this PNL delivery nanosystem could be used as the first standardized cannabinoid nanoformulation for oral administration, overcoming the benefits of conventional formulations for oral delivery of cannabinoids such as Sativex® [18, 19]. Moreover, the encapsulation of Δ(9)-THC in PLGA nanoparticles demonstrated a higher in vitro and in vivo anticancer activity of this phytocannabinoid compared to Δ(9)-THC in free form. Additionally, the bioactivity and biodistribution of this nanoformulation could be improved through its surface functionalization with biodegradable polymers. For instance, the speed rate of the sustained release of Δ(9)-THC from the nanoparticles may be increased or decreased by using PEG or chitosan, respectively. Biocompatibility studies showed an adequate in vivo safety profile of these nanoformulations, while protein adsorption tests demonstrated the protective role of PEGylation against opsonization and plasma clearance by reticuloendothelial system [20, 21]. Likewise, other studies have also shown a great antitumoral activity of polymeric microparticles, loaded with Δ(9)-THC in lung and other types of cancer [22, 23]. Similar results were obtained when the chemotherapeutic activity of CBD incorporated into microparticles of ε-polycaprolactone (PCL) was assessed. The enhancement of its therapeutic properties in comparison with the free drug was also demonstrated [24]. Solid lipid nanoparticles carrier of Δ9-THC-valine-hemisuccinate and Δ9-THC were tested and compared with an emulsion of these drugs in free form and with marketed formulations of timolol maleate and pilocarpine HCl. It was done in order to obtain comparative results about their efficacy in the treatment of glaucoma in a normotensive rabbit model. The cannabinoid nanoformulation caused an intraocular pressure drop more prolonged and more intense than that provoked by both these cannabinoids formulated in free form and the tested conventional marketed formulations. Therefore, the assessed Δ9-THC-valine-hemisuccinate nanoformulation has more promising therapeutic effects in the treatment of glaucoma than conventional pharmacotherapeutic formulations [25].

The therapeutic potential of the endogenous cannabinoid anandamide (AEA) has also been underestimated over time because of its pharmacokinetic and pharmacodynamic limitations related to unfavorable physico-chemical properties and—in some circumstances—undesirable psychoactive effects. In this regard, it has been demonstrated that the encapsulation of AEA in polymeric nanoparticles of PCL/Pluronic® F127 allowed overcoming the disadvantages related to its administration in free form. Of interest, this nanoformulation was able to reverse all altered cardiovascular markers and parameters in an in vivo model of cardiovascular remodeling caused by hypertension (spontaneously hypertensive rats) [26]. The incorporation of AEA in polymeric nanoparticles of PCL has also allowed its stable encapsulation for at least 4 months at different temperatures, which is of special interest considering that free AEA is stable for only about 24 h at room temperature. Likewise, the improvement of physicochemical properties of AEA encapsulated in polymeric nanoparticles has allowed exploring new biological applications of this endocannabinoid that cannot be exploited using AEA in free form. For instance, nanoformulated AEA has proved to have optimal bioactivity at different biological levels, including natriuretic activity on human renal proximal tubule cells [27]. In addition, nanoformulated AEA was able to reduce systolic blood pressure, inflammatory/oxidative markers both at the peripheral and central levels, and central apoptosis, punctually at the brain cortex in spontaneously hypertensive rats. This nanoformulated endocannabinoid stimulated neuroprotective signaling pathways that would involve the Wilms tumor transcription factor 1, the type I angiotensin II receptor, the inducible isoform of nitric oxide synthase, and the intracellular heat shock protein 70. Likewise, AEA encapsulated in polymeric nanoparticles allowed to reverse the abnormal behaviors observed in this animal model (exacerbated hyperactivity and lowered anxiety levels) without producing the classical adverse effects of AEA in free form at the CNS level [28].

Conclusion and Prospects

Nanotechnology may significantly help to highlight the therapeutic potential of cannabinoids in multiple diseases, including addiction disorders. However, it is necessary to analyze different factors and carefully evaluate which cannabinoid and which nanotechnological strategies will be used when developing the most appropriate treatment for each particular addiction problem.

The fast advance of nanotechnology and nanomedicine—especially in the last two decades—has allowed the development of multiple biocompatible cannabinoid nanocarriers useful in various therapeutic applications. They are able to prevent and treat different complex pathologies, thus significantly promoting the progress of medical knowledge. Nevertheless, cannabinoid delivery through pharmacotherapeutic nanoformulations for addictions treatment is a field not explored so far. Scientific evidence has proved that pharmacotherapeutic nanoformulations may offer considerable advantages compared to current/traditional therapies, which could not only be complemented but also even replaced by these nanotherapeutic alternatives in the near future. However, to transfer these achievements into clinical practice, it is needed to carry out an initial assessment of these novel nanoplatforms in extensive in vivo clinical trials. It may lead to obtain detailed data about the pharmacologic effects of administered nanomaterials in terms of their efficacy, optimal doses, and toxicity levels. Notably, the transferring of nanomedicines from the basic and preclinical research to clinical phase in patients requires a great investment of time and money, but it has been demonstrated that the huge benefits of nanomedicine may compensate all performed endeavors. Another important aspect to take into account is that the mentioned benefits of nanotechnology and nanomedicine, at many times, are clouded by long-term safety worries, regulatory issues, limitations related to scale-up and ineffective patent protection which have hampered their commercialization. Therefore, future efforts should be oriented to overcome these obstacles.

References

1. Suzuki J, Weiss RD. Cannabinoids for the treatment of opioid use disorder: where is the evidence? J Addict Med. 2021;15(2):91–2. https://doi.org/10.1097/ADM.0000000000000711.
2. Nance E. Careers in nanomedicine and drug delivery. Adv Drug Deliv Rev. 2019;144:180–9. https://doi.org/10.1016/j.addr.2019.06.009.
3. Pathak K, Akhtar N. Nose to brain delivery of nanoformulations for neurotherapeutics in Parkinson's disease: defining the preclinical, clinical and toxicity issues. Curr Drug Deliv. 2016;13:1205–21.
4. Gilani SJ, Jahangir MA, Chandrakala, Rizwanullah M, Taleuzzaman M, Shahab MS, Shakeel K, Aqil M, Imam SS. Nano-based therapy for treatment of skin cancer. Recent Pat Antiinfect Drug Discov. 2018;13(2):151–63. https://doi.org/10.2174/1574891X13666180911095440.
5. Uppal S, Italiya KS, Chitkara D, Mittal A. Nanoparticulate-based drug delivery systems for small molecule anti-diabetic drugs: an emerging paradigm for effective therapy. Acta Biomater. 2018;81:20–42. https://doi.org/10.1016/j.actbio.2018.09.049.
6. Sunoqrot S, Hamed R, Abdel-Halim H, Tarawneh O. Synergistic interplay of medicinal chemistry and formulation strategies in nanotechnology—from drug discovery to nanocarrier design and development. Curr Top Med Chem. 2017;17(13):1451–68. https://doi.org/10.2174/1568026616666161222111656.
7. Al-Lawati H, Binkhathlan Z, Lavasanifar A. Nanomedicine for the effective and safe delivery of non-steroidal anti-inflammatory drugs: a review of preclinical research. Eur J Pharm Biopharm. 2019;142:179–94. https://doi.org/10.1016/j.ejpb.2019.06.025.
8. Punyamurthula NS, Adelli GR, Gul W, Repka MA, ElSohly MA, Majumdar S. Ocular disposition of Δ^8-tetrahydrocannabinol from various topical ophthalmic formulations. AAPS PharmSciTech. 2017;18(6):1936–45. https://doi.org/10.1208/s12249-016-0672-2.
9. Nouar A. Cannabinoid encapsulating nanoparticles for atherosclerosis therapy. An in vitro study Master's thesis, Delft University of Technology. 2017.
10. Conte R, Marturano V, Peluso G, Calarco A, Cerruti P. Recent advances in nanoparticle-mediated delivery of anti-inflammatory phytocompounds. Int J

Mol Sci. 2017;18(4):709. https://doi.org/10.3390/ijms18040709.

11. Grottkau BE, Cai X, Wang J, Yang X, Lin Y. Polymeric nanoparticles for a drug delivery system. Curr Drug Metab. 2013;14(8):840–6. https://doi.org/10.2174/138920021131400105.
12. Ngwa W, Kumar R, Moreau M, Dabney R, Herman A. Nanoparticle drones to target lung cancer with radiosensitizers and cannabinoids. Front Oncol. 2017;7:208. https://doi.org/10.3389/fonc.2017.00208.
13. Durán-Lobato M, Muñoz-Rubio I, Holgado MA, Alvarez-Fuentes J, Fernández-Arévalo M, Martín-Banderas L. Enhanced cellular uptake and biodistribution of a synthetic cannabinoid loaded in surface-modified poly(lactic-co-glycolic acid) nanoparticles. J Biomed Nanotechnol. 2014;10(6):1068–79. https://doi.org/10.1166/jbn.2014.1806.
14. Martín-Banderas L, Alvarez-Fuentes J, Durán-Lobato M, Prados J, Melguizo C, Fernández-Arévalo M, Holgado MÁ. Cannabinoid derivate-loaded PLGA nanocarriers for oral administration: formulation, characterization, and cytotoxicity studies. Int J Nanomedicine. 2012;7:5793–806. https://doi.org/10.2147/IJN.S34633.
15. Berrocoso E, Rey-Brea R, Fernández-Arévalo M, Micó JA, Martín-Banderas L. Single oral dose of cannabinoid derivate loaded PLGA nanocarriers relieves neuropathic pain for eleven days. Nanomedicine. 2017;13(8):2623–32. https://doi.org/10.1016/j.nano.2017.07.010.
16. Xian S, Parayath NN, Nehoff H, Giles NM, Greish K. The use of styrene maleic acid nanomicelles encapsulating the synthetic cannabinoid analog WIN55,212-2 for the treatment of cancer. Anticancer Res. 2015;35(9):4707–12.
17. Greish K, Mathur A, Al Zahrani R, Elkaissi S, Al Jishi M, Nazzal O, Taha S, Pittalà V, Taurin S. Synthetic cannabinoids nano-micelles for the management of triple negative breast cancer. J Control Release. 2018;291:184–95. https://doi.org/10.1016/j.jconrel.2018.10.030.
18. Cherniakov I, Izgelov D, Barasch D, Davidson E, Domb AJ, Hoffman A. Piperine-pro-nanolipospheres as a novel oral delivery system of cannabinoids: pharmacokinetic evaluation in healthy volunteers in comparison to buccal spray administration. J Control Release. 2017;266:1–7. https://doi.org/10.1016/j.jconrel.2017.09.011.
19. Atsmon J, Cherniakov I, Izgelov D, Hoffman A, Domb AJ, Deutsch L, Deutsch F, Heffetz D, Sacks H. PTL401, a new formulation based on pro-nano dispersion technology, improves oral cannabinoids bioavailability in healthy volunteers. J Pharm Sci. 2018;107(5):1423–9. https://doi.org/10.1016/j.xphs.2017.12.020.
20. Martín-Banderas L, Muñoz-Rubio I, Prados J, Álvarez-Fuentes J, Calderón-Montaño JM, López-Lázaro M, Arias JL, Leiva MC, Holgado MA, Fernández-Arévalo M. In vitro and in vivo evaluation of Δ9-tetrahidrocannabinol/PLGA nanoparticles for cancer chemotherapy. Int J Pharm. 2015;487(1-2):205–12. https://doi.org/10.1016/j.ijpharm.2015.04.054.
21. Martín-Banderas L, Muñoz-Rubio I, Álvarez-Fuentes J, Durán-Lobato M, Arias JL, Holgado MÁ, Fernández-Arévalo M. Engineering of Δ9-tetrahydrocannabinol delivery systems based on surface modified-PLGA nanoplatforms. Colloids Surf B: Biointerfaces. 2014;123:114–22. https://doi.org/10.1016/j.colsurfb.2014.09.002.
22. Hernán Pérez de la Ossa D, Gil-Alegre ME, Ligresti A, Aberturas Mdel R, Molpeceres J, Torres AI, Di Marzo V. Preparation and characterization of Δ(9)-tetrahydrocannabinol-loaded biodegradable polymeric microparticles and their antitumoral efficacy on cancer cell lines. J Drug Target. 2013;21(8):710–8. https://doi.org/10.3109/1061186X.2013.809089.
23. Hernán Pérez de la Ossa D, Lorente M, Gil-Alegre ME, Torres S, García-Taboada E, Aberturas Mdel R, Molpeceres J, Velasco G, Torres-Suárez AI. Local delivery of cannabinoid-loaded microparticles inhibits tumor growth in a murine xenograft model of glioblastoma multiforme. PLoS One. 2013;8(1):e54795. https://doi.org/10.1371/journal.pone.0054795.
24. Hernán Pérez de la Ossa D, Ligresti A, Gil-Alegre ME, Aberturas MR, Molpeceres J, Di Marzo V, Torres Suárez AI. Poly-ε-caprolactone microspheres as a drug delivery system for cannabinoid administration: development, characterization and in vitro evaluation of their antitumoral efficacy. J Control Release. 2012;161(3):927–32. https://doi.org/10.1016/j.jconrel.2012.05.003.
25. Taskar PS, Patil A, Lakhani P, Ashour E, Gul W, ElSohly MA, Murphy B, Majumdar S. Δ9-tetrahydrocannabinol derivative-loaded nanoformulation lowers intraocular pressure in normotensive rabbits. Transl Vis Sci Technol. 2019;8(5):15. https://doi.org/10.1167/tvst.8.5.15.
26. Martín Giménez VM, Díaz-Rodríguez P, Sanz RL, Vivero-Lopez M, Concheiro A, Diez E, Prado N, Enrique Kassuha D, Alvarez-Lorenzo C, Manucha W. Anandamide-nanoformulation obtained by electrospraying for cardiovascular therapy. Int J Pharm. 2019;566:1–10. https://doi.org/10.1016/j.ijpharm.2019.05.047.
27. Martín Giménez VM, Russo MG, Narda GE, Fuentes LB, Mazzei L, Gamarra-Luques C, Kassuha DE, Manucha W. Synthesis, physicochemical characterisation and biological activity of anandamide/ε-polycaprolactone nanoparticles obtained by electrospraying. IET Nanobiotechnol. 2020;14(1):86–93. https://doi.org/10.1049/iet-nbt.2019.0108.
28. Martín Giménez VM, Mocayar Marón FJ, García S, Mazzei L, Guevara M, Yunes R, Manucha W. Central nervous system, peripheral and hemodynamic effects of nanoformulated anandamide in hypertension. Adv Med Sci. 2020;66(1):72–80. https://doi.org/10.1016/j.advms.2020.12.003.

Cannabis: A Drug of Addiction 20

Michel Bourin

Introduction

Cannabis (or hemp) is a plant native to equatorial regions, present in most regions of the globe. Among the various species of cannabis that exist, we must first distinguish the species intended for industry (containing little Tetra-Hydro-Cannabinol, THC) whose production is generally supervised by the States. Hemp fiber has, in fact, been used for several millennia in the textile, paper, and cordage industry because of its resistance. Hemp seeds have been used as feed for farm animals. Second, the species consumed for their psychotropic effects come from the Cannabis sativa family (including Cannabis indica, native to the Indian subcontinent). Certain parts of the plant—where Tetra-Hydro-Cannabinol (THC) is concentrated—can be consumed—either ingested or inhaled—for their psychotropic properties. Marijuana corresponds to the flowers of the plant and contains between 0.1% and 25% THC; hashish is a resin prepared from the plant (10–30% THC) and cannabis oil obtained after dissolving in a solvent contains 60–80% THC [1].

There is a new category of psychoactive substances which occupies an important place among the 98 new synthetic products (New psychoactive substances, NPS) detected for the first time in 2015 and notified in the early warning system of the European Union. Among these are the synthetic cannabinoids (SC) [2]. SC were detected in the drug market in the early 2000s. Most are manufactured by chemical companies located in Asia (China, South Korea) and are presented in powder form. SC are often presented as a smoking mixture. The preparation consists of dissolving a few tens of milligrams of SC with an industrial solvent such as acetone or methanol, then mixing or spraying them on plant materials. The mixture is then dried and packaged. Turnera diffusa as well as damiana (an herbal medicine known to increase sexual activity), lemon balm, mint, and thyme are commonly used as an herbal base in the preparation of smoking mixes. Other presentations of SC, imitating cannabis resin or incorporated into e-cigarette liquid cartridges, have also been identified. Given the growing public acceptance of recreational and medical marijuana, coupled with negative perceptions and increasing regulation of synthetic cannabinoid compounds, botanical marijuana is likely to remain more available and more popular than synthetic cannabinoids [3]. Cannabinoids are constituents of the marijuana plant (cannabis sativa plant). The main psychoactive ingredient is delta-9-tetrahydrocannabinol, known as THC. Marijuana effects vary based on individual factors and are produced by binding to the brain's specific receptors called cannabinoid receptors [4].

M. Bourin (✉)
Neurobiologie de l'anxiété et de la dépression, Université de Nantes, Nantes, France
e-mail: michel.bourin@univ-nantes.fr

P. Á. Gargiulo, H. L. Mesones-Arroyo (eds.), *Psychiatry and Neuroscience Update – Vol. V*,
https://doi.org/10.1007/978-3-031-72219-6_20

The Psychological Effects of Cannabis (THC)

Cannabis has many effects on perception, thoughts, and mood. Generally speaking, smoking cannabis induces a slight euphoria often accompanied by a feeling of relaxation. Some people feel more socially at ease, more uninhibited, and are able to communicate more easily. But the reverse is also described [5].

What Could Explain These Differences?

The effects may vary depending on the amount and concentration of THC in the product, the consumer's expectations, or their mental and physical dispositions. The frequency of consumption, its mode (smoked or ingested), and its context (for example, the atmosphere linked to a place) also play a decisive role [6].

Consumer Expectations

The effects are also dependent on the expectations of the consumer in relation to the product. For example, if a person anticipates that smoking a joint will relax them, this expectation of a relaxing effect will increase the possibility of actually achieving the desired state [7]. On the contrary, a fear related to consumption can precipitate an anxious state.

Frequency of Consumption

During the first experiments, cannabis has a stronger euphoric effect. On the other hand, more consumers that are regular describe a "habituation" which leads to a decrease in the euphoric and relaxing effects [8]. Habituation is also called tolerance. Regular consumption can lead to a drop in mood, motivation to do activities, and short-term memory (a memory system that allows you to temporarily retain information, such as a phone number) [9].

Amplifier of Emotions

Clinically, some patients describe emotional amplification. This is why they sometimes advise against using cannabis when the mood is low or when a person is anxious as it can also increase the intensity of these emotions and possibly lead to a feeling of anxiety, depression, or, at worst, produce a "bad trip" [10].

Acute Psychic Effects

The acute effects of cannabis on cognitive functioning have been tested in detail in various studies. The main result is an effect of amnesia on short-term memory [11]. In more regular consumers, the following phenomena are also observed: drowsiness, moderate euphoria, feeling of well-being, impaired perception of time, short-term memory problems and inability to perform several tasks simultaneously [12]. Heavy drinking associated with cannabis consumption can cause language or movement coordination problems, increased reaction time (slowness in reactions) as well as irritability or sadness [13]. Certain clinical observations have described an amotivational syndrome (decrease in cravings and social, academic or professional activities as well as a decrease or slowing down of ideas and emotional indifference) in very heavy consumers [14]. People are less affected by their surroundings. People who consume heavily and for a long time are also at risk of developing anxiety disorders, including panic attacks [15].

Rather, some people will have "interpretative ideas of reference" (feel they are in the center of the interest of others, or targeted by others) and threat [16]. Normally, if this is a substance-induced psychological disorder, it should go away after you stop using it. Otherwise, a psychiatric consultation is recommended to identify and manage any associated disorder.

What Is *Cannabis Addiction*?

It is common to distinguish between physical and psychological dependence. In general, physical addiction to THC is considered rather minor and psychological (emotional) addiction as more difficult to overcome. Nevertheless, 5–10% of regular cannabis users develop a physical dependence and the severity of this depends on the extent of the use [17].

In short, we talk about addiction when, on a lasting and daily basis, a person can no longer do without consuming a substance while the use of the product has harmful consequences on his life or creates real suffering. It means a loss of control over consumption behavior (notion of craving = irresistible impulse to consume). It is observed as a continued consumption despite the harmful effects on the consumer and his entourage. Criteria also include notions of tolerance (getting used to the substance and needing to take more to get the same effect) and withdrawal symptoms (symptoms related to stopping use) [18].

Who says dependence on a psychotropic substance says the need to take the drug regularly: when you stop, so-called withdrawal symptoms appear [19]. From the list below, two symptoms typically appear in more than half of the smokers trying to quit [20]:

- irritability, aggressiveness, stress;
- anxiety;
- sadness, inner discomfort, disturbed mood;
- sleeping trouble, seeing an excessive need to sleep;
- decreased appetite and weight loss;
- sweating or nausea;
- milder symptoms such as fatigue, weakness, yawning, psychomotor slowing down.

These symptoms are not very specific but are present in almost all drugs withdrawal.

Most symptoms begin 24–48 h after stopping consumption, reach their maximum intensity between the fourth and sixth day and generally last between 1 and 3 weeks, but they can go beyond in the case of very high consumption. Many of these symptoms are hindrances to withdrawal—potential causes of relapse [21].

The intensity of these symptoms is related to particular consumption habits and the amounts used. Stopping cannabis can be difficult to overcome and may lead to the recurrence of "discomfort" or psychological symptoms that the use of the drug was intended to alleviate. Deciding to quit is more than a matter of willpower, and may require outside help. 5–10% of regular consumers of cannabis are dependent. In fact, it all depends on the definition of addiction. We will approach this question from two angles. The first refers to the theories of learning (conditioning). The second meets the official diagnostic criteria of the "DSM IV" manual [22].

Addiction and Conditioning

Overall, a person who uses a substance seeks two types of rewards: a direct positive effect, for example, pleasure, or a decrease in psychological or internal discomfort [18]. Addiction occurs when the person loses control over their consumption despite negative consequences on their life or the associated suffering. In more detail, the maintenance of consumption can be explained by the theory of conditioning (which conditions us to repeat a behavior). For example, if a person produces a behavior that has positive consequences (a reward), they will naturally tend to reproduce it. However, smoking cannabis is associated in some people with a feeling of pleasure or a reduction in discomfort ("relaxing" effect, illustrated by a thought such as "ah, that relaxes me"). The use will therefore have a good chance of being repeated [23].

If the initiation to Cannabis results in a positive experience (e.g., sense of well-being), then a person will be tempted to reproduce the experience and, therefore, consume again (this is Skinner's operant conditioning) [24]. In addition, when a person finds themselves in a similar context (for example, going back to a place where they bought cannabis), the memory of the past experience will automatically come back to them and this will increase the risk of developing a craving, to consume, or even promote consumption (conditioning in the sense of Pavlov).

Addiction may be present when repeated use becomes such a necessity that it takes up a significant amount of space in a person's mind and generally in a person's life. In this sense, addiction arguably corresponds to the expression "to be addicted." This phenomenon could sometimes be favored by the occurrence of difficult events or series of events. This could promote the establishment of certain conditioning, by the relief felt, for example [25].

Clinical, Pathophysiological and Statistical Aspects of Cannabis Withdrawal Syndrome

The withdrawal syndrome has already been described for several years in several studies [26, 27], but it was not until the fifth version of the DSM that it appeared. It appears in more than half of patients about 3 days after stopping cannabis. Symptoms have a maximum intensity between 2 and 6 days off, most often disappear between 4 and 14 days and are sometimes present for up to 45 days [27].

DSM 5 describes the cannabis withdrawal syndrome in patients who have stopped massive and prolonged cannabis use (daily or more, for several months). The symptoms found are: irritability, anxiety, sleep disorders such as insomnia or strange dreams, decreased appetite with weight loss, restlessness, depressed mood, as well as physical symptoms such as tremors, abdominal pain, sweating, fever, chills, or headaches. These symptoms significantly alter the social or professional functioning of the patient and no other diagnosis explains the disorders [20].

If it is not systematic, the withdrawal syndrome can lead to a resumption of the use of cannabis or another substance. The greater the consumption, the more numerous and varied the symptoms of withdrawal syndrome [28]. The prevalence of withdrawal syndrome is higher in women [29]. While the symptoms are the same in both sexes, they are more intense in women. These differences may be related to the different expression of the endocannabinoid system according to the sexes [30, 31]. There is no correlation between serum THC levels and the intensity of craving symptoms, according to a study in hospitalized patients [32]. During isolated cannabis withdrawal, the appearance of psychiatric symptoms such as anxiety and depression is independent of serum THC levels. Only motor and cognitive disorders are associated with it. However, a drastic drop in serum THC levels may well lead to withdrawal symptoms in a regular smoker [33].

The architecture of sleep is disrupted during cannabis withdrawal, but its mechanisms remain, to this day, unknown [34]. In opioid users, sleep disturbances during cannabis withdrawal are more important than in patients who do not consume opiates, this being explained by the interactions of the endocannabinoid system and that of opiates in the mechanisms of sleep.

The Standardized Assessment of Withdrawal Syndrome

To fully understand the intensity of the symptoms that characterize the withdrawal syndrome that patients present, caregivers must be able to benefit from specific assessment tools to put in place the most appropriate treatment. Currently, health professionals have at their disposal seven specific standardized assessment grids or scales and eight subscales for the assessment of problematic cannabis use, to which are added eight other scales not specific to cannabis but adapted or used and tested for this drug. These specific standardized assessments can assess abuse of consumption, dependence on the product, disorders linked to cannabis use or the severity of the consequences of such consumption. To date, there is only one standardized assessment in the English language, validated for clinical practice, to assess the intensity of the withdrawal syndrome. An Australian team developed this tool, the Cannabis Withdrawal Scale [35]. This standardized self-assessment includes 19 items and assesses the intensity of the different symptoms rated from 0 to 10 during the last 24 h. The score adds up the results of the items. It ranges from 0 to 190 points and can be broken down into two subcategories: one, assessing the intensity of the withdrawal syndrome and the other, its negative impact.

For this, according to the DSMV classification, three additional criteria among the following seven, must be present:

- Develop tolerance to the product, or more simply get used to it, that is, gradually needing more of the substance to achieve the desired effect.
- Experience unpleasant symptoms when the substance is withdrawn (stopping or not being available).
- Cannabis withdrawal syndrome (CWS) is a criterion of cannabis use disorders (CUDs) (Diagnostic and Statistical Manual of Mental Disorders—Fifth Edition) and cannabis dependence (International Classification of Diseases [ICD]-10).

Patients describe irritability, nervousness or anxiety, trouble sleeping, and changes in appetite. Some people also evoke depression or a certain discomfort, but these symptoms are sometimes pre-existing to consumption in the sense that consumption was used to manage them. The substance is used more often, for longer, or in larger amounts than the person would like [27].

- A person wishes but fails to reduce or control his consumption. Much time is spent on activities necessary to obtain the substance (e.g., finding a supplier), using the product (e.g., continuously smoking), or recovering from its effects.
- Important social or professional activities are abandoned or reduced because of the use of the substance. For example, going much less often to see people around you or doing much less sport to focus on using cannabis.
- A person realizes that their use has caused or worsened a persistent problem (social, psychological, or physical) but continues it anyway (e.g., continuing to use cannabis even though the person admits to lack of motivation or depression related to this one).

Psychiatric Disorders Induced

Acute or chronic poisoning by cannabis is mainly due to the effects of delta 9 tetrahydrocannabinol (THC). The induced neuropsychic effects exhibit interindividual variability (difference between chronic and occasional users), as well as variability according to the quantity consumed and the mode of consumption [12]. In its minor form, acute poisoning results in mild, euphoric, dream-like intoxication associated with drowsiness. The duration of intoxication is quite short. There are cognitive effects during acute poisoning, mainly affecting memory, impaired psychomotor functions, with slower reaction time and impaired decision-making [12, 36]. These cognitive effects can last for up to 24 h after consumption [37].

It can also cause psychiatric symptoms. A state of anxiety can be induced. It mainly presents in the form of a panic attack and is spontaneously resolved with the elimination of delta 9 THC [38]. In chronic users, numerous studies have made it possible to associate this mode of consumption with cognitive disorders, mainly memory disorders [39]. There is an effect dose, cognitive impairment depending on the dose consumed, frequency of consumption, early onset (before 15 years) and duration of consumption and serum delta 9 THC level [40]. After a month's weaning, the disorders disappear (working memory and disorders attentional), while others persist (semantic memory, procedural memory, and decision making). In addition, regular consumers who started before the age of 18 do not fully recover their cognitive functions after a 1-year stoppage [41]. Consumers can suffer from an amotivational syndrome, which causes them to following symptoms: anhedonia, loss of interest, emotional detachment, loss of initiative, apragmatism and social withdrawal [42].

Particularity of Induced Psychotic Disorders

During acute consumption, approximately 15% of subjects free from psychiatric pathology who have consumed cannabis present positive psychotic symptoms in the form of delusional ideas interpretative of persecution, suspicion, or grandeur [43]. These psychotic symptoms are more frequent in chronic consumers during acute poisoning. They appear an hour and a half after consumption, last 2–4 h, then decrease and disappear at 12 or 24 h [7, 10, 44]. Other, rarer symptoms exist. Chronic consumption increases the risk of developing psychotic disorders. The increase in this risk is linked to several factors, such as the earliness of consumption (before 15 years), a dose effect, the cannabinoid level, consumption in predisposed subjects (family history of psychosis, schizotypal personality, etc.) and genetic and environmental factors. Cannabis is also a precipitating factor in schizophrenic disorders. Cannabis use is associated with an earlier onset of the disorders by around 2.5 years compared to never-consuming schizophrenic patients [45].

A neurodevelopmental disorder affecting the mesolimbic dopaminergic pathway appears to be associated with certain forms of schizophrenia [46]. In adolescence, at the stage of maturation of the systems already in place, mesocortical hypodopaminergy appears. It could encourage the consumption of cannabis in order to compensate for certain deficit expressions [47]. THC stimulation of CB1 receptors in the area of the ventral tegmentum increases the electrical activity of mesocortical neurons, which are reportedly insufficiently active. In doing so, it increases the release of dopamine in the cortex [48]. But simultaneously, it stimulates the activity of mesolimbic neurons (which are said to be already hyperactive), in relation to D2-type receptors, which would then trigger positive expressions (delusions, hallucinations, etc.) [49]. At the stage of brain maturation (in adolescence), THC is believed to worsen pre-existing disturbances. Behavioral disturbances evoking schizophrenic expressions have been observed after administration of cannabis, especially disruption of social interactions [50]. We know that the resumption of cannabis use in psychotics is often associated with a recurrence of the disorders. It has been established that the average length of hospital stay, in relation to resistance to antipsychotic therapy, is increased in patients who continue to use cannabis during hospitalization [51].

Various other indexes link cannabis and schizophrenia, such as overrepresentation of cannabis use in schizophrenics similarities between the effects developed by cannabis and certain disorders seen in schizophrenics, changes in anandamide levels in cerebrospinal fluid, correlated with psychotic expressions, abnormalities in the expression of CB1 receptors, and so on [52]. It should be noted that the antipsychotic, reputed to be the most active of all, clozapine, is the only one that possesses CB1 receptor antagonist activity, which could give it a grip on psychotic disorders that resist treatment, because of cannabis use [53].

Adolescents' marked sensitivity to the onset of psychosis in response to cannabis is because THC disrupts the maturation of certain brain systems at this time of life [54]. This maturation is made of a balance between the constitution of new synapses, in relation with a process of proliferation of the cylindrical ramifications of the neurons (the sprouting) and, simultaneously, the pruning of the synapses which are not stabilized by the function (the pruning) [55]. THC not only disrupts this balance but allows the formation of aberrant connections. Desensitization of CB1 receptors—induced by THC abuse—disrupts the role that these receptors play in these maturation phenomena [56].

Unfortunately, little is known about the factors explaining why some smoke cannabis while others do not. We know that genetic factors influence the risk of consuming cannabis (significant influence, estimated at 45%). However, so far, little information was available on the genetic factors in question. A recent study, involving a considerable number of subjects identified 16 genetic regions (14 of which have not been identified so far) associated with the risk of consuming cannabis (simple consumption, abuse, or addiction) [57].

The new genes identified not only provide information on the mechanisms involved in cannabis use (for example, the NCAM1 gene is involved in neurogenesis and dopaminergic transmission) but they also suggest that cannabis use should be considered as a relevant reflection of an individual's level of vulnerability for different psychiatric disorders or substance use [58]. Thus, the CADM2 gene (the most significant result of the study) is also associated with alcohol consumption and risk-taking behaviors [59]. The study also confirms the existence of an overlap between the genetic factors associated with cannabis consumption and those associated with personality traits (risk-taking behavior, extraversion), psychiatric disorders (ADHD, bipolarity, autism, schizophrenia) or substance abuse (tobacco, alcohol).

These studies also shed light on an old but still unresolved question: do you develop schizophrenia from using cannabis? Or is cannabis used to improve some symptoms of schizophrenia? The results strongly support a causal influence of schizophrenia. In other words, having a schizophrenic disorder would greatly increase the risk of using cannabis. This is consistent with the hypothesis that individuals at risk of developing schizophrenia experience prodromes and resort to cannabis for self-medication. Surprisingly, the results do not support cannabis use as a causative risk factor for schizophrenic disorders. However, these latter results should be taken with caution as the analysis performed lacked power.

References

1. Asati AK, Sahoo HB, Sahu S, Dwivedi A. Phytochemical and pharmacological profile of Cannabis sativa L. Int J Ind Herbs Drugs. 2017;2:37–45.
2. Hondebrink L, Nugteren-van Lonkhuyzen JJ, Hunault CC, van den Berg J, van der Gouwe D, van Riel AJHP. New psychoactive substances (NPS) in the Netherlands: occurrence in forensic drug samples, consumer drug samples and poisons center exposures between 2013 and 2017. Addiction. 2020;115:716–25.
3. Lauritsen KJ, Rosenberg H. Comparison of outcome expectancies for synthetic cannabinoids and botanical marijuana. Am J Drug Alcohol Abuse. 2016;42:377–84.
4. Atakan Z. Cannabis, a complex plant: different compounds and different effects on individuals. Ther Adv Psychopharmacol. 2012;2:241–54.
5. Stuyt E. The problem with the current high potency THC marijuana from the perspective of an addiction psychiatrist. Mo Med. 2018;115:482–6.
6. Volkow ND, Baler RD, Compton WM, Weiss SR. Adverse health effects of marijuana use. N Engl J Med. 2014;370:2219–27.
7. Bourin M, Chagraoui A. Abuse and misuse. In: Emilien G, Weikunat R, Lüdicke F, editors. Consumer perception of product risks and benefits. Dordrecht: Springer; 2017. p. 429–53.
8. Pesta DH, Angadi SS, Burtscher M, Roberts CK. The effects of caffeine, nicotine, ethanol, and tetrahydrocannabinol on exercise performance. Nutr Metab (Lond). 2013;10:71.
9. Stern CA, Gazarini L, Takahashi RN, Guimaraes FS, Bertoglio LJ. On disruption of fear memory by reconsolidation blockade: evidence from cannabidiol treatment. Neuropsychopharmacology. 2012;37:2132–42.
10. Mangot AG. Bad trip due to anticholinergic effect of cannabis. Gen Hosp Psychiatry. 2013;35:682.e5–6.
11. Schoeler T, Bhattacharyya S. The effect of cannabis use on memory function: an update. Subst Abus Rehabil. 2013;4:11–27.
12. Crean RD, Crane NA, Mason BJ. An evidence-based review of acute and long-term effects of cannabis use on executive cognitive functions. J Addict Med. 2011;5:1–8.
13. Subbaraman MS, Kerr WC. Simultaneous versus concurrent use of alcohol and cannabis in the National Alcohol Survey. Alcohol Clin Exp Res. 2015;39:872–9.
14. Kupfer DJ, Detre T, Koral J, Fajans P. A comment on the "amotivational syndrome" in marijuana smokers. Am J Psychiatry. 1973;130:1319–22.
15. Kedzior KK, Laeber LT. A positive association between anxiety disorders and cannabis use or cannabis use disorders in the general population—a meta-analysis of 31 studies. BMC Psychiatry. 2014;14:136.
16. Radhakrishnan R, Wilkinson ST, D'Souza DC. Gone to pot—a review of the association between cannabis and psychosis. Front Psychiatry. 2014;5:54.
17. Budney AJ, Roffman R, Stephens RS, Walker D. Marijuana dependence and its treatment. Addict Sci Clin Pract. 2007;4:4–16.
18. Goodman A. Addiction: definition and implications. Br J Addict. 1990;85:1403–8.
19. McLellan AT. Substance misuse and substance use disorders: why do they matter in healthcare? Trans Am Clin Climatol Assoc. 2017;128:112–30.
20. Bonnet U, Preuss UW. The cannabis withdrawal syndrome: current insights. Subst Abus Rehabil. 2017;8:9–37.
21. Connor JP, Stjepanović D, Le Foll B, Hoch E, Budney AJ, Hall WD. Cannabis use and cannabis use disorder. Nat Rev Dis Primers. 2021;7(1):16.

22. Karila L, Roux P, Rolland B, Benyamina A, Reynaud M, Aubin HJ, Lançon C. Acute and long-term effects of cannabis use: a review. Curr Pharm Des. 2014;20:4112–8.
23. Kogan NM, Mechoulam R. Cannabinoids in health and disease. Dialogues Clin Neurosci. 2007;9:413–30.
24. Köpetz CE, Lejuez CW, Wiers RW, Kruglanski AW. Motivation and self-regulation in addiction: a call for convergence. Perspect Psychol Sci. 2013;8:3–24.
25. Volkow ND, Wang GJ, Fowler JS, Tomasi D, Telang F, Baler R. Addiction: decreased reward sensitivity and increased expectation sensitivity conspire to overwhelm the brain's control circuit. Bioessays. 2010;32:748–55.
26. Vandrey R, Budney AJ, Kamon JL, Stanger C. Cannabis withdrawal in adolescent treatment seekers. Drug Alcohol Depend. 2005;78:205–10.
27. Budney AJ, Hughes JR. The cannabis withdrawal syndrome. Curr Opin Psychiatry. 2006;19(3):233–8.
28. Levin KH, Copersino ML, Heishman SJ, Liu F, Kelly DL, Boggs DL, Gorelick DA. Cannabis withdrawal symptoms in non-treatment-seeking adult cannabis smokers. Drug Alcohol Depend. 2010;111:120–7.
29. Herrmann ES, Weerts EM, Vandrey R. Sex differences in cannabis withdrawal symptoms among treatment-seeking cannabis users. Exp Clin Psychopharmacol. 2015;23:415–21.
30. Castelli MP, Fadda P, Casu A, Spano MS, Casti A, Fratta W, et al. Male and female rats differ in brain cannabinoid CB1 receptor density and function and in behavioural traits predisposing to drug addiction: effect of ovarian hormones. Curr Pharm Des. 2014;20:2100–13.
31. Craft RM, Marusich JA, Wiley JL. Sex differences in cannabinoid pharmacology: a reflection of differences in the endocannabinoid system? Life Sci. 2013;92:476–81.
32. Bonnet U, Borda T, Scherbaum N, Specka M. Abstinence phenomena of chronic cannabis-addicts prospectively monitored during controlled inpatient detoxification (Part II): psychiatric complaints and their relation to delta-9-tetrahydrocannabinol and its metabolites in serum. Drug Alcohol Depend. 2015;155:302–6.
33. Laprevote V, Gambier N, Cridlig J, Savenkoff B, Scala-Bertola J, Hingray C, Schwan R. Early withdrawal effects in a heavy cannabis smoker during hemodialysis. Biol Psychiatry. 2015;77:e25–6.
34. Gates P, Albertella L, Copeland J. Cannabis withdrawal and sleep: a systematic review of human studies. Subst Abus. 2016;37:255–69.
35. Allsop DJ, Norberg MM, Copeland J, Fu S, Budney AJ. The Cannabis Withdrawal Scale development: patterns and predictors of cannabis withdrawal and distress. Drug Alcohol Depend. 2011;119:123–9.
36. Morrison PD, Zoys V, McKeown DA, Lee TD, Holt DW, Powell JF, et al. The acute effects of synthetic intravenous Delta9-tetrahydrocannabinol on psychosis, mood and cognitive functioning. Psychol Med. 2009;39:1607–16.
37. Haney M, Comer SD, Ward AS, Foltin RW, Fischman MW. Factors influencing marijuana self-administration by humans. Behav Pharmacol. 1997;8:101–12.
38. Kamal BS, Kamal F, Lantela DE. Cannabis and the anxiety of fragmentation-A systems approach for finding an anxiolytic cannabis chemotype. Front Neurosis. 2018;12:730.
39. Klugman A, Gruzelier J. Chronic cognitive impairment in users of 'ecstasy' and cannabis. World Psychiatry. 2003;2:184–90.
40. Calabrese EJ, Rubio-Casillas A. Biphasic effects of THC in memory and conditioner. J Clin Invest. 2018;48(5):e12920.
41. Solowij N, Battisti R. The chronic effects of cannabis on memory in humans: a review. Curr Drug Abuse Rev. 2008;1:81–98.
42. De Aquino JP, Sherif M, Radhakrishnan R, Cahill JD, Ranganathan M, D'Souza DC. The psychiatric consequences of cannabinoids. Clin Ther. 2018;40:1448–56.
43. Pearson NT, Berry JH. Cannabis and psychosis through the lens of DSM-5. Int J Environ Res Public Health. 2019;16:4149.
44. Lowe DJE, Sasiadek JD, Coles AS, George TP. Cannabis and mental illness: a review. Eur Arch Psychiatry Clin Neurosis. 2019;269:107–20.
45. Sewell RA, Skosnik PD, Garcia-Sosa I, Ranganathan M, D'Souza D. Behavioral, cognitive and psychophysiological effects of cannabinoids: relevance to psychosis and schizophrenia. Braz J Psychiatry. 2010;32(Suppl 1):S15–30.
46. Patel KR, Cherian J, Gohil K, Atkinson D. Schizophrenia: overview and treatment options. P T. 2014;39:638–45.
47. Jacobus J, Tapert SF. Effects of cannabis on the adolescent brain. Curr Pharm Des. 2014;20:2186–93.
48. French ED. Delta9-Tetrahydrocannabinol excites rat VTA dopamine neurons through activation of cannabinoid CB1 but not opioid receptors. Neurosci Lett. 1997;226:159–62.
49. Li P, Snyder GL, Vanover KE. Dopamine targeting drugs for the treatment of schizophrenia: past, present and future. Curr Top Med Chem. 2016;16:3385–403.
50. Bossong MG, Niesink RJ. Adolescent brain maturation, the endogenous cannabinoid system and the neurobiology of cannabis-induced schizophrenia. Prog Neurobiol. 2010;92:370–85.
51. Patel R, Wilson R, Jackson R, Ball M, Shetty H, Broadbent M, Stewart R, McGuire P, Bhattacharyya S. Association of cannabis use with hospital admission and antipsychotic treatment failure in first episode psychosis: an observational study. BMJ Open. 2016;6(3):e009888.
52. Patel S, Khan SMS, Hamid P. The association between cannabis use and schizophrenia: causative or curative? A systematic review. Cureus. 2020;12(7):e9309.
53. Asenjo Lobos C, Komossa K, Rummel-Kluge C, Hunger H, Schmid F, Schwarz S, Leucht S. Clozapine

versus other atypical antipsychotics for schizophrenia. Cochrane Database Syst Rev. 2010;11:CD006633.

54. Squeglia LM, Jacobus J, Tapert SF. The influence of substance use on adolescent brain development. Clin EEG Neurosci. 2009;40:31–8.
55. Tau GZ, Peterson BS. Normal development of brain circuits. Neuropsychopharmacology. 2010;35:147–68.
56. Huestis MA, Gorelick DA, Heishman SJ, Preston KL, Nelson RA, Moolchan ET, Frank RA. Blockade of effects of smoked marijuana by the CB1-selective cannabinoid receptor antagonist SR141716. Arch Gen Psychiatry. 2001;58:322–8.
57. Demontis D, Rajagopal VM, Thorgeirsson TE, Als TD, Grove J, Leppälä K, Gudbjartsson DF, Pallesen J, Hjorthøj C, Reginsson GW, Tyrfingsson T, Runarsdottir V, Qvist P, Christensen JH, Bybjerg-Grauholm J, Bækvad-Hansen M, Huckins LM, Stahl EA, Timmermann A, Agerbo E, Børglum AD. Genome-wide association study implicates CHRNA2 in cannabis use disorder. Nat Neurosci. 2019;22:1066–74.
58. Prom-Wormley EC, Ebejer J, Dick DM, Bowers MS. The genetic epidemiology of substance use disorder: a review. Drug Alcohol Depend. 2017;180:241–59.
59. Arends RM, Pasman JA, Verweij KJH, Derks EM, Gordon SD, Hickie I, Thomas NS, Aliev F, Zietsch BP, van der Zee MD, Mitchell BL, Martin NG, Dick DM, Gillespie NA, de Geus EJC, Boomsma DI, Schellekens AFA, Vink JM. Associations between the CADM2 gene, substance use, risky sexual behavior, and self-control: a phenome-wide association study. Addict Biol. 2021;18:e13015.

21 Endocannabinoid System as an Important Cross-Talk Mechanism Related to Neurosciences and Psychiatry

Ali Ahmadalipour, Saeid Charsouei, Maryam Homaei, Siamak Razavi, Leila Hosseinzadeh Anvar, Adel Kashefi, and Carlos Tomaz

Endocannabinoid System

The present chapter reviews the latest information on the potential implication and the pharmacological modulation of the endocannabinoid system in psychiatric disorders. The very first findings of the endocannabinoid system, which is a widespread neuromodulatory and complex cell-signaling system, occurred in 1964 by scientists who were exploring Tetrahydrocannabinol (THC) [1], the most potent psychoactive component of cannabis. This system exists and is active in the body even if the individual does not use cannabis. More than 60 exogenous cannabis Sativa plant-based cannabinoids (phytocannabinoids) have been identified and structurally characterized, the most famous of which are THC, cannabidiol (CBD), and cannabinol (CBN).

Cannabis sativa has been used for several thousands of years both recreationally or for its psychotropic properties, while medicinal application of cannabis was because of some effects such as analgesia, incitement of appetite, and anti-emesis. In fact, reports of the medicinal effect of cannabis can be traced back to 2700 BC, and even at that time, the reports indicated the neuroprotective effect of this plant [2]. Parts of dried flower tops and leaves are smoked in the form of cigarettes, known as a 'joint' or a 'reefer'. The strongest form of the plant extracts' hash oil is a liquid, and the dried resins, called 'hashish'. Medicinal properties of the cannabis sativa from which marijuana (leaves, stems, seeds) is derived have been known for millennia [3]. The proposed uses included pain control, muscle spasms, antinausea, and epileptic seizures. In the past decades, synthetic cannabinoids, which are human-made mind-altering synthetic molecules acting as agonists of CB1 and/or CB2 receptors and mimic the

A. Ahmadalipour (✉) · M. Homaei · S. Razavi
Research Center of Psychiatry and Behavioral Sciences, Tabriz University of Medical Sciences, Tabriz, Iran
e-mail: alipoura@tbzmed.ac.ir

S. Charsouei · L. Hosseinzadeh Anvar
Department of Neurology, Faculty of Medicine, Tabriz University of Medical Sciences, Tabriz, Iran

A. Kashefi
Laboratory of Neuroscience and Behavior, Institute of Biology, University of Brasília, Brasilia, DF, Brazil

C. Tomaz
Laboratory of Neuroscience and Behavior and Graduate Program in Environment, University CEUMA, São Luís, MA, Brazil
e-mail: ctomaz@ceuma.br

P. Á. Gargiulo, H. L. Mesones-Arroyo (eds.), *Psychiatry and Neuroscience Update – Vol. V*,
https://doi.org/10.1007/978-3-031-72219-6_21

action of both endocannabinoids and phytocannabinoids, are produced.

To date, it is shown that the endocannabinoid system plays modifying role in wide-ranging physiological processes and functions such as sleep, mood, memory, appetite, reproduction, and fertility. The endocannabinoid system is composed of three central components: endocannabinoid neurotransmitters (agonists), receptors, and enzymes (Fig. 21.1).

Neurotransmitters (Agonists) of Endocannabinoid System

Endocannabinoids, also called endogenous cannabinoids, are lipid-based retrograde neurotransmitters that are similar to external cannabinoids, but they are synthesized by the organism. Two main endocannabinoids that are most studied include anandamide, also known as N-arachidonoylethanolamine (AEA) and

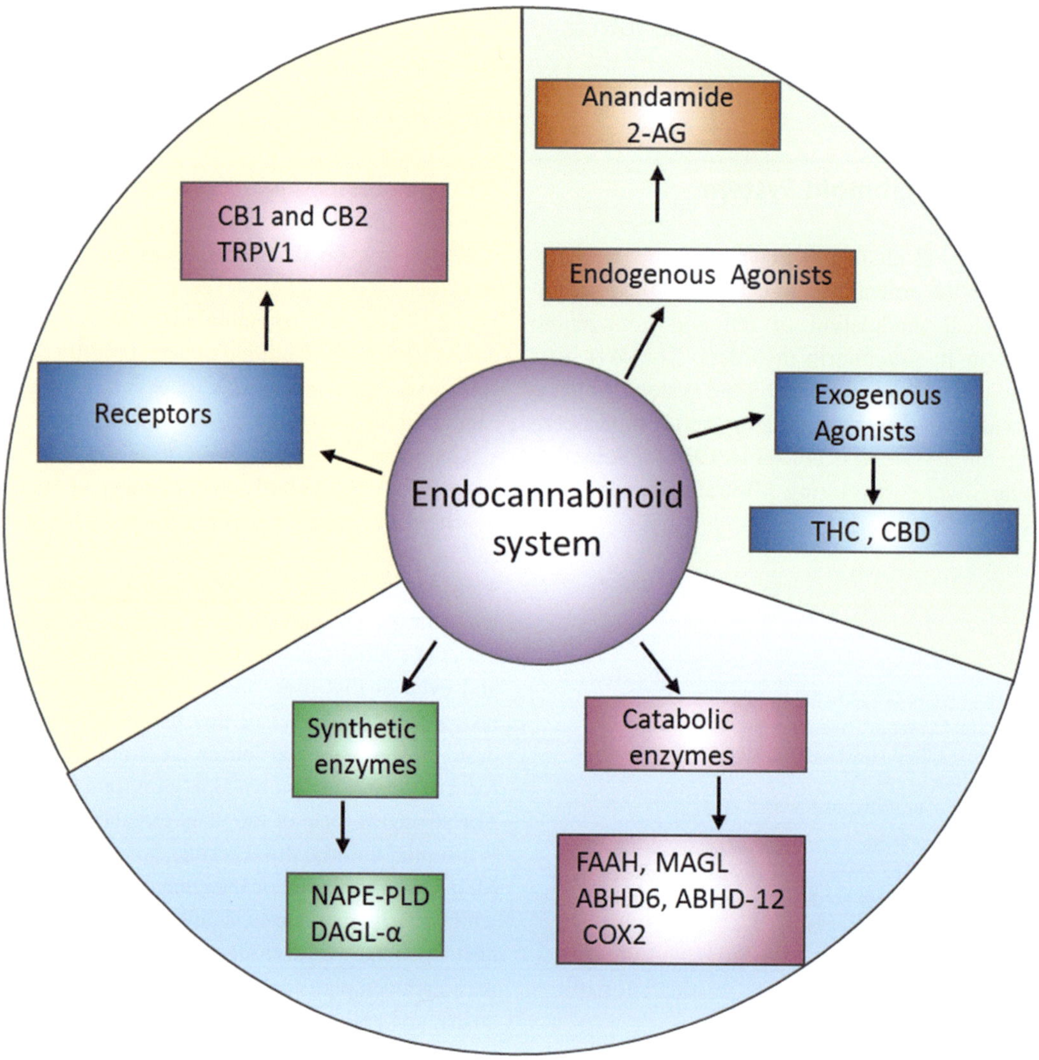

Fig. 21.1 Endocannabinoid system and its three central components: endocannabinoid neurotransmitters (agonists), receptors, and enzymes

2-arachidonoylglyerol (2-AG). Due to endocannabinoid's lipid nature, anandamide and 2AG are not stored in vesicles but are synthesized in the body as needed (on demand) by cleavage of membrane lipid precursors and are released from cells immediately through Ca^{2+}dependent mechanisms after their production. Therefore, it is hard to know what the typical levels are for each.

Receptors of Endocannabinoid System

The two main types of cannabinoid receptors identified and cloned are cannabinoid receptors 1 (CB1), which are typically found in the central nervous system (CNS), and cannabinoid receptors 2 (CB2), which are generally found in immune cells and the peripheral nervous system. They show about 44% overall identity to CB1 [4]. Preliminary studies showed that CB2 was not present in the brain [5, 6]. However, several later studies have shown the expression of CB2 receptors in brain cells, including astrocytomas, astrocytes, and microglia in Alzheimer's disease [6, 7]. The expression in microglia, T cells, and astrocytes in multiple sclerosis (MS) has been reported [8].

These receptors are encoded by *CNR1* and *CNR2* genes, respectively. In terms of number, CB1 receptors have the largest number of G protein-coupled receptors in the brain. They are particularly expressed in areas with known involvement in emotion and reward, addiction, and cognitive, motor and appetitive functions. They include brain areas such as the amygdala, cingulate cortex, substantia nigra, forebrain cortex (PFC), ventral pallidum, caudal putamen, nucleus accumbens (NAc), ventral tegmental area (VTA), and the lateral hypothalamus [9, 10].

Although CB2R is primarily expressed by immune cells, recent evidence suggests that such receptors are also found in neurons, endothelial cells, and glia in the brain. The similarity in the homology of amino acid sequences in humans and rodents is 97% and 81% for CB1 and CB2, respectively. CB1Rs and CB2Rs are associated with a similar transport system primarily through the regulation of intracellular levels of cAMP by interacting with G-protein-coupled receptors family (Gi/o, Gs–CB1R; Gi/o–CB2R) [11].

The effects of endocannabinoids depend on the location of the receptor and the kind of endocannabinoid which binds to it. For instance, endocannabinoids form an important endogenous mechanism in the spinal cord that modifies nociceptive transmission primarily through targeting CB1 receptors [12]. On the other hand, in immune cells, they might bind to a CB2 receptor to signal that the body is experiencing inflammation, a common sign of autoimmune disorders. CB1Rs directly inhibit the release of GABA, glutamate, and acetylcholine, which have broad effects on neuronal signaling in many neurotransmitter systems. Anandamide is an agonist to both CB1 and CB2 receptors with slightly greater affinity to CB1 and low efficacy as an agonist at both receptors [13]. Potent agonist effects at transient receptor potential (TRP) ion vanilloid channels (TRPV1) by anandamide are also reported [14]. Control of the intensity and duration of anandamide signaling is done by a two-step elimination process: the first stage is the internalization of anandamide by the cells [15] and the second stage is its hydrolysis by the intracellular membrane-bound amidases, mostly by fatty acid amide hydrolase (FAAH) [14, 16]. 2-AG binds with the same affinity at CB1 and CB2 and shows larger agonist efficacy than anandamide (Fig. 21.2).

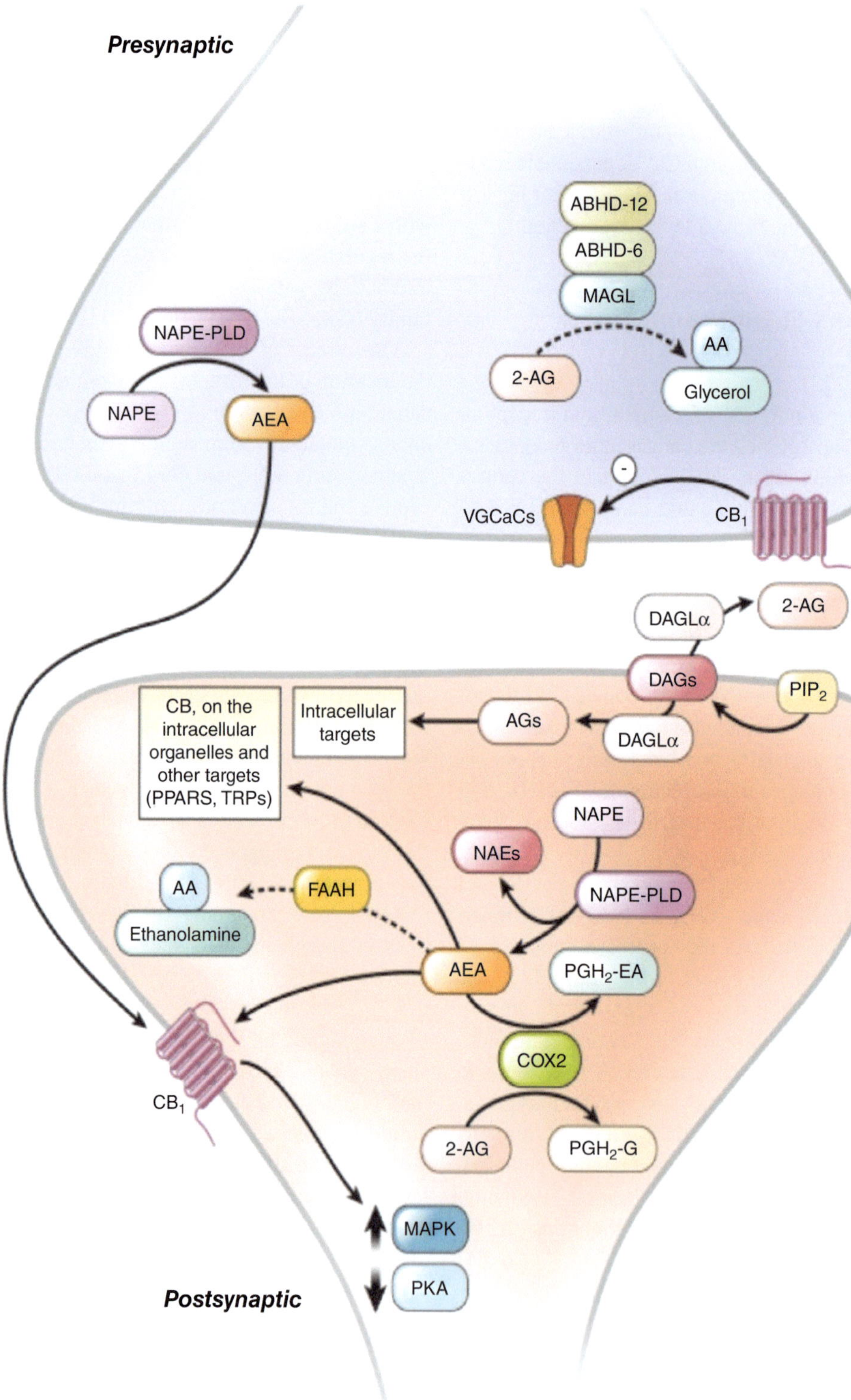

Fig. 21.2 Endocannabinoid system components and enzymes involved in the synthesis and break down of endocannabinoids in the nervous system. (Figure is used with permission from Ref. [16])

Enzymes of Endocannabinoid System

Anandamide is derived from Narachidonoyl-phosphatidylethanolamine (NAPE), a membrane phospholipid precursor. NAPEspecific phospholipase D (NAPEPLD) is likely to have a key role in anandamide formation, although the detailed mechanisms for this process are not yet well understood. 2AG derives mainly from the hydrolytic cleavage of arachidonic acid-esterified diacylglycerols (DAGs) by the DAG lipases (DAGLs) DAGLα and DAGLβ. They are members of serine hydrolase superfamily that use a catalytic serine for calcium-dependent cleavage of DAGs in a sn-1 selective manner [17]. There are two key enzymes responsible for breaking down endocannabinoids once they've done their function. They are FAAH, which breaks down anandamide, and monoacylglycerol acid lipase (MAGL), which typically breaks down 2-AG. 2-AG is also partly catabolized by α, β-hydrolase 6 (ABHD6), cyclooxygenase 2 (COX2), and FAAH (Fig. 21.3).

The Functions of the Endocannabinoid System

The endocannabinoid system is a complicated and versatile system that plays a modulatory role in many physiological functions that contribute to homeostasis, which refers to the stability of the internal environment, including:

- Mood and behaviors
- Learning and memory
- Motor control
- Sleep
- Digestion and appetite
- Metabolism
- Immune system responses such as inflammation
- Cardiovascular system function
- Reproductive system function
- Muscle function
- Liver function
- Bone growth and remodeling
- Skin and nerve function

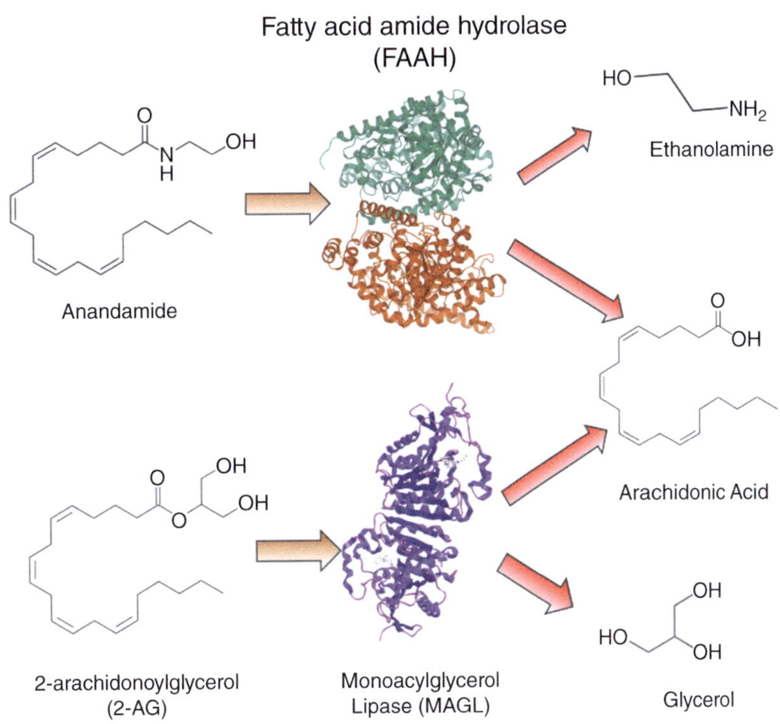

Fig. 21.3 Two important and most studied enzymes responsible for catabolism of endocannabinoids: fatty acid amide hydrolase (FAAH), which breaks down anandamide, and monoacylglycerol acid lipase (MAGL), which typically breaks down 2-AG

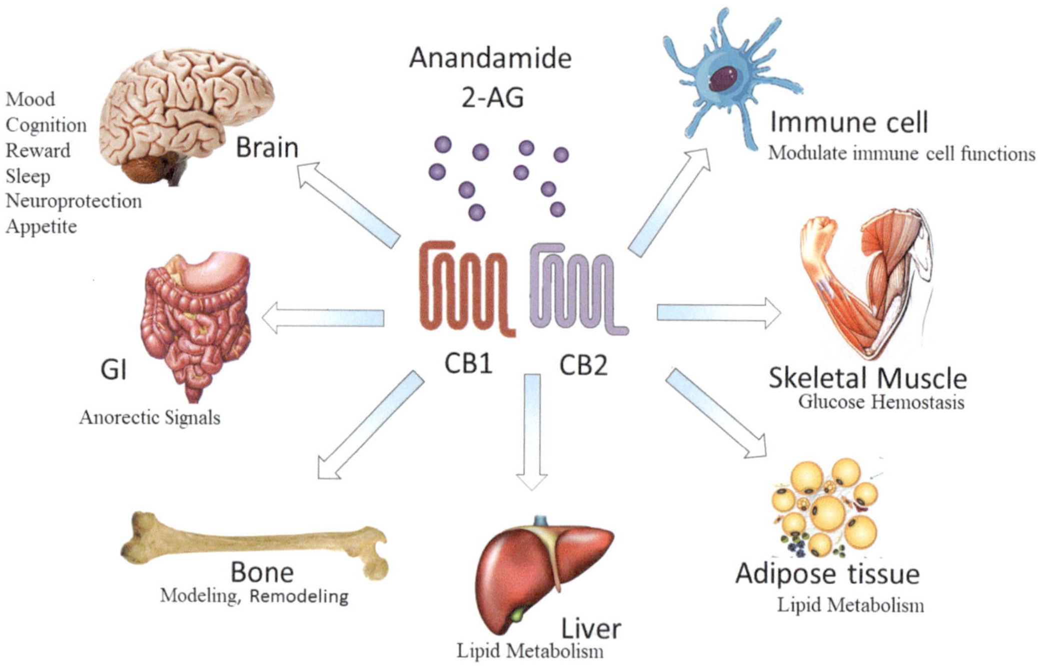

Fig. 21.4 Some functions of the endocannabinoid system mediated by CB1 and CB2 receptors

In addition, dysfunction of this system has been involved in:

- Stress and anxiety disorders
- Neurologic and psychiatric disorders
- Chronic pain
- Obesity (Fig. 21.4)

Clinical Endocannabinoid Deficiency (CECD) Theory

Clinical endocannabinoid deficiency (CECD) theory was presented in 2001 [18], but more thoroughly explored in 2004 [19]. This theory proposes that dysfunction in the endocannabinoid system or low endocannabinoid levels in the body can lead to the development of certain conditions. CECD theory is based on the concept that some neurotransmitter deficiencies are related to several CNS disorders, e.g., dopamine in parkinsonian syndromes, acetylcholine in Alzheimer's disease, and norepinephrine and serotonin in depression. A similar deficiency in endocannabinoid levels may be equally evident in certain disorders that show predictable clinical features as a consequence of this deficiency. A review article in 2016 proposed that CECD theory could clarify why some people develop fibromyalgia, migraine, and irritable bowel syndrome due to the common feature in the symptomatology of these conditions, demonstrating central sensitization and hyperalgesia with probable common causal pathophysiology [20]. In certain conditions, due to acquired or congenital reasons, endocannabinoid signaling tone becomes defective and may lead to pathophysiological syndromes. It has been documented that there was a statistically significant difference (lower) in cerebrospinal fluid anandamide levels in migraineurs [21], and other studies in people with post-traumatic stress disorder, using advanced imaging, have revealed endocannabinoid system hypofunction [20]. Clinical data have also made evidence for improved sleep, decreased pain, and other advantages to cannabinoid treatment and approaches in lifestyle affecting the endocannabinoid system. If CECD does play any kind of role in these conditions, targeting the endocannabinoid system could be the missing key to treatment, but more research is needed.

Endocannabinoid System and Depression

A number of potential mechanisms have been extensively documented as contributing factors to the cause of depression. The depression monoamine hypothesis based on antidepressant therapies on monoamine systems (including the serotonin, dopamine, and noradrenaline systems) has been a critical focus in the research and treatment of depression for the last decades and has dominated available information on the pathophysiology of depression for a long time. However, there is now a common agreement about the etiology of this psychiatric disorder that is much more complex and drug discovery needs to move beyond the monoamine systems to progress patient outcomes.

Other studies in this field that confirmed mood improvement in marijuana smokers and its antidepressant-like actions made a new idea about the etiology of major depressive disorder (MDD) and new goals for new antidepressant drugs [22]. THC mediates most of marijuana's mood-related and psychoactive effects. Though high-dose cannabis use is associated with increased risks for psychosis, anxiety disorders, depression, and cognitive deficiency, particularly among teenagers, a great number of depressed patients (30–64%) utilize cannabis as a method of self-medication. This effort to control depressive symptoms using cannabis suggests possible therapeutic benefits for depression [22].

It has been shown that several specific genetic polymorphisms in CB1 and CB2 receptors are associated with major depression and bipolar disorder [22, 23] and resistance to treatment was found in depression patients having a single nucleotide polymorphism in the CNR1 gene (CB1 receptor) [24, 25]. The potent effects of the endocannabinoid system on neurotransmission, neuroendocrine, and inflammatory processes, which are known to be deranged in depression, are suggested by extensive evidence [26]. Cannabidiol (CBD) has been shown to exert some antidepressant effects in animal models of depression. These effects may be due to CBD's facilitation of 5HT1A receptor activity, facilitation of endocannabinoid activity, and/or facilitation of hippocampal neurogenesis.

Inhibitors of FAAH are addressed for capable antianxiety drugs, but human studies on stress and affective phenotypes and genetically reduced FAAH activity are scarce. In a related study in 2016 by Lazary et al., the effect of a functional polymorphism of FAAH (FAAH C385A or rs324420), in which the A allele is associated with low FAAH activity and high anandamide concentration, was investigated together with childhood adversity on the depressive and anxious phenotypes in 858 individuals from the general population and Childhood Adversity Questionnaire (CHA). It was used to evaluate early life traumas [27]. They found that the frequency of the A allele was greater among subjects with high Zung Self-Rating Depression Scale (ZSDS) scores in comparison with the CC genotype. Additionally, the CHA and FAAH C385A have shown a strong gene-environment interaction, namely, significantly higher depression, and anxiety scores were demonstrated in the A allele carriers if they had high CHA scores in comparison with the CC genotype (Fig. 21.5).

C385A (rs324420) is the most studied and functional polymorphism of *FAAH* and has been reported to be related to several functions, phenotypes, and disorders such as biopsychosocial disorder, mental diseases, obesity, etc. [28, 29]. Some of other SNPs include: rs324420, rs932816, rs324419, rs324418, rs2295632, rs2295633, rs3766246, rs6429600, rs932816, rs4141964, and others mentioned in table (Table 21.1). The association between these SNPs and lots of neurological and psychiatric disorders are studied in the past two decades. Some of these studies reported an association and some of them reported no association (30–44).

It is shown that the activity of common antidepressants, such as selective serotonin reuptake inhibitor-escitalopram, the tricyclic imipramine, and selective inhibitor of noradrenaline reuptake-

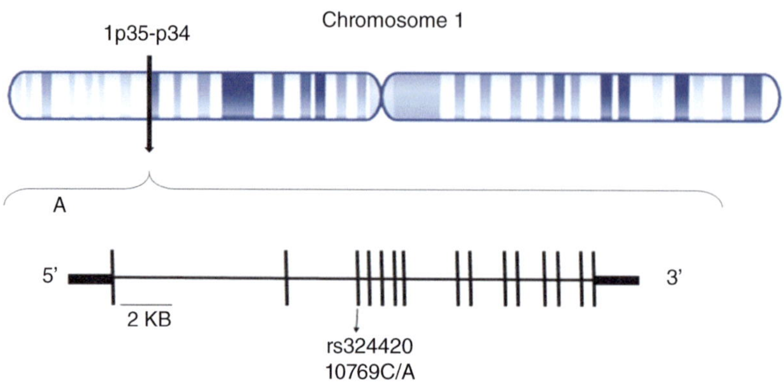

Fig. 21.5 Location of the human FAAH (or FAAH1) gene is on the short (p) arm of chromosome 1 at section 3 band 3, and its length is 20 kb. It comprises 15 exons with much conserved intron-exon borders. The rs324420 or C385A polymorphism on the coding region at position 385 of this gene is a missense mutation with the nucleotide cysteine replacement to adenine

Table 21.1 Summary of some of *FAAH* gene SNPs with their relationships

Phenotypes	Related	Unrelated	References
Parkinson-related pain	rs324419		Greenbaum et al. [30]
Post-traumatic stress disorder	–	rs324419, rs913168, rs3766246, rs6703669, rs7524148	Pardini et al. [31]
Pain	rs932816, rs2295633, rs3766246, rs4141964	rs324419, rs2295632	Kim et al. [32] and Cajanus et al. [33]
Eating disorder	–	rs324419, rs873978, rs932816, rs2295632	Müller et al. [34]
Obesity	rs324418, rs873978, rs2295632, rs2295633, rs6429600	rs3766246, rs6703669, rs12029329, rs41305628, rs41309147, rs2295633	Lieb et al. [35], Durand et al. [36] and Müller et al. [37]
Addiction	rs2295633, rs4141964	rs4141964, rs6703669, rs11576941	Palmer et al. [38], Bidwell et al. [39] and Melroy-Greif et al. [40]
Fatigue	rs2295633, rs3766246	rs6703669	Hillard et al. [41] and Dlugos et al. [42]
Schizophrenia	rs2295633, rs6429600	–	Si et al. [43]
ADHD	rs2295633	–	Ahmadalipour et al. [44]

reboxetine, can be potentiated by cannabinoid (CB) receptor ligands [45, 46].

The neurobiological basis of the antidepressant effects of rapid-acting therapeutic interventions in the treatments of depression within a few days or even hours including sleep deprivation (SD), deep brain stimulation (DBS), transcranial magnetic stimulation (TMS), electroconvulsive therapy (ECT), exercise, intravenous infusion of N-methyl-D-aspartate antagonist ketamine, and intravenous administration of Thyrotropin Releasing Hormone (TRH) is most likely different from today's first-line treatments and not sufficiently understood up to now. Interestingly, all these fast-acting interventions share a common feature which is the activation of the endocannabinoid system.

Endocannabinoid System and Psychosis

Some evidence for the role of the endocannabinoid system in both mood and psychotic disorders is provided by postmortem, cerebrospinal fluid, peripheral, and in vivo imaging studies. The endocannabinoid system seems to be unusual in studies with people with symptoms of psychosis and offers a valuable target for illness treatment and measurement. The relevance of the endocannabinoid system to psychosis is through the association between cannabis use and the onset and course of the disorder and the antipsychotic properties of CBD.

Animal research that focused on the relationship between the endocannabinoid system and schizophrenia relies on the assessment of sensorimotor gating deficits by the prepulse inhibition (PPI) paradigm [47–49]. The CB1 receptor was found to be critically involved in schizophrenia. It is shown that the activation of CB1 receptors induces psychotic-like effects, while the blockade of these receptors presents opposite actions [50]. Phencyclidine-induced disruption of PPI was eliminated significantly with the administration of AM251 (CB1 antagonist) in a similar way to clozapine [51], and counteract deficits in recognition memory or increased behavioral despair in the FST in the phencyclidine model of psychosis [52].

Elevated anandamide was detected in the peripheral blood in treated and untreated patients withschizophrenia compared to healthy controls [53, 54]. These alterations in anandamide were detected when measured in whole blood, plasma, and serum [53, 55]. Contrary to patients with schizophrenia, elevation in serum anandamide was not detected in antipsychotic-naïve patients with first-episode psychosis [56, 57]. Three of four studies that measured other *N*-acylethanolamines detected elevated levels of either oleoylethanolamide (OEA) or palmitoylethanolamide (PEA) in patients with schizophrenia who were treated or clinically stable [55], or of both OEA and PEA in patients with comorbid substance use disorders [54]. Finally, 2-AG levels in plasma did not differ significantly between healthy individuals and patients with schizophrenia, with or without comorbid substance use disorders [55].

In a recent meta-analysis performed to identify the differences in the endocannabinoid system markers between healthy controls and people with schizophrenia, from a total of 18 studies, five of them, including 226 patients and 385 controls, reported significantly higher concentrations of anandamide in the CSF of patients than controls. In 9 studies involving 411 controls and 344 patients, anandamide levels were significantly higher in the blood of patients compared to controls. Additionally, in 3 studies with 179 controls and 88 patients, a significantly higher expression of CB1 on peripheral immune cells was reported in schizophrenia patients compared to controls [58]. Higher endocannabinoid system tone was found at an early stage of the disorder in individuals who were antipsychotic-naïve or free and it had an inverse association with symptom severity and was normalized after successful treatment. Moderate to a high level of heterogeneity in methods was found between studies.

Endocannabinoid System and Epilepsy

Epilepsy is the most common chronic neurological disease that can have an emotional and psychological impact on people with this disorder and their families and statistics show that about 65 million people worldwide have epilepsy [59]. Epilepsy affects mental and physical function and is defined as when a patient has two or more seizures without a reversible underlying stimulus. Seizures occur when a group of nerve cells undergoes an abnormal electrical discharge that alters person's level of consciousness, movements, and reactions. Despite medication and other available treatments, many patients continue to have seizures that severely limit their education, occupation, and other activities in life. Each type of epilepsy has its own characteristics and response to its own treatment.

It is generally accepted that complete seizure control with drugs is reported in 50% of patients and a significant improvement is seen in 25% of patients [60]. About one-third of epileptic patients show drug resistance. Drug resistance in epilepsy is defined as the patient receiving at least two appropriate drug treatments and seizures persisting [61]. In these patients, existing drug therapies are ineffective in controlling seizures [62]. There is a great desire to develop new drugs with anticonvulsant properties, especially the factors that affect new receptors, in the hope that it will help patients with drug resistance to anticonvulsants [63].

The use of cannabis has received a lot of attention in recent years. Evidence for the use of cannabis to treat seizures dates back to 2900 BC, which was common among the Sumerians and was used among the Arabs in the twelfth century. Cannabis has been used in the United States since 1854 to treat depression, pain, muscle cramps, insomnia, and anorexia. Gowers reported a disease controlled by cannabis in his seizures in the mid-nineteenth century [64]. Devinsky et al. [65] found that patients receiving cannabidiol (a component of cannabis) had fewer seizures than placebo and that about 5% of patients had their seizures completely controlled. Some recent studies show that facilitating or activating the endocannabinoid (EC) system in rodents has antiepileptic effects.

In simple models of acute seizures, anticonvulsant effects of acute CB1R agonism are shown in rodents, whereas converse effects are induced by CB1R antagonists in the same models [66]. However, when more complex models of epilepsy, neuroprotection, and epileptogenesis are examined using such ligands, a less simplistic narrative emerges. In 2017, CB1 (Cnr1) and CB2 (Cnr2) single-knockout mice have been generated by Shane Rowley et al. [67]. Provoked behavioral seizures were found in 30% of double-knockout mice, and following 24/7 electroencephalographic and video monitoring, 80% of animals were found to be epileptic [67]. The importance of the endocannabinoid system in maintaining the stability of the neural network is determined based on these findings.

Among important phytocannabinoids, CBD has a more consistent antiepileptic efficacy than THC [68]. Although CBD does not activate cannabinoid receptors, it does interact with a number of other signaling systems such as transient receptor potential vanilloid type 1 (TRPV1)-mediated signaling which may be the most relevant pathway in the anticonvulsant effect of CBD [2, 68]. In 2016, Devinsky and colleagues examined the safety and tolerability of CBD and in 214 patients, their findings showed that CBD could reduce seizure frequency and might have an adequate safety profile in children and young adults with highly treatment-resistant epilepsy [69].

Endocannabinoid System and Stress

A growing body of evidence suggests an important and integral regulator role for the endocannabinoid system in the stress response. The association between stress-induced regulation of endocannabinoid system signaling and the consequential role changes in its signaling and many effects of stress have been indicated in many studies. Findings within human populations have shown that cannabis use typically causes an improvement in relaxation, a dampening of perceived stress, and a reduction of feelings of anxiety [70]. Considering that activation of CB1 receptors is responsible for the physiological actions of cannabis, it makes sense that the endocannabinoid system's normal function might dampen or buffer against the effects of stress.

Through a wide range of stress models, it is mostly shown that stress results in bidirectional alterations in the two endocannabinoid agonists, anandamide and 2-AG, with stress exposure increasing 2-AG levels and reducing anandamide levels. Additionally, a loss or downregulation in the expression of CB1 receptors has been shown in almost every brain region examined by various studies in the animal models exposed to chronic stress paradigms. Considering the functional role of alterations in the signaling of endocannabinoids during stress, studies have shown that the reduction of anandamide levels might play some role as a part of the stress response, such as increases in anxiety behavior and activation of the hypothalamic-pituitary-adrenal (HPA) axis. Inversely, the increased signaling of 2-AG may play a role in adaptation and termination of the HPA axis, as well as potentially contributing to modifications in pain perception, synaptic plasticity, and memory. Translational studies have demonstrated that the signaling of endocannabinoids may play an important role in the regulation of many similar animal domains and appears to be a central constituent in the regulation of various aspects of the stress response. Deficiencies in this system might increase the vulnerability to stress-related psychiatric disorders, including depression, anxiety, and post-traumatic stress disorder (PTSD). Collectively, these data create a compelling argument that eCB signaling is an important regulatory system in the brain; especially, the areas of the brain that largely function to buffer against many of the effects of stress. Therefore, the dynamic changes in this system contribute to different aspects of the stress response (Fig. 21.6).

Endocannabinoid System and Drug Addiction

One of the most important recurrent chronic disorders in the modern world is drug addiction, which has created a huge health burden around the world. There is currently no effective treatment available to control this complex disorder due to difficulties in finding new treatment targets. Therefore, there is a serious need to find new therapeutic approaches in this field. Several studies suggest that the endocannabinoid system plays an essential role in the neurological context underlying opioid addiction [71]. The mesocorticolimbic system, which is very important in initiating and sustaining drug use and compulsion and losing behavioral control during drug addiction, is one of the parts of the brain where endocannabinoids and cannabinoid receptors are widely distributed.

Given the identification of the essential role that CB1 receptors play in addiction disorder, the theory of the production and possible use of a commercial CB1 receptor antagonist in the treatment of addiction has been strengthened. However, the numerous side effects of these drugs, especially in the field of psychiatry, led to the withdrawal of these drugs from the market, and numerous research programs in this field, which were being carried out by various companies, were stopped. On the other hand, the use of the endocannabinoid system to develop new drugs in the field of addiction treatment is being considered with new research strategies that have

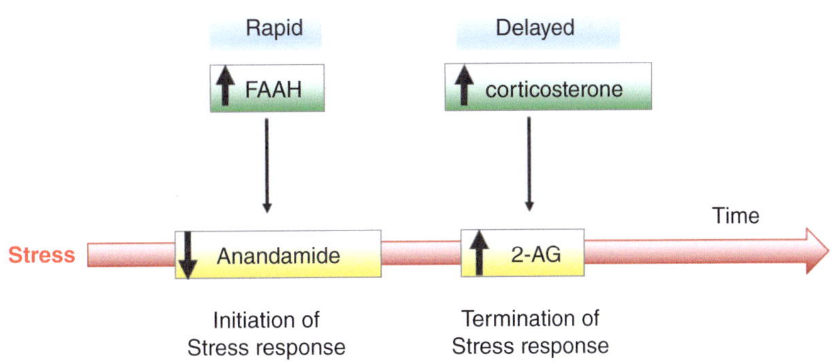

Fig. 21.6 Temporal dynamics of anandamide and 2-arachidonoyl glycerol (2-AG) alterations following stress exposure

fewer side effects. For example, allosteric negative modulators of CB1 receptors as well as substances that target CB2 receptors are such research strategies. Given the important role of CB2 receptors in addiction, high hopes have been raised for the development of new therapeutic approaches for addiction.

Neuropsychiatric Disorders and Probiotic; Possible Role of the Endocannabinoid System

Almost 1800 different phyla and 40,000 bacterial species live in the human gastrointestinal system hosts [72], collectively known as microbiota. A large body of evidence indicates a link between brain function and gut microbiota.

In a recent study about the cross-talk between gut microbiota and neuropsychiatric disorders, Pearson-Leary et al. reported that gut microbiota contributes to the depressive-like behavior and inflammatory processes in the hippocampus of stress vulnerable rodents [73]. Another recent study revealed the potential pathway by which targeting the gut microbiota with probiotics (nutrients for intestinal bacteria) can modify the peripheral immune response and alter neuroinflammation in middle age [74].

The increase in the number of microbiota in the large intestine has anxiolytic and cognitive improving effects in both humans and rodents [75]. Extensive evidence shows that dysregulation and abnormalities in the brain-gut axis contribute to the etiology of a variety of neuropsychiatric disorders [76].

Brain-derived neurotrophic factor (BDNF) and N-methyl-d-aspartate (NMDA) receptor of glutamate are suggested as key factors in the effects of probiotics and the gut-brain axis interaction [75]. Probiotic feeding raises central BDNF and modulates NMDA receptors. It seems that not only BDNF and NMDA receptors, but also other players have an important role in the neurobehavioral effects of probiotics and the gut-brain axis communication. Here we hypothesize that the modulation of the EC system is most likely associated with improvement of neuropsychiatric disorders by probiotic administration. EC system is a modulatory neurotransmission system that is a very important signaling system not only in the brain but also in peripheral tissues [77]. The EC system has been called one of the most widespread and multifunctional signaling systems ever discovered. The role of the EC system in the pathophysiology of neuropsychiatric disorders is well documented in recent years [78]. There are several lines of evidence suggesting that the EC system may be an important regulator of various aspects of probiotic responses.

First, recent evidence suggests that one of the mechanisms by which the intestinal microbiota affects the host is regulating the gut EC system. For example, the intestinal microbiota has been shown to regulate the EC tone in intestinal and adipose tissues and the intestinal microbiota controls anandamide content, its degrading enzyme FAAH, and receptor expression in intestinal and adipose tissues [79]. Changing intestinal microbiota leads to increased EC system activity with higher expression of CB1R (cannabinoid receptor 1) mRNA and anandamide [80].

Second, elevating the levels of intrinsic gut Lactobacilli with selective antimicrobials increases brain BDNF concentrations in mice [81]. BDNF functions are mediated by several mechanisms, and one of the most important of them is mutual interaction with the EC system. In fact, a positive correlation between the EC system and BDNF levels is demonstrated [82]. It is shown that BDNF attenuates inhibitory transmission by inducing the postsynaptic release of ECs that act retrogradely to suppress GABA release in the somatosensory cortex [83].

Furthermore, probiotic feeding modulates NMDA receptors. It has been shown that EC signaling is triggered by NMDA receptor-mediated calcium entry into rat hippocampal neurons [84]. Also, the activation of NMDA receptors can directly contribute to the generation of EC signaling through elevating postsynaptic Ca^{2+} concentration. Strong activation of NMDA receptors alone induced endocannabinoid release and suppressed the cannabinoid-sensitive synaptic transmission. Mild activation of NMDA receptors, which by itself caused the little effect, enhanced the endocannabinoid release driven by muscarinic receptors or I-mGluRs (Fig. 21.7).

Therefore, increasing the growth of gut microbiota with probiotics may afford greater benefits to the brain. Most studies focus on the influence of the BDNF and NMDA receptors in mediating neurobehavioral improvements of probiotics as these are believed to be involved in synaptic plasticity and cognitive function. BDNF is an important trigger for ECs synthesis and release [85]. Strong activation of NMDA receptors alone induced ECs release [84]. In addition, modulating gut microbiota with prebiotics changes the EC system tone [80].

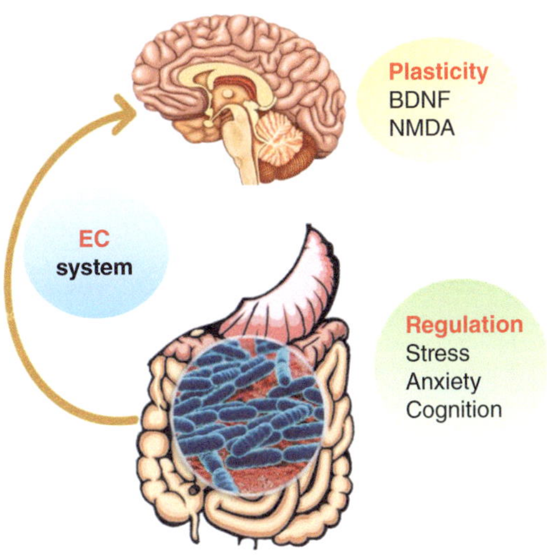

Fig. 21.7 Possible role of the endocannabinoid system in the relationship between neuropsychiatric disorders and probiotic

Therefore, finding the pathways and mechanisms by which the GI microbiota contribute to the modulation of the EC system activity could generate new insights relevant to the development of new therapies for neuropsychiatric disorders.

In a recent study in an animal model, the results showed that microbiome changes are associated with reduced endocannabinoid signaling and reduced adult neurogenesis in the hippocampus. To explain this association, it is suggested that stress-induced alterations in the gut microbiome resulted in a reduction of some fatty acid metabolites which are precursors of endocannabinoids. This proposes a direct pathway by which bacteria in the GI tract can probably cause mood disorders and might be the mechanism, at least in part, that associates mood disorders to microbiota dysbiosis, which in turn might influence the composition of the gut microbiota through modulation of the immune system and physiological regulations. It is also shown that in humans suffering from depression, Lactobacillus microbiome strains are lower than normal levels. Additionally, dysregulations in hippocampal endocannabinoid systems have been linked to several human neurological disorders. However, these findings make no claim to propose that newly discovered pathway is the only gut-brain mechanism that affects mood. Instead, this may be one of the many ways that environmental stress can lead to depression, and hopefully these gut-brain connections will be revealed in the future studies and lead to novel treatments for a variety of mood disorders (Fig. 21.8).

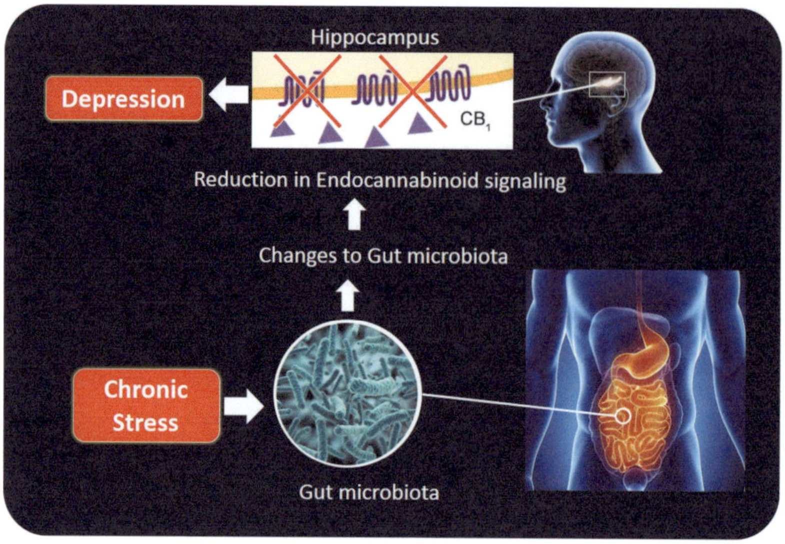

Fig. 21.8 Microbiome alterations due to chronic stress are associated with reduced endocannabinoid signaling and reduced adult neurogenesis in the hippocampus which can lead to many situations such as depression

Conclusion

Based on the topics discussed in this chapter, it seems that the endocannabinoid system is one of the attractive subjects for research in various fields of medicine, especially in the field of numerous mental diseases and psychiatric disorders. The Endocannabinoid system is known later than systems like the sympathetic and parasympathetic systems; the serotonergic system, the dopaminergic system, and so on, and therefore, less research has been done about the function of this system compared to other physiological systems. Therefore, it is necessary to design and conduct various research in the field of this system.

References

1. Gaoni Y, Mechoulam R. Isolation, structure, and partial synthesis of an active constituent of Hashish. J Am Chem Soc. 1964;86(8):1646–7.
2. Perucca E. Cannabinoids in the treatment of epilepsy: hard evidence at last? J Epilepsy Res. 2017;7(2):61–76.
3. Kompoliti K, Metman LV. Encyclopedia of movement disorders. 2010:1–1632.
4. Munro S, Thomas KL, Abu-Shaar M. Molecular characterization of a peripheral receptor for cannabinoids. Nature. 1993;365(6441):61–5.
5. Griffin G, Wray EJ, Tao Q, McAllister SD, Rorrer WK, Aung M, et al. Evaluation of the cannabinoid CB2 receptor-selective antagonist, SR144528: further evidence for cannabinoid CB2 receptor absence in the rat central nervous system. Eur J Pharmacol. 1999;377(1):117–25.
6. Scotter EL, Abood ME, Glass M. The endocannabinoid system as a target for the treatment of neurodegenerative disease. Br J Pharmacol. 2010;160:480–98.
7. Benito C, Núñez E, Tolón RM, Carrier EJ, Rábano A, Hillard CJ, et al. Cannabinoid CB2 receptors and fatty acid amide hydrolase are selectively overexpressed in neuritic plaque-associated glia in Alzheimer's disease brains. J Neurosci. 2003;23(35):11136–41.
8. Benito C, Romero JP, Tolón RM, Clemente D, Docagne F, Hillard CJ, et al. Cannabinoid CB1 and CB2 receptors and fatty acid amide hydrolase are specific markers of plaque cell subtypes in human multiple sclerosis. J Neurosci. 2007;27(9):2396–402.
9. Parsons LH, Hurd YL. Endocannabinoid signalling in reward and addiction. Nat Rev Neurosci [Internet]. 2015;16(10):579–94. https://doi.org/10.1038/nrn4004.
10. Adamczyk P, Papp M. On the role of the endocannabinoid system in cocaine addiction. In: Neuropathology of drug addictions and substance misuse. 2016. p. 48–62.
11. Preedy VR. Neuropathology of drug addictions and substance misuse. 2016;2:1–1143.
12. Yang F, Xu Q, Shu B, Tiwari V, He SQ, Vera-Portocarrero LP, et al. Activation of cannabinoid CB1 receptor contributes to suppression of spinal nociceptive transmission and inhibition of mechanical hypersensitivity by Aβ-fiber stimulation. Pain. 2016;157(11):2582–93.
13. Laredo SA, Marrs WR, Parsons LH. Endocannabinoid signaling in reward and addiction: from homeostasis

to pathology. Endocannabinoids Lipid Mediat Brain Funct. 2017;16(10):257–318.
14. Vaughn LK, Denning G, Stuhr KL, De Wit H, Hill MN, Hillard CJ. Endocannabinoid signalling: has it got rhythm? Br J Pharmacol. 2010;160(3):530–43.
15. Fu J, Bottegoni G, Sasso O, Bertorelli R, Rocchia W, Masetti M, et al. A catalytically silent FAAH-1 variant drives anandamide transport in neurons. Nat Neurosci. 2012;15(1):64–9.
16. Sharkey KA, Wiley JW. The role of the endocannabinoid system in the brain–gut axis. Gastroenterology. 2016;151:252–66.
17. Shin M, Ware TB, Hsu KL. DAGL-beta functions as a PUFA-specific triacylglycerol lipase in macrophages. Cell Chem Biol. 2020;27(3):314–21.e5.
18. Russo E. Hemp for headache: an in-depth historical and scientific review of cannabis in migraine treatment. J Cannabis Ther. 2001;1(2):21–92.
19. Russo EB. Clinical endocannabinoid deficiency (CECD): can this concept explain therapeutic benefits of cannabis in migraine, fibromyalgia, irritable bowel syndrome and other treatment-resistant conditions? Neuroendocrinol Lett. 2004;25:31–9.
20. Russo EB. Clinical endocannabinoid deficiency reconsidered: current research supports the theory in migraine, fibromyalgia, irritable bowel, and other treatment-resistant syndromes. Cannabis Cannabinoid Res. 2016;1:154–65.
21. Sarchielli P, Pini LA, Coppola F, Rossi C, Baldi A, Mancini ML, et al. Endocannabinoids in chronic migraine: CSF findings suggest a system failure. Neuropsychopharmacology. 2007;32(6):1384–90.
22. Smaga I, Bystrowska B, Gawlinski D, Przegalinski E, Filip M. The endocannabinoid/endovanilloid system and depression. Curr Neuropharmacol [Internet]. 2014;12(5):462–74. Available from: http://www.eurekaselect.com/openurl/content.php?genre=article&issn=1570-159X&volume=12&issue=5&spage=462
23. Monteleone P, Bifulco M, Maina G, Tortorella A, Gazzerro P, Proto MC, et al. Investigation of CNR1 and FAAH endocannabinoid gene polymorphisms in bipolar disorder and major depression. Pharmacol Res. 2010;61(5):400–4.
24. Minocci D, Massei J, Martino A, Milianti M, Piz L, Di Bello D, et al. Genetic association between bipolar disorder and 524A>C (Leu133Ile) polymorphism of CNR2 gene, encoding for CB2 cannabinoid receptor. J Affect Disord. 2011;134(1–3):427–30.
25. Domschke K, Dannlowski U, Ohrmann P, Lawford B, Bauer J, Kugel H, et al. Cannabinoid receptor 1 (CNR1) gene: impact on antidepressant treatment response and emotion processing in Major Depression. Eur Neuropsychopharmacol. 2008;18(10):751–9.
26. Huang WJ, Chen WW, Zhang X. Endocannabinoid system: role in depression, reward and pain control (Review). Mol Med Rep. 2016;14(4):2899–903.
27. Lazary J, Eszlari N, Juhasz G, Bagdy G. Genetically reduced FAAH activity may be a risk for the development of anxiety and depression in persons with repetitive childhood trauma. Eur Neuropsychopharmacol. 2016;26(6):1020–8.
28. Behl T, Chadha S, Sachdeva M, Sehgal A, Kumar A, Dhruv, et al. Understanding the possible role of endocannabinoid system in obesity. Prostagland Other Lipid Mediat. 2021;152:1–10.
29. Ibarra-Lecue I, Pilar-Cuéllar F, Muguruza C, Florensa-Zanuy E, Díaz Á, Urigüen L, et al. The endocannabinoid system in mental disorders: evidence from human brain studies. Biochem Pharmacol. 2018;157:97–107.
30. Greenbaum L, Tegeder I, Barhum Y, Melamed E, Roditi Y, Djaldetti R. Contribution of genetic variants to pain susceptibility in Parkinson disease. Eur J Pain (United Kingdom). 2012;16(9):1243–50.
31. Pardini M, Krueger F, Koenigs M, Raymont V, Hodgkinson C, Zoubak S, et al. Fatty-acid amide hydrolase polymorphisms and post-traumatic stress disorder after penetrating brain injury. Transl Psychiatry [Internet]. 2012;2(1):e75-5. https://doi.org/10.1038/tp.2012.1.
32. Kim H, Mittal DP, Iadarola MJ, Dionne RA. Genetic predictors for acute experimental cold and heat pain sensitivity in humans. J Med Genet. 2006;43(8):1–8.
33. Cajanus K, Holmström EJ, Wessman M, Anttila V, Kaunisto MA, Kalso E. Effect of endocannabinoid degradation on pain: role of FAAH polymorphisms in experimental and postoperative pain in women treated for breast cancer. Pain. 2016;157(2):361–9.
34. Müller TD, Reichwald K, Brönner G, Kirschner J, Nguyen TT, Scherag A, et al. Lack of association of genetic variants in genes of the endocannabinoid system with anorexia nervosa. Child Adolesc Psychiatry Ment Health. 2008;2:33.
35. Lieb W, Manning AK, Florez JC, Dupuis J, Cupples LA, McAteer JB, et al. Variants in the CNR1 and the FAAH genes and adiposity traits in the community. Obesity. 2009;17(4):755–60.
36. Durand E, Lecoeur C, Delplanque J, Benzinou M, Degraeve F, Boutin P, et al. Evaluating the association of FAAH common gene variation with childhood, adult severe obesity and type 2 diabetes in the French population. Obes Facts. 2008;1(6):305–9.
37. Müller TD, Brönner G, Wandolski M, Carrie J, Nguyen TT, Greene BH, et al. Mutation screen and association studies for the fatty acid amide hydrolase (FAAH) gene and early onset and adult obesity. BMC Med Genet. 2010;11(1).
38. Palmer RHC, McGeary JE, Knopik VS, Bidwell LC, Metrik JM. CNR1 and FAAH variation and affective states induced by marijuana smoking. Am J Drug Alcohol Abuse. 2019;45(5):514–26.
39. Cinnamon Bidwell L, Metrik J, Mcgeary J, Palmer RHC, Francazio S, Knopik VS. Impulsivity, variation in the cannabinoid receptor (CNR1) and fatty acid amide hydrolase (FAAH) Genes, and marijuana-related problems. J Stud Alcohol Drugs. 2013;74(6):867–78.
40. Melroy-Greif WE, Wilhelmsen KC, Ehlers CL. Genetic variation in FAAH is associated with cannabis use disorders in a young adult sample

of Mexican Americans. Drug Alcohol Depend. 2016;166:249–53.
41. Hillard CJ, Weinlander KM, Stuhr KL. Contributions of endocannabinoid signaling to psychiatric disorders in humans: genetic and biochemical evidence. Neuroscience. 2012;204:207–29.
42. Dlugos AM, Hamidovic A, Hodgkinson CA, Goldman D, Palmer AA, De Wit H. More aroused, less fatigued: fatty acid amide hydrolase gene polymorphisms influence acute response to amphetamine. Neuropsychopharmacology. 2010;35:613–22.
43. Si P, Liu S, Tong D, Cheng M, Wang L, Cheng X. Association of polymorphisms of NAPE-PLD and FAAH genes with schizophrenia in Chinese Han population. Chin J Med Genet. 2018.
44. Ahmadalipour A, Mehdizadeh Fanid L, Zeinalzadeh N, Alizadeh M, Vaezi H, Hassanpour Aydinlou Z, et al. The first evidence of an association between a polymorphism in the endocannabinoid-degrading enzyme FAAH (FAAH rs2295633) with attention deficit hyperactivity disorder. Genomics. 2020;112(2):1330–4.
45. Poleszak E, Wośko S, Sławińska K, Wyska E, Szopa A, Doboszewska U, et al. Influence of the CB1 cannabinoid receptors on the activity of the monoaminergic system in the behavioural tests in mice. Brain Res Bull. 2019;150:179–85.
46. Poleszak E, Wośko S, Sławińska K, Wyska E, Szopa A, Świąder K, et al. Influence of the endocannabinoid system on the antidepressant activity of bupropion and moclobemide in the behavioural tests in mice. Pharmacol Rep. 2020;72(6):1562–72.
47. Powell SB, Zhou X, Geyer MA. Prepulse inhibition and genetic mouse models of schizophrenia. Behav Brain Res. 2009;204(2):282–94.
48. Braff DL. Prepulse inhibition of the startle reflex: a window on the brain in schizophrenia. Curr Top Behav Neurosci. 2010;4:349–71.
49. Saletti PG, Tomaz C. Cannabidiol effects on prepulse inhibition in nonhuman primates. Rev Neurosci. 2019;30(1):95–105.
50. Navarrete F, García-Gutiérrez MS, Jurado-Barba R, Rubio G, Gasparyan A, Austrich-Olivares A, et al. Endocannabinoid system components as potential biomarkers in psychiatry. Front Psychiatry. 2020;11:1–30.
51. Ballmaier M, Bortolato M, Rizzetti C, Zoli M, Gessa G, Heinz A, et al. Cannabinoid receptor antagonists counteract sensorimotor gating deficits in the phencyclidine model of psychosis. Neuropsychopharmacology. 2007;32(10):2098–107.
52. Guidali C, Viganò D, Petrosino S, Zamberletti E, Realini N, Binelli G, et al. Cannabinoid CB1 receptor antagonism prevents neurochemical and behavioural deficits induced by chronic phencyclidine. Int J Neuropsychopharmacol. 2011;14(1):17–28.
53. De Gómez Dumm NT, Giammona AM, Touceda LA. Variations in the lipid profile of patients with chronic renal failure treated with pyridoxine. Lipids Health Dis. 2003;2:1–6.
54. Potvin S, Kouassi É, Lipp O, Bouchard RH, Roy MA, Demers MF, et al. Endogenous cannabinoids in patients with schizophrenia and substance use disorder during quetiapine therapy. J Psychopharmacol. 2008;22(3):262–9.
55. Koethe D, Pahlisch F, Hellmich M, Rohleder C, Mueller JK, Meyer-Lindenberg A, et al. Familial abnormalities of endocannabinoid signaling in schizophrenia. World J Biol Psychiatry. 2019;20(2):117–25.
56. Giuffrida A, Leweke FM, Gerth CW, Schreiber D, Koethe D, Faulhaber J, et al. Cerebrospinal anandamide levels are elevated in acute schizophrenia and are inversely correlated with psychotic symptoms. Neuropsychopharmacology. 2004;29(11):2108–14.
57. Reuter AR, Bumb JM, Mueller JK, Rohleder C, Pahlisch F, Hanke F, et al. Association of anandamide with altered binocular depth inversion illusion in schizophrenia. World J Biol Psychiatry. 2017;18(6):483–8.
58. Minichino A, Senior M, Brondino N, Zhang SH, Godwlewska BR, Burnet PWJ, et al. Measuring disturbance of the endocannabinoid system in psychosis: a systematic review and meta-analysis. JAMA Psychiatry. 2019;76:914–23.
59. Mehndiratta MM, Wadhai SA. International epilepsy day—a day notified for global public education & awareness. Indian J Med Res. 2015;142:143–4.
60. Goldenberg MM. Overview of drugs used for epilepsy and seizures etiology, diagnosis, and treatment. P T. 2010;35(7):392–415.
61. Kwan P, Arzimanoglou A, Berg AT, Brodie MJ, Hauser WA, Mathern G, et al. Definition of drug resistant epilepsy: consensus proposal by the ad hoc Task Force of the ILAE Commission on Therapeutic Strategies. Epilepsia. 2010;51:1069–77.
62. Mohanraj R, Brodie MJ. Diagnosing refractory epilepsy: response to sequential treatment schedules. Eur J Neurol. 2006;13(3):277–82.
63. Rosenberg EC, Tsien RW, Whalley BJ, Devinsky O. Cannabinoids and epilepsy. Neurotherapeutics. 2015;12(4):747–68.
64. Gowers WR. Epilepsy and other chronic convulsive diseases: their causes, symptoms and treatment. By Sir William R. Gowers, M. D., F. R. C. P., F. R. S., Consulting Physician to University College Hospital, etc., etc. Second edition. (Philadelphia, P. Blakiston's Sons & Co., 1012 Walnut St., 1901.). Am J Psychiatry. 1901;58(2):346–7.
65. Devinsky O, Cross JH, Laux L, Marsh E, Miller I, Nabbout R, et al. Trial of cannabidiol for drug-resistant seizures in the dravet syndrome. N Engl J Med. 2017;376(21):2011–20.
66. Rosenberg EC, Patra PH, Whalley BJ. Therapeutic effects of cannabinoids in animal models of seizures, epilepsy, epileptogenesis, and epilepsy-related neuroprotection. Epilepsy Behav. 2017;70:319–27.
67. Rowley S, Sun X, Lima IV, Tavenier A, de Oliveira ACP, Dey SK, et al. Cannabinoid receptor 1/2 double-knockout mice develop epilepsy. Epilepsia. 2017;58(12):e162–6.

68. Silva GD, Del Guerra FB, de Oliveira LM, Pinto LF. Cannabidiol in the treatment of epilepsy: a focused review of evidence and gaps. Front Neurol. 2020;11:1–20.
69. Devinsky O, Marsh E, Friedman D, Thiele E, Laux L, Sullivan J, et al. Cannabidiol in patients with treatment-resistant epilepsy: an open-label interventional trial. Lancet Neurol. 2016;15(3):270–8.
70. Green B, Kavanagh D, Young R. Being stoned: a review of self-reported cannabis effects. Drug Alcohol Rev. 2003;22:453–60.
71. Manzanares J, Cabañero D, Puente N, García-Gutiérrez MS, Grandes P, Maldonado R. Role of the endocannabinoid system in drug addiction. Biochem Pharmacol. 2018;157:108–21.
72. Lv F, Chen S, Wang L, Jiang R, Tian H, Li J, et al. The role of microbiota in the pathogenesis of schizophrenia and major depressive disorder and the possibility of targeting microbiota as a treatment option. Oncotarget. 2017;8(59):100899–907.
73. Pearson-Leary J, Zhao C, Bittinger K, Eacret D, Luz S, Vigderman AS, et al. The gut microbiome regulates the increases in depressive-type behaviors and in inflammatory processes in the ventral hippocampus of stress vulnerable rats. Mol Psychiatry. 2020;25(5):1068–79.
74. Boehme M, van de Wouw M, Bastiaanssen TFS, Olavarría-Ramírez L, Lyons K, Fouhy F, et al. Mid-life microbiota crises: middle age is associated with pervasive neuroimmune alterations that are reversed by targeting the gut microbiome. Mol Psychiatry. 2020;25(10):2567–83.
75. Savignac HM, Corona G, Mills H, Chen L, Spencer JPE, Tzortzis G, et al. Prebiotic feeding elevates central brain derived neurotrophic factor, N-methyl-d-aspartate receptor subunits and d-serine. Neurochem Int. 2013;63(8):756–64.
76. Cenit MC, Sanz Y, Codoñer-Franch P. Influence of gut microbiota on neuropsychiatric disorders. World J Gastroenterol. 2017;23(30):5486–98.
77. Matias I, Bisogno T, Di Marzo V. Endogenous cannabinoids in the brain and peripheral tissues: regulation of their levels and control of food intake. Int J Obes. 2006;30:S7–12.
78. Marco EM, García-Gutiérrez MS, Bermúdez-Silva FJ, Moreira FA, Guimarães F, Manzanares J, et al. Endocannabinoid system and psychiatry: in search of a neurobiological basis for detrimental and potential therapeutic effects. Front Behav Neurosci. 2011;5(OCTOBER):1–23.
79. Muccioli GG, Naslain D, Bäckhed F, Reigstad CS, Lambert DM, Delzenne NM, et al. The endocannabinoid system links gut microbiota to adipogenesis. Mol Syst Biol. 2010;6:1–15.
80. Cani PD, Osto M, Geurts L, Everard A. Involvement of gut microbiota in the development of low-grade inflammation and type 2 diabetes associated with obesity. Gut Microbes. 2012;3:279–88.
81. Denou E, Jackson W, Lu J, Blennerhassett P, McCoy K, Verdu EF, et al. The intestinal microbiota determines mouse behavior and brain BDNF levels. Gastroenterology. 2011, 140(5):S-57.
82. Heyman E, Gamelin FX, Goekint M, Piscitelli F, Roelands B, Leclair E, et al. Intense exercise increases circulating endocannabinoid and BDNF levels in humans-possible implications for reward and depression. Psychoneuroendocrinology. 2012;37(6):844–51.
83. Zhao L, Li-Wen Yeh M, Levine ES. Role for endogenous BDNF in endocannabinoid-mediated long-term depression at neocortical inhibitory synapses. eNeuro [Internet]. 2015;2(2). Available from: http://eneuro.sfn.org/cgi/doi/10.1523/ENEURO.0029-14.2015
84. Ohno-shosaku T, Hashimotodani Y, Ano M, Takeda S, Tsubokawa H, Kano M. Endocannabinoid signalling triggered by NMDA receptor-mediated calcium entry into rat hippocampal neurons. J Physiol. 2007:407–18.
85. Yeh ML, Selvam R, Levine ES. BDNF-induced endocannabinoid release modulates neocortical glutamatergic neurotransmission. Synapse. 2017;71(5):1–10.

22 Melatonin and the Chronobiology of Drug Abuse

Daniel P. Cardinali

Introduction

Chronobiology, the science studying rhythmic phenomena, is in a phase of increasing expansion not only on basic data, but also on its application for both therapeutic and preventive approaches in remarkably diverse clinical fields. Cardiology and oncology are just two examples of medical specialties that currently benefit from the knowledge provided by chronopharmacology [1, 2]. In the case of drug abuse, and although the interest in the study of the relationships between rhythmic expression and the consumption of psychoactive substances is in its beginning, current knowledge already supports its importance [3–5].

The chronobiology of addiction is a rapid developing field of study based on relevant results derived from both basic and clinical research. It has been long known that drug consumption has a negative effect on the expression of circadian rhythmicity, generally producing a flattening of amplitude, and/or a phase delay of rhythms and eventually irregularity with disappearance of rhythms [6, 7]. Moreover, polymorphisms of circadian clock genes, e.g., clock and Per2, are associated with vulnerability to addiction. Overall, the evening circadian phenotype is a major individual difference to be taken into account as a risk factor in the development of drug addiction [8, 9]. Therefore, the reorganization of circadian rhythmicity with regular daily schedules adjusted to the environmental cycle of light-dark by exposure to natural or artificial light in the morning and to the administration of chronobiotics, e.g., melatonin, in the evening can be useful strategies to improve efficacy of treatments in drug addictions [3, 10].

Circadian Rhythmicity as Indicator of Health

There is a multiplicity of biological rhythms, although the most studied both for their interest in relation to socio-labor performance and in the clinic are the circadian or 24-h rhythms. Briefly, the central circadian system comprises three main elements: an endogenous oscillator, which in mammals is located in the hypothalamic suprachiasmatic nuclei (SCN), an entrainment agent (zeitgeber), and pathways that couple the internal clock to rhythms in physiology and behavior [11]. The SCN controls a number of peripheral oscillators throughout the body, which are otherwise autonomous in terms of their rhythmic properties [12]. Under normal conditions, circadian rhythmic expression is synchronized with environmental rhythmic information, among which the solar light-dark cycle is the principal

D. P. Cardinali (✉)
Faculty of Medical Sciences, Pontificia Universidad Católica Argentina, Buenos Aires, Argentina
e-mail: daniel_cardinali@uca.edu.ar

P. Á. Gargiulo, H. L. Mesones-Arroyo (eds.), *Psychiatry and Neuroscience Update – Vol. V*,
https://doi.org/10.1007/978-3-031-72219-6_22

one [11]. The endogenous clock controls the rhythmic expression of our organism with extreme precision and shows a relevant capacity for plasticity to adjust its phase to environmental changes, such as a transmeridian air travel which abruptly transports us to another time zone.

At a molecular level, circadian clocks are based on clock genes, some of which encode proteins able to feedback and inhibit their transcription. These cellular oscillators consist of interlocked transcriptional and posttranslational feedback loops that involve a small number of core clock genes (about 12 genes identified currently) [13]. The negative and positive transcriptional/translational feedback loops to form the core clockwork have been characterized in rodents by transgenic gene deletion methodology. Clock gene expression oscillates because of the delay in the feedback loops, regulated in part by phosphorylation of the clock proteins that control their stability, nuclear reentry, and transcription complex formation [13].

As a consequence, most biological and behavioral parameters show circadian rhythmicity, among which central temperature and melatonin stand out as rhythmic markers widely studied and having important clinical implications. The central temperature, with a sinusoidal function whose daily maximum occurs between 1700 and 2000 h and its minimum between 0300 and 0500 h, is considered an estimator of brain activity and its disorganization is evident in various mood disorders like endogenous major depression [14]. The pineal hormone melatonin is the body's chemical code of darkness and exhibits a marked nocturnal peak of secretion and minimum values during wakefulness depending on the duration of the environmental photoperiod [15].

The compromise of rhythmic behavior like that found in drug abuse can occur in various ways, although the most common is by flattening of the amplitude of rhythm, i.e., by lowering the maximum and increasing the minimum values [3]. Eventually, desynchronization leads to disappearance of rhythm. Thus, in the case of temperature, this means less activation during wakefulness and less ability to fall asleep and to maintain a night's sleep. The loss of the melatonin peak results in a clear detriment to the quantity and quality of sleep, which can even be disorganized, while the endogenous antioxidant activity of the organism and the immunological activity decrease [16–18]. Adequate rhythmic expression is thus the quintessence of health and quality of life in all phases of the life cycle.

Association of Circadian Rhythm Disruption with Drug Abuse

Reward-related behavior, fundamental for drug addiction, is mediated by a group of brain structures connected through the mesolimbic dopaminergic pathway that originates in the ventral tegmental area of the midbrain (VTA) and projects into the nucleus accumbens (NAc), the medial prefrontal cortex (mPFC), the amygdala, and the hippocampus [19]. Two circuits, mesolimbic and mesocortical, are involved in addictive behavior. The mesolimbic circuit (projections of DA neurons from the VTA to the NAc, amygdala, and hippocampus) is involved in acute reinforcing effects, memory, conditioned responses, and emotional changes of withdrawal syndrome. The mesocortical circuit (projections of the VTA to the mPFC, orbitofrontal cortex, and cingulate cortex) is involved in the conscious experience of the effects of drugs, "craving", and the compulsive use of drugs [19].

The mPFC is a modulator of daily drug-seeking rhythms. The mPFC sends glutamatergic projections to NAc and VTA and has been implicated in drug screening in a variety of contexts [20]. This structure exhibits a diurnal rhythm in neural activation, circadian clock gene expression, and dendritic complexity [21]. The transient pharmacological inhibition of mPFC during the acquisition or expression phases of addictive behavior induced by amphetamines attenuates the diurnal rhythm in the search for the drug. mPFC provides a top-down rhythmic control of the mesolimbic reward system [20].

Dopamine (DA) is the main neurotransmitter in the neural pathway linked to drug abuse. Drugs of abuse stimulate the brain reward system by increasing DA release from the NAc [22]. DA (acting via D_1 receptors) activates the striatal pathway, whereas it inhibits the striatocortical pathway through D_2 receptors. Iterative drug use is associated with neuroplastic changes involving the glutamatergic inputs to the striatum and midbrain DA neurons, thus enhancing the way the brain reacts to drug cues, weakening self-regulation, reducing sensitivity to nondrug rewards, and increasing sensitivity to stress [23]. DA neurotransmission, which is also important for motor control at the basal ganglia, has been implicated at several levels in the circadian system, starting with the photic input pathway to the clock [24]. In the retina and the SCN, DA plays a role in circadian photoentrainment [24].

Circadian fluctuations in extracellular DA levels have been reported in the striatum and nucleus accumbens, with maximal levels during the active phase [25]. In mice, DA and its metabolite, dihydroxyphenylacetic acid, exhibit opposite rhythms, the former peaking at night [26]. Tyrosine hydroxylase and cholecystokinin mRNA were upregulated in ventral tegmental area and the substantia nigra in the course of the day [27]. In the caudate and putamen, the mRNA levels for DA D_2 and adenosine 2A receptor, dynorphin, and substance P were lower during the day than during the night, whereas the expression of DA D_1 receptor, encephalin, and somatostatin was stable. These neurotransmitters are part of the indirect basal ganglia pathway [28]. Some results indicate that such DA circadian variations are regulated directly by the SCN [29]. Other observations indicate that DA might also regulate the expression of PER2 clock gen in the striatum of the rat, without overt effects on the SCN [24, 25].

The daily rhythm in positive affect in humans has been observed in constant routine chronobiological protocols such as forced desynchronization, indicating its mediation by the circadian system [3–5]. Daily rhythms in response to reward have also been reported in humans. For example, both the heart rate and the activation of the ventral striatum in response to a monetary reward are elevated in the afternoon as compared to the morning. Taken together, these data suggest that mesolimbic dopaminergic activity and reward responsiveness vary diurnally in humans.

In the initial phase of drug addiction, circadian regulation of DA neurotransmission can alter drug-induced reward in the dopaminergic pathways [30]. Hence, DA signaling has been implicated in the regulation of biological rhythms as an important non-photic signal for circadian entrainment [4, 24].

Compelling evidence suggests that drug use follows a circadian pattern [7]. Preclinical studies have shown that motivation to seek rewarding stimuli varies throughout the day [21]. Daily rhythms in drug self-administration occur in various species with increased intake generally in the activity period. Drug self-administration and brain self-stimulation rhythms persist under constant conditions, indicating their circadian origin [21].

Several studies have identified diurnal rhythms in the craving of abstinent users [31]. Moderate diurnal rhythm of nicotine craving in abstinent smokers with a low point in the early morning that increases throughout waking hours has been reported. Daily rate of signal-induced craving in abstinent heroin addicts with a noon nadir and peaks during the morning and afternoon hours also occurs [21]. These results suggest that people who abstain from drugs may be more likely to relapse at certain times of the day.

The chronic use of psychoactive substances negatively affects circadian rhythmic expression. This produces a flattening of the periodic function and a delay in the maximum and may even lead to a state of desynchronization of endogenous control [32]. Alcohol is one of the most examined substances in this respect. Chronic alcohol consumption decreases the rhythmic amplitude of both body temperature and melatonin, observing a maximization of this during the withdrawal syndrome [33]. Thus, the production of hypothermia during wakefulness and hyperthermia in the night hours has been observed together with a considerable decrease in nocturnal melatonin secretion and increased diurnal values [34]. The impact on alcohol consumption the circadian rhythm of melatonin is verified in young and healthy individuals. The data acquire a special relevance in the case of intensive intermittent alcohol consumption ("binging") in adolescents and young people [35, 36]. Accordingly, the negative consequences of drug use also vary in intensity depending on the time of the day, e.g., an increase in emergency hospitalizations related to drug use is observed during the night [37].

Preclinical studies have shown that motivation to seek rewarding stimuli varies throughout the day. Daily rhythms in drug self-administration occur in various species with increased intake generally in the period of activity. Drug self-administration and brain self-stimulation rhythms persist under constant conditions, indicating a circadian origin [33].

Polymorphisms of clock genes have been associated with a variety of psychopathological disorders, including drug addiction [3, 38, 39]. Mice carrying a mutant clock gene responsible for the activation of various circadian genes [40] were much more active both before the administration of cocaine and after its administration as compared to the wild type control. Likewise, the response of the reward system to the drug was much higher, with a greater rise in the levels of DA and its synthesizing enzyme. The results point to the clock gene as a direct regulator of dopaminergic activity in reward areas of the brain [38].

The circadian gene Per2 has been shown to be essential to inhibit sensitivity to the effects of cocaine [41], alcohol [32], or methamphetamine [42]. Genetically manipulated animals with absence of the expression of Per 2 gene show an increased response to the effects of both drugs and the loss of the known diurnal variation of sensitivity. Variations in the Per2 gene have also been found in humans associated with high alcohol consumption [43]. In addition, drug use can influence gene expression and modify circadian gene expression, establishing permanent functional changes associated with ingestion of varying magnitude depending on the individual's vulnerability [3].

Circadian expression of clock genes is very well documented in the VTA and substantia nigra [24, 33]. Mutations or knock-down of specific clock genes in these areas lead to changes in DA signaling-dependent phenotypes related to drug addiction and mental disorders and even result in altered SCN function. Therefore, there is a bidirectional link between dopaminergic signaling and the circadian system, with circadian systems regulating dopaminergic signaling and the activation of the dopaminergic system resulting in circadian disturbances.

During the transition from the early stages to the advanced phases of addiction, individuals tend to show a shift in the time of day in which drugs are used. For example, in healthy human volunteers, the desire for and the intake of alcohol are more frequently reported in the early evening. However, individuals with alcohol use disorder report a peak in craving during the early morning, suggesting a circadian disruption in the control of the desire to drink [34]. In clock gene knock-out or mutant animals, changes in the daily rhythms of alcohol sensitivity [44] and in the tolerance and withdrawal signs induced by morphine have been reported [45].

Circadian disruption as a consequence of chronic drug use causes a misalignment of the biological rhythms with the environment, resulting in insomnia, anhedonia, and fatigue [46]. Because during the advance stages of addiction relapse is often observed to alleviate negative effects, circadian disruption is suggested as one of the major contributors to relapse [38]. Moreover, a polymorphism in the clock gene PER3 (related to evening chronotype and insomnia) is associated with the severity of sleep disturbances in alcoholic patients, suggesting that a genetic component related to circadian system also could contribute to relapse [47]. Therefore, clock gene functions are not limited to circadian regulation and may also be involved in other processes and behaviors, such as those related to drug addiction [48].

The Circadian Evening Typology as a Risk Factor

Not all individuals have identical circadian rhythmic expression. This is very important concerning addictive behavior because the evening chronotype is consistently associated with an increased risk of impulsive behavior, including alcohol and drug abuse [8, 49, 50].

The circadian typology is an individual difference about which much information has been gathered in the last two decades [51, 52]. Individuals are classified into three circadian typologies (morning, intermediate or "no type", and evening) based on their self-evaluations to specific questionnaires [53]. The morning people go to bed and get up early and place their best time to develop physical and mental activities in the early hours of the day, while the evening ones get up and go to bed late manifesting their optimum at the end of the day and even in the early hours of the night. The lags in the circadian rhythmic functions of the extreme groups oscillate between 2 and 10 h, depending on the parameter examined. The group of "no type" usually presents an intermediate position and belongs to about 60% of the young adult population, while the extreme groups account for 20%. Morning and evening not only differ in rhythmic expression, but also in personality traits and habits, contributing to different lifestyles [8, 49, 50].

Initial studies reported differences in the consumption of legal psychoactive substances (nicotine, alcohol, and caffeine) between circadian typologies, with evening subjects consuming more of all of them [54]. Subsequent studies have confirmed the observation, which is particularly relevant in the adolescent population. While the morning circadian typology seems to be a protective factor in the initiation and maintenance of drug use, the evening typology can be considered a risk factor. The evening type may consume stimulants, perhaps to adjust their level of daytime activation to socio-environmental demands when their state is deficient and depressants at the end of the day when their level of activation exceeds that required at that time. Thus, evening individuals obtain superior reinforcement, which promotes behavior maintenance [51, 52]. If consumption becomes habitual, the well-known stress spiral will occur and its magnitude is greater in the evening phenotype [55].

An extreme evening typology also supposes a risk factor in the development of other psychopathological disorders, highlighting those of humor [8, 49, 50]. Although there are many other elements that also participate in the initiation and maintenance of drug use, the circadian typology is a principal one. Preventive approaches to drug addiction should incorporate the promotion of habits that benefit the circadian rhythmic organization with special emphasis on channeling the hourly patterns of individuals with an extreme evening pattern, much more frequent during adolescence.

Sleep disruption in adolescence is a major problem. Indeed, drug abuse and a disrupted sleep are interconnected phenomena [56]. Acute exposure to drugs of abuse disrupts sleep by lengthening sleep onset latency, reducing total sleep time, increasing the frequency of nighttime awakenings, and decreasing rapid eye movement (REM) sleep and slow wave, non-REM sleep [57]. On the other hand, sleep disorders are a risk factor for drug abuse [58]. With chronic consumption of the drug, sleep disruption becomes more severe, and during abstinence, insomnia with a negative effect prevails, which drives drug craving and contributes to impulsivity and relapse. One of the problems is that current medication therapies for opioid, alcohol, or nicotine addiction do not reverse sleep dysfunctions, and this may be an obstacle to recovery [59, 60]. In this context, the importance of melatonin as a medication emerges. Due to the hypnotic and chronobiotic properties of melatonin, its use for the treatment of insomnia has been recommended. Several meta-analyses and consensuses support such a therapeutic role [61–67].

Basic Biology of Melatonin Relevant to Drug Abuse

"Chronobiotics" are drugs that synchronize or increase the amplitude of circadian rhythms, melatonin being their natural prototype [68, 69]. The essential role of melatonin as a chronobiotic is defined by its prominent light/dark rhythm in circulation. Melatonin inhibits the wakefulness-facilitating activity of the SCN in the late afternoon, triggering sleep [70, 71]. As the secretion of pineal melatonin is proportional to the length of the night, it provides the neuroendocrine apparatus with fundamental information on the time of year regulating seasonality [72].

Although more than 90% of circulating melatonin derives from the pineal gland [73], there is ample evidence that it is synthesized locally in most cells, tissues, and organs [74]. Indeed, the idea is held that melatonin is produced in all animal cells that have mitochondria [75] and that a mitochondrial protective function is critical for cytoprotection [76].

Melatonergic receptors (MT_1 and MT_2) are responsible for the chronobiotic function of melatonin. Both receptors are members of the superfamily of membrane receptors associated with G proteins (G-protein-coupled receptors, GPCR) [77]. A third member of the melatonin receptor family, GPR50, displays high sequence homology with MT_1 and MT_2, but rather than binding melatonin or any other known ligand, it forms homo and heteromers with MT_1 and MT_2 as well as with other GPCRs [78].

MT_1 and MT_2 receptors have been identified in SCN and in several CNS areas, including the cerebral and cerebellar cortex and the midbrain [79]. In the midbrain, MT_1 and MT_2 receptors are related to modulation of the nigrostriatal and mesocorticolimbic dopaminergic pathways. Functional melatonin receptors have been localized in substantia nigra, NAc, VTA, and caudate-putamen [80].

Due to its amphiphilic properties, melatonin crosses readily cell membranes. Calmodulin and tubulin are among the cytoplasmic proteins that interact with melatonin [81]. Melatonin also enters the cell nucleus and interacts indirectly with orphan RZR / ROR superfamily of receptors [76] through the activation of sirtuin-1, which affects the circadian accessory oscillator RORα 1 [82].

The cytoprotective activity of melatonin cannot be explained by interaction with MT_1 and MT_2 receptors only. As mentioned, the amounts of intracellular melatonin greatly exceed those found in circulation [74]. Intramitochondrially synthesized melatonin is retained within the organelle and the melatonin doses capable to modify the intracellular melatonin concentration are much higher than those used clinically as a chronobiotic [83].

Although in cell cultures, some physiologically relevant effects of melatonin are revealed at doses in the range of 10^{-8} to 10^{-9} M [84] for most studies on cytoprotective effects in animals, pharmacological doses that clearly exceed receptor saturation were employed [85].

For recent reviews related to the activity of melatonin to reverse altered signaling mechanisms in neurodegeneration, including impaired autophagic integrity, proteostasis dysfunction, and abnormalities in Notch, Wnt/ß, and insulin signaling pathways, see [86–88].

The melatonin antioxidant and scavenging effects on free radicals occurring in both the cytoplasm and the cell nucleus are largely independent of receptors. Besides being a free radical scavenger itself, there is an oxidation-drive conversion of melatonin to compounds with higher antioxidant activity. In addition, melatonin displays a strong indirect antioxidant effect by stimulating the synthesis of antioxidant enzymes and by inhibiting that of prooxidant enzymes. In protecting against oxidative damage, melatonin is more effective that vitamin C and E [89]. Moreover, melatonin facilitates the effects of other antioxidants, like Trolox or vitamin C. A stabilizing activity of melatonin on mitochondrial membrane explains several cytoprotective and antiapoptotic effects exerted by melatonin under ischemic conditions (not related to free radicals) [75].

Immunomodulation by melatonin includes pro-inflammatory and anti-inflammatory effects [90, 91]. Anti-inflammatory actions of melatonin have been demonstrated in low-grade inflammation, like neurodegenerative processes or aging as well as in high-grade inflammation such as sepsis, ischemia / reperfusion, or brain injury.

Melatonin anti-inflammatory properties are related to the inhibition of nuclear factor κB (NF κB) binding to DNA and of cyclooxygenase (Cox) [92] (mainly Cox-2) [93]), as well as to downregulation of inducible nitric oxide synthase receptors [76]. Other signaling pathways include upregulation of nuclear factor erythroid 2-related factor 2 and of toll-like receptor-4 activation and high-mobility group box-1 signaling receptors and prevention of NLRP3 inflammasome activation by melatonin [76]. Collectively, these effects of melatonin result in increased production of anti-inflammatory cytokines and reduced levels of pro-inflammatory cytokines [90, 91].

The GABAergic system is involved in melatonin-mediated neuroprotection. In fact, melatonin exerts anti-excitatory and sedative effects [94, 95] and there is information that melatonin protects neurons from ß-amyloid peptide toxicity through the activation of GABAergic receptors [96]. An allosteric modulation of $GABA_A$ receptors by melatonin was indicated by the efficacy of the benzodiazepine antagonist flumazenil, and the lack of activity of the melatonin receptor antagonist luzindole, to modify upregulation of GABA activity by melatonin [97].

The anti-excitotoxic activity of melatonin should be also considered. For example, melatonin administration protects CA1 neurons in the hippocampus from transient ischemia [98] or from death due to high doses of glucocorticoids [99]. Kainate, an agonist of the ionotropic glutamate receptor, induces neuronal death, an effect also prevented by melatonin [100]. As revealed by the lack of effects of specific blockers, melatonin receptors do not participate in the anti-excitotoxic activity of melatonin [101].

There is an antagonizing relationship between DA and melatonin [102]. Inhibition of DA release by melatonin has been demonstrated in mammalian central nervous system (hypothalamus, hippocampus, brainstem, and retina). Antidopaminergic activities of melatonin have been demonstrated in the striatum of normal mice [103]. Melatonin MT_1 and MT_2 receptors have been found to be expressed in human dopaminergic areas [104].

Melatonin in Drug Abuse. Experimental Studies

The capacity of melatonin to affect neurobiological aspects of drug abuse is now documented by several experimental studies [10]. Table 22.1 summarizes the information obtained in experimental models of drug-seeking behavior. Melatonin has been shown effective in withdrawal/relapse and behavioral sensitization. It also prevented several indicators of neurodegeneration, like autophagy, apoptosis, oxidative stress, and neurotoxic injury in brain areas linked to reward and emotionality (Table 22.1).

From the doses of melatonin used in the experiment listed in Table 22.1, the human equivalent dose (HED) of melatonin for a 75 kg adult was calculated by normalization of body surface area [105] . Body surface area correlates well across several mammalian species with several parameters of biology, including oxygen utilization, caloric expenditure, basal metabolism, blood volume, circulating plasma proteins, and renal function and has been advocated as a factor to be used when converting a dose for translation from animals to humans. Noteworthy, theoretical human equivalent doses calculated from Table 22.1's results ranged from 2- to 3-orders of magnitude greater than those usually employed in humans, as shown in Table 22.2.

Table 22.1 In vivo effect of melatonin in animal models of drug abuse. The human equivalent dose of melatonin for a 75 kg adult is calculated by normalization of body surface area [105]

Reference	Design	Results	Melatonin human daily equivalent dose for a 75 kg adult
[106]	Four dosages (5, 20, 40, 80 mg/kg) of melatonin were administered to mice i.p. 30 min prior to the injections of methamphetamine	The higher doses (40 or 80 mg/kg) of melatonin significantly attenuated methamphetamine-induced toxic effects on both dopamine and serotonin systems	240 or 480 mg
[107]	Swiss Webster mice were administered with methamphetamine (5 mg/kg) and/or melatonin (10 mg/kg)	Pretreatment with melatonin at 10 mg/kg body weight prevented the development of methamphetamineinduced depletion of dopamine and/or its metabolites and depletion of dopamine transporter-binding sites. It also attenuated methamphetamineinduced behaviors and diminished hyperthermia, although it did not reverse fully developed methamphetamine-induced behavioral sensitization	60 mg
[108]	A physical-dependent model in mice was established by s.c. injection of morphine. Melatonin was given in 25, 50, 100, or 200 mg/kg doses	The physical withdrawal syndrome was inhibited partly by the four different doses (25, 50, 100, 200 mg/kg) in a dose-dependent manner. The increased concentration of serum norepinephrine and dopamine in morphine-dependent mice was reduced by 100 mg/kg of melatonin	150, 300, 600 or 1200 mg
[109]	Morphine-induced tolerance and dependence was studied in mice. A 10-day repeated injection regimen was followed to induce morphine tolerance and dependence. Melatonin (1–10 mg/kg) was administered i.p.	Co-administration of melatonin with morphine during the induction phase (day 1–9) reversed the development of opioid tolerance and dependence tested on 10th day. Acute administration of melatonin (on the 10th day, i.e., during the expression phase of morphine dependence) reduced the incidence of naloxone-induced withdrawal jumps without affecting the tolerance to analgesic effect	6–60 mg
[110]	Morphine-induced tolerance and dependence was studied in mice. Melatonin (1–5 mg/kg) was administered i.p.	Melatonin-induced reversal of morphine tolerance and dependence may involve its ability to suppress nitric oxide synthase activity. Further, the melatonin-induced reversal of morphine tolerance and dependence is not mediated through its actions via putative melatonin receptors. The agonistic activity of melatonin towards peripheral benzodiazepine receptors may contribute to the suppression of morphine dependence but not to the reversal of tolerance to the analgesic activity of morphine	6–30 mg
[111]	Adult male Sprague–Dawley rats injected daily with cocaine were given two melatonin injections of 30 mg/kg	Rats injected daily with melatonin prior to cocaine injections failed to elicit cocaine sensitization. These behavioral effects of melatonin do not completely mimic those of other NOS inhibitors	720 mg

(continued)

Table 22.1 (continued)

Reference	Design	Results	Melatonin human daily equivalent dose for a 75 kg adult
[112]	Sprague Dawley rats drinking a solution of melatonin (200 ng/ml) at night or pretreated with 200 ng/kg i.p.)	Rats drinking melatonin either during repeated cocaine administration or during its withdrawal showed less anxiety-like behavior. Pretreatment with melatonin attenuated the augmentation of cAMP levels in nucleus accumbens following cocaine administration	0.2 mg (p.o.), 0.02 mg (i.p.)
[113]	A physical-dependent model in mice was established by s.c. injection of morphine. Melatonin (4 daily injections of 15 mg/kg) was given by intragastric infusion for three days. Withdrawal syndromes were induced by intraperitoneal injection of naloxone	The physical withdrawal syndrome and the content of NO in plasma and brain tissue in morphine-dependent mice were inhibited by melatonin	360 mg
[114]	Male Kunming mice received s.c. morphine to establish morphine dependence model. Withdrawal response was induced by naloxone preinjected or not with 80 mg/kg of melatonin	Melatonin inhibited the naloxone-precipitated withdrawal responses, increased the content of β-EP in the PAG of midbrain and attenuated the intensity of β-EP-like immunoreactivity in the arcuate nucleus	480 mg
[115, 116]	Male Sprague Dawley albino rats subjected to heroin addiction or heroin withdrawal were used. Dose used for melatonin was 10 mg/kg (i.p.)	Exogenous melatonin relieved bio-element status and antioxidant enzyme activities caused by heroin	120 mg
[117]	Murine model of morphine addiction. Pretreatment with melatonin (0.5 mg/kg and 5 mg/kg)	In mice, coadministration of melatonin with morphine ameliorated morphine-induced behavioral sensitization, analgesic tolerance and mtDNA content reduction	3 y 30 mg
[118]	To evaluate the protective effect of exogenous melatonin in rats and their offspring on neurotoxicity caused by chronic alcohol consumption during pregnancy pregnant Wistar rats under ethanol treatment were treated with melatonin (10 mg/kg/day).	Ethanol induced in cerebellum lipid peroxidation, decreased antioxidants activities, increased homocysteine level. Ethanol also disrupted locomotor activities in offsprings. All these effects were counteracted by melatonin	120 mg
[119]	Male C57BL/6 mice were divided into four groups, including the control, methamphetamine-treated, melatonin-pretreated + methamphetamine-treated, and melatonin-treated groups. Melatonin was injected at a dose of 5 mg/kg/daily	Melatonin attenuates methamphetamine-induced inhibition of hippocampal neurogenesis and reduction of MAPK kinase signaling in the hippocampus. Melatonin attenuates the methamphetamine-induced decrease in NR2A but increase in NR2B in the hippocampus	30 mg
[120]	Male Wistar rats were subjected to long-term voluntary alcohol consumption with repeated abstinence phases. Each animal received three daily injections of melatonin (50 mg/kg) or agomelatine (30 mg/kg)	Both drugs caused a phase advance in the diurnal drinking pattern when compared with the control vehicle-treated group and a reduced frequency of approaches to alcohol bottles	1800 mg

(continued)

Table 22.1 (continued)

Reference	Design	Results	Melatonin human daily equivalent dose for a 75 kg adult
[121]	To explore the possible mechanism of melatonin in diminishing morphine tolerance, intrathecal catheters were implanted in male Wistar rats for drug delivery. One was linked to a mini-osmotic pump for morphine or saline infusion. On the seventh day, 50 μg of melatonin or vehicle was injected through the other catheter instantly after discontinuation of morphine or saline infusion. The antinociceptive response was then measured using the tail-flick test every 30 min for 120 min	Chronic morphine infusion elicited antinociceptive tolerance and upregulated heat shock protein 27 expression in the dorsal horn of the rat spinal cord. Melatonin pretreatment partially restored morphine's antinociceptive effect in morphine-tolerant rats and reversed morphine-induced protein upregulation. In addition, chronic morphine infusion induced microglial cell activation and was reversed by melatonin treatment	600 μg intrathecally
[122]	Male Kunming mice were treated with melatonin (10 mg/kg) for 14 consecutive days during behavior sensitization, a long-lasting enhancement of locomotor activity after exposure to psychostimulants	Melatonin significantly attenuated the expression of methamphetamine sensitization. Neuronal expression of MeCP2, an X-linked transcription factor, was attenuated by melatonin	60 mg
[123]	Male Sprague-Dawley rats were submitted to long-term cocaine self-administration training. Melatonin, 25 or 50 mg/kg, was injected 3–4 h after the dark phase onset, 30 min prior to each test	Both doses of melatonin decreased the cocaine-seeking behavior and the motivation to work for cocaine	300 y 600 mg
[124]	To evaluate the protective effect of exogenous melatonin in rats and their offspring on the genotoxic response induced by chronic alcohol consumption during pregnancy pregnant Wistar rats under ethanol treatment were treated with melatonin (10 and 15 mg/kg/day)	Treatments with melatonin reduced the genotoxicity caused by ethanol in the blood of dams and neonates (males and females), liver of dams and male offsprings, and in the brain of female offsprings	120 and 180 mg
[125]	The differentially expressed genes in the process of morphine tolerance and altered gene expression subsequent to melatonin treatment in chronic were examined in morphine-infused spinal cords of Wistar rats. Morphine tolerance was induced by intrathecal morphine infusion. Melatonin was administered intrathecally (50 μg in 5 μl of 10% ethanol) 30 min later	In rat expression microarrays principal component analysis and clustering analysis revealed that the overall gene profiles were different in morphine and melatonin treatments. A panel of genes exclusively expressed following melatonin treatment and another panel of genes with inverse expression between both groups were also established. The expression levels of genes of interest were also confirmed using a reverse transcription-quantitative polymerase chain reaction	600 μg intrathecally
[126]	Male ICR mice were randomly assigned to control and treatment groups pretreated with methamphetamine (3 mg/kg) or melatonin (2.5, 5, 10 mg/kg) plus methamphetamine	Acute methamphetamine administration decreased latency to initial attacks of aggression and thereby increased the number and duration of attacks in male ICR mice. Medium melatonin pretreatment dose could significantly reverse acute MA-induced aggressive behavior accompanied by increases in DA, HVA, and 5-HIAA levels, and 5-HIAA/5-HT ratios in the hippocampus	7.5, 15, 30 or 60 mg

(continued)

Table 22.1 (continued)

Reference	Design	Results	Melatonin human daily equivalent dose for a 75 kg adult
[127]	Naïve and pinealectomized Wistar rats received cocaine at different times of day, melatonin (30 mg/kg) being administered 30 min before cocaine; luzindole was administered 15 min prior to melatonin	Continuous lighting and pinealectomy increased cocaine-induced locomotor activity. Melatonin administration decreased cocaine-induced locomotor activity in control and pinealectomized rats at different times of day. Luzindole blocked the melatonin-induced reduction in cocaine-induced locomotor activity in pinealectomized rats	360 mg
[128]	Wistar rats were subjected to neuropathic pain induction by chronic constriction injury. An intrathecal osmotic pump was used for continued drug delivery to induce morphine tolerance. Continued i.v. infusion of 3 μg/h of melatonin was made	Melatonin attenuated morphine tolerance in both neuropathic and naïve rats. This protective effect was independent of melatonin receptors. The transcriptional profile of pro-inflammatory and pain-related receptor genes in morphine-tolerant rats was blocked by melatonin. Melatonin increased antioxidative enzymes in the spinal cord of morphine-tolerant rats	0.2 mg/h
[129]	To assess the protective effects of melatonin on methamphetamine-induced alterations of blood brain barrier integrity Wistar underwent melatonin pretreatment (10 mg/kg) before escalating-high doses of methamphetamine treatment	Melatonin recovered tight junction loss; attenuated excessive MMP-9, NOX2, and cell adhesion molecule expression; and reduced serum albumin in the brain. Protective effects of melatonin against methamphetamine neurotoxic characterized by reactive gliosis: microglia (integrin-αM) and astrocyte (GFAP); an excessive upregulation of primary pro-inflammatory cytokines: interleukin-1β, interleukin-6, and tumor necrosis factor-α; activation of nuclear factor-kappa B; and suppression of nuclear factor erythroid 2-related factor, were found	120 mg
[130]	Male Wistar rats received cocaine during the induction and expression of locomotor sensitization. Melatonin (30 mg/kg) was administered 30 min before cocaine	Melatonin decreased cocaine-induced locomotor sensitization and intracellular dopamine levels, as well as cocaine conditioned place preference. Luzindole blocked the melatonin-induced decrease in the expression of locomotor sensitization	360 mg
[131]	Male ICR Mice were treated with either methamphetamine (1 mg/kg) or saline for 7 days, followed by melatonin (10 mg/kg) or saline for another 14 days	Methamphetamine impaired learning and memory in mice, an effect counteracted by melatonin probably through the changes in hippocampal BDNF, NMDA receptors, TrkB receptors, CaMKII, βIII tubulin and synaptophysin	60 mg

Table 22.2 Clinical studies of melatonin application in drug abuse

References	Subjects	Design	Treatment	Measured	Results
[132]	A 43 year old woman who had suffered from insomnia for the past 11 years	Case report	1 mg of controlled release melatonin p.o./daily at bed time	Subjective evaluation of sleep quality. Urinary 6-sulphatoxymelatonin measurement	Treatment with melatonin enabled the patient to cease any benzodiazepine (BZD) use within two days, with an improvement in sleep quality and no side effects. Before the melatonin treatment that the levels urinary 6-sulphatoxymelatonin were very low and lacked the typical circadian rhythm of excretion. During melatonin treatment a normal circadian rhythm of melatonin excretion occurred
[133]	41 patients with sleep disturbance including insomniacs, depressed and demented patients	Open-label study	3 mg melatonin p.o./daily at bed time	Daily logs of sleep and wake quality completed by the patients or their caretakers	Four (31%) of the 13 insomniac patients who were receiving BZD reduced BZD use by 50–75% and 4 (31%) discontinued it. Of the 7 depressed and 7 demented patients who were receiving BZD, 2 (29%) in each group reduced BZD use by up to 50%
[134]	34 primary insomnia outpatients who took BZD and had low urinary 6-sulphatoxy melatonin levels	Randomized double-blind, placebo-controlled study followed by a single blind period	Patients received melatonin (2 mg controlled release p.o.) or placebo for 6 weeks. On day 14 of treatment, BZD dose was reduced by half and on day 28, it was halted	Sleep diary and recording of BZD use	14 of 18 subjects who had received melatonin, but only 4 of 16 in the placebo group, discontinued BZD therapy. Sleep-quality scores were higher in the melatonin group
[135]	41 insomniac patients. Twenty of 22 patients were on BZD treatment	Open-label study	3 mg melatonin p.o./daily at bed time	Sleep diary and recording of BZD use. Serum concentrations of prolactin, TSH, FSH, and estradiol and urinary 6-sulphatoxymelatonin excretion were measured by RIA	In 13 of 20 patients taking BZD together with melatonin, BZD use could be stopped, and in another 4 patients, BZD dose could be decreased to 25–66% of the initial dose. Urinary 6-sulphatoxymelatonin correlated negatively with age, but not with the intensity of sleep disorder or the outcome of treatment

[136]	45 patients regularly taking anxiolytic BZD in low doses were studied	Randomized double-blind, placebo-controlled study	3 mg melatonin p.o./ daily at bed time. On day 14 of treatment, BZD dose was reduced by half and on day 28, it was halted	Sleep diary and recording of BZD use. Urinary 6-sulphatoxymelatonin measurement	No significant modifications of sleep or wakefulness were detected after BZD withdrawal. As compared to basal, there was a general lack of changes in quality of wakefulness or sleep in patients taking melatonin or placebo. Melatonin advanced sleep onset and decreased significantly the variability of sleep onset time. The urinary concentration of 6-sulphatoxymelatonin prior to the study did not correlate with any parameter examined
[137]	Of 503 long-term users of BZD asked to participate in a discontinuation program, 38 patients agreed	Placebo-controlled trial	5 mg melatonin or placebo p.o. 4 h before patients went to bed	Participants received 4 questionnaires about their use of BZD medication. The urine was tested for the presence of BZD	After one year 40% had stopped their BZD use, both in the intervention group on melatonin and in the placebo control group. Comparing stoppers and non-stoppers did not reveal significant differences in BZD use, or awareness of problematic use
[138]	60 mild cognitive impairment (MCI) out patients	Open-label, retrospective study	35 patients received daily 3–9 mg of a fast-release melatonin preparation p.o. at bedtime. Melatonin was given in addition to the standard medication	Daily logs of sleep and wake quality. Initial and final neuropsychological assessment	Beck Depression Inventory score improved in melatonin-treated patients, concomitantly with an improvement in wakefulness, sleep quality and neuropsychological assessment. Twenty-one out of 25 MCI patients not treated with melatonin received BZD treatment vs. 6 out 25 patients in the melatonin group

(continued)

Table 22.2 (continued)

References	Subjects	Design	Treatment	Measured	Results
[139]	80 patients enrolled at a community methadone maintenance clinic recruited to a BDZ withdrawal program	Double-blind cross-over control study to evaluate the effectiveness of melatonin in attenuating sleep difficulties during BZD withdrawal	Fast release melatonin (5 mg/day, p.o.) or placebo: 6 weeks one arm, 1 week washout, 6 weeks other arm	Urine BZD; self-reported Pittsburgh Sleep Quality Index (PSQI) and the Center for Epidemiologic Studies Depression questionnaires administered at baseline, and at 6, 7 and 13 weeks	Sixty-one patients (77.5% in the 'melatonin first' condition and 75% in the 'placebo first' condition) completed 6 weeks of treatment, showing a similar BZD discontinuation rate. Sleep quality in patients who continued abusing BZD improved more in the 'melatonin first' group than in the 'placebo first' group, with no differences in sleep quality improvement in patients who stopped BZD. Although melatonin did not enhance BDZ discontinuation, it improved sleep quality, especially in patients who did not stop BDZ
[140]	22 older adults with a history of sleep disorder complaints; 14 were receiving BZD treatment	Randomized, double-blind, placebo-controlled, crossover study	Participants received 2 months of fast release melatonin (5 mg/day) and 2 months of placebo	Sleep disorder evaluation with the Northside Hospital Sleep Medicine Institute test, discarding secondary insomnia and evaluating sleep quality. Behavioral disorders were evaluated with the Yesavage Geriatric Depression Scale and Goldberg Anxiety Scale.	Melatonin treatment significantly improved sleep quality scores. Depression and anxiety also improved significantly after melatonin. Nine out of 14 subjects receiving BZD drugs were able to discontinue this treatment
[141]	5 alcohol-dependent patients with chronic sleep disorders	Open observational study	Ramelteon (8 mg at bedtime) for 4 weeks	Insomnia Index, actigraphy	Ramelteon improved insomnia over a 4-week period, and exerted some of its effect by increasing total sleep time by more than 1 h and decreasing sleep onset latency by nearly half an hour on average
[142]	96 MCI outpatients	Open-label, retrospective study	61 patients received daily 3–24 mg of a fast-release melatonin preparation p.o. at bedtime. Melatonin was given in addition to the standard medication	Daily logs of sleep and wake quality. Initial and final neuropsychological assessment	Beck Depression Inventory score improved in melatonin-treated patients, concomitantly with an improvement in wakefulness, sleep quality and neuropsychological assessment; 6 out of 61 patients treated with melatonin needed concomitant BZD treatment vs. 22 out of 35 MCI patients not receiving melatonin

[143]	112 insomniac outpatients classified according to their use of hypnotic BZD or BZD-like drugs	Retrospective study from a longitudinal database	melatonin (2 mg controlled release) p.o.	Discontinuation rate of BZD	31% of patients discontinued BZD after melatonin initiation. The discontinuation rate was higher in patients receiving two or three melatonin prescription rounds
[144]	Pharmaco-epidemiologic analysis and evaluation of the impact of anti-BZD/Z-drugs campaigns in face of the availability of alternative pharmacotherapy (melatonin)		Annual sales data from 9 European countries were extracted from the IMS sales database	To determine whether trends in use of treatment options were attributed to campaigns and/or availability and affordability of safer alternatives on the market	Campaigns aiming to reduce the use of BZD/Z-drugs failed when they were not associated with the availability and market uptake of melatonin. The reimbursement of melatonin supports better penetration rates and a higher reduction in sales for BZD/Z-drugs
[145]	45 alcohol-dependent patients with sleep and mild affective disorders	Open label study	Fast release melatonin (3–6 mg/day, p.o.) for 3 weeks	A battery of psychometric scales (a subjective sleep quality questionnaire, the Epworth sleepiness scale, a sleep apnea screening questionnaire, HAM-A, HAM-D, an alcohol consumption questionnaire) was used	Melatonin improved sleep latency, quality and duration of sleep, and breathing during sleep. The drug decreased daily sleepiness and affective disorders, particularly, anxiety
[146]	9 alcohol-dependent patients with chronic sleep disorders	Open observational study	Agomelatine (25 mg daily) at bedtime. After 3 weeks, in 6 of 9 patients, the dosage of agomelatine was increased to 50 mg/day. Assessment of sleep quality was made after 6 weeks of treatment	PSQI	Sleep quality improved significantly in the agomelatine group
[147]	92 patients with primary insomnia and chronic BZD use in a primary health care outpatient clinic	Double-blind, placebo-controlled, randomized trial	Controlled release melatonin 2 mg or placebo during the 1 month withdrawal from BZDs. Follow-up continued for up to 6 months	Successful BZD withdrawal by the end of 1 month was confirmed by BZD in plasma	Reduction in BZD use was similar or even more rare in the melatonin than in the placebo group. Withdrawal symptoms did not differ between the groups

(continued)

Table 22.2 (continued)

References	Subjects	Design	Treatment	Measured	Results
[148]	597 insomniac outpatients classified according to their use of hypnotic BZD or BZD-like drugs (68% previously treated with hypnotics)	Post-marketing surveillance study in Germany	melatonin (2 mg controlled release) p.o.	Sleep diary and recording of BZD use	Most of the patients (77%) who used traditional hypnotics before melatonin treatment had stopped using them and only 5.6% of naive patients started such drugs after melatonin discontinuation
[149]	48 patients with severe mental illness (schizophrenia or bipolar disorder)	Randomized, double-blinded clinical trial with 24 weeks follow-up	controlled-release melatonin (2 mg p.o.)	BZD dosage was gradually tapered; 72 h of actigraphic assessment of activity-rest cycles performed pre and post tapering	Melatonin significantly increased the interdaily stability and decreased the intradaily variability compared with placebo. BZD dose reduction was not associated with circadian rhythm parameters
[150]	Patients with severe mental illness (schizophrenia or bipolar disorder)	Randomized, double-blinded clinical trial with 24 weeks follow-up	controlled-release melatonin (2 mg p.o.)	Subsample of 23 patients underwent polysomnography and 55 patients participated in subjective sleep quality ratings	Melatonin had no effect on objective sleep efficiency, but significantly improved self-reported sleep quality
[151]	86 patients with severe mental illness (schizophrenia or bipolar disorder)	Randomized, double-blinded clinical trial with 24 weeks follow-up	Controlled-release melatonin (2 mg p.o.)	The primary outcome was mean BZD daily dosage at 24 weeks. Secondary outcomes included pattern of BZD dosage over time, BZD cessation proportion, and BZD withdrawal symptoms	BZD cessation proportion was similar in the melatonin group and the placebo group. Prolonged-release melatonin had no effect on BZD withdrawal symptoms
[152]	86 patients with severe mental illness (schizophrenia or bipolar disorder)	Randomized, double-blinded clinical trial with 24 weeks follow-up	Controlled-release melatonin (2 mg p.o.)	The Brief Assessment of Cognition in Schizophrenia (BACS) was used to assess neurocognitive performance with additional assessments of subjective well-being and psychosocial functioning	BACS composite and sub scale scores (except motor speed) significantly improved in parallel with BZD dose reduction, but there was no additional effect of melatonin

[153]	70 males 18 years of age and older in recovery from substance use at a residential program in South-Western Pennsylvania	Double-blind, placebo-controlled, randomized trial	Melatonin (5 mg) of a fast-release preparation or placebo p.o. at bedtime	The primary outcome measures were changes in severity of anxiety; depression; stress; sleep complaints; and how sleep is affecting daily life as assessed by Generalized Anxiety Disorder Scale , Personal Health Questionnaire Depression Scale, Perceived Stress Scale and PSQI questionnaires	No statistically significant between-group differences were detected for baseline characteristics. Even though the proportion of individuals reporting an adverse event between groups was not significantly different, the frequency of reported adverse events was greater in the melatonin group. Intention-to-treat analysis for all the measured outcomes revealed no statistically significant between-group differences for same day comparisons
[154]	92 patients with primary insomnia and chronic BZD use in a primary health care outpatient clinic	Double-blind, placebo-controlled, randomized trial	Controlled release melatonin 2 mg or placebo during the 1 month withdrawal from BZDs. Sleep hygiene counselling and psychosocial support were provided. Three years later, use of BZDAs and other medications was determined by interview and confirmed from medical records	Of the original 92 outpatients, 90% participated in the 3-year survey. The number of BZD-free participants decreased from 37% at 6 months to 28%; intention-to-treat at 3 years. That of irregular BZD users decreased from 48% at 6 months to 29% at 3 years, while that of regular users increased from 12% at 6 months to 33% at 3 years. At 3 years, compared to baseline, use of antidepressants, dopamine agonists, melatonin, and NSAIDs/paracetamol was significantly more common in the whole cohort	Randomization to melatonin or placebo during BZD withdrawal was unrelated to BZD-withdrawal result

(continued)

Table 22.2 (continued)

References	Subjects	Design	Treatment	Measured	Results
[155]	54 patients under methadone maintenance treatment (MMT)	Randomized, double-blind, placebo-controlled trial	10 mg (n = 26) or placebo (n = 28) once a day, 1 h before bedtime for 12 weeks	Sleep quality (PSQI), Beck Depression Inventory and Beck Anxiety Inventory indexes, International Index of Erectile Functions, serum insulin levels, homeostasis model of assessment-insulin resistance, insulin sensitivity check index, and serum HDL-cholesterol, high sensitivity C-reactive protein, malondialdehyde and protein carbonyl levels	Melatonin supplementation significantly decreased PSQI, Beck Depression Inventory and Beck Anxiety Inventory indexes and significantly increased International Index of Erectile Functions Subjects who received melatonin supplements had significantly lower serum insulin levels, homeostasis model of assessment-insulin resistance and higher quantitative insulin sensitivity check index and HDL-cholesterol levels. Additionally, melatonin intake resulted in a significant reduction in serum high sensitivity C-reactive protein. malondialdehyde and protein carbonyl levels
[156]	60 outpatients diagnosed with alcohol use disorder and suffering from sleep problems	Double blind randomized placebo-controlled trial with two arms	Melatonin (5 mg) or placebo at bedtime for 4 weeks	Change in sleep quality was the primary outcome assessed by PSQI scale	In linear mixed models used to statistically analyze the difference in scores before and after 4 weeks of treatment there was a reduction in the global PSQI score in both groups with no significant drug effect between groups
[157]	52 patients with intracerebral hemorrhage were selected; 26 patients were randomly assigned to two groups of melatonin and control	Double-blind, randomized, placebo-controlled study with a parallel assignment of patients	Melatonin (3 mg) or placebo was administered at 9:00 p.m vía de nasogastric tube	Primary outcome was the amount of the most used sedative drug (midazolam, fentanyl, methadone, and morphine sulfate) during the melatonin/placebo treatment). Secondary outcomes were mechanical ventilation time;ICU staying time; Glasgow Coma Scale (GCS) and hemodynamic parameters	Morphine consumption and mechanical ventilation time were significantly lower in the melatonin group. The rise in GCS was faster in the melatonin group

Melatonin in Drug Abuse. Clinical Studies

Table 22.2 summarizes the clinical data available on melatonin activity to improve sleep in human drug abuse. Information is scant, the number of studies reported being low except for benzodiazepine (BDZ) abuse.

Melatonin use in alcohol addicts has been supported by studies on low plasma melatonin levels in this group of substance users [158, 159]. In an open label study of 45 alcohol-dependent patients with sleep and mild affective disorders, a fast release preparation of melatonin (3–6 mg/day, p.o.) for 3 weeks improved sleep latency, quality, and duration of sleep. Melatonin decreased daily sleepiness and affective disorders, particularly anxiety [145]. In a double blind randomized placebo-controlled trial of 60 outpatients diagnosed with alcohol use disorder and suffering from sleep problems, melatonin (5 mg daily) improved sleep as shown subjectively by using the Pittsburgh sleep quality index (PSQI) [156].

Concerning BZD addiction, melatonin has been shown, as listed in Table 22.2, to be effective for BZD-related drugs withdrawal in a number of studies but not in all (see a systematic review for discussion, [160]). Generally, sleep and anxiety improved and a meta-analysis concluded that melatonin given as premedication reduces preoperative anxiety as the standard treatment with midazolam [161].

The involvement of the endogenous opioid system is relevant in drug abuse. Brain imaging studies have shown an increase in opioid receptors density in persons experiencing withdrawal not only from opioids [162] but also from alcohol [163] and cocaine [164]. In a randomized, double-blind, placebo-controlled trial of 54 patients under methadone maintenance treatment, melatonin (10 mg daily) decreased PSQI, Beck Depression Inventory, and Beck Anxiety Inventory indexes and showed lower serum insulin levels, higher quantitative insulin sensitivity check index, and increased HDL-cholesterol levels [155]. Additionally, melatonin intake resulted in a significant reduction in serum high sensitivity C-reactive protein, malondialdehyde, and protein carbonyl levels. However, a lower melatonin dose (5 mg/day) was ineffective to improve recovery from substance use at a residential program in South-Western Pennsylvania [153]. A number of studies support the efficacy of melatonin to reduce the use of sedative drug (midazolam, fentanyl, methadone, morphine sulfate) in intensive care unit patients [157, 165] as well as to decrease the necessity of morphine analgesia [95, 166, 167].

Other studies have examined the efficacy of melatonergic analogs in mitigating addiction-related sleep disorders. In an examination of the capacity of the melatonin MT_1/MT_2 receptor agonist ramelteon to attenuate insomnia in recovering alcoholics, an improvement in sleep quality and quantity was reported [141]. Another study using agomelatine (a melatonergic agonist at MT_1 and MT_2 receptors and a 5¬HT_{2C} antagonist) reported improved sleep in alcohol-dependent subjects with insomnia [146].

Circadian Clocks and Addiction: Considerations for Treatment

Evidence thus shows that there are complex two-way interactions between the circadian and reward systems [3, 4]. The time of day is clearly a risk factor for relapse. Circadian desynchronization and vulnerability to addiction occur. For example, inappropriate exposure to light, as can occur with shift work or transmeridian travel, can cause a state of internal desynchrony which, when chronic, can act as a biological stressor. Lack of sleep and circadian desynchronization reduce the activity of the prefrontal cortex and increase the activity of the ventral striatum in anticipation of reward in adolescents [33]. This leads to poor executive function with poor academic performance, increased impulsivity, and risk-taking behavior. In turn, drug administration can also influence the expression of circadian clock genes in mesocorticolimbic structures. Therefore, the use of chronobiological therapies to promote circadian organization could be beneficial in the clinical management of addiction [3].

Strategies to reorganize rhythmic circadian expression during detoxification and cessation are an excellent measure of support for patients. This is well-known by professionals, who, regardless of the therapeutic approach, recommend stable sleep-wake schedules, meals, and daily activities to be carried out. Maintaining these habits after discharge from the clinic is not only advisable, but highly recommended to improve the quality of life and avoid relapses, although longitudinal studies are required to explore and objectively quantify this [3, 4].

Simple control measures on hourly habits may not always be sufficient in recovering a rhythmicity within homeostatic or health-related values. It is also very convenient to take care that patients are exposed to natural daylight in the morning. Between half an hour or an hour of daily light (the presence of sun is not necessary), during the morning hours, is a therapy with a powerful chronobiological effect [15]. This promotes that the pineal produces an adequate peak of nocturnal melatonin for a better quality sleep and reduces both the risk of suffering from mood disorders and the presence of dysphoric symptoms so frequent in drug withdrawal phases [3].

The administration of exogenous melatonin is a chronopharmacological therapeutic possibility to be considered in the field of drug addiction. It has an organizing effect on circadian rhythmicity (hypnotic and daytime activator), which is why it is a more conservative and first-option treatment compared to the traditionally used BZD hypnotics. Melatonin is not addictive, does not produce tolerance, and has an excellent safety profile, which give it added value for long-term treatments. Its powerful cytoprotective activity provides additional benefit both during detoxification and cessation treatment and in dependent patients who do not stop consumption to minimize the risk of neurodegeneration and the appearance of neuropsychiatric pathology [168].

As discussed in this chapter, studies using 2–10 mg of melatonin/day are not adequate to provide an adequate comparison with data on the protection derived from animal studies on drug abuse. Hence, clinical trials with doses in the 50–100 mg/day range are urgently needed. It should be noted that melatonin is remarkably nontoxic, and its safety is remarkably high. The lethal dose 50 for the intraperitoneal injection of melatonin was determined for rats (1168 mg/kg) and mice (1131 mg/kg), but the oral administration of melatonin (tested up to 3200 mg/kg in rats) could not be determined, like neither for melatonin subcutaneous injection (tested up to 1600 mg/kg in rats and mice) [169]. In humans, melatonin has a high safety profile and, in general, is very well tolerated [170].

Unfortunately, the pharmaceutical industry is refractive to support costly RTC studies for melatonin because of the lack of protective patents for a natural compound. Hence, only with the involvement of governmental and non-profit organizations, such a goal can be achieved. At present, the only option for the attending physician interested in the use of melatonin as a cytoprotective is the off-label indication of the drug.

The question of whether melatonin has a therapeutic value in the prevention or treatment of drug abuse deserves further analysis. Multicenter double-blind studies are needed to explore and further investigate the potential and utility of melatonin. The doses of melatonin used should be reevaluated in view of the equivalent human doses of melatonin derived from preclinical data. Unfortunately, of the 594 clinical trials related to drug abuse (recruitment and non-recruitment) listed in PubMed (ClinicalTrials.gov) search results (10/22/2024), none is directed to chronobiology or melatonin.

Regulating hourly habits, exposure to natural or artificial light, and the prescription of melatonin, in order to reorganize the circadian rhythmic expression, are strategies that can be greatly beneficial in the clinical management of drug-dependent patients. These can improve the response to treatments, avoiding the need to prescribe certain psychotropic drugs whose management in these patients is more complex due to contraindications and greater risk of adverse reactions or development of dependence. Finally, their excellent safety allows them to be used for long periods of time and even for life and may be a protective measure against relapses or the appearance of neuropsychiatric symptoms and the appearance of neuropsychiatric pathology.

Acknowledgment The author is an Emeritus Superior Investigator from the Argentine National Research Council (CONICET) and Emeritus Professor, University of Buenos Aires.

Conflict of Interest The author declares that there are no commercial or financial relationships that could be construed as a potential conflict of interest.

References

1. Ohdo S. Chrono-drug discovery and development based on circadian rhythm of molecular, cellular and organ level. Biol Pharm Bull. 2021;44:747–61. https://doi.org/10.1248/bpb.b21-00277.
2. Ayyar VS, Sukumaran S. Circadian rhythms: influence on physiology, pharmacology, and therapeutic interventions. J Pharmacokinet Pharmacodyn. 2021;48:321–38. https://doi.org/10.1007/s10928-021-09751-2.
3. Tamura EK, Oliveira-Silva KS, Ferreira-Moraes FA, Marinho EAV, Guerrero-Vargas NN. Circadian rhythms and substance use disorders: a bidirectional relationship. Pharmacol Biochem Behav. 2021;201. https://doi.org/10.1016/j.pbb.2021.173105.
4. Gillman AG, Rebec GV, Pecoraro NC, Kosobud AEK. Circadian entrainment by food and drugs of abuse. Behav Process. 2019;165:23–8. https://doi.org/10.1016/j.beproc.2019.05.017.
5. Taylor BJ, Hasler BP. Chronotype and mental health: recent advances. Curr Psychiatry Rep. 2018;20. https://doi.org/10.1007/s11920-018-0925-8.
6. Logan RW, Williams WP, McClung CA. Circadian rhythms and addiction: mechanistic insights and future directions. Behav Neurosci. 2014;128:387–412. https://doi.org/10.1037/a0036268.
7. Kosobud AEK, Gillman AG, Leffel JK, Pecoraro NC, Rebec GV, Timberlake W. Drugs of abuse can entrain circadian rhythms. ScientificWorldJournal. 2007;7:203–12. https://doi.org/10.1100/tsw.2007.234.
8. Adan A, Archer SN, Hidalgo MP, Di Milia L, Natale V, Randler C. Circadian typology: a comprehensive review. Chronobiol Int. 2012;29:1153–75. https://doi.org/10.3109/07420528.2012.719971.
9. Facer-Childs ER, Middleton B, Bagshaw AP, Skene DJ. Human circadian phenotyping and diurnal performance testing in the real world. J Vis Exp. 2020;2020. https://doi.org/10.3791/60448.
10. Onaolapo OJ, Onaolapo AY. Melatonin in drug addiction and addiction management: exploring an evolving multidimensional relationship. World J Psychiatry. 2018;8:64–74. https://doi.org/10.5498/wjp.v8.i2.64.
11. Foster RG. Sleep, circadian rhythms and health. Interface Focus. 2020;10. https://doi.org/10.1098/rsfs.2019.0098.
12. Hastings MH, Maywood ES, Brancaccio M. Generation of circadian rhythms in the suprachiasmatic nucleus. Nat Rev Neurosci. 2018;19:453–69. https://doi.org/10.1038/s41583-018-0026-z.
13. Welz PS, Benitah SA. Molecular connections between circadian clocks and aging. J Mol Biol. 2020;432. https://doi.org/10.1016/j.jmb.2019.12.036.
14. Micic G, de Bruyn A, Lovato N, Wright H, Gradisar M, Ferguson S, et al. The endogenous circadian temperature period length (tau) in delayed sleep phase disorder compared to good sleepers. J Sleep Res. 2013;22:617–24. https://doi.org/10.1111/jsr.12072.
15. Arendt J. Melatonin: countering chaotic time cues. Front Endocrinol (Lausanne). 2019;10. https://doi.org/10.3389/fendo.2019.00391.
16. Manchester LC, Coto-Montes A, Boga JA, Andersen LPH, Zhou Z, Galano A, et al. Melatonin: an ancient molecule that makes oxygen metabolically tolerable. J Pineal Res. 2015;59:403–19. https://doi.org/10.1111/jpi.12267.
17. Bondy SC, Campbell A. Melatonin and regulation of immune function: impact on numerous diseases. Curr Aging Sci. 2020;13. https://doi.org/10.2174/1874609813666200711153223.
18. Besedovsky L, Lange T, Haack M. The sleep-immune crosstalk in health and disease. Physiol Rev. 2019;99:1325–80. https://doi.org/10.1152/physrev.00010.2018.
19. Bart CP, Titone MK, Ng TH, Nusslock R, Alloy LB. Neural reward circuit dysfunction as a risk factor for bipolar spectrum disorders and substance use disorders: a review and integration. Clin Psychol Rev. 2021;87:102035. https://doi.org/10.1016/j.cpr.2021.102035.
20. Xu P, Chen A, Li Y, Xing X, Lu H. Medial prefrontal cortex in neurological diseases. Physiol Genomics. 2019;51:432–42. https://doi.org/10.1152/physiolgenomics.00006.2019.
21. Webb IC. Circadian rhythms and substance abuse: chronobiological considerations for the treatment of addiction. Curr Psychiatry Rep. 2017;19. https://doi.org/10.1007/s11920-017-0764-z.
22. Di Chiara G. Nucleus accumbens shell and core dopamine: differential role in behavior and addiction. Behav Brain Res. 2002;137:75–114. https://doi.org/10.1016/S0166-4328(02)00286-3.
23. Volkow ND, Morales M. The brain on drugs: from reward to addiction. Cell. 2015;162:712–25. https://doi.org/10.1016/j.cell.2015.07.046.
24. Grippo RM, Güler AD. Dopamine signaling in circadian photoentrainment: consequences of desynchrony. Yale J Biol Med. 2019;92:271–81.
25. Hood S, Cassidy P, Cossette MP, Weigl Y, Verwey M, Robinson B, et al. Endogenous dopamine regulates the rhythm of expression of the clock protein PER2 in the rat dorsal striatum via daily activation of D2 dopamine receptors. J Neurosci. 2010;30:14046–58. https://doi.org/10.1523/JNEUROSCI.2128-10.2010.

26. Khaldy H, Escames G, León J, Bikjdaouene L, Acuña-Castroviejo D. Synergistic effects of melatonin and deprenyl against MPTP-induced mitochondrial damage and DA depletion. Neurobiol Aging. 2003;24:491–500. https://doi.org/10.1016/S0197-4580(02)00133-1.
27. Weber M, Lauterburg T, Tobler I, Burgunder JM. Circadian patterns of neurotransmitter related gene expression in motor regions of the rat brain. Neurosci Lett. 2004;358:17–20. https://doi.org/10.1016/j.neulet.2003.12.053.
28. Grace AA. Physiology of the normal and dopamine-depleted basal ganglia: insights into levodopa pharmacotherapy. Mov Disord. 2008;23 https://doi.org/10.1002/mds.22020.
29. Mendoza J, Challet E. Circadian insights into dopamine mechanisms. Neuroscience. 2014;282:230–42. https://doi.org/10.1016/j.neuroscience.2014.07.081.
30. Freyberg Z, Logan RW. The intertwined roles of circadian rhythms and neuronal metabolism fueling drug reward and addiction. Curr Opin Physiol. 2018;5:80–9. https://doi.org/10.1016/j.cophys.2018.08.004.
31. Chandra S, Scharf D, Shiffman S. Within-day temporal patterns of smoking, withdrawal symptoms, and craving. Drug Alcohol Depend. 2011;117:118–25. https://doi.org/10.1016/j.drugalcdep.2010.12.027.
32. Perreau-Lenz S, Spanagel R. The effects of drugs of abuse on clock genes. Drug News Perspect. 2008;21:211–7. https://doi.org/10.1358/dnp.2008.21.4.1213350.
33. Gulick D, Gamsby JJ. Racing the clock: the role of circadian rhythmicity in addiction across the lifespan. Pharmacol Ther. 2018;188:124–39. https://doi.org/10.1016/j.pharmthera.2018.03.003.
34. Danel T, Touitou Y. Chronobiology of alcohol: from chronokinetics to alcohol-related alterations of the circadian system. Chronobiol Int. 2004;21:923–35. https://doi.org/10.1081/CBI-200036886.
35. Haynie DL, Lewin D, Luk JW, Lipsky LM, O'Brien F, Iannotti RJ, et al. Beyond sleep duration: bidirectional associations among chronotype, social jetlag, and drinking behaviors in a longitudinal sample of US high school students. Sleep. 2018;41 https://doi.org/10.1093/sleep/zsx202.
36. Crego A, Holguín SR, Parada M, Mota N, Corral M, Cadaveira F. Binge drinking affects attentional and visual working memory processing in young university students. Alcohol Clin Exp Res. 2009;33:1870–9. https://doi.org/10.1111/j.1530-0277.2009.01025.x.
37. Miró Ò, Waring WS, Dargan PI, Wood DM, Dines AM, Yates C, et al. Variation of drugs involved in acute drug toxicity presentations based on age and sex: an epidemiological approach based on European emergency departments. Clin Toxicol. 2021. https://doi.org/10.1080/15563650.2021.1884693.
38. Depoy LM, McClung CA, Logan RW. Neural mechanisms of circadian regulation of natural and drug reward. Neural Plast. 2017;2017. https://doi.org/10.1155/2017/5720842.
39. Forde LA, Kalsi G. Addiction and the role of circadian genes. J Stud Alcohol Drugs. 2017;78:645–53. https://doi.org/10.15288/jsad.2017.78.645.
40. McClung CA, Sidiropoulou K, Vitaterna M, Takahashi JS, White FJ, Cooper DC, et al. Regulation of dopaminergic transmission and cocaine reward by the Clock gene. Proc Natl Acad Sci USA. 2005;102:9377–81. https://doi.org/10.1073/pnas.0503584102.
41. Abarca C, Albrecht U, Spanagel R. Cocaine sensitization and reward are under the influence of circadian genes and rhythm. Proc Natl Acad Sci USA. 2002;99:9026–30. https://doi.org/10.1073/pnas.142039099.
42. Kim M, Jeon SJ, Custodio RJ, Lee HJ, Sayson LV, Ortiz DMD, et al. Gene expression profiling in the striatumof per2 komice exhibiting more vulnerable responses against methamphetamine. Biomol Ther. 2021;29:135–43. https://doi.org/10.4062/biomolther.2020.123.
43. Spanagel R. Alcoholism: a systems approach from molecular physiology to addictive behavior. Physiol Rev. 2009;89:649–705. https://doi.org/10.1152/physrev.00013.2008.
44. Perreau-Lenz S, Spanagel R. Clock genes×stress×reward interactions in alcohol and substance use disorders. Alcohol. 2015;49:351–7. https://doi.org/10.1016/j.alcohol.2015.04.003.
45. Perreau-Lenz S, Sanchis-Segura C, Leonardi-Essmann F, Schneider M, Spanagel R. Development of morphine-induced tolerance and withdrawal: involvement of the clock gene mPer2. Eur Neuropsychopharmacol. 2010;20:509–17. https://doi.org/10.1016/j.euroneuro.2010.03.006.
46. Siemann JK, Grueter BA, McMahon DG. Rhythms, reward, and blues: consequences of circadian photoperiod on affective and reward circuit function. Neuroscience. 2021;457:220–34. https://doi.org/10.1016/j.neuroscience.2020.12.010.
47. Brower KJ, Wojnar M, Sliwerska E, Armitage R, Burmeister M. PER3 polymorphism and insomnia severity in alcohol dependence. Sleep. 2012;35:571–7. https://doi.org/10.5665/sleep.1748.
48. Roehrs T, Sibai M, Roth T. Sleep and alertness disturbance and substance use disorders: a bi-directional relation. Pharmacol Biochem Behav. 2021;203 https://doi.org/10.1016/j.pbb.2021.173153.
49. Martin JS, Gaudreault MM, Perron M, Laberge L. Chronotype, light exposure, sleep, and daytime functioning in high school students attending morning or afternoon school shifts: an actigraphic study. J Biol Rhythm. 2016;31:205–17. https://doi.org/10.1177/0748730415625510.
50. Hasler BP, Pedersen SL. Sleep and circadian risk factors for alcohol problems: a brief overview and proposed mechanisms. Curr Opin Psychol. 2020;34:57–62. https://doi.org/10.1016/j.copsyc.2019.09.005.
51. Montaruli A, Castelli L, Mulè A, Scurati R, Esposito F, Galasso L, et al. Biological rhythm and chrono-

type: new perspectives in health. Biomolecules. 2021;11. https://doi.org/10.3390/biom11040487.
52. Logan RW, Hasler BP, Forbes EE, Franzen PL, Torregrossa MM, Huang YH, et al. Impact of sleep and circadian rhythms on addiction vulnerability in adolescents. Biol Psychiatry. 2018;83:987–96. https://doi.org/10.1016/j.biopsych.2017.11.035.
53. Caci H, Deschaux O, Adan A, Natale V. Comparing three morningness scales: age and gender effects, structure and cut-off criteria. Sleep Med. 2009;10:240–5. https://doi.org/10.1016/j.sleep.2008.01.007.
54. Adan A. Chronotype and personality factors in the daily consumption of alcohol and psychostimulants. Addiction. 1994;89:455–62. https://doi.org/10.1111/j.1360-0443.1994.tb00926.x.
55. Chen SA, O'Dell LE, Hoefer ME, Greenwell TN, Zorrilla EP, Koob GF. Unlimited access to heroin self-administration: independent motivational markers of opiate dependence. Neuropsychopharmacology. 2006;31:2692–707. https://doi.org/10.1038/sj.npp.1301008.
56. Angarita GA, Emadi N, Hodges S, Morgan PT. Sleep abnormalities associated with alcohol, cannabis, cocaine, and opiate use: a comprehensive review. Addict Sci Clin Pract. 2016;11. https://doi.org/10.1186/s13722-016-0056-7.
57. Reid-Varley WB, Ponce Martinez C, Khurshid KA. Sleep disorders and disrupted sleep in addiction, withdrawal and abstinence with focus on alcohol and opioids. J Neurol Sci. 2020;411. https://doi.org/10.1016/j.jns.2020.116713.
58. Tripathi R, Rao R, Dhawan A, Jain R, Sinha S. Opioids and sleep—a review of literature. Sleep Med. 2020;67:269–75. https://doi.org/10.1016/j.sleep.2019.06.012.
59. Dunn KE, Finan PH, Andrew Tompkins D, Strain EC. Frequency and correlates of sleep disturbance in methadone and buprenorphine-maintained patients. Addict Behav. 2018;76:8–14. https://doi.org/10.1016/j.addbeh.2017.07.016.
60. Ashare RL, Lerman C, Tyndale RF, Hawk LW, George TP, Cinciripini P, et al. Sleep disturbance during smoking cessation: withdrawal or side effect of treatment? J Smok Cessat. 2017;12:63–70. https://doi.org/10.1017/jsc.2016.11.
61. Ferracioli-Oda E, Qawasmi A, Bloch MH. Meta-analysis: melatonin for the treatment of primary sleep disorders. Focus (Madison). 2018;16:113–8. https://doi.org/10.1176/appi.focus.16101.
62. Auld F, Maschauer EL, Morrison I, Skene DJ, Riha RL. Evidence for the efficacy of melatonin in the treatment of primary adult sleep disorders. Sleep Med Rev. 2017;34:10–22. https://doi.org/10.1016/j.smrv.2016.06.005.
63. Li T, Jiang S, Han M, Yang Z, Lv J, Deng C, et al. Exogenous melatonin as a treatment for secondary sleep disorders: a systematic review and meta-analysis. Front Neuroendocrinol. 2019;52:22–8. https://doi.org/10.1016/j.yfrne.2018.06.004.
64. Wilson SJ, Nutt DJ, Alford C, Argyropoulos SV, Baldwin DS, Bateson AN, et al. British Association for Psychopharmacology consensus statement on evidence-based treatment of insomnia, parasomnias and circadian rhythm disorders. J Psychopharmacol. 2010;24:1577–600. https://doi.org/10.1177/0269881110379307.
65. Palagini L, Manni R, Aguglia E, Amore M, Brugnoli R, Girardi P, et al. Expert opinions and consensus recommendations for the evaluation and management of insomnia in clinical practice: joint statements of five Italian scientific societies. Front Psychiatry. 2020;11. https://doi.org/10.3389/fpsyt.2020.00558.
66. Vecchierini MF, Kilic-Huck U, Quera-Salva MA. Melatonin (MEL) and its use in neurological diseases and insomnia: recommendations of the French Medical and Research Sleep Society (SFRMS). Rev Neurol (Paris). 2020. https://doi.org/10.1016/j.neurol.2020.06.009.
67. Geoffroy PA, Micoulaud Franchi JA, Lopez R, Schroder CM. The use of melatonin in adult psychiatric disorders: expert recommendations by the French institute of medical research on sleep (SFRMS). Encéphale. 2019;45:413–23. https://doi.org/10.1016/j.encep.2019.04.068.
68. Dawson D, Armstrong SM. Chronobiotics—drugs that shift rhythms. Pharmacol Ther. 1996;69:15–36. https://doi.org/10.1016/0163-7258(95)02020-9.
69. Cardinali DP, Pandi-Perumal SR, Srinivasan V, Spence DW, Trakht I. Therapeutic potential of melatonin agonists. Expert Rev Endocrinol Metab. 2008;3 https://doi.org/10.1586/17446651.3.2.269.
70. Lavie P. Melatonin: role in gating nocturnal rise in sleep propensity. J Biol Rhythm. 1997;12:657–65. https://doi.org/10.1177/074873049701200622.
71. Lewy A, Emens J, Jackman A, Yuhas K. Circadian uses of melatonin in humans. Chronobiol Int. 2006;23:403–12. https://doi.org/10.1080/07420520500545862.
72. Pandi-Perumal SR, Trakht I, Srinivasan V, Spence DW, Maestroni GJM, Zisapel N, et al. Physiological effects of melatonin: role of melatonin receptors and signal transduction pathways. Prog Neurobiol. 2008;85 https://doi.org/10.1016/j.pneurobio.2008.04.001.
73. Claustrat B, Leston J. Melatonin: physiological effects in humans. Neurochirurgie. 2015;61:77–84. https://doi.org/10.1016/j.neuchi.2015.03.002.
74. Acuña-Castroviejo D, Escames G, Venegas C, Díaz-Casado ME, Lima-Cabello E, López LC, et al. Extrapineal melatonin: sources, regulation, and potential functions. Cell Mol Life Sci. 2014;71:2997–3025. https://doi.org/10.1007/s00018-014-1579-2.
75. Tan D-X, Reiter RJ. Mitochondria: the birth place, battle ground and the site of melatonin metabolism in cells. Melatonin Res. 2019;2:44–66. https://doi.org/10.32794/mr11250011.
76. Hardeland R, Cardinali DP, Srinivasan V, Spence DW, Brown GM, Pandi-Perumal SR. Melatonin-A

pleiotropic, orchestrating regulator molecule. Prog Neurobiol. 2011;93. https://doi.org/10.1016/j.pneurobio.2010.12.004.

77. Dubocovich ML, Delagrange P, Krause DN, Sugden D, Cardinali DP, Olcese J. International union of basic and clinical pharmacology. LXXV. Nomenclature, classification, and pharmacology of G protein-coupled melatonin receptors. Pharmacol Rev 2010;62. https://doi.org/10.1124/pr.110.002832.
78. Cecon E, Oishi A, Jockers R. Melatonin receptors: molecular pharmacology and signalling in the context of system bias. Br J Pharmacol. 2018;175:3263–80. https://doi.org/10.1111/bph.13950.
79. Ng KY, Leong MK, Liang H, Paxinos G. Melatonin receptors: distribution in mammalian brain and their respective putative functions. Brain Struct Funct. 2017;222:2921–39. https://doi.org/10.1007/s00429-017-1439-6.
80. Uz T, Arslan AD, Kurtuncu M, Imbesi M, Akhisaroglu M, Dwivedi Y, et al. The regional and cellular expression profile of the melatonin receptor MT1 in the central dopaminergic system. Mol Brain Res. 2005;136:45–53. https://doi.org/10.1016/j.molbrainres.2005.01.002.
81. Jiménez-Rubio G, Ortíz-López L, Benítez-King G. Melatonin modulates cytoskeletal organization in the rat brain hippocampus. Neurosci Lett. 2012;511:47–51. https://doi.org/10.1016/j.neulet.2012.01.040.
82. Hardeland R. Recent findings in melatonin research and their relevance to the CNS. Cent Nerv Syst Agents Med Chem. 2018;18:102–14. https://doi.org/10.2174/1871524918666180531083944.
83. Venegas C, García JA, Doerrier C, Volt H, Escames G, Lõpez LC, et al. Analysis of the daily changes of melatonin receptors in the rat liver. J Pineal Res. 2013;54:313–21. https://doi.org/10.1111/jpi.12019.
84. Zemková H, Vaněček J. Inhibitory effect of melatonin on gonadotropin-releasing hormone-induced Ca2+ Oscillations in pituitary cells of newborn rats. Neuroendocrinology. 1997;65:276–83. https://doi.org/10.1159/000127185.
85. Cardinali DP. Are melatonin doses employed clinically adequate for melatonin-induced cytoprotection? Melatonin Res. 2019;2:106–32. https://doi.org/10.32794/mr11250025.
86. Shukla M, Chinchalongporn V, Govitrapong P, Reiter RJ. The role of melatonin in targeting cell signaling pathways in neurodegeneration. Ann N Y Acad Sci. 2019;1443:75–96. https://doi.org/10.1111/nyas.14005.
87. Tan HY, Ng KY, Koh RY, Chye SM. Pharmacological effects of melatonin as neuroprotectant in rodent model: a review on the current biological evidence. Cell Mol Neurobiol. 2020;40:25–51. https://doi.org/10.1007/s10571-019-00724-1.
88. Tamtaji OR, Reiter RJ, Alipoor R, Dadgostar E, Kouchaki E, Asemi Z. Melatonin and Parkinson disease: current status and future perspectives for molecular mechanisms. Cell Mol Neurobiol. 2020;40:15–23. https://doi.org/10.1007/s10571-019-00720-5.
89. Reiter RJ, Rosales-Corral S, Tan DX, Jou MJ, Galano A, Xu B. Melatonin as a mitochondria-targeted antioxidant: one of evolution's best ideas. Cell Mol Life Sci. 2017;74:3863–81. https://doi.org/10.1007/s00018-017-2609-7.
90. Hardeland R. Melatonin and inflammation—story of a double-edged blade. J Pineal Res 2018;65. https://doi.org/10.1111/jpi.12525.
91. Carrillo-Vico A, Lardone PJ, Álvarez-Śnchez N, Rodrĩguez-Rodrĩguez A, Guerrero JM. Melatonin: buffering the immune system. Int J Mol Sci. 2013;14:8638–83. https://doi.org/10.3390/ijms14048638.
92. Cardinali DP, Ritta MN, Fuentes AM, Gimeno MF, Gimeno AL. Prostaglandin E release by rat medial basal hypothalamus in vitro. Inhibition by melatonin at submicromolar concentrations. Eur J Pharmacol. 1980;67 https://doi.org/10.1016/0014-2999(80)90025-4.
93. Deng WG, Tang ST, Tseng HP, Wu KK. Melatonin suppresses macrophage cyclooxygenase-2 and inducible nitric oxide synthase expression by inhibiting p52 acetylation and binding. Blood. 2006;108:518–24. https://doi.org/10.1182/blood-2005-09-3691.
94. Golombek DA, PéVet P, Cardinali DP. Melatonin effects on behavior: possible mediation by the central GABAergic system. Neurosci Biobehav Rev. 1996;20. https://doi.org/10.1016/0149-7634(95)00052-6.
95. Caumo W, Levandovski R, Hidalgo MPL. Preoperative anxiolytic effect of melatonin and clonidine on postoperative pain and morphine consumption in patients undergoing abdominal hysterectomy: a double-blind, randomized, placebo-controlled study. J Pain. 2009;10:100–8. https://doi.org/10.1016/j.jpain.2008.08.007.
96. Louzada PR, Lima ACP, Mendonca-Silva DL, Noël F, De Mello FG, Ferreira ST. Taurine prevents the neurotoxicity of β-amyloid and glutamate receptor agonists: activation of GABA receptors and possible implications for Alzheimer's disease and other neurological disorders. FASEB J. 2004;18:511–8. https://doi.org/10.1096/fj.03-0739com.
97. Cheng XP, Sun H, Ye ZY, Zhou JN. Melatonin modulates the GABAergic response in cultured rat hippocampal neurons. J Pharmacol Sci. 2012;119:177–85. https://doi.org/10.1254/jphs.11183FP.
98. Cho S, Joh TH, Baik HH, Dibinis C, Volpe BT. Melatonin administration protects CA1 hippocampal neurons after transient forebrain ischemia in rats. Brain Res. 1997;755:335–8. https://doi.org/10.1016/S0006-8993(97)00188-1.
99. Furio AM, Fontao R, Falco N, Ruiz JI, Caccuri R, Cardinali DP. Neuroprotective effect of melatonin on glucocorticoid toxicity in the rat hippocampus. Open

Physiol J. 2014;1:23–7. https://doi.org/10.2174/1874360900901010023.
100. Giusti P, Upartiti M, Franceschini D, Schiavo N, Floreani M, Manev H. Neuroprotection by melatonin from kainate-induced excitotoxicity in rats. FASEB J. 1996;10:891–6. https://doi.org/10.1096/fasebj.10.8.8666166.
101. Escames G, León J, López LC, Acuña-Castroviejo D. Mechanisms of N-methyl-D-aspartate receptor inhibition by melatonin in the rat striatum. J Neuroendocrinol. 2004;16:929–35. https://doi.org/10.1111/j.1365-2826.2004.01250.x.
102. Zisapel N, Egozi Y, Laudon M. Inhibition of dopamine release by melatonin: regional distribution in the rat brain. Brain Res. 1982;246:161–3. https://doi.org/10.1016/0006-8993(82)90157-3.
103. Khaldy H, León J, Escames G, Bikjdaouene L, García JJ, Acuña-Castroviejo D. Circadian rhythms of dopamine and dihydroxyphenyl acetic acid in the mouse striatum: effects of pinealectomy and of melatonin treatment. Neuroendocrinology. 2002;75:201–8. https://doi.org/10.1159/000048238.
104. Adi N, Mash DC, Ali Y, Singer C, Shehadeh L, Papapetropoulos S. Melatonin MT1 and MT2 receptor expression in Parkinson's disease. Med Sci Monit. 2010;16:BR61–7.
105. Reagan-Shaw S, Nihal M, Ahmad N. Dose translation from animal to human studies revisited. FASEB J. 2008;22:659–61. https://doi.org/10.1096/fj.07-9574lsf.
106. Hirata H, Asanuma M, Cadet JL. Melatonin attenuates methamphetamine-induced toxic effects on dopamine and serotonin terminals in mouse brain. Synapse. 1998;30:150–5. https://doi.org/10.1002/(SICI)1098-2396(199810)30:2<150::AID-SYN4>3.0.CO;2-B.
107. Itzhak Y, Martin JL, Dean Black M, Ali SF. Effect of melatonin on methamphetamine- and 1-methyl-4-phenyl-1,2,3,6- tetrahydropyridine-induced dopaminergic neurotoxicity and methamphetamine- induced behavioral sensitization. Neuropharmacology. 1998;37:781–91. https://doi.org/10.1016/S0028-3908(98)00067-7.
108. Qiu Y, Kang L, Qiu X. [The inhibitory effect of melatonin on morphine withdrawal syndromes and serum monoamines in morphine dependent mice]. Zhonghua Yi Xue Za Zhi. 1998;78:704–6.
109. Raghavendra V, Kulkarni SK. Reversal of morphine tolerance and dependence by melatonin: possible role of central and peripheral benzodiazepine receptors. Brain Res. 1999;834:178–81. https://doi.org/10.1016/S0006-8993(99)01520-6.
110. Raghavendra V, Kulkarni SK. Possible mechanisms of action in melatonin reversal of morphine tolerance and dependence in mice. Eur J Pharmacol. 2000;409:279–89. https://doi.org/10.1016/S0014-2999(00)00849-9.
111. Sircar R. Effect of melatonin on cocaine-induced behavioral sensitization. Brain Res. 2000;857:295–9. https://doi.org/10.1016/S0006-8993(99)02460-9.
112. Zhdanova IV, Giorgetti M. Melatonin alters behavior and cAMP levels in nucleus accumbens induced by cocaine treatment. Brain Res. 2002;956:323–31. https://doi.org/10.1016/S0006-8993(02)03565-5.
113. Zhou YH, Huo ZY, Qiu XC. Inhibitory effect of melatonin on morphine withdrawal syndromes and the content of no in plasma and brain tissue in morphine dependent mice. Yaoxue Xuebao. 2002;37:175–7.
114. Wei YM, Xu Y, Yu CX, Han J. Melatonin enhances the expression of β-endorphin in hypothalamic arcuate nucleus of morphine-dependent mice. Sheng Li Xue Bao. 2009;61:255–62.
115. Cemek M, Büyükokuroğlu ME, Hazman Ö, Konuk M, Bulut S, Birdane YO. The roles of melatonin and vitamin E plus selenium in prevention of oxidative stress induced by naloxone-precipitated withdrawal in heroin-addicted rats. Biol Trace Elem Res. 2011;142:55–66. https://doi.org/10.1007/s12011-010-8744-8.
116. Cemek M, Büyükokuroğlu ME, Hazman Ö, Bulut S, Konuk M, Birdane Y. Antioxidant enzyme and element status in heroin addiction or heroin withdrawal in rats: effect of melatonin and vitamin E plus se. Biol Trace Elem Res. 2011;139:41–54. https://doi.org/10.1007/s12011-010-8634-0.
117. Feng YM, Jia YF, Su LY, Wang D, Lv L, Xu L, et al. Decreased mitochondrial DNA copy number in the hippocampus and peripheral blood during opiate addiction is mediated by autophagy and can be salvaged by melatonin. Autophagy. 2013;9:1395–406. https://doi.org/10.4161/auto.25468.
118. Bagheri F, Goudarzi I, Lashkarbolouki T, Elahdadi SM. Melatonin prevents oxidative damage induced by maternal ethanol administration and reduces homocysteine in the cerebellum of rat pups. Behav Brain Res. 2015;287:215–25. https://doi.org/10.1016/j.bbr.2015.03.022.
119. Singhakumar R, Boontem P, Ekthuwapranee K, Sotthibundhu A, Mukda S, Chetsawang B, et al. Melatonin attenuates methamphetamine-induced inhibition of neurogenesis in the adult mouse hippocampus: an in vivo study. Neurosci Lett. 2015;606:209–14. https://doi.org/10.1016/j.neulet.2015.09.011.
120. Vengeliene V, Noori HR, Spanagel R. Activation of melatonin receptors reduces relapse-like alcohol consumption. Neuropsychopharmacology. 2015;40:2897–906. https://doi.org/10.1038/npp.2015.143.
121. Lin SH, Huang YN, Kao JH, Tien LT, Tsai RY, Wong CS. Melatonin reverses morphine tolerance by inhibiting microglia activation and HSP27 expression. Life Sci. 2016;152:38–43. https://doi.org/10.1016/j.lfs.2016.03.032.
122. Wu J, Zhu D, Zhang J, Li G, Liu Z, Sun J. Melatonin treatment during the incubation of sensitization attenuates methamphetamine-induced locomotor sensitization and MeCP2 expression. Prog Neuro-Psychopharmacol Biol Psychiatry. 2016;65:145–52. https://doi.org/10.1016/j.pnpbp.2015.09.008.

123. Takahashi TT, Vengeliene V, Spanagel R. Melatonin reduces motivation for cocaine self-administration and prevents relapse-like behavior in rats. Psychopharmacology. 2017;234:1741–8. https://doi.org/10.1007/s00213-017-4576-y.
124. Sousa Coelho IDD, Lapa Neto CJC, Souza TGS, Silva MA, Chagas CA, Santos KRP, et al. Protective effect of exogenous melatonin in rats and their offspring on the genotoxic response induced by the chronic consumption of alcohol during pregnancy. Mutat Res Genet Toxicol Environ Mutagen. 2018;832–833:52–60. https://doi.org/10.1016/j.mrgentox.2018.06.018.
125. Cheng YC, Tsai RY, Sung YT, Chen IJ, Tu TY, Mao YY, et al. Melatonin regulation of transcription in the reversal of morphine tolerance: microarray analysis of differential gene expression. Int J Mol Med. 2019;43:791–806. https://doi.org/10.3892/ijmm.2018.4030.
126. Wang Y, Wang X, Chen J, Li S, Zhai H, Wang Z. Melatonin pretreatment attenuates acute methamphetamine-induced aggression in male ICR mice. Brain Res. 2019;1715:196–202. https://doi.org/10.1016/j.brainres.2019.04.002.
127. Barbosa-Méndez S, Salazar-Juárez A. Melatonin decreases cocaine-induced locomotor activity in pinealectomized rats. Braz J Psychiatry. 2020;42:295–308. https://doi.org/10.1590/1516-4446-2018-0400.
128. Chen IJ, Yang CP, Lin SH, Lai CM, Wong CS. The circadian hormone melatonin inhibits morphine-induced tolerance and inflammation via the activation of antioxidative enzymes. Antioxidants. 2020;9:1–20. https://doi.org/10.3390/antiox9090780.
129. Namyen J, Permpoonputtana K, Nopparat C, Tocharus J, Tocharus C, Govitrapong P. Protective effects of melatonin on methamphetamine-induced blood–brain barrier dysfunction in rat model. Neurotox Res. 2020;37:640–60. https://doi.org/10.1007/s12640-019-00156-1.
130. Barbosa-Méndez S, Pérez-Sánchez G, Becerril-Villanueva E, Salazar-Juárez A. Melatonin decreases cocaine-induced locomotor sensitization and cocaine-conditioned place preference in rats. J Psychiatr Res. 2021;132:97–110. https://doi.org/10.1016/j.jpsychires.2020.09.027.
131. Veschsanit N, Yang JL, Ngampramuan S, Viwatpinyo K, Pinyomahakul J, Lwin T, et al. Melatonin reverts methamphetamine-induced learning and memory impairments and hippocampal alterations in mice. Life Sci 2021;265. https://doi.org/10.1016/j.lfs.2020.118844.
132. Dagan Y, Zisapel N, Nof D, Laudon M, Atsmon J. Rapid reversal of tolerance to benzodiazepine hypnotics by treatment with oral melatonin: a case report. Eur Neuropsychopharmacol. 1997;7:157–60. https://doi.org/10.1016/S0924-977X(96)00381-1.
133. Fainstein I, Bonetto AJ, Brusco LI, Cardinali DP. Effects of melatonin in elderly patients with sleep disturbance: a pilot study. Curr Ther Res—Clin Exp 1997;58. https://doi.org/10.1016/S0011-393X(97)80066-5.
134. Garfinkel D, Zisapel N, Wainstein J, Laudon M. Facilitation of benzodiazepine discontinuation by melatonin: a new clinical approach. Arch Intern Med. 1999;159:2456–60. https://doi.org/10.1001/archinte.159.20.2456.
135. Siegrist C, Benedetti C, Orlando A, Beltrán JM, Tuchscherr L, Noseda CMJ, et al. Lack of changes in serum prolactin, FSH, TSH, and estradiol after melatonin treatment in doses that improve sleep and reduce benzodiazepine consumption in sleep-disturbed, middle-aged, and elderly patients. J Pineal Res 2001;30. https://doi.org/10.1034/j.1600-079X.2001.300105.x.
136. Cardinali DP, Brusco LI, Pérez Lloret S, Furio AM. Melatonin in sleep disorders and jet-lag. Neuroendocrinol Lett 2002; Suppl 1:9–13.
137. Vissers FHJA, Knipschild PG, Crebolder HFJM. Is melatonin helpful in stopping the long-term use of hypnotics? A discontinuation trial. Pharm World Sci. 2007;29:641–6. https://doi.org/10.1007/s11096-007-9118-y.
138. Furio AM, Brusco LI, Cardinali DP. Possible therapeutic value of melatonin in mild cognitive impairment: a retrospective study. J Pineal Res. 2007;43. https://doi.org/10.1111/j.1600-079X.2007.00491.x.
139. Peles E, Hetzroni T, Bar-Hamburger R, Adelson M, Schreiber S. Melatonin for perceived sleep disturbances associated with benzodiazepine withdrawal among patients in methadone maintenance treatment: a double-blind randomized clinical trial. Addiction. 2007;102:1947–53. https://doi.org/10.1111/j.1360-0443.2007.02007.x.
140. Garzón C, Guerrero JM, Aramburu O, Guzmán T. Effecf of melatonin administration on sleep, behavioral disorders and hypnotic drug discontinuation in the elderly: a randomized, double-blind, placebo-controlled study. Aging Clin Exp Res. 2009;21:38–42. https://doi.org/10.1007/BF03324897.
141. Brower KJ, Conroy DA, Kurth ME, Anderson BJ, Stein MD. Ramelteon and improved insomnia in alcohol-dependent patients: a case series. J Clin Sleep Med. 2011;7:274–5. https://doi.org/10.5664/JCSM.1070.
142. Cardinali DP, Vigo DE, Olivar N, Vidal MF, Furio AM, Brusco LI. Therapeutic application of melatonin in mild cognitive impairment. Am J Neurodegener Dis. 2012;1(3):280–91.
143. Kunz D, Bineau S, Maman K, Milea D, Toumi M. Benzodiazepine discontinuation with prolonged-release melatonin: hints from a German longitudinal prescription database. Expert Opin Pharmacother. 2012;13:9–16. https://doi.org/10.1517/14656566.2012.638284.
144. Clay E, Falissard B, Moore N, Toumi M. Contribution of prolonged-release melatonin and anti-benzodiazepine campaigns to the reduction of benzodiazepine and z-drugs consumption in nine European countries. Eur J Clin

Pharmacol. 2013;69:1–10. https://doi.org/10.1007/s00228-012-1424-1.
145. Eryshev OF, Anipchenko A V., Andreeva NE, Andrianov F V. An open-label non-comparative study of the efficacy and safety of melaxen in treatment of sleep disorders in alcohol dependent patients during the period of abstinence. Zhurnal Nevrol i Psihiatr Im SS Korsakova. 2013;113.
146. Grosshans M, Mutschler J, Luderer M, Mann K, Kiefer F. Agomelatine is effective in reducing insomnia in abstinent alcohol-dependent patients. Clin Neuropharmacol. 2014;37:6–8. https://doi.org/10.1097/WNF.0000000000000007.
147. Lähteenmäki R, Puustinen J, Vahlberg T, Lyles A, Neuvonen PJ, Partinen M, et al. Melatonin for sedative withdrawal in older patients with primary insomnia: a randomized double-blind placebo-controlled trial. Br J Clin Pharmacol. 2014;77:975–85. https://doi.org/10.1111/bcp.12294.
148. Hajak G, Lemme K, Zisapel N. Lasting treatment effects in a postmarketing surveillance study of prolonged-release melatonin. Int Clin Psychopharmacol. 2015;30:36–42. https://doi.org/10.1097/YIC.0000000000000046.
149. Baandrup L, Fasmer OB, Glenthøj BY, Jennum PJ. Circadian rest-activity rhythms during benzodiazepine tapering covered by melatonin versus placebo add-on: data derived from a randomized clinical trial. BMC Psychiatry 2016;16. https://doi.org/10.1186/s12888-016-1062-8.
150. Baandrup L, Glenthøj BY, Jennum PJ. Objective and subjective sleep quality: melatonin versus placebo add-on treatment in patients with schizophrenia or bipolar disorder withdrawing from long-term benzodiazepine use. Psychiatry Res. 2016;240:163–9. https://doi.org/10.1016/j.psychres.2016.04.031.
151. Baandrup L, Lindschou J, Winkel P, Gluud C, Glenthoj BY. Prolonged-release melatonin versus placebo for benzodiazepine discontinuation in patients with schizophrenia or bipolar disorder: a randomised, placebo-controlled, blinded trial. World J Biol Psychiatry. 2016;17:514–24. https://doi.org/10.3109/15622975.2015.1048725.
152. Baandrup L, Fagerlund B, Glenthoj B. Neurocognitive performance, subjective well-being, and psychosocial functioning after benzodiazepine withdrawal in patients with schizophrenia or bipolar disorder: a randomized clinical trial of add-on melatonin versus placebo. Eur Arch Psychiatry Clin Neurosci. 2017;267:163–71. https://doi.org/10.1007/s00406-016-0711-8.
153. Bondi CD, Kamal KM, Johnson DA, Witt-Enderby PA, Giannetti VJ. The effect of melatonin upon postacute withdrawal among males in a residential treatment program (M-PAWS): a randomized, double-blind, placebo-controlled trial. J Addict Med. 2018;12:201–6. https://doi.org/10.1097/ADM.0000000000000386.
154. Puustinen J, Lähteenmäki R, Nurminen J, Vahlberg T, Aarnio P, Partinen M, et al. Long-term persistence of withdrawal of temazepam, zopiclone, and zolpidem in older adults: a 3-year follow-up study. BMC Geriatr. 2018;18. https://doi.org/10.1186/s12877-018-0829-9.
155. Ghaderi A, Banafshe HR, Mirhosseini N, Motmaen M, Mehrzad F, Bahmani F, et al. The effects of melatonin supplementation on mental health, metabolic and genetic profiles in patients under methadone maintenance treatment. Addict Biol. 2019;24:754–64. https://doi.org/10.1111/adb.12650.
156. Gendy MNS, Lagzdins D, Schaman J, Le Foll B. Melatonin for Treatment-Seeking Alcohol Use Disorder patients with sleeping problems: a randomized clinical pilot trial. Sci Rep. 2020;10. https://doi.org/10.1038/s41598-020-65166-y.
157. Soltani F, Salari A, Javaherforooshzadeh F, Nassajjian N, Kalantari F. The effect of melatonin on reduction in the need for sedative agents and duration of mechanical ventilation in traumatic intracranial hemorrhage patients: a randomized controlled trial. Eur J Trauma Emerg Surg. 2020. https://doi.org/10.1007/s00068-020-01449-3.
158. Kühlwein E, Hauger RL, Irwin MR. Abnormal nocturnal melatonin secretion and disordered sleep in abstinent alcoholics. Biol Psychiatry. 2003;54:1437–43. https://doi.org/10.1016/S0006-3223(03)00005-2.
159. Wetterberg L, Aperia B, Gorelick DA, Gwirtzman HE, McGuire MT, Serafetinides EA, et al. Age, alcoholism and depression are associated with low levels of urinary melatonin. J Psychiatry Neurosci. 1992;17:215–24.
160. Morera-Fumero AL, Fernandez-Lopez L, Abreu-Gonzalez P. Melatonin and melatonin agonists as treatments for benzodiazepines and hypnotics withdrawal in patients with primary insomnia. A systematic review. Drug Alcohol Depend. 2020;212. https://doi.org/10.1016/j.drugalcdep.2020.107994.
161. Madsen BK, Zetner D, Møller AM, Rosenberg J. Melatonin for preoperative and postoperative anxiety in adults. Cochrane Database Syst Rev. 2020;2020. https://doi.org/10.1002/14651858.CD009861.pub3.
162. Williams TM, Daglish MRC, Lingford-Hughes A, Taylor LG, Hammers A, Brooks DJ, et al. Brain opioid receptor binding in early abstinence from opioid dependence: positron emission tomography study. Br J Psychiatry. 2007;191:63–9. https://doi.org/10.1192/bjp.bp.106.031120.
163. Heinz A, Reimold M, Wrase J, Hermann D, Croissant B, Mundle G, et al. Correlation of stable elevations in striatal μ-opioid receptor availability in detoxified alcoholic patients with alcohol craving: a positron emission tomography study using carbon 11-labeled carfentanil. Arch Gen Psychiatry. 2005;62:57–64. https://doi.org/10.1001/archpsyc.62.1.57.
164. Zubieta JK, Gorelik DA, Stauffer R, Ravert HT, Dannals RF, Frost JJ. Increased mu opioid receptor binding detected by PET in cocaine-dependent

men is associated with cocaine craving. Nat Med. 1996;2:1225–9. https://doi.org/10.1038/nm1196-1225.

165. Mistraletti G, Umbrello M, Miori S, Taverna M, Cerri B, Mantovani E, et al. Melatonin reduces the need for sedation in ICU patients: a randomized controlled trial. Minerva Anestesiol. 2015;81:1298–310.

166. Tunay DL, Ilgınel MT, Ünlügenç H, Tunay M, Karacaer F, Biricik E. Comparison of the effects of preoperative melatonin or vitamin c administration on postoperative analgesia. Bosn J Basic Med Sci. 2020;20:117–24. https://doi.org/10.17305/bjbms.2019.4379.

167. Javaherforooshzadeh F, Amirpour I, Janatmakan F, Soltanzadeh M. Comparison of effects of melatonin and gabapentin on post operative anxiety and pain in lumbar spine surgery: a randomized clinical trial. Anesthesiol Pain Med 2018;8. https://doi.org/10.5812/aapm.68763.

168. Cardinali DP. Melatonin and healthy aging. Vitamins and Hormones, 2021,115, 67-88. https://doi.org/10.1016/bs.vh.2020.12.004.

169. Sugden D. Psychopharmacological effects of melatonin in mouse and rat. J Pharmacol Exp Ther. 1983;227.

170. Cardinali DP. Melatonin: clinical perspectives in neurodegeneration. Front Endocrinol (Lausanne). 2019;10. https://doi.org/10.3389/fendo.2019.00480.

23 Psychotropic Substances and Sleep

Vinícius Dokkedal Silva

Introduction

A common definition for psychotropic substances would be "a class of substances with significant central effects, paired with strong reinforcing properties and liable of self-administration" [1]. Such definition encapsulates most of the drugs that are misused nowadays and every drug used for recreational purposes. Delving deeper in this concept, it is possible to define different classes of psychotropic substances depending on their action on the central nervous system. Therefore, three large groups are defined: the stimulants, which are known to accelerate mental processes; the depressants, which can slow down mental processes; and the hallucinogens, which promote qualitative changes in such mental processes [2]. These three categories, while separated due to their fundamental qualities, share common traits that are ubiquitous and resonate directly with the functioning of the individual. These functions would include feeding, social interaction, professional activities, sexual activity, and sleep. Focusing on the latter, it is of common knowledge that substances pertaining to a specific class would cause disturbances in sleep in a way that is particular to that entire class (e.g., stimulants would reduce sleep, depressants would promote it, and so on). However, particularities about each substance can be overlooked if a simplistic approach is adopted. Alcohol would be a prime example of a substance that has many different effects on behavior and sleep, warranting a cautious approach to its classification and to the study of its risks. In this sense, it is necessary that in-depth analysis is undertaken to evaluate each substance and its impact on the sleep-wake cycle. The present chapter focuses on bringing to light current evidence and recent findings respective of the three main classes of psychotropic substances (stimulant, depressant, and hallucinogenic) and addressing the main characteristics of the more prominent substances in each of these categories. It must be remembered that this body of evidence is by no means exhaustive, due to the high research output in this field.

Stimulants

Stimulants are a class of substances that act on acceleration of mental processes. Table 23.1 briefly summarizes the main effects substances of this class have on sleep.

V. D. Silva (✉)
Departamento de Psicobiologia, Escola Paulista de Medicina, Universidade Federal de São Paulo, São Paulo, SP, Brazil

P. Á. Gargiulo, H. L. Mesones-Arroyo (eds.), *Psychiatry and Neuroscience Update – Vol. V*,
https://doi.org/10.1007/978-3-031-72219-6_23

Table 23.1 Listing of commonly observed effects on sleep caused by popular stimulant substances

Substance	Effect on sleep
Cocaine	↓ REM sleep
	↓ N3 (slow-wave) sleep
	↑ Sleep onset latency
	Occult insomnia
Amphetamines	↓ REM sleep
	↑ Variability in sleep duration
Methylphenidate	↑ Sleep onset latency
	↓ Total sleep time
Nicotine	↓ REM sleep
	↓N3 (slow-wave) sleep
	↑ Sleep onset latency
	↑ REM sleep onset latency
	↑ Sleep fragmentation

It must be remembered that peculiarities in the observed effects may be reported in selected articles, and that this table encompasses common findings in regard to these drugs

Cocaine

Cocaine is a well-studied and well-known illicit stimulant whose distribution worldwide is the focus of concern of health regulating agencies and governments. As an exclusively recreational drug nowadays, cocaine is known to significantly affect a multitude of mechanisms and systems in the organism.

On sleep, cocaine provokes marked dysregulation, with decreases in total sleep time, REM sleep suppression, slow-wave sleep (SWS) reduction, and increase in sleep onset latency [3]. A previous study showed that cocaine, among several substances assessed, was the one to which every single sleep parameter evaluated was associated [4]. One of the staples cocaine use leaves on sleep is the phenomenon called "occult insomnia". In this scenario, individuals complain about worsening of sleep during the first days without cocaine. Commonly, users report hypersomnia, fatigue, nightmares, agitation, and depressed mood, which are reflected in objective evaluation of sleep, carried out with polysomnographic exams (PSG) [3]. In the following weeks, it is common that patients report a marked improvement in sleep quality, which may become statistically similar to the self-reported sleep quality of non-cocaine users during this period of time. Simultaneously, objective assessments indicate that sleep parameters continue to worsen during this period, reaching a nadir about 14–17 days after discontinuation of cocaine [5]. At this point, total sleep time may be as little as 300 min during a night [3]. This characterizes a dissonance between subjective and objective evaluation of sleep that defines occult insomnia.

The objective impairment of sleep observed in cocaine abstinence does not become apparent immediately following discontinuation. Evidence points to a rebound of REM sleep following cocaine cessation, as well as an improvement in sleep onset latency [6]. These are short-lived, however, as in the following weeks REM sleep presents a marked decrease and mean sleep onset latency reaches 60 min.

Some considerations must be made in regard to the subjective sleep of these individuals. One would think that subjective sleep should at least receive a degree of attention during the abstinence period. However, the presence of cognitive deficits in these patients favors the follow-up of objective sleep parameters, which may have a crucial connection to these impairments [3]. It must also be pondered if the improvement of sleep reported by the ex-users is not biased, since their sleep has been disrupted by a substantial amount of time [3].

Mechanistically speaking, hypotheses regarding how occult insomnia operates include a possible impairment of homeostatic sleep mechanisms. They confer the capacity of adequately self-evaluate sleep quality and the rebound of delta waves that is observed in patients following cocaine cessation [5]. This could possibly induce the subjective sleep improvement [5].

In regard to the cognitive deficits observed following cocaine cessation, it has been observed that they may be partially reverted with administration of cocaine during this period [5, 7, 8]. This raises the possibility that the cognitive deficit could be a player in the relapse of cocaine, one of the major challenges in the treatment of this substance use disorder. Sleep would integrate this pathway as, besides the well-known impact poor sleep has on cognition, studies show that quantified decreases in total sleep time and REM sleep time predicted the amount of cocaine an individual would consume [9]. Conversely, better sleep was associated with more favorable clinical outcomes and reduced amount of consumed cocaine. In preclinical studies, sleep restriction protocols elicit a higher craving for cocaine, further supporting this connection [10].

Co-use of cocaine and cannabis is one of the strategies users may experiment with the intent of improving sleep. In a study by Wheeler and colleagues, the contrary is shown to actually happen, with sleep of co-users of cocaine and cannabis being worse than that of sole cocaine users [11]. Formally, treatment of sleep during cocaine abstinence has a few options that were considered throughout history: lisuride, a D2-receptor agonist that can reduce REM sleep latency [12]; tiagabin, a GABA reuptake inhibitor [13], and modafinil [14], a stimulant that shares traits with cocaine, but does not impair REM sleep and has low abuse potential.

Amphetamines

Being a large class of substances, amphetamines are stimulants that are both used as recreational drugs and as treatment for ADHD and other disorders. Amphetamines are known for the dependence and tolerance they may elicit in its users [15], and therefore, impacts in different aspects of the organism are ubiquitous in regard to these drugs.

Amphetamines are known to negatively affect both subjective and objective sleep quality. In one of the first studies conducted in this sense, Rechtschaffen et al. [16] showed that volunteers, after consuming amphetamine, presented a marked reduction in REM sleep duration, with a complete suppression of the first expected episodes of this sleep phase. In order to eliminate any doubts that the suppression of REM was caused by the amphetamine administration, a second experiment was performed, in which volunteers ingested pentobarbital alongside amphetamine; this would reduce body movements, which were abundant in the first experiment and could have interfered with the results [16]. Comparing 2 experimental nights, one in which users received amphetamine and pentobarbital, and another in which placebo and pentobarbital were administered, differences in REM sleep were still maintained, proving amphetamine directly affected sleep architecture. In a final experiment, Rechtschaffen and coworkers saw that participants in the study presented a rebound REM sleep after several days receiving both amphetamine and pentobarbital [16].

In another instance, it has been shown that chronic amphetamine use, when discontinued, elicits alterations in sleep parameters in a similar fashion to cocaine. Patients would present rebound sleep in the first days, which would then be replaced by marked worsening across all parameters that were evaluated by the end of the first week, a change that persisted for the following 20 days of protocol. Those participating in this study would also have great variability in the total sleep time between one night and another [17].

A recent and interesting data involves the impact amphetamine may have on the secretion of melatonin, the endogenous substance that regulates the sleep-wake cycle [18]. When compared to opioid users and controls, amphetamine users presented markedly lower levels of melatonin by the end of the afternoon, at 16:00. The same group presented higher levels of melatonin at 00:00, when compared to opioid users; controls had a better performance in melatonin measures at all timepoints. While it is still early to qualitatively determine what these fluctuations mean, the results of this study show that an imbalance in melatonin levels does exist in amphetamine nonmedical users [18].

The impact caused by amphetamines on sleep seems to be particularly associated with psychiatric symptoms. A study by Crouse and colleagues [19] found that stress and depressed mood had a link to self-reported poor sleep among amphetamine users already diagnosed with a psychiatric condition. This may be a common trait observed in this population and a useful finding for future treatment of sleep disorder among amphetamine misusers.

In respect of treatment of poor sleep associated to amphetamine use disorder, nonpharmacological alternatives have been investigated [20]. A study has shown that practice of Tai Chi has improved sleep and mood in abstinent amphetamine individuals. This also impacted the chance of relapse, which was of 9% in the practicing group, against 26% in non-practitioners. Evidences in this direction may suggest that improvement of mood and sleep is a crucial point of concern to increase odds of success at amphetamine discontinuation [20].

Methylphenidate

Structurally similar to amphetamines, methylphenidate (MPD) deserves mention in a separate section due to its long history as a treatment for ADHD in pediatric patients and its status as a licit drug (in contrast to the large number of amphetamines that are illicit).

In its trajectory as a medication for ADHD symptoms, evidence supports methylphenidate usage with findings of improved cognitions in patients, as pointed by a meta-analysis [21]. In this instance, no effect of MPD was seen on higher cognitive functions, such as executive memory. In lower cognitive functions, a dose-response effect of MPD was detected. Although no negative effect was detected in this meta-analysis respective of MPD usage, authors admit that the effect size of each dose over the parameters that were assessed varies widely, which indicates the need of further, more thorough analyses [21].

Efforts to map possible repercussions of MPD in sleep have focused in one of the populations of higher interest, pediatric patients with ADHD [22, 23]. In an investigation conducted with 85 children, atomoxetine and MPD were compared, with MPD increasing sleep onset latency. Children treated with this substance also reported higher difficulty to fall asleep, reduced appetite, and more insomnia complaints [22]. Conversely, awakenings during the night diminished under MPD administration. Impairment of sleep was also found in another study with 27 children, who had lower sleep efficiency and total sleep time and increased sleep onset latency. MPD, however, did not affect sleep architecture [23]. Finally, a Brazilian systematic review found a higher occurrence of sleep bruxism events in adolescent patients making use of MPD [24].

In a trial conducted with adults, an increased N2 sleep time was observed, but apart from this, alterations in sleep were nonsignificant [25]. Authors advert, however, that the reduced sample of the study and its open-label nature indicated need of caution when weighing the presented results.

Nicotine

The main active principle of tobacco products constitutes one of the most popular recreational substances around the world, together with alcohol. Contrary to other substances deemed as stimulants, nicotine acts on cholinergic receptors, which have been previously a source of research in regard to its alertness inducing properties [26]. Another peculiarity would be that, in higher doses, nicotine starts to exert sedative activity instead of the stimulation observed at a lower dosage, something called "Nesbitt's Paradox" [27].

Effects of nicotine consumption on the organism are well-described. Tobacco consumption, specifically, has been linked to higher cardiovascular risk [28] and pulmonary diseases [29]. As expected from this widely available drug, studies of its implications on sleep are abundant. A consensus on the effects of nicotine on sleep, however, has surprisingly not been reached, not to a point that causes a change in the paradigm of treating nicotine dependence while considering the importance of sleep.

A study with 405 young adults self-reporting sleep quality and tobacco consumption found a correlation between subjective poor sleep and presence of tobacco craving, amount of cigarettes, higher tolerance and dependence scores in the modified Fagerstrom Tolerance Questionnaire and ICD-10, respectively, and withdrawal symptoms. Prevalence of poor sleep quality among this sample was 36% [30].

A clinical review by Jaehne et al. [31] has mapped effects of nicotine and tobacco during the acute stage of use and during discontinuation. Acute effects of nicotine included reduction in total sleep time, REM sleep time, sleep efficiency and increase in sleep onset latency, REM sleep onset latency, sleep fragmentation, and excessive daytime sleepiness. In the opposite direction, poor sleep, alongside depressed mood, predicted lower success rates during abstinence. Worsening of breathing-related events during the night was also reported in this review. Authors are aware, however, that the heterogeneity of methodologies in the included studies demands caution when analyzing conclusions of the review [31].

Together with the standard cigarette consumption, popularization of e-cigarettes is another trend that has caught the attention of the scientific community. In an evaluation of 227 people who used regular cigarettes and e-cigarettes, each was found to predict specific outcomes. Regular cigarettes were associated with shorter sleep duration, while e-cigarettes were linked with more severe daytime dysfunction due to poor sleep. They had a combined effect on the odds of using sleep medications [32].

In an in-depth study which aimed to evaluate the role of the prefrontal cortex cholinergic nuclei in arousal and sleep regulation, nicotine was directly injected into the brain or rodent models. Nicotine provoked reduction of latency to wakefulness and increased REM sleep onset latency. No changes in architecture were detected [26].

Evidence on the relationship between nicotine and sleep can be conflicting. In a study aimed at evaluating whether pure nicotine could improve sleep breathing disorders, volunteers spent a night with a transdermal patch of nicotine [33]. They presented reduced total sleep time, REM sleep time, sleep efficiency, and increase in REM sleep onset latency. Snoring index (number of snoring events) did not present a significant difference, but intensity of snoring and oxygen desaturation were attenuated and duration of breathing events decreased. At the same time, qualitative changes were noticed in the brain wave patterns, with increase in alpha patterns during the entire first sleep cycle, and slow-wave activity decrease in N2 and REM sleep phases [33]. In this sense, it becomes clear that the relationship of nicotine with sleep is multidimensional and still needs further research.

In regard to treatment of dependence, nicotine replacement therapy has been considered one of the most prominent alternatives. On patients with depressive mood disorder, nicotine patches exerted the same effect as antidepressants [31]. Another promising alternative is the non-pharmacological option of performing exercises [34]. A trial in which individuals under smoking cessation performed exercise routines found an expressive improvement of sleep maintenance and reduced arousal episodes. Individuals presenting the most severe withdrawal symptoms and sleep complaints were those who also presented the most expressive attenuation of these symptoms [34].

Cathinone and Synthetic Cathinones

This large group of molecules has risen to prominence in recent years. Synthetic cathinones receive this name due to being based on the structure of cathinone, the main psychoactive component found in *Catha edulis*, or khat, a plant commonly consumed in Africa and Asia due to its stimulant properties. Synthetic cathinones have become popular as, by being only recently introduced in the market, they had no specific laws that controlled or prohibited their use and sale, thus fulfilling the role of "legal highs" [35]. Legislation controlling the circulation of these substances has been approved in the past few years. However, the dissemination of this substance class has already become widespread and the scientific community is pursuing a better understanding of this wide array of compounds [36]. Since they are a very recent class of drug, studies that have evaluated their effects on sleep (as well as on many different functions and systems) are scarce. Birhanu and colleagues [37] have suggested that consumption of khat in their Ethiopian sample may explain the sleep impairments observed in their study, but did not pursue this any further [37]. Assi and colleagues had a similar opinion on their findings, but also did not carry on with a specific investigation, limiting themselves to notice a combination of sleep aid medications and cathinones in their sample. The authors also mention that other reports indicate that cathinones are frequently found in combination with other substances, such as benzodiazepines and alcohol, which may warrant attention from health agencies [38].

Two substances deserve an in-depth literature revision, methylenedioxypyrovalerone (MDPV) and mephedrone, two of the most popular synthetic cathinones in the market. MDPV has been assessed in animal studies, having cognitive deficits attributed to its administration in such cases [39, 40]. Perirhinal and entorhinal cortex degradation was also noted, together with worse performance in novel object recognition tasks. Even though sleep was not the outcome of interest in this study, authors strongly believe that sleep impairment caused by the binge-like MDPV administration protocol may have caused the deficits and neurotoxic effects they found [39]. Combination of MDPV with benzodiaepines was shown in an anecdotal report covering a patient who was admitted presenting hallucinations and delirium, which authors ponder may have been brought about due to the combination of both substances [41]. Once again, this assumption deserves caution as it is based on a case report rather than a larger-scale study.

In regard to mephedrone, a comparison with MDMA found that the synthetic cathinone was more consistently associated with the apparition of paranoia, irritability, and negative mood [42]. Alterations of sleep were reported by the participants, as well as increased anxiety, but objective evaluation did not find a significant difference between mephedrone and MDMA [42]. Another investigation compared active users with abstainers of mephedrone [43]. Users complained of worse mood, fatigue, and physical problems. This study had a sample largely reporting nonrestorative sleep and cannabis use, which were treated as covariates at the occasion. Although investigating sleep in this case would have been interesting, controlling for report of nonrestorative sleep allowed authors to identify that effects on mood and fatigue were indeed caused by mephedrone [43]. These evidences are starting points that indicate the necessity of investigating not only mephedrone and MDPV, but also other popular synthetic cathinones, as an impact on sleep is a solid possibility as implied by these preliminary findings. Diversification of studies on this class may bring important evidence that will be able to direct treatment of users and detection of synthetic cathinone consumption in clinical evaluations in the future. Table 23.2 lists some of the observed effects on sleep caused by synthetic cathinones, together with drugs from the phenethylamine and tryptamine class, which also lack a better clarification of its effects on sleep. Since studies on the connection between sleep alteration and consumption of these substances are still scarce, these findings must be assumed cautiously and would be greatly benefitted by future studies.

Table 23.2 Listing of sleep effects of cathinones, phenethylamines and tryptamines

Substance	Effects observed
Synthetic Cathinones	Reports indicate sleep impairment and fatigue
Mescaline	Qualitative changes in brain wave patterns
MDMA	↓ N2 sleep
	↑ Wakefulness
	Circadian disruption
Psilocin	Qualitative changes in brain wave patterns
DMT	↑ REM sleep onset latency
	↓ REM sleep
LSD	Qualitative changes in brain wave patterns

Effects listed below mainly originate from scarce studies or animal experiments, and therefore, encapsulate what limited evidence is currently available concerning these substances. Caution in assuming occurrence and frequency of these effects among users is strongly recommended. Further studies to improve the current body of evidence in respect of these drugs are mandatory

Depressants

Depressants are a class of substances known to slow down mental processes in users. Table 23.3 summarizes the most commonly observed effects substances of this class can cause.

Barbiturates

Barbiturates are a class of medication used for treatment of sleep disorders in the early 20th century. At the time, they rose to popularity by repre-

Table 23.3 Listing of commonly observed effects on sleep caused by popular depressant substances

Substance	Effect on sleep
Barbiturates	↑ Total sleep time
	↑ REM sleep onset latency
	↓ REM sleep
Benzodiazepines	↓ N3 (slow-wave) sleep
	↓ REM sleep
	↑ Benzodiazepine spindles
	↑ Obstructive events
Opioids	↑ N2 sleep
	↓ N3 (slow-wave) sleep
	↓ REM sleep
	↑ Central sleep apnea events
	↑ Obstructive events
Z-Drugs	No significant sleep alterations detected
Ethanol	↓ Sleep onset latency (healthy)
	↑ Sleep onset latency (AUD)
	↓ N3 (slow-wave) sleep
	↓ REM sleep
	↑ Obstructive events

It must be remembered that peculiarities in the observed effects may be reported in selected articles, and that this table encompasses common findings in regard to these drugs

senting a novelty in the treatment of sleep complaints. However, risks originating from their use were rapidly uncovered. Barbiturates can be classified as psychotropic substances, but more importantly, presented a very thin line separating therapeutic and toxic doses. In this sense, barbiturate overdose was commonly reported [44]. Nowadays, this class of medication has a very restricted presence in the clinical scenario, among which phenobarbital is one of the more prominent molecules, being used as an anticonvulsant.

The effects of barbiturates on sleep mainly include increase in total sleep time and architectural changes, which, according to a study by Evans and colleagues, amount to a reduction in REM sleep time and an increase in REM sleep onset latency [45].

On another instance, evaluation of different anticonvulsants used on pediatric patients and their risk for eliciting sleep bruxism was performed. Barbiturates, when assessed separately, had a positive correlation to sleep bruxism occurrence in children [24]. Another investigation found that phenobarbital caused worsening of sleep in children, but its effect size on Pittsburgh Sleep Quality Index (PSQI) scores was low, implying a low predictive power for this evaluation [46].

Benzodiazepines

Discovered by Leo Sternbach in 1955, benzodiazepines represented a leap in the treatment of sleep and psychiatric disorders. When compared to barbiturates, they had a much higher safety margin and therefore revolutionized the pharmacological scenario at the time [47].

Benzodiazepines can have a diversity of approved uses according to each molecule, mainly fulfilling the role of hypnotics, anticonvulsants, anxiolytics, and sedatives [47].

Although there is a difference of specific effects between benzodiazepines approved for different uses, their action still shares similarities due to all having a common mechanism of action. Benzodiazepines are allosteric modulators that increase the frequency of openings of the Cl- channels in the GABA-A receptor, thus regulating the action of GABA in the neuronal activity [48]. They bind to the benzodiazepine receptors that are present at the intersection of α and γ subunits of the GABA-A receptor. There are several types of α subunits, numbered 1 to 6. Benzodiazepines can successfully bind to benzodiazepine receptors which present a histidine residue (the α1, 2, 3, and 5 subunits) [49, 50]. Benzodiazepines vary according to the higher or lower binding affinity to each of the α subunit types, and this is what confers each substance a different therapeutic action: benzodiazepines with higher affinity to receptors containing α1 subunits have a more pronounced hypnotic effect, while those with affinity to α2 and α3 subunits present greater anxiolytic effects [50]. Nonetheless, since all of them can still bind to the benzodiazepine site, their effects are not mutually exclusive, e.g., a benzodiazepine that is approved for hypnotic use can be also approved for use as anxiolytic, and vice-versa.

Concern may arise from the fact that benzodiazepines can be prescribed for treating conditions for which they are not approved for, and therefore their features can lead to unwanted effects during treatment. An example was provided by the study of Contreras-Gonzalez et al., [51], which evaluated the impairments on executive function caused by clonazepam, due to this molecule, normally approved for use as anticonvulsant and anxiolytic, being prescribed as a sleep aid medication. In this study, executive impairment was observed and was significantly correlated to clonazepam usage. The "mis-prescription" of benzodiazepines has become, henceforth, a source of interest for health regulating agencies.

As benzodiazepines share pharmacological traits that allow their use for conditions they were not approved, another point of concern has surfaced: the un-prescribed use of benzodiazepines, which may be of recreational or self-medication nature [52–55]. In the first scenario, benzodiazepines can be used by substance misusers, such as those who consume opioids recreationally, as a replacement drug in case the preferred substance is not available [52, 53]. In the second case, benzodiazepines are obtained without a prescription (sold through illicit means) or are used in a way that diverts from the initial prescription purpose, with individuals frequently using them to self-medicate conditions without medical follow-up [54, 55]. Complaints normally reported by self-medication benzodiazepine users include anxiety and poor sleep.

It is necessary to clarify that, although benzodiazepines represented a significant advance in the treatment of sleep disorders and are commonly misused by those seeking to self-medicate their sleep complaints, their effects on sleep are not without consequences. Benzodiazepines are known to provoke marked REM sleep suppression, reduction of SWS, and promote appearance of the so-called benzodiazepine spindles in the EEG recording [56]. They elicit tolerance on its users, and in order to continue exerting effects on sleep, it is commonly necessary to increase the dose constantly [57]. Eventually, the need of maintaining satisfactory effects induces users to increase dosage above recommended levels. Together with the development of tolerance, benzodiazepines are prone to causing dependence. Their use is normally recommended to last for a maximum of 4 weeks to avoid establishment of dependence symptoms [57]. When patients discontinue usage of benzodiazepines, the process needs to be carefully conducted. It is recommended that benzodiazepine doses are tapered down gradually during this period [57], rather than an abrupt cessation of use. It can involve replacement of a more potent benzodiazepine by a less potent one, such as diazepam or chlordiazepoxide. If cessation is performed inadequately, a rebound of symptoms for which benzodiazepines were being used is commonly reported, paired with increased chance of convulsions and psychotic states [57, 58]. Complaints in these cases include anxiety and depression symptoms, as well as a significant worsening of sleep quality [58]. Recovery may not be straightforward, as some parameters still present a deficit, such as sleep efficiency, but after 2 weeks of discontinuation from benzodiazepines, improvements can be seen in sleep [59]. Clinical follow-up is of utmost importance during this period, due to the severity of withdrawal symptoms potentially becoming very high during discontinuation.

Opioids

Opioids constitute a class of substances derived from opium, a drug that was popular during the 19th century and is extracted from the opium poppy plant (*Papaver somniferum*). Opiates constitute a subclass of opioids that includes compounds directly extracted from opium poppy, such as morphine. Opioids are not prescribed as sleep aid medications, rather being potent analgesics with a multitude of utilities in the clinical scenario [60]. Besides morphine, others, such as oxycodone, codeine, and fentanyl, are either sold as painkillers in pharmacies or administered in hospital settings to treat acute pain caused by cancer or severe fractures.

Although their utility has been proven extensively throughout the decades, their usage is well-known to imply substantial risks. Opioids are prone to developing severe dependence and tolerance in their users [61]. Their nonmedical use, paired with cases of inadequate and indiscriminate prescription, made opioid consumption a health issue worldwide, with the prime example being the opioid crisis undergoing in the United States [62].

Opioid use is tightly connected to the appearance of sleep disorders and their impact on breathing regulation contributes directly to sleep impairment. On sleep architecture, opioids promote sleep superficialization, with significant increase of N2 sleep time and REM sleep and SWS reduction [63]. In regard to the respiratory problems that surface from opioid use, they cause dysregulation in the response to hypoxia and hypercapnia in the organism, especially as an acute effect [64]. Central sleep apnea (CSA) is a particularly common consequence of this dysregulation, with studies finding prevalence of 30% and as high as 55% of CSA in patients under opioid treatment [65, 66]. Obstructive sleep apnea (OSA) is also commonly reported with one study (reporting a prevalence of 39% among opioid users), as opioid usage may reduce tone in the pharyngeal and airway dilation muscles, encompassed by impairment in the motor response of hypoglossum [67]. Guilleminault and colleagues [68] found that patients undergoing opioid treatment and CPAP therapy for OSA tended to present an increase in the number of central apnea events when compared to controls. Conversely, the number of obstructive events on this same group became greatly reduced in the same period [68].

Z-Drugs

Nonbenzodiazepine drugs, benzodiazepine receptor agonists, or more colloquially z-drugs are names to a relatively novel class of substances that represented the next advance in pharmacological sleep therapy. They receive this designation due to acting on the benzodiazepine site of GABAergic receptors. Substances in this class include zolpidem, zopiclone, eszopiclone, and zaleplon. Among them, zolpidem is commonly regarded as the gold standard in pharmacotherapy of sleep. Due to the key difference to benzodiazepines in having a higher specificity on the α1 subunit, zolpidem has a more focused action as hypnotics and a decreased chance of causing dependence and being misprescribed or used recreationally [69]. Another advantage they represent is the few alterations they provoke on sleep continuity and architecture, with users exhibiting a sleep pattern that is closer to the normal sleep than that caused by benzodiazepines [70].

However, anecdotal evidence has already found that z-drugs, specially zolpidem, seem to have some abuse potential, even if to a lower degree than benzodiazepines. Side-effects are also reported and include amnesia and hallucinations [71, 72]. Nonetheless, there is a lack of large-scale studies to support these claims, and z-drugs remain as the main pharmacological option for treatment of sleep disorders.

Ethanol

Ethanol remains the most widely consumed psychotropic substance in the world, being part of the culture of several nations. With its commercialization being allowed in many countries, repercussions of its indiscriminate use are the focus of extensive research and attention from governments and health regulating agencies, and these impacts are of utmost social importance. Alcohol use disorder (AUD) was considered the most prevalent substance use disorder, afflicting more than 100 million individuals worldwide [73] in a recent assessment, and consequences to health are well-described.

Regarding its effects on sleep, it can be said that ethanol might have a dual effect. While commonly associated to sleepiness (and in some cases, consumed for this reason), ethanol actually can lead to differing effects depending on the health state of the user. Although healthy individuals experience reduction of sleep latency, those with AUD tend to present an increase in this same parameter [3]. Alcohol consumption also leads to reduced SWS and total sleep time among AUD individuals (intensified during abstinence). Concerning those with AUD, certain parameters, such as amount of SWS and total sleep time, tend to present improvements over time with abstinence [3]. Evidence regarding REM sleep and REM sleep latency tends to be more conflicting, as although there are studies showing that decreases in REM sleep and increase in REM sleep latency are expected in AUD, a few studies did not find a difference in these patients when compared to controls [3]. Ethanol consumption is also associated with the increase in the occurrence of OSA episodes [74, 75].

Hallucinogens

Cannabis

Cannabis is a particular case in which it is difficult to determine its category precisely. While well-known for its relaxing, depressant-like effects [76], certain components of cannabis appear to exert hallucinogen effects, a property that becomes more apparent in higher doses [77]. The multitude of different effects caused by cannabis is attributed to the high number of different chemical substances found within it, the cannabinoids. Among these, Δ9-Tetra-Hydro-Cannabinol (Δ9-THC) and cannabidiol are the most widely studied.

General knowledge of cannabis normally is that of a psychotropic substance that induces relaxation with few side-effects and risks. Nonetheless, extensive evidence demonstrates that it can generate dependence [78], besides the capability of eliciting psychotic effects and cognitive impairment [79, 80].

Effects on sleep follow this heterogeneous trend, also due to the great variety of centrally acting molecules found in cannabis. The effect of specific cannabinoids on sleep has been a focus of extensive research for clinical purposes. Δ9-THC, one of the 2 more prominent molecules found in plants of the Cannabis genus, is now credited as the one responsible for their main psychotomimetic effects, which seem to be counteracted by cannabidiol [81]. THC might reduce latency to sleep onset, but undesired effects, including delayed sleep onset on the following day and reduced nighttime sleep, have also been observed. CBD, conversely, seems to improve total sleep time, decrease number of arousals, and might have therapeutic effects on REM sleep behavior disorder, a prodromal condition to Parkinson, while there is report about it decreasing Stage 3 sleep. This great heterogeneity of data shows how extensive is the work still to be done regarding the investigation of these 2 molecules [82]. Besides this frontier of research, it is known that there are about 118 different cannabinoid compounds found in the species of the *Cannabis* genus, which remain largely unexplored. Table 23.4 describes some of the main perceptions about sleep effects of the 2 mainly studied cannabinoids, Δ9-THC and CBD.

Table 23.4 Listing of selected reported effects on sleep caused by the two mainly studied cannabinoids

Cannabinoid	Effects on sleep
Δ9-THC	↑ Sleep onset latency (in the following day)
	↓ Total sleep time
CBD	↓ Number of awakenings
	↑ Total sleep time

It must be remembered that there is a non-exhaustive evidence listing, and that studies concerning these substances are still needed before a consensus is reached

Phenethylamines

Phenethylamine is an alkaloid monoamine produced by many different lifeforms, ranging from unicellular organisms to humans. The chemical structure of phenethylamine is the basis for the greater group called substituted phenethylamines, encompassing both synthetic and natural molecules. Amphetamines may also be included on this group, but are normally treated separately.

One of the more famous natural compounds of this class is the hallucinogen mescaline, found in the Mexican cactus peyote (*Lophophora williamsii*). Mescaline preparations were consumed throughout the centuries with shamanic and entheogen purposes [83]. It is known to provoke visual hallucinations. Despite its long trajectory of use by different civilizations, gaps in the knowledge of mescaline effects still exist, among which are potential impacts on sleep quality. What little information there is about mescaline activity on sleep originates from animal studies. In one instance, it has been shown that coupling mescaline and sleep deprivation in rodents did not elicit any significant behavioral change, contrary to what may be observed following treatment with amphetamine [84]. In another investigation [85], qualitative changes in neuronal signaling patterns were noticed following mescaline treatment in mice, with loss of brain connectivity, but not in power of the brain waves. A rebound of theta occipital waves was detected, however. It was also reported that mice receiving mescaline in this experiment displayed intense locomotor stimulation. Authors of this study advocate that their findings regarding loss of neural connectivity have robust translational validity, based on similar findings in human experiments concerning other hallucinogens [85].

Another widely consumed phenethylamine is 3,4-Methylenedioxymethamphetamine (MDMA), the active principle found in ecstasy tables consumed in electronic music parties and raves. MDMA is known for its empathogen properties (that is, its capability of causing strong feelings of empathy) [86], and for being a potent stimulant. Hallucinations are reported, but are not the most commonly reported effect and may not be classified as actual hallucinations, rather being distortions of perception [86]. MDMA provokes accentuated reduction in somnolence, increases vigilance, and disrupts sleep architecture, with evidence pointing to reduction of NREM sleep, primarily stage 2 sleep [87]. Preclinical evidence has also suggested a role of MDMA in circadian disruption [87].

Apart from these 2 substances, the substituted phenethylamines present a wide array of different molecules, many of which have only recently been created. In the same fashion as synthetic cathinones, the structure of phenethylamines can be manipulated and presents a great number of sites for substitute groups. Therefore, creation of psychotropic substances with stimulant and hallucinogenic properties has become a popular strategy to avoid "legal highs" and has filled the market with many novel and scarcely studied molecules [88]. Due to being recently created molecules, there is still need to map their effects on different aspects of the organism, including sleep. Table 23.2 encompasses effects on sleep that have been observed for selected phenethylamines, mescaline and MDMA.

Tryptamines

Tryptamine is an indolamine, a precursor to the essential amino-acid tryptophan. As with phenethylamine, the chemical structure of tryptamine is the basis for a much larger group of substances, the substituted tryptamines. Among these, several potent serotonergic agonists with hallucinogenic properties are counted, as well as the hormone melatonin.

Melatonin has become one of the most prominently studied substances in the previous decades. Although it does not have any psychotropic nor hallucinogenic effects, its importance in the class of tryptamines warrants discussion. Produced in the pineal gland, it is known as the hormonal regulator and signaling agent of the sleep-wake cycle. Evidence has shown that exogenous melatonin can aid in a multitude of sleep disorders [89]. Other than that, melatonin has demonstrated itself to be useful as an antioxidant and neuroprotective agent [90], which could indirectly have positive effects in the treatment of neurodegenerative disorders, although this possibility still needs further investigation. Research on these topics is still underway and clearer answers regarding whether melatonin can aid in these conditions are bound to be found in the future.

Psilocybin is a hallucinogen found in mushrooms such as *Psilocybe cubensis* (colloquially known as "magical mushrooms"). When consumed, psilocybin is quickly metabolized into psilocin, an active compound that binds to 5HT1A receptors and exerts potent psychedelic effects [91].

Vejmola and colleagues have also investigated psilocin effects on brain wave patterns, having found loss of brain connectivity, decrease of neuronal activity, and reduced power. Effects were intense during the first epoch that was analyzed but, due to psilocin having a short biological half-life, no identifiable effects were present by the last evaluated epoch. In another animal experiment, psilocin was found to increase REM sleep onset latency and reduce NREM sleep maintenance for the 3 h following administration [85]. Finally, when paired with a sleep deprivation protocol, psilocin slowed recovery of wave patterns in selected areas of the brain, implying an impact on local sleep rather than general sleep [92]. Its possible connection with sleep has been hypothesized by Froese et al. [93], who proposed it could act in tandem to sleep regulating functions to improve cognitive performance. By revisiting findings of a previous study, the authors believe that psilocin administration, paired with sleep, caused improvements in performance of rodents, and that such results could be pursued in the clinical scenario [93].

Dimethyltryptamine (DMT) is another highlighted tryptamine. Found in ayahuasca and Santo Daime preparations, it is another drug used for religious purposes. By itself, DMT is a small molecule that is quickly degraded by primary metabolism. However, when mixed with beta-carbolines present in these beverages, its degradation takes longer, and its potent hallucinogenic effects surface [94]. Ayahuasca is one of the few hallucinogenic drugs that has been studied directly regarding its effects on sleep. Volunteers of the investigation conducted by Barbanoj and colleagues [95] did not present alterations in the onset and maintenance of sleep, although REM sleep onset latency was increased and REM sleep duration was significantly decreased [95]. Changes in power of high-frequency brain waves were also found. Another interesting finding in this instance was the increase of power in slow waves during the first sleep cycle, an indicator of augmented sleep pressure. In comparison, volunteers treated with dextroamphetamine had a reduction of this same parameter [95].

Lysergic acid (LSD) is the last tryptamine that deserves to be covered in particular. LSD is a lysergamide, a class of substance derived from tryptamines. It is an extremely potent and long-lasting hallucinogen, being active at doses in the order of micrograms. Vejmola and colleagues identified similarities in action between LSD and mescaline, the only 2 substances they tested that caused a rebound of theta occipital waves in the third epoch they evaluated [85]. In a rare study evaluating its effects directly in human volunteers, LSD administration, paired with a sleep deprivation protocol, presented a significant cognitive impairment that was not identified in control individuals [96].

As with phenethylamines, there is a great number of synthetic tryptamines that were popularized in the market in the past years. Tryptamine is another molecule that is easy to manipulate in the laboratory, with a plethora of sites for substitute groups, generating a great number of analogues to evade regulation and prohibition in the market [88]. In this sense, there is a wide array of tryptamines available that have not been thoroughly studied. As with many other hallucinogens, studies regarding their impact on the organism and furthermore, their effects on the sleep-wake cycle still remain to be seen. Table 23.2 reunites some of the main findings for more commonly studied tryptamines. It must be highlighted that, since information on sleep effects of recreational tryptamines are scarce, these findings must be assumed cautiously and would benefit from future studies to better characterize the relationship between tryptamines and sleep.

Conclusions

Although this chapter has extensively covered information pertinent to the general effects of several psychotropic substances on sleep, it must not be treated as an exhaustive document. From this affirmation, a conclusion can be drawn: many questions regarding the relationship between psychotropic substances and sleep remain to be answered. This is especially egregious when considering the vast amount of novel molecules, namely the synthetic cathinones, phenethylamines and tryptamines, that have entered the drug market in the recent years. Added to that are the many gaps in the understanding of how sleep is affected by (or affects) the action of well-described drugs, such as LSD and mescaline and the ever-growing evidence supporting the role of drugs whose effects on sleep are well-known. Another conclusion that can be reached is that sleep is one of the aspects of the organism most prominently affected by psychotropic substance misuse. Conversely, it is increasingly believed that a bidirectional relationship exists in many cases, and sleep quality may be a key factor in the success of discontinuation and in the therapy of patients with dependence symptoms. In light of these conclusions, much remains to be done. With the popularization of recreational use of certain medication classes, such as benzodiazepines and opioids, it is fundamental that updates and further research on the impact of these drugs on sleep (and vice-versa) will be one of the leading pillars in substance use disorder therapy.

References

1. Carlini EA, Nappo SA, Galduróz JCF, Noto AR. Drogas psicotrópicas: o que são e como agem. Revista Imesc. 2001;3:9–35.
2. Chaloult L. Une nouvelle classification des drogues toxicomanogènes. Toxicomanies. 1971;4(4):371–5.
3. Angarita GA, Emadi N, Hodges S, Morgan PT. Sleep abnormalities associated with alcohol, cannabis, cocaine, and opiate use: a comprehensive review. Addict Sci Clin Pract. 2016;11(1):9.
4. Dolsen MR, Harvey AG. Life-time history of insomnia and hypersomnia symptoms as correlates of alcohol, cocaine and heroin use and relapse among adults seeking substance use treatment in the United States from 1991 to 1994. Addiction. 2017;112(6):1104–11.
5. Morgan PT, Pace-Schott EF, Sahul ZH, Coric V, Stickgold R, Malison RT. Sleep, sleep-dependent procedural learning and vigilance in chronic cocaine users: evidence for occult insomnia. Drug Alcohol Depend. 2006;82(3):238–49.
6. Johanson CE, Roehrs T, Schuh K, Warbasse L. The effects of cocaine on mood and sleep in cocaine-dependent males. Exp Clin Psychopharmacol. 1999;7(4):338–46.
7. Morgan PT, Pace-Schott EF, Sahul ZH, Coric V, Stickgold R, Malison RT. Sleep architecture, cocaine and visual learning. Addiction. 2008;103(8):1344–52.
8. Pace-Schott EF, Morgan PT, Malison RT, Hart CL, Edgar C, Walker M, Stickgold R. Cocaine users differ from normals on cognitive tasks which show poorer performance during drug abstinence. Am J Drug Alcohol Abuse. 2008;34(1):109–21.
9. Angarita GA, Canavan SV, Forselius E, Bessette A, Pittman B, Morgan PT. Abstinence-related changes in sleep during treatment for cocainedependence. Drug Alcohol Depend. 2014;134:343–7.
10. Chen B, Wang Y, Liu X, Liu Z, Dong Y, Huang YH. Sleep regulates incubation of cocaine craving. J Neurosci. 2015;35(39):13300–10.
11. Wheeler PB, Dogan JN, Stevens-Watkins D, Stoops WW. Sleep time differs among people who co-use cocaine and cannabis compared to people who only use cocaine. Pharmacol Biochem Behav. 2021;201:173109.
12. Gillin JC, Pulvirenti L, Withers N, Golshan S, Koob G. The effects of lisuride on mood and sleep during acute withdrawal in stimulant abusers: a preliminary report. Biol Psychiatry. 1994;35(11):843–9.
13. Walsh JK, Randazzo AC, Stone K, Eisenstein R, Feren SD, Kajy S, et al. Tiagabine is associated with sustained attention during sleep restriction: evidence for the value of slow-wave sleep enhancement? Sleep. 2006;29(4):433–43.
14. Mereu M, Bonci A, Newman AH, Tanda G. The neurobiology of modafinil as an enhancer of cognitive performance and a potential treatment for substance use disorders. Psychopharmacology. 2013;229(3):415–34.
15. Malenka RC, Nestler EJ, Hyman SE, Holtzman DM. Chapter 16: Reinforcement and addictive disorders. In: Molecular neuropharmacology: a foundation for clinical neuroscience, 3rd edn. New York: McGraw-Hill Medical; 2015.
16. Rechtschaffen A, Maron L. The effect of amphetamine on the sleep cycle. Electroencephalogr Clin Neurophysiol. 1964;16:438–45.
17. Gossop MR, Bradley BP, Brewis RK. Amphetamine withdrawal and sleep disturbance. Drug Alcohol Depend. 1982;10(2-3):177–83.
18. Khazaie H, Ahmadi HR, Kiani A, Ghadami MR. Circadian melatonin profile in opium and amphetamine dependent patients: a preliminary study. Neurobiol Sleep Circadian Rhythms. 2019;7:100046.
19. Crouse JJ, Lee RSC, White D, Moustafa AA, Hickie IB, Hermens DF. Distress and sleep quality in young amphetamine-type stimulant users with an affective or psychotic illness. Psychiatry Res. 2018;262:254–61.
20. Zhu D, Dai G, Xu D, Xu X, Geng J, Zhu W, Jiang X, Theeboom M. Long-term effects of Tai Chi intervention on sleep and mental health of female individuals with dependence on amphetamine-type stimulants. Front Psychol. 2018;9:1476.
21. Vertessen K, Luman M, Staff A, Bet P, de Vries R, Twisk J, Oosterlaan J. Meta-analysis: dose-dependent effects of methylphenidate on neurocognitive functioning in children with attention-deficit/hyperactivity disorder. J Am Acad Child Adolesc Psychiatry. 2021;S0890-8567(21)01709-3.
22. Sangal RB, Owens J, Allen AJ, Sutton V, Schuh K, Kelsey D. Effects of atomoxetine and methylphenidate on sleep in children with ADHD. Sleep. 2006;29(12):1573–85.
23. Galland BC, Tripp EG, Taylor BJ. The sleep of children with attention deficit hyperactivity disorder on and off methylphenidate: a matched case-control study. J Sleep Res. 2010;19(2):366–73.
24. Melo G, Dutra KL, Rodrigues Filho R, Ortega AOL, Porporatti AL, Dick B, Flores-Mir C, De Luca Canto G. Association between psychotropic medications and presence of sleep bruxism: a systematic review. J Oral Rehabil. 2018;45(7):545–54.
25. Fredriksen M, Golparian N, Beiske K, Stavem K. Impact of methylphenidate on sleep problems in adults with ADHD: a pilot polysomnography study. Nord J Psychiatry. 2021;75(3):234–8.

26. Parkar A, Fedrigon DC, Alam F, Vanini G, Mashour GA, Pal D. Carbachol and nicotine in prefrontal cortex have differential effects on sleep-wake states. Front Neurosci. 2020;14:567849.
27. Parrott AC. Nesbitt's Paradox resolved? Stress and arousal modulation during cigarette smoking. Addiction. 1998;93(1):27–39.
28. Winniford MD. Smoking and cardiovascular function. J Hypertens Suppl. 1990;8(5):S17–23.
29. Burns DM. Tobacco-related diseases. Semin Oncol Nurs. 2003;19(4):244–9. https://doi.org/10.1053/j.soncn.2003.08.001.
30. Dugas EN, Sylvestre MP, O'Loughlin EK, Brunet J, Kakinami L, Constantin E, O'Loughlin J. Nicotine dependence and sleep quality in young adults. Addict Behav. 2017;65:154–60.
31. Jaehne A, Loessl B, Bárkai Z, Riemann D, Hornyak M. Effects of nicotine on sleep during consumption, withdrawal and replacement therapy. Sleep Med Rev. 2009;13(5):363–77.
32. So CJ, Meers JM, Alfano CA, Garey L, Zvolensky MJ. Main and interactive effects of nicotine product type on sleep health among dual combustible and e-cigarette users. Am J Addict. 2021;30(2):147–55.
33. Davila DG, Hurt RD, Offord KP, Harris CD, Shepard JW Jr. Acute effects of transdermal nicotine on sleep architecture, snoring, and sleep-disordered breathing in nonsmokers. Am J Respir Crit Care Med. 1994;150(2):469–74.
34. Soreca I, Conklin CA, Vella EJ, Salkeld RP, Joyce CJ, Mumma JM, Jakicic JM, Kupfer DJ. Can exercise alleviate sleep disturbances during acute nicotine withdrawal in cigarette smokers? Exp Clin Psychopharmacol. 2020;29. https://doi.org/10.1037/pha0000390.
35. Karila L, Megarbane B, Cottencin O, Lejoyeux M. Synthetic cathinones: a new public health problem. Curr Neuropharmacol. 2015;13(1):12–20.
36. Gonçalves JL, Alves VL, Aguiar J, Teixeira HM, Câmara JS. Synthetic cathinones: an evolving class of new psychoactive substances. Crit Rev Toxicol. 2019;49(7):549–66.
37. Birhanu TE, Getachew B, Gerbi A, Dereje D. Prevalence of poor sleep quality and its associated factors among hypertensive patients on follow up at Jimma University Medical Center. J Hum Hypertens. 2021;35(1):94–100.
38. Assi S, Gulyamova N, Kneller P, Osselton D. The effects and toxicity of cathinones from the users' perspectives: a qualitative study. Hum Psychopharmacol. 2017;32(3).
39. Sewalia K, Watterson LR, Hryciw A, Belloc A, Ortiz JB, Olive MF. Neurocognitive dysfunction following repeated binge-like self-administration of the synthetic cathinone 3,4-methylenedioxypyrovalerone (MDPV). Neuropharmacology. 2018;134(Pt A):36–45.
40. Alegre-Zurano L, López-Arnau R, Luján MÁ, Camarasa J, Valverde O. Cannabidiol modulates the motivational and anxiety-like effects of 3,4-methylenedioxypyrovalerone (MDPV) in mice. Int J Mol Sci. 2021;22(15):8304.
41. Bertol E, Mari F, Boscolo Berto R, Mannaioni G, Vaiano F, Favretto D. A mixed MDPV and benzodiazepine intoxication in a chronic drug abuser: determination of MDPV metabolites by LC-HRMS and discussion of the case. Forensic Sci Int. 2014;243:149–55.
42. Jones L, Reed P, Parrott A. Mephedrone and 3,4-methylenedioxy-methamphetamine: comparative psychobiological effects as reported by recreational polydrug users. J Psychopharmacol. 2016;30(12):1313–20.
43. Homman L, Seglert J, Morgan MJ. An observational study on the sub-acute effects of mephedrone on mood, cognition, sleep and physical problems in regular mephedrone users. Psychopharmacology. 2018;235(9):2609–18.
44. López-Muñoz F, Ucha-Udabe R, Alamo C. The history of barbiturates a century after their clinical introduction. Neuropsychiatr Dis Treat. 2005;1(4):329–43. PMID: 18568113; PMCID: PMC2424120.
45. Evans JI, Lewis SA, Gibb IA, Cheetham M. Sleep and birbiturates: some experiments and observations. Br Med J. 1968;4(5626):291–3.
46. Liguori C, Toledo M, Kothare S. Effects of anti-seizure medications on sleep architecture and daytime sleepiness in patients with epilepsy: a literature review. Sleep Med Rev. 2021;60:101559.
47. Longo LP, Johnson B. Addiction: part I. Benzodiazepines—side effects, abuse risk and alternatives. Am Fam Physician. 2000;61:2121–8.
48. Johnston GA. GABAA receptor pharmacology. Pharmacol Ther. 1996;69(3):173–98.
49. Wafford KA, Macaulay AJ, Fradley R, O'Meara GF, Reynolds DS, Rosahl TW. Differentiating the role of gamma-aminobutyric acid type A (GABAA) receptor subtypes. Biochem Soc Trans. 2004;32(Pt3):553–6.
50. Hevers W, Lüddens H. The diversity of GABAA receptors. Pharmacological and electrophysiological properties of GABAA channel subtypes. Mol Neurobiol. 1998;18(1):35–86.
51. Contreras-González N, Téllez-Alanís B, Haro R, JiménezCorrea U, Poblano A. Executive dysfunction in patients with chronic primary insomnia treated with clonazepam. Neurol Res. 2015;37:1047–53.
52. di Giannantonio M, Negri A, Schiavone S, Vannini C, Pettorruso M, De-Giorgio F, Verrastro V, Trabace L, Corbo M, Gottardo R, Camuto C, Mazzarino M, Barra A, De Berardis D, Lopez JI, Del Villar CM, Schifano F, Martinotti G. Prescription drug misuse in "clubbers" and disco goers in Ibiza. Front Psychiatry. 2020;11:592594.
53. Murphy KD, Lambert S, McCarthy S, Sahm LJ, Byrne S. "You don't feel": the experience of youth benzodiazepine misuse in Ireland. J Psychoactive Drugs. 2018;50(2):121–8.
54. Cole JO, Chiarello RJ. The benzodiazepines as drugs of abuse. J Psychiatr Res. 1990;24(suppl 2):135–44.
55. Votaw VR, Geyer R, Rieselbach MM, McHugh RK. The epidemiology of benzodiazepine mis-

use: a systematic review. Drug Alcohol Depend. 2019;200:95–114.
56. Dujardin S, Pijpers A, Pevernagie D. Prescription drugs used in insomnia. Sleep Med Clin. 2018;13(2):169–82.
57. Ashton H. The diagnosis and management of benzodiazepine dependence. Curr Opin Psychiatry. 2005;18(3):249–55.
58. Pétursson H. The benzodiazepine withdrawal syndrome. Addiction. 1994;89(11):1455–9.
59. Poyares D, Guilleminault C, Ohayon MM, Tufik S. Chronic benzodiazepine usage and withdrawal in insomnia patients. J Psychiatr Res. 2004;38(3):327–34.
60. Clausen RP, Hansen HS. 19 Opioid and cannabinoid receptors. In: Strømgaard K, Krogsgaard-Larsen P, Madsen U, editors. Textbook of drug design and discovery. Boca Raton: CRC Press; 2016.
61. Drug facts: Prescription opioids. NIDA. 2019.
62. Vadivelu N, Kai AM, Kodumudi V, Sramcik J, Kaye AD. The opioid crisis: a comprehensive overview. Curr Pain Headache Rep. 2018;22(3):16.
63. Dimsdale JE, Norman D, DeJardin D, Wallace MS. The effect of opioids on sleep architecture. J Clin Sleep Med. 2007;3(1):33–6.
64. Wang D, Teichtahl H. Opioids, sleep architecture and sleep-disordered breathing. Sleep Med Rev. 2007;11(1):35–46.
65. Wang D, Teichtahl H, Drummer OH, Goodman C, Cherry G, Cunnington D, et al. Central sleep apnea in stable methadone maintenance treatment patients. Chest. 2005;128:1348–56.
66. Farney RJ, McDonald AM, Boyle KM, Snow GL, Nuttall RT, Coudreaut MF, Wander TJ, Walker JM. Sleep disordered breathing in patients receiving therapy with buprenorphine/naloxone. Eur Respir J. 2013;42(2):394–403.
67. Sharkey KM, Kurth ME, Anderson BJ, Corso RP, Millman RP, Stein MD. Obstructive sleep apnea is more common than central sleep apnea in methadone maintenance patients with subjective sleep complaints. Drug Alcohol Depend. 2010;108(1-2):77–83.
68. Guilleminault C, Cao M, Yue HJ, Chawla P. Obstructive sleep apnea and chronic opioid use. Lung. 2010;188:459–68.
69. Sanger DJ. The pharmacology and mechanisms of action of new generation, non-benzodiazepine hypnotic agents. CNS Drugs. 2004;18(Suppl 1):9–15; discussion 41, 43–5.
70. Wagner J, Wagner ML. Non-benzodiazepines for the treatment of insomnia. Sleep Med Rev. 2000;4(6):551–81.
71. Stone JR, Zorick TS, Tsuang J. Dose-related illusions and hallucinations with zaleplon. Clin Toxicol (Phila). 2008;46(4):344–5.
72. Tsai JH, Yang P, Chen CC, Chung W, Tang TC, Wang SY, Liu JK. Zolpidem-induced amnesia and somnambulism: rare occurrences? Eur Neuropsychopharmacol. 2009;19(1):74–6.
73. GBD 2016 Alcohol and Drug Use Collaborators. The global burden of disease attributable to alcohol and drug use in 195 countries and territories, 1990–2016: a systematic analysis for the Global Burden of Disease Study 2016. Lancet Psychiatry. 2018;5(12):987–1012.
74. Scrima L, Broudy M, Nay KN, Cohn MA. Increased severity of obstructive sleep apnea after bedtime alcohol ingestion: diagnostic potential and proposed mechanism of action. Sleep. 1982;5(4):318–28.
75. Taveira KVM, Kuntze MM, Berretta F, de Souza BDM, Godolfim LR, Demathe T, De Luca CG, Porporatti AL. Association between obstructive sleep apnea and alcohol, caffeine and tobacco: a meta-analysis. J Oral Rehabil. 2018;45(11):890–902.
76. Block RI, Erwin WJ, Farinpour R, Braverman K. Sedative, stimulant, and other subjective effects of marijuana: relationships to smoking techniques. Pharmacol Biochem Behav. 1998;59(2):405–12.
77. Ibarra-Lecue I, Mollinedo-Gajate I, Meana JJ, Callado LF, Diez-Alarcia R, Urigüen L. Chronic cannabis promotes pro-hallucinogenic signaling of 5-HT2A receptors through Akt/mTOR pathway. Neuropsychopharmacology. 2018;43(10):2028–35.
78. Zehra A, Burns J, Liu CK, Manza P, Wiers CE, Volkow ND, Wang GJ. Cannabis addiction and the brain: a review. J NeuroImmune Pharmacol. 2018;13(4):438–52.
79. Hasan A, von Keller R, Friemel CM, Hall W, Schneider M, Koethe D, Leweke FM, Strube W, Hoch E. Cannabis use and psychosis: a review of reviews. Eur Arch Psychiatry Clin Neurosci. 2020;270(4):403–12.
80. Kroon E, Kuhns L, Cousijn J. The short-term and long-term effects of cannabis on cognition: recent advances in the field. Curr Opin Psychol. 2021;38:49–55.
81. Sainz-Cort A, Jimenez-Garrido D, Muñoz-Marron E, Viejo-Sobera R, Heeroma J, Bouso JC. Opposite roles for cannabidiol and δ-9-tetrahydrocannabinol in psychotomimetic effects of cannabis extracts: a naturalistic controlled study. J Clin Psychopharmacol. 2021;41(5):561–70.
82. Babson KA, Sottile J, Morabito D. Cannabis, cannabinoids, and sleep: a review of the literature. Curr Psychiatry Rep. 2017;19(4):23.
83. Freye E. Peyote, a mescaline-containing cactus. In: Freye E, Levy JV, editors. Pharmacology and abuse of cocaine, amphetamines, ecstasy and related designer drugs. Dordrecht: Springer; 2009.
84. Alves CN, Goyos AC, Carlini EA. Aggressiveness induced by marihuana and other psychotropic drugs in REM sleep deprived rats. Pharmacol Biochem Behav. 1973;1(2):183–9.
85. Vejmola Č, Tylš F, Piorecká V, Koudelka V, Kadeřábek L, Novák T, Páleníček T. Psilocin, LSD, mescaline, and DOB all induce broadband desynchronization of EEG and disconnection in rats with robust translational validity. Transl Psychiatry. 2021;11(1):506.
86. Mauri MC, Paletta S, Di Pace C. Hallucinations in the substance-induced psychosis. In: Brambilla P, Mauri

M, Altamura A, editors. Hallucinations in psychoses and affective disorders. Cham: Springer; 2018.
87. McCann UD, Ricaurte GA. Effects of (+/–) 3,4-me thylenedioxymethamphetamine (MDMA) on sleep and circadian rhythms. ScientificWorldJournal. 2007;7:231–8.
88. Scherbaum N, Schifano F, Bonnet U. New psychoactive substances (NPS)—a challenge for the addiction treatment services. Pharmacopsychiatry. 2017;50(3):116–22.
89. Zisapel N. New perspectives on the role of melatonin in human sleep, circadian rhythms and their regulation. Br J Pharmacol. 2018;175(16):3190–9.
90. Gupta YK, Gupta M, Kohli K. Neuroprotective role of melatonin in oxidative stress vulnerable brain. Indian J Physiol Pharmacol. 2003;47(4):373–86.
91. Dinis-Oliveira RJ. Metabolism of psilocybin and psilocin: clinical and forensic toxicological relevance. Drug Metab Rev. 2017;49(1):84–91.
92. Thomas CW, Blanco-Duque C, Breant B, Sharp T, Goodwin G, Bannerman D, Vyazovskiy, VV. Psilocin acutely disrupts sleep and affects local but not global sleep homeostasis in laboratory mice. bioRxiv. 2021.
93. Froese T, Leenen I, Palenicek T. A role for enhanced functions of sleep in psychedelic therapy? Adapt Behav. 2018;26:129–35.
94. Domínguez-Clavé E, Soler J, Elices M, Pascual JC, Álvarez E, de la Fuente RM, Friedlander P, Feilding A, Riba J. Ayahuasca: pharmacology, neuroscience and therapeutic potential. Brain Res Bull. 2016;126:89–101.
95. Barbanoj MJ, Riba J, Clos S, Giménez S, Grasa E, Romero S. Daytime Ayahuasca administration modulates REM and slow-wave sleep in healthy volunteers. Psychopharmacology. 2008;196:315–26.
96. Safer DJ. The effect of LSD on sleep-deprived men. Psychopharmacologia. 1970;17(5):414–24.

24

Nicotinic Acetylcholine Receptors, Cannabinoid Receptors, and Their Interplay in Drug Addiction

Ana Sofía Vallés and Francisco J. Barrantes

Introduction

Neuronal nicotinic acetylcholine receptors (nAChRs) are ligand-gated ion channels that are widely expressed throughout the nervous system [1, 2]. They are part of the cholinergic receptor system and can be found pre-, post-, and perisynaptically in axon terminals, axons, dendrites, and somata [3–6]. nAChRs are pentameric proteins permeable to small cations. Ion permeation is the epiphenomenon of the activation of the receptor protein upon binding of the natural neurotransmitter, acetylcholine (ACh), a step that can be mimicked by a wide variety of natural or synthetic ligands [7, 8]. nAChRs are comprised of five different subunits, each containing an extracellular N-terminus that contributes to ligand-binding, three hydrophobic transmembrane domains (M1–M3), an intracellular loop, a fourth hydrophobic transmembrane domain (M4), and an extracellular C-terminus. In vertebrates, 12 homologous nAChRs subunits have been described. nAChR subtypes can be classified as homopentameric or heteropentameric. In the former case all five subunits are identical, whereas the latter consists of a combination of subunits. The blend of nine α-subunits (α2–10) and three β-subunits (β2–4) gives rise to the multiple homologous isoforms of native nAChRs, each with potentially different roles [9].

In the brain the most abundant homomeric nAChR is the α7 subtype, whereas α4β2 is most commonly expressed among heteromeric receptor subunit combinations [10–13]. Heteromeric α7β2 nAChRs have been described in subpopulations of basal forebrain, hippocampal, and cortical neurons [14–17].

nAChRs can adopt multiple conformational states. In the closed state the channel can be activated by ligand exposure. In the open state the receptor protein allows the influx of small cations, resulting in changes in membrane potential that lead to the depolarization of the postsynaptic membrane. The open channel can return to a closed state or adopt a desensitized (and closed) state that is unable to be activated by ligand binding. The kinetics of these conformational stages are governed by the subunit composition of the nAChR. Likewise, the subunit composition affects the selective cationic permeability of the channel and the pharmacological affinities of various agonists [18–21]. When nAChRs are activated in presynaptic terminals, Ca^{2+} influx depolarizes the presynaptic cell and triggers a cascade of intracellular signaling events that facilitate neurotransmitter release into the synaptic clef. At

A. S. Vallés
Instituto de Investigaciones Bioquímicas de Bahía Blanca (UNS-CONICET), Buenos Aires, Argentina
e-mail: svalles@criba.edu.ar

F. J. Barrantes (✉)
Biomedical Research Institute (BIOMED), UCA-CONICET, Buenos Aires, Argentina
e-mail: francisco_barrantes@uca.edu.ar

P. Á. Gargiulo, H. L. Mesones-Arroyo (eds.), *Psychiatry and Neuroscience Update – Vol. V*,
https://doi.org/10.1007/978-3-031-72219-6_24

postsynaptic sites, nAChR activation also modulates neuronal excitability and activity-dependent long-term potentiation (LTP), a form of synaptic plasticity.

The effects of drugs of abuse in the brain impinge upon a number of anatomical structures that have been implicated in the neurobiology of drug dependence. Many of these drugs activate dopamine neurons in the ventral tegmental area (VTA) that project to the nucleus accumbens (NAc) [22–24]. The resulting dopamine efflux in the NAc is associated with reward-based learning and with the addiction mechanisms [23, 25]. Some nAChR subtypes are present in the VTA and on axon terminals of afferents from other brain regions, therefore being able to participate in the rewarding effects of drug addiction.

Drug addiction involves learning associations between the rewarding effects of drugs and the environmental cues that predict the availability of drugs, which further leads to compulsive drug use and the propensity to relapse even after long periods of drug withdrawal [10]. Neuroadaptations in the hippocampus and amygdala are believed to underlie these drug-related learning and memory processes. Furthermore, the neuroadaptations that occur in the brain as a consequence of drug exposure are of key importance for the development of dependence. Gaining new insights related to the involvement of nAChR and cannabis receptors in drug addiction will contribute to open new avenues for future interventions.

This short review is concerned with the central nervous system and the addictive effects of nicotine and cannabis. The reader is referred to other works on the effects of cannabinoids on the peripheral nervous system and on nociception [26–28] and on new potential therapeutic avenues, e.g., in pancreatic adenocarcinomas [29–31].

Nicotine

Nicotine, a naturally occurring alkaloid (1-methyl-2-[3-pyridyl] pyrrolidine) used by plants as protection against nicotine-sensitive insects, is a tertiary amine containing a pyridine and a pyrrolidine [32]. In tobacco, it can be present in the form of (S)-nicotine, whereas when tobacco is heated during smoking, small quantities of the (S)-nicotine isomer can be transformed into the (R)-isomer, as is found in cigarette smoke. The (S)- nicotine isomer binds to many nAChR subtypes and is a full agonist of this receptor, whereas the (R)- isomer is a weak agonist of nAChRs. Nicotine ($pK_a = 8.0$) is a weak base and can exist in both a charged and an uncharged form. It can permeate cell membranes and enter the brain when it is in the uncharged state, although in its charged form it can also bind to nAChRs [2, 25].

In terms of drug administration, the gas phase of smoking provides a highly efficient and rapid vehicle to reach the lungs and ultimately the brain within seconds, precluding the first-pass intestinal and hepatic metabolism and ensuring fast absorption of nicotine.

Absorption through buccal mucosa, by chewing tobacco or nicotine gums, cannot bypass the hepatic metabolism. When nicotine reaches the liver, it is extensively transformed into its catabolite cotinine by the enzymes CYP2A6, CYP2B6, and CYP2E1 [33]. The half-life of nicotine is ~2 h, whereas the half-life of cotinine is ~16 h. Therefore, cotinine levels are mostly stable throughout the day in smokers. Recently, cotinine was shown to act as a positive allosteric modulator of the α7 subtype nAChR [34, 35]. Nicotine and cotinine are further metabolized by glucuronidation, the latter process being the major determining factor of nicotine clearance. In regular smokers, the amount of nicotine in the central nervous system (CNS) is about 4 times higher than in occasional smokers [36]. Permanent exposure to nicotine in brain can induce changes in the expression (stoichiometries or receptor number) and function of nAChRs as well as in the intracellular processes undergone by these receptors [37, 38].

Unlike ACh, nicotine is not hydrolyzed by any enzyme at the synapse [19, 25, 38, 39]. Hence, the long-lasting presence of nicotine at the synapse promotes the desensitized state of the nAChRs. This functional inhibition of nAChRs [19, 40–42] leads to its subtype-specific upregulation [4] through changes in receptor assembly, trafficking, and degradation [4, 43–45] to maintain brain homeostasis [10, 18, 46, 47].

Studies using brain imaging techniques have shown that nicotine can increase the activity in prefrontal cortex, thalamus, and visual system, consistent with activation of corticobasal ganglia-thalamic brain circuits [48].

As shown in Fig. 24.1, activation of nAChRs by nicotine results in the release of other neurotransmitters in brain, including the release of dopamine (DA) from dopaminergic neurons in the VTA of the midbrain [49–51]. Importantly, the release of DA in the shell of the NAc has been described as a critical pathway in drug-induced reward mechanisms [52, 53].

Nicotine also promotes the release of ACh, serotonin, γ-aminobutyric acid (GABA), glutamate, and endorphins by activating nAChR from different neurons, modulating various brain circuits [48] and thus contributing to the mediation of different behaviors. Common to many drugs of abuse, the release of DA by dopaminergic terminals results in the perception of pleasure that is critical to the reinforcing effects of nicotine [53]. In rats, the chemical or anatomical lesion of dopaminergic neurons precludes nicotine self-administration [54].

The nAChRs that contain the α4 and β2 subunits, and also those that include the α6 subunit, have been described as particularly important for nicotine's ability to increase midbrain DA neuron firing rates and phasic burst firing [55], thus playing an essential role in mediating the rewarding effects of nicotine [38, 52]. Indeed, studies using mice that lack the β2 subunit show no increase in their extracellular DA after the administration of nicotine [56]. Furthermore, the reexpression of β2 subunits into dopaminergic neurons of the VTA of mice carrying β2 subunit deletions restores both nicotine modulation of VTA neuron activity and nicotine self-administration behavior [57]. These data suggest that the rewarding effects of nicotine appear to be mediated by the β2 subunit [58, 59].

The role that α7 nAChRs play in the reinforcing properties of nicotine has not been fully elucidated since deletion of the α7 subunit does not affect nicotine self-administration [60]. Studies using the α7 nAChR antagonist methyllycaconitine have shown that the animals exhibit attenuated nicotine self-administration [61] and diminished rewarding responses to nicotine when the ligand is applied directly into the VTA [62]. Acute systemic injection of nicotine into VTA neurons has been shown to activate nAChRs, increasing not only dopaminergic [57, 63, 64] but also GABAergic activity [64]. DA release is also facilitated by nicotine-mediated augmentation of glutamate release. While β2 subunit-containing nAChRs directly excite DA and GABA neurons, α7 nAChRs promote the release of glutamate

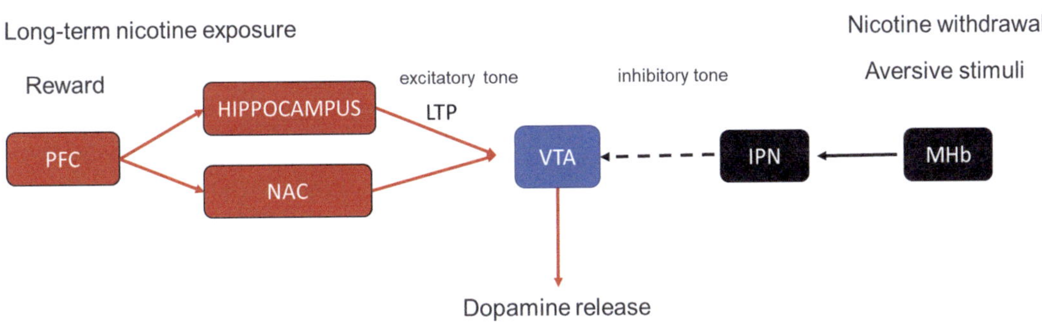

Fig. 24.1 During long-term nicotine exposure, glutamatergic projections that excite dopaminergic neurons of the VTA can initiate long-term potentiation (LTP) and enhance DA release, promoting reward-related behavior. Negative (aversive) reinforcement mechanisms such as nicotine withdrawal are mediated by the habenulo-interpeduncular pathway. The medial habenula (MHb) projects cholinergic and glutamatergic afferents to GABAergic neurons in the interpeduncular nucleus (IPN), therefore conferring their inhibitory nature on the VTA dopaminergic neurons of the mesolimbic pathway, while increased DA levels are hypothesized to confer the hedonistic properties ultimately responsible for the reward mechanisms associated with delivery of the drug [22]

from glutamatergic terminals [65–67]. In fact, α7 nAChRs are mainly concentrated on presynaptic glutamatergic in the VTA, rather than on cholinergic terminals [68, 69]. While α4β2 nAChRs desensitize rapidly when exposed to nicotine, α7 nAChRs desensitize less rapidly [42, 65, 70] since they have a much lower affinity for nicotine compared with β2-containing nAChRs [71–73]. Thus, nicotine exposure activates α4β2 nAChRs and enhances DA release in the NAc. In parallel, nicotine acting on α4β2 nAChRs on GABAergic neurons induces a transient inhibition of DA activity. However, these receptors also rapidly desensitize, consequently reducing the inhibitory control of GABA on dopaminergic neurons [65]. Additionally, nicotine will bind to α7 nAChRs present on glutamatergic terminals in the VTA and induce glutamate release. NMDA- type glutamate receptors located on dopaminergic cell bodies will be activated and consequently increase the frequency of spontaneous excitatory postsynaptic currents (sEPSCs) [66, 74–76]. In summary, upon nicotine exposure GABAergic inputs to the DA neurons are inhibited, while glutamatergic inputs are enhanced, with a net increase in the excitation of DA neurons [65, 76] (Fig. 24.2). Moreover, behavioral reinforcement is associated with inhibition of GABAergic transmission.

Studies in which rodent self-administered $GABA_A$ receptor antagonist is focally infused into the VTA show that VTA neuronal activity is increased as well as DA-dependent behaviors [77, 78]. Since DA increases in the NAc after $GABA_A$ receptor blockade in the VTA, it is likely that the reduced GABAergic transmission induced by nAChR desensitization in the VTA contributes to the reinforcing effects of nicotine. Furthermore, this enhanced activity of dopaminergic neurons has been suggested to promote Hebbian long-term potentiation (LTP) of glutamatergic afferents onto the midbrain dopaminergic neurons and has been proposed to be a critical step in the initiation of addiction [66, 79–81].

Nicotine exposure reduces GABAergic transmission in a time scale of minutes [82], whereas nicotine-induced LTP of excitatory transmission may last for hours [66]. Therefore, limited expo-

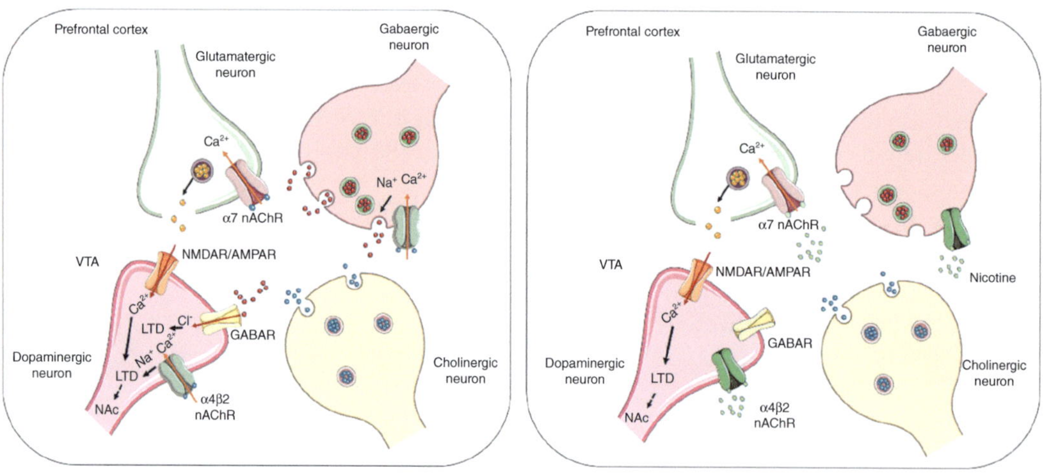

Fig. 24.2 nAChRs regulate neuronal excitability of dopaminergic neurons in the ventral tegmental area (VTA). Dopaminergic neurons in the VTA receive excitatory inputs from glutamatergic and cholinergic terminals. These excitatory inputs are decoded by NMDAR/AMPAR and α4β2 nAChRs, respectively, leading to burst firing that promotes long-term potentiation (LTP) in the VTA. LTP is subsequently propagated to the nucleus accumbens (NAc). Acetylcholine release from cholinergic neurons activates α4β2 nAChRs localized on GABAergic neurons, promoting GABA release and long-term depression (LTD) of dopaminergic neurons. Nicotine rapidly desensitizes α4β2 nAChRs, thereby inhibiting GABAergic inputs to dopaminergic neurons. α7 nAChRs desensitize to a lesser degree and hence glutamatergic inputs are amplified, leading to a net increase in the excitation of dopaminergic neurons

sure to nicotine should suffice to induce profound and long-lasting modifications to the mesolimbic reward system circuitry.

Neuromodulation upon nicotine administration has been reported to increase dendritic spine density in the NAc and prefrontal cortex of adult rats [83] as well as increase the dendritic length and branch number in the NAc shell of adolescent rats [84].

The prefrontal cortex (PFC) is the area of the brain that regulates executive cognitive function, attention, and working memory. Nicotine in the PFC enhances DA overflow by acting on both β2- and α7-containing nAChRs [85]. By activating D1 and D2 receptors, DA can result in long-term depression (LTD) independently of NMDAR activation [86, 87] or in LTP through cooperative actions of D1 and NMDA receptors [88, 89]. Of critical importance for the direction of synaptic plasticity (LTD or LTP) is the relative timing of action potentials in pre- and postsynaptic neurons or spike-timing-dependent plasticity (STDP) [90–92]. LTP is induced when the presynaptic spike occurs prior to the postsynaptic spike, whereas LTD is induced if the postsynaptic spike precedes the presynaptic spike. Couey and collaborators [90] found that nicotine increases the threshold for induction of STDP in pyramidal neurons by reducing dendritic calcium signaling in these cells through nicotine-induced augmentation of GABAergic inhibition. These authors speculate that nicotine may improve cognition by increasing the signal-to-noise ratio during PFC neural processing [90].

Nicotine Withdrawal

The inability to halt cigarette use, or relapse, is linked to the hedonically positive rewarding effects but also to the avoidance of negative states associated with withdrawal. Nicotine-withdrawal symptoms are associated with a negative emotional state, frequently including depressed mood, anxiety, irritability, and craving in dependent subjects, constituting a key component of nicotine addiction [93, 94]. The duration of nicotine withdrawal symptoms can vary from a couple of weeks of abstinence [95, 96] to more than a month [97, 98]. The severity of the symptoms predicts increased risk of relapse [99–103]. The expression of these withdrawal symptoms depends on the α2, α3, α5, and β4 nAChR subunits in the epithalamic habenular complex and its target regions [55]. Nicotine withdrawal depresses activity of mesolimbic DA neurons, with anhedonic consequences [104]. In animal model studies the knockout of the nAChR β4 subunit can prevent somatic signs (e.g., shaking, paw tremors, or scratching) of nicotine withdrawal in mice [105] and also prevent withdrawal-induced anhedonia [106]. Other nAChRs, including the α7, α3 [107], α5 [108, 109], β4 [105–107], and α2 [109, 110] subunits, have been implicated in the somatic signs of nicotine withdrawal [55, 111, 112]. In contrast, knockout of the nAChR β2 subunit has no effect on somatic withdrawal signs compared with controls [105]. These animals show, however, a reduction in the affective components of withdrawal [108, 112]. α6 subunit-containing nAChRs have also been associated with the affective components of nicotine withdrawal [113].

Neural circuits mediate nicotine withdrawal and maintain addiction-related behaviors. The maintenance of chronic nicotine intake is facilitated through both positive (rewarding) reinforcement mechanisms by activation of the mesolimbic DA pathway and negative (aversive) reinforcement mechanisms mediated by the habenulo-interpeduncular pathway [111, 114, 115]. The habenula mediates different forms of negative affections such as fear, anxiety, and depression [25, 116–119]. Located close to the third ventricle, the habenula is anatomically divided into medial (MHb) and lateral (LHb) nuclei; the former, mainly associated with nicotine withdrawal [111, 115, 120], receives primary inputs from the limbic system and projects cholinergic and glutamatergic afferents to the interpeduncular nucleus (IPN) (see Fig. 24.1 in preceding section) [121, 122]. Almost all neuronal types of nAChR are expressed in the MHb-IPN axis [123, 124] and cholinergic habenular signaling is implicated in nicotine withdrawal [125]. Furthermore, in rats, spontaneous nicotine withdrawal results in a significant decrease in brain reward functions determined by elevations in brain reward thresholds [93]. Similarly, administration of nAChR antagonist leads to a dose-dependent increase in brain reward thresholds in chronic nicotine-treated rats.

Increased nAChR activity in the MHb has been shown to produce anxiety-related symptoms of nicotine withdrawal [114]. Additionally, human genetic data point to the nAChR expressed in the MHb-IPN as a critical mediator of nicotine withdrawal mechanisms [126]. A considerable number of genome-wide association studies (GWAS) have linked single nucleotide polymorphisms in the *CHRNA5-CHRNA3-CHRNB4* nAChR-coding genes to tobacco use [126–129] and nicotine addiction [130].

Nicotine withdrawal is also associated with the extrahypothalamic corticotropin-releasing factor (CRF) system [131]. Activation of this system leads to anxiety behavior. It has also been suggested that activation of the CRF system promotes relapse to smoking [37]. Additionally, nicotine withdrawal has been shown to cause elevations of intracranial self-stimulation thresholds in rats [93]. Nicotine conditioning also becomes an important element of smoking addiction. The association between smoking and certain environmental situations becomes a powerful cue for the urge to smoke [37, 132, 133]. Nicotine addiction is thus a consequence of the combined positive reinforcements (DA outflow) and the avoidance of withdrawal symptoms. The neurobiological mechanisms through which cues mediate drug-seeking behavior have been extensively studied using animal models [134]. Environmental stimuli can induce drug craving, increasing the probability of relapse to drug use [135]. It has been suggested that conditioned reinforcers could be the primary motivation to smoke during periods when desensitization of nAChRs prevents the reinforcing effects of nicotine resulting from smoking [22].

Fu and coworkers [136] demonstrated that nicotine activation of nAChRs in the brainstem stimulates the release of norepinephrine in both the amygdala and the hippocampus. They further suggested that α3 subunit-containing nAChRs are responsible for this effect. Norepinephrine release contributes to memory function and stress response [137, 138] and to reward-related learning [10].

Cannabinoids

Cannabis is one of the most widely used addictive drugs; its increasing consumption in the United States [139] and elsewhere, particularly in the form of smoking dried *Cannabis sativa* leaves, makes it today's most used illicit drug. The two main constituents of cannabis are Δ^9-tetrahydracannabinol (THC) and cannabidiol (CBD). The addictive potential of cannabis has been attributed to THC because of its psychoactive properties and associated effects on brain dopaminergic function. In animal and human studies, acute THC administration produces striatal DA release [140–143].

Cannabinoids mediate their effects through the activation of cannabinoid receptors and their downstream effectors. The two cannabinoid receptors identified to date have been termed cannabinoid-1 receptor (CB1) and cannabinoid-2 receptor (CB2), two G-protein coupled receptors (GPCRs) belonging to the $G_{i/o}$ subtype. The downstream mechanisms triggered by this type of G proteins are the inhibition of adenylate cyclase activity and associated cAMP cascade and inhibition of voltage-gated Ca^{2+} channels. CB1s also inhibit voltage-activated Ca^{2+} channels, promote inwardly rectifying K^+ currents, and activate both phospholipase C and PI-3-kinase [144]. The two cannabinoid receptors share 44% amino acid sequence homology [145, 146]. CB1 constitutes the most abundant GPCR in the CNS [147], particularly in cerebral cortex, hippocampus, cerebellum, and basal ganglia, whereas CB2 is localized preferentially in immune cells and peripheral immune tissues [146] and to a lesser extent in the brainstem, cortex, hippocampus, and cerebellar neurons and microglia [148, 149]. Conversely, CB1s in the periphery constitute a mere 1% of the number of CB2s.

The endocannabinoid system modulates neurotransmitter release and maintains homeostasis in health and disease through the regulation of neuronal activity in the CNS. This is mainly accomplished through two endogenous substances (endocannabinoids), anandamide (N-arachidonoylethanolamide, AEA) and 2-arachidonoylglycerol (2-AG). The two are lipophilic molecules that act as ligands on the cannabinoid receptors, previously considered orphan receptors. Endocannabinoids serve as retrograde synaptic messengers [150, 151]. CB1s mediate the inhibition of perpetual release of different excitatory and inhibitory neurotransmitters [152–154]. At postsynaptic terminals, the increase in intracellular Ca^{2+} induced by certain neurotransmitters triggers endocannabinoid biosynthesis and release, allowing endocannabinoids to act on presynaptic CB1s to inhibit the release of both excitatory and inhibitory neurotransmitters. Thus, endocannabinoids act as fine tuners of excitatory and inhibitory signaling activity.

Growing evidence supports the key role of the endocannabinoid system in the modulation of the addiction-related effects of nicotine [155]. The overlapping distribution of cannabinoid receptors and nAChRs is not fortuitous. They share a close anatomical overlap in brain areas such as the midbrain, the hippocampus, and the amygdala. As previously mentioned, these structures are important in mediating the reinforcing properties of nicotine and nicotine-associated memory [156–158].

In experimental model systems that heterologously express α7-type nAChR in *Xenopus* oocytes [159, 160], the natural endocannabinoid AEA reversibly inhibits nicotine-induced currents in a concentration-dependent manner without significantly affecting its half maximal effective concentration (EC50) value, indicating that AEA exerts noncompetitive antagonism on α7 nAChRs. In support of the noncompetitive action of AEA on this neuronal nAChR is the observation that AEA does not inhibit specific [^{3}H]nicotine binding in human frontal cortex membranes [161]. Additionally, AEA inhibits the peak amplitudes of α4β2 nAChR-mediated currents in SH-EP1 cells [162] as well as in myenteric neurons [163, 164].

THC acts as a partial agonist on both CB1 and CB2 [165]. The magnitude of the responses it elicits is strongly influenced by the expression level and signaling efficiency of cannabinoid receptors, as well as by background endogenous cannabinoid release [165]. THC exerts complex effects on the dopaminergic system and disrupts the finely tuned endogenous endocannabinoid system, thereby contributing to the drug's recreational and harmful effects [143]. THC elicits its acute psychoactive effects via CB1. Although THC has been linked to the rewarding aspects of cannabis use, it has also been associated with the induction of symptoms of mental illnesses and cognitive impairment [143]. Acute THC use increases DA release and neuronal activity, while long-term use has been associated with blunting of the dopaminergic system [143]. Low doses of THC increase the conversion of tyrosine into DA, while high doses result in decreased DA synthesis [166]. In vivo microdialysis studies have demonstrated that acute THC administration increases DA efflux in the PFC, striatum, and NAc [140, 167, 168]. In animal studies, overlapping pharmacological effects have been reported between the primary psychoactive ingredients in cannabis (THC) and tobacco (nicotine), including induction of antinociception, hypothermia, rewarding effects, dependence, and impairment of locomotion [169–175]. Some studies also report that nicotine can facilitate many of the acute pharmacological and biochemical effects of THC [176, 177]. When administered together at subthreshold doses, THC and nicotine potentiate their anxiolytic effects in a synergistic manner [176, 178–180]. Synthetic cannabinoids and THC have been reported to modulate cholinergic neurotransmission in the hippocampus [181–183].

Cannabinoid Withdrawal

Withdrawal syndrome in humans is observed after abrupt discontinuation following chronic exposure to smoked cannabis or oral THC. Withdrawal symptoms involve sleep disturbances, disrupted cognition, decreased appetite, restlessness, irritability, sweating, chills, and nausea [184, 185]. Increased craving and desire to resume use is also observed [186]. Preclinical and clinical studies concur in that THC effectively ameliorates cannabinoid withdrawal signs [187, 188] . However, to date there are no approved pharmacological treatments for treating cannabis use disorder [189].

Recent work by Donvito and collaborators [190] suggests that $\alpha3\beta4^*$ and $\alpha6\beta4^*$ nAChR subtypes (asterisk indicates the presence of additional subunits) represent viable targets for the development of medications to counteract THC dependence.

Their study shows that multiple nAChRs contribute to the development and/or expression of THC withdrawal [190]. Additionally, they suggest that $\alpha3\beta4^*$ and $\alpha6\beta4^*$ nAChR subtypes in the MHb-IPN pathway may contribute to the mediation of THC withdrawal responses. Another study also points to involvement of the $\alpha2$ nAChR subunit in cannabis use disorder with decreased expression of *CHRNA2* in the cerebellum and other brain regions [191].

Cannabidiol

Cannabidiol (CBD), the other most abundant cannabinoid found in cannabis extracts [192], has no psychoactive properties [193, 194]. CBD has shown potential to be effective in several syndromic forms of epilepsy [195, 196]. Zhang and coworkers have suggested that at submicromolar concentrations, CBD could act as an effective antiepileptic drug by shifting the voltage dependence of Kv7.2/7.3 channels in the hyperpolarizing direction, thus reducing neuronal hyperexcitability [197].

CBD has been reported to inhibit $\alpha7$ nAChR currents in a concentration-dependent manner (IC50 value of 12.7 mM) expressed in *Xenopus* oocytes and rat hippocampal neurons [198]. These authors propose that CBD interacts with the closed state of the receptor; that CBD does not interact with the acetylcholine binding site on the receptor; and that the CBD-binding site is not affected by the transmembrane electric field [198]. They further suggest that because of the lipophilic nature of CBD, it must first dissolve into the lipid membrane and then diffuse into a non-annular lipid space to inhibit the ion channel-receptor complex.

Concluding Remarks

Chronic use of cannabis and tobacco is associated with symptoms of dependence, withdrawal, and great difficulties in ceasing consumption [199]. Preference for multiple rather than single drug use is common in these addictions [200] and co-use of cannabis and tobacco is frequent among addicted users. The obvious appeal to addicted individuals of combined substance use warrants further research into the underlying neurobiological mechanism(s) for this preference. Tobacco is considered to be a gateway drug because its use tends to precede other addictions, but there are also reports indicating that prior cannabis use increases the likelihood of becoming dependent on tobacco [201]. In addition to a common route of administration, synergistic and compensatory effects that favor cannabis and tobacco co-use have been proposed [199]. Current evidence suggests that simultaneous tobacco and cannabis abstinence predicts better therapeutical outcomes [199].

Synergistic and compensatory mechanisms are mediated within the neurocircuitry of the brain mesolimbic dopaminergic system. These mechanisms involve the modification of physiological processes such as reward and aversion learning [155, 202].

A deeper understanding of the biological mechanisms linking the cholinergic and cannabinoid systems in the brain is necessary for future intervention in drug addiction, most particularly at times of increasing worldwide trends toward cannabis legalization. Both systems show structural and functional overlap within the brain and mediate the rewarding and aversive effects of nicotine and cannabis.

Acknowledgments Figures were created using Servier Medical Art Commons Attribution 3.0 Unported License. (http://smart.servier.com). Servier Medical Art by Servier is licensed under a Creative Commons Attribution 3.0 Unported License.

Conflicts of Interest Authors declare no conflicts of interest.

Author Contributions F.J.B. and A.S.V. conceived the work, searched the literature, and wrote the manuscript.

Funding No funding is associated with this review.

References

1. Papke RL. Merging old and new perspectives on nicotinic acetylcholine receptors. Biochem Pharmacol. 2014;89:1–11. https://doi.org/10.1016/j.bcp.2014.01.029.
2. Dani JA, Bertrand D. Nicotinic acetylcholine receptors and nicotinic cholinergic mechanisms of the central nervous system. Annu Rev Pharmacol Toxicol. 2007;47:699–729. https://doi.org/10.1146/annurev.pharmtox.47.120505.105214.
3. Grady SR, Salminen O, Laverty DC, Whiteaker P, McIntosh JM, Collins AC, Marks MJ. The subtypes of nicotinic acetylcholine receptors on dopaminergic terminals of mouse striatum. Biochem Pharmacol. 2007;74:1235–46. https://doi.org/10.1016/j.bcp.2007.07.032.
4. Henderson BJ, Lester HA. Inside-out neuropharmacology of nicotinic drugs. Neuropharmacology. 2015;96:178–93. https://doi.org/10.1016/j.neuropharm.2015.01.022.
5. McGehee DS, Heath MJ, Gelber S, Devay P, Role LW. Nicotine enhancement of fast excitatory synaptic transmission in CNS by presynaptic receptors. Science. 1995;269:1692–6. https://doi.org/10.1126/science.7569895.
6. Nashmi R, Lester HA. CNS localization of neuronal nicotinic receptors. J Mol Neurosci. 2006;30:181–4. https://doi.org/10.1385/JMN:30:1:181.
7. Cooper E, Couturier S, Ballivet M. Pentameric structure and subunit stoichiometry of a neuronal nicotinic acetylcholine receptor. Nature. 1991;350:235–8. https://doi.org/10.1038/350235a0.
8. Morales-Perez CL, Noviello CM, Hibbs RE. X-ray structure of the human α4β2 nicotinic receptor. Nature. 2016;538:411–5. https://doi.org/10.1038/nature19785.
9. Caton M, Ochoa ELM, Barrantes FJ. The role of nicotinic cholinergic neurotransmission in delusional thinking. npj Schizophr. 2020;6:16. https://doi.org/10.1038/s41537-020-0105-9.
10. Feduccia, A.; Chatterjee, S.; Bartlett, S. Neuronal nicotinic acetylcholine receptors: neuroplastic changes underlying alcohol and nicotine addictions. Front Mol Neurosci. 2012;5. https://doi.org/10.3389/fnmol.2012.00083.
11. Gotti C, Zoli M, Clementi F. Brain nicotinic acetylcholine receptors: native subtypes and their relevance. Trends Pharmacol Sci. 2006;27:482–91. https://doi.org/10.1016/j.tips.2006.07.004.
12. Chen D, Patrick JW. The alpha-bungarotoxin-binding nicotinic acetylcholine receptor from rat brain contains only the alpha7 subunit. J Biol Chem. 1997;272:24024–9. https://doi.org/10.1074/jbc.272.38.24024.
13. Drisdel RC, Green WN. Neuronal alpha-bungarotoxin receptors are alpha7 subunit homomers. J Neurosci. 2000;20:133–9. https://doi.org/10.1523/JNEUROSCI.20-01-00133.2000.
14. Liu Q, Huang Y, Xue F, Simard A, DeChon J, Li G, Zhang J, Lucero L, Wang M, Sierks M, et al. A novel nicotinic acetylcholine receptor subtype in basal forebrain cholinergic neurons with high sensitivity to amyloid peptides. J Neurosci. 2009;29:918–29. https://doi.org/10.1523/JNEUROSCI.3952-08.2009.
15. Liu Q, Huang Y, Shen J, Steffensen S, Wu J. Functional α7β2 nicotinic acetylcholine receptors expressed in hippocampal interneurons exhibit high sensitivity to pathological level of amyloid β peptides. BMC Neurosci. 2012;13:155. https://doi.org/10.1186/1471-2202-13-155.
16. Azam L, Winzer-Serhan U, Leslie FM. Co-expression of alpha7 and beta2 nicotinic acetylcholine receptor subunit mRNAs within rat brain cholinergic neurons. Neuroscience. 2003;119:965–77. https://doi.org/10.1016/s0306-4522(03)00220-3.
17. Thomsen MS, Zwart R, Ursu D, Jensen MM, Pinborg LH, Gilmour G, Wu J, Sher E, Mikkelsen JD. α7 and β2 nicotinic acetylcholine receptor subunits form heteromeric receptor complexes that are expressed in the human cortex and display distinct pharmacological properties. PLoS One. 2015;10:e0130572. https://doi.org/10.1371/journal.pone.0130572.
18. Giniatullin R, Nistri A, Yakel JL. Desensitization of nicotinic ACh receptors: shaping cholinergic signaling. Trends Neurosci. 2005;28:371–8. https://doi.org/10.1016/j.tins.2005.04.009.
19. Picciotto MR, Addy NA, Mineur YS, Brunzell DH. It is not "either/or": activation and desensitization of nicotinic acetylcholine receptors both contribute to behaviors related to nicotine addiction and mood. Prog Neurobiol. 2008;84:329–42. https://doi.org/10.1016/j.pneurobio.2007.12.005.
20. Wang J, Lindstrom J. Orthosteric and allosteric potentiation of heteromeric neuronal nicotinic acetylcholine receptors. Br J Pharmacol. 2018;175:1805–21. https://doi.org/10.1111/bph.13745.
21. Zoli M, Pucci S, Vilella A, Gotti C. Neuronal and extraneuronal nicotinic acetylcholine receptors. Curr Neuropharmacol. 2018;16:338–49. https://doi.org/10.2174/1570159X15666170912110450.

22. Balfour DJK. The neurobiology of tobacco dependence: a preclinical perspective on the role of the dopamine projections to the nucleus accumbens [corrected]. Nicotine Tob Res. 2004;6:899–912. https://doi.org/10.1080/14622200412331324965.
23. Di Chiara G, Imperato A. Drugs abused by humans preferentially increase synaptic dopamine concentrations in the mesolimbic system of freely moving rats. Proc Natl Acad Sci USA. 1988;85:5274–8. https://doi.org/10.1073/pnas.85.14.5274.
24. Clarke PB, Fu DS, Jakubovic A, Fibiger HC. Evidence that mesolimbic dopaminergic activation underlies the locomotor stimulant action of nicotine in rats. J Pharmacol Exp Ther. 1988;246:701–8.
25. De Biasi M, Dani JA. Reward, addiction, withdrawal to nicotine. Annu Rev Neurosci. 2011;34:105–30. https://doi.org/10.1146/annurev-neuro-061010-113734.
26. Hone AJ, McIntosh JM. Nicotinic acetylcholine receptors in neuropathic and inflammatory pain. FEBS Lett. 2018;592:1045–62. https://doi.org/10.1002/1873-3468.12884.
27. Agarwal N, Pacher P, Tegeder I, Amaya F, Constantin CE, Brenner GJ, Rubino T, Michalski CW, Marsicano G, Monory K, et al. Cannabinoids mediate analgesia largely via peripheral type 1 cannabinoid receptors in nociceptors. Nat Neurosci. 2007;10:870–9. https://doi.org/10.1038/nn1916.
28. Modesto-Lowe V, Bojka R, Alvarado C. Cannabis for peripheral neuropathy: the good, the bad, and the unknown. Cleve Clin J Med. 2018;85:943 LP–949. https://doi.org/10.3949/ccjm.85a.17115.
29. Falasca V, Falasca M. Targeting the endocannabinoidome in pancreatic cancer. Biomolecules. 2022;12. https://doi.org/10.3390/biom12020320.
30. Sharafi G, He H, Nikfarjam M. Potential use of cannabinoids for the treatment of pancreatic cancer. J Pancreat cancer. 2019;5:1–7. https://doi.org/10.1089/pancan.2018.0019.
31. Adamska A, Domenichini A, Capone E, Damiani V, Akkaya BG, Linton KJ, Di Sebastiano P, Chen X, Keeton AB, Ramirez-Alcantara V, et al. Pharmacological inhibition of ABCC3 slows tumour progression in animal models of pancreatic cancer. J Exp Clin Cancer Res. 2019;38:312. https://doi.org/10.1186/s13046-019-1308-7.
32. Dani J, Kosten T, Benowitz N. Chapter 14, The pharmacology of nicotine and tobacco. In: Miller SC, Fiellin DA, Rosenthal RN, Saitz R, editors. The ASAM principles of addiction medicine, 6th edn. Wolters Kluwer/Lippincott Williams & Wilkins; 2019. p. 190–207.
33. Hukkanen J, Jacob P 3rd, Benowitz NL. Metabolism and disposition kinetics of nicotine. Pharmacol Rev. 2005;57:79–115. https://doi.org/10.1124/pr.57.1.3.
34. Grizzell JA, Patel S, Barreto GE, Echeverria V. Cotinine improves visual recognition memory and decreases cortical Tau phosphorylation in the Tg6799 mice. Prog Neuro-Psychopharmacol Biol Psychiatry. 2017;78:75–81. https://doi.org/10.1016/j.pnpbp.2017.05.010.
35. Echeverria V, Yarkov A, Aliev G. Positive modulators of the α7 nicotinic receptor against neuroinflammation and cognitive impairment in Alzheimer's disease. Prog Neurobiol. 2016;144:142–57. https://doi.org/10.1016/J.PNEUROBIO.2016.01.002.
36. Heishman SJ, Kleykamp BA, Singleton EG. Meta-analysis of the acute effects of nicotine and smoking on human performance. Psychopharmacology. 2010;210:453–69. https://doi.org/10.1007/s00213-010-1848-1.
37. Benowitz NL. Pharmacology of nicotine: addiction, smoking-induced disease, and therapeutics. Annu Rev Pharmacol Toxicol. 2009;49:57–71. https://doi.org/10.1146/annurev.pharmtox.48.113006.094742.
38. Nashmi R, Xiao C, Deshpande P, McKinney S, Grady SR, Whiteaker P, Huang Q, McClure-Begley T, Lindstrom JM, Labarca C, et al. Chronic nicotine cell specifically upregulates functional α4* nicotinic receptors: basis for both tolerance in midbrain and enhanced long-term potentiation in perforant path. J Neurosci. 2007;27:8202–18. https://doi.org/10.1523/JNEUROSCI.2199-07.2007.
39. Baker LK, Mao D, Chi H, Govind AP, Vallejo YF, Iacoviello M, Herrera S, Cortright JJ, Green WN, McGehee DS, et al. Intermittent nicotine exposure upregulates nAChRs in VTA dopamine neurons and sensitises locomotor responding to the drug. Eur J Neurosci. 2013;37:1004–11. https://doi.org/10.1111/ejn.12114.
40. Dani JA, Radcliffe KA, Pidoplichko VI. Variations in desensitization of nicotinic acetylcholine receptors from hippocampus and midbrain dopamine areas. Eur J Pharmacol. 2000;393:31–8. https://doi.org/10.1016/s0014-2999(00)00003-0.
41. Pidoplichko VI, DeBiasi M, Williams JT, Dani JA. Nicotine activates and desensitizes midbrain dopamine neurons. Nature. 1997;390:401–4. https://doi.org/10.1038/37120.
42. Wooltorton JRA, Pidoplichko VI, Broide RS, Dani JA. Differential desensitization and distribution of nicotinic acetylcholine receptor subtypes in midbrain dopamine areas. J Neurosci. 2003;23:3176–85. https://doi.org/10.1523/JNEUROSCI.23-08-03176.2003.
43. Henderson BJ, Srinivasan R, Nichols WA, Dilworth CN, Gutierrez DF, Mackey EDW, McKinney S, Drenan RM, Richards CI, Lester HA. Nicotine exploits a COPI-mediated process for chaperone-mediated up-regulation of its receptors. J Gen Physiol. 2014;143:51–66. https://doi.org/10.1085/jgp.201311102.
44. Mazzo F, Pistillo F, Grazioso G, Clementi F, Borgese N, Gotti C, Colombo SF. Nicotine-modulated subunit stoichiometry affects stability and trafficking of α3β4 nicotinic receptor. J Neurosci. 2013;33:12316–28. https://doi.org/10.1523/JNEUROSCI.2393-13.2013.
45. Rezvani K, Teng Y, De Biasi M. The ubiquitin-proteasome system regulates the stability of neu-

ronal nicotinic acetylcholine receptors. J Mol Neurosci. 2010;40:177–84. https://doi.org/10.1007/s12031-009-9272-x.
46. Fenster CP, Whitworth TL, Sheffield EB, Quick MW, Lester RA. Upregulation of surface alpha-4beta2 nicotinic receptors is initiated by receptor desensitization after chronic exposure to nicotine. J Neurosci. 1999;19:4804–14. https://doi.org/10.1523/JNEUROSCI.19-12-04804.1999.
47. Fenster CP, Hicks JH, Beckman ML, Covernton PJ, Quick MW, Lester RA. Desensitization of nicotinic receptors in the central nervous system. Ann N Y Acad Sci. 1999;868:620–3. https://doi.org/10.1111/j.1749-6632.1999.tb11335.x.
48. Brody AL. Functional brain imaging of tobacco use and dependence. J Psychiatr Res. 2006;40:404–18. https://doi.org/10.1016/j.jpsychires.2005.04.012.
49. Cooper SY, Henderson BJ, The impact of electronic nicotine delivery system (ENDS) flavors on nicotinic acetylcholine receptors and nicotine addiction-related behaviors. Molecules. 2020;25. https://doi.org/10.3390/molecules25184223.
50. Engle SE, Shih P-Y, McIntosh JM, Drenan RM. α4α6β2* nicotinic acetylcholine receptor activation on ventral tegmental area dopamine neurons is sufficient to stimulate a depolarizing conductance and enhance surface AMPA receptor function. Mol Pharmacol. 2013;84:393–406. https://doi.org/10.1124/mol.113.087346.
51. Liu L, Zhao-Shea R, McIntosh JM, Gardner PD, Tapper AR. Nicotine persistently activates ventral tegmental area dopaminergic neurons via nicotinic acetylcholine receptors containing α4 and α6 subunits. Mol Pharmacol. 2012;81:541–8. https://doi.org/10.1124/mol.111.076661.
52. Dani JA, De Biasi M. Cellular mechanisms of nicotine addiction. Pharmacol Biochem Behav. 2001;70:439–46. https://doi.org/10.1016/s0091-3057(01)00652-9.
53. Nestler EJ. Is there a common molecular pathway for addiction? Nat Neurosci. 2005;8:1445–9. https://doi.org/10.1038/nn1578.
54. Cryan JF, Bruijnzeel AW, Skjei KL, Markou A. Bupropion enhances brain reward function and reverses the affective and somatic aspects of nicotine withdrawal in the rat. Psychopharmacology. 2003;168:347–58. https://doi.org/10.1007/s00213-003-1445-7.
55. Wittenberg RE, Wolfman SL, De Biasi M, Dani JA. Nicotinic acetylcholine receptors and nicotine addiction: a brief introduction. Neuropharmacology. 2020;177:108256. https://doi.org/10.1016/j.neuropharm.2020.108256.
56. Picciotto MR, Zoli M, Rimondini R, Léna C, Marubio LM, Pich EM, Fuxe K, Changeux JP. Acetylcholine receptors containing the beta2 subunit are involved in the reinforcing properties of nicotine. Nature. 1998;391:173–7. https://doi.org/10.1038/34413.
57. Maskos U, Molles BE, Pons S, Besson M, Guiard BP, Guilloux J-P, Evrard A, Cazala P, Cormier A, Mameli-Engvall M, et al. Nicotine reinforcement and cognition restored by targeted expression of nicotinic receptors. Nature. 2005;436:103–7. https://doi.org/10.1038/nature03694.
58. Yan Y, Beckley NA, Kim VJ, Drenan RM. Differential nicotinic modulation of glutamatergic and GABAergic VTA microcircuits. eneuro. 2019;6:ENEURO.0298-19.2019. https://doi.org/10.1523/ENEURO.0298-19.2019.
59. Yan Y, Peng C, Arvin MC, Jin X-T, Kim VJ, Ramsey MD, Wang Y, Banala S, Wokosin DL, McIntosh JM, et al. Nicotinic cholinergic receptors in VTA glutamate neurons modulate excitatory transmission. Cell Rep. 2018;23:2236–44. https://doi.org/10.1016/j.celrep.2018.04.062.
60. Pons S, Fattore L, Cossu G, Tolu S, Porcu E, McIntosh JM, Changeux JP, Maskos U, Fratta W. Crucial role of alpha4 and alpha6 nicotinic acetylcholine receptor subunits from ventral tegmental area in systemic nicotine self-administration. J Neurosci. 2008;28:12318–27. https://doi.org/10.1523/JNEUROSCI.3918-08.2008.
61. Markou A, Paterson NE. The nicotinic antagonist methyllycaconitine has differential effects on nicotine self-administration and nicotine withdrawal in the rat. Nicotine Tob Res. 2001;3:361–73. https://doi.org/10.1080/14622200110073380.
62. Laviolette SR, van der Kooy D. The motivational valence of nicotine in the rat ventral tegmental area is switched from rewarding to aversive following blockade of the α7-subunit-containing nicotinic acetylcholine receptor. Psychopharmacology. 2003;166:306–13. https://doi.org/10.1007/s00213-002-1317-6.
63. Mameli-Engvall M, Evrard A, Pons S, Maskos U, Svensson TH, Changeux J-P, Faure P. Hierarchical control of dopamine neuron-firing patterns by nicotinic receptors. Neuron. 2006;50:911–21. https://doi.org/10.1016/j.neuron.2006.05.007.
64. Tolu S, Eddine R, Marti F, David V, Graupner M, Pons S, Baudonnat M, Husson M, Besson M, Reperant C, et al. Co-activation of VTA DA and GABA neurons mediates nicotine reinforcement. Mol Psychiatry. 2013;18:382–93. https://doi.org/10.1038/mp.2012.83.
65. Mansvelder HD, McGehee DS. Cellular and synaptic mechanisms of nicotine addiction. J Neurobiol. 2002;53:606–17. https://doi.org/10.1002/neu.10148.
66. Mansvelder HD, McGehee DS. Long-term potentiation of excitatory inputs to brain reward areas by nicotine. Neuron. 2000;27:349–57. https://doi.org/10.1016/s0896-6273(00)00042-8.
67. Dani JA. Neuronal nicotinic acetylcholine receptor structure and function and response to nicotine. Int Rev Neurobiol. 2015;124:3–19. https://doi.org/10.1016/bs.irn.2015.07.001.
68. Klink R, de Kerchove d'Exaerde A, Zoli M, Changeux JP. Molecular and physiological diversity of nicotinic acetylcholine receptors in the midbrain dopaminer-

gic nuclei. J Neurosci. 2001;21:1452–63. https://doi.org/10.1523/JNEUROSCI.21-05-01452.2001.
69. Jones IW, Wonnacott S. Precise localization of α7 nicotinic acetylcholine receptors on glutamatergic axon terminals in the rat ventral tegmental area. J Neurosci. 2004;24:11244–52. https://doi.org/10.1523/JNEUROSCI.3009-04.2004.
70. Quick MW, Lester RAJ. Desensitization of neuronal nicotinic receptors. J Neurobiol. 2002;53:457–78. https://doi.org/10.1002/neu.10109.
71. Alkondon M, Albuquerque EX. Initial characterization of the nicotinic acetylcholine receptors in rat hippocampal neurons. J Recept Res. 1991;11:1001–21. https://doi.org/10.3109/10799899109064693.
72. Alkondon M, Albuquerque EX. Nicotinic acetylcholine receptor α7 and α4β2 subtypes differentially control GABAergic input to CA1 neurons in rat hippocampus. J Neurophysiol. 2001;86:3043–55. https://doi.org/10.1152/jn.2001.86.6.3043.
73. Jensen AA, Frølund B, Liljefors T, Krogsgaard-Larsen P. Neuronal nicotinic acetylcholine receptors: structural revelations, target identifications, and therapeutic inspirations. J Med Chem. 2005;48:4705–45. https://doi.org/10.1021/jm040219e.
74. Schilström, B.; Fagerquist, M. V; Zhang, X.; Hertel, P.; Panagis, G.; Nomikos, G.G.; Svensson, T.H. Putative role of presynaptic alpha7* nicotinic receptors in nicotine stimulated increases of extracellular levels of glutamate and aspartate in the ventral tegmental area. Synapse 2000, 38, 375–383, doi:https://doi.org/10.1002/1098-2396(20001215)38:4<375::AID-SYN2>3.0.CO;2-Y.
75. Marchi M, Risso F, Viola C, Cavazzani P, Raiteri M. Direct evidence that release-stimulating alpha7* nicotinic cholinergic receptors are localized on human and rat brain glutamatergic axon terminals. J Neurochem. 2002;80:1071–8. https://doi.org/10.1046/j.0022-3042.2002.00805.x.
76. Pidoplichko VI, Noguchi J, Areola OO, Liang Y, Peterson J, Zhang T, Dani JA. Nicotinic cholinergic synaptic mechanisms in the ventral tegmental area contribute to nicotine addiction. Learn Mem. 2004;11:60–9. https://doi.org/10.1101/lm.70004.
77. Ikemoto S, Murphy JM, McBride WJ. Self-infusion of GABA(A) antagonists directly into the ventral tegmental area and adjacent regions. Behav Neurosci. 1997;111:369–80. https://doi.org/10.1037/0735-7044.111.2.369.
78. David V, Durkin TP, Cazala P. Self-administration of the GABAA antagonist bicuculline into the ventral tegmental area in mice: dependence on D2 dopaminergic mechanisms. Psychopharmacology. 1997;130:85–90. https://doi.org/10.1007/s002130050214.
79. Saal D, Dong Y, Bonci A, Malenka RC. Drugs of abuse and stress trigger a common synaptic adaptation in dopamine neurons. Neuron. 2003;37:577–82. https://doi.org/10.1016/s0896-6273(03)00021-7.
80. Ostroumov A, Dani JA. Convergent neuronal plasticity and metaplasticity mechanisms of stress, nicotine, and alcohol. Annu Rev Pharmacol Toxicol. 2018;58:547–66. https://doi.org/10.1146/annurev-pharmtox-010617-052735.
81. Mao D, Gallagher K, McGehee DS. Nicotine potentiation of excitatory inputs to ventral tegmental area dopamine neurons. J Neurosci. 2011;31:6710–20. https://doi.org/10.1523/JNEUROSCI.5671-10.2011.
82. Mansvelder HD, Keath JR, McGehee DS. Synaptic mechanisms underlie nicotine-induced excitability of brain reward areas. Neuron. 2002;33:905–19. https://doi.org/10.1016/S0896-6273(02)00625-6.
83. Brown RW, Kolb B. Nicotine sensitization increases dendritic length and spine density in the nucleus accumbens and cingulate cortex. Brain Res. 2001;899:94–100. https://doi.org/10.1016/S0006-8993(01)02201-6.
84. McDonald CG, Eppolito AK, Brielmaier JM, Smith LN, Bergstrom HC, Lawhead MR, Smith RF. Evidence for elevated nicotine-induced structural plasticity in nucleus accumbens of adolescent rats. Brain Res. 2007;1151:211–8. https://doi.org/10.1016/j.brainres.2007.03.019.
85. Livingstone PD, Srinivasan J, Kew JNC, Dawson LA, Gotti C, Moretti M, Shoaib M, Wonnacott S. α7 and non-α7 nicotinic acetylcholine receptors modulate dopamine release in vitro and in vivo in the rat prefrontal cortex. Eur J Neurosci. 2009;29:539–50. https://doi.org/10.1111/j.1460-9568.2009.06613.x.
86. Otani S, Blond O, Desce J-M, Crépel F. Dopamine facilitates long-term depression of glutamatergic transmission in rat prefrontal cortex. Neuroscience. 1998;85:669–76. https://doi.org/10.1016/S0306-4522(97)00677-5.
87. Law-Tho D, Desce JM, Crepel F. Dopamine favours the emergence of long-term depression versus long-term potentiation in slices of rat prefrontal cortex. Neurosci Lett. 1995;188:125–8. https://doi.org/10.1016/0304-3940(95)11414-R.
88. Gurden H, Tassin J-P, Jay TM. Integrity of the mesocortical dopaminergic system is necessary for complete expression of in vivo hippocampal–prefrontal cortex long-term potentiation. Neuroscience. 1999;94:1019–27. https://doi.org/10.1016/S0306-4522(99)00395-4.
89. Gurden H, Takita M, Jay TM. Essential role of D1 but not D2 receptors in the NMDA receptor-dependent long-term potentiation at hippocampal-prefrontal cortex synapses in vivo. J Neurosci. 2000;20:RC106. https://doi.org/10.1523/JNEUROSCI.20-22-j0003.2000.
90. Couey JJ, Meredith RM, Spijker S, Poorthuis RB, Smit AB, Brussaard AB, Mansvelder HD. Distributed network actions by nicotine increase the threshold for spike-timing-dependent plasticity in prefrontal cortex. Neuron. 2007;54:73–87. https://doi.org/10.1016/j.neuron.2007.03.006.
91. Bi GQ, Poo MM. Synaptic modifications in cultured hippocampal neurons: dependence on spike

timing, synaptic strength, and postsynaptic cell type. J Neurosci. 1998;18:10464–72. https://doi.org/10.1523/JNEUROSCI.18-24-10464.1998.
92. Markram H, Lübke J, Frotscher M, Sakmann B. Regulation of synaptic efficacy by coincidence of postsynaptic APs and EPSPs. Science. 1997;275:213–5. https://doi.org/10.1126/science.275.5297.213.
93. Epping-Jordan MP, Watkins SS, Koob GF, Markou A. Dramatic decreases in brain reward function during nicotine withdrawal. Nature. 1998;393:76–9. https://doi.org/10.1038/30001.
94. Hughes JR, Hatsukami D. Signs and symptoms of tobacco withdrawal. Arch Gen Psychiatry. 1986;43:289–94. https://doi.org/10.1001/archpsyc.1986.01800030107013.
95. Hughes JR. Effects of abstinence from tobacco: valid symptoms and time course. Nicotine Tob Res. 2007;9:315–27. https://doi.org/10.1080/14622200701188919.
96. Shiffman S. Reflections on smoking relapse research. Drug Alcohol Rev. 2006;25:15–20. https://doi.org/10.1080/09595230500459479.
97. Gilbert DG, McClernon FJ, Rabinovich NE, Plath LC, Masson CL, Anderson AE, Sly KF. Mood disturbance fails to resolve across 31 days of cigarette abstinence in women. J Consult Clin Psychol. 2002;70:142–52. https://doi.org/10.1037/0022-006x.70.1.142.
98. Gilbert DG, McClernon FJ, Rabinovich NE, Dibb WD, Plath LC, Hiyane S, Jensen RA, Meliska CJ, Estes SL, Gehlbach BA. EEG, physiology, and task-related mood fail to resolve across 31 days of smoking abstinence: relations to depressive traits, nicotine exposure, and dependence. Exp Clin Psychopharmacol. 1999;7:427–43. https://doi.org/10.1037/1064-1297.7.4.427.
99. Piasecki TM, Jorenby DE, Smith SS, Fiore MC, Baker TB. Smoking withdrawal dynamics: I. Abstinence distress in lapsers and abstainers. J Abnorm Psychol. 2003;112:3–13.
100. Piasecki TM, Jorenby DE, Smith SS, Fiore MC, Baker TB. Smoking withdrawal dynamics: II. Improved tests of withdrawal-relapse relations. J Abnorm Psychol. 2003;112:14–27.
101. Piasecki TM, Jorenby DE, Smith SS, Fiore MC, Baker TB. Smoking withdrawal dynamics: III. Correlates of withdrawal heterogeneity. Exp Clin Psychopharmacol. 2003;11:276–85. https://doi.org/10.1037/1064-1297.11.4.276.
102. West RJ, Hajek P, Belcher M. Severity of withdrawal symptoms as a predictor of outcome of an attempt to quit smoking. Psychol Med. 1989;19:981–5. https://doi.org/10.1017/s0033291700005705.
103. al' Absi M, Hatsukami D, Davis GL, Wittmers LE. Prospective examination of effects of smoking abstinence on cortisol and withdrawal symptoms as predictors of early smoking relapse. Drug Alcohol Depend. 2004;73:267–78. https://doi.org/10.1016/j.drugalcdep.2003.10.014.
104. Kenny PJ, Markou A. Neurobiology of the nicotine withdrawal syndrome. Pharmacol Biochem Behav. 2001;70:531–49. https://doi.org/10.1016/s0091-3057(01)00651-7.
105. Salas R, Pieri F, De Biasi M. Decreased signs of nicotine withdrawal in mice null for the beta4 nicotinic acetylcholine receptor subunit. J Neurosci. 2004;24:10035–9. https://doi.org/10.1523/JNEUROSCI.1939-04.2004.
106. Stoker AK, Olivier B, Markou A. Role of α7- and β4-containing nicotinic acetylcholine receptors in the affective and somatic aspects of nicotine withdrawal: studies in knockout mice. Behav Genet. 2012;42:423–36. https://doi.org/10.1007/s10519-011-9511-0.
107. Jackson KJ, Sanjakdar SS, Muldoon PP, McIntosh JM, Damaj MI. The α3β4* nicotinic acetylcholine receptor subtype mediates nicotine reward and physical nicotine withdrawal signs independently of the α5 subunit in the mouse. Neuropharmacology. 2013;70:228–35. https://doi.org/10.1016/j.neuropharm.2013.01.017.
108. Jackson KJ, Martin BR, Changeux JP, Damaj MI. Differential role of nicotinic acetylcholine receptor subunits in physical and affective nicotine withdrawal signs. J Pharmacol Exp Ther. 2008;325:302–12. https://doi.org/10.1124/jpet.107.132977.
109. Salas R, Sturm R, Boulter J, De Biasi M. Nicotinic receptors in the habenulo-interpeduncular system are necessary for nicotine withdrawal in mice. J Neurosci. 2009;29:3014–8. https://doi.org/10.1523/JNEUROSCI.4934-08.2009.
110. Lotfipour S, Byun JS, Leach P, Fowler CD, Murphy NP, Kenny PJ, Gould TJ, Boulter J. Targeted deletion of the mouse α2 nicotinic acetylcholine receptor subunit gene (Chrna2) potentiates nicotine-modulated behaviors. J Neurosci. 2013;33:7728–41. https://doi.org/10.1523/JNEUROSCI.4731-12.2013.
111. McLaughlin I, Dani JA, De Biasi M. Nicotine withdrawal. Curr Top Behav Neurosci. 2015;24:99–123. https://doi.org/10.1007/978-3-319-13482-6_4.
112. De Biasi M, Salas R. Influence of neuronal nicotinic receptors over nicotine addiction and withdrawal. Exp Biol Med (Maywood). 2008;233:917–29. https://doi.org/10.3181/0712-MR-355.
113. Jackson KJ, McIntosh JM, Brunzell DH, Sanjakdar SS, Damaj MI. The role of alpha6-containing nicotinic acetylcholine receptors in nicotine reward and withdrawal. J Pharmacol Exp Ther. 2009;331:547–54. https://doi.org/10.1124/jpet.109.155457.
114. Pang X, Liu L, Ngolab J, Zhao-Shea R, McIntosh JM, Gardner PD, Tapper AR. Habenula cholinergic neurons regulate anxiety during nicotine withdrawal via nicotinic acetylcholine receptors. Neuropharmacology. 2016;107:294–304. https://doi.org/10.1016/j.neuropharm.2016.03.039.
115. McLaughlin I, Dani JA, De Biasi M. The medial habenula and interpeduncular nucleus circuitry is

critical in addiction, anxiety, and mood regulation. J Neurochem. 2017;142(Suppl):130–43. https://doi.org/10.1111/jnc.14008.
116. Lecca S, Meye FJ, Mameli M. The lateral habenula in addiction and depression: an anatomical, synaptic and behavioral overview. Eur J Neurosci. 2014;39:1170–8. https://doi.org/10.1111/ejn.12480.
117. Meye FJ, Trusel M, Soiza-Reilly M, Mameli M. Neural circuit adaptations during drug withdrawal—spotlight on the lateral habenula. Pharmacol Biochem Behav. 2017;162:87–93. https://doi.org/10.1016/j.pbb.2017.08.007.
118. Winter C, Vollmayr B, Djodari-Irani A, Klein J, Sartorius A. Pharmacological inhibition of the lateral habenula improves depressive-like behavior in an animal model of treatment resistant depression. Behav Brain Res. 2011;216:463–5. https://doi.org/10.1016/j.bbr.2010.07.034.
119. Ikemoto S. Brain reward circuitry beyond the mesolimbic dopamine system: a neurobiological theory. Neurosci Biobehav Rev. 2010;35:129–50. https://doi.org/10.1016/j.neubiorev.2010.02.001.
120. Dao DQ, Perez EE, Teng Y, Dani JA, De Biasi M. Nicotine enhances excitability of medial habenular neurons via facilitation of neurokinin signaling. J Neurosci. 2014;34:4273–84. https://doi.org/10.1523/JNEUROSCI.2736-13.2014.
121. Hikosaka O. The habenula: from stress evasion to value-based decision-making. Nat Rev Neurosci. 2010;11:503–13. https://doi.org/10.1038/nrn2866.
122. Ren J, Qin C, Hu F, Tan J, Qiu L, Zhao S, Feng G, Luo M. Habenula "cholinergic" neurons co-release glutamate and acetylcholine and activate postsynaptic neurons via distinct transmission modes. Neuron. 2011;69:445–52. https://doi.org/10.1016/j.neuron.2010.12.038.
123. Marks MJ, Pauly JR, Gross SD, Deneris ES, Hermans-Borgmeyer I, Heinemann SF, Collins AC. Nicotine binding and nicotinic receptor subunit RNA after chronic nicotine treatment. J Neurosci. 1992;12:2765–84. https://doi.org/10.1523/JNEUROSCI.12-07-02765.1992.
124. Grady SR, Moretti M, Zoli M, Marks MJ, Zanardi A, Pucci L, Clementi F, Gotti C. Rodent habenulo-interpeduncular pathway expresses a large variety of uncommon nAChR subtypes, but only the alpha3beta4* and alpha3beta3beta4* subtypes mediate acetylcholine release. J Neurosci. 2009;29:2272–82. https://doi.org/10.1523/JNEUROSCI.5121-08.2009.
125. Frahm S, Antolin-Fontes B, Görlich A, Zander J-F, Ahnert-Hilger G, Ibañez-Tallon I. An essential role of acetylcholine-glutamate synergy at habenular synapses in nicotine dependence. elife. 2015;4:e11396. https://doi.org/10.7554/eLife.11396.
126. Dani JA, De Biasi M. Mesolimbic dopamine and habenulo-interpeduncular pathways in nicotine withdrawal. Cold Spring Harb Perspect Med. 2013;3:a012138. https://doi.org/10.1101/cshperspect.a012138.
127. Amos CI, Wu X, Broderick P, Gorlov IP, Gu J, Eisen T, Dong Q, Zhang Q, Gu X, Vijayakrishnan J, et al. Genome-wide association scan of tag SNPs identifies a susceptibility locus for lung cancer at 15q25.1. Nat Genet. 2008;40:616–22. https://doi.org/10.1038/ng.109.
128. Berrettini W, Yuan X, Tozzi F, Song K, Francks C, Chilcoat H, Waterworth D, Muglia P, Mooser V. Alpha-5/alpha-3 nicotinic receptor subunit alleles increase risk for heavy smoking. Mol Psychiatry. 2008;13:368–73. https://doi.org/10.1038/sj.mp.4002154.
129. Thorgeirsson TE, Geller F, Sulem P, Rafnar T, Wiste A, Magnusson KP, Manolescu A, Thorleifsson G, Stefansson H, Ingason A, et al. A variant associated with nicotine dependence, lung cancer and peripheral arterial disease. Nature. 2008;452:638–42. https://doi.org/10.1038/nature06846.
130. Bühler K-M, Giné E, Echeverry-Alzate V, Calleja-Conde J, de Fonseca FR, López-Moreno JA. Common single nucleotide variants underlying drug addiction: more than a decade of research. Addict Biol. 2015;20:845–71. https://doi.org/10.1111/adb.12204.
131. George O, Ghozland S, Azar MR, Cottone P, Zorrilla EP, Parsons LH, O'Dell LE, Richardson HN, Koob GF. CRF-CRF1 system activation mediates withdrawal-induced increases in nicotine self-administration in nicotine-dependent rats. Proc Natl Acad Sci USA. 2007;104:17198–203. https://doi.org/10.1073/pnas.0707585104.
132. Rose JE, Behm FM, Levin ED. Role of nicotine dose and sensory cues in the regulation of smoke intake. Pharmacol Biochem Behav. 1993;44:891–900. https://doi.org/10.1016/0091-3057(93)90021-k.
133. Rose JE, Behm FM, Westman EC, Johnson M. Dissociating nicotine and nonnicotine components of cigarette smoking. Pharmacol Biochem Behav. 2000;67:71–81. https://doi.org/10.1016/s0091-3057(00)00301-4.
134. Perry CJ, Zbukvic I, Kim JH, Lawrence AJ. Role of cues and contexts on drug-seeking behaviour. Br J Pharmacol. 2014;171:4636–72. https://doi.org/10.1111/bph.12735.
135. Fuchs RA, Lasseter HC, Ramirez DR, Xie X. Relapse to drug seeking following prolonged abstinence: the role of environmental stimuli. Drug Discov Today Dis Model. 2008;5:251–8. https://doi.org/10.1016/j.ddmod.2009.03.001.
136. Fu Y, Matta SG, James TJ, Sharp BM. Nicotine-induced norepinephrine release in the rat amygdala and hippocampus is mediated through brainstem nicotinic cholinergic receptors. J Pharmacol Exp Ther. 1998;284:1188–96.
137. Liang KC, McGaugh JL, Yao HY. Involvement of amygdala pathways in the influence of post-training intra-amygdala norepinephrine and peripheral epinephrine on memory storage. Brain Res. 1990;508:225–33. https://doi.org/10.1016/0006-8993(90)90400-6.

138. Bremner JD, Krystal JH, Southwick SM, Charney DS. Noradrenergic mechanisms in stress and anxiety: I. Preclinical studies. Synapse. 1996;23:28–38. https://doi.org/10.1002/(SICI)1098-2396(199605)23:1<28::AID-SYN4>3.0.CO;2-J.
139. Carliner H, Brown QL, Sarvet AL, Hasin DS. Cannabis use, attitudes, and legal status in the U.S.: a review. Prev Med (Baltim). 2017, 104:13–23. https://doi.org/10.1016/j.ypmed.2017.07.008.
140. Ng Cheong Ton JM, Gerhardt GA, Friedemann M, Etgen AM, Rose GM, Sharpless NS, Gardner EL. The effects of delta 9-tetrahydrocannabinol on potassium-evoked release of dopamine in the rat caudate nucleus: an in vivo electrochemical and in vivo microdialysis study. Brain Res. 1988;451:59–68. https://doi.org/10.1016/0006-8993(88)90749-4.
141. Stokes PRA, Egerton A, Watson B, Reid A, Breen G, Lingford-Hughes A, Nutt DJ, Mehta MA. Significant decreases in frontal and temporal [11C]-raclopride binding after THC challenge. NeuroImage. 2010;52:1521–7. https://doi.org/10.1016/j.neuroimage.2010.04.274.
142. Bossong MG, Mehta MA, van Berckel BNM, Howes OD, Kahn RS, Stokes PRA. Further human evidence for striatal dopamine release induced by administration of Δ9-tetrahydrocannabinol (THC): selectivity to limbic striatum. Psychopharmacology. 2015;232:2723–9. https://doi.org/10.1007/s00213-015-3915-0.
143. Bloomfield MAP, Ashok AH, Volkow ND, Howes OD. The effects of Δ(9)-tetrahydrocannabinol on the dopamine system. Nature. 2016;539:369–77. https://doi.org/10.1038/nature20153.
144. Di Marzo V, De Petrocellis L. Plant, synthetic, and endogenous cannabinoids in medicine. Annu Rev Med. 2006;57:553–74. https://doi.org/10.1146/annurev.med.57.011205.135648.
145. Matsuda LA, Lolait SJ, Brownstein MJ, Young AC, Bonner TI. Structure of a cannabinoid receptor and functional expression of the cloned cDNA. Nature. 1990;346:561–4. https://doi.org/10.1038/346561a0.
146. Munro S, Thomas KL, Abu-Shaar M. Molecular characterization of a peripheral receptor for cannabinoids. Nature. 1993;365:61–5. https://doi.org/10.1038/365061a0.
147. Herkenham M, Lynn AB, Little MD, Johnson MR, Melvin LS, de Costa BR, Rice KC. Cannabinoid receptor localization in brain. Proc Natl Acad Sci USA. 1990;87:1932–6. https://doi.org/10.1073/pnas.87.5.1932.
148. Van Sickle MD, Duncan M, Kingsley PJ, Mouihate A, Urbani P, Mackie K, Stella N, Makriyannis A, Piomelli D, Davison JS, et al. Identification and functional characterization of brainstem cannabinoid CB2 receptors. Science. 2005;310:329–32. https://doi.org/10.1126/science.1115740.
149. Núñez E, Benito C, Pazos MR, Barbachano A, Fajardo O, González S, Tolón RM, Romero J. Cannabinoid CB2 receptors are expressed by perivascular microglial cells in the human brain: an immunohistochemical study. Synapse. 2004;53:208–13. https://doi.org/10.1002/syn.20050.
150. Kreitzer AC. Neurotransmission: emerging roles of endocannabinoids. Curr Biol. 2005;15:R549–51. https://doi.org/10.1016/j.cub.2005.07.005.
151. Vaughan CW, Christie MJ. Retrograde signalling by endocannabinoids. Handb Exp Pharmacol. 2005:367–83. https://doi.org/10.1007/3-540-26573-2_12.
152. Howlett AC, Barth F, Bonner TI, Cabral G, Casellas P, Devane WA, Felder CC, Herkenham M, Mackie K, Martin BR, et al. International Union of Pharmacology. XXVII. Classification of cannabinoid receptors. Pharmacol Rev. 2002;54:161–202. https://doi.org/10.1124/pr.54.2.161.
153. Pertwee RG, Ross RA. Cannabinoid receptors and their ligands. Prostaglandins Leukot Essent Fat Acids. 2002;66:101–21. https://doi.org/10.1054/plef.2001.0341.
154. Szabo B, Schlicker E. Effects of cannabinoids on neurotransmission. Handb Exp Pharmacol. 2005:327–65. https://doi.org/10.1007/3-540-26573-2_11.
155. Scherma M, Muntoni A, Melis M, Fattore L, Fadda P, Fratta W, Pistis M. Interactions between the endocannabinoid and nicotinic cholinergic systems: preclinical evidence and therapeutic perspectives. Psychopharmacology. 2016;233:1765–77. https://doi.org/10.1007/S00213-015-4196-3.
156. Picciotto MR, Caldarone BJ, King SL, Zachariou V. Nicotinic receptors in the brain. Links between molecular biology and behavior. Neuropsychopharmacology. 2000;22:451–65. https://doi.org/10.1016/S0893-133X(99)00146-3.
157. Schlicker E, Kathmann M. Modulation of transmitter release via presynaptic cannabinoid receptors. Trends Pharmacol Sci. 2001;22:565–72. https://doi.org/10.1016/s0165-6147(00)01805-8.
158. Le Foll B, Goldberg SR. Cannabinoid CB1 receptor antagonists as promising new medications for drug dependence. J Pharmacol Exp Ther. 2005;312:875–83. https://doi.org/10.1124/jpet.104.077974.
159. Oz M, Ravindran A, Diaz-Ruiz O, Zhang L, Morales M. The endogenous cannabinoid anandamide inhibits alpha7 nicotinic acetylcholine receptor-mediated responses in Xenopus oocytes. J Pharmacol Exp Ther. 2003;306:1003–10. https://doi.org/10.1124/jpet.103.049981.
160. Oz M, Zhang L, Ravindran A, Morales M, Lupica CR. Differential effects of endogenous and synthetic cannabinoids on alpha7-nicotinic acetylcholine receptor-mediated responses in Xenopus Oocytes. J Pharmacol Exp Ther. 2004;310:1152–60. https://doi.org/10.1124/jpet.104.067751.
161. Lagalwar S, Bordayo EZ, Hoffmann KL, Fawcett JR, Frey WH. 2nd Anandamides inhibit binding to the muscarinic acetylcholine receptor. J Mol Neurosci. 1999;13:55–61. https://doi.org/10.1385/JMN:13:1-2:55.

162. Spivak CE, Lupica CR, Oz M. The endocannabinoid anandamide inhibits the function of α4β2 nicotinic acetylcholine receptors. Mol Pharmacol. 2007;72:1024–32. https://doi.org/10.1124/mol.107.036939.
163. Oz M. Receptor-independent effects of endocannabinoids on ion channels. Curr Pharm Des. 2006;12:227–39. https://doi.org/10.2174/138161206775193073.
164. Oz M. Receptor-independent actions of cannabinoids on cell membranes: focus on endocannabinoids. Pharmacol Ther. 2006;111:114–44. https://doi.org/10.1016/j.pharmthera.2005.09.009.
165. Pertwee RG. The diverse CB1 and CB2 receptor pharmacology of three plant cannabinoids: delta9-tetrahydrocannabinol, cannabidiol and delta9-tetrahydrocannabivarin. Br J Pharmacol. 2008;153:199–215. https://doi.org/10.1038/sj.bjp.0707442.
166. Poddar MK, Dewey WL. Effects of cannabinoids on catecholamine uptake and release in hypothalamic and striatal synaptosomes. J Pharmacol Exp Ther. 1980;214:63–7.
167. Chen JP, Paredes W, Li J, Smith D, Lowinson J, Gardner EL. Delta 9-tetrahydrocannabinol produces naloxone-blockable enhancement of presynaptic basal dopamine efflux in nucleus accumbens of conscious, freely-moving rats as measured by intracerebral microdialysis. Psychopharmacology. 1990;102:156–62. https://doi.org/10.1007/BF02245916.
168. Pistis M, Ferraro L, Pira L, Flore G, Tanganelli S, Gessa GL, Devoto P. Delta(9)-tetrahydrocannabinol decreases extracellular GABA and increases extracellular glutamate and dopamine levels in the rat prefrontal cortex: an in vivo microdialysis study. Brain Res. 2002;948:155–8. https://doi.org/10.1016/s0006-8993(02)03055-x.
169. Jackson KJ, Marks MJ, Vann RE, Chen X, Gamage TF, Warner JA, Damaj MI. Role of alpha5 nicotinic acetylcholine receptors in pharmacological and behavioral effects of nicotine in mice. J Pharmacol Exp Ther. 2010;334:137–46. https://doi.org/10.1124/jpet.110.165738.
170. Howlett AC, Bidaut-Russell M, Devane WA, Melvin LS, Johnson MR, Herkenham M. The cannabinoid receptor: biochemical, anatomical and behavioral characterization. Trends Neurosci. 1990;13:420–3. https://doi.org/10.1016/0166-2236(90)90124-s.
171. Lichtman AH, Cook SA, Martin BR. Investigation of brain sites mediating cannabinoid-induced antinociception in rats: evidence supporting periaqueductal gray involvement. J Pharmacol Exp Ther. 1996;276:585–93.
172. Sañudo-Peña MC, Romero J, Seale GE, Fernandez-Ruiz JJ, Walker JM. Activational role of cannabinoids on movement. Eur J Pharmacol. 2000;391:269–74. https://doi.org/10.1016/s0014-2999(00)00044-3.
173. Justinova Z, Goldberg SR, Heishman SJ, Tanda G. Self-administration of cannabinoids by experimental animals and human marijuana smokers. Pharmacol Biochem Behav. 2005;81:285–99. https://doi.org/10.1016/j.pbb.2005.01.026.
174. Ahsan HM, de la Peña JBI, Botanas CJ, Kim HJ, Yu GY, Cheong JH. Conditioned place preference and self-administration induced by nicotine in adolescent and adult rats. Biomol Ther (Seoul). 2014;22:460–6. https://doi.org/10.4062/biomolther.2014.056.
175. Vallés AS, Barrantes FJ. Nanoscale subcompartmentalization of the dendritic spine compartment. Biomolecules. 2021;11 https://doi.org/10.3390/biom11111697.
176. Valjent E, Mitchell JM, Besson M-J, Caboche J, Maldonado R. Behavioural and biochemical evidence for interactions between Delta 9-tetrahydrocannabinol and nicotine. Br J Pharmacol. 2002;135:564–78. https://doi.org/10.1038/sj.bjp.0704479.
177. Viveros M-P, Marco EM, File SE. Nicotine and cannabinoids: parallels, contrasts and interactions. Neurosci Biobehav Rev. 2006;30:1161–81. https://doi.org/10.1016/j.neubiorev.2006.08.002.
178. Scherma M, Justinová Z, Zanettini C, Panlilio LV, Mascia P, Fadda P, Fratta W, Makriyannis A, Vadivel SK, Gamaleddin I, et al. The anandamide transport inhibitor AM404 reduces the rewarding effects of nicotine and nicotine-induced dopamine elevations in the nucleus accumbens shell in rats. Br J Pharmacol. 2012;165:2539–48. https://doi.org/10.1111/j.1476-5381.2011.01467.x.
179. Balerio GN, Aso E, Berrendero F, Murtra P, Maldonado R. Delta9-tetrahydrocannabinol decreases somatic and motivational manifestations of nicotine withdrawal in mice. Eur J Neurosci. 2004;20:2737–48. https://doi.org/10.1111/j.1460-9568.2004.03714.x.
180. Balerio GN, Aso E, Maldonado R. Role of the cannabinoid system in the effects induced by nicotine on anxiety-like behaviour in mice. Psychopharmacology. 2006;184:504–13. https://doi.org/10.1007/s00213-005-0251-9.
181. Acquas E, Pisanu A, Marrocu P, Goldberg SR, Di Chiara G. Δ9-tetrahydrocannabinol enhances cortical and hippocampal acetylcholine release in vivo: a microdialysis study. Eur J Pharmacol. 2001;419:155–61. https://doi.org/10.1016/S0014-2999(01)00967-0.
182. Pisanu A, Acquas E, Fenu S, Di Chiara G. Modulation of Δ9-THC-induced increase of cortical and hippocampal acetylcholine release by μ opioid and D1 dopamine receptors. Neuropharmacology. 2006;50:661–70. https://doi.org/10.1016/j.neuropharm.2005.11.023.
183. Tzavara ET, Wade M, Nomikos GG. Biphasic effects of cannabinoids on acetylcholine release in the hippocampus: site and mechanism of action. J Neurosci. 2003;23:9374–84. https://doi.org/10.1523/JNEUROSCI.23-28-09374.2003.
184. Haney M, Ward AS, Comer SD, Foltin RW, Fischman MW. Abstinence symptoms following

smoked marijuana in humans. Psychopharmacology. 1999;141:395–404. https://doi.org/10.1007/s002130050849.
185. Haney M, Ward AS, Comer SD, Foltin RW, Fischman MW. Abstinence symptoms following oral THC administration to humans. Psychopharmacology. 1999;141:385–94. https://doi.org/10.1007/s002130050848.
186. Budney AJ, Vandrey RG, Hughes JR, Thostenson JD, Bursac Z. Comparison of cannabis and tobacco withdrawal: severity and contribution to relapse. J Subst Abus Treat. 2008;35:362–8. https://doi.org/10.1016/j.jsat.2008.01.002.
187. Lichtman AH, Fisher J, Martin BR. Precipitated cannabinoid withdrawal is reversed by Delta(9)-tetrahydrocannabinol or clonidine. Pharmacol Biochem Behav. 2001;69:181–8. https://doi.org/10.1016/s0091-3057(01)00514-7.
188. Haney M, Hart CL, Vosburg SK, Nasser J, Bennett A, Zubaran C, Foltin RW. Marijuana withdrawal in humans: effects of oral THC or divalproex. Neuropsychopharmacology. 2004;29:158–70. https://doi.org/10.1038/sj.npp.1300310.
189. Balter RE, Cooper ZD, Haney M. Novel pharmacologic approaches to treating cannabis use disorder. Curr Addict Rep. 2014;1:137–43. https://doi.org/10.1007/s40429-014-0011-1.
190. Donvito G, Muldoon PP, Jackson KJ, Ahmad U, Zaveri NT, McIntosh JM, Chen X, Lichtman AH, Damaj MI. Neuronal nicotinic acetylcholine receptors mediate Δ(9) -THC dependence: mouse and human studies. Addict Biol. 2020;25:e12691. https://doi.org/10.1111/adb.12691.
191. Demontis D, Rajagopal VM, Thorgeirsson TE, Als TD, Grove J, Leppälä K, Gudbjartsson DF, Pallesen J, Hjorthøj C, Reginsson GW, et al. Genome-wide association study implicates CHRNA2 in cannabis use disorder. Nat Neurosci. 2019;22:1066–74. https://doi.org/10.1038/s41593-019-0416-1.
192. Mechoulam R, Hanuš L. Cannabidiol: an overview of some chemical and pharmacological aspects. Part I: chemical aspects. Chem Phys Lipids. 2002;121:35–43. https://doi.org/10.1016/S0009-3084(02)00144-5.
193. Izzo AA, Borrelli F, Capasso R, Di Marzo V, Mechoulam R. Non-psychotropic plant cannabinoids: new therapeutic opportunities from an ancient herb. Trends Pharmacol Sci. 2009;30:515–27. https://doi.org/10.1016/j.tips.2009.07.006.
194. Yang K-H, Galadari S, Isaev D, Petroianu G, Shippenberg TS, Oz M. The nonpsychoactive cannabinoid cannabidiol inhibits 5-hydroxytryptamine3A receptor-mediated currents in Xenopus laevis oocytes. J Pharmacol Exp Ther. 2010;333:547–54. https://doi.org/10.1124/jpet.109.162594.
195. Miller I, Scheffer IE, Gunning B, Sanchez-Carpintero R, Gil-Nagel A, Perry MS, Saneto RP, Checketts D, Dunayevich E, Knappertz V, et al. Dose-ranging effect of adjunctive oral cannabidiol vs placebo on convulsive seizure frequency in Dravet syndrome: a randomized clinical trial. JAMA Neurol. 2020;77:613–21. https://doi.org/10.1001/jamaneurol.2020.0073.
196. Devinsky O, Cross JH, Laux L, Marsh E, Miller I, Nabbout R, Scheffer IE, Thiele EA, Wright S. Trial of cannabidiol for drug-resistant seizures in the Dravet syndrome. N Engl J Med. 2017;376:2011–20. https://doi.org/10.1056/NEJMoa1611618.
197. Zhang H-XB, Heckman L, Niday Z, Jo S, Fujita A, Shim J, Pandey R, Al Jandal H, Jayakar S, Barrett LB, et al. Cannabidiol activates neuronal Kv7 channels. elife. 2022;11:e73246. https://doi.org/10.7554/eLife.73246.
198. Mahgoub M, Keun-Hang SY, Sydorenko V, Ashoor A, Kabbani N, Al Kury L, Sadek B, Howarth CF, Isaev D, Galadari S, et al. Effects of cannabidiol on the function of α7-nicotinic acetylcholine receptors. Eur J Pharmacol. 2013;720:310–9. https://doi.org/10.1016/j.ejphar.2013.10.011.
199. Rabin RA, George TP. A review of co-morbid tobacco and cannabis use disorders: possible mechanisms to explain high rates of co-use. Am J Addict. 2015;24:105–16. https://doi.org/10.1111/ajad.12186.
200. Smart RG, Ogborne AC. Drug use and drinking among students in 36 countries. Addict Behav. 2000;25:455–60. https://doi.org/10.1016/S0306-4603(99)00013-1.
201. Panlilio, L. V; Zanettini, C.; Barnes, C.; Solinas, M.; Goldberg, S.R. Prior exposure to THC increases the addictive effects of nicotine in rats. Neuropsychopharmacology 2013, 38, 1198–1208, doi:https://doi.org/10.1038/npp.2013.16.
202. Kandel D, Kandel E. The Gateway Hypothesis of substance abuse: developmental, biological and societal perspectives. Acta Paediatr. 2015;104:130–7. https://doi.org/10.1111/apa.12851.

Linking the Neurobiological Basis and Behavioral Features of Craving

25

Augusto Pascual Ítalo Gargiulo,
Antonella Ariela Trovato, Ana Paula Colombini,
Mercedes María Lucrecia Gargiulo,
and Ángel José Martín Gargiulo

Introduction

The term craving has been used since the late 1980s by both ordinary people and scientists. Etymologically, craving derives from Carfian, an old English word that means to beg, implore, demand, or request. The concept changed over the last 30 years, and scientists tried to understand its biology and link it to all patterns of addictive behavior [1]. A Consensus that took place in 1991, sponsored by the Addiction Research Center (ARC) of the National Institute on Drug Abuse (NIDA), defined craving as a subjective state in humans that is associated with drug dependence [1]. Furthermore, many experts in this consensus agreed that this component is a significant factor that helps establish the prognosis of addiction and relapse. This meeting came about because everyone at the time, scientists or not, was using this term without a rigorous definition. The objective was to unify the concept to use a common language and be able to measure it. Moreover, in a later step, test the hypothesis of the craving-relapse phenomenon. However, this definition was far from precise. It is a typical issue in mental health.

To date, the research community has a core concept agreed upon by all, drive and search behavior [2]. However, different researchers use craving in many ways, and there seems to be disagreement among experts from several disciplines about its definition and usefulness. Some focus only on the consumption impulse and explain that it is craving only when the desire is intense [3]. They would agree that the subjective state is the most critical component of craving. Others emphasize the phenomenon of worry/anticipation [4] or the problem of loss of self-control [5]. There is an ongoing trend of looking at craving as a seeking behavior with many con-

A. P. Í. Gargiulo (✉)
Researcher in Laboratorio de Neurociencias y Psicología Experimental, Fundación Corporación Tecnológica Latinoamericana (FUCOTEL. CONICET), Universidad Católica Argentina (UCA), Universidad Nacional de Cuyo (UNCuyo), Buenos Aires, Argentina

CISMA (Centro Integral de Salud Mental Argentino), Buenos Aires, Argentina

A. A. Trovato · M. M. L. Gargiulo
CISMA (Centro Integral de Salud Mental Argentino), Buenos Aires, Argentina

A. P. Colombini
CISMA (Centro Integral de Salud Mental Argentino), Buenos Aires, Argentina

Hospital Bernardino Rivadavia, Buenos Aires, Argentina

Á. J. M. Gargiulo
CISMA (Centro Integral de Salud Mental Argentino), Buenos Aires, Argentina

Facultad de Medicina, IBCN (Instituto de Biología Celular y Neurociencias)-CONICET, UBA (Universidad de Buenos Aires), Buenos Aires, Argentina

P. Á. Gargiulo, H. L. Mesones-Arroyo (eds.), *Psychiatry and Neuroscience Update – Vol. V*,
https://doi.org/10.1007/978-3-031-72219-6_25

scious and unconscious components. Its triggering depends on many variables and neural pathways [6].

What Is Craving?

"Use Drive" was central in analyzing addictive behavior from the first models and scientific studies. Jellinek began studying the etiology of alcoholism in the late 1940s, and one of the critical events he proposed in his models was craving [7, 8]. He argued that this was the central feature of alcoholism and could be used to explain the onset and maintenance of this diagnosis. Also, it explains relapse after a long period of abstinence [3]. A classic view of addiction observed avoiding withdrawal as the motivation to continue using drugs. It is clear that today when the withdrawal syndrome disappears in a few weeks, the craving is still present in people with problematic consumption [2].

Craving and the urge to consume stopped being the central concept of addiction models in the early 1970s. It happened due to two phenomena. The first was that loss of control became significant, and in Jellinek's laboratory settings, people with alcoholism could drink low doses without the need to drink excessively. The second was the emergence of behaviorism in clinical practice. In those years, this paradigm did not focus on mental processes [3]. Tiffany, in the 1990s, proposed a cognitive model that focuses on an automatic schema of action that interconnects various cognitive functions by associative learning that automatically and effortlessly executes the skills to pursue drug use. All these behaviors are stored in implicit memory [3]. Added to this, Tiffany and Carter, in 1998, proposed with substantial scientific evidence that craving is the origin of compulsive drug use. Many researchers remain attached to subjective mood. Drummond, in 2001, defines craving as a conscious experience of the desire to consume [9]. It is widely accepted that craving is a complex behavior that various stimuli can trigger, has a conscious and unconscious mechanism, and depends on contingencies [10]. It means that depending on whether or not the drug is reached, the craving will be reinforced or punished.

Paradigms

Behaviorism, neurobiology, and neural networks are the paradigms of our definition. The first is radical behaviorism taking into account the post-Skinnerian version. The behavioral worldview establishes a ground that promotes precise concepts and individualization of behaviors. These are essential to measure and predict. According to this paradigm, all actions a human being can perform are behaviors, including all mental processes, for example, overt behaviors, emotions, feelings, consciousness, thinking, salivation, and sweating. Furthermore, all of them are under the influence of classical and operant conditioning systems [11–13]. Associative learning and behavior followed by consequences are at the core of this theoretical approach. Language and cognitions are explained by "Relational Frame Theory" (RFT), a functional and behavioral approach to verbal events [14]. This theory is the post-Skinnerian version. It suggests that verbal language and thoughts occur in humans thanks to the fact that we are the only species to generate direct, inverse, and indirect relationships between stimuli or events: direct training, mutual linkage, and combinatorial linkage. We make equivalence stimulate [15, 16]. Even in chimpanzees trained in human language for years, it has not been achieved. Humans generate relationships between stimuli without being specifically learned or trained (relationships derived from stimuli). The generation of "relational frameworks" developed between stimuli is arbitrary, automatic, and mostly unconscious. If they are reinforced, they will be maintained over time. According to RFT, these frames of relationships or verbal behavior are to put stimuli or events in relation and act or react according to the resulting relationships. This way of relating is not primarily controlled by the nonarbitrary relationships between the related stimuli, but by other contextual cues. The stimuli that function as such cues are mainly combinations of sounds that we usually call words. However, additional contextual factors, such as gestures or even features of the nonsocial environment, may also play this role. To be more precise, the language functions as medium and long-term contingencies.

The second paradigm is neurobiology, from subcellular mechanisms to neural circuits. We consider the neurobiological influences on behavior, taking neuronal plasticity, long-term potentiation mechanisms, neurotransmitter-receptor dynamics, and limbic system circuits as the central axis [4, 17–20]. All these information provide the ability to predict how long behavioral changes take and which drugs could aggravate the craving when addictions present as dual disorders.

The third is Neural Networks, which explain how complex these circuits are and how all the information are used and analyzed in the mind, like intelligent software. Each neuron is a computational device capable of receiving thousands of synaptic stimuli (excitatory or inhibitory post-potentials-information). If these reach the threshold, said neuron fires an action potential. The connection between neurons is not just simple circuits that go from one nucleus to another. These connections form a network of networks that generate the ability to analyze millions of stimuli and information constantly and simultaneously [21]. There is currently much basic scientific research on neural networks, and little by little, they are beginning to be behavioral models of craving that analyze behavior as computational systems [22](Fig. 25.1).

A Possible Current Definition

Craving can be defined as brain programming to address intensely reinforced behaviors that promote the search for substance use or the perfor-

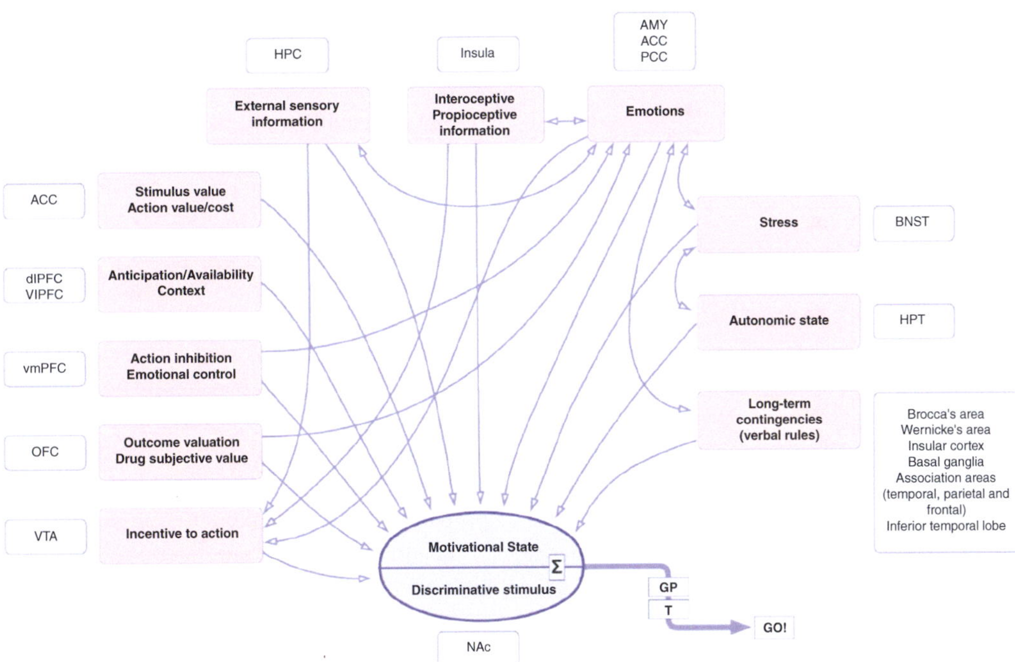

Fig. 25.1 This image shows how neural networks interconnect with each other. The behavior will depend on the result of the total sum of stimuli. Stimuli are mediated and analyzed through inhibitory and excitatory neuronal post-potentials. *NAc* nucleus accumbens, *VTA* ventral tegmental area, *OFC* orbito-frontal cortex, *vmPFC* ventro-medial prefrontal cortex, *dlPFC* dorso-lateral prefrontal cortex, *vlPFC* ventro-lateral prefrontal cortex, *ACC* anterior cingulate cortex, *PCC* posterior cingulate cortex, *HPC* hippocampus, *AMY* amygdala, *BNST* bed nucleus of stria terminalis, *HPT* hypothalamus

mance of a specific behavior (within an addictive behavior pattern). This brain programming is also behavior since it is sensitive to contingencies. Their frequency and intensity are modified depending on whether they are punished or reinforced. This behavior is dependent on contextual cues (environmental or mental). This programming will start depending on the total sum of pro or anti-craving stimuli registered and analyzed as computations [22]. These are thousands of pieces of information that are evaluated unconsciously and simultaneously. Craving, like all behavior, is learned, and this learning is unconscious [13].

This programming has four components:

1. Specific cognitive bias: language, thoughts, and words.
2. Autonomic response
3. Specific drive: impulse action.
4. Perception: awareness of autonomic and impulse response.

We will describe it later.

When Do People Have an Addiction?

People have an addiction when they cannot stop a pattern of behavior or substance use, despite harmful consequences and their best efforts to quit [23].

Traditionally, scientists have limited the term "addiction" to substances that promote physical dependence. However, that is changing. New insights suggest that, as far as the brain is concerned, a reward is a reward, regardless of whether it comes from a chemical or experience. So, where there is a reward, there is a risk of getting caught in a compulsion [24]. However, once people become addicted, the pleasure of the addictive behavior may decrease, but the urge to engage in the addictive behavior will remain and increase. At that point, the addictive behavior may be reinforced not by pleasure but by relief from intense and unpleasant urges. Some people say that when they engage in addictive behaviors, they feel "normal" again. In these cases, a behavior that may have started with positive reinforcement (that is, it gives pleasure) is maintained with negative reinforcement (that is, the anguish ceases to be unbearable).

Addictions are not conceptualized as a will problem since, if this were correct, we would all be perfect. We think of addictions as a particular sensitivity to the behavioral pattern at a biological level, an evident lack of ability to tolerate discomfort and meet goals within an environment that plays a fundamental role. It is mainly a contingency problem that makes an individual unable to postpone the reward [25].

The presence or absence of craving in an individual with a pattern of addiction could be helpful for diagnosis. However, there is no evidence that it can predict relapse or that it should be diminished for a successful treatment [26].

Withdrawal Syndrome and Craving

Commonly, the word abstinence is confused with withdrawal syndrome and craving. Abstinence is colloquially defined as not consuming a substance. The withdrawal syndrome can concomitantly have craving, but it is not this. Withdrawal syndrome is the sign-symptom derived from the abrupt decrease or cessation of the consumption of a substance in an individual who chronically consumes it [27]. This symptomatology occurs because of neuronal changes due to chronic consumption, primarily up/downregulation of different receptors. Therefore, if there is a decrease in the plasma levels of the substance and it is no longer in a steady state, the person begins feeling symptoms that are usually opposite to the effects of the drug. For example, alcohol withdrawal starts with anxiety, irritability, and tremors and could lead to severe cases of delirium tremens. Cocaine withdrawal is often manifested by hypersomnia and irritability. Caffeine withdrawal is also with hypersomnia. Cocaine withdrawal usually manifests with hypersomnia, hyperphagia, and irritability [28]. The abrupt cessation of opium consumption by dependent consumers generates a syndrome characterized by diarrhea, generalized pain, nausea, and insomnia [29]. Marijuana withdrawal syndrome usually has several components: anxiety, irritability, hotness, and decreased appetite, among others [30]. The craving in these circumstances is triggered by the negative affective state and would function as negative reinforcement [19].

The time it takes to start a withdrawal syndrome depends on the drug's half-life in question since steady-state plasma levels will be affected after five half-lives have elapsed without drug ingestion or with continued minor ingestion. For example, alcohol withdrawal starts in 6–24 h, marijuana withdrawal in 2–5 days, tobacco at 8 h, and cocaine at 8 h [27, 28, 30, 31].

Neurobiology

Molecular Aspects of Drug Consumption

Chronic drug consumption leads to several molecular and cellular modifications through altering gene and protein expression. This causes long-term alterations in neural circuits and, therefore, long-term alterations in behavior. One of the most studied transcription factors related to learning and memory is cyclic adenosine monophosphate response-element binding protein (CREB) (Fig. 25.2). CREB is activated through its phosphorylation by several kinases such as protein kinase A, CaM-kinases, or growth factor-associated kinases, therefore being at a point of convergence for different neurotransmitter-intracellular signaling pathways. In addition, CREB regulates gene expression binding to CRE sites situated in promoter regions of different genes [4, 32, 33].

Acute and chronic consumption of stimulant drugs and opiates can lead to phosphorylation and activation of CREB in brain structures related to reward, such as the VTA, amygdala, and frontal cortex [34–36], although other drugs (such as nicotine and alcohol) do not cause this effect. Stimulant drugs induce the activation of CREB in the NAc partly through D1 signaling. In animal models, the increased expression and activation

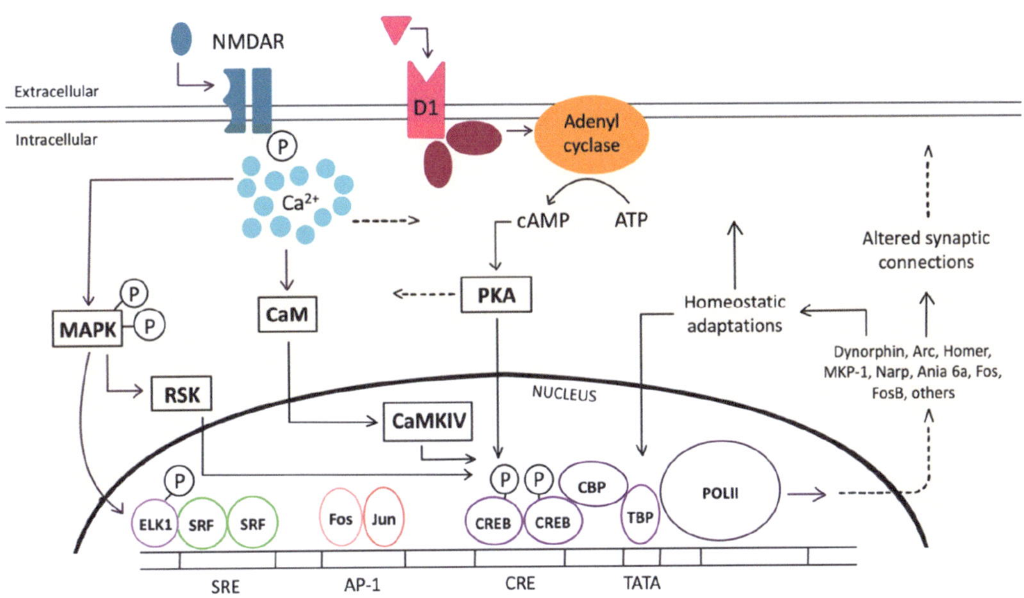

Fig. 25.2 *SRE* serum response element, *AP-1* activator protein-1 element, *CRE:* cyclic AMP (cAMP) response element, *CBP:* CREB binding protein, *CREB:* cAMP response element binding protein, *MAPK:* MAP kinase, *NMDAR:* NMDA receptor, *PKA:* protein kinase A, *TBP:* TATA binding protein. (Modified from Ref. [33]).

of CREB reduces the animal's sensitivity to the rewarding effects of drugs such as cocaine, while on the contrary, the decreased expression and activity of CREB causes the opposite [37]. One of the pathways by which CREB decreases reward sensitivity is inducing the expression of dynorphin peptides, decreasing DA release in VTA neurons, and dopaminergic activity in the NAc. With chronic drug consumption, the continuous activation of CREB and induction of dynorphin could explain processes such as tolerance and dependence, causing the negative emotional states seen in withdrawal, such as dysphoria [4, 33].

Other transcription factors also induced by addictive drugs are those of the Fos family. Together with Jun family proteins, Fos family members form heterodimers that unite with activator protein-1 (AP-1) sites present in the promoters of certain genes. Acute administration of addictive drugs increases the expression of Fos and Jun families' proteins in the NAc and DS [38]. The genes that encode Fos proteins have a rapid but short-lived induction following certain stimuli. With the acute administration of addictive drugs, there is a rapid but transient increase in the expression of these genes in the NAc. However, DFosB, a highly stable member of the Fos family, accumulates with repeated drug administration over more extended periods of time. Animals with increased DFosB activity have a higher sensitivity to the rewarding effects of addictive drugs. This way, the sustained induction of DFosB could act as a molecular switch to initiate and sustain prolonged aspects of drug addiction [4, 33, 38].

Together these data indicate that the alteration of cellular signaling pathways in the NAc neurons, because of drug consumption, leads to the regulation of gene expression through the activation of different transcription factors. Initially, drug exposure activates CREB and Fos-Jun proteins, and eventually, with repeated drug exposure, other transcription factors, such as DFosB, are induced. This way, these transcription factors can remodel chromatin in specific genes and therefore alter protein expression, leading to altered synaptic connections and structural modifications in the brain that are translated into the behavioral alterations related to addiction [4, 33].

Reward Circuit and Goal-Directed Behavior

The brain's reward system involves several structures; however, the trajectory with the lower thresholds and hence the most sensitive to reward is the mesolimbic dopaminergic system, which involves projections from ventral tegmental area (VTA) dopaminergic (DAp) neurons to the ventral striatum through the medial forebrain bundle. The projections of VTA DAp neurons onto the ventral striatum reach the nucleus accumbens (NAc), the major component of the ventral striatum (VS), the olfactory tubercle, and other limbic structures, including the hippocampus and basolateral amygdala [4, 33, 39]. All rewards, including addictive drugs, increase dopamine synapsis in the NAc from the VTA [33].

The ability of a stimulus to produce a reward is related to the type of dopamine (DA) release generated when presented. This is because low-affinity D1 receptors are activated in the presence of fast and intense release of DA and are crucial for the rewarding effect of a stimulus and for establishing conditioned responses. In contrast, low and tonic release of DA activates D2 receptors, which are not enough to produce a rewarding effect. This explains why the initial rewarding effects of most drugs of abuse rely on the induction of significant and rapid increases in the level of DA in the NAc [5, 19, 40].

Other areas related to the reward system include the prefrontal cortex (PFC) and the amygdala. The PFC is another important projection site from VTA DA neurons. It is associated with assigning value to rewards and the representation of goals. Limbic structures, including the hippocampus (HPC) and amygdala, also receive projections from the VTA DA neurons and establish reward-associated memories. The consolidation of action repertories directed towards obtaining a specific reward and habit forming depends on the dorsal striatum, which receives

DA projections from the substantia nigra in the midbrain [33].

Glutamate also plays an essential role in the reward systems of the brain. Both VTA and NAc receive numerous glutamatergic afferents. VTA receives glutamatergic afferents from different structures such as the amygdala, PFC, lateral habenula, lateral hypothalamus, ventral pallidum, and brainstem structures such as laterodorsal tegmental and pedunculopontine tegmental nucleus [41–43]. The glutamatergic afferents that reach VTA DA neurons have a modulating effect on DA cells and DA release, regulating the burst firing of DA and thus regulating the rewarding effects of a stimulus [44].

The NAc also receives extensive glutamatergic projections from the PFC, amygdala, hippocampus, insula, and thalamic nuclei [45]. Glutamate can regulate DA cells' reactivity in the NAc and DA release, further supporting its crucial role in the process of reward [17, 46]. Glutamatergic afferents from the hippocampus and amygdala to the NAc are of particular importance because they have a "gating" effect on PFC projections to the NAc, meaning they can regulate the responsiveness of the NAc to PFC afferents [47].

The NAc sends projections to the ventral pallidum (VP). VP then sends projections to the thalamus, particularly to the mediodorsal nucleus. This one has interconnections with the PFC. It regulates this activity. In this way, the "gating" effect of the hippocampus and amygdala can determine what information travels from the PFC to the NAc and VP to activate thalamocortical circuits. The importance of this "gating" effect by the hippocampus and the amygdala lies in the function of these two structures in modulating stimuli and response concerning context (hippocampus) and the affective state (amygdala). In a practical sense, the PFC provides the NAc with multiple motor plans, driving goal-oriented behavior. Moreover, the "gating" effect of the hippocampus and amygdala can, therefore, facilitate the responsiveness of the NAc neurons to the most effective plan based on context (HPC) and affect (amygdala) [47].

Reward and Learning

The role of reward in learning is associated with DA release. As previously mentioned, DA is released throughout the mesolimbic-dopaminergic system when presented with a reward. However, DA release happens at a different moment when a cue is repeatedly associated with a reward. Once a cue is associated with a reward, DA release no longer occurs when the reward itself is presented but rather when the cue is. If the reward is not presented following the cue, then DA release is paused, whereas if the reward presented is unexpected (greater or earlier than expected), there is a burst in DA release [48, 49].

On the other hand, if the reward is as expected, the tonic firing of DA continues without a burst in its release, suggesting that there is nothing new to learn about the environment since the reward presented was as expected. This finding suggests that the release of DA works as a way of learning about the environment and establishing learned associations. It also suggests that DA release can work as a signal to recruit a specific behavior in response to a stimulus. This way, the release of DA can initiate an adaptative behavior in response to a rewarding stimulus and establish an association between the event and the response, making it easier to reproduce the adaptative behavioral response in case the event reoccurs [46, 48, 49].

Negative Affect/Withdrawal-Induced Craving Circuit

During withdrawal, addicted individuals often experience a set of negative affect and experiences which can generate craving. This process is related to many neurobiological adaptations and changes that occur during this stage. These changes include a decreased DA signaling in response to rewards and greater sensitivity of the brain's stress systems, involving the extended amygdala [17].

Concerning DA system alterations, modifications occur in the mesolimbic dopamine system responsible for reward and the acute positive reinforcement of drugs. This system shows decreased DA reactivity during withdrawal, resulting in a lowered sensitivity for non-drug-related stimuli. It generates a decreased response to non-drug-related rewards producing anhedonia while also creating a motivational deficit for non-drug-related goals [4] (Fig. 25.3).

The extended amygdala is also involved in the negative emotional state seen in withdrawal. This anatomical structure processes the negative emotional experience that produces negative reinforcement mechanisms in addiction, meaning it processes the negative affect during withdrawal that drives the reinstatement of a drug-seeking behavior to escape this state [4].

The extended amygdala includes the central nucleus of the amygdala (CeA), the bed nucleus of the stria terminalis, and the shell of the NAc. It receives afferents from the basolateral amygdala (BLA) and HPC. Also, it sends efferents to the medial part of the ventral pallidum, the brainstem, and the lateral hypothalamus. During withdrawal, brain stress systems, including corticotrophin-releasing factor (CRF), norepinephrine, and dynorphin, are recruited in the extended amygdala and are associated with the negative emotional states of abstinence and withdrawal [4, 19].

In this stage, there is an increased activity of the hypothalamic-pituitary-adrenal axis and the brain stress/aversive system mediated by CRF, which is secreted by the bed nucleus of the stria terminalis (BNST). These systems are activated during acute withdrawal from chronic administration of drugs of abuse, resulting in elevated levels of adrenocorticotropic hormone (ACTH), corticosterone, and amygdala CRF. This could be

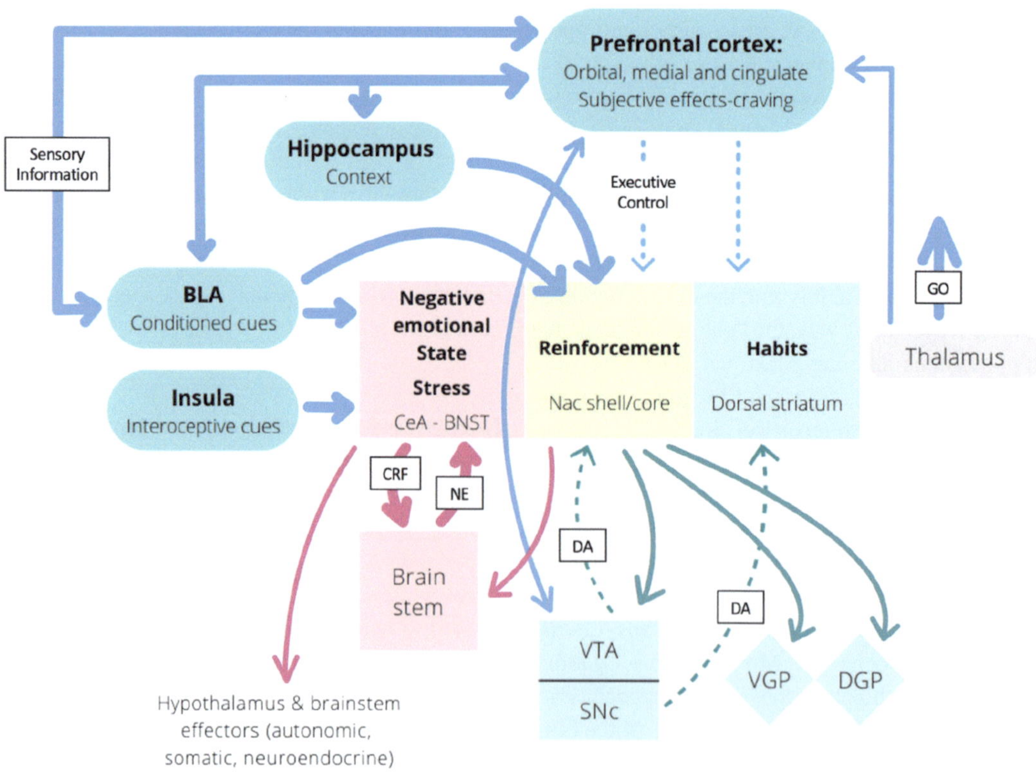

Fig. 25.3 *NE* norepinephrine, *CRF:* corticotrophin-releasing factor, *DA:* dopamine, *VTA:* ventral tegmental area, *SNc:* substantia nigra pars compacta, *VGP:* ventral globus pallidus, *DGP:* dorsal globus pallidus, *BNST:* bed nucleus of the stria terminalis, *CeA:* central nucleus of the amygdala. (Modified from Ref. [4])

responsible for the aversive or anxiety-like state seen during acute withdrawal and the association between stress and its inductive role in the reinstatement of drug-seeking behavior, as seen in animal models [4, 17].

Norepinephrine is also related to the process of withdrawal-induced craving. As previously mentioned, during this stage, there is a more significant activity in the BNST, with a greater secretion of CRF. This neurotransmitter can then modulate norepinephrine secretion in the brainstem. Norepinephrine, in return, modulates the activity of the CeA, which then induces further secretion of CRF, creating a loop [4].

Dynorphin is also involved in the alterations produced in reward systems since decreases in the release of DA in the NAc can be observed in response to increases in dynorphin activity in the NAc. The decrease of DA release in the NAc could also be associated with increases in CRF activity in the VTA, further integrating these circuits [19].

The activation of all these stress systems in the extended amygdala, including CRF, norepinephrine, and dynorphin, creates a significant emotional dysregulation leading to craving and the reinstatement of drug-seeking behavior [4].

Cue-Induced Craving Circuit

As addiction evolves, more stimuli become conditioned to the drug, becoming drug-related cues. Drug-related cues can induce craving in addicted individuals partly because they produce a fast and intense release of DA in the NAc, which is an essential driver of goal-oriented actions. This phenomenon redirects attention to the cue and creates the drive and motivation to seek the drug [17].

The significant reactivity to drug-related cues in addiction appears to be associated with an alteration in the balance of D1 receptors (D1R) and D2 receptors (D2R) signaling in the NAc, where the strengthening of D1R-expressing medium spiny neurons (D1R-MSNs) enhances cocaine reward and strengthening of D2R-expressing medium spiny neurons (D2R-MSNs) suppresses it. Animal studies have shown that cue-induced reinstatement can be intensified by activating D1R-MSNs or reducing the activity of D2R-MSNs [50]. In addition, a previous study showed that chronic cocaine uses in mice shifted the balance between D1R and D2R signaling, with D1R predominating over D2R [51]. This could increase the amount of DA burst firing and D1R signaling in response to cues, eliciting and increasing cue-induced craving leading to drug-seeking behavior while simultaneously diminishing tonic DA firing and D2R opposition [17].

The orbitofrontal cortex (OFC) and cingulate gyrus (CG) are also activated by drug-related cues, triggering craving [19]. Their involvement in cue-related craving can be associated with these structures' role in attributing salience and motivational value to a stimulus. Through glutamatergic efferences to the NAc, these regions can regulate DA release in the NAc, modulating the value of a given stimulus. In drug addiction, these circuits are altered, resulting in an increased burst firing of DA in response to reward and reward-predictive cues in the VS, possibly enhancing the incentive motivational value of drugs (and drug-related cues) for addicted individuals and increasing the impulse to engage in drug-seeking when presented with cues [17, 19, 52, 53]. The insula also activates during craving, probably serving as a source of interoceptive cues that are conditioned to the drug and induce the desire for drug-seeking [19].

The BLA and hippocampus also intervene. The BLA has glutamatergic projections to the NAc and PFC and processes learned associations with neutral stimuli and motivationally relevant events [46]. The hippocampus is crucial for processing contextual information and contextual cues, which can also trigger craving. This is also regulated by the hippocampus' glutamatergic projections to the NAc, through which ability it modulates DA release in this nucleus (Fig. 25.3).

The dorsal striatum (DS) is also related to these processes, given its relevance in stimulus-response habit learning. DA neurons from the SN project to the DS, leading reward signals to turn into habitual actions that, over time, are selected over others based on prior experience of the association of the reward with that particular action. The repetition of the reward-associated behavior can then lead to the development of habits [17]. In addition, drug-associated cues cause the increase of DA in the DS, which is correlated to self-reports of craving [19]. This way, the encounter with these cues can also lead to further consolidation in the dorsal striatum of such habit learning, thus enhancing the behavioral response of drug-seeking when presented with conditioned cues [17].

Drug-Induced Craving

In addicted individuals, a small dosage of the addictive drug can elicit craving. This can be explained by the drug's ability to cause persistent DA stimulation, driving the impulse to continue self-administration of the drug. Upon drug consumption, the sudden and intense increase of DA caused by the drug's effect stimulates D1R causing the activation of D1R-MSNs in the NAc, leading to further desire and attention towards taking the drug, often resulting in a binging episode [19].

The DS is also involved similarly to cue-induced craving mechanisms via its role in habit learning and the development of compulsive drug-taking. During the initial stages of addiction, the enhanced DA release in the NAc during drug-taking elicits the desire to continue consumption through positive reinforcement and establishes action-outcome learning. The information also flows from the NAc to the DS, then the VP, and finally reaches the frontal motor cortex, activating a motor response to further engage in drug-seeking behavior. However, after repeated drug use, the association between stimulus and response is established in the DS, creating a habit. This indicates a shift from goal-oriented behavior to habitual behavior that denotes a shift in control from the VS to the DS and is impulsed by the self-administration of the addicted drug, promoting the development of continuous drug-seeking habits and leading to the compulsive intake of the addicted drug [54].

Animal studies suggest that drug-induced reinstatement also involves a circuit consisting of glutamatergic projections from the PFC to the NAc, which are modulated by DA through D1 and D2 receptors in the frontal cortex. DA afferents from the VTA innervate interneurons and pyramidal neurons in the PFC, modulating their projections to the NAc. Pyramidal neurons in the PFC have biphasic states, with a "down state" where the membrane potential is hyperpolarized and an "up state" where it is depolarized. Cocaine-induced increase in DA promotes the up state, which increases excitatory transmission through the glutamatergic to the NAc, increasing its activity [19, 54] (Fig. 25.3).

Cognitive Components of Craving

Human behavior can be influenced by direct experiences, like every living being, and by verbal language that predicts potential consequences. Verbal information achieves the mind and evokes a conscious experience that emulates the contingencies. Stimuli in the human brain and mind have stimulus equivalence. This mental process has its root in the Relational Frame Theory. This feature is an evolutionary advantage because we can learn by talking. We do not need to cross by every trouble to learn how to behave against adversities.

Most classical psychotherapies intensely focus on what patients say. Commonly, radical behaviorists did not center on the potential role of the client's verbal behavior in influencing the establishment, maintenance, and modification of adult psychopathology. A contributing factor to this neglect has been the lack of a basic research database from which applied strategies and principles can be derived. Behavior analysts rarely published basic research on instructional control, stimulus equivalence, rule-governed behavior, verbal behavior, and related topics until 1980. However, recent efforts in the basic, applied, and conceptual dimensions of rule-governed behavior have produced findings relevant to patient verbal behavior and behavioral approaches to psychotherapy [55].

Words can have several functions. One is that thoughts (words and language) can play as a discriminative stimulus [56]. Verbal events can indicate to the person that the search behavior, consumption, or addictive behavior will be reinforcing. For example, a person at a roulette wheel who has just bet and lost says, "I just lost, and now I am sure I am going to win." This verbal stimulus predicts the reinforcing effect of a specific behavior. Another kind of function is the motivational stimulus. In this case, many stimuli reach the nucleus accumbens and influence to generate a specific motivational state. One of these motivational pieces of information is Values. Language constructs values, which in concrete and technical terms are contingencies of the long term ("the father/mother I want to be"; "the scientist I want to become"; e.g.). People can have experience of the future while thinking or talking. It is an indirect way of interacting with contingencies that have not occurred.

An additional type of role that language can play is establishment operation. In this case, the rule does not describe a relationship between behavior and contingency but instead potentially alters the value of reinforcing the addictive behavior. For example, what happens in Vegas stays in Vegas. These kinds of rule-driven behaviors are called Augmentals. It is essential to be in contact with these concepts since messing with the content of these thoughts only puts the person with addictive patterns on the defensive since they have the function of approaching search or consumption behaviors. They feel controlled by confronting these ideas, and control measures have paradoxical effects.

Language can serve to enter the context of "giving reasons" [57]. People give reasons for their behavior, and the context expects some reciprocity. It promotes that people do not make changes and regulate the response of those around them. "The craving I felt was unbearable"; "I used it because I felt very depressed." These behaviors can influence the environment so that they do not severely punish their conduct. In this situation, they have the function of operant behavior (relational frames are operant behaviors with unique characteristics). To avoid the suffering of not being able to consume, an individual can give himself reasons to continue consuming and thus prevent the loss of the possibility of a pleasant moment. Some examples could be "I am a better driver when I drink," "later, I am going to quit," "everyone drinks something," "I am an alcoholic, I am like that," and "I cannot take this craving anymore."

On the other hand, on many occasions, the consultants refer that when they begin to have a craving and thoughts of future negative contingencies of what will happen if they consume appear in mind, the craving increases. They enter into a pattern similar to compulsive thoughts (mental controls), and this craving becomes more and more intense [58]. Control measures of thoughts or mental events have paradoxical effects [59]. "The more I try to make something disappear from my mind, it will come back with more frequency and intensity." Rumination about consumption markedly increases cravings [60]. This point of cognitive control over the craving is a fundamental factor in maintaining addictions. It happens because verbal contingencies are given more importance than short-term contingencies (contingency management), and there is an overestimation of the influence of cognitive control on the person's global behavior. The evidence of Contingency Management as the best treatment option for every addictive pattern supports this premise.

Conclusion

It is highly relevant, in our opinion, to consider that problematic substance use depends on multiple variables, whether neurobiological, personal, contextual, or socio-cultural. Therefore, verbally asking someone not to consume or with classical psychotherapy or stop with drug therapy alone is a clear example of an invalidating environment. The scientific and clinical community is slowly getting closer to understanding the behavioral phenomena associated with addictions. Approaching this could generate more efficient proposals for treatments, prevention policies, and cultural awareness.

References

1. Pickens RW, Johanson CE. Craving: consensus of status and agenda for future research. Drug Alcohol Depend. 1992;30(2):127–31.
2. Alcaro A, Brennan A, Conversi D. The seeking drive and its fixation: a neuro-psycho-evolutionary approach to the pathology of addiction. Front Hum Neurosci. 2021;15(August):1–12.
3. Tiffany ST. A cognitive model of drug urges and drug-use behavior: role of automatic and nonautomatic processes. Psychol Rev. 1990;97(2):147–68.
4. Koob GF, Volkow ND. Neurocircuitry of addiction. Neuropsychopharmacology [Internet]. 2010;35(1):217–38. https://doi.org/10.1038/npp.2009.110.
5. Baler RD, Volkow ND. Drug addiction: the neurobiology of disrupted self-control. Trends Mol Med. 2006;12(12):559–66.
6. Lueptow LM, Shashkova EC, Miller MG, Evans CJ, Cahill CM. Insights into the neurobiology of craving in opioid use disorder. Curr Anesthesiol Rep. 2020;10(4):378–87.
7. Jellinek EM. Phases in the drinking history of alcoholics. Am J Psychol. 1949;62:606–7.
8. Jellinek EM. Alcoholism, a genus and some of its species. Can Med Assoc J. 1960;83:1341–5.
9. Drummond DC. Theories of drug craving, ancient and modern. Addiction. 2001;96(1):33–46.
10. Heyman GM. Do addicts have free will? An empirical approach to a vexing question. Addictive Behav Rep [Internet]. 2017;5:85–93. https://doi.org/10.1016/j.abrep.2017.02.001.
11. Skinner BF. Science and human behavior. Science and human behavior. Oxford: Macmillan; 1953. p. 461.
12. Skinner BF. About behaviorism. About behaviorism. Alfred A. Knopf: Oxford; 1974. p. 256.
13. Skinner BF. Contingencies of reinforcement: a theoretical analysis. New York: Appleton-Century-Crofts; 1969.
14. Barnes-Holmes Y, Hayes SC, Barnes-Holmes BR. Relational frame theory: a post-Skinnerian account of human language and cognition. 2001;28:101–38.
15. Sidman M, Tailby W. Conditional discrimination vs. matching to sample: an expansion of the testing paradigm. J Exp Anal Behav. 1982;37(1):5–22.
16. Hayes SC. Nonhumans have not yet shown stimulus equivalence. J Exp Anal Behav. 1989;51(3):385–92.
17. Volkow ND, Michaelides M, Baler R. The neuroscience of drug reward and addiction. Physiol Rev. 2019;99(4):2115–40.
18. Koob GF. The neurobiology of addiction: a neuroadaptational view relevant for diagnosis. Addiction. 2006;101(SUPPL. 1):23–30.
19. Koob GF, Volkow ND. Neurobiology of addiction: a neurocircuitry analysis. Lancet Psychiatry [Internet]. 2016;3(8):760–73. https://doi.org/10.1016/S2215-0366(16)00104-8.
20. Volkow ND, Koob GF, McLellan AT. Neurobiologic advances from the brain disease model of addiction. N Engl J Med. 2016;374(4):363–71.
21. Kriegeskorte N, Golan T. Neural network models and deep learning. Curr Biol. 2019;29:R231–6.
22. Grasman J, Grasman RPPP, van der Maas HLJ. The dynamics of addiction: craving versus self-control. PLoS One. 2016;11(6):1–11.
23. Linehan MM. DBT® skills training manual, 2nd edn. Guilford Press; 2015.
24. Holden C. 'Behavioral' addictions: do they exist? Science (1979). 2001;294(November).
25. Petry NM. Contingency management for substance abuse treatment: a guide to implementing this evidence-based practice. Routledge/Taylor & Francis Group; 2012.
26. Tiffany ST, Wray JM. The clinical significance of drug craving. Ann N Y Acad Sci. 2012;1248(1):1–17.
27. Wolf C, Curry A, Nacht J, Simpson SA. Management of alcohol withdrawal in the emergency department: current perspectives. Open Access Emerg Med. 2020;12:53–65.
28. LAGO JA, KOSTEN TR. Stimulant withdrawal. Addiction. 1994;89(11):1477–81.
29. Rahimi-Movaghar A, Gholami J, Amato L, Hoseinie L, Yousefi-Nooraie R, Amin-Esmaeili M. Pharmacological therapies for management of opium withdrawal. Cochr Database Syst Rev. 2018;2018(6).
30. Bonnet U, Preuss UW. The cannabis withdrawal syndrome: current insights. Subst Abuse Rehabil. 2017.
31. Mirijello A, D'Angelo C, Ferrulli A, Vassallo G, Antonelli M, Caputo F, et al. Identification and management of alcohol withdrawal syndrome. Drugs. 2015;75(4):353–65.
32. Impey S, McCorkle SR, Cha-Molstad H, Dwyer JM, Yochum GS, Boss JM, et al. Defining the CREB regulon: a genome-wide analysis of transcription factor regulatory regions. Cell. 2004;119(7):1041–54.
33. Hyman SE, Malenka RC, Nestler EJ. Neural mechanisms of addiction: the role of reward-related learning and memory. Annu Rev Neurosci. 2006;29:565–98.
34. Cole RL, Konradi C, Douglass J, Hyman SE. Neuronal adaptation to amphetamine and dopamine: molecular mechanisms of prodynorphin gene regulation in rat striatum. Neuron. 1995;14(4):813–23.
35. Shaw-Lutchman TZ, Impey S, Storm D, Nestler EJ. Regulation of CRE-mediated transcription in mouse brain by amphetamine. Synapse. 2003;48(1):10–7.
36. Olson VG, Zabetian CP, Bolanos CA, Edwards S, Barrot M, Eisch AJ, et al. Regulation of drug reward by cAMP response element-binding protein: evidence for two functionally distinct subregions of the ventral tegmental area. J Neurosci. 2005;25(23):5553–62.

37. McClung CA, Nestler EJ. Regulation of gene expression and cocaine reward by CREB and DeltaFosB. Nat Neurosci. 2003;6(11):1208–15.
38. McClung CA, Nestler EJ. Neuroplasticity mediated by altered gene expression. Neuropsychopharmacology. 2008;33(1):3–17.
39. Goto Y, Grace AA. The dopamine system and the pathophysiology of schizophrenia: a basic science perspective. Int Rev Neurobiol. 2007;78(6):41–68.
40. Grace AA, Floresco SB, Goto Y, Lodge DJ. Regulation of firing of dopaminergic neurons and control of goal-directed behaviors. Trends Neurosci. 2007;30(5):220–7.
41. Geisler S, Zahm DS. Afferents of the ventral tegmental area in the rat-anatomical substratum for integrative functions. J Comp Neurol. 2005;490(3):270–94.
42. Watabe-Uchida M, Zhu L, Ogawa SK, Vamanrao A, Uchida N. Whole-brain mapping of direct inputs to midbrain dopamine neurons. Neuron. 2012;74(5):858–73.
43. Geisler S, Wise RA. Functional implications of glutamatergic projections to the ventral tegmental area. Rev Neurosci. 2008;19(4–5):227–44.
44. Taber MT, Das S, Fibiger HC. Cortical regulation of subcortical dopamine release: mediation via the ventral tegmental area. J Neurochem. 1995;65(3):1407–10.
45. Brog JS, Salyapongse A, Deutch AY, Zahm DS. The patterns of afferent innervation of the core and shell in the "Accumbens" part of the rat ventral striatum: Immunohistochemical detection of retrogradely transported fluoro-gold. J Comp Neurol. 1993;338(2):255–78.
46. Kalivas PW, Volkow ND. The neural basis of addiction: a pathology of motivation and choice. Am J Psychiatry. 2005;162(8):1403–13.
47. Grace AA. Gating of information flow within the limbic system and the pathophysiology of schizophrenia. Brain Res Rev. 2000;31(2–3):330–41.
48. Schultz W. Predictive reward signal of dopamine neurons. J Neurophysiol. 1998;80(1):1–27.
49. Schultz W. Behavioral theories and the neurophysiology of reward. Annu Rev Psychol. 2006;57:87–115.
50. Heinsbroek JA, Neuhofer DN, Griffin WC, Siegel GS, Bobadilla AC, Kupchik YM, et al. Loss of plasticity in the D2-accumbens pallidal pathway promotes cocaine seeking. J Neurosci. 2017;37(4):757–67.
51. Park K, Volkow ND, Pan Y, Du C. Chronic cocaine dampens dopamine signaling during cocaine intoxication and unbalances D1 over D2 receptor signaling. J Neurosci. 2013;33(40):15827–36.
52. D'Souza MS. Glutamatergic transmission in drug reward: Implications for drug addiction. Front Neurosci. 2015;9(NOV).
53. Wolf ME, Ferrario CR. AMPA receptor plasticity in the nucleus accumbens after repeated exposure to cocaine. Neurosci Biobehav Rev. 2010;35(2):185–211.
54. McFarland K, Kalivas PW. The circuitry mediating cocaine-induced reinstatement of drug-seeking behavior. J Neurosci. 2001;21(21):8655–63.
55. Zettle RD, Hayes SC. Dysfunctional control by client verbal behavior: the context of reason-giving. Anal Verbal Behav. 1986;4(1):30–8.
56. Dixon M. Analysis of gambling behavior. 2007;1(1):1.
57. Wilson KG, Hayes SC. Why it is crucial to understand thinking and feeling: an analysis and application to drug abuse. Behav Anal. 2000;23(1):25–43.
58. Bernard L, Cyr L, Bonnet-Suard A, Cutarella C, Bréjard V. Drawing alcohol craving process: a systematic review of its association with thought suppression, inhibition and impulsivity. Heliyon. 2021;7(1).
59. Wegner DM, Schneider DJ, Carter SR, White TL. Paradoxical effects of thought suppression. J Pers Soc Psychol. 1987;53(1):5–13.
60. Caselli G, Gemelli A, Querci S, Lugli AM, Canfora F, Annovi C, et al. The effect of rumination on craving across the continuum of drinking behaviour. Addictive Behav [Internet]. 2013;38(12):2879–83. https://doi.org/10.1016/j.addbeh.2013.08.023.

26 Psychoneurobiology of Dopaminergic Pathways and the Reward System

Gustavo E. Tafet and Tomás Ortiz Alonso

The Concept of Reward

Reward constitutes an affective experience characterized by pleasant or positive feelings. A rewarding experience may be triggered by certain environmental stimuli or desirable events, which may be perceived as positive or pleasant, which in turn may lead to a conscious experience of subjective pleasure [1]. Noteworthy, rewarding experiences may be elicited, not only by perceiving positive environmental stimuli, but also by evoking gratifying memories, such as the pleasurable experience elicited by remembering positive life experiences [2]. The concept of reward was also associated with that of motivated behavior. In this regard, reward has been also defined as something that may lead a living organism to perform an arbitrary behavior to get it, while the opposite, defined as a punishment, is something that may lead a living organism to perform a behavior to escape or avoid it [3]. Hence, a successful behavior may lead to a rewarding outcome, associated with approaching positive or avoiding negative stimuli, which in turn becomes the necessary positive reinforcer of the previous behavior, as it was described in certain forms of learning, such as instrumental conditioning [4].

Therefore, the concept of reward constitutes a complex affective experience that includes a hedonic component, which is associated with subjective feelings of liking and pleasure [4], as well as a behavioral component. This behavioral component, in turn, involves a learning process that may allow the association between certain behaviors and the positive experience elicited by a rewarding outcome. Interestingly, the rewarding value of certain outcomes, which motivate the repetition of behaviors aimed at attaining specific goals, is mostly learned through experience, although, in certain cases, it may be also innately determined, such as those related to natural resources associated with survival.

It has been shown that perceived stimuli are processed in the central nervous system (CNS), where new information, transiently held in the short-term memory, may be integrated with old related information, which has been previously incorporated into cognitive schemas, stored in the long-term memory. This cognitive processing may lead to the development of new relationships between new and old cognitions, which in turn may lead to further changes or consolidation of these long-term memories. Environmental information may be perceived

G. E. Tafet (✉)
Fundacion Internacional para el Desarroillo de las Neurociencias, Buenos Aires, Argentina

Department of Psychiatry and Behavioral Sciences, Texas A&M University, Bryan, TX, USA
e-mail: getafet@fidn.org

T. Ortiz Alonso
Department of Psychiatry, Universidad Complutense de Madrid, Madrid, Spain
e-mail: tortiz@ucm.es

P. Á. Gargiulo, H. L. Mesones-Arroyo (eds.), *Psychiatry and Neuroscience Update – Vol. V*,
https://doi.org/10.1007/978-3-031-72219-6_26

during different life experiences, including rewarding experiences or stressful life events, where certain stimuli may be associated with various characteristics, such as the intensity and length of their impact, or the context where they were perceived, which in turn may provide them with certain emotional relevance. This subjective relevance may allow perceived information to be incorporated into long-term memories, to influence cognitive processing, to provoke emotional reactions, and to shape behavioral responses. Emotional relevance is characterized by certain salience and valence.

Salience refers to the possibility that certain stimuli may be more perceptible, to result detectable or to stand out from the context. Salience may be strongly influenced by certain factors attributed to environmental stimuli, such as intensity or sensory characteristics, but mainly depends on subjective emotional and cognitive factors, which may provide perceived stimuli with a particular significance and importance. Hence, salience may enhance focused attention on certain stimuli, which may be subjectively interpreted as relevant or important, while ignoring other cues, which may be out of the attentional focus but may provide additional contextual information. Salience may be also understood as the property of certain stimuli to increase the chance an organism will elicit certain behavioral responses, either approaching or withdrawing, according to the perceived valence of those stimuli. Hence, salience is closely associated with valence, which may depend on subjective cognitive and emotional processes, and also the potential arousal provoked by perceived stimuli. Valence refers to positive or negative characteristics of perceived stimuli, which in turn may strongly influence emotional states. In this regard, positive valence is associated with the need or desires of approaching certain stimuli, which in turn may be associated with subjective feelings of reward and pleasure, while negative valence is associated with the tendency to avoid or escape it, which in turn may be associated with negative emotions, such as fear and anxiety. Therefore, in order to be perceived as rewarding, environmental stimuli should be characterized by certain salience and a positive valence, which in turn may be associated with subjective feelings of pleasure and reward.

Dopaminergic Pathways and the Reward System

It has been demonstrated that DA plays a critical role in the neurobiology of positive emotions, such as reward. In addition, DA is also involved in the psycho-neuro-endocrinological mechanisms of adaptive responses to stress, including the regulation of the hypothalamic-pituitary-adrenal (HPA) axis, and in the pathophysiological mechanisms associated with the origin and development of depression [5, 6]. As it was described in different aminergic systems, DA is stored in synaptic vesicles, in presynaptic terminals of dopaminergic neurons, and may be released into the synaptic cleft, where it may bind to specific dopaminergic receptors, mainly located in postsynaptic terminals. Dopaminergic receptors are specific transmembrane proteins, classified as "D1-like", including the D_1 and D_5 receptors, and "D2-like", including the D_2, D_3, and D_4 receptors. All of them are coupled to G proteins, and therefore are known as the DA G-protein-coupled-receptors (DA-GPCRs) family. The "D1-like" receptors are known to be coupled to G_s proteins, which, upon binding of DA, the first messenger molecule in this molecular chain of events, may lead to the activation of adenylyl cyclase (AC), with the consequent formation of a second messenger, known as cyclic AMP (cAMP). The "D2-like" receptors are coupled to G_i or G_o proteins, which are known to induce the opposite effect [7]. At the molecular level, dopaminergic neurotransmission is regulated by a different kind of transmembrane protein, responsible for the reuptake of DA from the synaptic cleft, hence known as the DA transporter (DAT) [8].

The neurobiology of reward involves specific pathways in the CNS, where dopamine (DA) plays a critical role. Dopaminergic neurons in the CNS are mainly located in specific nuclei, such as the retro-rubro field (also identified as A8), the substantia nigra pars compacta (SNc, also identified as A9), and the ventral tegmental area (VTA, also identified as A10), located in the brainstem. Among these, the VTA represents the main source of dopaminergic projections in the CNS, critically involved in cognitive and emotional processes, such as the mesolimbic (M-L) and the mesocortical (M-C) pathways [5, 9, 10].

One of the most important achievements in affective neuroscience was the identification of a mesolimbic network, a group of neural structures that responded to anticipated or received positive incentives [11]. These neural structures included the midbrain [12], containing the main dopaminergic nuclei, the ventral striatum (VS), which contains the Nucleus Accumbens (NAc) [13], the dorsal striatum (DS) [14] and different areas of the prefrontal cortex (PFC), including the orbitofrontal cortex (OFC) [15] and areas of the mesial PFC [16], mainly overlapping with the anterior cingulate cortex (ACC). This network constitutes the "reward pathway", which has been shown to be activated in the presence of rewarding stimuli [17].

The NAc constitutes one of the most important components of the reward pathway. Activation of the NAc has been associated with anticipation of positive incentives, and it has been shown to play a critical role in the assessment to distinguish between positive and negative valence [13, 18]. Hence, the subjective perception of a positive valence may increase with the obtained reward magnitude, or probability to receive a reward [17]. In this regard, it has been observed that there is an increased activation of the NAc in response to increased magnitude of anticipated rewards [13] and increased positive arousal [19]. In contrast, a decreased activation of the NAc in response to potential losses has been observed [20]. In addition, it has been shown that activation of midbrain dopaminergic neurons, which project to the NAc, may lead to reward anticipation [21]. These studies suggested that dopaminergic input from midbrain nuclei to the NAc may constitute a predictive learning signal, which may direct behavioral responses toward rewards [17]. It has been also proposed that activation of the NAc may direct attention towards relevant and unexpected events, based on the salience of perceived stimuli, rather than their positive or negative valence [22]. In this regard, it has been shown that the NAc may be activated by the relative importance and novelty of perceived events, as well as the contingency of behavioral responses, associated with the expected outcome of these responses [17].

The M-L pathway conveys dopaminergic output from the VTA to the VS, mainly to the NAc, as well as other limbic structures, such as the hippocampal formation and the extended amygdala, which includes the central nucleus of the amygdala (CNA) and the bed nucleus of the stria terminalis (BNST). The NAc and the extended amygdala represent the main neural structures involved in the processing of reward and motivation in the CNS [23, 24]. As it has been shown, the NAc represents the central hub of the reward system. Accordingly, the NAc receives dopaminergic projections from the VTA, as well as glutamatergic projections from the basolateral nucleus of the amygdala (BLA), the hippocampal formation, through the ventral subiculum, and certain areas of the PFC, including the OFC and the ACC [25, 26]. These glutamatergic excitatory projections participate in the detection and assessment of salience and valence of perceived stimuli, detection and anticipation and cue-related environmental signals, associated with reward information. More specifically, it has been shown that certain neurons in the ventromedial PFC (VMPFC), including areas of the OFC and the ACC, are involved in the assessment of rewarding value, error prediction, and decision making between short- and long-term outcomes. In this regard, the OFC receives sensory information of different modalities, as well as emotional and motivational information from different limbic structures, which may be integrated to allow the OFC to discriminate rewarding stimuli and to regulate their responses according to their motivational value [3]. It has been shown that some neurons may be activated by reward-predicting stimuli, while others may be activated after detection of rewarding stimuli. Moreover, neurons in the OFC share reciprocal connections with certain nuclei of the amygdala, particularly with the BLA, which are involved in the continuous assessment of associations between perceived stimuli and potential rewards. Neurons in the ACC participate in the selection of potential responses to rewarding stimuli and the continuous assessment of action-consequences contingencies. Some neurons in the ACC, particularly located in BA 25 and 32, send projections to certain areas of the NAc, which participate in the hedonic component of reward.

The NAc may be divided into two different regions, known as the shell, which is mainly connected to limbic structures, and the core, mainly connected to cortical areas [27]. It has been shown that the shell participates in emotion and motivation, novelty detection, hedonic sensitivity, and the rewarding effect of different substances [28]. The core participates in the expression of behaviors involved in processing of incentive salience and tolerance to delayed rewards [29].

As it was described previously, the BLA shares connections with the OFC and the ACC, as well as different sensory and association cortices, and sends projections to the NAc. The CNA is closely connected with the BNST, constituting the extended amygdala. The BLA and the CNA participate in reward-based emotional learning, where the BLA has been shown to be involved in potential associations between sensory stimuli and rewards, which in turn may lead to instrumental conditioning and the resulting adaptive behaviors. In addition, the connections between the BLA and the NAc have been shown to be involved in the activation of appetitive behaviors. The CNA is connected with the hypothalamus and different aminergic nuclei in the brainstem, including the VTA, serotonergic neurons in the raphe nuclei (RN), and noradrenergic neurons in the locus coeruleus (LC), hence contributing to orient behavioral responses toward reward [29]. The CNA and the BNST are connected with the dopaminergic system, through projections to the shell of the NAc and the VTA, where they may contribute to affective processing, incentive motivation, and visceral responses [23].

Therefore, neurons in the NAc receive excitatory glutamatergic input from the VMPFC, the BLA, and the hippocampal formation, and dopaminergic input from the VTA, through the M-L pathway, which participate in the detection of salience and valence associated with rewarding stimuli. Other neurons in the NAc are involved in reward detection and anticipation, and the integration between new environmental information and long-term memory information is related to previous experiences. Neurons located in the shell of the NAc, which are mainly GABAergic, send projections to the VTA, the ventromedial pallidum (VMP), the lateral hypothalamus, the central nucleus of the amygdala (CNA), and the BNST. These projections are involved in the regulation of emotional and motivational value-related responses [30]. In response to stressful events, DA may be released in the M-L pathway, and this may be conditioned by the intensity and extent of the impact, as well as the potential to avoid ability, predictability, and controllability of perceived stressors. Mild and moderate stressors, which may be perceived as brief, novel, avoidable, or controllable stimuli, may stimulate DA release, while the sustained and prolonged impact of chronic stressors, which may be perceived as unavoidable or uncontrollable, may inhibit DA release. Moreover, acute or short-term stressors may induce DA release in the NAc and the VMPFC, which has been associated with rewarding activity, while chronic or long-term stressors may decrease DA release in these structures, which has been associated with anhedonia and depression. Furthermore, the impact of certain environmental stressors may lead to activation of the amygdala, which has been associated with increased DA release in the M-C pathway, more specifically in the OFC and the ACC, which in turn may be translated into the assigning of excessive salience to negative events, hence contributing to negative biases in cognitive processing [5]. In this regard, the M-C pathway is not directly involved in behavioral responses, but may participate in neural processing of rewarding information through connections with the OFC and the ACC [31].

Since the M-L pathway sends dopaminergic projections from the VTA to the VS, it has been closely associated with the processing and reinforcement of rewarding stimuli, motivation, and the subjective experience of pleasure, therefore constituting the core of the "reward pathway" [5]. In addition to these neural structures, the dorsal striatum (DS) is connected with the VMPFC, which is involved in a neural circuit associated with goal-directed behaviors and, more specifically, perceived control over stressful events. In addition, this neural circuit is associated with the hippocampal formation and dopaminergic projections from the VTA, as well as the SNc. The interactions between these neural structures, with their reciprocal connections, play a critical role in the rewarding experience of subjective control, which in turn is critically involved in the development of active coping strategies, necessary to implement successful responses to stressful events. Moreover, these active coping strategies may be translated into active responses, hence contributing to prevent passive responses, associated with learned helplessness and the development of depression.

The Role of the Reward System in Controllability

It has been shown that activation of the dopaminergic system may be associated with the presence of rewarding stimuli, as well as the impact of adverse events, when these are perceived as predictable and controllable [30, 32].

It has been shown that the impact of environmental stressors may lead to different responses in the M-L pathway, depending on the potential controllability on perceived stressors [33], the subjective appraisal of stressful events, and the available resources to cope with them. Hence, the impact of acute and controllable stressors may lead to increased DA release in the NAc, whereas the sustained and prolonged impact of increasingly uncontrollable stressors may lead to decreased DA release in the M-L pathway [33]. Moreover, the impact of unavoidable or uncontrollable stressors may lead to decreased DA release in the NAc and impaired response to environmental stimuli, which in turn have been associated with depressive symptoms after exposure to chronic stressful conditions [34]. Hence, the difficulty to experience pleasure, associated with subjective lack of interest and motivation, represents the typical symptoms of anhedonia observed in depressed subjects [6], which has been associated with impaired dopaminergic function and altered reward processing [35, 36]. It has been shown that the NAc plays a critical role in the processing of rewarding and hedonic experiences in association with the OFC, which in turn participates in the subjective assessments of hedonic and rewarding value [37]. In this regard, the OFC is closely associated with the ACC, in the VMPFC, and both PFC structures are also associated with the dorsolateral PFC (DLPFC), therefore allowing the interaction between emotional and cognitive processing. The NAc receives dopaminergic projections from the VTA and glutamatergic projections from the amygdala, hence enhancing the DA input and increasing motivation [37]. Dopaminergic activity in the VTA may be also modulated by serotonergic projections from the RN, where reciprocal connections, particularly between the dorsal RN (DRN) and the VTA, has been shown.

The M-L system shares connections with different nuclei of the extended amygdala. It has been shown that the VTA receives projections from the CNA and the BNST, particularly from the dorsolateral (DL-BNST) and the ventrolateral (VL-BNST). These nuclei send corticotrophin releasing factor (CRF) stimulatory projections, which activate CRF_1 and CRF_2 receptors in the VTA, therefore stimulating DA neurons. Indirect stimulatory pathways, mediated by glutamatergic terminals and GABAergic interneurons, have been also described. Additional regulatory mechanisms may also include release of GABA by projections from the CNA and the DL-BNST, while projections from the VL-BNST may also release glutamate. Therefore, DA release from the VTA into the NAc and PFC may be regulated by CRF, as well as other neurotransmitters, which in turn may exert influence on appetitive and aversive behaviors associated with anxiety. The VTA also is reciprocally connected with the extended amygdala, where it has been shown that excitatory DA projections may reach CRF neurons in the CNA and the BNST, hence providing a positive feedback circuit. In response to stressful events, activation of these mechanisms may lead to increased release of DA by neurons in the VTA, with the consequent increased concentrations of DA in the NAc and the PFC. The stimulatory effects of CRF may also reach the dopaminergic system through serotonergic projections from the DRN, which also receive stimulatory CRF projections from the amygdala and the BNST. It has been shown that increased dopaminergic activity in the M-L pathway may be associated with the perception of rewarding stimuli, as well as aversive situations which may be perceived as controllable and escapable. In this regard, the subjective perception of controllability may be highly relieving and rewarding.

The Role of Controllability in the Development of Resilience

Adaptive responses to stress involve cognitive, affective, and goal-directed behavioral responses, which in turn involve the availability of necessary resources to assess potential reawards and risks, as well as predictability and controllability to succesfully cope with stressful events. These processes are strongly conditioned by incoming environmental information as well as long-term memory information associated with previous experiences, which may be evoked in response to perceived stressful situations. In this regard, affective cognitive and emotional processing may lead to successful coping strategies, which may enhance subjective perception of predictability and controllability, which in turn may be perceived and interpreted as rewarding experiences. Hence, the reward system is critically involved in the implementation of adaptive responses and the development of resilience.

In order to succesfully cope with stressful events, it is necessary to develop certain skills, such as the ability to recognize threatening or adverse situations, to avoid potentially dangerous stimuli, to learn about the characteristics of these stimuli, and to develop resources to successfully cope with them [38, 39]. Successful coping also requires the ability to recognize rewarding stimuli, to learn about their characteristics, and potential strategies to approach them. Among rewarding stimuli, it is possible to define a category of primary or natural rewards, such as those associated with survival and satisfaction of basic needs, which may be clearly observed in those behaviors associated with the search for food and sex. Secondary rewards require abstract cognitive representations, which are not directly associated with survival, but may lead to facilitate survival and may significantly improve quality of life. This category of secondary or cognitive rewards includes money, power, and challenging experiences [28, 40, 41]. The reward system, as it was previously described, includes the VTA and the NAc, among other neural structures, and reciprocal connections between the NAc, the hippocampus, the amygdala, and the VM-PFC, where the NAc has been shown to play a critical role in anticipation of positive and rewarding stimuli [18]. It has been shown that anticipated perception of rewards, characterized by their positive valence, may be associated with activation of the NAc, which participate in the recognition of positive and negative valence [18]. The perception of a positive valence may be enhanced by the reward magnitude or probability, therefore, activation of the NAc has been associated with anticipatory reward and the consequent approach behavior, with the resulting positive emotional experience. The NAc has been also involved in the assessment of salience of perceived stimuli, which in turn may enhance attention towards relevant stimuli and unexpected events [22]. The amygdala also participates in this process, particularly the BLA, which is involved in reward-stress modulation [42]. Moreover, it has been shown that rewarding stimuli may enhance neuroplasticity in the NAc and the BLA, which in turn have been associated with reduced HPA reactivity [42]. In this regard, rewarding stimuli may moderate subsequent responses to stressful events, which have been reflected through decreased HPA reactivity, with the resulting decrease in cortisol release, and enhanced coping strategies, including problem-solving abilities [43], which in turn may lead to an increased feeling of controllability. A subjective perception of controllability, even an illusion of control, is relieving and highly rewarding, hence representing a critical condition for the development of resilience. In this regard, it has been demonstrated that a subjective perception of controllability plays a critical role in this process [44], which may contribute to "learned resilience", as well as the opposite, a subjective perception of decreased controllability, may lead to develop learned helplessness [45], especially during early periods of life. Exposure to uncontrollable early adverse experiences may lead to dysregulation of the HPA axis [46], with the resulting increased levels of CRF and cortisol. However, exposure to mild or moderate stressors, which may be perceived as controllable, may contribute to develop resilience in response to different stressful situations in later periods of life [44, 47]. This potential immunity has been identified as "stress inoculation" [48] and has been associated with successful adaptive responses, which in turn may lead to subjective perception of controllability and higher tolerance to adverse situations [49]. This process has been associated with increased neuroplasticity, particularly in the PFC [49], which has been also associated with improved cognitive control and increased volume of the VM-PFC [50, 51]. Therefore, it has been proposed that stress inoculation may result in a process of "learned controllability"; likewise, the impact of early traumatic experiences may result in a process of learned helplessness. Therefore, psychological and neurobiological processes are closely integrated in the development of resilience, which is necessary to successfully cope with stressful events, as well as the implementation of potential changes that may contribute to transform negative distressful events into positive and rewarding experiences.

Conclusion

The dopaminergic system plays a critical role in rewarding experiences, which in turn are critical in the development of resilience. Chronic stressful events, which are perceived as unpredictable and uncontrollable, may lead to the development of learned helplessness, which is associated with an imbalance between limbic activity, mainly mediated by hyperactivation of the amygdala, and cortical activity, mainly mediated by the DL-PFC and the VM-PFC.

The possibility to improve a subjective sense of controllability on stressful situations, which involve cognitive and emotional processes, may lead to rewarding experiences, which in turn are associated with dopaminergic activity.

References

1. Berridge KC, Robinson TE, Aldridge JW. Dissecting components of reward: 'liking', 'wanting', and learning. Curr Opin Pharmacol. 2009;9(1):65–73.
2. Speer ME, Bhanji JP, Delgado MR. Savoring the past: positive memories evoke value representations in the striatum. Neuron. 2014;84(4):847–56.
3. Rolls ET. The brain and emotion. Oxford: Oxford University Press; 1999.
4. Schultz W. Behavioral theories and the neurophysiology of reward. Annu Rev Psychol. 2006;57:87–115.
5. Dunlop BW, Nemeroff CB. The role of dopamine in the pathophysiology of depression. Arch Gen Psychiatry. 2007;64(3):327–37.
6. Nestler EJ, Carlezon WA Jr. The mesolimbic dopamine reward circuit in depression. Biol Psychiatry. 2006;59(12):1151–9.
7. Missale C, Nash SR, Robinson SW, Jaber M, Caron MG. Dopamine receptors: from structure to function. Physiol Rev. 1998;78(1):189–225.
8. Chen N, Reith ME. Structure and function of the dopamine transporter. Eur J Pharmacol. 2000;405(1-3):329–39.
9. Smelik PG. Adaptation and brain function. Prog Brain Res. 1987;72:3–9.
10. Cabib S, Puglisi-Allegra S. Stress, depression and the mesolimbic dopamine system. Psychopharmacology. 1996;128:331–42.
11. Olds J, Milner P. Positive reinforcement produced by electrical stimulation of septal area and other regions of rat brain. J Comp Physiol Psychol. 1954;47:419–27.
12. Schultz W. Predictive reward signal of dopamine neurons. J Neurophysiol. 1998;80:1–27.
13. Knutson B, Adams CM, Fong GW, Hommer D. Anticipation of increasing monetary reward selectively recruits nucleus accumbens. J Neurosci. 2001;21(16):RC159.
14. Zald DH, Boileau I, El-Dearedy W, Gunn R, McGlone F, Dichter GS, Dagher A. Dopamine transmission in the human striatum during monetary reward tasks. J Neurosci. 2004;24(17):4105–12.

15. Rolls ET. The functions of the orbitofrontal cortex. Brain Cogn. 2004;55(1):11–29.
16. Knutson B, Fong GW, Bennett SM, Adams CM, Hommer D. A region of mesial prefrontal cortex tracks monetarily rewarding outcomes: characterization with rapid event-related fMRI. NeuroImage. 2003;18(2):263–72.
17. Cooper JC, Knutson B. Valence and salience contribute to nucleus accumbens activation. NeuroImage. 2008;39(1):538–47.
18. Ikemoto S, Panksepp J. The role of nucleus accumbens dopamine in motivated behavior: a unifying interpretation with special reference to reward-seeking. Brain Res Brain Res Rev. 1999;31(1):6–41.
19. Drevets WC, Price JL, Furey ML. Brain structural and functional abnormalities in mood disorders: implications for neurocircuitry models of depression. Brain Struct Funct. 2008;213(1-2):93–118.
20. Tom SM, Fox CR, Trepel C, Poldrack RA. The neural basis of loss aversion in decision-making under risk. Science. 2007;315(5811):515–8.
21. Schultz W, Dayan P, Montague PR. A neural substrate of prediction and reward. Science. 1997;275(5306):1593–9.
22. Berridge KC, Robinson TE. What is the role of dopamine in reward: hedonic impact, reward learning, or incentive salience? Brain Res Brain Res Rev. 1998;28(3):309–69.
23. McGinty JF. Advancing from the ventral striatum to the extended amygdale. Ann N Y Acad Sci. 1999;877:12–5.
24. Heimer L. A new anatomical framework for neuropsychiatric disorders and drug abuse. Am J Psychiatry. 2003;160:1726–39.
25. Haber SN, McFarland NR: The concept of the ventral striatum in nonhuman primates. Ann N Y Acad Sci. 1999;877:33–48.
26. Haber SN, Knutson B. The reward circuit: linking primate anatomy and human imaging. Neuropsychopharmacology. 2010 Jan;35(1):4–26.
27. Chau DT, Roth RM, Green AI. The neural circuitry of reward and its relevance to psychiatric disorders. Curr Psychiatry Rep. 2004;6(5):391–9.
28. Berridge KC, Robinson TE. Parsing reward. Trends Neurosci. 2003;26:507–13.
29. Cardinal RN, Parkinson JA, Hall J, et al. Emotion and motivation: the role of the amygdala, ventral striatum, and prefrontalcortex. Neurosci Biobehav Rev. 2002;26:321–52.
30. Baik JH. Stress and the dopaminergic reward system. Exp Mol Med. 2020;52(12):1879–90.
31. Tzschentke TM. Pharmacology and behavioral pharmacology of the mesocortical dopamine system. Prog Neurobiol. 2001;63:241–320.
32. Cabib S, Latagliata C, Orsini C. Role of stress-related dopamine transmission in building and maintaining a protective cognitive reserve. Brain Sci. 2022;12(2):246.
33. Suridjan I, Boileau I, Bagby M, Rusjan PM, Wilson AA, Houle S, Mizrahi R. Dopamine response to psychosocial stress in humans and its relationship to individual differences in personality traits. J Psychiatr Res. 2012;46(7):890–7.
34. Cabib S, Puglisi-Allegra S. The mesoaccumbens dopamine in coping with stress. Neurosci Biobehav Rev. 2012;36(1):79–89.
35. Krishnan V, Nestler EJ. Linking molecules to mood: new insight into the biology of depression. Am J Psychiatry. 2010;167(11):1305–20.
36. Bogdan R, Nikolova YS, Pizzagalli DA. Neurogenetics of depression: a focus on reward processing and stress sensitivity. Neurobiol Dis. 2013;52:12–23.
37. Der-Avakian A, Markou A. The neurobiology of anhedonia and other reward-related deficits. Trends Neurosci. 2012;35(1):68–77.
38. LeDoux J, Daw ND. Surviving threats: neural circuit and computational implications of a new taxonomy of defensive behaviour. Nat Rev Neurosci. 2018;19(5):269–82.
39. Sapolsky RM. Why zebras don't get ulcers. New York: Holt Paperbacks; 2004.
40. Schultz W. Neuronal reward and decision signals: from theories to data. Physiol Rev. 2015;95(3):853–951.
41. Sescousse G, Caldú X, Segura B, Dreher JC. Processing of primary and secondary rewards: a quantitative meta-analysis and review of human functional neuroimaging studies. Neurosci Biobehav Rev. 2013 May;37(4):681–96.
42. Ulrich-Lai YM, Christiansen AM, Ostrander MM, Jones AA, Jones KR, Choi DC, Krause EG, Evanson NK, Furay AR, Davis JF, Solomon MB, de Kloet AD, Tamashiro KL, Sakai RR, Seeley RJ, Woods SC, Herman JP. Pleasurable behaviors reduce stress via brain reward pathways. Proc Natl Acad Sci USA. 2010;107(47):20529–34.
43. Dutcher JM, Creswell JD. The role of brain reward pathways in stress resilience and health. Neurosci Biobehav Rev. 2018;95:559–67.
44. Feder A, Charney DS, Collins K. Neurobiology of resilience. In: Southwick SM, Litz BT, Charney DS, Friedman MJ, editors. Resilience and mental health. New York: Cambridge University Press; 2011.
45. Overmier JB, Seligman ME. Effects of inescapable shock upon subsequent escape and avoidance responding. J Comp Physiol Psychol. 1967;63:28–33.
46. Heim C, Newport DJ, Mletzko T, Miller AH, Nemeroff CB. The link between childhood trauma and depression: insights from HPA axis studies in humans. Psychoneuroendocrinology. 2008 Jul;33(6):693–710.
47. Russo SJ, Murrough JW, Han MH, Charney DS, Nestler EJ. Neurobiology of resilience. Nat Neurosci. 2012;15(11):1475–84.

48. Rutter M. Resilience: some conceptual considerations. J Adolesc Health. 1993;14(626–631):690–6.
49. Southwick SM, Charney DS. The science of resilience: implications for the prevention and treatment of depression. Science. 2012;338(6103):79–82.
50. Parker KJ, Buckmaster CL, Justus KR, Schatzberg AF, Lyons DM. Mild early life stress enhances prefrontal-dependent response inhibition in monkeys. Biol Psychiatry. 2005;57:848–55.
51. Lyons DM, Parker KJ, Katz M, Schatzberg AF. Developmental cascades linking stress inoculation, arousal regulation, and resilience. Front Behav Neurosci. 2009;3:32.

Methylphenidate and Reward: Functional Role of Neurotransmitters in Relapse Process and Drug-Seeking Behavior

27

Adel Kashefi and Carlos Tomaz

Introduction

MPH is a medication used to manage and help reduce symptoms of ADHD in children, adolescents, and adults [1]. Since the 1970s, MPH has been increasingly used as the first treatment of ADHD and sales in the United States have been increased during 1991–1999. Interestingly, the United Nations reports that 85% of the world's total MPH production and consumption occur in this country [2]. In recent years, MPH abuse has increased markedly among college students. The oral route of administration has been said to be the most common and convenient. Additionally, the prescription use of the stimulants MPH and amphetamine increased by 35.5% in the United States from 2008 to 2012 among adolescents and adults [3]. There are reports of using the MPH for the treatment of autistic, depression, and neurodegenerative disorders [4, 5]. Despite the treatment properties of MPH, there has widespread speculation regarding the potential abuse of this psychostimulant drug [6].

The prefrontal cortex (PFC) and hippocampus are two important and main parts in continued attention and memory formation, respectively [7]. Furthermore, the mesolimbic pathway is recognized as a major component in processing responses to drugs of abuse. Dopamine (DA) projection neurons from the Ventral Tegmental Area (VTA) to the Nucleus Accumbens (NAc) lead to reward facilitation [8, 9].

The specific properties of MPH, including enhanced alertness, elevation in mood, facilitation of concentration, and euphoria induction, have led to these drugs being considered as an effective treatment for many diseases [10]. Unfortunately, long-term or recreational use of these stimulant medications is common and associated with abuse that can cause serious problems. They include cognitive, behavioral, and physiological symptoms and psychosis. It demonstrates that the continued use of the substance leads to significant substance-related problems. Current evidence suggests that MPH use in children diagnosed with ADHD may increase the risk of future substance abuse [11].

A. Kashefi
Laboratory of Neurosciences and Behavior, Department of Physiological Sciences, University of Brasilia, Brasília, Brazil

Laboratory of learning and Memory, Research Center and Department of Physiology, School of Medicine, Semnan University of Medical Sciences, Semnan, Iran

C. Tomaz (✉)
Laboratory of Neuroscience and Behavior, Post-Graduate Program in Environment, University CEUMA, São Luís, Maranhão, Brazil
e-mail: ctomaz@ceuma.br

P. Á. Gargiulo, H. L. Mesones-Arroyo (eds.), *Psychiatry and Neuroscience Update – Vol. V*,
https://doi.org/10.1007/978-3-031-72219-6_27

Effects of MPH

MPH and Attention-Deficit/Hyperactivity Disorder

ADHD is one of the most common mental disorders in children and adolescents, with approximately 3–10% of school children in the United States affected by this diagnosis [12].

This chronic psychiatric disorder has a high rate of comorbid diagnosis such as learning disability, impulsivity, conduct disorder, anxiety disorder, and inattention. Hence, the incidence of ADHD can be an intricate process because of the subjective nature of teacher and parent accounts of a kid's behavior [13].

Concerns about the possible abuse of MPH in young children have been disseminated in the media [14–16]. They are the result of the rapid increase in MPH usage, an increase in the number of preschool-aged children diagnosed with ADHD and treated with MPH, and a lack of information on the long-term consequences of psychostimulants on brain development [14, 17, 18]. Moreover, there are controversial reports on whether MPH treatment has the potential to elicit drug dependence as it occurs with other psychostimulants, such as cocaine and amphetamine [15, 19]. Additional concerns are the possible adverse effects produced by such psychopharmacological intervention in a developing brain [20]. During childhood, vital neurodevelopment happens with the production and elimination of many neuronal connections, i.e., synaptic pruning. Repeated treatment with psychostimulants can result in the initiation and intensification of biochemical and behavioral manifestations that ultimately lead to modulation of these critical developmental processes and produce plasticity in the cellular components of the central nervous system (CNS) and thus cause dependence of the drug and behavioral sensitization [21]. Behavioral sensitization refers to the progressive augmentation of behavioral responses to the repetitive use of psychostimulants that develop as a result of enduring drug responses [22–24].

MPH and Brain-Derived Neurotrophic Factors (BDNF)

BDNF is another vital member of the neurotrophins family and can cross the blood-brain barrier. There is a positive relationship between plasma and brain BDNF protein concentrations. It is suggested that circulating BDNF levels might originate from the neurons and glial cells of CNS [25, 26]. Brain-derived neurotrophic factor (BDNF) is associated with increased reward response to substance abuse. BDNF acts through binding to TrkB (tyrosine receptor kinase B) receptor, increasing the growth and maintenance of several monoamine neuronal systems, performing as a modulator of learning-related synaptic plasticity and rewarding drug memories [27]. The findings indicate that mesocorticolimbic BDNF was effective in cocaine craving, so that observed boost BDNF expression levels in VTA, accumbens, and amygdala subsequently promote an increase in cue-induced cocaine-seeking after withdrawal [28].

BDNF levels enhanced in MPH-treated animals after 6 weeks. Rats exposed to MPH (5 mg/kg) exhibited significantly increased BDNF in the brain regions related to drug addiction and reward [29, 30]. Also during adolescence, MPH significantly increased dorsal hippocampal BDNF in both males and females [31]. It also produced a significant increase in accumbal BDNF levels [32]. Infusion of BDNF into the mesolimbic DA system significantly increased both cocaine-induced locomotion and facilitation of termed conditioned reinforcers in male rats [33]. Studies have shown that SCH-23390 or eticlopride can reduce BDNF in MPH-induced CPP. The effects of MPH on the BDNF appear to be mediated by Dopaminergic D1 (DAD1) and dopaminergic D2 (DAD2) receptors [29].

BDNF is an important factor for the reward system in the mesolimbic DA system. Drugs of abuse activate this system. It is the case of opioids and psychostimulants. The activation induces an increase in BDNF. BDNF-TrkB transmission contributes to cocaine CPP. Cocaine self-administration in the accumbens enhances

BDNF-TrkB signaling in specific areas of the brain, such as the VTA. It also improves the CPP induced by cocaine and morphine [34, 35]. Also, BDNF-TrkB transmission in the hippocampus contributes to amphetamine CPP [36]. The above research shows that the effects of BDNF vary depending on the area of the brain and the type of task [37].

MPH and Reward Mechanism

The reward system is defined as a group of neural structures that are critically implicated in mediating the effects of reinforcement in specific regions of the brain. Research has found that MPH is a powerful reinforcer that can cause various side effects [38]. In our laboratory, we showed that various exposures to different doses of MPH (1 and 2.5 mg/kg; i.p.) in rats and (5 mg/kg; i.p.) in monkeys produced CPP. The animals following the conditioning period showed a significant difference in the time spent on post-conditioning and reinstatement. Also, we demonstrated that the rewarding properties of MPH play a crucial role in drug-seeking behavior that persists long after a withdrawal period in the CPP model [39, 40]. Most relevant to our work, Wooters et al. demonstrated that MPH has a rewarding effect and can establish CPP in male rats [41].

It has been shown that the long-term MPH exposure in both male and female rats may lead to long-lasting alterations in brain structure, natural reward systems, and induce a CPP [29]. In another study, the effects of MPH doses on young and old rats showed that a high dose (5 mg/kg) of MPH but not 1 mg/kg resulted in a significant preference that was more robust in younger adolescent males. These results demonstrate that the rewarding aspects of MPH are probably mediated by neurotransmitters' release [42].

In humans, MPH can produce behavioral and subjective effects similar to those of cocaine and amphetamine [43–45]. However, the expression of such effects depends on several of variables such as route of administration, prior drug history, and diagnostic status [15, 46]. For example, the reinforcing effects of MPH and its ability to induce a subjectively rated 'high' are more prominent after intravenous than after oral administration [46]. Such differences have been attributed to the more rapid elevation in serum levels of the drug and presumably extracellular DA following intravenous administration [47, 48].

The major mechanism of MPH is well recognized to inhibit the dopamine transporter (DAT) and norepinephrine transporter (NET) [49]. MPH has a similar function to cocaine, blocks the reuptake of the DAT and norepinephrine (NE) transporter, resulting in elevated synaptic extracellular DA and NE levels in the reward pathway [50].

MPH and Conditioned Place Preference (CPP)

The CPP task is one of the most common and validated tests for measuring the rewarding effects of drugs. Recently, we have extensively investigated the effects of drug and food addiction on reward-related behaviors in the acquisition, expression, extinction, and reinstatement of CPP. According to this, it is well established that repeated cocaine administrations in marmoset monkeys led to the acquisition of a CPP [51]. To determine the behavioral effects of food-induced CPP, it was found that monkeys treated repeatedly with chocolate in a specific environment induced a CPP response for this area. In addition, significant differences were observed in the time spent in the chocolate-paired compartment in post-CPP, compared to pre-CPP levels [52]. It was also identified in monkeys subsequently and repeatedly exposed to a high versus low fat/sugar (palatable) food; each at different parts of the chamber developed a remarkable CPP response for the former item. The time spent in the food-paired chamber during post-conditioning increased significantly compared to the preconditioning level [53].

However, our two recent studies show that MPH enhances the pleasurable effects and produces CPP in both monkeys and rats. We showed daily administration of MPH during the conditioning phase; induced CPP during the post-conditioning and reinstatement period in subjects [39, 40]. Most animals initially preferred the drug-paired chamber of the CPP. We used here Cannabidiol (CBD). In other studies, we used CBD to test the involvement of the endocannabinoid system in the modulation of MPH effects. It seems that CBD is able to reduce the reinstatement of psychostimulant drugs [54, 55]. We used CBD as a new candidate in the prevention and treatment of MPH relapse. CBD injection facilitated the extinction, while had no effect on reinstatement of MPH-induced CPP in marmoset monkeys [40]. In contrast, intracerebroventricular (ICV) microinjection of CBD (50 or 10 μg/5 μl) suppressed priming-induced reinstatement of MPH CPP. Also, the ICV injected of CBD (10 and 50 μg/5 μl) showed a shorter latency for the extinction period than Naïve and/or DMSO control group in rats [39].

Neurotransmitters and MPH

Dopamine

The neurotransmitter DA has an important role in reward-motivated behavior. To motivate actions that cause rewards, DA release is essential during rewarding experiences. DA is vital in the rewarding properties of drugs of abuse. All psychostimulant drugs including amphetamine, cocaine, and methamphetamine activate the mesolimbic DA pathway. Furthermore, it has been shown that drugs of abuse increase DA release within brain's reward pathway [56]. In our recent studies, the mesolimbic dopamine system also appears to be largely responsible for the reward system induced by MPH administration. It is important to realize that chronic exposure to MPH during the developmental periods in childhood and adolescence has exhibited changes in the structure of brain DA cells, behavioral disorders, and future vulnerability to drug abuse [57–60].

DAD1 and DAD2 receptors are well known as the most prominent expressed DA receptors in the brain and related to emotional behaviors, memory, and motivation learning, as well as control of reward-related behaviors [61]. Research has demonstrated that rewarding aspects of MPH and the most addictive substance are regulated by both D1 and D2 receptors and contribute to reinforcement behavior [62]. Also, these receptors are involved in the development and expression of behavioral sensitization to the rewarding property of other drugs of abuse such as MPH [63]. The activity of DA D1 and D2 receptors can be different on reward functions. It is the case of a high-dose MPH-induced CPP. It is blocked by D1-receptor antagonist, SCH23390, but not by raclopride, a D2-receptor antagonist, indicating the key role of the D1 receptor in the MPH-induced rewarding effects [62]. It has been established that the MPH administration enhanced the learning of cue-reward via D1 receptor-dependent mechanisms and impaired via a DA D2 receptor-dependent mechanism. These results reveal essential and distinct roles for dopamine receptor subtypes in mediating MPH-induced enhancements of synaptic transmission and learning performance [64].

Norepinephrine

Previous research showed that NE is known as another important neurotransmitter in the reward system and plays an important role in executive functions involved in higher-level behavior including the pathophysiology of ADHD and its treatment [65].

It is well established that noradrenergic transmission is involved in drug craving, reinstatement, and withdrawal. Zarrindast and collaborators showed a main involvement of brain NE in the behavioral and central effects of opiates. This study pointed to the key role of α2-adrenoceptors in morphine-induced CPP [66]. Another study showed decreases in accumbal DA-related morphine-induced locomotor hyperactivity by the local injection of the adrenergic antagonist into the PFC [67]. NE appears to play an influential role in the reward function and mesoaccumbens DA synthesis. Eventually, a major role of NE in the medial prefrontal cortex (mpFC) has been identified in other reinforces such as amphetamine and cocaine [68–70].

Serotonin

5-HT is also involved in the hedonic experience, mood, and higher cognitive functions including consciousness or self-reflection [71]. 5-HT depletion suppressed instrumental reward-based reinforcement learning in rats [72]. Likewise, depletion of 5-HT impaired the acquisition of responding to appetitive conditioned reinforcement, but not extinction in the frontal cortex of marmoset monkeys [73]. Recent studies have shown that a previous injection of a 5-HT7 agonist could have a direct modulatory impact on rewarding and stimulant MPH effects [74]. In another study, the results showed that the 5-HT7R selective antagonist, SB-269970, significantly decreased amphetamine-induced hyperactivity in both rats and mice [75, 76].

It is interesting to know that there is a strong association between serotonin and dopamine [77]. DA neurons are important for driving motivation (i.e., wanting). Also, 5-HT neurons may play a pivotal role in other aspects of the reward systems including consolidation of positive emotion and predictions via context evaluation. It is acceptable that serotonin impairs dopamine actions in some motivational behaviors by signaling reward satiety, but the two systems synergistically promote other elements of reward processing such as attention, pleasure, learning, and memory. Finally, DA and 5-HT could provide a combined reward signal, so that its dissociation in the absence or decline of DA may encode punishment [70].

Brain Reward Sites

Ventral Tegmental Area

The VTA is another important part of the brain in mediating reinforcing properties, hedonics, behavioral adaptation, and reward-related processes [78]. VTA is a modulation site of behavioral sensitization after repetitive psychostimulant exposure. Intra-VTA infusions of amphetamine result in a sensitized behavioral response to subsequent systemic administration of amphetamine, morphine, and cocaine [79–81]. Similar results in animals displayed the development of sensitization by chronically being exposed to MPH in the VTA [82].

Preclinical studies indicated a significant enhancement of cocaine self-administration after amphetamine intra-VTA administration [83]. VTA-NAc pathway is a key region of a rewarding stimulus. MPH produces an increase of DA signaling in VTA and projects to the NAC [84]. Brain imaging studies of drug-dependent individuals have shown exposure to cues in addicted people associated with increased activation of VTA and NAc [85], which could be potentially attributed to acute increases of dopamine in several other regions. The other regions that are co-activated during cue exposure are PFC, cerebellum, limbic regions, and insula [84]. It seems that strengthening of dopaminergic neurotransmission between VTA and NAc increases locomotor activity in behaviorally sensitized animals [86].

VTA neuronal plasticity is essential for appropriate action of learning and extinction [87]. The new study involving mice demonstrated that early postnatal Shank3 downregulation in the VTA induces synaptic excitatory shortages related to social preference [88].

Prefrontal Cortex

The PFC is a major part of the brain and plays an essential role in brain reward processing, regions involved in processes relevant to substance abuse such as compulsive drug use, impulse inhibition, decision-making, regulation, and maintenance of addictive behavior [89]. Animal studies point to the PFC as the most important target of MPH. MPH injection increased neuronal activity and dopamine release in the PFC [90]. It has been reported that oral administration of MPH in monkeys increased DA levels in both PFC and striatum [91, 92]. High dose of MPH but not a low dose increases dopamine synthesis 1 hour after PFC injection [90]. In addition, patients with ADHD symptoms display decreased PFC function and MPH administration related to remarkable increased neural activity in this region [93]. Preclinical studies have shown a decreased global DNA methylation of cocaine-induced CPP in the PFC [94]. Similarly, cognitive impairment following chronic cocaine exposure is mediated by altered PFC activity [95].

It has also been confirmed that MPH dose-dependently augmented dopamine and noradrenaline concentration in the NAc and PFC. However, MPH had significantly smaller effects on dopamine concentration in the NAc, and it produced considerably larger noradrenaline than dopamine concentration in the PFC [96].

Nucleus Accumbens

The NAc is a section of the ventral striatum from the rostral basal forebrain to the preoptic area of the hypothalamus [97]. The NAc is strongly linked with various types of neurological illnesses, including obsessive-compulsive disorder [98], obesity [99], anxiety disorders [100], depression [101], bipolar disorder [102], Huntington's disease [103], Parkinson's disease [104], and Alzheimer's disease [105, 106]. Thorough understanding of the structure and anatomy of the NAc can help discover and develop appropriate therapies [106]. Overall, studies on animals highlight the key role of NAc in the brain's circuitry that is responsible for translating motivation into action [107].

NAc is also known as one of the main components of the reward and pleasure behavior that is necessary for other activities including reinforcement learning, aggression, addiction, and the placebo effect [108–111]. It is well established that therapeutic doses of MPH increase dopamine (DA) levels in the NAc [38]. For example, lower alcohol-induced CPP is related to reduced extracellular levels of DA by alcohol in the NAc [112].

The NAc seems to play important roles in the learning-related processes, including avoidance [113, 114] and CPP (an animal model of reward learning) [115, 116]. Recently, our studies have shown that the NAc is probably a major part in the reinstatement of reward-induced CPP [39, 40]. In another study, electrical activation of the NAc blocks morphine-induced CPP and shows impairment of learning and memory formation [117]. In support of this, microinjection of DA receptor antagonist into the nucleus accumbens and/or NAc lesion reduces the reinforcing effect of drug substance. This evidence suggests a direct relationship between suppression of dopamine transmission in NAc and decreasing reinforcing effect of drugs [118].

In rodents, it has been observed that the NAc is essential for regulating locomotor activity and stereotyped behaviors [119]. Injection of psychostimulant drugs, including cocaine [120], and amphetamine [121], within the NAc demonstrated significantly increased locomotor activity via release of dopamine [122]. Activation D1 and inhibition of D2 neurons increased locomotor activity, while the opposite results were observed after activation of D2 neurons in the NAc [122].

Hippocampus

The hippocampus is an area of the brain that plays a fundamental role in formation, organization, and storage of new memories and spatial memories [123]. Hippocampus is also involved in spatial memory and consolidating memories during sleep [124]. The ventral hippocampus is an effective structure to regulate the mesoaccumbal dopamine in responding to the reward system. Animal studies also showed that psychostimulants induce enhanced hippocampal long-term potentiation (LTP) and, in opposite, decreased hippocampal neurogenesis and memory in animal models [125].

Long-term psychostimulant drug misuse (such as MPH, amphetamine, methamphetamine, and cocaine) has negative physical and mental health consequences. Drug abuse actions on the hippocampus induce long-term changes in these systems and impact adult hippocampal neurogenesis-related processes, which may promote drug dependence by changing emotional and learning processes' drug-related cues [126].

Substance abuse can produce an acute and protracted withdrawal syndrome and also a number of adverse effects including psychosis, dysphoria, anxiety, intense drug craving, and stress hypersensitivity [127–132]. These symptoms can occur in the form of cravings and relapse in both animals [133, 134] and humans [129, 135, 136]. It is thought that enable stress-sensitive experiences following exposure to psychostimulants in the withdrawal phase can lead to relapse. Recent studies show that psychostimulants have a profound effect on hippocampal synaptic plasticity and memory performance. There is a major concern that the substances can cause a host of changes to the mesolimbic system and other parts involved in reward-based learning, including the hippocampus [126].

Amygdala

The amygdala is definitely one of the most important parts of the brain involved in learning and memory, attention, emotion, arousal, and reward. Amygdala is essential in regulation of motivational behaviors, such as reward-seeking motivation as well as appetitive and aversive motivational behaviors [137]. Past and recent studies have widely referred to the vital role of the amygdala in many different mechanisms of the brain, such as attention and conditioned reinforcer learning. The results of a study show that psychostimulant drugs such as MPH facilitate learning-induced amygdala plasticity [64].

The specialization and interaction of the amygdala in emotion and the hippocampus in declarative or episodic memory are necessary for reacting and adapting to biologically and socially significant stimuli [138]. Brain imaging studies have also shown a relationship between the activation of amygdala and the hippocampus during emotional memory retrieval [139–141]. The correlation between the two regions can influence the process of sensitizing reward-related motivations [142]. Amygdala is associated with the acquisition of cocaine-induced and food-induced CPP [143] and also with the acquisition or expression of a sucrose and amphetamine CPP [144]. In concurrent studies, it has been found that post-training intra-amygdala microinjections of lidocaine disrupt the consolidation of food-related memory in a CPP task [145]. In another study, intra-amygdala injection of muscarinic cholinergic agonists increased memory in contextual fear conditioning, inhibitory avoidance, and changes in reward magnitude [146]. In addition, the basolateral amygdala (BLA) is a region of the amygdala necessary in making significant experiences memorable. A recent study involving mice showed that neurons that are activated in NAc core and BLA are crucial foundation of cocaine context-related reward memory [147].

Conclusion

MPH is undoubtedly the most effective stimulant medication for the treatment of ADHD and commonly abused drug among young people that its abuse has increased sharply in recent years. Unfortunately, there is still currently no definitive test to diagnose ADHD. ADHD misdiagnosis and wrong medication can be very dangerous and lead to the development of drug abuse. Recent studies show that MPH treatment has the dependence potential to other psychostimulants, such as cocaine and amphetamine [148]. MPH abuse can change the brain's structure as well as neurotransmitter release and neural circuits that are long-lasting and permanent. MPH increases extracellular levels of dopamine and noradrenaline in the key parts of the brain's major parts (striatum and NAc) primarily by inhibiting the reuptake of these catecholamines by their respective transporters. Self-administration of MPH enhances reward-seeking behaviors and increases motivation to administer amphetamine. Psychostimulants such as MPH participate in a set of molecular mechanisms usually involved in learning and memory. As described above, the striatum, NAc, amygdala, and hippocampus are important parts involved in learning-related changes in protein synthesis. Release of dopamine following MPH injection by activating common signal transduction pathways may modify learning-related molecular changes.

The inference from the literature mentioned in this review is that regions involved in central representations of predictive reward are a subset of those that really participate in associative learning.

References

1. Storebø OJ, Ramstad E, Krogh HB, Nilausen TD, Skoog M, Holmskov M, et al. Methylphenidate for children and adolescents with attention deficit hyperactivity disorder (ADHD). Cochrane Database Syst Rev. 2015;15(11):CD009885.
2. Elzein R, Abdelrahman S, Hay M, Lopez M, Bondy M, Morris D, et al. Cytogenetic effects in children treated with methylphenidate. Cancer Lett. 2005;230(2):284–91.
3. Faraone SV, Rostain AL, Montano CB, Mason O, Antshel KM, Newcorn JH. Systematic review: nonmedical use of prescription stimulants: risk factors, outcomes, and risk reduction strategies. J Am Acad Child Adolesc Psychiatry. 2019;59(1).
4. Sturman N, Deckx L, van Driel ML. Methylphenidate for children and adolescents with autism spectrum disorder. Cochrane Database Syst Rev. 2017;11(11):CD011144.
5. Pae CU, Marks DM, Masand PS, Peindl K, Hooper-Wood C, Han C, Mannelli P, Ciccone P, Patkar AA. Methylphenidate extended release (OROS MPH) for the treatment of antidepressant-related sexual dysfunction in patients with treatment-resistant depression. Clin Neuropharmacol. 2009;32(2):85–8.
6. Morton WA, Stockton GG. Methylphenidate abuse and psychiatric side effects. Prim Care Companion CNS Disord. 2000;2(5):159–64.
7. Sheridan MA, Hinshaw S, D'Esposito M. Efficiency of the prefrontal cortex during working memory in attention-deficit/hyperactivity disorder. J Am Acad Child Adolesc Psychiatry. 2007;46(10):1357–66.
8. Koob G, Bloom F. Cellular and molecular mechanisms of drug dependence. Science. 1988;242(4879):715–23.
9. Wise RA, Bozarth MA. Brain mechanisms of drug reward and euphoria. Psychiatr Med. 1985;3(4):445–60.
10. Rapoport JL, Buchsbaum MS, Zahn TP, Weingartner H, Ludlow C, Mikkelsen EJ. Dextroamphetamine: cognitive and behavioral effects in normal prepubertal boys. Science. 1978;199(4328):560–3.
11. Lee C-T, McClernon FJ, Kollins SH, Fuemmeler BF. Childhood ADHD symptoms and future illicit drug use: the role of adolescent cigarette use. J Pediatr Psychol. 2017;43(2):162–71.
12. Buitelaar JK. Epidemiological aspects: what have we learned over the last decade. Hyperact Atten Disord Child. 2002;2:30–63.
13. Rowland AS, Lesesne CA, Abramowitz AJ. The epidemiology of attention-deficit/hyperactivity disorder (ADHD): a public health view. Ment Retard Dev Disabil Res Rev. 2002;8(3):162–70.
14. Accardo P, Blondis TA. What's all the fuss about Ritalin? J Pediatr. 2001;138(1):6–9.
15. Kollins SH. Comparing the abuse potential of methylphenidate versus other stimulants: a review of available evidence and relevance to the ADHD patient. J Clin Psychiatry. 2003;64(Suppl 11):14–8.
16. Kollins SH, MacDonald EK, Rush CR. Assessing the abuse potential of methylphenidate in nonhuman and human subjects: a review. Pharmacol Biochem Behav. 2001;68(3):611–27.
17. Adriani W, Chiarotti F, Laviola G. Elevated novelty seeking and peculiar d-amphetamine sensitization in periadolescent mice compared with adult mice. Behav Neurosci. 1998;112(5):1152–66.
18. Aizenstein ML, Segal DS, Kuczenski R. Repeated amphetamine and fencamfamine: sensitization and reciprocal cross-sensitization. Neuropsychopharmacology. 1990;3(4):283–90.
19. JAFFE SL. Intranasal abuse of prescribed methylphenidate by an alcohol and drug abusing adolescent with ADHD. J Am Acad Child Adolesc Psychiatry. 1991;30(5):773–5.
20. Levin FR, Kleber HD. Attention-deficit hyperactivity disorder and substance abuse: relationships and implications for treatment. Harv Rev Psychiatry. 1995;2(5):246–58.
21. Fernandez-Espejo E, Rodriguez-Espinosa N. Psychostimulant drugs and neuroplasticity. Pharmaceuticals. 2011;4(7):976–91.
22. Kalivas PW, Duffy P, DuMars LA, Skinner C. Behavioral and neurochemical effects of acute and daily cocaine administration in rats. J Pharmacol Exp Ther. 1988;245(2):485–92.
23. Robinson TE. Behavioral sensitization: characterization of enduring changes in rotational behavior produced by intermittent injections of amphetamine in male and female rats. Psychopharmacology. 1984;84(4):466–75.
24. Wolf ME. The role of excitatory amino acids in behavioral sensitization to psychomotor stimulants. Prog Neurobiol. 1998;54(6):679–720.
25. Pan W, Banks WA, Fasold MB, Bluth J, Kastin AJ. Transport of brain-derived neurotrophic factor across the blood–brain barrier. Neuropharmacology. 1998;37(12):1553–61.
26. Sartorius A, Hellweg R, Litzke J, Vogt M, Dormann C, Vollmayr B, et al. Correlations and discrepancies between serum and brain tissue levels of neurotrophins after electroconvulsive treatment in rats. Pharmacopsychiatry. 2009;42(06):270–6.
27. Andero R, Choi DC, Ressler KJ. BDNF–TrkB receptor regulation of distributed adult neural plas-

ticity, memory formation, and psychiatric disorders. Prog Mol Biol Transl Sci. 2014;122:169–92.

28. Grimm JW, Lu L, Hayashi T, Hope BT, Su TP, Shaham Y. Time-dependent increases in brain-derived neurotrophic factor protein levels within the mesolimbic dopamine system after withdrawal from cocaine: implications for incubation of cocaine craving. J Neurosci. 2003;23(3):742–7.
29. Cummins ED, Griffin SB, Duty CM, Peterson DJ, Burgess KC, Brown RW. The role of dopamine D1 and D2 receptors in adolescent methylphenidate conditioned place preference: sex differences and brain-derived neurotrophic factor. Dev Neurosci. 2014;36(3–4):277–86.
30. Fumagalli F, Cattaneo A, Caffino L, Ibba M, Racagni G, Carboni E, et al. Sub-chronic exposure to atomoxetine up-regulates BDNF expression and signalling in the brain of adolescent spontaneously hypertensive rats: comparison with methylphenidate. Pharmacol Res. 2010;62(6):523–9.
31. Chong SL, Claussen CM, Dafny N. Nucleus accumbens neuronal activity in freely behaving rats is modulated following acute and chronic methylphenidate administration. Brain Res Bull. 2012;87(4–5):445–56.
32. Cummins ED, Leedy KK, Dose JM, Peterson DJ, Kirby SL, Hernandez LJ, et al. The effects of adolescent methylphenidate exposure on the behavioral and brain-derived neurotrophic factor response to nicotine. J Psychopharmacol. 2016;31(1):75–85.
33. Horger BA, Iyasere CA, Berhow MT, Messer CJ, Nestler EJ, Taylor JR. Enhancement of locomotor activity and conditioned reward to cocaine by brain-derived neurotrophic factor. J Neurosci. 1999;19(10):4110–22.
34. Routtenberg A. Reverse piedpiperase: is the knockout mouse leading neuroscientists to a watery end? Trends Neurosci. 1996;19(11):471–2.
35. Vargas-Perez H, Ting-A-Kee R, Walton CH, Hansen DM, Razavi R, Clarke L, et al. Ventral tegmental area BDNF induces an opiate-dependent–like reward state in naïve rats. Science. 2009;324(5935):1732–4.
36. Shen W, Wu B, Zhang Z, Dou Y, Rao Z, Chen Y, et al. Activity-induced rapid synaptic maturation mediated by presynaptic Cdc42 signaling. Neuron. 2006;50(3):401–14.
37. Ghitza UE, Zhai H, Wu P, Airavaara M, Shaham Y, Lu L. Role of BDNF and GDNF in drug reward and relapse: a review. Neurosci Biobehav Rev. 2010;35(2):157–71.
38. dela Peña I, Kim H, Sohn A, Kim B-N, Han D, Ryu J, et al. Prefrontal cortical and striatal transcriptional responses to the reinforcing effect of repeated methylphenidate treatment in the spontaneously hypertensive rat, animal model of attention-deficit/hyperactivity disorder (ADHD). Behav Brain Funct. 2014;10(1):17.
39. Kashefi A, Tomaz C, Jamali S, Rashidy-Pour A, Vafaei AA, Haghparast A. Cannabidiol attenuated the maintenance and reinstatement of extinguished methylphenidate-induced conditioned place preference in rats. Brain Res Bull. 2021;166:118–27.
40. Kashefi A, Duarte RB, Jesus FM, Jamali S, Haghparast A, Tomaz C. Methylphenidate produces conditioned place preference, and cannabidiol exposure during extinction does not inhibit the reinstatement of methylphenidate in the marmoset monkeys. Int J Adv Eng Res Sci. 2019;6(7):66–72.
41. Wooters TE, Walton MT, Bardo MT. Oral methylphenidate establishes a conditioned place preference in rats. Neurosci Lett. 2011;487(3):293–6.
42. Freeman ED. Methylphenidate conditioned place preference in juvenile and adolescent male and female rats [Electronic Theses]. East Tennessee State University; 2013.
43. Rush CR, Essman WD, Simpson CA, Baker RW. Reinforcing and subject-rated effects of methylphenidate and d-amphetamine in non–drug-abusing humans. J Clin Psychopharmacol. 2001;21(3):273–86.
44. Rush CR, Baker RW. Behavioral pharmacological similarities between methylphenidate and cocaine in cocaine abusers. Exp Clin Psychopharmacol. 2001;9(1):59–73.
45. Volkow ND, Ding Y-S, Fowler JS, Wang G-J, Logan J, Gatley JS, et al. Is methylphenidate like cocaine? Studies on their pharmacokinetics and distribution in the human brain. Arch Gen Psychiatry. 1995;52(6):456–63.
46. Volkow ND, Swanson JM. Variables that affect the clinical use and abuse of methylphenidate in the treatment of ADHD. Am J Psychiatry. 2003 Nov;160(11):1909–18.
47. Swanson JM, Volkow ND. Serum and brain concentrations of methylphenidate: implications for use and abuse. Neurosci Biobehav Rev. 2003;27(7):615–21.
48. Swanson JM, Volkow ND. Pharmacokinetic and pharmacodynamic properties of stimulants: implications for the design of new treatments for ADHD. Behav Brain Res. 2002;130(1–2):73–8.
49. Bymaster F. Atomoxetine increases extracellular levels of norepinephrine and dopamine in prefrontal cortex of rat A potential mechanism for efficacy in attention deficit/hyperactivity disorder. Neuropsychopharmacology. 2002;27(5):699–711.
50. Tilley MR, Cagniard B, Zhuang X, Han DD, Tiao N, Gu HH. Cocaine reward and locomotion stimulation in mice with reduced dopamine transporter expression. BMC Neurosci. 2007;8(1):42.
51. Barros M, Dempster EL, Illott N, Chabrawi S, Maior RS, Tomaz C, et al. Decreased methylation of the NK3 receptor coding gene (TACR3) after cocaine-induced place preference in marmoset monkeys. Addict Biol. 2013;18(3):452–4.
52. Duarte RBM, Patrono E, Borges AC, César AAS, Tomaz C, Ventura R, et al. Consumption of a highly palatable food induces a lasting place-conditioning memory in marmoset monkeys. Behav Process. 2014;107:163–6.

53. Duarte RBM, Patrono E, Borges AC, Tomaz C, Ventura R, Gasbarri A, et al. High versus low fat/sugar food affects the behavioral, but not the cortisol response of marmoset monkeys in a conditioned-place-preference task. Physiol Behav. 2015;139:442–8.
54. Mahmud A, Gallant S, Sedki F, D'Cunha T, Shalev U. Effects of an acute cannabidiol treatment on cocaine self-administration and cue-induced cocaine seeking in male rats. J Psychopharmacol. 2017;31(1):96–104.
55. Yang G, Liu L, Zhang R, Li J, Leung C-K, Huang J, et al. Cannabidiol attenuates methamphetamine-induced conditioned place preference via the Sigma1R/AKT/GSK-3β/CREB signaling pathway in rats. Toxicol Res (Camb). 2020;9(3):202–11.
56. Volkow ND, Wang G-J, Fowler JS, Logan J, Gatley SJ, Hitzemann R, et al. Decreased striatal dopaminergic responsiveness in detoxified cocaine-dependent subjects. Nature. 1997;386(6627):830–3.
57. Bolanos CA, Barrot M, Berton O, Wallace-Black D, Nestler EJ. Methylphenidate treatment during pre-and periadolescence alters behavioral responses to emotional stimuli at adulthood. Biol Psychiatry. 2003;54(12):1317–29.
58. Brandon CL, Steiner H. Repeated methylphenidate treatment in adolescent rats alters gene regulation in the striatum. Eur J Neurosci. 2003;18(6):1584–92.
59. Brandon CL, Marinelli M, Baker LK, White FJ. Enhanced reactivity and vulnerability to cocaine following methylphenidate treatment in adolescent rats. Neuropsychopharmacology. 2001;25(5):651–61.
60. Brandon CL, Marinelli M, White FJ. Adolescent exposure to methylphenidate alters the activity of rat midbrain dopamine neurons. Biol Psychiatry. 2003;54(12):1338–44.
61. Baik J-H. Dopamine signaling in reward-related behaviors. Front Neural Circuits. 2013;7:152.
62. Meririnne E, Kankaanpää A, Seppälä T. Rewarding properties of methylphenidate: sensitization by prior exposure to the drug and effects of dopamine D1-and D2-receptor antagonists. J Pharmacol Exp Ther. 2001;298(2):539–50.
63. Robinson TE, Berridge KC. The neural basis of drug craving: an incentive-sensitization theory of addiction. Brain Res Rev. 1993;18(3):247–91.
64. Tye KM, Tye LD, Cone JJ, Hekkelman EF, Janak PH, Bonci A. Methylphenidate facilitates learning-induced amygdala plasticity. Nat Neurosci. 2010;13(4):475.
65. Sengupta SM, Grizenko N, Thakur GA, Bellingham J, DeGuzman R, Robinson S, et al. Differential association between the norepinephrine transporter gene and ADHD: role of sex and subtype. J Psychiatry Neurosci. 2012;37(2):129.
66. Zarrindast M-R, Bahreini T, Adl M. Effect of imipramine on the expression and acquisition of morphine-induced conditioned place preference in mice. Pharmacol Biochem Behav. 2002;73(4):941–9.
67. Drouin C, Darracq L, Trovero F, Blanc G, Glowinski J, Cotecchia S, et al. α1b-Adrenergic receptors control locomotor and rewarding effects of psychostimulants and opiates. J Neurosci. 2002;22(7):2873–84.
68. Ventura R, Cabib S, Alcaro A, Orsini C, Puglisi-Allegra S. Norepinephrine in the prefrontal cortex is critical for amphetamine-induced reward and mesoaccumbens dopamine release. J Neurosci. 2003;23(5):1879–85.
69. Guzman D, Moscarello JM, Ettenberg A. The effects of medial prefrontal cortex infusions of cocaine in a runway model of drug self-administration: evidence of reinforcing but not anxiogenic actions. Eur J Pharmacol. 2009;605(1–3):117–22.
70. Fischer AG, Ullsperger M. An update on the role of serotonin and its interplay with dopamine for reward. Front Hum Neurosci. 2017;11:484.
71. Faulkner P, Deakin JFW. The role of serotonin in reward, punishment and behavioural inhibition in humans: insights from studies with acute tryptophan depletion. Neurosci Biobehav Rev. 2014;46:365–78.
72. Izquierdo A, Carlos K, Ostrander S, Rodriguez D, McCall-Craddolph A, Yagnik G, et al. Impaired reward learning and intact motivation after serotonin depletion in rats. Behav Brain Res. 2012;233(2):494–9.
73. Walker SC, Robbins TW, Roberts AC. Differential contributions of dopamine and serotonin to orbitofrontal cortex function in the marmoset. Cereb Cortex. 2009;19(4):889–98.
74. Carbone C, Lo Russo SLM, Lacivita E, Frank A, Alleva E, Stark H, et al. Prior activation of 5-HT7 receptors modulates the conditioned place preference with methylphenidate. Front Behav Neurosci. 2019;13:208.
75. Galici R, Boggs JD, Miller KL, Bonaventure P, Atack JR. Effects of SB-269970, a 5-HT7 receptor antagonist, in mouse models predictive of antipsychotic-like activity. Behav Pharmacol. 2008;19(2):153–9.
76. Waters KA, Stean TO, Hammond B, Virley DJ, Upton N, Kew JNC, et al. Effects of the selective 5-HT7 receptor antagonist SB-269970 in animal models of psychosis and cognition. Behav Brain Res. 2012;228(1):211–8.
77. Yagishita S. Transient and sustained effects of dopamine and serotonin signaling in motivation-related behavior. Psychiatry Clin Neurosci. 2020;74(2):91–8.
78. Mantsch JR, Baker DA, Funk D, Lê AD, Shaham Y. Stress-induced reinstatement of drug seeking: 20 years of progress. Neuropsychopharmacology. 2016;41(1):335–56.
79. Kalivas PW, Weber B. Amphetamine injection into the ventral mesencephalon sensitizes rats to peripheral amphetamine and cocaine. J Pharmacol Exp Ther. 1988;245(3):1095–102.
80. Vezina P, Stewart J. Amphetamine administered to the ventral tegmental area but not to the nucleus accumbens sensitizes rats to systemic morphine: lack of conditioned effects. Brain Res. 1990;516(1):99–106.

81. Hooks MS, Jones GH, Liem BJ, Justice JB Jr. Sensitization and individual differences to IP amphetamine, cocaine, or caffeine following repeated intracranial amphetamine infusions. Pharmacol Biochem Behav. 1992;43(3):815–23.
82. Karim TJ, Reyes-Vazquez C, Dafny N. Comparison of the VTA and LC response to methylphenidate: a concomitant behavioral and neuronal study of adolescent male rats. J Neurophysiol. 2017;118(3):1501–14.
83. Suto N, Austin JD, Tanabe LM, Kramer MK, Wright DA, Vezina P. Previous exposure to VTA amphetamine enhances cocaine self-administration under a progressive ratio schedule in a D 1 dopamine receptor dependent manner. Neuropsychopharmacology. 2002;27(6):970–9.
84. Volkow N, Morales M. The brain on drugs: from reward to addiction. Cell. 2015;162(4):712–25.
85. Goudriaan AE, Veltman DJ, van den Brink W, Dom G, Schmaal L. Neurophysiological effects of modafinil on cue-exposure in cocaine dependence: a randomized placebo-controlled cross-over study using pharmacological fMRI. Addict Behav. 2013;38(2):1509–17.
86. Wanchoo SJ. Role of dopamine of nucleus accumbens in behavioral sensitization to methylphenidate. UT Grad Sch Biomed Sci Houst Diss Theses. 2010;14.
87. Salinas-Hernández XI, Duvarci S. Dopamine in Fear Extinction. Front Synaptic Neurosci. 2021;13:10.
88. Bariselli S, Contestabile A, Tzanoulinou S, Bellone C. SHANK3 downregulation in the VTA accelerates the extinction of contextual associations induced by non-familiar conspecific interaction. Front Mol Neurosci. 2018;342295.
89. Perry JL, Joseph JE, Jiang Y, Zimmerman RS, Kelly TH, Darna M, et al. Prefrontal cortex and drug abuse vulnerability: translation to prevention and treatment interventions. Brain Res Rev. 2011;65(2):124–49.
90. Kodama T, Kojima T, Honda Y, Hosokawa T, Tsutsui K, Watanabe M. Oral administration of methylphenidate (ritalin) affects dopamine release differentially between the prefrontal cortex and striatum: a microdialysis study in the monkey. J Neurosci. 2017;37(9):2387–94.
91. Jedema HP, Narendran R, Bradberry CW. Amphetamine-induced release of dopamine in primate prefrontal cortex and striatum: striking differences in magnitude and timecourse. J Neurochem. 2014;130(4):490–7.
92. Narendran R, Jedema HP, Lopresti BJ, Mason NS, Gurnsey K, Ruszkiewicz J, et al. Imaging dopamine transmission in the frontal cortex: a simultaneous microdialysis and [11 C] FLB 457 PET study. Mol Psychiatry. 2014;19(3):302–10.
93. Devilbiss DM, Berridge CW. Cognition-enhancing doses of methylphenidate preferentially increase prefrontal cortex neuronal responsiveness. Biol Psychiatry. 2008;64(7):626–35.
94. Tian W, Zhao M, Li M, Song T, Zhang M, Quan L, et al. Reversal of cocaine-conditioned place preference through methyl supplementation in mice: altering global DNA methylation in the prefrontal cortex. PLoS One. 2012;7(3):e33435.
95. Pena-Bravo JI, Reichel CM, Lavin A. Abstinence from cocaine-induced conditioned place preference produces discrete changes in glutamatergic synapses onto deep layer 5/6 neurons from prelimbic and infralimbic cortices. Eneuro. 2017;4(6).
96. Engert V, Pruessner JC. Dopaminergic and noradrenergic contributions to functionality in ADHD: the role of methylphenidate. Curr Neuropharmacol. 2008;6(4):322–8.
97. Zarrindast M-R, Izadi M, Nasehi M, Paktinat A, Hoseinpourfard M. Reward system on dopaminergic pathway. Int J Med Rev. 2015;2(3):261–4.
98. Denys D, Mantione M, Figee M, Van Den Munckhof P, Koerselman F, Westenberg H, et al. Deep brain stimulation of the nucleus accumbens for treatment-refractory obsessive-compulsive disorder. Arch Gen Psychiatry. 2010;67(10):1061–8.
99. García-García I, Morys F, Dagher A. Nucleus accumbens volume is related to obesity measures in an age-dependent fashion. J Neuroendocrinol. 2020;32(12):e12812.
100. Strasser A, Xin L, Gruetter R, Sandi C. Nucleus accumbens neurochemistry in human anxiety: a 7 T 1H-MRS study. Eur Neuropsychopharmacol. 2019;29(3):365–75.
101. Ma K, Zhang H, Wang S, Wang H, Wang Y, Liu J, Song X, Dong Z, Han X, Zhang Y, Li H, Rahaman A, Wang S, Baloch Z. The molecular mechanism underlying GABAergic dysfunction in nucleus accumbens of depression-like behaviours in mice. J Cell Mol Med. 2019;23(10):7021–8.
102. Whittaker JR, Foley SF, Ackling E, Murphy K, Caseras X. The functional connectivity between the nucleus accumbens and the ventromedial prefrontal cortex as an endophenotype for bipolar disorder. Biol Psychiatry. 2018;84(11):803–9.
103. Hirano M, Iritani S, Fujishiro H, Torii Y, Habuchi C, Sekiguchi H, Yoshida M, Ozaki N. Clinicopathological differences between the motor onset and psychiatric onset of Huntington's disease, focusing on the nucleus accumbens. Neuropathology. 2019;39(5):331–41.
104. Carriere N, Besson P, Dujardin K, Duhamel A, Defebvre L, Delmaire C, Devos D. Apathy in Parkinson's disease is associated with nucleus accumbens atrophy: a magnetic resonance imaging shape analysis. Mov Disord. 2014;29(7):897–903.
105. Cordella A, Krashia P, Nobili A, Pignataro A, La Barbera L, Viscomi MT, Valzania A, Keller F, Ammassari-Teule M, Mercuri NB, Berretta N, D'Amelio M. Dopamine loss alters the hippocampus-nucleus accumbens synaptic transmission in the Tg2576 mouse model of Alzheimer's disease. Neurobiol Dis. 2018;116:142–54.

106. Salgado S, Kaplitt MG. The nucleus accumbens: a comprehensive review. Stereotact Funct Neurosurg. 2015;93(2):75–93.
107. Klawonn AM, Malenka RC. Nucleus accumbens modulation in reward and aversion. Cold Spring Harb Symp Quant Biol. 2018;83:119–29.
108. Schwienbacher I, Fendt M, Richardson R, Schnitzler HU. Temporary inactivation of the nucleus accumbens disrupts acquisition and expression of fear-potentiated startle in rats. Brain Res. 2004;1027(1–2):87–93.
109. Basar K, Sesia T, Groenewegen H, Steinbusch HW, Visser-Vandewalle V, Temel Y. Nucleus accumbens and impulsivity. Prog Neurobiol. 2010;92(4):533–57.
110. Hopkin M. Revealed: how the mind processes placebo effect. Nature. 2007.
111. Di Chiara G, Bassareo V, Fenu S, De Luca MA, Spina L, Cadoni C, Acquas E, Carboni E, Valentini V, Lecca D. Dopamine and drug addiction: the nucleus accumbens shell connection. Neuropharmacology. 2004;47:227–41.
112. Arefin TM. GPR88 signatures in mouse neuronal connectivity and behavior: a potential therapeutic target for psychiatric disorders [Theses]. Albert-Ludwigs-Universität Freiburg; 2017.
113. Wadenberg ML, Ericson E, Magnusson O, Ahlenius S. Suppression of conditioned avoidance behavior by the local application of (−)sulpiride into the ventral, but not the dorsal, striatum of the rat. Biol Psychiatry. 1990;28(4):297–307.
114. McCullough LD, Sokolowski JD, Salamone JD. A neurochemical and behavioral investigation of the involvement of nucleus accumbens dopamine in instrumental avoidance. Neuroscience. 1993;52(4):919–25. Disponível em: https://doi.org/10.1016/0306-4522(93)90538-q.
115. Everitt BJ, Morris KA, O'Brien A, Robbins TW. The basolateral amygdala-ventral striatal system and conditioned place preference: further evidence of limbic-striatal interactions underlying reward-related processes. Neuroscience. 1991;42(1):1–18.
116. Carr GD, White NM. Conditioned place preference from intra-accumbens but not intra-caudate amphetamine injections. Life Sci. 1983;33(25):2551–7.
117. Karimi S, Radahmadi M, Fazilati M, Azizi-Malekabadi H, Alaei H. Roles of the nucleus accumbens (shell) in the acquisition and expression of morphine-induced conditioned behavior in freely moving rats. Int J Prev Med. 2014;5(3):262.
118. Taber M, Fibiger H. Electrical stimulation of the prefrontal cortex increases dopamine release in the nucleus accumbens of the rat: modulation by metabotropic glutamate receptors. J Neurosci [Internet]. 1 maio 1995 [citado 18 nov 2022];15(5):3896–904. Disponível em: https://doi.org/10.1523/jneurosci.15-05-03896.1995.
119. McEwen BS, Chao HM, Angulo JA. Glucocorticoid and estrogen effects on the nigrostriatal and mesolimbic dopaminergic systems. In: Trophic regulation of the basal ganglia. Neuroscience Biobehavioural Review; 1994. p. 67–88.
120. Delfs J, Schreiber L, Kelley A. Microinjection of cocaine into the nucleus accumbens elicits locomotor activation in the rat. J Neurosci. 1990;10(1):303–10.
121. Essman WD, McGonigle P, Lucki I. Anatomical differentiation within the nucleus accumbens of the locomotor stimulatory actions of selective dopamine agonists andd-amphetamine. Psychopharmacology. 1993;112(2–3):233–41.
122. Zhu X, Ottenheimer D, DiLeone RJ. Activity of D1/2 receptor expressing neurons in the nucleus accumbens regulates running, locomotion, and food intake. Front Behav Neurosci. 2016;10:66.
123. Izquierdo I, Cammarota M, Da Silva WC, Bevilaqua LRM, Rossato JI, Bonini JS, et al. The evidence for hippocampal long-term potentiation as a basis of memory for simple tasks. An Acad Bras Cienc. 2008;80(1):115–27.
124. Peigneux P, Laureys S, Fuchs S, Collette F, Perrin F, Reggers J, et al. Are spatial memories strengthened in the human hippocampus during slow wave sleep? Neuron. 2004;44(3):535–45.
125. Heysieattalab S, Naghdi N, Hosseinmardi N, Zarrindast M-R, Haghparast A, Khoshbouei H. Methamphetamine-induced enhancement of hippocampal long-term potentiation is modulated by NMDA and GABA receptors in the shell-accumbens. Synapse. 2016;70(8):325–35.
126. Barr JL, Bray B, Forster GL. The hippocampus as a neural link between negative affect and vulnerability for psychostimulant relapse. In: Stuchlik A, editor. Hippocampus—plasticity functions. London: UK IntechOpen Limited; 2018. p. 127–67.
127. Gawin F. Cocaine addiction: psychology and neurophysiology. Science. 1991;251(5001):1580–6.
128. Gawin FH. Abstinence symptomatology and psychiatric diagnosis in cocaine abusers. Arch Gen Psychiatry. 1986;43(2):107.
129. Gossop M. Review: limited evidence to support pharmacological therapy for amphetamine withdrawal. Evid Based Ment Health. 2009;12(4):122.
130. Resnick RB, Resnick EB. Cocaine abuse and its treatment. Psychiatr Clin North Am. 1984;7(4):713–28.
131. Romanelli F, Smith KM. Clinical effects and management of methamphetamine abuse. Pharmacotherapy. 2006;26(8):1148–56.
132. Shoptaw SJ, Kao U, Heinzerling K, Ling W. Treatment for amphetamine withdrawal. Cochrane Database Syst Rev. 2009;2:CD003021.
133. Barr AM, Markou A. Psychostimulant withdrawal as an inducing condition in animal models of depression. Neurosci Biobehav Rev. 2005;29(4–5):675–706.
134. Cryan JF, Hoyer D, Markou A. Withdrawal from chronic amphetamine induces depressive-like behavioral effects in rodents. Biol Psychiatry. 2003;54(1):49–58.
135. Kishi T, Matsuda Y, Iwata N, Correll CU. Antipsychotics for cocaine or psycho-

stimulant dependence. J Clin Psychiatry. 2013;74(12):e1169–80.
136. Pérez-Mañá C, Castells X, Torrens M, Capellà D, Farre M. Efficacy of psychostimulant drugs for amphetamine abuse or dependence. Cochrane Database Syst Rev. 2013;9:CD009695.
137. Everitt BJ, Cardinal RN, Parkinson JA, Robbins TW. Appetitive behavior: impact of amygdala-dependent mechanisms of emotional learning. Ann N Y Acad Sci. 2003;985(1):233–50.
138. Smith APR, Stephan KE, Rugg MD, Dolan RJ. Task and content modulate amygdala-hippocampal connectivity in emotional retrieval. Neuron. 2006;49(4):631–8.
139. Maratos EJ, Dolan RJ, Morris JS, Henson RNA, Rugg MD. Neural activity associated with episodic memory for emotional context. Neuropsychologia. 2001;39(9):910–20.
140. Phelps EA, O'Connor KJ, Gatenby JC, Gore JC, Grillon C, Davis M. Activation of the left amygdala to a cognitive representation of fear. Nat Neurosci. 2001;4(4):437–41.
141. Smith APR, Henson RNA, Dolan RJ, Rugg MD. fMRI correlates of the episodic retrieval of emotional contexts. NeuroImage. 2004;22(2):868–78.
142. Becker S, Navratilova E, Nees F, Van Damme S. Emotional and motivational pain processing: current state of knowledge and perspectives in translational research. Pain Res Manag. 2018;2018:1–12.
143. Brown EE, Fibiger HC. Differential effects of excitotoxic lesions of the amygdala on cocaine-induced conditioned locomotion and conditioned place preference. Psychopharmacology. 1993;113(1):123–30.
144. Hiroi N, White N. The lateral nucleus of the amygdala mediates expression of the amphetamine-produced conditioned place preference. J Neurosci. 1991;11(7):2107–16.
145. Hsu EH, Schroeder JP, Packard MG. The amygdala mediates memory consolidation for an amphetamine conditioned place preference. Behav Brain Res. 2002;129(1–2):93–100.
146. McGaugh J. Amygdala modulation of memory consolidation: interaction with other brain systems. Neurobiol Learn Mem. 2002;78(3):539–52.
147. Wang J-J, Yao W-Q, Chen Y-J, Ma L, Tao Y-Z. Neurons in NAc core and BLA are activated during cocaine context-associated reward memory retrieval in mice. Sheng Li Xue Bao Acta Physiol Sin. 2014;66(5):545–58.
148. Calipari ES, Ferris MJ, Salahpour A, Caron MG, Jones SR. Methylphenidate amplifies the potency and reinforcing effects of amphetamines by increasing dopamine transporter expression. Nat Commun. 2013;4:2720.

The Neuroesteroids and Its Association with Carcinogenesis and Drug Use. Impact on the Reproductive Axis

28

Myriam Raquel Laconi,
Antonella Rosario Ramona Cáceres,
María de los Ángeles Sanhueza,
and Daniela Alejandra Cardone

Introduction

The hypothalamic-pituitary-gonadal (HPG) axis is critical for reproduction and includes neuroendocrine networks that integrate a wide range of internal and external inputs to coordinate reproductive competence. Gonadotropin-releasing hormone (GnRH) is a decapeptide and the main regulator of reproduction. It controls gonadotropin secretion and, subsequently, gonadal function [1].

Authors Myriam Raquel Laconi and Antonella Rosario Ramona Cáceres have contributed equally to this chapter.

M. R. Laconi (✉) · A. R. R. Cáceres · D. A. Cardone
Laboratorio de Fisiopatología ovárica, Instituto de Medicina y Biología Experimental de Cuyo IMBECU- CONICET, Mendoza, Argentina

Cátedra de Fisiología y Biofísica. Facultad de Ingeniería y Facultad de Ciencias Médicas, Universidad de Mendoza, Mendoza, Argentina
e-mail: mlaconi@mendoza-conicet.gob.ar; acaceres@mendoza-conicet.gob.ar

María de los Ángeles Sanhueza
Laboratorio de Fisiopatología ovárica, Instituto de Medicina y Biología Experimental de Cuyo IMBECU- CONICET, Mendoza, Argentina
e-mail: msanhueza@mendoza-conicet.gob.ar

It is known that a group of kisspeptin neurons in the arcuate nucleus of the hypothalamus are in charge of GnRH pulsatile release [2]. The pulses are regulated by a gonadotropin feedback system. GnRH acts on gonadotropic cells of the adenohypophysis, which in turn release gonadotropins, luteinizing hormone (LH), and follicle stimulating hormone (FSH). Fast pulsatile release stimulates LH and slow release FSH. Alteration of these patterns induces reproductive pathologies. In the ovary, LH and FSH bind to granulosa and theca cells to stimulate folliculogenesis, sex steroid, and gonadal peptide production.

The regulation of GnRH secretion is a complex process involving different stimulatory and inhibitory factors such as γ-amino butyric acid (GABA) and neurosteroids [3]. Feleder et al. [4] suggested that the receptors for GnRH are in the axon terminals in the median eminence of the hypothalamus and in glutamatergic and GABAergic neurons. Also, GnRH could perform as an ultra-short auto inhibitory or stimulatory feedback of its own secretion. It is well established that gonadotropin-releasing hormone (GnRH) neurons do not express critical receptors for reproduction (oestrogen receptor alpha, ER-α-, or classical progesterone receptor, PGR). Control of reproduction in the central nervous system (CNS), such as sexual maturation,

P. Á. Gargiulo, H. L. Mesones-Arroyo (eds.), *Psychiatry and Neuroscience Update – Vol. V*,
https://doi.org/10.1007/978-3-031-72219-6_28

requires signalling between progesterone (P4) synthesizing astrocytes, kisspeptin, and GnRH neurons [5].

The role of neurosteroids in the CNS is well known, whereas in gonadal functions they have not yet been fully explored. In this chapter we will focus on the effects of P4, allopregnanolone or 3α,5α-tetrahydroprogesterone (ALLO), pregnenolone or 3α,5β-tetrahydroprogesterone (P5), and dehydroepiandrosterone (DHEA) on the hypothalamic-pituitary-gonadal axis and reproductive pathophysiological processes, such as carcinogenesis. We will also discuss the association with drug use and its possible effects.

Neurosteroids and the Hypothalamic-Pituitary-Gonadal Axis

The term "neurosteroids" was introduced by Baulieu, and it refers to biologically active steroids generated in the brain [6–8]. They are involved in the neuroendocrine control of reproduction and in the control of sexual behaviour and sexual differentiation in the brain. It has been found that even after depletion of peripheral steroids by procedures such as adrenalectomy, castration, and hypophysectomy, several steroids and their sulphated and lipid esters were found to be accumulated in the brains of several mammalian species [9–12]. Therefore, steroids can be synthesised locally de novo from cholesterol in the brain.

The nervous system expresses the two proteins that initiate steroidogenesis, steroidogenesis acute regulatory protein (StAR) and cholesterol side-chain cleavage enzyme (P450scc) [13–15]. Schwann cells and type 1 astrocytes can produce neurosteroids, such as P4, DHEA, 17β-oestradiol, and steroids reduced to 5α-3α,5α-tetrahydrodeoxycorticosterone (THDOC), ALLO, and P5 [6]. In this review, we chose to focus on the neurosteroids P4, P5, ALLO, and DHEA since they have been the most studied in recent years. In particular, ALLO has gained relevance in clinical pharmacology as a molecule of interest in various psychiatric and neurological pathologies [16–19].

The mechanisms of action of neurosteroids involve two kinds of responses: a fast response, via membrane or surface effects that entail modulation of ion-channel receptors, and a slow response, via cytosolic receptors, through traditional genomic expression [20]. Rapid membrane-initiated signalling can affect neuronal responsiveness and alter reproductive physiological processes [21, 22]. Classical steroid receptors can be "trafficked" to the plasma membrane [23–26] and interact with G proteins and signalling kinases to mediate rapid effects [27]. A "ligand-independent activation" of PR has been described, where not only the cognate ligand (P4), but also nitric oxide [28], and dopamine [29], can elicit P4-like effects in reproductive behaviour [30]. The action of neurosteroids on the HPG axis can be also exerted through interaction with various neurotransmission systems, such as the gabaergic, dopaminergic [31, 32], noradrenergic [22], and glutamatergic systems [33, 34]. GABA acts on the axis at different levels (brain, pituitary, and gonadal), and these actions are mediated by binding to its specific $GABA_{A/C}$ and/or $GABA_B$ receptors [35].

Little is known about the role of neurosteroids in male reproduction and sexual differentiation of the brain. Male rats do have higher cerebellar levels of StAR, P450scc, and mRNA aromatase [36]. It is currently uncertain to what extent neurosteroids such as 3α-dihydroprogesterone may affect FSH or LH secretion. In contrast to females, oestrogen does not induce hypothalamic P4 production to stimulate GnRH release in castrated adrenalectomised males [37]. However, recent findings demonstrate that male aromatase neurons convert testosterone to oestradiol (E2) to regulate kisspeptin neuron activity [38].

The release of GnRH for an LH surge requires P4 acting through hypothalamic P4 receptors [39, 40]. The astrocytes that synthesise P4 are first stimulated by activation of oestrogen-sensitive membrane receptors. It has been shown that the administration of supraphysiological amounts of oestrogen (50 μg subcutaneous, unique dose) to ovariectomised/adrenalectomised rats induces de novo synthesis of P4 in the medial basal hypothalamus, in addition to LH surge via the release of GnRH [37, 41]. Oestrogen treatment increases the conversion of P5 to P4 through the increase of 3β-HSD mRNA [41]. LH induces neuronal P5 production through the modulation of LH receptor expression, increased mitochondrial cholesterol transport, and increased P450scc-mediated cholesterol cleavage [42]. Furthermore, it has been shown that the LH surge does not occur if hypothalamic P4 synthesis is blocked in female rats, demonstrating the importance of P4 signalling [37, 43, 44].

The relevance of neurosteroids in male reproduction is revealed following pharmacological treatments that inhibit 5α-reductases (Type 1 and 2). Treatments based on dutasteride/finasteride cause a reduction of ALLO concentrations in blood and brain, which also affect the composition of $GABA_A$ receptor subunits. The above-mentioned effects are associated with post-finasteride syndromes, e.g. induced mood swings up to suicide [45]. The post-finasteride syndrome causes loss of libido, erectile dysfunction, decreased arousal, and difficulty in reaching orgasm, as side effects that persist despite withdrawal of the drug [46, 47].

Allopregnanolone

Allopregnanolone is the most studied regarding its actions on the HPG axis, as a potent positive allosteric modulator of GABA action on the $GABA_A$ receptor [31, 48]. At low nanomolar concentrations, ALLO enhances GABA currents by acting allosterically on the $GABA_A$ receptor, whereas in a sub-micromolar-to-micromolar range it activates the $GABA_A$ receptor channel complex [49].

ALLO, through GABAergic allosteric agonism, inhibits GnRH and LH release in 30-day-old female rats, postponing their sexual maturation [50–52]. The same effect is repeated on the day of oestrus causing an inhibitory effect on the pituitary LH surge release, altering ovulation and female sexual receptivity [34, 53]. ALLO under natural or stressful situations has an inhibitory effect over the HPG of luteal-phase sheep [54]. Also, Laconi et al. [55] established the participation of ALLO in the control of pituitary hormone secretion which causes modifications in the synthesis and release of steroid and protein hormones at both hypothalamic and gonadal levels [33, 56, 57].

ALLO inhibits dopaminergic and noradrenergic neurons located in the hypothalamus through both types of receptors ($GABA_A$ and $GABA_B$) [55, 58–63]. Magnaghi et al. [64] suggested that ALLO controls $GABA_B$ receptor expression through $GABA_A$ receptors and reveals a complex mechanism involving both receptors in Schwann cell biology. Akema and Kimura [65] proposed that the $GABA_B$ receptor is involved in the LH response to oestrogens in castrated female rats, while other authors attribute sexual differences in post-castration gonadotropin increase, together with $GABA_A$ receptors [66, 67].

ALLO intracerebroventricularly (i.c.v) administered in cycling female rats inhibits pituitary LH release and increases serum P4 concentration, without altering oestrogen concentrations. Both effects are mediated by the $GABA_A$ receptor since, when inhibited with bicuculline, the effect was lost [22, 55]. ALLO central actions thus delayed ovarian corpus luteum luteolysis evidenced by an increase in the enzymatic activity of 3-β-hydroxysteroid dehydrogenase and serum P4 [22, 57].

Studies in women showed the utility of P4 derivatives for the modulation of postpartum depression [68–70], peri-menopausal syndrome [71, 72], to decrease anxiety and to facilitate recognition memory in adulthood [48, 60, 73, 74]. In female rats, the substitutive hormonal treatment with P4 and ALLO reverted the cognitive deficit caused by long-term ovariectomy. Both treatments increased the number of dendritic spines and induced a structural reorganisation of the basal dendritic trees in the *stratum oriens* [73, 75].

The i.c.v administration of ALLO in a dose similar to concentrations under stress conditions can induce the dysregulation of the HPG axis altering ovarian morphophysiology and thus inhibiting ovulation and female sexual receptivity, probably by modifying the activity of central GABA and dopamine [32, 55, 57, 76]. On the other hand, ALLO central administration exerted a protective effect on luteal cells and was involved in anti-luteolytic effects [57]. In gonadectomised rats ALLO induced a decrease in the DA/DOPAC turnover index in the preoptic area and in the basal mid-hypothalamus (MBH). These changes could be responsible for the inhibition of sexual receptivity and/or the release of gonadotropins [32, 60] (Fig. 28.1).

ALLO in male rats potentiates $GABA_A$ channel activity in the medial preoptic area, a region essential for sexual interest, erection, copulation, and ejaculation [78–80]. Pregnenolone sulphate (PS) opposes the effects of ALLO.

Currently, the actions of ALLO are being studied in parallel at four levels (CNS, peripheral nervous system, ovary, and granulosa cells). The results (not yet published) indicate that there are notable effects in the regulation of apoptosis, angiogenesis, and proliferation depending on the concentration and the route of administration used [81].

Other types of receptors abundant in the CNS are glutamate receptors, ionotropic or metabotropic, which can be found in the hypothalamic nuclei and are critical for reproductive functions. It is proposed that glutamate exerts fundamental functions in the control of processes such as puberty, pulsatility, and the preovulatory peak of gonadotropins, reproductive behaviour

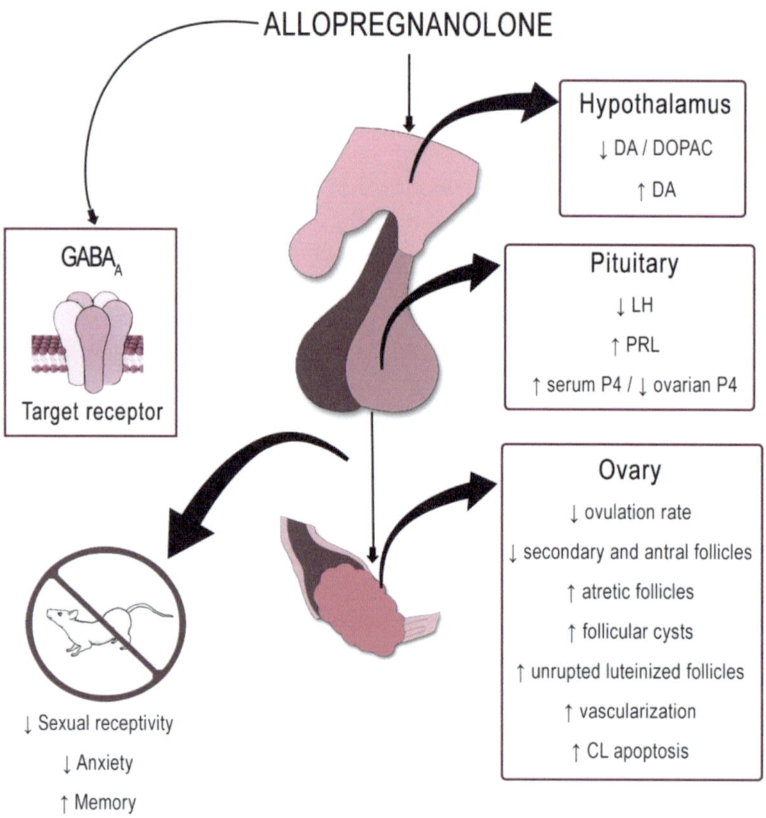

Fig. 28.1 Effects of ALLO through the hypothalamic-pituitary-ovarian axis. ALLO acts at the hypothalamic level decreasing the DA/DOPAC turnover rate in the preoptic area and increasing DA at the basal mid-hypothalamus [31, 32]. It acts as a positive allosteric modulator of $GABA_A$ by increasing hypothalamic activity and thereby inhibiting GnRH and LH release in female rats and increasing serum PRL levels [33, 34, 48, 55]. ALLO-administered i.c.v caused an increase in serum P4 and a decrease at the ovarian level [55, 57, 76]. ALLO inhibits female rat sexual behaviour, as well as reducing anxiety levels and improving memory [48, 60, 73, 77]. *DA* dopamine, *DOPAC* 3, 4-Dihydroxyphenylacetic acid, *PRL* prolactin, *P4* progesterone, *LH* luteinizing hormone

[82–86], and ageing [87–89]. ALLO has been associated with the NMDA and GABA receptor in relation to puberty processes and specific actions in the oestrous cycle of the female rat [33, 34]. The sulphated forms of some neurosteroids, allopregnanolone sulphate and PS, have been effectively shown to be positive allosteric modulators of the NMDA receptor [90–92]. Direct actions of ALLO and P5 on sexual behaviour in female rats have also been reported. Their effects can be inhibitory [48, 60] or stimulatory, depending on the dose and the route of administration [93, 94].

Dehydroepiandrosterone

Dehydroepiandrosterone (DHEA-3β-hydroxyandrost-5-en-17-one) is another neurosteroid produced by the adrenal gland and the CNS, and the precursor of oestrogens and androgens. Baulieu [95] mentioned DHEA as one of the neurosteroids with the ability to beneficially influence some deficits associated with ageing in rats. The ageing process is accompanied by a decrease in GnRH expression, a decrease in the adrenal production of DHEA and its sulphated ester (DHEA-S), as well as a decrease in the plasma levels of both steroids [96]. DHEA-S inhibits postsynaptic $GABA_A$ receptor activation in GnRH neurons of diestrous female mice [97].

Subcutaneous administration of DHEA in old rats restored GnRH expression levels [98]. In females, there are lower GnRH concentrations in the MBH of middle-aged animals in constant oestrus stage compared to those observed in cyclic young rats. In young adult females, DHEA produced an increase in GnRH mRNA in both intact and ovariectomised animals [98–100]. In the sheep, DHEA stimulates primordial follicle initiation and early preantral to antral follicular development in the gonadotropin-responsive stages, enhanced granulosa cell proliferation, and modulated local growth factors [101]. In vivo studies demonstrate that DHEA treatment has stimulating effects on folliculogenesis [102]. A subcutaneous injection of DHEA to rats in the pre- and post-pubertal period induced an increase in ovarian weight, the number of ovarian cysts, and the thickness of the uterus [103]. DHEA inhibits proliferation and promotes apoptosis of ovarian granulosa cells through down-regulation of human *Interferon-γ* (IFN-γ) expression in rats with polycystic ovary syndrome [104].

The use of systemic DHEA therapy improves sexual function in peri- and postmenopausal women and those with adrenal insufficiency [105]. In a primary culture study of rat Leydig cells, DHEA prevented oxidative damage and inhibited early apoptosis of cells, previously induced by hydrogen peroxide (H_2O_2) [106]. DHEA supplementation in women with poor ovarian response improved their reaction to *in vitro* fertilisation [107]. Vaginal administration of DHEA has recently been approved by the Food and Drug Administration (FDA) as effective and safe for relieving genitourinary symptoms in menopausal women [108].

Pregnenolone

Pregnenolone (P5-pregn-5-en-3β-ol-20-one) is synthesised in glial cells and neurons. P5 appears altered frequently in cerebral pathological conditions and has been reported as a biomarker of schizophrenia, anxiety-depressive disorders, stress, and cognitive alterations [109–111]. Low levels of P5 can contribute to headaches or cognitive dysfunctions in patients with migraine during menstruation [112]. P5 also promotes recovery from fatigue, has neuroprotective effects, and promotes myelination in brain neurons [109, 110, 113]. In its sulphated form, pregnenolone sulphate (PS) can directly potentiate GnRH release through the NMDA receptor in hypothalamic neurons and through an autocrine excitatory loop by also increasing the local production of glutamate [114].

PS acts as an endogenous neuroactive steroid, although its mechanisms and functions have not yet been well established. PS regulates PRL synthesis and secretion in vivo and in vitro through mitogen-activated protein kinase (MAPK) signalling, suggesting that it could be used as a therapy to treat PRL-related disorders [115].

As for P5, it activates oestrogen receptor (ER)-related signalling through oestrogen receptor-beta (ERβ) without being converted to other steroid hormones in uterine cells. Activation of ERβ by P5 can regulate cell proliferation and functions in reproductive organs that express ERβ. P5 was found to decrease ovarian cell proliferation and viability [116]. P5, in a cell culture model of antral follicles, restored the steroidogenesis of hormones except oestradiol, but was not able to prevent growth inhibition. It also increases follicle atresia generated by a metabolite of the pesticide methoxychlor [117]. An ICV administration of PS reduces female pheromone odour cues relevant to male sexual interest [118]. Han et al. [119] blocked testicular steroidogenesis with an active immunisation method against P5. This, in turn, reduced hypothalamic GnRH synthesis and pituitary LH synthesis by abrogating the action of sex steroids on hypothalamic GnRH neurons. Thus, it synergistically suppresses spermatogenesis and induces testicular atrophy.

In mice, LH induces the production of neuronal P5 through modulation of the expression of the LH receptor [42]. These studies suggest that P5 and its sulphated form are capable of altering male and female steroidogenesis and reproductive physiology.

Neurosteroids and Carcinogenesis in Reproductive Tissues

Neurosteroids have a neuroprotective effect on glioma genesis [120]. High concentrations of oestrogens in the female brain could bind to nuclear or membrane receptors and potentially stimulate different interconnected signalling pathways [120]. In rat pituitary adenoma cells, PS significantly increases PRL mRNA and protein levels [115].

Neurosteroids can also affect carcinogenic processes in reproductive tissues. In ovarian cancer cell culture, P4 may act as an anti-tumour molecule, reducing cell migration, invasion, and proliferation. These processes might be occurring via the P4 receptor (PR) or via modulation of the protein kinase pathway, as a decrease in FAK and Src phosphorylation was observed [121–124]. In contrast, Pelegrina et al. [125] showed that both P4 and ALLO, in ovarian epithelial carcinoma-derived cells, increased migration in a concentration-dependent manner, producing the maximum effect at the lowest concentration (10^{-11}M), while ALLO alone increased both cell proliferation and migration at physiological concentrations (10^{-11}M) at higher concentrations (10^{-5}M).

Neurosteroid levels were measured in postmenopausal women with ovarian and endometrial cancer. In this study, the risk of ovarian and endometrial cancer was not associated with circulating P4 levels, but an increased P4-E2 ratio was inversely associated for endometrial cancer. An increase in 17-hydroxypregnenolone levels was positively associated with ovarian cancer and conversely associated with endometrial cancer [126]. P4 was also significantly elevated in postmenopausal women with mucinous ovarian tumours [127].

P4 and progestins have also been associated with breast cancer risk. Trabert et al. [126] have measured circulating concentrations of P4 and its major metabolites in patients with breast cancer diagnosed during 12 years of follow-up and in postmenopausal women not using exogenous hormones. Increased levels of circulating P4 were linked to a moderately increased risk of breast cancer. Wiebe et al. [128] found in breast cancer-derived cell lines that P4 4-pregnene derivatives may have anti-tumour effects, whereas 5-alpha-pregnene derivatives are pro-tumourigenic. In addition, P4 receptors have been used as prognostic markers of breast cancer and ERα function, and as a predictive marker of response to endocrine therapy [129, 130]. RPs have been linked to the spread of breast cancer stem cells postulating that they are the principal reactive cells in hidden or latent disease [131–133].

The effects of P5 on cancer cells are controversial. Sometimes they have pro-tumour effects and in some cases an anti-tumour effect [134, 135]. In prostate cancer, P5 was shown to stimulate cell proliferation and xenograft tumour growth in mice [134].

In breast cancer, DHEA inhibits cell proliferation and migration and the expression of

MET proteins and reduces the growth of xenografts in mice. The underlying molecular mechanisms have not yet been fully elucidated [136, 137]. DHEA promotes the proliferation of ovarian cancer cells in a dose-dependent manner. It also inhibits necrosis and proliferation in endothelial cells [138]. In prostate cancer, DHEA has been shown to reduce apoptosis of tumour cells by activating the TrkA receptor [139]. A study in hormone-naïve prostate cancer patients shows that low serum DHEA concentrations are associated with a poor prognosis [140].

Neuroesteroids and Drugs of Abuse

As previously described, neuroesteroids play an important role in the modulation of various physiological responses as well as in the regulation of moods. There are studies that evaluate the role of neuroesteroids and its association with drug use, as well as their effects. In the following section, some of the most common drugs of abuse are analysed.

Cannabis

There is scarce evidence on the association of P4 with cannabis use. General findings from human and animal studies suggest that cannabis and its active component tetrahydrocannabinol (THC) is capable of decreasing circulating P4 levels [141, 142]. Chronic and sub-chronic exposures to THC during the follicular phase in rhesus monkeys decreased P4 production [143]. In female and gonadectomised male Sprague-Dawley rats, P4 may contribute to an increased dependence in females following THC effects, whereas testosterone may protect against dependence in males [144].

Acute administration of the main classes of drugs of abuse (THC, cocaine, morphine, alcohol, nicotine) increased brain levels of P5 without altering plasma levels. However, THC induced a greater increase. P5 appears to counteract the effects of THC by acting as a specific inhibitor of CB1 receptor signaling, for which THC has the highest affinity [145].

As for ALLO, no evidence related to cannabis use has been found.

On the other hand, in a clinical study cannabis was found to have the highest percentage as a consumption habit in humans, and this was associated with a significant concentration of urinary DHEA in women and testosterone for men [146]. There are heterogeneous studies regarding the association between cannabis use and testosterone. Some in vitro and in vivo studies in mice show an increase in testosterone levels after cannabis exposure [147, 148], while other studies find no associations in serum levels between cannabis users and non-users [149–151]. However, recent findings in men showed that cannabis use reduced serum and urine levels of testosterone [152, 153].

Cocaine

As for smoked cocaine, it has been shown in women that its effects were diminished in the luteal phase (when P4 levels are highest) compared to the follicular phase [154–156]. The results of a previous study [157] indicated that women treated with P4 showed a decrease in the positive subjective effects of smoked cocaine compared to those treated with placebo. Elevated plasma P4 levels have also been associated with stress-induced cocaine cravings [158]. These results show concordance with research in other mammals, such as monkeys [159] and rodents [160, 161], where cocaine self-administration was higher during phases with high P4 levels.

In a behavioural study in mice P4 inhibited cocaine-induced place preference, while DHEA and P5 potentiated it. These effects would be mediated by the σ_1 receptor [162]. On the other hand, Wu et al. (2012) [163] observed that after prenatal cocaine exposure maternal and fetal rat plasma P4 and P5 concentrations were decreased, as well as P450scc protein and mRNA expression.

It has been shown that cocaine increases plasma levels of P4 and its metabolite ALLO in females, but not in males [164]. ALLO attenuated the pro-convulsant and sensitizing properties of cocaine [165]. In female rats, ALLO was able to attenuate the reinstatement of cocaine-seeking behaviour induced by a stressful stimulus [166]. When injected alone, ALLO did not restore cocaine-seeking behaviour but decreased it [167].

On the other hand, rats administered with DHEA before and during cocaine self-administration attenuated cocaine-seeking behaviour [168]. A recent study supports these findings by showing that the effect is maintained in the long term [169].

These findings show that there is an association between neuroesteroids and drug use in both women and men. The influence of neuroesteroids on drug-induced behavioural responses, as well as their effect on neuroesteroid levels, could be considered an important target when investigating potential therapeutic applications for drug use.

Conflict of Interest Statement The authors declare no conflict of interest.

Funding Information Universidad de Mendoza, Grant/Award Number: 113/10; Consejo Nacional de Investigaciones Científicas y Técnicas, Grant/Award Number: PIP N° 5942.

References

1. Plant TM. The hypothalamo-pituitary-gonadal axis. J Endocrinol. 2015;226:T41–54. https://doi.org/10.1530/JOE-15-0113.
2. Terasawa E. Mechanism of pulsatile GnRH release in primates: unresolved questions. Mol Cell Endocrinol. 2019;498:110578. https://doi.org/10.1016/J.MCE.2019.110578.
3. Giorgio D, Paula N. GABA y receptores GABA B en el eje reproductivo : su relación con GnRH y kisspeptinas GABA y receptores GABA B en el eje reproductivo : su relación con GnRH y kisspeptinas Tesis presentada para optar por el título de Doctor de la 2013.
4. Feleder C, Ginzburg M, Wuttke W, Moguilevsky JA, Arias P. GABAergic activation inhibits the hypothalamic-pituitary-ovaric axis and sexual development in the immature female rat. Associated changes in hypothalamic glutamatergic and taurinergic systems. Dev Brain Res. 1999;116:151–7. https://doi.org/10.1016/S0165-3806(99)00087-5.
5. Sinchak K, Mohr MA, Micevych PE. Hypothalamic astrocyte development and physiology for neuroprogesterone induction of the luteinizing hormone surge. Front Endocrinol (Lausanne). 2020;11:420. https://doi.org/10.3389/fendo.2020.00420.
6. Compagnone NA, Mellon SH. Neurosteroids: biosynthesis and function of these novel neuromodulators. Front Neuroendocrinol. 2000;21:1–56. https://doi.org/10.1006/frne.1999.0188.
7. Paul SM, Purdy RH. Neuroactive steroids. FASEB J. 1992;6:2311–22. https://doi.org/10.1096/fasebj.6.6.1347506.
8. Baulieu EE, Robel P. Neurosteroids: a new brain function? J Steroid Biochem Mol Biol. 1990;37:395–403. https://doi.org/10.1016/0960-0760(90)90490-C.
9. Corpéchot C, Young J, Calvel M, Wehrey C, Veltz JN, Touyer G, et al. Neurosteroids: 3 alpha-hydroxy-5 alpha-pregnan-20-one and its precursors in the brain, plasma, and steroidogenic glands of male and female rats. Endocrinology. 1993;133:1003–9.
10. Corpéchot C, Synguelakis M, Talha S, Axelson M, Sjövall J, Vihko R, et al. Pregnenolone and its sulfate ester in the rat brain. Brain Res. 1983;270:119–25. https://doi.org/10.1016/0006-8993(83)90797-7.
11. Corpechot C, Robel P, Axelson M, Sjövall J, Baulieu EE. Characterization and measurement of dehydroepiandrosterone sulfate in rat brain. Proc Natl Acad Sci USA. 1981;78:4704–7. https://doi.org/10.1073/pnas.78.8.4704.
12. Robel P, Bourreau E, Corpéchot C, Dang DC, Halberg F, Clarke C, et al. Neuro-steroids: 3β-hydroxy-δ5-derivatives in rat and monkey brain. J Steroid Biochem. 1987;27:649–55. https://doi.org/10.1016/0022-4731(87)90133-6.
13. Mellon SH, Deschepper CF. Neurosteroid biosynthesis: genes for adrenal steroidogenic enzymes are expressed in the brain. Brain Res. 1993;629:283–92. https://doi.org/10.1016/0006-8993(93)91332-M.
14. King SR, Manna PR, Ishii T, Syapin PJ, Ginsberg SD, Wilson K, et al. An essential component in steroid synthesis, the steroidogenic acute regulatory protein, is expressed in discrete regions of the brain. J Neurosci. 2002;22:10613–10620. https://doi.org/10.1523/JNEUROSCI.22-24-10613.2002.
15. King SR, Ginsberg SD, Ishii T, Smith RG, Parker KL, Lamb DJ. The steroidogenic acute regulatory protein is expressed in steroidogenic cells of the day-old brain. Endocrinology. 2004;145:4775–80. https://doi.org/10.1210/en.2003-1740.
16. Powell JG, Garland S, Preston K, Piszczatoski C. Brexanolone (Zulresso): finally, an FDA-approved treatment for postpartum depression. Ann Pharmacother. 2020;54:157–63. https://doi.org/10.1177/1060028019873320.
17. Boero G, Porcu P, Morrow AL. Neurobiology of Stress Pleiotropic actions of allopregnanolone underlie therapeutic benefits in stress-related disease. Neurobiol Stress. 2020;12:100203. https://doi.org/10.1016/j.ynstr.2019.100203.

18. Chew L, Sun KL, Sun W, Wang Z, Rajadas J, Flores RE, et al. Association of serum allopregnanolone with restricted and repetitive behaviors in adult males with autism. Psychoneuroendocrinology. 2021;123:105039. https://doi.org/10.1016/J.PSYNEUEN.2020.105039.
19. Paul SM, Pinna G, Guidotti A. Allopregnanolone: from molecular pathophysiology to therapeutics. A historical perspective. Neurobiol Stress. 2020;12:100215. https://doi.org/10.1016/J.YNSTR.2020.100215.
20. McEwen BS. Non-genomic and genomic effects of steroids on neural activity. Trends Pharmacol Sci. 1991;12:141–7. https://doi.org/10.1016/0165-6147(91)90531-v.
21. Mittelman-Smith MA, Rudolph LM, Mohr MA, Micevych PE. Rodent models of non-classical progesterone action regulating ovulation. Front Endocrinol (Lausanne). 2017;8:165. https://doi.org/10.3389/fendo.2017.00165.
22. Cáceres ARR, Vega Orozco AS, Cabrera RJ, Laconi MR. Rapid actions of the neurosteroid allopregnanolone on ovarian and hypothalamic steroidogenesis: central and peripheral modulation. J Neuroendocrinol. 2020;32:1–13. https://doi.org/10.1111/jne.12836.
23. Micevych PE, Mermelstein PG. Membrane estrogen receptors acting through metabotropic glutamate receptors: an emerging mechanism of estrogen action in brain. Mol Neurobiol. 2008;38:66–77. https://doi.org/10.1007/s12035-008-8034-z.
24. Schwartz N, Verma A, Bivens CB, Schwartz Z, Boyan BD. Rapid steroid hormone actions via membrane receptors. Biochim Biophys Acta. 1863;2016:2289–98. https://doi.org/10.1016/j.bbamcr.2016.06.004.
25. Rudolph LM, Cornil CA, Mittelman-Smith MA, Rainville JR, Remage-Healey L, Sinchak K, et al. Actions of steroids: new neurotransmitters. J Neurosci. 2016;36:11449–11458. https://doi.org/10.1523/JNEUROSCI.2473-16.2016.
26. Micevych PE, Wong AM, Mittelman-Smith MA. Estradiol membrane-initiated signaling and female reproduction. Compr Physiol. 2015;5:1211–22. https://doi.org/10.1002/cphy.c140056.
27. Mani SK, Mermelstein PG, Tetel MJ, Anesetti G. Convergence of multiple mechanisms of steroid hormone action. Horm Metab Res = Horm Und Stoffwechselforsch = Horm Metab. 2012;44:569–76. https://doi.org/10.1055/s-0032-1306343.
28. González-Flores O, Gómora-Arrati P, Garcia-Juárez M, Gómez-Camarillo MA, Lima-Hernández FJ, Beyer C, et al. Nitric oxide and ERK/MAPK mediation of estrous behavior induced by GnRH, PGE2 and db-cAMP in rats. Physiol Behav. 2009;96:606–12. https://doi.org/10.1016/j.physbeh.2008.12.019.
29. Mani SK, Allen JM, Lydon JP, Mulac-Jericevic B, Blaustein JD, DeMayo FJ, et al. Dopamine requires the unoccupied progesterone receptor to induce sexual behavior in mice. Mol Endocrinol. 1996;10:1728–37. https://doi.org/10.1210/mend.10.12.8961281.
30. Chu HP, Morales JC, Etgen AM. Cyclic GMP may potentiate lordosis behaviour by progesterone receptor activation. J Neuroendocrinol. 1999;11:107–13. https://doi.org/10.1046/j.1365-2826.1999.00298.x.
31. Laconi MR, Reggiani PC, Penissi A, Yunes R, Cabrera RJ. Allopregnanolone modulates striatal dopamingergic activity of rats under different gonadal hormones conditions. Neurol Res. 2007;29:622–7. https://doi.org/10.1179/016164107X166281.
32. Laconi MR, Cabrera RJ. Effect of centrally injected allopregnanolone on sexual receptivity, luteinizing hormone release, hypothalamic dopamine turnover, and release in female rats. Endocrine. 2002;17:77–83. https://doi.org/10.1385/endo:17:2:077.
33. Giuliani FA, Escudero C, Casas S, Bazzocchini V, Yunes R, Laconi MR, et al. Allopregnanolone and puberty: modulatory effect on glutamate and GABA release and expression of 3α-hydroxysteroid oxidoreductase in the hypothalamus of female rats. Neuroscience. 2013;243:64–75. https://doi.org/10.1016/j.neuroscience.2013.03.053.
34. Giuliani FA, Yunes R, Mohn CE, Laconi M, Rettori V, Cabrera R. Allopregnanolone induces LHRH and glutamate release through NMDA receptor modulation. Endocrine. 2011;40:21–6. https://doi.org/10.1007/s12020-011-9451-8.
35. Chebib M, Johnston GAR. The "ABC" of GABA receptors: a brief review. Clin Exp Pharmacol Physiol. 1999;26:937–40. https://doi.org/10.1046/j.1440-1681.1999.03151.x.
36. Lavaque E, Mayen A, Azcoitia I, Tena-Sempere M, Garcia-Segura LM. Sex differences, developmental changes, response to injury and cAMP regulation of the mRNA levels of steroidogenic acute regulatory protein, cytochrome p450scc, and aromatase in the olivocerebellar system. J Neurobiol. 2006;66:308–18. https://doi.org/10.1002/neu.20221.
37. Micevych P, Sinchak K, Mills RH, Tao L, LaPolt P, Lu JKH. The luteinizing hormone surge is preceded by an estrogen-induced increase of hypothalamic progesterone in ovariectomized and adrenalectomized rats. Neuroendocrinology. 2003;78:29–35. https://doi.org/10.1159/000071703.
38. Wartenberg P, Farkas I, Csillag V, Colledge WH, Hrabovszky E, Boehm U. Sexually dimorphic neurosteroid synthesis regulates neuronal activity in the murine brain. J Neurosci. 2021;41:9177–9191. https://doi.org/10.1523/JNEUROSCI.0885-21.2021.
39. Chappell PE, Schneider JS, Kim P, Xu M, Lydon JP, O'Malley BW, et al. Absence of gonadotropin surges and gonadotropin-releasing hormone self-priming in ovariectomized (OVX), estrogen (E2)-treated, progesterone receptor knockout (PRKO) mice*. Endocrinology. 1999;140:3653–8. https://doi.org/10.1210/endo.140.8.6895.

40. Chappell PE, Lee J, Levine JE. Stimulation of gonadotropin-releasing hormone surges by estrogen. II. Role of cyclic adenosine 3′,5′-monophosphate. Endocrinology. 2000;141:1486–92. https://doi.org/10.1210/endo.141.4.7427.
41. Soma KK, Sinchak K, Lakhter A, Schlinger BA, Micevych PE. Neurosteroids and female reproduction: estrogen increases 3β-HSD mRNA and activity in rat hypothalamus. Endocrinology. 2005;146:4386–90. https://doi.org/10.1210/en.2005-0569.
42. Liu T, Wimalasena J, Bowenà RL, Atwood CS, Bowen RL, Atwood CS. Luteinizing hormone receptor mediates neuronal pregnenolone production via up-regulation of steroidogenic acute regulatory protein expression. J Neurochem. 2007;100:1329–39. https://doi.org/10.1111/j.1471-4159.2006.04307.x.
43. Kuo J, Hamid N, Bondar G, Prossnitz ER, Micevych P. Membrane estrogen receptors stimulate intracellular calcium release and progesterone synthesis in hypothalamic astrocytes. J Neurosci. 2010;30:12950–7. https://doi.org/10.1523/JNEUROSCI.1158-10.2010.
44. Micevych P, Bondar G, Kuo J. Estrogen actions on neuroendocrine glia. Neuroendocrinology. 2010;91:211–22. https://doi.org/10.1159/000289568.
45. Diviccaro S, Melcangi RC, Giatti S. Post-finasteride syndrome: an emerging clinical problem. Neurobiol Stress. 2019;12:100209. https://doi.org/10.1016/j.ynstr.2019.100209.
46. Pinna G. Allopregnanolone, the neuromodulator turned therapeutic agent: thank you, next? Front Endocrinol (Lausanne). 2020;11:236. https://doi.org/10.3389/fendo.2020.00236.
47. Traish AM, Mulgaonkar A, Giordano N. The dark side of 5α-reductase inhibitors' therapy: sexual dysfunction, high gleason grade prostate cancer and depression. Kor J Urol. 2014;55:367–79.
48. Pelegrina L, Escudero C, Giuliani F, Cabrera R, Laconi M. Pharmacological effect of one icv dose of allopregnanolone in the female rat: behavioral profile. Braz J Biol Sci. 2015;2:39–50.
49. Callachan H, Cottrell GA, Hather NY, Lambert JJ, Nooney JM, Peters JA. Modulation of the GABAA receptor by progesterone metabolites. Proc R Soc Lond Ser B Biol Sci. 1987;231:359–69. https://doi.org/10.1098/rspb.1987.0049.
50. Arias P, Feleder C, Rodríguez M, Ginzburg M, Refojo D, Szwarcfarb B, et al. Repeated intracerebroventricular administration of taurine lowers LH levels and postpones vaginal opening in peripubertal female rats. Dev Brain Res. 1995;85:137–9. https://doi.org/10.1016/0165-3806(94)00188-6.
51. Calogero AE, Palumbo MA, Bosboom AMJ, Burrello N, Ferrara E, Palumbo G, et al. The neuroactive steroid allopregnanolone suppresses hypothalamic gonadotropin-releasing hormone release through a mechanism mediated by the gamma-aminobutyric acid(A) receptor. J Endocrinol. 1998;158:121–5. https://doi.org/10.1677/joe.0.1580121.
52. Halász B. Neuroendocrinology in 1992. Neuroendocrinology. 1993;57:1196–207. https://doi.org/10.1159/000126486.
53. Moguilevsky JA, Wuttke W. Changes in the control of gonadotrophin secretion by neurotransmitters during sexual development in rats. Exp Clin Endocrinol Diabetes. 2001;109:188–95. https://doi.org/10.1055/s-2001-15105.
54. Młotkowska P, Marciniak E, Roszkowicz-Ostrowska K, Misztal T. Effects of allopregnanolone on central reproductive functions in sheep under natural and stressful conditions. Theriogenology. 2020;158:138–47. https://doi.org/10.1016/j.theriogenology.2020.09.010.
55. Laconi MR, Chavez C, Cavicchia JC, Fóscolo M, Sosa Z, Yunes RF, et al. Allopregnanolone alters the luteinizing hormone, prolactin, and progesterone serum levels interfering with the regression and apoptosis in rat corpus luteum. Horm Metab Res. 2012;44:632–8. https://doi.org/10.1055/s-0032-1314834.
56. Nanfaro F, Cabrera R, Bazzocchini V, Laconi M, Yunes R. Pregnenolone sulfate infused in lateral septum of male rats impairs novel object recognition memory. Pharmacol Rep. 2010;62:265–72. https://doi.org/10.1016/S1734-1140(10)70265-6.
57. Asensio JA, Cáceres ARR, Pelegrina LT, Sanhueza M, Scotti L, Parborell F, et al. Allopregnanolone alters follicular and luteal dynamics during the estrous cycle. Reprod Biol Endocrinol. 2018;16:1–12. https://doi.org/10.1186/s12958-018-0353-y.
58. Lamberts R, Vijayan E, Graf M, Mansky T, Wuttke W. Involvement of preoptic-anterior hypothalamic GABA neurons in the regulation of pituitary LH and prolactin release. Exp Brain Res. 1983;52:356–62. https://doi.org/10.1007/BF00238029.
59. Fuchs E, Mansky T, Stock KW, Vijayan E, Wuttke W. Involvement of catecholamines and glutamate in GABAergic mechanism regulatory to luteinizing hormone and prolactin secretion. Neuroendocrinology. 1984;38:484–9. https://doi.org/10.1159/000123937.
60. Laconi MR, Casteller G, Gargiulo PA, Bregonzio C, Cabrera RJ. The anxiolytic effect of allopregnanolone is associated with gonadal hormonal status in female rats. Eur J Pharmacol. 2001;417:111–6. https://doi.org/10.1016/S0014-2999(01)00865-2.
61. Hartman RD, He JR, Barraclough CA. γ-aminobutyric acid-A and -B receptor antagonists increase luteinizing hormone-releasing hormone neuronal responsiveness to intracerebroventricular norepinephrine in ovariectomized estrogen-treated rats. Endocrinology 1990;127:1336–1345. https://doi.org/10.1210/endo-127-3-1336.
62. Donoso AO, Seltzer AM, Navarro CE, Cabrera RJ, López FJ, Negro-Vilar A. Regulation of luteinizing hormone-releasing hormone and luteinizing hormone secretion by hypothalamic amino acids. Braz

J Med Biol Res = Rev Bras Pesqui Medicas e Biol. 1994;27:921–32.

63. Adler BA, Crowley WR. Evidence for γ-aminobutyric acid modulation of ovarian hormonal effects on luteinizing hormone secretion and hypothalamic catecholamine activity in the female rat. Endocrinology. 1986;118:91–7. https://doi.org/10.1210/endo-118-1-91.
64. Magnaghi V, Parducz A, Frasca A, Ballabio M, Procacci P, Racagni G, et al. GABA synthesis in Schwann cells is induced by the neuroactive steroid allopregnanolone. J Neurochem. 2010;112:980–90. https://doi.org/10.1111/j.1471-4159.2009.06512.x.
65. Akema T, Kimura F. Modulation of pulsatile LH secretion by baclofen, a selective $GABA_B$ receptor agonist, in ovariectomized rats. Neuroendocrinology. 1992;56:141–7. https://doi.org/10.1159/000126221.
66. Gay VL, Midgley ARJ. Response of the adult rat to orchidectomy and ovariectomy as determined by LH radioimmunoassay. Endocrinology. 1969;84:1359–64. https://doi.org/10.1210/endo-84-6-1359.
67. Luderer U, Schwartz NB. Acute changes in pulsatile LH and FSH secretion after ovariectomy in rats: treatment with oestradiol for 24 h suppresses LH, but not FSH, for at least 48 h. J Reprod Fertil. 1994;100:613–21. https://doi.org/10.1530/jrf.0.1000613.
68. Payne JL. Evaluating brexanolone for the treatment of postpartum depression. Expert Opin Pharmacother. 2021;22:959–64. https://doi.org/10.1080/14656566.2021.1897105.
69. Morrow AL, Balan I, Boero G. Mechanisms underlying recovery from postpartum depression following brexanolone therapy. Biol Psychiatry. 2022;91:252–3. https://doi.org/10.1016/j.biopsych.2021.11.006.
70. Walton N, Maguire J. Allopregnanolone-based treatments for postpartum depression: why/how do they work? Neurobiol Stress. 2019;11:100198. https://doi.org/10.1016/j.ynstr.2019.100198.
71. Slopien R, Pluchino N, Warenik-Szymankiewicz A, Sajdak S, Luisi M, Drakopoulos P, et al. Correlation between allopregnanolone levels and depressive symptoms during late menopausal transition and early postmenopause. Gynecol Endocrinol. 2018;34:144–7. https://doi.org/10.1080/09513590.2017.1371129.
72. Standeven LR, Olson E, Leistikow N, Payne JL, Osborne LM, Hantsoo L. Polycystic ovary syndrome, affective symptoms, and neuroactive steroids: a focus on allopregnanolone. Curr Psychiatry Rep. 2021;23 https://doi.org/10.1007/s11920-021-01244-w.
73. Escudero C, Giuliani F, Bernedo MM, Yunes R, Cabrera R. Allopregnanolone reversion of estrogen and progesterone memory impairment: interplay with serotonin release. J Neural Transm. 2019;126:1321–8. https://doi.org/10.1007/s00702-019-02052-6.
74. Accioly NE, Guedes RCA. Topical cortical application of ovarian hormones and modulation of brain electrical activity: analysis of spreading depression in well-nourished and malnourished female rats. Nutr Neurosci. 2020;23:887–95. https://doi.org/10.1080/1028415X.2019.1575574.
75. Barreto-Cordero LM, Ríos-Carrillo J, Roldán-Roldán G, Rasia-Filho AA, Flores G, Bringas ME, et al. Cyclic changes and actions of progesterone and allopregnanolone on cognition and hippocampal basal (stratum oriens) dendritic spines of female rats. Behav Brain Res. 2020;379 https://doi.org/10.1016/j.bbr.2019.112355.
76. Pelegrina LT, Cáceres ARR, Giuliani FA, Asensio JA, Parborell F, Laconi MR. A single dose of allopregnanolone affects rat ovarian morphology and steroidogenesis. Reproduction. 2017;153:75–83. https://doi.org/10.1530/REP-16-0463.
77. Cabrera RJ, Bregonzio C, Laconi M, Mampel A. Allopregnanolone increase in striatal N-methyl-D-aspartic acid evoked [3H]dopamine release is estrogen and progesterone dependent. Cell Mol Neurobiol. 2002;22:445–54. https://doi.org/10.1023/A:1021015705597.
78. Haage D, Bäckström T, Johansson S. Interaction between allopregnanolone and pregnenolone sulfate in modulating GABA-mediated synaptic currents in neurons from the rat medial preoptic nucleus. Brain Res. 2005;1033:58–67. https://doi.org/10.1016/J.BRAINRES.2004.11.020.
79. Haage D, Johansson S. Neurosteroid modulation of synaptic and GABA-evoked currents in neurons from the rat medial preoptic nucleus. 1999.
80. Uchida S, Noda E, Kakazu Y, Mizoguchi Y, Akaike N, Nabekura J. Allopregnanolone enhancement of GABAergic transmission in rat medial preoptic area neurons. 2002. https://doi.org/10.1152/ajpendo.00049.2002.%2D%2DAminobutyric.
81. A.R.R.C. Effects of allopregnanolone on the reproductive physiology of the female rat. PROBIOL, Universidad Nacional de Cuyo; 2022.
82. Casteller G, Laconi M, Fraile M, Landa A, Cabrera RGP. Disinhibitory effect of allopregnanolone within the medial prefrontal cortex of male rats on the plus maze test. Int J Neuroprotect Neuroregen. 2006;2:120–6.
83. Gargiulo PA, Muñoz V, Donoso AO. Inhibition by N-methyl-D-aspartic acid (NMDA) receptor antagonist of lordosis behavior induced by estrogen followed by progesterone or luteinizing hormone-releasing hormone (LHRH) in the rat. Physiol Behav. 1992;52:737–9. https://doi.org/10.1016/0031-9384(92)90407-s.
84. Gargiulo PA, Donoso AO. Interaction between glutamate and luteinizing hormone-releasing hormone (LHRH) in lordosis behavior and luteinizing hormone release (LH): further studies on NMDA receptor mediation. Physiol Behav. 1995;58:169–73. https://doi.org/10.1016/0031-9384(95)00040-p.

85. Landa AI, Cabrera RJ, Gargiulo PA. Prazosin blocks the glutamatergic effects of N-methyl-D-aspartic acid on lordosis behavior and luteinizing hormone secretion in the estrogen-primed female rat. Braz J Med Biol Res = Rev Bras Pesqui Medicas e Biol. 2006;39:365–70. https://doi.org/10.1590/s0100-879x2006000300007.
86. Landa AI, Gargiulo AJM, Gargiulo MML, Cabrera RJ, Bregonzio C, Lafuente Sánchez JV, et al. Alpha and beta noradrenergic mediation of NMDA glutamatergic effects on lordosis behaviour and plasmatic LH concentrations in the primed female rat. J Neural Transm. 2009;116:551–7. https://doi.org/10.1007/s00702-009-0217-x.
87. Otero Losada ME. Acute stress and GABAergic function in the rat brain. Br J Pharmacol. 1989;96:507–12. https://doi.org/10.1111/j.1476-5381.1989.tb11846.x.
88. Brann DW, Mahesh VB. Excitatory amino acids: evidence for a role in the control of reproduction and anterior pituitary hormone secretion. Endocr Rev. 1997;18:678–700. https://doi.org/10.1210/edrv.18.5.0311.
89. Dhandapani KM, Brann DW. The role of glutamate and nitric oxide in the reproductive neuroendocrine system. Biochem Cell Biol. 2000;78:165–79.
90. Johansson T, Le Grevès P. The effect of dehydroepiandrosterone sulfate and allopregnanolone sulfate on the binding of [3H]ifenprodil to the N-methyl-d-aspartate receptor in rat frontal cortex membrane. J Steroid Biochem Mol Biol. 2005;94:263–6. https://doi.org/10.1016/j.jsbmb.2005.01.020.
91. Chisari M, Wilding TJ, Brunwasser S, Krishnan K, Qian M, Benz A, et al. Visualizing pregnenolone sulfate-like modulators of NMDA receptor function reveals intracellular and plasma-membrane localization. Neuropharmacology. 2019;144:91–103. https://doi.org/10.1016/j.neuropharm.2018.10.015.
92. Krausova BH, Kysilov B, Cerny J, Vyklicky V, Smejkalova T, Ladislav M, et al. Site of action of brain neurosteroid pregnenolone sulfate at the N-methyl-D-aspartate receptor. J Neurosci. 2020;40:5922–36. https://doi.org/10.1523/JNEUROSCI.3010-19.2020.
93. Genazzani AR, Palumbo MA, de Micheroux AA, Artini PG, Criscuolo M, Ficarra G, et al. Evidence for a role for the neurosteroid allopregnanolone in the modulation of reproductive function in female rats. Eur J Endocrinol. 1995;133:375–80. https://doi.org/10.1530/eje.0.1330375.
94. Frye CA. Novel substrates for, and sources of, progestogens for reproduction. J Neuroendocrinol. 2011;23:961–73. https://doi.org/10.1111/j.1365-2826.2011.02180.x.
95. Baulieu EE. Neurosteroids: a novel function of the brain. Psychoneuroendocrinology. 1998;23:963–87. https://doi.org/10.1016/s0306-4530(98)00071-7.
96. Baulieu EE. Neurosteroids: of the nervous system, by the nervous system, for the nervous system. Recent Prog Horm Res. 1997;52:1–32.
97. Sullivan SD, Moenter SM. Neurosteroids alter γ-aminobutyric acid postsynaptic currents in gonadotropin-releasing hormone neurons: a possible mechanism for direct steroidal control. Endocrinology. 2003;144:4366–75. https://doi.org/10.1210/en.2003-0634.
98. Li S, Garcia de Yebenes E, Pelletier G. Effects of dehydroepiandrosterone (DHEA) on GnRH gene expression in the rat brain as studied by in situ hybridization. Peptides. 1995;16:425–30. https://doi.org/10.1016/0196-9781(94)00201-g.
99. Wise PM, Ratner A. Effect of ovariectomy on plasma LH, FSH, estradiol, and progesterone and medial basal hypothalamic LHRH concentrations old and young rats. Neuroendocrinology. 1980;30:15–9. https://doi.org/10.1159/000122968.
100. Gruenewald DA, Matsumoto AM. Age-related decreases in serum gonadotropin levels and gonadotropin-releasing hormone gene expression in the medial preoptic area of the male rat are dependent upon testicular feedback. Endocrinology. 1991;129:2442–50. https://doi.org/10.1210/endo-129-5-2442.
101. Narkwichean A, Jayaprakasan K, Maalouf WE, Hernandez-Medrano JH, Pincott-Allen C, Campbell BK. Effects of dehydroepiandrosterone on in vivo ovine follicular development. Hum Reprod. 2014;29:146–54. https://doi.org/10.1093/humrep/det408.
102. Narkwichean A, Maalouf W, Baumgarten M, Polanski L, Raine-Fenning N, Campbell B, et al. Efficacy of Dehydroepiandrosterone (DHEA) to overcome the effect of ovarian ageing (DITTO): a proof of principle double blinded randomized placebo controlled trial. Eur J Obstet Gynecol Reprod Biol. 2017;218:39–48. https://doi.org/10.1016/j.ejogrb.2017.09.006.
103. Kim E-J, Jang M, Choi JH, Park KS, Cho I-H. An improved dehydroepiandrosterone-induced rat model of polycystic ovary syndrome (PCOS): post-pubertal improve PCOS's features. Front Endocrinol (Lausanne). 2018;9:735. https://doi.org/10.3389/fendo.2018.00735.
104. Li Y, Zheng Q, Sun D, Cui X, Chen S, Bulbul A, et al. Dehydroepiandrosterone stimulates inflammation and impairs ovarian functions of polycystic ovary syndrome. J Cell Physiol. 2019;234:7435–47. https://doi.org/10.1002/jcp.27501.
105. Greaves RF, Wudy SA, Badoer E, Zacharin M, Hirst JJ, Quinn T, et al. A tale of two steroids: the importance of the androgens DHEA and DHEAS for early neurodevelopment. J Steroid Biochem Mol Biol. 2019;188:77–85. https://doi.org/10.1016/j.jsbmb.2018.12.007.
106. Ding X, Yu L, Ge C, Ma H. Protective effect of DHEA on hydrogen peroxide-induced oxidative damage and apoptosis in primary rat Leydig cells. 2017;8.
107. Kushnir VA, Darmon SK, Barad DH, Weghofer A, Gleicher N. Effects of dehydroepiandros-

terone (DHEA) supplementation on sexual function in premenopausal infertile women. Endocrine. 2019;63:632–8. https://doi.org/10.1007/s12020-018-1781-3.

108. Labrie F, Archer DF, Koltun W, Vachon A, Young D, Frenette L, et al. Efficacy of intravaginal dehydroepiandrosterone (DHEA) on moderate to severe dyspareunia and vaginal dryness, symptoms of vulvovaginal atrophy, and of the genitourinary syndrome of menopause. Menopause. 2016;23:243–56. https://doi.org/10.1097/GME.0000000000000571.
109. Vallée M. Neurosteroids and potential therapeutics: focus on pregnenolone. J Steroid Biochem Mol Biol. 2016;160:78–87. https://doi.org/10.1016/j.jsbmb.2015.09.030.
110. Vallée M, Purdy RH, Mayo W, Koob GF, Le Moal M. Neuroactive steroids: new biomarkers of cognitive aging. J Steroid Biochem Mol Biol. 2003;85:329–35. https://doi.org/10.1016/s0960-0760(03)00227-9.
111. Weng J-H, Chung B-C. Nongenomic actions of neurosteroid pregnenolone and its metabolites. Steroids. 2016;111:54–9. https://doi.org/10.1016/j.steroids.2016.01.017.
112. Rustichelli C, Bellei E, Bergamini S, Monari E, Lo Castro F, Baraldi C, et al. Comparison of pregnenolone sulfate, pregnanolone and estradiol levels between patients with menstrually-related migraine and controls: an exploratory study. J Headache Pain. 2021;22:13. https://doi.org/10.1186/s10194-021-01231-9.
113. Marcinkowska E, Wiedłocha A. Steroid signal transduction activated at the cell membrane: from plants to animals. Acta Biochim Pol. 2002;49:735–45.
114. El-Etr M, Akwa Y, Baulieu E-E, Schumacher M. The neuroactive steroid pregnenolone sulfate stimulates the release of gonadotropin-releasing hormone from GT1-7 hypothalamic neurons, through N-methyl-d-aspartate receptors. Endocrinology. 2006;147:2737–43. https://doi.org/10.1210/en.2005-1191.
115. Kang E-J, Hong S-H, Lee J-E, Kim SC, Yang H-S, Yi PI, et al. Pregnenolone sulfate regulates prolactin production in the rat pituitary. J Endocrinol. 2016;230:339–46. https://doi.org/10.1530/JOE-16-0088.
116. Shin YY, Kang E-J, Jeong JS, Kim MJ, Jung E-M, Jeung E-B, et al. Pregnenolone as a potential candidate for hormone therapy for female reproductive disorders targeting ERβ. Mol Reprod Dev. 2019;86:109–17. https://doi.org/10.1002/mrd.23086.
117. Craig ZR, Hannon PR, Flaws JA. Pregnenolone cotreatment partially restores steroidogenesis, but does not prevent growth inhibition and increased atresia in mouse ovarian antral follicles treated with monohydroxy methoxychlor. Toxicol Appl Pharmacol. 2013;272:780–6. https://doi.org/10.1016/j.taap.2013.08.002.
118. Kavaliers M, Kinsella DM. Male preference for the odors of estrous female mice is reduced by the neurosteroid pregnenolone sulfate. Brain Res. 1995;682:222–6. https://doi.org/10.1016/0006-8993(95)00335-N.
119. Han X, Cheng W, Chen Z, Du X, Cao X, Zeng X. Active immunisation against pregnenolone reduces testicular steroidogenesis and GnRH synthesis in rabbits. Anim Reprod Sci. 2014;145:161–9. https://doi.org/10.1016/j.anireprosci.2014.01.016.
120. Hirtz A, Rech F, Dubois-Pot-Schneider H, Dumond H. Astrocytoma: a hormone-sensitive tumor? Int J Mol Sci. 2020;21 https://doi.org/10.3390/ijms21239114.
121. Lima MA, da Silva SV, Freitas VM. Progesterone acts via the progesterone receptor to induce adamts proteases in ovarian cancer cells. J Ovarian Res. 2016;9:9. https://doi.org/10.1186/s13048-016-0219-x.
122. Lima MA, Silva SV, Jaeger RG, Freitas VM. Progesterone decreases ovarian cancer cells migration and invasion. Steroids. 2020;161:108680. https://doi.org/10.1016/j.steroids.2020.108680.
123. Pedernera E, Gómora MJ, Morales-Vásquez F, Pérez-Montiel D, Mendez C. Progesterone reduces cell survival in primary cultures of endometrioid ovarian cancer. J Ovarian Res. 2019;12:15. https://doi.org/10.1186/s13048-019-0486-4.
124. Kim O, Park EY, Kwon SY, Shin S, Emerson RE, Shin YH, et al. Targeting progesterone signaling prevents metastatic ovarian cancer. Proc Natl Acad Sci USA. 2020;117:31993–2004. https://doi.org/10.1073/pnas.2013595117.
125. Pelegrina LT, de los Ángeles Sanhueza M, Ramona Cáceres AR, Cuello-Carrión D, Rodriguez CE, Laconi MR. Effect of progesterone and first evidence about allopregnanolone action on the progression of epithelial human ovarian cancer cell lines. J Steroid Biochem Mol Biol. 2020;196:105492. https://doi.org/10.1016/j.jsbmb.2019.105492.
126. Trabert B, Bauer DC, Buist DSMM, Cauley JA, Falk RT, Geczik AM, et al. Association of circulating progesterone with breast cancer risk among postmenopausal women. JAMA Netw Open. 2020;3:e203645. https://doi.org/10.1001/jamanetworkopen.2020.3645.
127. Matsuoka A, Tate S, Nishikimi K, Ishikawa H, Shozu M. Elevated serum progesterone levels in postmenopausal women with mucinous ovarian tumors. Menopause. 2016;23:544–9. https://doi.org/10.1097/GME.0000000000000587.
128. Wiebe JP, Lewis MJ, Cialacu V, Pawlak KJ, Zhang G. The role of progesterone metabolites in breast cancer: potential for new diagnostics and therapeutics. J Steroid Biochem Mol Biol. 2005;93:201–8. https://doi.org/10.1016/j.jsbmb.2004.12.003.
129. Mohammed H, Russell IA, Stark R, Rueda OM, Hickey TE, Tarulli GA, et al. Progesterone receptor modulates ERα action in breast cancer. Nature. 2015;523:313–7. https://doi.org/10.1038/nature14583.

130. Singhal H, Greene ME, Zarnke AL, Laine M, Abosy RA, Chang YF, et al. Progesterone receptor isoforms, agonists and antagonists differentially reprogram estrogen signaling. Oncotarget. 2018;9:4282. https://doi.org/10.18632/ONCOTARGET.21378.
131. Truong TH, Dwyer AR, Diep CH, Hu H, Hagen KM, Lange CA. Phosphorylated progesterone receptor isoforms mediate opposing stem cell and proliferative breast cancer cell fates. Endocrinology. 2019;160:430–46. https://doi.org/10.1210/en.2018-00990.
132. Axlund SD, Sartorius CA. Progesterone regulation of stem and progenitor cells in normal and malignant breast. Mol Cell Endocrinol. 2012;357:71–9. https://doi.org/10.1016/j.mce.2011.09.021.
133. Joshi PA, Jackson HW, Beristain AG, Di Grappa MA, Mote PA, Clarke CL, et al. Progesterone induces adult mammary stem cell expansion. Nature. 2010;465:803–7. https://doi.org/10.1038/nature09091.
134. Grigoryev DN, Long BJ, Njar VC, Brodie AH. Pregnenolone stimulates LNCaP prostate cancer cell growth via the mutated androgen receptor. J Steroid Biochem Mol Biol. 2000;75:1–10. https://doi.org/10.1016/s0960-0760(00)00131-x.
135. Roy S, Sipthorp J, Mahata B, Pramanik J, Hennrich ML, Gavin A-C, et al. CLICK-enabled analogues reveal pregnenolone interactomes in cancer and immune cells. BioRxiv. 2019. https://doi.org/10.1101/800649.
136. Colín-Val Z, González-Puertos VY, Mendoza-Milla C, Gómez EO, Huesca-Gómez C, López-Marure R. DHEA increases epithelial markers and decreases mesenchymal proteins in breast cancer cells and reduces xenograft growth. Toxicol Appl Pharmacol. 2017;333:26–34. https://doi.org/10.1016/J.TAAP.2017.08.002.
137. Colín-Val Z, López-Díazguerrero NE, López-Marure R. DHEA inhibits proliferation, migration and alters mesenchymal-epithelial transition proteins through the PI3K/Akt pathway in MDA-MB-231 cells. J Steroid Biochem Mol Biol. 2021;208 https://doi.org/10.1016/J.JSBMB.2021.105818.
138. Gündoğan Gİ, Kig C, Karacan M, Doğruman H. Investigation of physiological effects induced by dehydroepiandrosterone in human endothelial cells and ovarian cancer cell line. Turk J Pharm Sci. 2021;18:185–91. https://doi.org/10.4274/TJPS.GALENOS.2020.58827.
139. Anagnostopoulou V, Pediaditakis I, Alkahtani S, Alarifi SA, Schmidt E-M, Lang F, et al. Differential effects of dehydroepiandrosterone and testosterone in prostate and colon cancer cell apoptosis: the role of nerve growth factor (NGF) receptors. 2013. https://doi.org/10.1210/en.2012-2249.
140. Miyoshi Y, Uemura H, Umemoto S, Sakamaki K, Taguri M, Suzuki K, et al. Low serum dehydroepiandrosterone examined by liquid chromatography-tandem mass spectrometry correlates with poor prognosis in hormone-naïve prostate cancer. Prostate. 2016;76:376–82. https://doi.org/10.1002/PROS.23129.
141. Almirez RG, Smith CG, Asch RH. The effects of marijuana extract and Δ9-tetrahydrocannabinol on luteal function in the rhesus monkey. Fertil Steril. 1983;39:212–7. https://doi.org/10.1016/S0015-0282(16)46821-4.
142. Smith CG, Besch NF, Smith RG, Besch PK. Effect of tetrahydrocannabinol on the hypothalamic-pituitary axis in the ovariectomized rhesus monkey. Fertil Steril. 1979;31:335–9. https://doi.org/10.1016/S0015-0282(16)43885-9.
143. Grace SC, Jeffrey B. Tolerance develops to the disruptive effects of Δ9-tetrahydrocannabinol on primate menstrual cycle. Science (80-). 1983;219:1453–5. https://doi.org/10.1126/science.6298938.
144. Marusich JA, Craft RM, Lefever TW, Wiley JL. The impact of gonadal hormones on cannabinoid dependence. Exp Clin Psychopharmacol. 2015;23:206–16. https://doi.org/10.1037/pha0000027.
145. Vallée M, Vitiello S, Bellocchio L, Hébert-Chatelain E, Monlezun S, Martin-Garcia E, et al. Pregnenolone can protect the brain from cannabis intoxication. Science. 2014;343:94–8. https://doi.org/10.1126/science.1243985.
146. Pichini S, De Luca R, Pellegrini M, Marchei E, Rotolo MC, Spoletini R, et al. Hair and urine testing to assess drugs of abuse consumption in couples undergoing assisted reproductive technology (ART). Forensic Sci Int. 2012;218:57–61. https://doi.org/10.1016/J.FORSCIINT.2011.10.011.
147. Dalterio S, Steger R, Mayfield D, Bartke A. Early cannabinoid exposure influences neuroendocrine and reproductive functions in male mice: I. Prenatal exposure. Pharmacol Biochem Behav. 1984;20:107–13. https://doi.org/10.1016/0091-3057(84)90110-2.
148. Dalterio SL, Bartke A, Mayfield D. Cannabinoids stimulate and inhibit testosterone production in vitro and in vivo. Life Sci. 1983;32:605–12. https://doi.org/10.1016/0024-3205(83)90205-9.
149. Belladelli F, Del Giudice F, Kasman A, Kold Jensen T, Jørgensen N, Salonia A, et al. The association between cannabis use and testicular function in men: a systematic review and meta-analysis. Andrology. 2021;9:503–10. https://doi.org/10.1111/andr.12953.
150. Thistle JE, Graubard BI, Braunlin M, Vesper H, Trabert B, Cook MB, et al. Marijuana use and serum testosterone concentrations among U.S. males. Andrology. 2017;5:732–8. https://doi.org/10.1111/andr.12358.
151. Shiff B, Blankstein U, Hussaen J, Jarvi K, Grober E, Lo K, et al. The impact of cannabis use on male sexual function: a 10-year, single-center experience. Can Urol Assoc J. 2021;15:E652–7. https://doi.org/10.5489/cuaj.7185.
152. Mousa A, Petrovic M, Fleshner NE. Prevalence and predictors of cannabis use among men receiving androgen-deprivation therapy for advanced prostate cancer. Can Urol Assoc J = J l'Association Des Urol

Du Canada. 2020;14:E20–6. https://doi.org/10.5489/cuaj.5911.
153. Moon JY, Kwon W, Suh S, Cheong JC, In MK, Chung BC, et al. Reference ranges for urinary levels of testosterone and epitestosterone, which may reveal gonadal function, in a Korean male population. J Steroid Biochem Mol Biol. 2014;140:100–5. https://doi.org/10.1016/J.JSBMB.2013.12.001.
154. Evans SM, Haney M, Foltin RW. The effects of smoked cocaine during the follicular and luteal phases of the menstrual cycle in women. Psychopharmacology. 2002;159:397–406. https://doi.org/10.1007/s00213-001-0944-7.
155. Evans SM, Foltin RW. Exogenous progesterone attenuates the subjective effects of smoked cocaine in women, but not in men. Neuropsychopharmacology. 2006;31:659–74. https://doi.org/10.1038/sj.npp.1300887.
156. Sofuoglu M, Dudish-Poulsen S, Nelson D, Pentel PR, Hatsukami DK. Sex and menstrual cycle differences in the subjective effects from smoked cocaine in humans. Exp Clin Psychopharmacol. 1999;7:274–83. https://doi.org/10.1037/1064-1297.7.3.274.
157. Sofuoglu M, Babb DA, Hatsukami DK. Effects of progesterone treatment on smoked cocaine response in women. Pharmacol Biochem Behav. 2002;72:431–5. https://doi.org/10.1016/S0091-3057(02)00716-5.
158. Sinha R, Fox H, Hong K-I, Sofuoglu M, Morgan PT, Bergquist KT. Sex steroid hormones, stress response, and drug craving in cocaine-dependent women: implications for relapse susceptibility. Exp Clin Psychopharmacol. 2007;15:445–52. https://doi.org/10.1037/1064-1297.15.5.445.
159. Mello NK, Knudson IM, Mendelson JH. Sex and menstrual cycle effects on progressive ratio measures of cocaine self-administration in cynomolgus monkeys. Neuropsychopharmacology. 2007;32:1956–66. https://doi.org/10.1038/sj.npp.1301314.
160. Feltenstein MW, See RE. Plasma progesterone levels and cocaine-seeking in freely cycling female rats across the estrous cycle. Drug Alcohol Depend. 2007;89:183–9. https://doi.org/10.1016/J.DRUGALCDEP.2006.12.017.
161. Lynch WJ. Acquisition and maintenance of cocaine self-administration in adolescent rats: effects of sex and gonadal hormones. Psychopharmacology. 2008;197:237–46. https://doi.org/10.1007/s00213-007-1028-0.
162. Romieu P, Martin-Fardon R, Bowen WD, Maurice T. Receptor-related neuroactive steroids modulate cocaine-induced reward. J Neurosci. 2003;23:3572–6. https://doi.org/10.1523/JNEUROSCI.23-09-03572.2003.
163. Wu L, Yan J, Qu SC, Feng YQ, Jiang XL. Abnormal regulation for progesterone production in placenta with prenatal cocaine exposure in rats. Placenta. 2012;33:977–81. https://doi.org/10.1016/J.PLACENTA.2012.10.001.
164. Quinones-Jenab V, Minerly ACE, Niyomchia T, Akahvan A, Jenab S, Frye C. Progesterone and allopregnanolone are induced by cocaine in serum and brain tissues of male and female rats. Pharmacol Biochem Behav. 2008;89:292–7. https://doi.org/10.1016/J.PBB.2007.12.024.
165. Kaminski RM, Gasior M, Carter RB, Witkin JM. Protective efficacy of neuroactive steroids against cocaine kindled-seizures in mice. Eur J Pharmacol. 2003;474:217–22. https://doi.org/10.1016/S0014-2999(03)02086-7.
166. Anker JJ, Carroll ME. Sex differences in the effects of allopregnanolone on yohimbine-induced reinstatement of cocaine seeking in rats. Drug Alcohol Depend. 2010;107:264–7. https://doi.org/10.1016/J.DRUGALCDEP.2009.11.002.
167. Anker JJ, Holtz NA, Zlebnik N, Carroll ME. Effects of allopregnanolone on the reinstatement of cocaine-seeking behavior in male and female rats. Psychopharmacology. 2009;203:63–72. https://doi.org/10.1007/s00213-008-1371-9.
168. Doron R, Fridman L, Gispan-Herman I, Maayan R, Weizman A, Yadid G. DHEA, a neurosteroid, decreases cocaine self-administration and reinstatement of cocaine-seeking behavior in rats. Neuropsychopharmacology. 2006;31:2231–6. https://doi.org/10.1038/sj.npp.1301013.
169. Ahdoot-Levi H, Croitoru O, Bareli T, Sudai E, Peér-Nissan H, Jacob A, et al. The effect of dehydroepiandrosterone treatment on neurogenesis, astrogliosis and long-term cocaine-seeking behavior in a cocaine self-administration model in rats. Front Neurosci. 2021;15. https://doi.org/10.3389/fnins.2021.773197.

Ketamine, from Anaesthetic to Drug Abuse

29

Manuel Alejandro Guevara, Iker Barrutieta-Arberas, Esteban Alejandro Romanowicz, Evelina Haralanova, Svetlozar Haralanov, Gabriel Walter Martínez, Luis Hernán Llano, Ángel José Martín Gargiulo, Augusto Pascual Ítalo Gargiulo, Ana Paula Colombini, Mercedes María Lucrecia Gargiulo, Marcos Constantino Josué Gargiulo, Andrés Acuña, Gonzalo Mesones, Humberto Luis Mesones-Arroyo, Norman Darío López Velásquez, José Vicente Lafuente Sánchez, Luis Enrique Echarte Alonso, Adriana Inés Landa de Gargiulo, and Pascual Ángel Gargiulo

M. A. Guevara (✉) · E. A. Romanowicz · G. W. Martínez · L. H. Llano · A. Acuña · G. Mesones · A. I. Landa de Gargiulo
Laboratorio de Neurociencias y Psicología Experimental, Fundación Corporación Tecnológica Latinoamericana (FUCOTEL). Cátedra de Psicopatología, Facultad de Humanidades y Ciencias Económicas, Universidad Católica Argentina (UCA), Área de Farmacología. Facultad de Ciencias Médicas, Universidad Nacional de Cuyo (UNCuyo), Consejo Nacional de Investigaciones Científicas y Técnicas (CONICET), Mendoza, Argentina

I. Barrutieta-Arberas · J. V. Lafuente Sánchez
LaNCE-Neuropharm Research Group, Dep Neurosciences, Facultad de Medicina y Enfermería, University of the Basque Country (UPV-EHU), Leioa, Spain
e-mail: onplasav@lg.ehu.es; josevicente.lafuente@ehu.eus

H. L. Mesones-Arroyo · P. Á. Gargiulo
Laboratory of Neurosciences and Experimental Psychology, Latin American Technological Corporation Foundation (FUCOTEL), Cathedra of Psychopathology, Catholic University of Argentina, Area of Pharmacology, Department of Pathology, National University of Cuyo, CONICET, Guaymallén, Mendoza, Argentina
e-mail: hlmesones@mesoneshumberto.com.ar

E. Haralanova · S. Haralanov
Department of Psychiatry and Medical Psychology, Medical University of Sofia, Sofia, Bulgaria

First Psychiatric Clinic, University Hospital for Neurology and Psychiatry "St. Naum", Sofia, Bulgaria

First Psychiatric Clinic, University Hospital for Neurology and Psychiatry "Sveti Naim", Sofia, Bulgaria

Á. J. M. Gargiulo · A. P. Í. Gargiulo · A. P. Colombini · M. M. L. Gargiulo · M. C. J. Gargiulo
Laboratorio de Neurociencias y Psicología Experimental, Fundación Corporación Tecnológica Latinoamericana (FUCOTEL). Cátedra de Psicopatología, Facultad de Humanidades y Ciencias Económicas, Universidad Católica Argentina (UCA), Área de Farmacología. Facultad de Ciencias Médicas,

P. Á. Gargiulo, H. L. Mesones-Arroyo (eds.), *Psychiatry and Neuroscience Update – Vol. V*,
https://doi.org/10.1007/978-3-031-72219-6_29

Introduction

Chemically, Ketamine is (2-(2-chlorophenyl)-2-methylamino)-cyclohexanone). Its chemical formula is $C_{13}H_{16}NClO$ (2-(2-chlorophenyl)-2-methylamino)-cyclohexanone) and Ketamine hydrochloride ($C_{13}H_{17}Cl_2NO$, see molecular structure in Fig. 29.1). The team directed by Calvin Stevens, Professor of Organic Chemistry in the Wayne State University and Parke Davis Laboratory Chemical Consultant, synthesized it [1]. Ketamine was patented in Belgium in 1963 and in the United States of America in 1966. It is a derivative of phencyclidine, a psychotogenic drug recognized as such [2, 3].

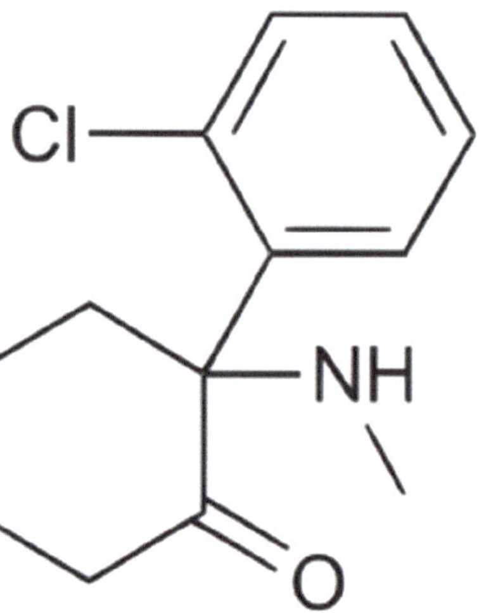

Fig. 29.1 Molecular structure of ketamine

Its chemical formula is $C_{13}H_{16}NClO$, and as a hydrochloride, it is $C_{13}H_{17}Cl_2NO$ (see molecular structure in Fig. 29.1). Ketamine hydrochloride occurs as white crystals soluble in water, with a pKa of 7.5; its free base is soluble in lipids and it contains a chiral centre at C-2 of the cyclohexanone ring. It has two enantiomers: S−(+)—ketamine and R−(−)—ketamine. The molecular weight for the free base is 237.73, and for the hydrochloride 274.18. Regarding equivalencies, 1.15 mg of ketamine hydrochloride is equivalent to 1 mg of free base. The melting point for the free base is 92-03 °C and for the hydrochloride it is 262–263 °C. Its metabolism is mainly in the liver by the cytochrome P450 family. More than 90% of its excretion is carried out by the kidney [4, 5].

It is considered a dissociative anaesthetic, since it produces functional and electrophysiological dissociation between the limbic and thalamo-neocortical systems, in which there is inhibition of association and thalamic areas, with excitation some regions of the limbic system and the hippocampus [6, 7]. The patient appears to be in a cataleptic state in which the eyes remain open with a fixed gaze. Different degrees of muscular hypertonia can be present. It is a particular anaesthetic state where there is marked sensory loss, analgesia, and amnesia that is not accompanied by actual loss of consciousness [8].

The neuropharmacological role of ketamine is relatively complex. It interacts with multiple binding sites such as NMDA and non-NMDA glutamate receptors, dopaminergic, serotonergic, adrenergic, cholinergic, opioid, and sigma receptors. It also acts on serotonin, norepinephrine, and dopamine reuptake transporters (SERT NET and DAT), respectively, and various channel ions such as voltage-gated ion channels and depolarization-gated cyclic nucleotides [9]. These interactions play a fundamental role in the pharmacology and clinic of ketamine. However, NMDA receptor antagonism accounts for most of

Universidad Nacional de Cuyo (UNCuyo), Consejo Nacional de Investigaciones Científicas y Técnicas (CONICET), Mendoza, Argentina

Centro Integral de Salud Mental Argentino (CISMA), Buenos Aires, Argentina

N. D. López Velásquez
Centro de Investigación e Innovación en Gerontología Aplicada (CIGAP), Facultad de Salud, Universidad Santo Tomas, Temuco, Chile

Carrera de Kinesiología, Facultad de Salud, Universidad Santo Tomás, Temuco, Chile
e-mail: nlopez17@cuc.edu.co; normanlopezve@santotomas.cl

L. E. Echarte Alonso
Humanities and Medical Ethics Unit, School of Medicine, University of Navarra, Pamplona, Spain
e-mail: lecharte@unav.es

its analgesic, amnesic, and psychotomimetic effect [10].

The hypnosis produced by ketamine is due to antagonism of excitatory transmission by blocking NMDA receptors, with inhibition of the actions of glutamate and aspartate activity. It also blocks the production of nitric oxide. On the other hand, it also inhibits the intracellular release of cGMP [11]. It interacts with all opioid receptors [12]; it is noteworthy that the sigma receptor would be involved in hallucinogenic and psychotomimetic effects [13]. Regarding nicotinic and muscarinic receptors, ketamine inhibits the release of acetylcholine mediated by NMDA receptors [14].

Apart from being used in human anaesthesiology for the induction and maintenance of the anaesthesia, its use as a general anaesthetic in veterinary medicine has been widely disseminated, including a great diversity of animal species, among them we find pets (canines, felines), farm animals (porcine, sheep, goats, horses), or wild and laboratory animals, including rodents [15, 16]. Over time, other types of uses were found (as analgesic, antidepressant, or inductor of pharmacological model of schizophrenia) [17].

As administration route, we can count intravenous, intraperitoneal, intramuscular, intranasal, oral, intrarectal, and intrathecal [6, 18]. The oral route has a large first-pass metabolism, producing a bioavailability of 17%, which would explain why this route is not routinely used [19]. The route of administration that has the highest bioavailability and fastest onset of action is intravenous [9].

The objective of the present paper is to share a rationale argument on the use of ketamine as a recreational drug and its adverse toxic effects.

Development

Ketamine is also known in the street as drug K, special k, super k, keta, ket, kit-kat, ck, psychedelic heroin, rave, super acid, deadly line (flatliners), and their combinations: Kalvin Clein (ketamine + cocaine), Mari-key and Maria-K (ketamine + marijuana). The chemical nomenclature according to the International Union of Pure and Applied Chemistry for ketamine is 2-(2-chlorophenyl)-2-(methylamino)-cyclohexanone ketamine [12].

Commercially available ketamine is a racemic mixture of the two optical enantiomers (s)-Ketamine and (R)-Ketamine, available as 1%, 5%, or 10% ketamine hydrochloride [20] prepared with bidistilled water. Benzalkonium chloride [21] or chlorobutanol [22] are used as a preservative.

According to a report by the Europol/European Monitoring Center for Drugs and Drug Addiction in the year 2000, in the European Union most of the ketamine used for recreational purposes comes from the diversion of the pharmaceutical industry, hospitals, veterinary clinics, or the distribution network of pharmaceutical products. Internet sources describe the synthesis of ketamine as very difficult. In rhodium.lycaeum.org, the synthesis described uses the precursors cyclopentyl bromide, o-chlorobenzonitrile, and methylamine [23].

Generally, the original pharmaceutical form is usually changed to powder for recreational use, since users do not like to use a needle. This process is carried out through evaporation and is sold in small plastic or paper bags. Tablets are even made for oral consumption. It is in these procedures that the drug can be adulterated with inactive ingredients or, worse still, with active ingredients, not knowing the actual dose of ketamine that is acquired to increase the risk of suffering an overdose [24].

The first record of recreational use was in 1965 [25] and it was increasing greatly. Studies in the United Kingdom indicated that the consumption of ketamine in nightclubs in the year 1993 was 25%, increasing in the year 2007 to 40% [26]. It has come to occupy the third place in choice of recreational drugs, ranking after cocaine and amphetamines [27]. In France, the first reports of its use as a drug of abuse were in 1992 [28]. Asia is not exempted from this phenomenon, where the generic pharmaceutical industry generates significant quantities, providing immediate supply. A 2003 study of people detained by the police in Taiwan indicated that 2% had used ketamine. In Hong Kong, ketamine is one of the most widely used recreational drugs on weekends and, since 2017, the use of analogues such as dechloro-N-atylketamine (2-oxo-PCE) has been reported [28]. In 2005, in Australia, 70% of "party drug" users reported having ever used ketamine [29].

The reason for its popularization as a recreational drug is not reliably known, although its low cost, the subjective belief that it is a "safer" drug [24], and its rapid onset of action tend to be strong arguments. We may mention as an example that 30 s are needed when it is administered intravenously and 5.30 min for the inhalation route. Its duration reaches up to 3 h, and the particular psychotropic effects [19] have been referred to as hallucinations, vivid dreams, various states of confusion, depersonalization, and dissociation. It has been described also as near-death experience [8, 30].

Corazza in his book "*Near-Death Experiences: Exploring the Mind-Body Connection*" recounts experiences of ketamine users where several stories stand out. In one of them, Mr. P. reported the effects after injecting 100 mg of ketamine intramuscularly while listening to a piece of music: "I have gradually lost my senses. The music was much distorted. I have tested myself by asking myself basic questions about mathematics, the names of the ones I love, etc., and suddenly I wasn't interested in it. So I tried to focus on "who I am" and lost interest again. There are visions that blur. It didn't mean that I was more, because I existed anyway. Then I tried the experience of death. I was going through a tunnel. I saw the planet Earth. I could feel the relationship between the human soul, the Earth and the planets. I thought I was a doll, do you know what the matryoshka is? I was the matryoshka of the whole system. I understood that the earth is inside something else. I felt its gravity. All this is embraced within a system. I was nothing, but I knew that my place was on Earth" [31]. These experiences should be considered very near of psychedelic experiences and may be a reason of misuse.

Main Adverse Reactions Associated with Misuse

Miss L. used ketamine only once in her life; she said: I felt a little paranoid. I felt that I was going to die. The first effects started very soon. I felt very confused and normal reality was just gone. She was dizzy and couldn't walk. I started running into the walls. I wanted to leave the room where I was, but it was very cold. I had no one around to help me [31]. The chances of suffering accidents, falls, and loss of consciousness are high, even suicidal ideas were mentioned [31].

Ketamine generates dependence and quickly tolerance, which leads to consuming more to obtain the same effect [27]. In the United Kingdom, cases of consumption for recreational purposes as high as 20 g per day were reported [29].

It has been known since the late 1990s that excess exposures to NMDA receptor antagonists such as MK801 and ketamine cause apoptosis in the brain of neonatal rats [32]. It was also shown that this neurotoxicity would affect the brain of developing prenatal and postnatal animals such as rats, mice, and even primates [33, 34]. Even today, ketamine is used in animal models to assess neuronal apoptosis in the retina [35]. Other studies indicate that ketamine produces neurotoxicity in the hippocampus of mice where tumour necrosis factor α is involved [36].

At a systemic level, urinary problems such as painful and small bladder, ureteral obstruction, incontinence, papillary necrosis, and liver dysfunction were detected [29, 37–39].

There are reports of weight loss and loss of appetite with heavy use. In very rare cases, respiratory and cardiac function can be suppressed, but most commonly these functions are stimulated. Apneas are more likely to occur when administered rapidly intravenously [27]. The risks of ketamine use increase when combined with other depressants such as alcohol [28], and when combined with stimulants such as amphetamines or substituted amphetamines (MDMA). There are reports suggesting that ketamine could be used as a drug for rape, since in some cases when using high doses, it has amnesiac effects while under the influence of the drug [19]. In addition, due to its lack of taste, smell, and high solubility in water, it is very difficult to be detected by the victim [28].

Studies carried out in human beings demonstrated that there is alteration in working, episodic, and semantic memory [40–42]. In our laboratory, we found preliminary results in rats showing alterations in rats in working memory, acquisition, and short-term memory in translational experiments [43].

There are results indicating that semantic memory problems associated with recreational use of ketamine are reversible with marked reduction in use. However, deficits in episodic memory seem long-lasting [44]. Some users experience schizophrenic symptoms and perceptual disturbances for short periods that persist after they stop using [27].

At the gastrointestinal level, it was found to produce epigastric pain, gallbladder problems, and liver toxicity [45]. There are reports of toxicity associated with urinary bladder problems, such as incontinence, painful bladder, and urethral obstruction [34, 46]. However, the mechanism by which these effects occur is not yet established, although it was shown in vitro that ketamine induces toxicity in urothelial cells by prolonged increase in cytosolic calcium concentration. This would induce mitochondrial stress and the release of cytochrome C. Consequently, caspases would be activated, thus starting cell apoptosis [47].

The lower urinary tract is affected more often than the upper urinary tract. This suggests that the longer contact time of the urinary ketamine metabolites with the bladder may be a contributing factor [37]. At the sperm level, tests produced in cats demonstrated a decrease in sperm concentration when the sample was obtained by electroejaculation under ketamine anaesthesia [48].

In human beings, studies carried out in vitro demonstrated a decrease in sperm viability and progressive motility [49]. In addition, sperm function would be altered by mechanisms related to calcium. These toxic effects are linked to the inhibition of channels called CatSper [50].

Erectile dysfunction was demonstrated in rats treated with long-term ketamine. This is due to the neuronal decrease in the enzyme nitric oxide-synthetase in the cavernous nerve and the increase in smooth muscle cell apoptosis [51].

The high safety profile of ketamine should be questioned since there are reports where the risk of death is analysed. According to the European Monitoring Centre for Drugs and Drug Addiction in 2002, 12 people died as a result of the misuse of ketamine. It is relevant to clarify that 3 cases were associated with the use of ketamine alone and 4 with the association with norketamine and tiletamine [23].

Ketamine Abuse Treatment

In most cases, people with symptoms of ketamine misuse only need supportive or symptomatic treatment, since the effects can last several hours, depending on the dose, metabolic capacity, and other factors [52].

At present, there are no specific antidotes approved by the U.S. Food and Drug Administration (FDA) to treat ketamine overdoses, but there are medications that are useful for treating agitation and psychosis. Benzodiazepines help by relieving agitation, psychotomimetic effects, hypertension, hyperthermia, and seizures [52]. Butyrophenones are used to treat psychotic episodes and agitation [12, 53].

Ketamine and Models of Schizophrenic Psychosis. Translational and Clinical Findings

The relationship between glutamatergic antagonists and schizophrenia dates back a long time. Particularly here, Ketamine, which is being used for the treatment of depression, can produce schizophreniform psychotic-like symptoms [54]. The magnitude of these signs and symptoms is today a matter of study. In a meta-analysis trial involving studies of healthy volunteers and patients with schizophrenia, it was observed that there is evidence that acute administration of ketamine induces psychotic symptoms of significant intensity. When a bolus injection is used, positive symptoms would clearly prevail over negative ones, which would be transitory [54].

The need has been pointed out for animal models of schizophrenia to be used in order to explain these effects of NMDA glutamatergic antagonism, mainly behavioural tasks in rodents [55]. Behavioural paradigms in animal models have been used to improve the design of new antipsychotic drugs for use in schizophrenia. Models based on behavioural tasks have thus been used to translationally reproduce positive, negative, and cognitive symptoms as a direct route for drug testing and mechanistic studies. Rodent models have been noted as very valuable methods for replicating aetiologies, brain pathologies, and cognitive and behavioural disorders of schizophrenia [56]. The use of numerous behavioural tests is required to evaluate the congruence of animal models with the numerous sign-symptom manifestations of schizophrenic psychoses [55, 56].

Models of schizophrenia started with dopamine hypothesis, and today glutamate hypothesis appears to fit better with recent evidences [2, 57]. This hypothesis started on the eighties of the previous cycle. It was proposed based on the fact that phencyclidine (PCP) and ketamine induced neurocognitive disorders and symptoms similar to those observed in schizophrenia. These facts led to a hypoglutamatergic deficit theory of schizophrenia. The dopaminergic dysregulation was proposed as secondary to NMDA alteration [2]. We proposed in our schizophrenia translational models that positive symptoms may be induced blocking NMDA receptors within Nucleus Accumbens Septi (NAS), and that dopamine was related to treatment effect, not to the induction of positive symptoms [58–60]. These preliminary findings relating NMDA glutamatergic transmission and schizophrenia led to some therapeutic trials. It was the case of the use of NMDA modulators. Using glycine, d-serine, and glycine transport inhibitors (GTIs), some initial interesting findings were observed. However, the results remain controversial [2, 3]. In this line, we proposed the blockade of the glutamate autoreceptor, since its improved efficiency in a visual task is used as a translational animal model of perceptual disturbances [59]. It may be a future line to be displayed [59]. These results were extensively reviewed by us [61–64].

These findings linking glutamate and schizophrenia have been validated in humans through clinical approaches. They consisted of the induction of schizophrenia-like symptoms using neurophysiological biomarkers and neuroimaging techniques [57].

Ketamine as Antidepressant

Ketamine and esketamine are considered novel alternatives in cases of treatment-resistant depression, being the first non-monoaminergic agents in major depressive disorder. Their safety and tolerability are still a matter of discussion. The appropriate position of these drugs in treatment algorithms is also unclear [65].

Although the antidepressant effect is observed with a single subanaesthetic dose, and the antidepressant actions are rapid and sustained, its use is still limited by its potential for abuse and its dissociative properties. Its effects have been reported to be mostly explainable by synaptic potentiation of the long-term potentiation (LTP) type and the actions of brain-derived neurotrophic factor (BDNF), as its main actions. Other convergent mechanisms have also been pointed out, which are not mutually exclusive and that can synergize these two main mechanisms [66, 67].

Ketamine Neurotoxicity

We have previously mentioned some relevant toxic effects of ketamine. Even having previously tangentially developed the topic of ketamine neurotoxicity, we thought it appropriate to make one last reflection on this point. We understand that this must be done based on the risk/benefit balance that is generated between the new therapeutic uses and their harmful effects.

The use of glutamate receptor antagonists has been an emerging line of treatment for several clinical entities. Their use has been proposed as anaesthetics, as preventives of neurodegeneration in brain trauma, stroke, epilepsy [68], and major depressive disorders (MDD) [69, 70].

Ketamine and some derivatives have antidepressant properties [69, 70]. Ketamine binds to and acts on human NMDA receptors. Through mechanisms related to these receptors, it produces its antidepressant effect. In this way, a single subanaesthetic dose of ketamine induces a rapid (in a matter of hours) and long-lasting antidepressant effect, particularly in patients refractory to other antidepressants. These evidences have generated expectations for the development of new antidepressant drugs [69].

Among the possible adverse effects after repeated administration of ketamine is the induction of Olney lesions. These were described for the first time in 1989 and are characterized by the appearance of vacuoles in the cytoplasmic compartment of neuronal populations, describing the lysis of mitochondria. It has been reported that various drugs, such as barbiturates and benzodiazepines, would prevent the morphological damage and psychotomimetic-type symptoms produced by ketamine [71, 72].

These effects have attracted attention, leading to questions about these compounds, given that NMDA antagonists induce neurotoxicity in rats and psychosis in humans [68]. This evidence has led to linking a state of hypofunction of the NMDA receptor in neurodegenerative (Alzheimer's disease) and psychotic (schizophrenia) conditions [68].

It has been proposed that the mechanism by which the neurotoxic and psychotomimetic effects of NMDA antagonists are induced is indirect, involving the alteration of a complex network that would involve glutamatergic, cholinergic, and catecholaminergic receptors. When NMDA receptors of inhibitory neurons are blocked, a disinhibition of glutamatergic and cholinergic projections to the cerebral cortex would occur [68].

These lesions with vacuolation of neurons occur mainly in the posterior cingulate cortex (PCC) and the retrosplenial region. They are observed after the administration of non-competitive antagonists of the NMDA receptor (ketamine, PCP, MK-801 and dextromethorphan) or competitive antagonists (CPP, CGS-19755 and CGP 37849) [71, 72]. Administration of dizocilpine (MK-801) produces cytoplasmic vacuolation as a manifestation of neuronal degeneration in the retrosplenial/posterior cingulate cortex (RS/PC), whereas the same is not observed with dextromethorphan [73].

After inoculation at low doses, this vacuolation appears to be reversed within 24 h after administration. This suggests that cellular damage is not permanent at clinically relevant doses in rats [71, 72, 74]. Studies in non-human primates show that repeated daily administration of ketamine affects white matter integrity. This phenomenon is observed in fronto-thalamo-temporal connections after a 3-month treatment [75]. When rats are subjected to treatment for more than 6 months, increased cell death is caused in the PFC [76].

Comparing the neurotoxic reactions of various NMDA receptor antagonists, differences are observed. Thus, with dizocilpine, it is observed that adult rats are more sensitive and that females have greater sensitivity than males. Nitric oxide exerts its action dependent on age, not sex. Finally, ketamine has the same age and sex dependence as dizocilpine [77]. As previously anticipated [71, 72], GABAmimetic drugs (propofol and thiopental sodium) protect against reversible neurotoxic changes in the brain of rats. Specifically, they prevent the irreversible neurodegenerative reaction induced by dizocilpine [78].

In ageing processes, hyper-phosphorylation of the tau protein is considered an early event in the ageing process and Alzheimer's disease. The presence of cells with hyperphosphorylated tau protein has been observed after the administration of ketamine for 6 months in the prefrontal cortical area (PFC) and entorhinal cortex of mice and monkeys compared to control animals. Ketamine was injected in bolus in primates and intraperitoneally in mice [79].

Exposure to ketamine causes very important neurotoxicity in the brain of rodents and primates when it acts in the critical period of synaptogenesis. This is related to lower subsequent cognitive performances. This would particularly affect the subiculum, affecting long-term potentiation (LTP) mechanisms. This suggests that cognitive deterioration would be linked to permanent alterations, which would have modifications of gamma waves as an electrophysiological correlate [80]. This neurotoxicity of ketamine is observed particularly during the embryonic period through the blood-placental barrier in rats, decreasing the levels of neurotrophic proteins such as, for example, Brain Derived Neurotrophic Factor (BDNF), due to the strong impact on the developing CNS [81].

It has been reported that both positive and negative and cognitive symptoms of schizophrenia can be produced through the application of acute and repeated administrations of ketamine. This has led to this treatment being proposed as a valid model of cognitive symptoms of schizophrenia. With this procedure, a set of alterations in the integrity of the white matter in the fronto-thalamo-temporal or striatothalamic connections has been observed. This has led to proposals for translational models not only of new antidepressants [81] but also of schizophrenia, such as those we have previously mentioned [75].

We can conclude by saying that the doses and administration time are key to maintaining a favourable therapeutic effect through the activation of neurotrophic factors mediated, among others, by BDNF. Possible adverse effects, such as dissociative symptoms, psychotomimetic, cognitive impairment, or abuse and addiction problems with higher or repeated doses, should be avoided.

Conclusions

The use of ketamine for recreational purposes is a public health problem. Consumption is associated with a large number of adverse effects and dangerous adverse reactions, including death. There are not many toxicological studies where consumption is evaluated for long periods of time. Many users mistakenly consider that it is a safe drug, therefore free of dangers. This paper has presented an overview of the problems associated with the misuse of ketamine, taking into account that numerous studies are in progress. We consider it very important to carry out new toxicological studies regarding the consumption of ketamine, with both acute and chronic schemes. Its experimental use as a tool to induce schizophrenic-like symptoms in animal models constitutes an interesting way to explain schizophrenia pathophysiology. Furthermore, its recent use as antidepressant is one interesting new line as new treatment for refractory depressive disorder. However, its use as an antidepressant needs further studies. We can conclude by saying that all the present considerations constitute an argument for continuing studying ketamine.

References

1. Dorandeu F. Happy 50th anniversary ketamine. CNS Neurosci Ther. 2013;19(6):369. https://doi.org/10.1111/cns.12074.
2. Javitt DC. Glutamate and schizophrenia: phencyclidine, N-methyl-D-aspartate receptors, and dopamine-glutamate interactions. Int Rev Neurobiol. 2007;78:69–108. https://doi.org/10.1016/S0074-7742(06)78003-5.
3. Javitt DC, Zukin SR, Heresco-Levy U, Umbricht D. Has an angel shown the way? Etiological and therapeutic implications of the PCP/NMDA model of schizophrenia. Schizophr Bull. 2012;38(5):958–66. https://doi.org/10.1093/schbul/sbs069.
4. Hakey P, Ouellette W, Zubieta J, Korter T. (S)-(+)-Ketamine hydro-chloride. Acta Crystallogr Sect E Struct Rep Online. 2008;64(Pt8):o1487. https://doi.org/10.1107/S1600536808021053.
5. Hansen KB, Wollmuth LP, Bowie D, Furukawa H, Menniti FS, Sobolevsky AI, Swanson GT, Swanger SA, Greger IH, Nakagawa T, McBain CJ, Jayaraman V, Low CM, Dell'Acqua ML, Diamond JS, Camp CR, Perszyk RE, Yuan H, Traynelis SF. Structure, function, and pharmacology of glutamate receptor ion channels. Pharmacol Rev. 2021;73(4):298–487. https://doi.org/10.1124/pharmrev.120.000131.
6. Reich DL, Silvay G Ketamine: an update on the first twenty-five years of clinical experience. Can J Anaesthesia = Journal Canadien D'anesthesie. 1989;36(2):186–97. https://doi.org/10.1007/BF03011442.
7. Miller RD, Eriksson LI, Fleisher LA, Wiener-Kronish JP, Cohen NH, Young WL. Miller's anesthesia e-book. Elsevier Health Sciences; 2014.
8. Bonta IL. Schizophrenia, dissociative anaesthesia and near-death experience; three events meeting at the

NMDA receptor. Med Hypotheses. 2004;62(1):23–8. https://doi.org/10.1016/S0306-9877(03)00307-4.
9. Kohtala S. Ketamine—50 years in use: from anesthesia to rapid antidepressant effects and neurobiological mechanisms. Pharmacol Rep. 2021;73(2):323–45. https://doi.org/10.1007/s43440-021-00232-4.
10. Zhang K, Yao Y, Hashimoto K. Ketamine and its metabolites: potential as novel treatments for depression. Neuropharmacology. 2023;222:109305. https://doi.org/10.1016/j.neuropharm.2022.109305.
11. Jonkman K, van der Schrier R, van Velzen M, Aarts L, Olofsen E, Sarton E, Niesters M, Dahan A. Differential role of nitric oxide in the psychedelic symptoms induced by racemic ketamine and esketamine in human volunteers. Br J Anaesth. 2018;120(5):1009–18. https://doi.org/10.1016/j.bja.2018.01.022.
12. Culp C, Kim HK, Abdi S. Ketamine use for cancer and chronic pain management. Front Pharmacol. 2021;11:599721. https://doi.org/10.3389/fphar.2020.599721.
13. Mori T, Yoshizawa K, Shibasaki M, Suzuki T. Discriminative stimulus effects of hallucinogenic drugs: a possible relation to reinforcing and aversive effects. J Pharmacol Sci. 2012;120(2):70–6. https://doi.org/10.1254/jphs.12r08cp.
14. Wohleb ES, Gerhard D, Thomas A, Duman RS. Molecular and cellular mechanisms of rapid-acting antidepressants ketamine and scopolamine. Curr Neuropharmacol. 2017;15(1):11–20. https://doi.org/10.2174/1570159X14666160309114549.
15. Serrano L, Guevara M, Gargiulo PA. Técnica neuroquirúrgica de estereotaxia en ratas para colocación de cánulas intracerebrales. Selecciones Veterinarias Revista de Neurología Veterinaria. 2014;3(1):105–16.
16. Guevara MA, Lorenzo Acquaro SA, Giai M, Gargiulo, PA. Comparison of two ketamine/xylazine anesthesic protocols in pigs (Sus scrofa domestica). Braz J Biol Sci. 2018;5(11):Art. 11. https://doi.org/10.21472/bjbs.051114.
17. Stefanovic A, Brandner B, Klaassen E, Cregg R, Nagaratnam M, Bromley LM, Das RK, Rossell SL, Morgan CJA, Curran HV. Acute and chronic effects of ketamine on semantic priming: modeling schizophrenia? J Clin Psychopharmacol. 2009;29(2):124. https://doi.org/10.1097/JCP.0b013e31819a4b91.
18. Clements JA, Nimmo WS, Grant IS. Bioavailability, pharmacokinetics, and analgesic activity of ketamine in humans. J Pharm Sci. 1982;71(5):539–42. https://doi.org/10.1002/jps.2600710516.
19. Corazza O, Assi S, Schifano F. From "Special K" to "Special M": the evolution of the recreational use of ketamine and methoxetamine. CNS Neurosci Ther. 2013;19(6):454–60. https://doi.org/10.1111/cns.12063.
20. Marland S, Ellerton J, Andolfatto G, Strapazzon G, Thomassen O, Brandner B, Weatherall A, Paal P. Ketamine: use in anesthesia. CNS Neurosci Ther. 2013;19(6):381–9. https://doi.org/10.1111/cns.12072.
21. Coates KM, Flood P. Ketamine and its preservative, benzethonium chloride, both inhibit human recombinant α7 and α4β2 neuronal nicotinic acetylcholine receptors in Xenopus oocytes. Br J Pharmacol. 2001;134(4):871–9. https://doi.org/10.1038/sj.bjp.0704315.
22. Errando CL, Mínguez A. Some misleadings about ketamine and their preservatives. Reg Anesth Pain Med. 1998;23(3):323–4. https://doi.org/10.1016/s1098-7339(98)90063-3.
23. European Monitoring Centre for Drugs and Drug Addiction. (Ed.). Report on the risk assessment of ketamine in the framework of the joint action on new synthetic drugs. Office for Official Publications of the European Communities; 2002.
24. Guevara M, Marquez Herrero S, Romanowicz E, Hernandez J, García Menéndez S, Gargiulo PA. El peligro del consumo de ketamina. Vet Argent. 2016;33(340):1–3.
25. Stevenson C. Ketamine: a review. Update in anaesthesia. 2005;20(20):5. https://www.semanticscholar.org/paper/KETAMINE%3A-A-REVIEW-Dr-Carl-Stevenson%2C-Medecins-Sans/1c0d09a56afb4b1d452b15353cc773984a940b3b.
26. McCambridge J, Winstock A, Hunt N, Mitcheson L. 5-year trends in use of hallucinogens and other adjunct drugs among uk dance drug users. Eur Addict Res. 2007;13(1):57–64. https://doi.org/10.1159/000095816.
27. Schifano F, Corkery J, Oyefeso A, Tonia T, Ghodse AH. Trapped in the "K hole". J Clin Psychopharmacol. 2008;28(1):114. https://www.academia.edu/19283787/Trapped_in_the_K_hole.
28. Daré BL, Pelletier R, Morel I, Gicquel T. Histoire de la kétamine: Une molécule ancienne qui a toujours la cote. Annales Pharmaceutiques Françaises, 2022;80(1):1. https://doi.org/10.1016/j.pharma.2021.04.005.
29. Wood D, Cottrell A, Baker SC, Southgate J, Harris M, Fulford S, Woodhouse C, Gillatt D. Recreational ketamine: from pleasure to pain. BJU Int. 2011;107(12):1881–4. https://doi.org/10.1111/j.1464-410X.2010.10031.x.
30. Jansen K. Near death experience and the NMDA receptor. Br Med J. 1989;298(6689):1708. https://www.ncbi.nlm.nih.gov/pmc/articles/PMC1836765/.
31. Corazza, O. Near-death experiences: exploring the mind-body connection. London: Routledge; 2008. https://doi.org/10.4324/9780203928905.
32. Ikonomidou C, Bosch F, Miksa M, Bittigau P, Vöckler J, Dikranian K, Tenkova TI, Stefovska V, Turski L, Olney JW. Blockade of NMDA receptors and apoptotic neurodegeneration in the developing brain. Science. 1999;283(5398):70–4. https://doi.org/10.1126/science.283.5398.70.
33. McGowan FXJ, Davis PJ. Anesthetic-related neurotoxicity in the developing infant: of mice, rats, monkeys and, possibly, humans. Anesthesia Analgesia. 2008;106(6):1599. https://doi.org/10.1213/ane.0b013e31817330cf.

34. Kalopita K, Armakolas A, Philippou A, Zarros A, Angelogianni P. Ketamine-induced neurotoxicity in neurodevelopment: a synopsis of main pathways based on recent in vivo experimental findings. J Anaesthesiol Clin Pharmacol. 2021;37(1):37–42. https://doi.org/10.4103/joacp.JOACP_415_19.
35. Zhang K, Wu L, Lin K, Zhang M, Li W, Tong X, Zheng J. Integrin-dependent microgliosis mediates ketamine-induced neuronal apoptosis during postnatal rat retinal development. Exp Neurol. 2021;340:113659. https://doi.org/10.1016/j.expneurol.2021.113659.
36. Zheng X, Zhou J, Xia Y. The role of TNF-α in regulating ketamine-induced hippocampal neurotoxicity. Arch Med Sci. 2015;11(6):1296–302. https://doi.org/10.5114/aoms.2015.56355.
37. Chu PSK, Ma W-K, Wong SC-W, Chu RW-H, Cheng C-H, Wong S, Tse JM, Lau F-L, Yiu M-K, Man CW. The destruction of the lower urinary tract by ketamine abuse: a new syndrome? BJU Int. 2008;102(11):1616–22. https://doi.org/10.1111/j.1464-410X.2008.07920.x.
38. Chu PSK, Kwok S, Lam K, Chu T, Chan S, Man C, Ma W, Chi K, Yiu M, Chan Y, Tse M, Lau F. 'Street ketamine'—associated bladder dysfunction: a report of ten cases. Hong Kong Med J. 2007;13:311–3. https://www.hkmj.org/abstracts/v13n4/311.htm.
39. Yang SSD, Jang MY, Lee KH, Hsu WT, Chen YC, Chen WS, Chang SJ. Sexual and bladder dysfunction in male ketamine abusers: a large-scale questionnaire study. PLoS One. 2018;13(11):e0207927. https://doi.org/10.1371/journal.pone.0207927.
40. Curran HV, Morgan C. Cognitive, dissociative and psychotogenic effects of ketamine in recreational users on the night of drug use and 3 days later. Addiction. 2000;95(4):575–90. https://doi.org/10.1046/j.1360-0443.2000.9545759.x.
41. Morgan CJA, Mofeez A, Brandner B, Bromley L, Curran HV. Ketamine impairs response inhibition and is positively reinforcing in healthy volunteers: a dose–response study. Psychopharmacology. 2004;172(3):298–308. https://doi.org/10.1007/s00213-003-1656-y.
42. Morgan CJA, Mofeez A, Brandner B, Bromley L, Curran HV. Acute effects of ketamine on memory systems and psychotic symptoms in healthy volunteers. Neuropsychopharmacology. 2004;29(1):Art. 1. https://doi.org/10.1038/sj.npp.1300342.
43. Guevara MA, Lorenzo S, Anselmi V, Romanowic E, Cabrera M, García Menéndez S, Barrutieta I, Baiardi G, La Fuente JV, Gargiulo PÁ. Nuevos aportes sobre alteraciones cognitivas y metabólico-cerebrales por la administración de ketamina en dosis subanestésicas en ratas Rattus norvegicus (estudio preliminar). II Congreso de Neurocirugía Veterinaria. VII Congreso Latinoamericano de Neurología Veterinaria. X Encuentro de Neurología Veterinaria del Cono Sur. Mendoza, argentina, 17 al 19 de setiembre de 2019. Revista Argentina de Neurología Veterinaria. 2020;8(1):45.
44. Morgan CJA, Monaghan L, Curran HV. Beyond the K-hole: a 3-year longitudinal investigation of the cognitive and subjective effects of ketamine in recreational users who have substantially reduced their use of the drug. Addiction. 2004;99(11):1450–61. https://doi.org/10.1111/j.1360-0443.2004.00879.x.
45. Bokor G, Anderson PD. Ketamine: an update on its abuse. J Pharm Pract. 2014;27(6):582–6. https://doi.org/10.1177/0897190014525754.
46. Wood DM, Davies S, Puchnarewicz M, Johnston A, Dargan PI. Acute toxicity associated with the recreational use of the ketamine derivative methoxetamine. Eur J Clin Pharmacol. 2012;68(5):853–6. https://doi.org/10.1007/s00228-011-1199-9.
47. Baker SC, Shabir S, Georgopoulos NT, Southgate J. Ketamine-induced apoptosis in normal human urothelial cells. Am J Pathol. 2016;186(5):1267–77. https://doi.org/10.1016/j.ajpath.2015.12.014.
48. Zambelli D, Cunto M, Prati F, Merlo B. Effects of ketamine or medetomidine administration on quality of electroejaculated sperm and on sperm flow in the domestic cat. Theriogenology. 2007;68(5):796–803. https://doi.org/10.1016/j.theriogenology.2007.06.008.
49. Absalan F, Ghannadi A, Zabihi A. The effects of different doses of ketamine on quality of normal ejaculated sperm. Int J Fertil Steril. 2014;8(2):207–14. https://www.ncbi.nlm.nih.gov/pmc/articles/PMC4107695/.
50. He Y, Zou Q, Li B, Chen H, Du X, Weng S, Luo T, Zeng X. Ketamine inhibits human sperm function by Ca2+-related mechanism. Biochem Biophys Res Commun. 2016;478(1):501–6. https://doi.org/10.1016/j.bbrc.2016.04.144.
51. Shang HS, Wu YN, Liao CH, Chiueh T, Lin YF, Chiang HS. Long-term administration of ketamine induces erectile dysfunction by decreasing neuronal nitric oxide synthase on cavernous nerve and increasing corporal smooth muscle cell apoptosis in rats. Oncotarget. 2016;8(43):73670-73683. https://doi.org/10.18632/oncotarget.10727.
52. Orhurhu VJ, Vashisht R, Claus LE, Cohen SP. Ketamine toxicity. In: StatPearls. StatPearls Publishing; 2022. http://www.ncbi.nlm.nih.gov/books/NBK541087/.
53. Moradi MM, Moradi MM, Safaie A, Baratloo A, Payandemehr P. Sub dissociative dose of ketamine with haloperidol versus fentanyl on pain reduction in patients with acute pain in the emergency department; a randomized clinical trial. Am J Emerg Med. 2022;54:165–71. https://doi.org/10.1016/j.ajem.2022.02.012.
54. Beck K, Hindley G, Borgan F, Ginestet C, McCutcheon R, Brugger S, Driesen N, Ranganathan M, D'Souza DC, Taylor M, Krystal JH, Howes OD. Association of ketamine with psychiatric symptoms and implications for its therapeutic use and for understanding schizophrenia: a systematic review and meta-analysis.

JAMA New Open. 2020;3(5):e204693. https://doi.org/10.1001/jamanetworkopen.2020.4693.
55. Ang MJ, Lee S, Kim JC, Kim SH, Moon C. Behavioral tasks evaluating schizophrenia-like symptoms in animal models: a recent update. Curr Neuropharmacol. 2021;19(5):641–64. https://doi.org/10.2174/1570159X18666200814175114.
56. Winship IR, Dursun SM, Baker GB, Balista PA, Kandratavicius L, Maia-de-Oliveira JP, Hallak J, Howland JG. An overview of animal models related to schizophrenia. Can J Psychiatr. 2019;64(1):5–17. https://doi.org/10.1177/0706743718773728.
57. Haaf M, Leicht G, Curic S, Mulert C. Glutamatergic deficits in schizophrenia—biomarkers and pharmacological interventions within the ketamine model. Curr Pharm Biotechnol. 2018;19(4):293–307. https://doi.org/10.2174/1389201019666180620112528.
58. Gargiulo PA, Siemann M, Delius JD. Visual discrimination in pigeons impaired by glutamatergic blockade of nucleus accumbens. Physiol Behav. 1998;63(4):705–9. https://doi.org/10.1016/s0031-9384(97)00516-7.
59. Gargiulo PA, Acerbo MJ, Krug I, Delius JD. Cognitive effects of dopaminergic and glutamatergic blockade in nucleus accumbens in pigeons. Pharmacol Biochem Behav. 2005;81(4):732–9. https://doi.org/10.1016/j.pbb.2005.05.009.
60. Acerbo MJ, Gargiulo PA, Krug I, Delius JD. Behavioural consequences of nucleus accumbens dopaminergic stimulation and glutamatergic blocking in pigeons. Behav Brain Res. 2002;136(1):171–7. https://doi.org/10.1016/s0166-4328(02)00109-2.
61. Gargiulo PA. Aproximaciones Experimentales a la Percepción Delirante (Experimental approaches to delusional perception). Alcmeón Revista Argentina de Neuropsiquiatría. 2001;37:18–30.
62. Gargiulo PA. Aproximaciones Experimentales a la Disfunción perceptual en la Esquizofrenia. (Experimental approaches to perceptual dysfunction in schizophrenia). Revista de Neurología. Rev Neurol. 2003;37(6):545–51.
63. Gargiulo PA, Landa de Gargiulo AI. Perception and psychoses: the role of glutamatergic transmission within the nucleus accumbens septi. Short Commun Behav Brain Sci. 2004;27(6):792–3.
64. Gargiulo PÁ, Landa De Gargiulo AI. Glutamate and modeling of schizophrenia symptoms: review of our findings: 1990–2014. Pharmacol Rep. 2014;66(3):343–52. https://doi.org/10.1016/j.pharep.2014.03.010.
65. McIntyre RS, Rosenblat JD, Nemeroff CB, Sanacora G, Murrough JW, Berk M, Brietzke E, Dodd S, Gorwood P, Ho R, Iosifescu DV, Lopez Jaramillo C, Kasper S, Kratiuk K, Lee JG, Lee Y, Lui LMW, Mansur RB, Papakostas GI, Subramaniapillai M, Thase M, Vieta E, Young AH, Zarate CA Jr, Stahl S. Synthesizing the evidence for ketamine and esketamine in treatment-resistant depression: an international expert opinion on the available evidence and implementation. Am J Psychiatry. 2021;178(5):383–99. https://doi.org/10.1176/appi.ajp.2020.20081251.
66. Zanos P, Gould TD. Mechanisms of ketamine action as an antidepressant. Mol Psychiatry. 2018;23(4):801–11. https://doi.org/10.1038/mp.2017.255.
67. Zanos P, Brown KA, Georgiou P, Yuan P, Zarate CA Jr, Thompson SM, Gould TD. NMDA receptor activation-dependent antidepressant-relevant behavioral and synaptic actions of ketamine. J Neurosci. 2023;43(6):1038–50. https://doi.org/10.1523/JNEUROSCI.1316-22.2022.
68. Farber NB, Kim SH, Dikranian K, Jiang XP, Heinkel C. Receptor mechanisms and circuitry underlying NMDA antagonist neurotoxicity. Mol Psychiatry. 2002;7(1):32–43. https://doi.org/10.1038/sj.mp.4000912.
69. Zhang Y, Ye F, Zhang T, Lv S, Zhou L, Du D, Lin H, Guo F, Luo C, Zhu S. Structural basis of ketamine action on human NMDA receptors. Nature. 2021; 596(7871):301–5. https://doi.org/10.1038/s41586-021-03769-9. Erratum in: Nature. 2021; 598(7882):E3.
70. Barrutieta-Arberas I, Ortuzar N, Vaquero-Rodríguez A, Picó-Gallardo M, Bengoetxea H, Guevara MA, Gargiulo PA, Lafuente JV. The role of ketamine in major depressive disorders: effects on parvalbumin-positive interneurons in hippocampus. Exp Biol Med (Maywood). 2023;248(7):588–95. https://doi.org/10.1177/15353702231170007.
71. Olney JW, Labruyere J, Price MT. Pathological changes induced in cerebrocortical neurons by phencyclidine and related drugs. Science. 1989;244(4910):1360–2. https://doi.org/10.1126/science.2660263.
72. Olney JW, Labruyere J, Wang G, Wozniak DF, Price MT, Sesma MA. NMDA antagonist neurotoxicity: mechanism and prevention. Science. 1991;254(5037):1515–8. https://doi.org/10.1126/science.1835799.
73. Carliss RD, Radovsky A, Chengelis CP, O'Neill TP, Shuey DL. Oral administration of dextromethorphan does not produce neuronal vacuolation in the rat brain. Neurotoxicology. 2007;28(4):813–8. https://doi.org/10.1016/j.neuro.2007.03.009.
74. Hargreaves RJ, Hill RG, Iversen LL. Neuroprotective NMDA antagonists: the controversy over their potential for adverse effects on cortical neuronal morphology. Acta Neurochir Suppl (Wien). 1994;60:15–9. https://doi.org/10.1007/978-3-7091-9334-1_4.
75. Li Q, Shi L, Lu G, Yu HL, Yeung FK, Wong NK, Sun L, Liu K, Yew D, Pan F, Wang DF, Sham PC. Chronic ketamine exposure causes white matter microstructural abnormalities in adolescent cynomolgus monkeys. Front Neurosci. 2017;11:285. https://doi.org/10.3389/fnins.2017.00285.

76. Sun WL, Coleman NT, Zelek-Molik A, Barry SM, Whitfield TW Jr, McGinty JF. Relapse to cocaine-seeking after abstinence is regulated by cAMP-dependent protein kinase A in the prefrontal cortex. Addict Biol. 2014;19(1):77–86. https://doi.org/10.1111/adb.12043.
77. Jevtovic-Todorovic V, Wozniak DF, Benshoff ND, Olney JW. A comparative evaluation of the neurotoxic properties of ketamine and nitrous oxide. Brain Res. 2001;895(1–2):264–7. https://doi.org/10.1016/s0006-8993(01)02079-0.
78. Jevtovic-Todorovic V, Wozniak DF, Powell S, Olney JW. Propofol and sodium thiopental protect against MK-801-induced neuronal necrosis in the posterior cingulate/retrosplenial cortex. Brain Res. 2001;913(2):185–9. https://doi.org/10.1016/s0006-8993(01)02800-1.
79. Yeung LY, Wai MS, Fan M, Mak YT, Lam WP, Li Z, Lu G, Yew DT. Hyperphosphorylated tau in the brains of mice and monkeys with long-term administration of ketamine. Toxicol Lett. 2010;193(2):189–93. https://doi.org/10.1016/j.toxlet.2010.01.008.
80. Manzella FM, Joksimovic SM, Orfila JE, Fine BR, Dietz RM, Sampath D, Fiedler HK, Tesic V, Atluri N, Raol YH, Jevtovic-Todorovic V, Herson PS, Todorovic SM. Neonatal ketamine alters high-frequency oscillations and synaptic plasticity in the subiculum but does not affect sleep macrostructure in adolescent rats. Front Syst Neurosci. 2020;14:26. https://doi.org/10.3389/fnsys.2020.00026.
81. Li Q, Qu FL, Gao Y, Jiang YP, Rahman K, Lee KH, Han T, Qin LP. Piper sarmentosum Roxb. produces antidepressant-like effects in rodents, associated with activation of the CREB-BDNF-ERK signaling pathway and reversal of HPA axis hyperactivity. J Ethnopharmacol. 2017;199:9–19. https://doi.org/10.1016/j.jep.2017.01.037.

Part III

Neurosciences, Learning, Teaching and the Role of Social Environment

30 Executive Functioning: The Necessity for a Contextualized and Ecologically Valid Evaluation

Mirta Susana Ison Zintilini
and Pascual Ángel Gargiulo

Introduction

Executive functioning (EF) is defined as a multidimensional construct, made up of a specific set of cognitive processes that intervene in the regulation of socio-emotional behavior in response to novel, complex situations and/or in the conscious resolution of problems aimed at specific objectives [1–9]. Thus, these executive skills allow us to initiate behaviors based on an objective, to inhibit the effect of irrelevant stimuli, to select relevant task objectives, to plan and organize the means to solve problems, and to analyze different perspectives of an event, mentally considering alternative solutions or approaches, flexibly changing strategies for achieving goals [10–12]. This executive functioning involves cognitive effort to analyze how different facts or ideas relate to each other, considering how past events can be related to future events, mentally establishing their relationship OR expanding the range of possible ways to understand a new situation and the changes associated with this functioning [13].

There is a consensus that the core of executive functioning is made up of working memory, inhibitory control, and cognitive flexibility, highly interrelated processes that share a common denominator, such as an underlying executive attention factor [7, 14–16]. Its harmonious functioning forms the basis for high-order processes, such as reasoning, problem-solving, and decision-making, functions that intervene in emotional self-regulation [1, 4, 11, 17, 18]. Neuroanatomical studies show that the seat of executive functions is found in the prefrontal cortex and its interconnections with other brain areas, such as the anterior cingulate cortex and the parietal cortex [9, 13, 19].

The executive functioning triad, composed of cognitive flexibility, working memory, and inhibitory control, is associated with distinct and partially overlapping networks involving dorsal, lateral, ventral, and medial regions of the prefrontal cortex. While hot EF, related to socio-emotional situations, depends more on the ventral and medial parts, cold EF, related to academic performance, rather depends more on the dorsal and lateral parts of the prefrontal cortex (PFC). PFC regions have been shown to be active in per-

M. S. Ison Zintilini (✉)
Human, Social and Environmental Science Institute of the National Scientific and Technical Research Council (INCIHUSA—CONICET), Technological Scientific Centre (CCT Mendoza- CONICET), Mendoza, Argentina

Faculty of Psychology, Aconcagua University, Mendoza, Argentina
e-mail: mison@uda.edu.ar; mison@mendoza-conicet.gob.ar

P. Á. Gargiulo
Laboratory of Neurosciences and Experimental Psychology, Latin American Technological Corporation Foundation (FUCOTEL), Cathedra of Psychopathology, Catholic University of Argentina, Area of Pharmacology, Department of Pathology, National University of Cuyo, CONICET, Guaymallén, Mendoza, Argentina

P. Á. Gargiulo, H. L. Mesones-Arroyo (eds.), *Psychiatry and Neuroscience Update – Vol. V*,
https://doi.org/10.1007/978-3-031-72219-6_30

haps hundreds of functional neuroimaging studies with adults when they complete tasks that involve holding information in mind, inhibiting one response in favor of another, and diverting attention from one set of tasks to another [19].

Connections of PFC with other brain areas occur primarily through white matter tracts, allowing for very rapid goal-directed, "top down" regulation of activity in multiple brain areas, such as those associated with attention, memory, motor responses, and language [9, 20]. Meta-analysis studies have highlighted that three periods stand out in which these processes develop more widely and coincide with peaks of intense metabolic activation of the frontal lobes: from 4-to-7 years, from 10-to-12 years of age, and from 16-to-19 years [13, 16, 21]. These are periods in which the strengthening of cognitive, social, and emotional skills plays a relevant role in the academic performance of children and adolescents [22–24].

Longitudinal studies provide consistent evidence of the interdependence between executive functioning, social competencies, and academic achievement. Good executive performance favors the development of social competencies and academic achievements and, in turn, the activities involved in learning strengthened executive functioning and performance in social competencies [24–27]. Given that the specific skills that make up the construct of executive functions go through a prolonged period of development spanning from childhood to early adulthood, it has been necessary to develop EF assessments, considering the different changes in development, from early childhood until old age [9, 10, 28, 29].

One of the most cited challenges in assessing EF is the problem of measurement impurity [7]. Measurement impurity refers to the idea that very few tests purely measure executive functioning skills. There are multiple processes that contribute to individual differences in performance on any EF task, and EF tasks require multiple executive processes to complete. The problem of impurity in the evaluation of EF and measures based on performance through highly structured tasks does not adequately characterize the real manifestation of EF skills in "everyday" life, considering the particularities of the different socio-environmental contexts of each evaluated person. This aspect is defined as ecological and contextualized validity in psychological and neuropsychological evaluation [9, 30].

In this chapter, some general considerations of executive functioning are presented, as well as the necessity of thinking contextualized ways of evaluating executive functions, providing greater ecological validity.

General Considerations of Executive Functions

In diverse circumstances, people face situations in which challenges are presented that should be addressed in new ways. To do this, a range of possible solutions should be considered for analyzing the consequences of actions and for making creative decisions, while self-regulating the emotional states in order to achieve solutions for situations according to the context. This is when a series of cognitive and emotional control processes called "executive functioning" are deployed. This functioning is closely related to information processing cognitive and socio-emotional speed. The information processing speed increases markedly throughout childhood, the speed gradually improving toward early adulthood [13]. Individual differences in information processing speed emerge in early childhood, and these differences predict later EF [31, 32].

As previously mentioned, the core of executive functioning is made up of working memory, inhibitory control, and cognitive flexibility, three highly interrelated and interdependent types of processes. These functions share a common denominator, which is underlying executive attention factor [7, 14, 15]. This triad is the basis of other more complex functions, such as planning, problem-solving, organization, fluency, and meta-cognition [7, 9, 14, 33]. Regarding attention, it is defined as a multidimensional construct in charge of regulating which stimuli address the perceptive resources, filtering irrelevant information to favor the retention of information during a period of time, before acting on it [34–36].

Following the model proposed by Mirsky and Duncan [37], attentional functioning results in the coordinated action of several elements linked to each other. These authors have proposed five elements of attention: Focusing/Execution, Sustained Attention, Shift of Attentional Focus, Codification, and Stability. These components represent significant aspects in the regulation of processing information.

Concerning details of these five components, first, *Focusing* represents the ability to select an objective of information and to execute a task in the presence of distracting stimuli. Selective functioning has been the focus of studies relating to ocular movement and visual selection [37]. Second, *Sustained Attention* represents the capacity to maintain focus and an alert state in the long term. An outstanding characteristic of this component is that the quality of sustained attention tends to decline with time. Maintained attentional focus involves the possibility of resisting distractor interference. Third, *Shifting* is the ability to change attentional focus in a flexible and adaptative way according to the requirements of the task. Fourth, *Stability* refers to the consistency and attentional effort over time in relation to the detection of the target stimuli. This component is defined, to a degree, by Misrky and Duncan [37]. Finally, *Codification* refers to the ability of internally representing and operating with this information, thus maintaining the information in memory during short periods of time to permit the execution of mental operations [37]. This concept is related to the definition of working memory [38].

The development of attention and working memory are very closely related. Attention plays an important role in successful performance of working memory and the development of the systems of attention that influence the development of working memory. Bidirectional effects are common control over development. Further, equally interesting is the potential influence of working memory in the development of the attention systems in infancy and early childhood [36].

Working memory (WM) is defined as a store of limited capacity that keeps information for a short period of time, thus maintaining and manipulating this information temporarily, but WM also processes and uses this information in an active way depending upon the objectives and tasks that the subject must solve [36, 39]. It involves keeping the information in mind and manipulating it in some way to understand and acquire more complex knowledge, using and integrating this information in a coherent whole [13, 40].

The classic work of Baddeley and Hitch [41] has pointed out that Working Memory constitutes a set of mental processes responsible for the temporary storage and manipulation of information with four differentiated subcomponents: the phonological loop, the visuospatial agenda, the central executive, and the episodic buffer.

First, the *phonological loop* refers to a control process based on articulatory review, being the repetition of information with subvocal language in relation to what is being read, a situation that helps process the information. Thus, the phonological loop is relevant for the transient storage of verbal material and for maintaining the inner speech involved in short-term memory.

Second, the *visuospatial agenda* manipulates and uses visual images, operating in a similar way to the phonological loop, only focusing on maintaining these images. It is important to clarify that the information that is processed can come from either of our sensory channels or from our long-term memory. WM also involves other mental activities, ranging from the simplest to the large-scale decision-making [42, 43].

Third, the *Supervisory Attentional System* (SAS) is activated when a situation is recognized as novel or nonroutine, which puts into action executive processes of anticipation, goal selection, planning, and monitoring. The SAS works with the information coming from the phonological loop and the visuospatial agenda simultaneously, and at the same time, it works on updating and maintaining the information [44]. That is, the attentional system is required to mediate the performance coming from both information channels.

Fourth, the *episodic buffer* refers to a system in which the phonological and visual information is integrated with current information, which comes from long-term memory. In other words, it is a system where information from the first two components and long-term memory are used, so that a multimodal and temporal representation of the current situation is created [44, 45].

Various studies show the bidirectionality between the development of attention systems and working memory performance in early childhood [15, 34, 36]. These bidirectional effects are common across development, and therefore, the potential influence of working memory on the later development of attention systems in infancy and early childhood is equally interesting. Given that some models emphasize the role of the prefrontal cortex and attentional control as a central component for working memory functioning [36, 39], it is logical to consider that the emergence of attentional control around 6 months of age contributes significantly to the development of working memory. This coincides with the improvements in working memory performance that occur from 5 to 6 months of age, probably influenced by the development of attention systems [34, 36, 46]. A review done by Canet-Juric et al. [17] has maintained that various studies have indicated that WM capacity increases constantly and progressively from 4 to 15 years.

WM is essential for the control of our cognitive activities and our behavior, regarding our intentions and objectives [47]. WM intervenes in important cognitive processes such as language comprehension, reading, reasoning and metacognition, among others.

Working Memory tasks also involve attentional control and inhibitory control, showing significant and prolonged development starting at 6 months of age [36]. Thus, WM tasks are associated with inhibitory control processes through the ability to stop unproductive responses to obtain greater efficiency in the manipulation of the information necessary to resolve various situations, preventing distractions from entering the active state [17, 48].

Inhibitory control, for its part, encompasses a series of cognitive processes that involve both selective attention and representations in working memory. This is defined as the multidimensional process responsible for regulating attention in order to ignore distracting stimuli, stop impulsive behavior, or stop unproductive responses. Thus, talking about inhibitory control implies thinking about voluntary control to inhibit stimuli, cognitions, and behavioral responses that are irrelevant to the proposed objective. Inhibitory control allows us both to focus attention and to regulate emotions and behavior for adequate coexistence [9, 49–52].

In the 1990s, Barkley suggested that inhibitory control should be considered a process somewhat separate from executive functions. This author has maintained that inhibitory control is a prerequisite for successful executive functioning, since it is the cognitive process on which executive functions pivot [53]. Barkley has maintained that inhibitory control brings together: (a) the ability to inhibit prepotent responses, such as inhibition of impulsivity; (b) the ability to inhibit ongoing responses in order to correct errors and redirect responses, also called cognitive flexibility; and, (c) control of interference from irrelevant stimuli. Current models consider inhibitory control as one of the central components of executive functioning, along with working memory and cognitive flexibility [9, 14]. Inhibitory control is also a fundamental process in human behavior and its effects, and its levels of sophistication differentiate us from animals.

Multidimensional approaches distinguish between 3 inhibitory control processes: perceptual, cognitive, and behavioral. Without a doubt, each of them implies, to a greater or lesser extent, the others.

Perceptual inhibition control refers to the ability to maintain attention focus by suppressing or controlling the interference generated by distracting or irrelevant stimuli to the ongoing tasks [14, 19]. This type of inhibitory process occurs at the perceptual level, in an initial stage of information processing and in situations of stimulus competition [49, 54]. A good functioning of perceptual inhibition would favor adequate performance in attentional focusing, by directing perceptual resources towards relevant stimuli in the environment.

Cognitive inhibition control refers to the control of automatic representations having a high degree of activation and emotional charge that strongly imposes themselves on other representations. It is related to attention since it favors attentional focusing, thus helping working memory not to be overloaded with irrelevant information [51, 52, 54]. One of the manifestations of cognitive inhibition is observed when there is resistance to proactive interference. Therefore, when previously learned information makes it difficult to retain recent information in working memory, we speak of proactive interference [54, 55]. In numerous situations of daily life, it is necessary for the person to flexibly use their attentional resources and implement a rapid attentional change, flexibly using cognitive resources to implement various ways of facing a task or activity, a situation which requires a certain amount of cognitive inhibition control.

Finally, behavioral inhibition control is also called response inhibition, referring to the process of stopping a prepotent motor response, and has generally been assessed using go/no-go stopping tasks and antisaccade (AI) tasks, both tasks requiring participants to intermittently suppress a given motor response [52, 55]. This response inhibition is related to the concept of self-control, as it refers to the management of our behaviors and the control of overbearing impulses, strongly related to the emotional world, in pursuit of a healthy coexistence in society. Response inhibition shows a long developmental trajectory, with rapid maturation in early childhood followed by gradual improvements throughout adolescence that continue into early adulthood [52, 56].

Finally, cognitive flexibility is the third function that makes up the executive triad. It is defined as the executive process that makes it possible both to change the attention focus from one perceptual paradigm to another, in a flexible and adaptive way, considering a situation from different perspectives, and to generate a new way of focusing on a situation ("shift"). Cognitive flexibility allows people to adapt mental activity and behavior according to the dynamic and fluctuating demands of the environment. Cognitive flexibility also allows an individual to correct actions or quickly adjust to change, depending on the context, thinking about various alternatives, or considering different points of view to solve a problem that implies different cognitive requirements [9, 56–59].

In addition, cognitive flexibility, like other cognitive control functions, follows a progressive development throughout childhood and adolescence, and the course of this trajectory will depend on multiple neuropsychological and socio-contextual factors. It clearly emerges during early childhood, around 3–4 years of age. At this age, children show a very important change in the basic processes of executive functioning, which brings with it a gradual increase in their abilities to make their thinking more flexible.

Several theoretical models have provided a conceptual basis to explain the cognitive processes of flexibility in children aged 3–5 years [9]. In this age range, flexibility of thinking is often assessed with card-sorting tasks, in which children have to sort two-dimensional cards, such as by color and shape, first, according to one dimension, such as by color, and, then, according to the other dimension, such as by shape. After sorting the cards according to the first dimension, children are asked to sort the cards according to the second dimension ("post-change phase") [9, 60]. Before age 4, the standard card-sorting task is characterized by consistent failure in the post-change phase. In other words, younger children persevere in sorting cards according to the first criterion, such as by color. Children aged 3 may not have sufficient reflection skills to manipulate rules and switch from one to another [16]. From the age of 4 onward, children manage to change to a new rule, since they no longer give perseverant responses based on the previous criterion.

Improvements in cognitive flexibility, analyzed through classification and task-switching paradigms, were observed in the groups of children aged 10–12 years, compared to younger children aged 7–9 years. A study carried out in the city of Mar del Plata, Argentina, investigated the relationships between the development of cognitive flexibility and working memory in a group of children aged 6–9 years. The results showed a significant correlation between cognitive flexibility and working memory. Nine-year-old children showed significant improvements compared to 6-year-old children, which provides evidence in favor of the concept that the key period for the development of these abilities is between 6 and 9 years of age [61]. In addition, in a study carried out by García Coni et al. [60], two categorization tasks were used to evaluate conceptual flexibility in primary school children aged 6–11 years in Mar del Plata. The findings indicate that conceptual flexibility increases at 8–9 years in the categorization task, with the lowest executive demand, and at 10–11 years in the categorization task, with the highest executive demand, due to the appearance of taxonomic responses. Around 12 years of age, it is observed that cognitive flexibility presents an important development, along with other cognitive functions, such as problem-solving and working memory, with intense development occurring between 15 and 19 years of age [13, 22, 45].

In summary, a close link is recognized between attention and the three basic components of executive functioning: working memory, inhibitory control, and cognitive flexibility [9, 62, 63]. This executive triad is the basis that supports other more complex cognitive functions, such as planning, organization, and metacognition [7, 9, 13, 14, 33]. Planning is a high-order cognitive process involved in problem-solving. It involves the ability to identify a goal, to sequence and organize the steps necessary to achieve it, to anticipate consequences, and to construct and evoke a mental map that serves to direct action to achieve an objective. Its adequate performance helps students to plan their school tasks and activities, to develop means-end thinking, and to predict the results of their actions [13].

The organization skill is described as a subprocess of the planning skill, as it involves ordering, sequencing, and prioritizing both thoughts and ideas, based on a previous work plan. This makes it possible to identify central ideas or concepts during the learning process [13].

Metacognition refers to a person's knowledge of their cognitive functioning and their attempts to control it. It is a superordinate processing, or second-order cognition, which allows monitoring, self-regulating, and developing strategies to enhance cognition. It is a key capacity for the student to learn to review and to control their learning processes and to rectify the situation if necessary, or "learning to learn" [64–66].

Although numerous studies have been carried out in relation to the skills that make up executive functioning, an aspect that is no less studied is the evaluation tests developed and used to investigate various processes of this construct. Even though there is a wide repertoire of batteries and specific tests to evaluate EFs, with good validity and reliability indices, there is one aspect that becomes increasingly relevant, and that is the need to complement this type of evaluation with those in which the actions of a subject are revealed in everyday-life situations [45, 67]. These contextual aspects associated with specific assessments of executive functioning allow for a more integrated understanding of a subject's capabilities and abilities in their context, providing greater ecological validity to the assessment process.

Contextualized Assessment of Executive Functions: Towards Increased Ecological Validity

Ecological validity in psychological and neuropsychological evaluation refers to the degree of correspondence between an individual's performance in a specific test, or set of tests, and its correlation to everyday-life situations [68]. In other words, it relates to what extent the results expressed in an evaluation of executive functioning are representative of individuals' strengths and weaknesses in real and every-day situations, manifested both through their academic performance and their socio-emotional skills.

The strategy usually followed for the evaluation of executive functioning has been the application of specific tests to evaluate the performance of some of the functions that make up this construct [45, 69]. Although in clinical, educational, or work practice, it is very common to identify which processes are preserved and which are below expectations, the truth is that one of the fundamental difficulties is the problem of impure measurements in the evaluation of executive functions. In other words, when evaluating some of these functions, other nonexecutive cognitive skills are also involved and indirectly evaluated, such as verbal, visuospatial skills, or motor speed. Thus, when evaluating any of the processes that make up executive functioning, it is difficult to analyze this information as a pure measurement of this process. If the aforementioned is analyzed in light of psychometric aspects, it is necessary to consider the random and systematic errors in the results of a test [45].

In addition, the evaluation of executive functioning performance should be able to reflect the performances that an individual has in their daily life. In other words, tests based on the execution of various tasks should be able to predict, with a certain degree of reliability, the performance of an individual in the various situations of daily life revealed in socio-affective relationships or in academic and work activities [69].

Despite the advantages reported by various studies on the need to include evaluation tests with ecological validity, integrated with traditional tests of executive functioning, this does not always happen when making a diagnosis. This situation is a limitation when formulating a prognosis, designing a therapeutic program, and analyzing its effectiveness [69–71].

There are two aspects to consider when identifying the degree of the ecological validity of an assessment instrument: verisimilitude and veracity [71, 72]. "*Verisimilitude*" reflects the extent to which there is correspondence between the theoretical foundations of an evaluation and the cognitive demands of everyday life. This concept indicates that tests with a higher degree of verisimilitude tend to be more sensitive to change in the performance of the Efs, evaluated as an individual's functional abilities increase. "*Veracity*" means the degree to which existing assessments are empirically related to measurements of everyday life. In psychometric terms, veracity is related to concurrent validity, analyzing how well a given test correlates with a previously recognized measurement. Thus, verisimilitude and veracity provide distinct, but complementary, methods for better understanding the complexities of ecological validity across all EF measurements.

All these aspects should allow the professional to avoid erroneous inferences regarding the functional capacity of the individual in their daily life. By virtue of this, it is necessary to have reliable and valid evaluation instruments that allow not only to evaluate executive functions, but also to predict to what extent this functioning is manifested through the psycho-social-emotional performance of children, adolescents, and adults in significant contexts of social interaction. The need for a more ecological orientation in the evaluation of executive functions would make it possible to analyze the clinical or educational usefulness of an evaluation in addition to the diagnostic utility [71, 73, 74]. Thus, the successful development of executive functioning assessment instruments with ecological validity allows for more precise and reliable diagnoses in order to establish prognoses with a higher degree of certainty and to carry out contextualized planning of interventions.

Conclusion

In this chapter, some general considerations were presented about executive functioning and its implication in the regulation of thought and emotional state, aspects that manifest themselves in people's behavior. Executive functioning largely predicts the degree of functional independence and psycho-social-emotional adjustment of healthy subjects and those with neuropsychological alterations [27, 69].

Over the last decades, there has been a growing interest in the study of EFs in the different stages of development because it is a significant predictor in the performance of both socio-emotional competencies [24, 25, 27, 75] and academic progress [76–78]. In particular, longitudinal studies provide consistent evidence of the interdependence between EFs and learning [79]. Thus, socio-cognitive functioning is fundamental for performance in many types of learning activities in children and adolescents [76–78]. Diverse studies have demonstrated that EFs have been predictors of long-term success in mathematics and literacy [23, 80–82].

However, executive functioning remains a complex construct to assess. One of the aspects to improve in the evaluation of executive functioning is to move towards contextualized modes of the information obtained, integrating the results of the specific tests with the performance of a subject in the activities of daily life, analyzing its functioning in different contexts of social interaction. Integrating these aspects adds ecological validity to the diagnostic evaluation, favors the accuracy of the prognosis, and allows therapeutic actions to be designed with a greater degree of effectiveness.

The contextualization of information implies having a deep knowledge of the socio-historical-cultural reality in which the subjects are immersed and adapting the forms and modalities of evaluation of executive functions considering their particularities. This would allow for better understanding and integration of the exploration findings. Adaptations of existing measures in combination with those carried out in naturalistic home and educational environments, as well as standardized virtual environments, could help to improve ecological validity in the measurement of EFs [83].

Reflecting on how to approach the exploration and measurement of executive functions challenges us to continue developing innovative and integrative evaluation proposals. Such proposals would better represent the performance of individuals in different contexts of social interaction, thus moving towards proposals with greater ecological validity.

Acknowledgment The authors gratefully acknowledge David Beach for the English version.

References

1. Baggetta P, Alexander PA. Conceptualization and operationalization of executive function. Mind Brain Educ. 2016;10(1):10–33.
2. Blair C, Diamond A. Biological processes in prevention and intervention: the promotion of self-regulation as a means of preventing school failure. Dev Psychopathol. 2008;20:899–911.
3. Carlson SM, Zelazo PD, Faja S. Executive function. In Zelazo PD, editor. Oxford handbook of developmental psychology, vol. 1. Oxford University Press; 2013. p. 706–42.
4. Clements DH, Sarama J, Germeroth C. Learning executive function and early mathematics: directions of causal relations. Early Child Res Q. 2016;36(3):79–90. https://doi.org/10.1016/j.ecresq.2015.12.009.
5. Hughes C. Changes and challenges in 20 years of research into the development of executive functions. Infant Child Dev. 2011;20:251–71. https://doi.org/10.1002/icd.736.
6. Meuwissen AS, Zelazo PD. Hot and cool executive function: foundations for learning and healthy development. Zero to Three. 2014;35(2):18–23.
7. Miyake A, Friedman NP, Emerson MJ, Witzki AH, Howerter A, Wager TD. The unity and diversity of executive functions and their contributions to complex "frontal lobe" tasks: a latent variable analysis. Cogn Psychol. 2000;41(1):49–100.
8. Romero López M, Álvarez Bernardo G, Justicia Arráez A, Alba Corredor G, Saforcada E, Fariña O. (Comp.). Neurociencias Aplicadas. Medioambiente, Desarrollo humano y Bienestar Comunitario. Ed. Nuevos Tiempos. 2017:93–143.
9. Zelazo PD, Blair CB, Willoughby MT. Executive function: implications for education (NCER 2017-2000). Washington, DC: National Center for Education Research, Institute of Education Sciences, U.S. Department of Education; 2016. This report is available on the Institute website at http://ies.ed.gov/.
10. Gioia GA, Espy KA, Isquith PK. BRIEF-P. Evaluación Conductual de la Función Ejecutiva-Versión Infantil. (E. Bausela y T. Luque, adaptadoras). TEA Ediciones; 2016.
11. Nyroosa M, Wiklund-Hörnqvistb C, Löfgrena K. Executive function skills and their importance in education: Swedish student teachers' perceptions. Think Skills Creat. 2018;27:1–12. https://doi.org/10.1016/j.tsc.2017.11.007.
12. Slattery EJ, Ryan P, Fortune DG, McAvinue LP. Contributions of working memory and sustained attention to children's reading achievement: a commonality analysis approach. Cogn Dev. 2021;58 https://doi.org/10.1016/j.cogdev.2021.101028.
13. Diamond A. Executive functions. In Gallagher A, Bulteau C, Cohen D, Michaud JL, editors. Handbook of clinical neurology. neurocognitive development: normative development. 2020;173:225–240. https://doi.org/10.1016/B978-0-444-64150-2.00020-4.
14. Diamond A. Executive functions. Annu Rev Psychol. 2013;64:135–68.
15. Posner MI, Rothbart MK. Attention to learning of school subjects. Trends Neurosci Educ. 2014. https://doi.org/10.1016/j.tine.2014.02.003i.

16. Zelazo PD. Executive function: reflection, iterative reprocessing, complexity, and the developing brain. Dev Rev. 2015;38:55–68. https://doi.org/10.1016/j.dr.2015.07.001.
17. Canet-Juric L, Introzzi I, Burin D. Desarrollo de la Capacidad de Memoria de Trabajo: Efectos de Interferencia Inter e Intra Dominio en Niños de Edad Escolar [Development of working memory capacity: the effects of inter- and intra-dominating interference in school-age children]. Revista Argentina de Ciencias del Comportamiento. 2015;7(1):26–37.
18. Lipina SJ, Evers K. Neuroscience of childhood poverty: evidence of impacts and mechanisms as vehicles of dialog with ethics. Front Psychol. 2017;8:61. https://doi.org/10.3389/fpsyg.2017.00061.
19. Friedman NP, Miyake A. Unity and diversity of executive functions: individual differences as a window on cognitive structure. Cortex. 2017;86:186–204.
20. Zelazo PD, Forston JL, Masten AS, Carlson SM. Mindfulness plus reflection training: effects on executive function in early childhood. Front Psychol. 2018;9:208. https://doi.org/10.3389/fpsyg.
21. Noble KG, Farah MJ. Neurocognitive consequences of socioeconomic disparities: the intersection of cognitive neuroscience and public health. Dev Sci. 2013;16(5):639–40. https://doi.org/10.1111/desc.12076.
22. Flores-Lázaro JC, Castillo-Preciado RE, Jiménez-Miramonte NA. Desarrollo de funciones ejecutivas de la niñez a la juventud [Development of executive functions from infancy to young adulthood]. Anales de Psicología. 2014;30(2):463–73.
23. Diamond A, Lee C, Senften P, Lam A, Abbott D. Randomized control trial of tools of the mind: marked benefits to kindergarten children and their teachers. PLoS ONE. 2019;14(9):e0222447. https://doi.org/10.1371/journal.pone.0222447.
24. Diamond A, Ling DS. Conclusions about interventions, programs, and approaches for improving executive functions that appear justified and those that, despite much hype, do not. Dev Cogn Neurosci. 2016;18:34–48. https://doi.org/10.1016/j.dcn.2015.11.005.
25. Benavides-Nieto A, Romero-López M, Quesada-Conde AB, Alba Corredor G. Basic executive functions in early childhood education and their relationship with social competence. Procedia Soc Behav Sci. 2017;2017(237):471–8. https://doi.org/10.1016/j.sbspro.2017.02.092.
26. González-Valenzuela MJ, Martín-Ruiz I. Rendimiento académico, lenguaje escrito y motivación en adolescentes españoles [Academic performance, written language and motivation in Spanish adolescents]. Universitas Psychologica. 2019;18(4):1–13. https://doi.org/10.11144/Javeriana.upsy18-4.rale.
27. McClelland MM, Cameron CE. Developing together: the role of executive function and motor skills in children's early academic lives. Early Child Res Q. 2019;46:142–51. https://doi.org/10.1016/j.ecresq.2018.03.014.
28. Anderson P. Assessment and development of executive function (EF) during childhood. Child Neuropsychol. 2002;8(2):71–82.
29. Howard SJ, Melhuish E. An early years toolbox for assessing early executive function, language, self-regulation, and social development: validity, reliability, and preliminary norms. J Psychoeduc Assess. 2017;35(3):255–75. https://doi.org/10.1177/0734282916633009.
30. Leibovich de Figueroa NB, Schmidt VI. Ecoevaluación psicológica del contexto familiar. Aspectos teóricos y empíricos. Adaptación Argentina de la Escala FACES III [Physchological Ecoevaluation of the family context. Argentinean Adaptation of PHASES Level III]. Editorial Guadalupe; 2010.
31. Muchiut AF, Vaccaro P, Pietto ML. Inteligencia, funciones ejecutivas y rendimiento académico [Intelligence, executive functions and academic performance]. Interdisciplinaria. 2021;38(3):83–102. https://doi.org/10.16888/interd.2021.38.3.5.
32. Sánchez-Escudero J, Medina-Gómez C, Gómez-Toro Y. Destrezas académicas y velocidad de procesamiento: modelos predictivos del rendimiento escolar en básica primaria [Academic skills and processing speed: predictive models of primary school achievement]. Psychologia. 2019;13(1):25–39. https://doi.org/10.21500/19002386.3754.
33. Miyake A, Friedman NP. The nature and organization of individual differences in executive functions, four general conclusions. Curr Dir Psychol Sci. 2012;21(1):8–14.
34. Amso D, Scerif G. The attentive brain: insights from developmental cognitive neuroscience. Nat Rev Neurosci. 2015;16(10):606–19. https://doi.org/10.1038/nrn4025.
35. Ison MS, Carrada M. Tipificación argentina del Test de Percepción de Diferencia (CARAS) [Argentinean classification of Perception Different Tests]. In: Thurstone LL, Yela M, editors. Test de Percepción de Diferencias Revisado (CARAS-R). TEA Ediciones; 2012. p. 37–63.
36. Reynolds GD, Romano AC. The development of attention systems and working memory in infancy. Front Syst Neurosci. 2016;10:15. https://doi.org/10.3389/fnsys.2016.00015.
37. Mirsky AF, Duncan CC. A nosology of disorders of attention. Ann N Y Acad Sci. 2001;931:17–32.
38. Fernández AL. Neuropsicología de la atención. Conceptos, alteraciones y evaluación [Neuropsychology of attention: Concepts, alterations and evaluations]. Revista Argentina de Neuropsicología. 2014;25:1–28.
39. Baddeley AD. Working memory. Oxford: Clarendon Press; 1986.
40. Ison MS. Attentional capacity in children: intervention programs for its development. In: Gargiullo PA, Mesones-Arroyo HL, editors. Psychiatry and neuroscience update. Springer; 2015. p. 243–52. https://doi.org/10.1007/978-3-319-17103-6.

41. Baddeley AD, Hitch GJ. Working memory. In: Bower GH, editor. The psychology of learning and motivation, vol. 8. Academic; 1974. p. 47–89.
42. Cowan N. The many faces of working memory and short-term storage. Psychon Bull Rev. 2017;24:1158–70. https://doi.org/10.3758/s13423-016-1191-6.
43. Espósito A. Estimulación cognitiva en escolares mendocinos: modalidades de intervención [Cognitive stimulation in Mendocinian schoolchildren: modalities of Intervention]. Tesis doctoral. Universidad Nacional de San Luis; 2017.
44. Tirapu-Ustárroz J, Cordero-Andrés P, Luna-Lario P, Hernáez-Goñi P. Propuesta de un modelo de funciones ejecutivas basado en análisis factoriales [Proposal for an executive function model based on factorial analysis]. Rev Neurol. 2017;64:75–84.
45. Tirapu-Ustárroz J, Bausela-Herreras E, Cordero-Andrés P. Modelo de funciones ejecutivas basado en análisis factoriales en población infantil y escolar: metaanálisis [Executive function model based on factorial analysis in infantile and school child population: metaanalysis]. Rev Neurol. 2018;2018(67):215–25.
46. Boen R, Ferschmann L, Vijayakumar N, Overbye K, Fjell AM, Espeseth T, Tamnes CK. Development of attention networks from childhood to young adulthood: a study of performance, intraindividual variability and cortical thickness. Cortex. 2021. https://doi.org/10.1016/j.cortex.2021.01.018.
47. Deleglise A, Cervigni M. Los códigos neurales de la percepción conciente y la memoria de trabajo [Neural codes of conscious perception and working memory]. Cuadernos de Neuropsicología/Panamerican J Neuropsychol. 2019;13(1):34–59.
48. Nutley SB. Development and training of higher order cognitive functions and their interrelations. The Department of Neuroscience, Karolinska Institute; 2011.
49. Aydmune Y, Lipina S, Introzzi I. Definiciones y métodos de entrenamiento de la inhibición en la niñez, desde una perspectiva neuropsicológica. Una revisión sistemática [Definitions and methods of training of inhibition in childhood: A systemic revision]. Revista Argentina de Ciencias del Comportamiento. 2017;3(9):104–41.
50. Nigg JT. On inhibition/disinhibition in developmental psychopathology: views from cognitive and personality psychology and a working inhibition taxonomy. Psychol Bull. 2000;126:220–46. https://doi.org/10.1037/0033-2909.126.2.220.
51. Nigg JT. Annual Research Review: on the relations among self-regulation, self-control, executive functioning, effortful control, cognitive control, impulsivity, risk-taking, and inhibition for developmental psychopathology. J Child Psychol Psychiatry. 2017;58(4):361–83. https://doi.org/10.1111/jcpp.12675.
52. Tiego J, Testa R, Bellgrove MA, Pantelis C, Whittle S. A hierarchical model of inhibitory control. Front Psychol. 2018;10:1339. https://doi.org/10.3389/fpsyg.2018.01339.
53. Barkley RA. Behavioral inhibition, sustained attention, and executive functions: constructing a unifying theory of ADHD. Psychol Bull. 1997;121(1):65–94.
54. Introzzi I, Canet Juric L, Aydmune Y, Stelzer F. Perspectivas teóricas y evidencia empírica sobre la inhibición [Theoretical perspectives and empirical evidence about inhibition]. Revista Colombiana de Psicología. 2016;25(2):351–68. https://doi.org/10.15446/rcp.v25n2.52011.
55. Aydmune Y, Introzzi I, Richards MM, Stelzer F, Krzemien D. Flexibilidad cognitiva y tres procesos inhibitorios durante los primeros años de la escolaridad primaria [Cognitive flexibility and three inhibitory processes during the first years of primary school]. Subjetividad y Procesos Cognitivos. 2019;23(2):186–202.
56. Luna B, Marek S, Larsen B, Tervo-Clemmens B, Chahal R. An integrative model of the maturation of cognitive control. Annu Rev Neurosci. 2015;38:151–70. https://doi.org/10.1146/annurev-neuro-071714-034054.
57. Brennan A, Bruderer A, Liu-Ambrose T, Handy TC, Enns JT. Lifespan changes in attention revisited: everyday visual search. Can Psychol Assoc. 2017;71(2):160–71. https://doi.org/10.1037/cep0000130.
58. Ison MS, Morelato GS. Habilidades socio-cognitivas implicadas en la solución de problemas interpersonales en la niñez [Socio-cognitive abilities implicated in the solution of interpersonal problems in early childhood]. Enciclopedia Argentina de Salud Mental. 8va Edición. 2022. http://www.enciclopediasaludmental.org.ar/trabajo.php?idt=165&idtt=246.
59. Joyce A, Hrin S. Attention: an evolving construct. Appl Neuropsychol Child. 2015;4(2):80–8. https://doi.org/10.1080/21622965.2015.1005476.
60. García Coni A, Ison MS, Vivas JR. Conceptual flexibility in school children: switching between taxonomic and thematic relations. Cogn Dev. 2019;52 https://doi.org/10.1016/j.cogdev.2019.100827.
61. Introzzi MI, Canet Juric L, Montes S, López S, Mascarello G. Procesos Inhibitorios y flexibilidad cognitiva: evidencia a favor de la Teoría de la Inercia Atencional [Inhibitory processes and cognitive flexibility: evidence in favour of the Theory of Attentional Inertia]. Int J Psychol Res. 2015;8(2):60–74.
62. Ariës RJ, Ghysels J, Groot W, Maassen van den Brink H. Combined working memory capacity and reasoning strategy training improves reasoning skills in secondary social studies education: Evidence from an experimental study. Think Skills Creat. 2016;22:233–46 https://doi.org/10.1016/j.tsc.2016.10.008.
63. Canet-Juric L, del-Valle MV, Gelpi-Trudo R, García-Coni A, Zamora EV, Introzzi I, Andrés ML. Desarrollo y validación del Cuestionario de Funciones Ejecutivas en niñosl de 9 a 12 años (CUFE) [Development and validation of the questionnaire on executive functions

of children between 9 and 12 years of age]. Avances en Psicología Latinoamericana. 2021;39(1):1–25. https://doi.org/10.12804/revistas.urosario.edu.co/apl/a.9892.
64. Kluwe-Schiavon B, Viola TW, Sanvicente-Vieira B, Malloy-Diniz LF, Grassi-Oliveira R. Front Psychol. Published online 2017 Jan 19;7:2067. https://doi.org/10.3389/fpsyg.2016.02067.
65. Korzeniowski C, Ison M. Escala de funcionamiento ejecutivo para escolares: análisis de las propiedades psicométricas [Scales of executive functions for students: analysis of the psychometric properties]. Educational Psychol. 2019;25(2):147–58. https://doi.org/10.5093/psed2019a4.
66. Schmeichel BJ, Tang D. Individual differences in executive functioning and their relationship to emotional processes and responses. Psychol Sci. 2015;24(2):93–8. https://doi.org/10.1177/0963721414555178.
67. Delgado-Reyes AC, Sánchez-López JV. Escenarios Virtuales para la Evaluación Neuropsicológica: una Revisión de Tema [Virtual scenarios for neuropyschological evaluation: a thematic review]. Cuadernos de Neuropsicología/Panamerican J Neuropsychol. 2021;15(2):196–213. https://doi.org/10.7714/CNPS/15.2.216.
68. Toscano Ferreira RC, Zanetti-Motta I, Torres Carrera L, Regina Kintschner N, Rodrigues Carreiro LR. Avaliação ecológica de funções executivas: um estudo de revisão integrativa [Ecological assessment of executive functions: an integrative review study]. Cadernos de Pós-Graduação em Distúrbios do Desenvolvimento. 2021;21(1):68–83. https://doi.org/10.5935/cadernosdisturbios.v21n1p68-83.
69. Bombín-González I, Cifuentes-Rodríguez A, Climent-Martínez G, Luna-Lario P, Cardas-Ibáñez J, Tirapu-Ustárroz J, et al. Validez ecológica y entornos multitarea en la evaluación de las funciones ejecutivas [Ecological validity and multitasking environments in the evaluation of executive functions]. Rev Neurol. 2014;59:77–87.
70. García-Molina A, Tirapu-Ustárroz J, Roig-Rovira T. Validez ecológica en la exploración de las funciones ejecutivas [Ecological validity in the exploration of executive functions]. Anales de psicología. 2007;23(2):289–99.
71. Wallisch A, Little LM, Dean E, Dunn W. Executive function measures for children: a scoping review of ecological validity. OTJR. 2018;38:6–14. https://doi.org/10.1177/1539449217727118.
72. Chaytor N, Schmitter-Edgecombe M. The ecological validity of neuropsychological tests: a review of the literature on everyday cognitive skills. Neuropsychol Rev. 2003;13:181–97. https://doi.org/10.1023/B:NERV.0000009483.91468.fb.
73. Souissi S, Chamari K, Bellaj T. Assessment of executive functions in school-aged children: a narrative review. Front Psychol. 2022;13:991699. https://doi.org/10.3389/fpsyg.2022.991699.
74. García Fernández T, González Castro P, Areces D, Cueli M, Rodríguez Pérez C. Funciones Ejecutivas en Niños y Adolescentes: Implicaciones del Tipo de Medidas de Evaluación Empleadas para su Validez en Contextos Clínicos y Educativos [Executive functions in children and adolescents: implications of the type of evaluation methods used for their validity in clinical and educational contexts]. Papeles del Psicólogo. 2014;35(3):215–23. http://www.papelesdelpsicologo.es.
75. Willoughby MT, Magnus B, Vernon-Feagans L, Blair CB, Family Life Project Investigators. Developmental delays in executive function from 3 to 5 years of age predict kindergarten academic readiness. J Learn Disabil. 2017;50:359–72. https://doi.org/10.1177/0022219415619754.
76. Ison MS. How to promote attentional efficacy and cognitive control processes: experience in argentine schoolchildren. Psychol Psychol Res Int J. 2020;5(4):000255.
77. Ison MS, González DF, Korzeniowski C. Strengthening socio-cognitive and emotional skills in early education through a school-based program: preliminary study. Eur J Psychol Educ Res. 2020;3(2):87–100. https://doi.org/10.12973/ejper.3.2.87.
78. Traverso L, Viterbori P, Usai MC. Effectiveness of an executive function training in italian preschool educational services and far transfer effects to pre-academic skills. Front Psychol. 2019;2019(10):2053. https://doi.org/10.3389/fpsyg.2019.02053.
79. Fuhs MW, Nesbitt KT, Farran DC, Dong N. Longitudinal associations between executive functioning and academic skills across content areas. Dev Psychol. 2014;50(6):1698–709. https://doi.org/10.1037/a0036633.
80. Blair C, Raver C. School readiness and self-regulation: a developmental psychobiological approach. Annu Rev Psychol. 2015;66:711–31. https://doi.org/10.1146/annurev-psych-010814-015221.
81. De Franchis V, Usai MC, Viterbori P, Traverso L. Preschool executive functioning and literacy achievement in Grades 1 and 3 of primary school: a longitudinal study. Learn Individ Differ. 2017;2017(54):184–95. https://doi.org/10.1016/j.lindif.2017.01.026.
82. Usai MC, Viterbori P, Traverso L. Preschool executive function profiles: implications for math achievement in grades 1 and 3. Eur Early Child Educ Res J. 2018;32(4):404–18. https://doi.org/10.1080/02568543.2018.1496957.
83. Diercks CM, Gunther KE, Teti DM, Lunkenheimer E. Ecological validity in measuring parents' executive function. Child Dev Perspect. 2022;16:208–14. https://doi.org/10.1111/cdep.12464.

Excessive Technological Consumption, Effects on Isolation and Stress

31

Eric Wainwright

Introduction

The Pandemic in 2020 made all of us conscious about the excess of consumption in unexpected situations. Two variables have been made evident by the pandemic, and both are hard to handle in any age group: *loneliness and uncertainty.* This unprecedented experience opened our eyes to a new challenge that was growing previously, but skyrocketed in 2020: *excessive technological consumption.* This includes all kind of screens, also news consumption in varied formats. It's deleterious effects were boosted by receiving news of varied reliability.

Social interaction and cooperation have driven the progress of human culture and civilization since the dawn of mankind. Thus, the most closely knit communities achieved greater growth than those with less cohesion. The difficulty that we see arises from the current trend, which will soon lead to more than 50% of the urban population living in single-person households.

E. Wainwright (✉)
Psychiatry Department, Buenos Aires British Hospital, Buenos Aires, Argentina

Psychiatry Department, Braulio Moyano Hospital, Buenos Aires, Argentina

Cathedra of Psychiatry, Faculty of Medical Sciences, Catholic University of Argentina, Buenos Aires, Argentina

Cathedra of Psychiatry, Faculty of Medical Sciences, Buenos Aires University, Buenos Aires, Argentina
e-mail: EWainwright@hbritanico.com.ar

Our culture has evolved in many different areas, but recent technological advances have presented a variety of difficulties, starting with the Japanese Hikikomori some years ago, to the current omnipresent smart phone use. The Hikikomori disorder included primarily adolescents or young adults who isolate themselves from the world. They do it in their rooms, in the house of their parents. They do it for an indefinite period, in some cases spending years isolated, rejecting most of face-to-face communication. Most interactions revolve around the use of the Internet. This trend has generalized thanks to the widespread use of new portable technologies. This disorder has developed into this new kind of addiction, on a mobile basis. Unfortunately, the new technologies don't seem to improve socialization, as media doesn't generally facilitate normal socialization.

Various studies report aggravation of different mental health conditions when an individual of various age groups is isolated for long periods.

The quality of the social relationships that people maintain with others has been directly related to psychological well-being. But this is not the only problem, since social isolation affects not only mental well-being, but also physical and CNS health.

Insufficient social stimulation affects:

(a) Reasoning and memory performance.
(b) Brain structure, connectivity, and function.

P. Á. Gargiulo, H. L. Mesones-Arroyo (eds.), *Psychiatry and Neuroscience Update – Vol. V*,
https://doi.org/10.1007/978-3-031-72219-6_31

(c) Hormonal functioning.
(d) Lower resistance to physical and mental illness.
(e) In older people it may precipitate Cognitive Decline.

Loneliness and social isolation, among other behavioral alterations, affect the immune system, reducing resistance to disease and infection [1, 2, 3]. A number of behavioral conditions influence social interaction, addictions being one of them. Prior to the arrival of the smartphone, extensive research had been conducted on addictive behavior involving exercise, videogames, online sex, food, shopping, work, gambling, gaming, and Internet [4].

The constant improving of mobile phones by expanding upon their functionalities, which in turn increase the likelihood of overuse and even addiction, is a fact. Internet addiction may affect the individual's physical and psychological health, academic and work performance, as well as social communication.

For practical and research ends, various definitions for Internet addiction have been proposed. Most are mainly based on criteria for substance abuse and impulse control disorders. Proposed criteria focus on such factors as preoccupation with Internet activities, inability to control Internet use, and distress when use is limited. Continued use is a key factor, despite interference with other essential activities in subject's lives such as working, learning, socializing, eating, or sleep [5].

Research has revealed the relationship between fiber abnormalities and behavioral measures of media addiction. Study results demonstrated that Smart Phone Dependence had significantly lower white matter integrity than controls in superior longitudinal fasciculus (SLF), superior corona radiata (SCR), internal capsule, external capsule, sagittal stratum, fornix/stria terminalis, and midbrain structures. Correlation analysis showed that the observed abnormalities in internal capsule and stria terminalis were correlated with the severity of dependence [6].

Other study results, in Internet Addiction Disorder patients, demonstrate that there is significant disruption in the functional connections, particularly in long-range and interhemispheric connections between regions located in the frontal, occipital, and parietal lobes. Although no difference in global network topology between addicted and healthy groups has been found, significant alterations have been observed in regional nodal metrics. In addition, correlation analysis demonstrated a correlation between the observed regional abnormalities, with the addiction severity and behavioral clinical assessments [7].

Other studies have found significant differences in orbitofrontal cortex, insula, anterior and posterior cingulate cortex, temporal and parietal regions, brain stem, and caudate nucleus. These regions are cortical and subcortical brain regions involved in cognitive control and reward processing. These areas have been previously associated to substance use disorder and are probably affecting young adults' brain functions in ways soon to be discovered [8].

"Fourth Industrial Revolution"

In most studies, subjects referred that the workplace was the preferred setting for Internet use among abusers. Lesser restrictions, colleagues, and access to unlimited Internet may have been the possible reasons for this observation.

Alcohol consumption and smoking have been associated with Internet addiction in various studies. Previous studies have made similar observations where pathological Internet use (PIU) or Internet addiction was associated with alcohol and smoking [9].

The accelerated development of new technologies has ushered a "Fourth Industrial Revolution" that modifies the nature and localization of workers. These changes generate new risks [5, 10]:

- Mounting stress associated to the impact of the increased control of the worker.
- Constant changes, and ubiquity of portable technologies, 24/7 availability.

- Unclear boundaries between work and private life, and the economy of online platforms.
- Increased ergonomic risks due to increased online working and use of mobile devices in out-of-office settings.
- Risks associated with new man-machine interfaces, in particular related to ergonomics and cognitive load.
- Increase in sedentary work, risk associated with obesity and noncommunicable diseases (cardiovascular and diabetes).
- Cybersecurity risks due to an increase in interconnection.
- Algorithmic work management, AI, monitoring technologies, even wearables.
- The Internet of Things and Big Data can lead to workers losing control over data protection, ethical issues, information inequality, and pressure on worker performance.
- Lack of the necessary skills to be able to use these technologies, adapt to change, and manage the balance between work and personal life [10].

Internet addiction and media overuse have been demonstrated to be more prevalent in postgraduate students than undergraduates. Some studies have reported that the incidence of Internet addiction increases as students' grades also do so. It is possibly due to Post-Graduate study being more demanding, including growing requirements to access the Internet and the increased affluence in this group allows students to bear the expenses of the Internet better than when Under-Graduate. We should highlight that, in general, subjects indicated that educational activity was the most common purpose for Internet use [9, 11].

Mental Health at Risk

The COVID-19 epidemic caused a parallel epidemic of fear, anxiety, and depression.

The population (especially those affected by psychiatric conditions) is more susceptible to influences by emotional responses during the epidemic. The main influencer being digital media. The uncertainty that accompanies these processes would be the cause of this situational susceptibility [12].

Excessive Consumption in the COVID-19 Quarantine:

Some authors use the term "Lack of Portion Control" to describe behavioral changes experienced during this unprecedented situation, including:

(i) Food, with the accompanying obesity risk.
(ii) Alcohol, and other substance abuse.
(iii) Media: Social Networks, news.

As an unexpected consequence of the prolonged quarantine or lockdown, unemployment has risen, particularly in emerging economies. This has been linked to loneliness, particularly as network and media use have proven unable to mitigate loneliness due mainly to their anonymity. Unemployment has been associated to increased stress and anxiety.

On the other hand, another consequence of the lockdown, rising home office, does not allow social work relations to evolve properly. All of these elements collude against socializing in the workplace, generating dissatisfaction in the employees.

With most of the world's population spending a significant amount of 2020 in lockdown, a media usage report, Digital 2021, reports that social media users have been shown to have grown exponentially over the last 3 years. There are now 4.2 billion social media users worldwide, representing a yearly growth of over 13% (490 million new users). The number of users of social networks is now equivalent to more than 53% of the world's population [13].

On the expansion of social networks use, Digital 2021 respondents said they spent roughly the same amount of time per day on social media as they did the previous year, 2 h and 25 min. Facebook remains the most used platform in the world, followed by YouTube and WhatsApp. The report informs that 45% of users between the ages of 16 and 64 look for information about brands on social networks and only 40% use them for work purposes. A key consideration is the growing popularity of messaging platforms, with 91% of Internet users aged 16–64 using chat apps each month. Messaging has overtaken the use of social media platforms, ranking second at 88% in 2021 [13].

Academy and Technology Abuse

Internet addiction among adolescents has also escalated abruptly, generating abuse-related problems, including refusal to attend school and health problems, such as loneliness, low self-esteem, insufficient sleep, fatigue, anxiety, and depression.

According to different researchers, students classified as addicted and possibly addicted could be considered "problematic" Internet users. The use of smartphones deserves special attention, as it is among the main factors that contribute to Internet addiction, as their versatility and connectivity facilitate addiction to their use [14].

The prevalence of pathological Internet use in Europe in 2016 varied from 1.2% in Italy to 11.8% in Israel. On the other hand, in Asia, it was reported: 13.8% in Taiwan, 10.7% in South Korea, between 3.0% and 6.7% in Hong Kong, and from 2.4% to 6.0% in Continental China [11].

In recent years, penetration has increased exponentially.

Consequences in Adolescence

Adolescence is a period of rapid psychological maturation, peer pressure, and great susceptibility to Internet attraction. Excessive Internet use was found to be detrimental to family relationships, self-esteem, feelings of satisfaction, and academic performance. This would usher an increase of social isolation. Incremental media usage would follow.

Adolescents with problematic Internet use experienced a higher incidence of suicidality and depression at the 9-month follow-up [11].

A study demonstrated the mental health sequelae of pathological use of the Internet for young people who were initially healthy. There was an increased risk of depression for pathological Internet users by 11/2 times compared with those who did not exhibit the pathological behaviors, but no such association was found for anxiety. The relationship of Internet abuse and mental health is probably bidirectional. It could be possible to understand the effect of smart phone abuse on the mental health of young people and its consequently greater involvement in pathological behaviors, triggering a vicious cycle that may spiral downward [15].

From a cognitive point of view, the exponential rise in media consumption has also increased the use of visual imagery relative to text and to auditory communication usually using short bursts of communication text rather than long sentences and paragraphs. The cognitive consequences of these communication changes are still unknown [15].

Media and mobile phone abuse have been suggested as a problematic behavior that presents signs and symptoms related to other recognized addictions since 1995s. While studies have initially indicated that individuals who pathologically use the Internet are mostly young men with introverted personalities, it has also been shown that the rates of these abuse among women have been increasing similarly. In recent years, with the greater availability of the Internet around the globe, pathological use of the Internet has become an increasing mental health issue among adolescents and children. Prevalence growth in adolescence has been reported by researchers in Taiwan and China to have increased from about 6% in 2000 to about 11% in 2004 [15].

These changes are particularly worrying in childhood, as years ago. Childhood activities mainly consisted of free play in group games, with only a minority socially withdrawn. Many children in recent years live in a world of web-based media that may be foreign to many parents, particularly to those educated in previous cultural paradigms [5].

In a Spanish student population, some elements could be concluded:

1. Individuals usually spend more time connected to electronic media than anticipated.
2. Patients prefer to be connected to device instead of most other option, except if this option involves going out with friends and acquaintances.
3. Users make "friends" on the network.
4. Individuals receive frequent complaints from parents or friends about excessive time online.
5. They think that life without electronic device would be boring.
6. Patients get irritated when interrupted while accessing web media.
7. They feel disconnected when not using electronic device.
8. They think about lengthening the connection time, when having to disconnect.
9. Patients occasionally try to reduce connection time but fail to do so.

As new technologies have been incorporated into children's media use, hours spent viewing TV have decreased. Trends in parent-reported TV viewing in children from 2 to 11 years of age, between 2001 and 2012 using data from the National Health and Nutrition Examination Survey (NHANES), demonstrated significant decreases in mean TV viewing over time, primarily for preschoolers and, to a lesser extent, for school-aged children [16].

In some South East Asian countries, study results show that the female population studied presented more symptoms of dependence to web media than the male population [17].

On the other hand, studies in India have shown that boys presented more Internet addiction symptoms or over use than girls did. Similar observations have been made in several other previous studies. Since boys are given more liberty in Indian society and have more frequent access to use the Internet in private than girls, it predisposes them to abuse it's use. Studies have also shown that males tend to play more online games and surf adult sites more often than females. Besides, males also tend to abuse illegal substances than girls, and it has also been reported in a meta-analysis of Internet addiction that subjects with a history of substance addiction is at higher risk of Internet addiction [9].

Other studies have detected a series of risk factors for Internet addiction, the most salient being: Male gender, continuous online availability, using the Internet for establishing friendships/relationships and less for work/academic use. Due to their higher computing skills and easy Internet access, young adults are at augmented risk for this kind of addiction.

Our culture has evolved in many different areas, but recent technological advances have presented a variety of difficulties, starting with the Japanese Hikikimori some years ago, to the current omnipresent smart phone use. The disorder includes primarily adolescents or young adults who isolate themselves from the world, in their rooms in the house of their parents for an indefinite period. In some cases, they spend years isolated, rejecting most of face to face communication, most interactions revolving around the use of Internet and new technologies. This disorder has developed into this new kind of addiction, on a mobile basis. Unfortunately, the new technologies do not seem to improve socialization, as media do not generally facilitate normal socialization.

Internet addiction among students has increased massively. Various parameters including female gender, time spent on electronic media, graduation level, place of Internet use, smoking, and alcohol have been associated with Internet addiction. Additionally, insomnia and depression are more common in Internet abusers, having a bidirectional causal relationship [9].

Studies have revealed a strong positive association between Internet addiction and insomnia. In a study of 984 undergraduate students, 35.4% of the study sample reported having poor sleep quality and Internet addiction as well. Another study including 719 Chinese adolescents in Hong Kong observed high comorbidity between Internet addiction and insomnia. In this study, 51.7% of students suffering Internet addiction also suffered insomnia [9, 16, 18].

Recreational electronic activities have become massively prevalent in youth, with a mean of approximately 3 h per day in the general population, and over 6 h per day in the psychiatric population. Youth with mental illness are particularly vulnerable to Internet addiction and overuse, with ADHD being the most common risk factor. High-risk youth may spend even more time in front of screens [5].

Risks of excessive media use include negative health effects on sleep, attention, learning, and depression. Exposure to inaccurate, inappropriate, or unsafe content and contacts and compromised privacy and confidentiality may also be included. In addition, physical problems may be conserved here, as associated to the increase in sedentarism, mainly a higher incidence of obesity. Patients may also experience a variety of physical discomforts or medical problems such as carpal tunnel syndrome, dry eyes, backaches, and severe headaches. Other eating irregularities have been reported, and many of them also suffer from other addictions, such as addiction to drugs, alcohol, gambling, pornography, or sex [7, 19].

In children, clinicians report that parents frequently refer difficulties managing their children's time on Internet, media, or gaming and the difficulty they experience in getting their child to comply with time limits to the game or Internet use. Children frequently overreact, who are not otherwise oppositional if career interrupts or suspends the use of the screen in the middle of a game, especially when a child is noncompliant with instructions to turn it off.

These findings clarify the negative consequences of Internet abuse on daily life in terms of behavioral components, psychosocial factors, symptom management, psychiatric comorbidity, clinical diagnosis, and treatment outcome [7]. Parents present many questions, regarding reasonable time limits, difficulties in socialization, sedentarism, other long-term consequences, etc. [5].

Adding to this worrying situation, the recent ubiquitous presence of smartphones has worsened the situation. Due to their versatility, they have now become a common choice for consumers both in business (initially intended mainly for business users) and general population. These mobile phones, with advanced features and functionality beyond traditional cell phone uses (making phone calls and sending text messages), have displaced most other portable technologies, (e.g., palm, and other portable electronic agendas, or gaming technologies) in most public places [20].

Several studies have reported that smartphone abuse was associated to subjective stress. Consistent with the stress-coping framework related to elevated perceived stress, abuse occurs when individuals are faced with a threatening situation, being unable to cope with it. Under these circumstances, the resource of smartphones as a coping mechanism would allow distraction from the stressful situation. From the existing studies, we expected that perceived stress would be positively associated with Problematic Smartphone Use. A perfectionism personality trait, defined as a person setting excessively high-performance standards, coupled with overly critical self, and other's evaluations, would also be a potential risk factor for this abuse, deserving further investigation [21].

As a Conclusion

Since the introduction of the term "Internet addiction" in 1995 by Dr. Ivan Goldberg for compulsive Internet use, excessive Internet use has been associated to pathological gambling. Young's Criteria have been adapted using DSM IV criteria to evaluate Internet use in the Internet addiction test (IAT), developed by her for this end [9].

Currently, the term Problematic Smartphone Use has gradually replaced other terms as Internet addiction disorder or problematic media use in daily life, as smartphones have occupied the leadership in the technology alternatives used by youth and adults alike.

The average youth is spending one-third of their day on screen activities and high-risk children are spending most of their leisure hours on screens. Risks and benefits must be evaluated, particularly for the benefit of parents, and the educative system. Investigators and parents agree in the worry about the effect of this massive degree of exposure on the development of brain functions on the long term.

In addition, what may be the effect of the loss of those activities that have been displaced by media entertainment, particularly in Problematic Smartphone Use? [19].

Our culture has developed thanks to interaction among people, not only in the playground, but also in the work place. We are currently witnessing accelerated changes in both populations, and no solid strategies have been deployed to normalize media use in youth, to stimulate a balanced time use further in life and preventing social isolation. Furthermore, electronic media use hasn't proved an adequate replacement to face-to-face social interaction.

Since the problem first went viral, with the Japanese Hikikomori some years ago, the situation hasn't improved due to the current smart phone availability. These disorders have developed into new kinds of mobile addictions. Unfortunately, media and social networks don't generally improve traditional socialization.

There is a clear association between Problematic Smartphone Use, Internet addiction, or problematic media use on sleep patterns. Increased time spent on the Internet, particularly in the evening, has been linked to a higher rate of sleep disturbance specially taking place among heavy Internet users due to a disruption of the sleep-wake schedule [9].

The deleterious impact of various online addictions on insomnia and depression has been studied in Hong Kong adolescents. The findings showed that digital media abuse was significantly associated with insomnia and depression. These data suggest complex associations exist between insomnia, Internet addiction, and depression. As previously depicted, overuse of the Internet has been linked with many conditions besides anxiety, depression, and insomnia. Several studies have shown that among users addicted to the Internet, depression has much higher prevalence than in normal users. Causal links have developed both ways, as depression and anxiety have been reported as predictors of Internet addiction in a study among Turkish students. It is worrying that these psychological and physical problems have been linked to academic decline, and with excessive alcohol and cigarette consumption, not only in adolescents. These findings have been associated to other substance abuses. As some studies have suggested, adolescents with Internet addiction may be vulnerable to other addictions and hence are at increased risk of substance abuse [9].

The long-term consequences of Internet abuse further than striatal activation are yet unknown. Measures may be required to keep media use within a balanced time frame. Coherent educative policies are necessary to stem the tide of digital media abuse in youthful users.

Hopefully, the benefits provided by rational media use will outweigh the problems presented above.

References

1. Kennedy D, Gläscher J, Tyszka J, et al. Personal space regulation by the human amygdala. Nat Neurosci. 2009;12:1226–7. https://doi.org/10.1038/nn.2381.
2. Kennedy D, Adolphs R. The social brain in psychiatric and neurological disorders. Trends Cogn Sci. 2012;16(11):559–72. ISSN 1364-6613
3. Madore KP, Khazenzon AM, Backes CW, et al. Memory failure predicted by attention lapsing and media multitasking. Nature. 2020;587:87–91.
4. De-Sola Gutiérrez J, Rodríguez de Fonseca F, Rubio G. Cell-phone addiction: a review. Front Psychiatry. 2016;7:art 175.
5. Weiss M, Baer S, Allan B, Saran K, Schibuk H. The screens culture: impact on ADHD. ADHD Atten Def Hyp Disord. 2011;3:327–34.
6. Hu Y, Long X, Lyu H, Zhou Y, Chen J. Alterations in white matter integrity in young adults with smartphone dependence. Front Hum Neurosci. 2017;11:532.
7. Wee C-Y, Zhao Z, Yap P-T, Wu G, Shi F, et al. Disrupted brain functional network in internet addic-

tion disorder: a resting-state functional magnetic resonance imaging study. PLoS One. 2014;9(9):e107306.
8. Sepede G, Tavino M, Santacroce R, Fiori F, Salerno RM, Di Giannantonio M. Functional magnetic resonance imaging of internet addiction in young adults. World J Radiol. 2016;8(2):210–25.
9. Jain A, Sharma R, Gaur KL, Yadav N, Sharma P, Sharma N, et al. Study of internet addiction and its association with depression and insomnia in university students. J Family Med Prim Care. 2020;9:1700–6.
10. Stacey N, Ellwood P, Bradbrook S, Reynolds J, Williams H, Lye D. Foresight on new and emerging occupational safety and health risks associated with digitalisation by 2025 European Agency for Safety and Health at Work (EU-OSHA). ISSN: 1831-9343.
11. Kawabe K, Horiuchi F, Ochi M, Oka Y, Ueno S. Internet addiction: prevalence and relation with mental states in adolescents. Psychiatry Clin Neurosci. 2016;70:405–12.
12. Yao H, Chen J-H, Xu Y-F. Patients with mental health disorders in the COVID-19 epidemic. 2020. www.thelancet.com/psychiatry.
13. Digital 2021—We Are Social in. https://wearesocial.com/uk/blog/2021/01/digitall-2021-uk/.
14. Kim K, Ryu E, Chon M, Yeun E, Choi S, Seo J, Nam B. Internet addiction in Korean adolescents and its relation to depression and suicidal ideation: a questionnaire survey. J Nurs Stud. 2006;43:185–92.
15. Lam L, Peng Z. Effect of pathological use of the internet on adolescent mental health, a prospective study arch. Pediatr Adolesc Med. 2010;164:901–6.
16. Bhandari PM, Neupane D, Rijal S, Thapa K, Mishra SR, Poudyal AK. Sleep quality, internet addiction and depressive symptoms among undergraduate students in Nepal. BMC Psychiatry. 2017;17:106–29.
17. Callejón Ferre A. Evaluación del uso de componentes electrónicos de los alumnos de 2° curso de eso. Universidad de Almeria; 2017.
18. Cheung LM, Wong WS. The effects of insomnia and internet addiction on depression in Hong Kong Chinese adolescents: an exploratory cross-sectional analysis. J Sleep Res. 2011;20:311–7.
19. Reid Chassiakos Y, Radesky J, Christakis D, et al. AAP council on communications and media. Children and adolescents and digital media. Pediatrics. 2016;138(5):e20162593.
20. Sarwar M, Soomro TR. Impact of smartphone's on society. 2013;98(2):216–26.
21. Long J, Liu T, Liao Y, Qi Ch, He H, Chen Sh, Billieux J. Prevalence and correlates of problematic smartphone use in a large random sample of Chinese undergraduates. BMC Psychiatry. 2016;16:408.

32 Addiction to New Technologies in Adolescents and Young People: Is Phubbing a New Digital Pandemic?

Santiago Resett, Belén Mesurado,
and María Emilia Oñate

Introduction

Technology has achieved unprecedented growth in recent decades. In Latin American countries, such as Argentina, the availability and fascination towards new technologies are remarkable with Argentinean adolescents, together with Chilean youth, being at the forefront of the "interactive generation" [1]. New information and communication technologies (ICT, for example, cell phones or tablets) have generated notable benefits, such as being more connected, more democratic access to knowledge, and greater diversity in entertainment. However, the advancement of ICT also brought negative behaviors [2], such as cyberbullying, trolling, or grooming, among others.

Another very frequent problem among adolescents and young people is addiction to new technologies due to the popularity of cell phones and computers among them. Especially among addictions, phubbing is the one that has attracted the most attention from scientists and professionals due to the psychosocial costs that it entails. This behavior is composed of cell phone addiction and impaired interpersonal communication. Despite this, its scientific study is incipient, especially in Latin American countries, such as Argentina. Therefore, in this chapter addiction to new technologies will be conceptualized, the concept and evolution of the term phubbing will be developed, scientific techniques for its measurement and data on its incidence in Argentinean adolescents and young people will be provided. Finally, it will finish with some guidelines for its detection and prevention.

S. Resett (✉) · B. Mesurado · M. E. Oñate
CONICET—Universidad Austral, Instituto de Filosofía, Pilar, Provincia de Buenos Aires, Argentina
e-mail: bmesurado@austral.edu.ar; MOnate@austral.edu.ar

New Technologies Among Adolescents and Young People

Information and communication technologies, known by their abbreviation as ICT, are nowadays a tool of permanent use. They refer to a set of technologies required for the storage, recovery, processing, and communication of information more efficiently [3], which are not conceived in isolation, but are more significant in an interactive and interconnected way.

In recent decades, the integration of ICT into our daily lives has revolutionized society in many aspects, causing drastic changes in the way we relate and communicate [4]. These digital technologies have changed access to information, facilitating learning and international interaction in educational or work settings, becoming a constitutive part of our lives [5, 6].

P. Á. Gargiulo, H. L. Mesones-Arroyo (eds.), *Psychiatry and Neuroscience Update – Vol. V*,
https://doi.org/10.1007/978-3-031-72219-6_32

ICT are increasingly present and influence the lives of children, adolescents, and young people who inhabit a world increasingly shaped by these innovations, since they have modified the way of accessing knowledge and the way of relating to others. In other words, they have not only influenced our lives by reforming the jobs we do, the way we learn, but also the social systems we inhabit since we are interconnected [7, 8].

The youngest ones who have access to ICT since they were born, and are considered digital natives, incorporate them as a lifestyle: surfing the Internet, using a smartphone, enjoying leisure time using video games, or interacting through virtual social networks [9]. This supposes a radical change in the way of using time, accessing information, and relating to others, since young people approach ICT in a more global way, incorporating them more naturally into their lives [10, 11].

According to the National Institute of Statistics of Spain (2020), the use of new technologies by minors is widespread. In this respect, 94.5% use the Internet, 91.5% have access to and use a computer, and from the age of 10 the possibility of having a personal smartphone begins to increase, and by the age of 15, 95.7% have one.

In Argentina, the National Institute of Statistics and Censuses [12] suggested that 90% of urban households have internet access and that 88 out of 100 people use a cell phone. The greatest use of the Internet is given by people who are between 13 and 29 years old; and more than 94 out of 100 people of those ages use it. The smartphone turns out to be the most widely used technology for the young and adult population. In the group that is between 4 and 17 years old, the use of the Internet exceeds that of the cell phone and the computer. Adolescents are the ones who use the computer the most (54.4%), while young people are the ones who use the cell phone the most [12].

New technologies have innumerable benefits that have made our lives easier in many areas, especially while we are going through the COVID-19 pandemic. They have collaborated in the continuity of work development, in the possibility of continuing to study, in being able to keep in touch with friends and relatives and in helping us to entertain ourselves during the free hours. However, ICT also have risks or negative aspects such as the limitation of physical contact or the lack of development of nonverbal communication [13, 14].

Specifically in the case of children and adolescents, the extension of the exposure time and the difficulty of families in setting limits around this issue can cause a greater probability of addictive behavior problems [15], low tolerance to frustration [16], problems with sleep [3], a greater tendency to immediate gratification with difficulties in achieving postponement [17], higher levels of depression, stress, and anxiety [18, 19], lower impulse control [20], self-harm [21], poor performance at school [22–24], as well as it can generate family tensions [25].

Addiction to New Technologies

The advancement of ICT, such as its greater accessibility and generalization and its use at increasingly younger ages, has brought about changes in our lives and daily customs that can be difficult to assimilate in a healthy way, so devices that can be useful also can carry risks associated with misuse [26, 27].

The scientific literature regarding the negative impact of ICT on mental health has increased, specifically discussing the possibility of behavioral addiction that they generate [10]. Even the adolescents themselves perceive it as a threat to their well-being in three aspects: as a cause of mood disorders, as a facilitator for cyberbullying, and because the use itself can become an addiction [28].

Addiction to new technologies is a pathology that still does not appear as such in the diagnostic manuals of mental disorders and illnesses, since there is a lack of scientific and academic consensus on the characteristic symptomatology and the intensity that it should have for its diagnosis. However, it is recognized as a public health problem [29] and a serious psychological and socio-family problem since it can lead to deterioration in the physical, mental, and/or social area of adolescents [30, 31]. In this sense, recently the

International Classification of Diseases in its latest version [32] included video game addiction as a mental disorder. Also, in Argentina, this problem is beginning to generate great concern. In a sample of 735 adolescents and young adults from Buenos Aires, Argentina, it was detected that almost 40% indicated that they felt "sometimes" or "often" that their behavior was that of a video game addict and 11% that it happened to them "very often".

Psychological, behavioral, or behavioral addictions emerge when a daily habit, such as surfing the internet or working, loses its original meaning and becomes a compulsive behavior and/or a reality avoidance strategy that as a consequence generates interference in other areas of life [27, 33] and can generate a distance from the closest people [14]. In other words, addictive behavior is not only evaluated based on the time invested in it and the frequency or intensity with which it is carried out, but the degree of affectation it produces in labor, social, and school relationships in all family members, as well [34].

For many years, research efforts were aimed at determining the specific amounts of time for children and adolescents to spend on new technologies without having to deal with the negative consequences [35]. But ultimately this value is only one of the criteria; what will be decisive is the degree of alteration it produces in daily life and it is considered that there is dependence on new technologies when there is a loss of control associated with excessive use. It may be also associated with anxiety, depression, or irritability. It is manifested, given the temporary impossibility of carrying out that behavior, when there is a rising need to increase that behavior to feel satiated and when a negative impact is generated in daily life with a decrease in sports activities or physical exercise [33]. In turn, the relationship between the use of new technologies and the development of these indicators will be mediated by other factors such as the type of digital technology used, the personality and motivations of the technology user, their environment, and their sociocultural context [8].

The excessive use of technology slowly and gradually leads to isolation, causes anxiety, and negatively affects personal esteem since the person has an increasing dependency that is detrimental to their ability to control, producing a narrowing in the breadth of their interests [33]. Initially, the addictive behavior is reinforced by positive aspects of the behavior, such as the pleasure it produces, but later it becomes reinforced by negative aspects, such as relieving tension and emotional discomfort, loneliness, boredom, or anger [36].

Addiction to new technologies is a matter of particular concern among adolescents, since the characteristics of this age group and the widespread presence of technology in their lives make them a risk group [37]. According to statistics, adolescents are the ones who connect the most to the Internet, are the most familiar with ICT, and are considered digital natives, added to the fact that due to the moment of life they are going through they tend to seek new and more strong sensations and have less impulse control [38, 39].

In order to show the magnitude of the problem, Table 32.1 presents the responses given by a group of adolescents and young adults ($N = 437$) from the Autonomous City of Buenos Aires and Gran Buenos Aires, Argentina, who responded to the Internet Addiction Scale [40]. This scale is made up of 11 questions which measure Internet addiction and presents two dimensions: behavioral symptomatology with eight questions (being online for a long time, spending more time on it than you should, feeling bad when not connected, among others) and dysfunctionality with three questions (problems associated with addiction: missing work or school due to being online for a long time, neglecting the home or housework, among others). Each item has Likert-type multiple choice responses with four options: *Very rarely* (1), *Rarely* (2), *Often* (3), and *Always* (4). This instrument showed adequate factorial structure and internal consistency [40]. It also retains its psychometric properties in Argentina [41].

There are certain signs that we can consider alarming to which parents and educators can be attentive, since they show a dependency on ICT; among them we can mention the following [42, 43]:

Table 32.1 Responses to the Internet Addiction Scale in Argentinean adolescents and young adults

Items	Very rarely	Rarely	Often	Always
1. When I am not connected, I imagine what it will be like the next time I am connected to the Internet	52%	32%	13%	3%
2. I feel worried or dream about connecting when I'm not	30%	40%	25%	5%
3. After going offline, I feel like I still want to be on the Internet	40%	35%	20%	4%
4. I feel depressed, moody, or nervous when I'm offline and it goes away when I'm back online	62%	28%	9%	1%
5. I spend more time on the Internet than I intended.	10%	22%	51%	17%
6. I often say "just a few more minutes" when online	18%	22%	48%	18%
7. I have tried to be connected less time but I have not been able	38%	35%	24%	3%
8. When I feel the urge to go online I can't control it	45%	30%	20%	5%
9. I have come to miss classes for being on the Internet	56%	22%	17%	5%
10. I have had problems at school for being on the Internet	62%	23%	12%	3%
11. I neglect housework to spend more time online	34%	26%	35%	6%

- Sleep fewer hours than usual to stay connected and/or have altered sleep patterns.
- Putting aside important activities, whether it's health care, schoolwork, social relationships, and family.
- That someone close, such as parents or siblings, complain about excessive use of the network.
- Constantly thinking about new technologies or the Internet when you are not connected and experience excessive irritability if the connection is very slow or fails.
- Having the desire and trying to reduce the amount of time dedicated to this behavior, but not being able to do so, losing track of the time dedicated to that end.
- Not telling the truth about the amount of time you are online.
- Have a lower academic performance compared to what he had before, be irritable and isolated on a social level.
- Experiencing unusual euphoria, joy, or activation when in front of the technological device.

When identifying some of these warning signs, it is very important to consult a psychology specialist, since it is necessary to carry out an evaluation of the adolescent in order to understand what his initial motivation was, what his function is, and what he has maintained it over time, while seeking to warn if there is also another concomitant or underlying pathology [35]. It is important to make it clear that not all subjects who make excessive use will suffer from addiction. This will depend, among other factors, on whether their personality is vulnerable, if their family has weak cohesion, and if their social relationships are poor. At the same time, it must be considered if he finds immediate rewards for his behaviors, if the addictive behavior is easy to carry out, if he feels social pressure to carry it out, or if he is under stressful circumstances or if he feels that his life is empty and lacks vital objectives [44].

This problem can be considered a public health problem, so it must be addressed from different institutions, such as family and educational institutes [45]. Parents, teachers, and educational institutions play a very important role in reducing the complexities that this situation presents, since they can guide them and offer them tools so that children and adolescents develop digital skills that give them the ability to function safely and appropriately [46].

When analyzing addiction to new technologies from the variables that surround the individual, it is essential to think about the context of development, either the peer group, the family, the school, or the community [47]. As we have mentioned, as a result of the gradual isolation that the person goes through, their relationships deteriorate and their school performance begins to decline, while the time they spend with their friends and family is reduced, at the same time that the family conflicts [48, 49]. Adolescents will have more chances of developing an addiction to new technologies in a conflictive and difficult family environment [50], while parental supervision and spending time together are inhibitory factors of said addiction [51, 52].

From all of the above, it can be seen that the use of ICT and their devices has generated the appearance of new behaviors, which can harm people's personal and family relationships [26]. Excessive use, dependence, or addiction to new technologies can generate problems in the affective, behavioral, and social spheres [53]. This is why the family and the context closest to adolescents have a fundamental role in detecting alarm signals and promoting the healthy use of technology, controlling the use they give to these media, increasing self-control and autonomy of children and teens [54]. And to achieve this, it is necessary for adults, whether parents or educators, to be trained in everything that ICT entail in order to carry out adequate supervision and accompaniment of their children and/or students [29].

Phubbing or Cell Phone Addiction in Adolescents and Young Adults

Technology has achieved unprecedented growth in recent decades [2, 41, 55]. Increasingly, mobile devices are used in different fields to facilitate the connection between people and solve different problems of daily life. However, the deployment of technology has brought new problems along with its use. Following the well-known dysfunctional phenomena such as trolling, cyberbullying, or sexting, one that has grown lately is phubbing. Phubbing—which is made up of the English words snubb and phone—is characterized as a behavior in which an individual ignores another for using a technology, such as a cell phone or tablet. Although it is a phenomenon that occurs in all people, it is more frequent in adolescents and young people due to the popularity of these devices in them; although it is also increasing in adult people, who even put their lives at risk due to the indiscriminate use of cell phones. This behavior, with the growth of battery life in devices, is occurring in several different settings, such as social gatherings, school, or work settings, among others.

With regard to the incidence of ICT -such as cell phones and computers- it is notably widespread, mainly among adolescents. For example, in our country there are almost two cell phones per person. Regarding the use of ICT in Argentinean adolescents, a survey indicates that 21% of adolescents manifest that they have a computer in their own room and 97% have a cell phone, even 22% affirm that their own parents bought it for them and the 67% play video games -mainly men. A central place has been occupied by social networks, such as Facebook, Instagram, Twitter, Tik Tok, or YouTube, which have changed the way of relating, working, studying, and entertainment. In this way, they generated positive aspects, such as being more communicated, informed, more democratic access to knowledge, and a great diversity of recreation.

In Argentina, mainly among the youngest, the use of social networks is widespread. Adolescents in Argentina have been called "the interactive generation" because they are one of the groups in Latin America that is most attracted to new technologies, as we pointed out. For example, in 2021 it is estimated that there were 36 million active social network users, with an increase of 2 million new users between 2020 and 2021. At the same time, an average of almost 3 and a half hours of time per day is used to be connected to them [56].

Conceptualizing Phubbing

But what is phubbing? We have all suffered at least once from phubbing during a meeting with friends, a work meeting, a family meal, or even in bed with a partner, as a consequence of the possibility of staying connected to the Internet at any time and in any place. As we said, this term formed from the English words, phone and snubbing. Its meaning began around 2012 thanks to the McCann advertising agency in Melbourne [57]. Phubbing occurs when people disapprove of or ignore other people in their company for focusing on their smartphone [58, 59]. Thus, phubbing is considered a multidimensional construction. For example, Karadağ et al. [60] point out that it can be explained by mobile phone addiction, SMS addiction, social media addiction, Internet addiction, and gaming addiction. Chotpitayasunondh and Douglas [61] revealed moderate correlations between phubbing behavior and smartphone and Internet addiction.

Thus, a phubber may experience an inability to monitor or control their smartphone; the inability to regulate mobile phone use and etiquette when tempted [61]. Despite the relevance of the subject, in Argentina, as in many Latin American countries, there are almost no studies on the matter. Due to the negative effects that phubbing can have, it is necessary to develop instruments to measure this construct.

Measuring Phubbing

Phubbing Scale by Karadag et al. [60] is one of the few instruments available in this regard. This scale is made up of 10 questions with five alternatives (1 = *Never* to 5 = ***Always***) that evaluate phubbing behaviors and other associated problm behaviors. Example of questions is: "When I am with my family, I am always busy with my cell phone". It consists of two dimensions which are behaviors that affect interpersonal communication and obsession with the cell phone. This scale has shown good psychometric properties, such as internal reliability and construct validity, such as the association of phubbing with the problematic use of new technologies and Internet addiction. It has shown good properties in Turkey, such as adequate factorial structure, internal consistency, and construct validity [60]. In Spain, it showed good properties as well [62]. In Argentina, this instrument demonstrated an adequate factorial structure of three factors and satisfactory internal consistency [41]. These three dimensions could be called interference due to the use of the cell phone (which refers to the problems that this generates in interpersonal relationships), obsession with the device (which refers to the addiction that it generates), and psychosocial problems (which points to how its use deteriorates the life of the subject). Although this structure was adequate in Argentina, it differed from the one postulated by the authors of the test, which is made up of only the first two. As it was the first time, it was used in our environment. The scale adapted to Spain was used. External judges only suggested the change from mobile phone to cell phone in our setting. First, it was taken in a pilot sample of 70 adolescents with the scale showing good internal consistency.

How Widespread Is Phubbing in Argentina?

The results of this problem will be reported below based on an intentional sample of adolescents and young adults of 1052 subjects in the Autonomous City of Buenos Aires (45%) and Paraná (55%), Argentina, with ages from 12 years to 40 (M age = 21.09, SD = 4.35), with 73% of women. A 60% of the sample had a cell phone before the age of 12 and 56% had a social network.

Table 32.2 shows the responses of the participants to the Karadag et al. phubbing scale.

As it may be seen in Table 32.2, the levels of phubbing were alarming. The questions referring to the obsession with regard to the cell phone "my cell phone is always near me" and "I feel that something is missing if I don't have my cell phone" were the ones indicated by almost 60% showing that it happened to them almost usually or always. On the other hand, in a question made by the present researchers, 10% said they had put their lives at risk due to misuse of cell phones, almost being hit by a car or almost crashing while driving.

Table 32.3 shows the phubbing scale scores, according to gender. The results indicated that there were no gender differences with the exception of cell phone addiction where males scored higher, but the difference was marginal $p < .06$, as shown in Table 32.3.

An association was also found between age and phubbing, suggesting that, at a younger age, there are higher phubbing scores at the level of interpersonal impairment, cell phone addiction,

Table 32.2 Responses to the Phubbing scale of Karadag et al. in Argentinean adolescents and young adults

Items	Never	Rarely	Sometimes	Usually	Always
1. My eyes start wandering on my phone when I'm together with others IC	6%	24%	44%	19%	7%
2. I am busy with my mobile phone when I'm with my friends IC	16%	46%	32%	5%	2%
3. People complain about me dealing with my mobile phone IC	40%	30%	22%	5%	3%
4. I'm busy with my mobile phone when I'm with my family IC	14%	39%	36%	10%	2%
5. I think that I annoy my partner when I'm busy with my mobile phone (or family, if you do not have a partner) IC	29%	25%	28%	9%	9%
6. My phone is within my reach OD	1%	2%	14%	35%	48%
7. When I wake up in the morning, I first check the messages on my phone OD	3%	5%	12%	23%	56%
8. I feel incomplete without my mobile phone OD	6%	10%	26%	22%	37%
9. My mobile phone use increases day by day PP	17%	27%	33%	12%	12%
10. The time allocated to social, personal, or professional activities decreases because of my mobile phone PP	26%	24%	28%	11%	12%

Note. *IC* interference due to cell phone use, *OD* obsession with the device, *PP* psychosocial problems

Table 32.3 Phubbing scores by gender

Dimension	Gender	*M*	*SD*
IC	Males	12.00	3.54
	Females	12.19	3.18
PP	Males	12.34	2.41
	Females	12.28	2.37
OD	Males	5.56	2.19
	Females	5.25	2.04

Note. *IC* interference due to cell phone use, *OD* obsession with the device, *PP* psychosocial problems

and psychosocial problems (rs = .12, .15, and .06, although in the latter case they were marginal, showing ps < .001, .001, and .08, respectively). These results indicated high phubbing results and some participants even confessed that they put their lives at risk by using the cell phone.

Gender did not introduce differences, except marginally on a scale, which can be explained by the fact that it is a widespread phenomenon in almost all people. The younger, the more phubbing, which can be explained by the use of cell phones at an early age, as well as the need young people have to show themselves on social networks and be accepted [63]. Finally, as some studies from first world countries point out [64], excessive phubbing affects interpersonal relationships with parents, mainly by increasing conflicts and fights, which was also detected in some Argentinean studies [41].

Future studies should examine this problem in randomly selected samples from various provinces of Argentina, as in other Latin American nations, in order to generalize the results and determine if it maintains its measurement invariance across the different provinces. A relevant issue is that future research should be longitudinal, both to examine its test/retest consistency and to determine how stable phubbing is over time-considering the rapid changes that occur in new technologies. In addition, the use of the cell phone (for example, its frequency) should be examined with more objective measurements, such as certain applications that evaluate daily the time each application is used, in order to have more precise measurements that do not depend on memory or the honesty of the participants.

Recommendations for a Healthy Use of Cell Phones and Social Networks

- Turn off the cell phone at night; in social or family gatherings or when working, keep it away; charge it outside the room where a person sleeps; and turn off cell phone notifications at all times.
- Responsible use of ICT: do not use them to attack or respond to aggression; be careful with the information or posts that are shared -there is a lot of fake news-; have the

networks configured in privacy; avoid using them at night or before going to bed—since they can cause difficulties in falling asleep-; do not share your current location or personal information.

- Having social networks, such as Facebook and Instagram, installed on the computer rather than on the cell phone. This prevents compulsive use of these and disturbance in social or family gatherings.
- Encourage healthy use in minors: do not enter social networks at an early age—for example, the pediatric society of England does not recommend exposure to screens before 2 years of age-; make supervised use of the it; prevent minors from having a computer or television in the room; use filters or parental control applications; avoid posting photos of children or their personal information on social networks; limit exposure to screens and consult a professional in case of any doubt.
- It is not about prohibiting the use in minors, but about supervising its use. To do this, you can make a routine of when to use them and when not -for example, not using them at lunchtime or at night. Sometimes, in specific circumstances or times, you have to turn off the cell phone. Schedule activities that are incompatible with the use, like to go out for a bike ride or go for a walk in the countryside, may be recommended. To teach a constructive use of them -to study, for example- is an interesting possibility. It must warn also that not all people are who they say they are on social networks. Do not do in the virtual world what is not done face to face, or that not everything that is shown in them is real.

References

1. Facio A, Resett S. Argentina. In: Arnett J, editor. Adolescent psychology around the world. EE. UU.: Psychological Press; 2012. p. 151–62.
2. Resett S, González Caino PC. Propiedades psicométricas de un Cuestionario de Trolling en una muestra argentina. Revista Argentina de Ciencias del Comportamiento. 2019;11(1):48–57.
3. Vallejo Hernández R. Efectos del mal uso de las Tecnologías de la Información y Comunicación en adolescentes: Ciberacoso. 2021.
4. Abellán Roselló L, Méndez Ballesteros E. Influencia de las nuevas tecnologías entre el alumnado de 10 a 12 años. Int J New Educ. 2021;7:193–210.
5. León M, Cerda C, Rehbein L, Saiz JL. Diseño y validación de un Escala de Inmersión Digital para Adolescentes. Estudios pedagógicos (Valdivia). 2021;47(3):229–49.
6. Plaza de la Hoz J. Ventajas y desventajas del uso adolescente de las TIC: visión de los estudiantes. Revista complutense de educación. 2018.
7. Hernández Ortiz ÁJ. Intervención social en la salud; uso de las nuevas tecnologías y su relación con la salud. 2021.
8. Orben A. Digital diet: A 21st century approach to understanding digital technologies and development. Infant Child Dev. 2022;31(1):e2228.
9. Patriarca A, Di Giuseppe G, Albano L, Marinelli P, Angelillo IF. Use of television, videogames, and computer among children and adolescents in Italy. BMC Public Health. 2009;9(1):1–10.
10. Muñoz-Miralles R, Ortega-González R, Batalla-Martínez C, López-Morón MR, Manresa JM, Torán-Monserrat P. Acceso y uso de nuevas tecnologías entre los jóvenes de educación secundaria, implicaciones en salud. Estudio JOITIC Atención Primaria. 2014;46(2):77–88.
11. Smith D, Leonis T, Anandavalli S. Belonging and loneliness in cyberspace: impacts of social media on adolescents' well-being. Aust J Psychol. 2021;73(1):12–23.
12. INDEC INdEyC. Acceso y uso de tecnologías de la información y la comunicación. EPH. Cuarto trimestre de 2020. Ciencia y tecnología, Informes técnicos. 2020. p. 89–115.
13. Espinar-Ruiz E, López Fernández C. Jóvenes y adolescentes ante las nuevas tecnologías: percepción de riesgos. 2009.
14. Guevara Cardeña L. Adolescentes y uso de las principales redes sociales. Teoría y Práctica: Revista Peruana de Psicología CPsP-CDR-I. 2021;3(2):e38-e.
15. Encinas FJL, González SMV. Menores y nuevas tecnologías: conductas indicadoras de posible problema de adicción. Psicothema. 2010;22(2):180–8.
16. Casey JE, Pennington LK, Lopez D. Increasing hispanic students' awareness and use of floor-robots through structured activities. Contemp Educ Technol. 2020;13(1):ep281.
17. Rosewell A, Shearman P, Ramamurthy S, Akers R. Transforming the health information system using mobile and geographic information technologies, Papua New Guinea. Bull World Health Organ. 2021;99(5):381.
18. Fondevila-Gascón J-F, Carreras Alcalde M, Mir Bernal P, Del Olmo Arriaga JL, Pesqueira Zamora MJ. El impacto de la mensajería instantánea en los estudiantes en forma de estrés y ansiedad para el apre-

ndizaje: Análisis empírico. Didáctica, innovación y multimedia. 2014(30):1–15.
19. Vuorre M, Orben A, Przybylski AK. There is no evidence that associations between adolescents' digital technology engagement and mental health problems have increased. Clin Psychol Sci. 2021;9(5):823–35.
20. Forzano L, Sorama M, O'Keefe M, Pizzonia K, Howard T, Dukic N. Impulsivity and self-control in elementary school children and adult females: using identical task and procedural parameters. Behav Process. 2021;188:104411.
21. Hollis C. Youth mental health: risks and opportunities in the digital world. World Psychiatry. 2022;21(1):81.
22. Malak MZ, Shuhaiber AH, Al-amer RM, Abuadas MH, Aburoomi RJ. Correlation between psychological factors, academic performance and social media addiction: model-based testing. Behav Inform Technol. 2022;41(8):1583–95.
23. Ortega FL, Gómez MF, de la Fuente Anuncibay R, del Río FP, del Burgo MR, de Albéniz GGP. Uso y abuso de las nuevas tecnologías. Elsevier Doyma; 2010. p. 2–4.
24. Quintas A, Bustamante J-C, Pradas F, Castellar C. Psychological effects of gamified didactics with exergames in physical education at primary schools: results from a natural experiment. Comput Educ. 2020;152:103874.
25. Barquero Madrigal A, Calderón Contreras F. Influencia de las nuevas tecnologías en el desarrollo adolescente y posibles desajustes. Revista Cúpula. 2016;30(2):11–25.
26. Jorquera Hernández AB. Violencia escolar, inteligencia emocional y uso de nuevas tecnologías en adolescentes de Educación Secundaria Obligatoria: Universidad de Murcia; 2021.
27. Soto A, De Miguel N, Díaz VP. Abordaje de adicciones a nuevas tecnologías: una propuesta de prevención en contexto escolar y tratamiento de rehabilitación. Papeles del Psicólogo. 2018;39(2):120–6.
28. O'reilly M, Dogra N, Whiteman N, Hughes J, Eruyar S, Reilly P. Is social media bad for mental health and wellbeing? Exploring the perspectives of adolescents. Clin Child Psychol Psychiatry. 2018;23(4):601–13.
29. Arab LE, Díaz GA. Impacto de las redes sociales e internet en la adolescencia: aspectos positivos y negativos. Rev Med Clin Condes. 2015;26(1):7–13.
30. Martín Perpiñá MdlM, Viñas Poch F, Malo Cerrato S. Media multitasking impact in homework, executive function and academic performance in Spanish adolescents. Psicothema. 2019.
31. Martín-Perpiñá MdlM, Poch FV, Cerrato SM. Personality and social context factors associated to self-reported excessive use of information and communication technology (ICT) on a sample of Spanish adolescents. Front Psychol. 2019;10:436.
32. Organization WH. International classification of diseases (ICD-11). World Health Organization; 2022.
33. Echeburúa E, De Corral P. Adicción a las nuevas tecnologías ya las redes sociales en jóvenes: un nuevo reto. Adicciones. 2010;22(2):91–5.
34. Przepiorka A, Blachnio A, Cudo A. The role of depression, personality, and future time perspective in internet addiction in adolescents and emerging adults. Psychiatry Res. 2019;272:340–8.
35. Matalí JL, Flores E. 3.¿ Cómo gestionamos el impacto de las nuevas tecnologías? Una mirada a la salud mental de los adolescentes. 75.
36. Potenza MN. Should addictive disorders include non-substance-related conditions? Addiction. 2006;101:142–51.
37. García-Oliva C, Piqueras JA, Marzo JC. Uso problemático de internet, el móvil y los videojuegos en una muestra de adolescentes alicantinos. Salud y drogas. 2017;17(2):189–200.
38. Sánchez Costas I. Adaptación y validación de la escala SAS (Smartphone Addiction Scale) en adolescentes españoles y factores asociados al uso de las nuevas tecnologías. Proyecto de investigación:. 2021.
39. Sánchez-Carbonell X, Beranuy M, Castellana M, Chamarro A, Oberst U. La adicción a Internet y al móvil:¿ moda o trastorno? Adicciones. 2008;20(2):149–59.
40. Lam-Figueroa N, Contreras-Pulache H, Mori-Quispe E, Nizama-Valladolid M, Gutiérrez C, Hinostroza-Camposano W, et al. Adicción a internet: desarrollo y validación de un instrumento en escolares adolescentes de Lima, Perú. Rev Peru Med Exp Salud Publica. 2011;28:462–9.
41. Resett SA, González PC. Propiedades psicométricas de una Escala de Phubbing en una muestra argentina. 2020.
42. Young K. Internet addiction: the emergence of a new clinical disorder. CyberPsychol Behav. 1998;1:237–44.
43. Young K. Internet addiction: diagnosis and treatment considerations. J Contemp Psychother. 2009;39(4):241–6.
44. Odriozola EE. Factores de riesgo y factores de protección en la adicción a las nuevas tecnologías y redes sociales en jóvenes y adolescentes. Revista española de drogodependencias. 2012;4:435–48.
45. Malak MZ, Khalifeh AH, Shuhaiber AH. Prevalence of Internet addiction and associated risk factors in Jordanian school students. Comput Hum Behav. 2017;70:556–63.
46. Valencia Ortiz R, Cabero Almenara J, Garay Ruiz U, Fernández Robles B. Problemática de estudio e investigación de la adicción a las redes sociales online en jóvenes y adolescentes. Revista Tecnología. Ciencia y Educación. 2021;18:99–125.
47. Oliva Delgado A, Hidalgo García MV, Moreno Rodríguez MdC, Jiménez García L, Jiménez Iglesias AM, Antolín Suarez L, et al. Uso y riesgo de adicciones a las nuevas tecnologías entre adolescentes y jóvenes andaluces. 2012.
48. Aponte Rueda DR, Castillo Chávez P, González Estrella JE. Prevalencia de adicción a internet y su relación con disfunción familiar en adolescentes. Revista Clínica de Medicina de Familia. 2017;10(3):179–86.

49. Kaya A, Dalgiç AI. How does internet addiction affect adolescent lifestyles? Results from a school-based study in the Mediterranean region of Turkey. J Pediatr Nurs. 2021;59:e38–43.
50. Yen J-Y, Yen C-F, Chen C-C, Chen S-H, Ko C-H. Family factors of internet addiction and substance use experience in Taiwanese adolescents. CyberPsychol Behav. 2007;10(3):323–9.
51. Jeong EJ, Kim DH. Social activities, self-efficacy, game attitudes, and game addiction. Cyberpsychol Behav Soc Netw. 2011;14(4):213–21.
52. Lin C-H, Lin S-L, Wu C-P. The effects of parental monitoring and leisure boredom on adolescents' internet addiction. Adolescence. 2009;44(176).
53. Gallimberti L, Buja A, Chindamo S, Terraneo A, Marini E, Rabensteiner A, et al. Problematic cell phone use for text messaging and substance abuse in early adolescence (11-to 13-year-olds). Eur J Pediatr. 2016;175(3):355–64.
54. Plaza de la Hoz J. Advantages and downsides of children ICT use in Spain: the parent's perspective. Int J Lifelong Educ Leadership. 2017;3(2):22–31.
55. Resett SA, Mesurado B, González Caino P, Oñate ME. Nuevas problemáticas relacionadas con el uso de las tecnologías en siglo XXI: unabordaje desde la prevención y el desarrollo psicosocial positivo enadolescentes. In: Ramos, del Río B, Martí Noguera JJ, editors. Experiencias en ciberpsicología: hacia una nueva era de la psicología. Universidad Nacional Autónoma de México: Facultad de Estudios Superiores Zaragoza; 2021. p. 165–98.
56. Alvino C. Estadísticas de la situación digital de Argentina en el 2020-2021. Branch. https://branch.com.co/marketing-digital/estadisticas-de….
57. Garrido E, Delgado S. Phubbing: conectados a la red y desconectados de la realidad: un análisis en relación al bienestar psicológico. Pixel-Bit. 2017.
58. Abramova O, Baumann A, Krasnova H, Lessmann S, editors. To phub or not to phub: understanding off-task smartphone usage and its consequences in the academic environment. ECIS; 2017.
59. Nazir T, Pişkin M. Phubbing: a technological invasion which connected the world but disconnected humans. Int J Indian Psychol. 2016;3(4):175–82.
60. Karadağ E, Tosuntaş ŞB, Erzen E, Duru P, Bostan N, Şahin BM, et al. Determinants of phubbing, which is the sum of many virtual addictions: a structural equation model. J Behav Addict. 2015;4(2):60–74.
61. Chotpitayasunondh V, Douglas KM. How "phubbing" becomes the norm: the antecedents and consequences of snubbing via smartphone. Comput Hum Behav. 2016;63:9–18.
62. Blanca MJ, Bendayan R. Spanish version of the Phubbing Scale: Internet addiction, Facebook intrusion, and fear of missing out as correlates. Psicothema. 2018;30(4):449–54.
63. Steinberg L. Adolescence. Boston: McGraw-Hill; 2008.
64. Stockdale LA, Coyne SM, Padilla-Walker LM. Parent and child technoference and socioemotional behavioral outcomes: a nationally representative study of 10-to 20-year-old adolescents. Comput Hum Behav. 2018;88:219–26.

Social Networks' Addiction in Adolescents and Young People: Effects and Possible Approaches

33

Elisa Mariajosé Martínez Canales,
Lucas Marcelo Rodriguez, and María José Zinoni

Social Networks and Their Influence on Mental Health

The way we live and develop has been transformed by modernization in this new digital age. Before modernization, the opportunities were different than today. Consequently, we could ask ourselves: *are these opportunities an advantage or a disadvantage for our mental health?* This new digital age allows people to connect with others, such as family, friends, and close relatives. Nevertheless, *this brings us closer or further away?* On one side, if someone moved to another city or country, their relatives and close people could communicate and keep in touch by video calls. At the same time, it prevents us from enjoying the here and the now. We can have everything and nothing at the same time; social networks have come to consume our valuable time. Another question emerged: do we really enjoy our present? We always yearn for more personal time to be with the family, go to the beach, read a book or rest, but we are so immersed in modernization that it becomes very difficult for us to disconnect from our cell phones. The way that we use cell phones does not allow us to share quality time with the people around us; we are together and far away at the same time. Actually, children are introduced to the virtual world from a very early age by their parents. So, adults give them the key to an unknown world that often separates them. Sometimes the distance is so great that the members of a family become complete strangers. They neither know tastes, perceptions, nor how it feels to be with each other. At family dinners, it has become common for everyone to have their cell phone in hand and be browsing social networks like Instagram, Facebook, Twitter, TikTok, etc.

Indeed, this study proposes a new question: how is mental health affected by the inappropriate use of social networks?

First of all, it is necessary to consider the concept of health:

"Health is a state of complete physical, mental and social well-being, and not just the absence of any disease or infirmity". The reference comes from the Preamble to the Constitution of the

E. M. Martínez Canales (✉)
National Autonomous University of Nicaragua at León (UNAN León – Universidad Nacional Autónoma de Nicaragua), León, Nicaragua

L. M. Rodriguez
Instituto de Filosofía - Facultad de Ciencias Biomédicas, Universidad Austral - Consejo Nacional de Investigaciones Científicas y Técnicas (CONICET), Pilar, Argentina

M. J. Zinoni
Instituto de Filosofía - Facultad de Ciencias Biomédicas, Universidad Austral - Consejo Nacional de Investigaciones Científicas y Técnicas (CONICET), Pilar, Argentina

Centro de Investigación interdisciplinar en Valores, Integración y Desarrollo Social, Universidad Católica Argentina - Consejo Nacional de Investigaciones Científicas y Técnicas (CONICET), Paraná, Argentina

P. Á. Gargiulo, H. L. Mesones-Arroyo (eds.), *Psychiatry and Neuroscience Update – Vol. V*,
https://doi.org/10.1007/978-3-031-72219-6_33

World Health Organization, which was adopted by the International Sanitary Conference that was held in New York from June 19 to July 22, 1946. It was signed on July 22, 1946, by the representatives of 61 States (Official records of the World Health Organization, No. 2, p. 100) and entered into force on April 7, 1948. The conceptual definition of health has not been modified since 1948.

The central question considers the influence on mental health; it is necessary to remember the following:

Mental and behavioral health problems are characterized by changes in thinking, behavior, and/or mood associated with distress or deterioration in general mental functioning. These problems are due to biological aspects associated with cultural and social factors. Besides, it could be intensified by an individual predisposition. Mental disorders, especially anxiety and depression, are one of the main causes of comorbidity in today's society. Both the daily activities of the individual and their social relationships are compromised. According to the World Health Organization (WHO), at least 350 million people worldwide live with depression [1].

Excessive use of social networks such as Instagram, Facebook, Twitter, and YouTube is a habit that has recently been strengthened. This is a recent phenomenon, so the possible effects and impacts on health of this new form of social interaction in different populations are still being studied. The increase in time dedicated to the use of different social networks is more related to the feeling of isolation from the real world. There are people who live submerged in their own world, which can contribute to developing mental disorders and other health problems. Although addiction to social networks is a phenomenon within Internet addiction, there is evidence that this addiction has maintained growth in the last two decades [2]. In this way, assessing the consequences of this type of addiction on mental health becomes relevant.

Definition of Social Networks in the Framework of ICTs

Defining the term social networks is not such a simple process. There are different author's approaches and several definitions have been given. Some of them are listed here: virtual social networks, such as Facebook, Tuenti, Hi5, etc. Despite being a recent communication system, this has been used by millions of users, many of whom have integrated these websites into their daily activity [3].

With the use of social networks, the term "Social Software" has appeared. This term is defined by Parameswaran and Whinston [4], as: "a category of applications and services that facilitate collective action and online social interaction with a rich exchange of multimedia information that generates knowledge evolution globally".

Social networks currently occupy a very important place in everyone's life. Not only they allow us to relate with our relatives and close people, but can also be used in the professional field to boost a career, for publicity to bring customers, etc. Social networks are tools that also help us to be updated on the news of daily events worldwide, which is why they have become an indispensable part of our daily routine.

Behavioral Addiction Applicable to Social Networks

The indiscriminate use of social networks has given rise to new addictive behaviors in this context. Historically, the term "addiction" has been used for drug addiction. However, it has been discovered that the principal element of all addictive disorders is the lack of control. Affected people lose the ability to control a specific behavior. At first, it can be pleasant but then other preferences are restricted and it becomes a dominant behavior [5].

Since the rise of the term "Internet addiction" [6], there have been many concerns and research projects aimed at categorizing this trend within the group of mental disorders. Psychologists and psychiatrists have pushed to include these behaviors in the DSM-5 (Diagnostic and Statistical Manual of Mental Disorders) as other addiction disorders. Defenders of the existence of this pathology mention that Internet is still a new area for research. They also mention that Internet user associations and companies do not accept this dependency because it would be against their model of business. Even so, they manifest symptoms such as "emotional shutdown", lack of concentration, and withdrawal. On the opposite side, experts and researchers in mental health affirm that these behaviors do not cause mental disorders. Instead, they express that these are temporary and transient problems but not disorders [7].

At present, it is more than clear that the different addictions are not only limited to behaviors generated by the uncontrollable consumption of substances (for example: cannabis, amphetamines, cocaine, opiates, caffeine, nicotine, or alcohol). In addition, there are behavioral habits that seem harmless but can become addictive and seriously interfere in the lives of the people involved [5].

When the addiction grows, the behaviors become automatic and are activated with impulses and emotions. Both cognitive control and self-criticism over these behaviors are poor. An addicted person expects immediate gratification and does not consider the possible negative consequences.

The different symptoms that are related to a behavioral addiction are as follows:

- Intense desire, anxiety, or uncontrollable urge to perform that pleasurable activity. In this case it is the urgent need to enter the virtual platforms, need to be recognized, and anxiety when the desired response is not obtained.
- Progressive loss of control over their own behavior, until reaching complete lack of control. Constant need to enter platforms whatever the situation. Responsibilities and obligations are set aside for the benefit of staying online.
- Absence in family, academic, work, or leisure activities.
- Inability to record indications relating to their behavior in the area of addiction. These negative characteristics presented by people with a behavioral addiction, particularly with an addiction to social networks, are usually noticed by close people and/or relatives. These people usually communicate this to the addict, although multiple warnings and calls for attention do not stop the activity and they become defensive. They often deny that they have a problem. Their anger can be so strong that it leads them to end relationships.
- Need to live constantly checking messages, networks, or simply entering social networks.
- Anger and irritability at the impossibility of performing the action that is addictive (abstinence), for example, when wifi or electricity is out of order so they cannot be online [5, 8].

Positive and Negative Effects of Using Social Networks

Actually, there are some positive and negative effects that can be listed on the use of social networks. They are mentioned here below.

Positive effects in the area of ***mental health***:

- The media and social communication networks can improve the mood of people who have had to move away from family. It also allows access to specialized information on different topics and even related to the axis of health.
- The use of social networks allows you to feel emotional support by staying in touch with other people and interacting with them.

Negative effects in the area of ***mental health***:

- Nowadays, the indiscriminate use of the different social network platforms can cause addiction to social media. Young people are the most affected.
- There has been an increase in the rates of anxiety and depression in people who use the different social networks for a long time. There is a search for acceptance by followers, number of likes and comments.
- The use of different social networks is related to difficulties in falling asleep and to self-image problems. It directly affects the self-esteem of people who spend their time on social networks.
- At present, there is another important term that is relevant. It is "cyberbullying or cyber bully-

ing". It is a growing problem since 7 out of 10 young people claim to have experienced it.
- Another problem that has been detected in different consumers of social networking platforms is the irrational fear of being ignored (missing out). It is characterized by the need to be constantly connected with other people's activities, so as not to "miss them" [9].

The development of information and communication technologies generated the emergence of addictions to virtual products such as Internet, games, and social networks and their effects among the population of adolescents and young people. These addictions have brought other negative effects. It is the case of data obtained from some research in adolescents. They found that social networks' addiction results in problems of depression, anxiety, insomnia, and psychological discomfort. Research shows a relationship between abusive use of social networks and externalizing problems in adolescents such as low emotional control, irritability, difficulties in interpersonal relationships, aggression, and attention deficit [10].

Meta-analysis studies not only focused on Internet addiction, but also exposed that addictive behavior is associated with a higher rate of mental health problems and a greater severity in the symptomatology. Among them, depression, anxiety, psychological inflexibility, low levels of self-concept, social withdrawal, etc. should be highlighted [11]. Another meta-analysis study showed a negative association between the problematic use of social networks and well-being indicators and anxiety [12]. This same study showed that the negative effect of problematic use of social networks on self-esteem is more serious in men.

Possible Ways of Intervention Against Addiction to Social Networks

A Latin American study carried out in Peru with an adolescent population affirmed that the risk of addiction to networks is greater when adolescents have low self-esteem and self-concept. In addition, those adolescents who share aspirations, values, and positive interactions with their parents and siblings have less risk of becoming addicted to social networks. On the other hand, this risk increases when relationships are conflictive; there are parents who are rigid, absent, or not very understanding [13]. These investigations allow us to trace a line of work for prevention of addiction to social networks, both at the individual level (working with self-esteem, self-concept, and personal assessment of adolescents and young people) as well as working with the family environment to achieve healthy interactions.

Monacis and others [14] emphasize the importance of certain protective factors such as those mentioned. In their empirical study [14], they evaluated addiction to Internet, online games, and social networks with identity and attachment. Of the identity styles proposed by Berzonsky [15, 16], the informational and diffuse-avoidant identity styles constitute risk factors for addictions. On the opposite way, the normative identity style acted as a protective factor. In addition, the secure attachment style constitutes another protective factor against this type of addiction while anxious and avoidant attachment are risk factors.

From this study, possible lines of interventions are traced to promote the development of protective factors. First, it is important to foster a normative identity style, in which individuals focus on the expectations, values, and prescriptions of their loved ones [15]. Second, it is important to promote types of secure attachment between parents and children, which allow optimal development of the potential of children.

Recent empirical studies have demonstrated the moderating role of mindfulness in anxiety and depression in smartphone addictions [17]. This also opens a way of working with mindfulness in adolescents and young people with the problem of addiction to social networks.

Conclusion

Social networks have mitigated feelings of loneliness and stress during the pandemic in the previous years [18]. It shows a positive aspect of these new technologies. However, the COVID-19 pandemic also exacerbated Internet addiction [1]. Addiction to the Internet and social networks has become a highly worrying phenomenon because there are more people who have access to different virtual platforms.

However, abuse in the use of the Internet may be a secondary manifestation of another addiction or psychopathology such as depression, social phobia, or other impulsive-compulsive problems [8, 19]. The principal characteristic of Internet addiction is that it occupies a central part of lives of people who are immersed in the cyberworld. The abuse of social networks may cause a loss of personal exchange skills (personal communication is learned by practicing) and this is precisely the area that has been deteriorating with the high consumption of social networks. At present, adolescents find it difficult to interact personally; they prefer texting by cell phone than to have a face-to-face conversation.

The problem of addiction to social networks is more important in adolescence as a key stage of the life cycle in which identity is consolidated. The abuse of social networks can play a key role in the need for acceptance (likes in publications), leading to the construction of identity being guided by trends in social networks and not by a true exploration of what is personal and the real possibilities of the environment. In this line of thought, Moya et al. [10] express that in the construction of identity through social networks, popularity and acceptance by the group prevail at the expense of freedom.

The therapeutic objective in drug-free addictions is the relearning controlled behaviors. One of the most important aspects is that the people who suffer from this addictive disorder must be aware of their problem and want to solve it. Then, they can get ahead, overcoming this problem.

This chapter does not intend to close this problem; on the contrary, there are still many factors to be considered in order to carry out an adequate initial therapeutic intervention. As behavioral control temporarily increases and the ability to cope successfully with the various situations is presented in daily life, the subject experiences a perception of control, which increases the expectation of success in the future [20, 21]. In a world where globalization is accelerating daily and new ways of communicating with social networks are emerging, it is important to promote the appropriate and responsible use of technologies.

References

1. World Health Organization. Prevention of Mental Disorders: effective interventions and policy options: summary report [Internet]. Geneva; 2004 [cited Aug 29 2019]. Available from: https://www.who.int/mental_health/evidence/en/prevention_of_mental_disorders_sr.pdf [Links].
2. Meng SQ, Cheng JL, Li YY, Yang XQ, Zheng JW, Chang XW, Sh J. Global prevalence of digital addiction in general population: a systematic review and meta-analysis. Clin Psychol Rev. 2022;92:102–28.
3. Boyd D, Ellison N. Social network sites: definition, history, and scholarship. J Comput-Mediat Commun. 2008;13(1)
4. Parameswaran M, Whinston A. Social computing: an overview. Commun Assoc Inf Syst. 2007;19:37.
5. Cía AH. Addictions not related to substances (DSM-5, APA, 2013): a first step towards the inclusion of behavioral addictions in current classifications. Revista de Neuro-Psiquiatria. 2014;76(4):210.
6. Goldberg I. Internet addiction disorder. Diagnostic criteria. Internet Addiction Support Group (IASG). 1995. Available at: http://www.iucf.indiana.edu/~brown/hyplan/addict.html
7. Prieto-Gutierrez JJ, Moreno-Cámara A. Internet social networks, a new addiction? Argentine. J Clin Psychol. 2015;XXIV(II):149–56.
8. Oliveros S. The impact of social networks on our health and mental well-being. Doctor Oliveros SL Group [Internet]. Available in https://www.grupodoctoroliveros.com/el-impacto-de-las-redes-sociales-en-nuestra-salud-y-bienestar-mental
9. StatusOfMind. Social media and young people's mental health and wellbeing, Young Health movement; Royal Society for Public Health (RSPH). London: Royal Society for Public Health; 2017. https://www.observatoriodelainfancia.es/oia/esp/documentos_ficha.aspx?id=5346
10. Moya GH, Garcia KNM, Soto KIP, Arias JAV, Palacios AAY. Network addiction in adolescents: systematic review. Reflect Social Work. 2022;2(3):46–56.
11. Lozano-Blasco R, Robres AQ, Sánchez AS. Internet addiction in young adults: a meta-analysis and systematic review. Comput Hum Behav. 2022;130:107201.
12. Huang C. A meta-analysis of the problematic social media use and mental health. Int J Soc Psychiatry. 2022;68(1):12–33.
13. Huaytalla KPC, Vega SR, Soncco JJ. Risk of addiction to social networks, self-esteem and self-control in high school students. J Health Sci. 2016;9(1):9–15.
14. Monacis L, de Palo V, Griffiths MD, et al. Exploring individual differences in online addictions: the

role of identity and attachment. Int J Ment Health Addiction. 2017;15:853–68. https://doi.org/10.1007/s11469-017-9768-5.
15. Berzonsky MD. Identity style: conceptualization and measurement. J Adolesc Res. 1989;4:267–81. https://doi.org/10.1177/074355488943002.
16. Berzonsky MD. Self-construction over the lifespan: a process perspective on identity formation. In: Neimeyer GJ, Neimeyer RA, editors. Advances in personal construct theory, vol. 1. Greenwich: JHA; 1990. p. 155–86.
17. Yang X, Zhou Z, Liu Q, Fan C. Mobile phone addiction and adolescents' anxiety and depression: the moderating role of mindfulness. In: Key topics in technology and behavior. Cham: Springer Nature; 2022. p. 21–9.
18. Marciano L, Ostroumova M, Schulz PJ, Camerini AL. Digital media use and Adolescents' mental health during the Covid-19 pandemic: a systematic review and meta-analysis. Front Public Health. 2022;9:793868. https://doi.org/10.3389/fpubh.2021.793868.
19. Echeburúa E. Risk factors and protection factors in addiction to new technologies and social networks in young people and adolescents. Spanish Mag Drug Addiction. 2012;37(4):435–47.
20. Echeburúa E, de Corral P. Addiction to new technologies and social networks in young people: a new challenge. Addictions. 2010;22(2):91–5.
21. Echeburua E, de Corral P. Addiction to new technologies and to online social networking in young people: a new challenge. Adicciones. 2010;22:91–5.

34 Educational Procedures for Patients with Alcohol Addiction: Considerations from Medicine and Nursing

Virginia Leonor Herbas Pacheco, Pascual Jiménez Aguilar, Ana María Arias, Ruth Ávila Herbas, Virginia Ramos Chuquimia, Yuliana Flórez, Norman Darío López Velásquez, Augusto Pascual Ítalo Gargiulo, Luis Echarte Alonso, and Pascual Ángel Gargiulo

Introduction

Alcohol is a drug with an extremely negative impact on the well-being of people and society in general. It is a depressant of the central nervous system and has a large number of addicts. This is attributed to the fact that drinks that contain it enjoy great social acceptance and its consumption is deeply rooted culturally. Alcohol also carries multiple symbolic values and is regularly used as false strategies against economic and psychosocial deprivation. Also add the "prestige", "security", or "affection" that its consumption grants according to the social position of the individual. All of these cause the problem to become complicated and cannot be addressed in a reductionist manner with approaches focused solely on the individual.

V. L. Herbas Pacheco (✉) · P. Jiménez Aguilar
A. M. Arias · R. Ávila Herbas · V. Ramos Chuquimia
Carrera de Enfermería. Facultad Ciencias de la Salud, Universidad Técnica de Oruro, Universidad Técnica de Oruro (UTO), Oruro, Bolivia

Y. Flórez
Yuliana Departamento de Ciencias Sociales, Universidad de La Costa, Barranquilla, Colombia
e-mail: yflorez1@cuc.edu.co

N. D. López Velásquez
Escuela de Kinesiología, Facultad de Salud, Universidad Santo Tomás, Temuco, Chile

Centro de Investigación en Gerontología Aplicada (CIGAP), Universidad Santo Tomás, Santiago, Chile
e-mail: normanlopezve@santotomas.cl; nlopez17@cuc.edu.co

A. P. Í. Gargiulo
Laboratorio de Neurociencias y Psicología Experimental, Fundación Corporación Tecnológica Latinoamericana (FUCOTEL), Cátedra de Psicopatología, Facultad de Humanidades y Ciencias Económicas, Universidad Católica Argentina (UCA), Área de Farmacología, Facultad de Ciencias Médicas, Universidad Nacional de Cuyo (UNCuyo), Consejo Nacional de Investigaciones Científicas y Técnicas (CONICET), Mendoza, Argentina

Centro Integral de Salud Mental Argentino (CISMA), Buenos Aires, Argentina

L. Echarte Alonso
Humanities and Medical Ethics Unit, School of Medicine, University of Navarra, Pamplona, Spain
e-mail: lecharte@unav.es

P. Á. Gargiulo
Laboratory of Neurosciences and Experimental Psychology, Latin American Technological Corporation Foundation (FUCOTEL), Cathedra of Psychopathology, Catholic University of Argentina, Area of Pharmacology, Department of Pathology, National University of Cuyo, CONICET, Guaymallén, Mendoza, Argentina

P. Á. Gargiulo, H. L. Mesones-Arroyo (eds.), *Psychiatry and Neuroscience Update – Vol. V*,
https://doi.org/10.1007/978-3-031-72219-6_34

Table 34.1 Alcohol-related deaths. Impact data on alcohol consumption

Risks	%	Causes
Due to injuries	28%	Road accidents. Self-harm and suicide. Interpersonal violence.
Due to diseases	21%	Deaths linked to alcohol due to digestive disorders.
	19%	Due to cardiovascular diseases

Source: Own elaboration, with data from BBC News Mundo and WHO Report, September 2018

Alcoholism is a form of dependence, characterized by an imminent need to consume alcohol for those who make it a habit. It reduces the ability to control one's own life and increases the risk of infections and accidents. All of these cause not only an increase in morbidity, but also mortality (Table 34.1).

Alcoholism is currently called alcohol dependence syndrome. However, although the term syndrome includes a set of signs and symptoms, alcoholism does not always show symptoms. This does not exclude obvious changes in the behaviour of the alcohol consumer.

The data we currently have reveal that of young people between 15 and 19 years old around the world, 27% drink alcohol. The highest consumption rates correspond to Europe (44%) followed by the Americas and the Western Pacific, both with 38% [1].

Conflict Situations

The literature does not allow us to identify defined causes for this major problem, but it is possible to determine several risk factors related to biopsychosocial aspects that we can classify into three broad categories: situations of family, work, and social conflict. And indeed, the social consequences of excessive alcohol consumption can be as harmful as the purely physiological adverse effects. Almost 20% of drinkers report having regular problems with friends, family, work, or the police due to their drinking [2].

Family Conflict

The relationship between individual health and family health is considered to be reciprocal, that is, any individual health problem can create a family health problem and vice versa. Therefore, an unhealthy family lifestyle can make family members sick [3].

Children are one of the main victims of alcoholism, who suffer situations of conflict and hostility. Parental responsibility translates into parental neglect in all areas. Home translates into an adverse space, not a warm shelter. The father stops being a care provider and loses authority, control, patience, and self-control. Communication is also lost, which hinders the adequate physical and psychological growth of children, adolescents, and young people, to the point of helplessness. The consequences of all this are low self-esteem, experiences of abandonment, rejection, and even abuse.

In the long term of this climate of insecurity, children run the risk of following in the same footsteps as their parents and falling into alcoholism. Likewise, couple relationships are bad; the couple can also fall into alcoholism and can be a victim of domestic violence. It translates into the most diverse patterns of abuse: physical, emotional, sexual, and even economic. It has been pointed out that family history linked to education and parental models can aggravate the risk of alcoholism. The age of initiation of alcohol consumption has been proposed as an aggravating indicator factor for the risk of consumption intensity [4].

Labour Conflict

Studies carried out in the general population and in the working population show that work problems (decreased work performance, absenteeism, dismissal, unemployment or unemployment, and work accidents) are frequent among alcohol consumers. In this sense, it seems that work problems are frequent among patients with alcohol dependence and that there is a significant decrease in them with the treatment of dependence. The available evidence suggests that workplace preventive programs to prevent and reduce alcohol-related problems among workers are effective and should be implemented. That is why the company can propose preventive information or screening programs to promote changes in attitudes about consumption, or intervene with assistance programs that facilitate the treatment of workers who have dependency problems and favour their subsequent labour and social reintegration [5].

Alcohol affects work productivity. The lack of job responsibility creates major work imbalances: decreased performance, absenteeism, work accidents, etc. This affects the company's profits: it reduces the employer's income, generates unfavourable working conditions, etc.

Social Conflict

Alcohol consumption brings with it worrying situations in which ethical and legal norms are affected, and ultimately, serious problems of social coexistence, leading to violence and physical or psychological aggression. Road accidents increase, as do violence, street fights, noise, assaults, and robberies to name a few. Alcoholism is universally accepted as one of the main public health problems throughout the world and represents a serious threat to the well-being and life of humanity, endangering both individual and social development [6].

Alcohol can be harmful to virtually all organs and systems in the body. It is psychoactive and can induce alterations in most, if not all, brain systems and structures. Its consumption contributes to more than 60 diseases and disorders, including chronic conditions such as alcohol dependence or liver cirrhosis and other acute health problems such as trauma. Likewise, the authors of this study state that since alcoholism was declared by the WHO as "An incurable, progressive and consequently fatal disease" in the middle of the last century, it has become completely clear that, as such, it can manifest itself on any person, regardless of age, sex, religion, or socioeconomic position. Finally, it will lead to death for those who suffer from it. Before death occurs, the person becomes ill, with a series of deteriorations in all aspects of their life, such as personal, family, and socioeconomic. There are serious effects on the physical and mental aspects. The individual ends up being a "human wreck." It eventually leads to death if the disease is not detected, stopped, and treated appropriately. A very peculiar situation of this disease is that it cannot be stopped if the patient is not completely willing to be helped [7].

Given the aforementioned background, it is a public health imperative to ensure that effective measures are taken to try to reduce alcohol consumption to the lowest possible level (according to the WHO motto "with regard to alcohol, the less, the better") [8].

Public Health and Essential Functions

One of the great fundamental pillars of public health to contribute to the decrease in cases of alcoholism is health promotion and disease prevention. It seems necessary, therefore, to contribute to the efforts carried out by both the PAHO and WHO, through joint work of all organizations and institutions, countries, and health professionals, related to health and not related, considering that this problem manifests itself worldwide. The Pan American Health Organization [PAHO] has accelerated its efforts in recent years to increase awareness of the harm caused by alcohol consumption and support countries' response to reduce its intake [8].

The harm caused by alcohol consumption affects the poor disproportionately, given their poor access to education, information, health services, and other social services [9]. The alcoholic patient is never cured, but his quality of life and health are determined by his ability to abstain, with educational work for patients and families playing a very important role in teaching the harmful effects of alcohol and its effects, consequences to avoid relapses, and direct attention from the family doctor [10].

The "Public Health in the Americas" initiative and its reason for existence establishes 11 essential public health functions. Of these we are particularly interested in the third, which consists of health promotion. This health promotion has been defined in various modalities, which in some way define specific objectives.

A first approach aims to define promotion as the promotion of lifestyles and environmental conditions to promote the development of a culture of health. In a second approach, the strengthening of alliances stands out. These intersectoral alliances aim to make health promotion actions more effective. A third objective is to carry out impact evaluations of public policies on health. Fourth, the relevance of the development of educational and social communication actions is highlighted in order to promote healthy lifestyles, conditions, behaviours, and environments. Fifth, the relevance of the reorientation of health services aimed at developing care models that lead to health promotion and favour health promotion is pointed out. Taken together, these objectives point out possible and concrete actions in the field of prevention [10].

These definitions support the need to promote education, commitment, and encouragement of professionals to health promotion actions and healthy lifestyles. They also help health professionals plan and develop disease prevention actions through education to achieve better lifestyles, behaviours, and healthy environments. Likewise, it allows us to know the effectiveness of the prevention of behavioural problems inherent to risks related to chronic diseases. Health responsibility in public health is effective for biopsychosocial well-being. This is one of its essential functions. The care of chronic diseases within its field of action through the monitoring and promotion of healthy behaviours in the population and the contribution to the development of its health benefits constitutes an essential element [11].

Educational Resources for Patients with Alcohol Addiction

Disease prevention represents a set of measures that avoid, delay, or reduce the effects of a certain disease. Thus, these interventions are carried out primarily (actions that make it possible to prevent the development of a disease) with the secondary ones (early detection of the disease) and the tertiary ones (manifest disease), corresponding to avoiding further damage or serious complications. According to the Specific Public Health Functions (SPHF), Primary Preventive Intervention (PPI) is what occurs before the disease appears and is aimed at protecting vulnerable populations against those factors that can generate the disease [12].

This being so, health educational measures are aimed at carrying out primary prevention interventions. These actions emphasize the promotion of education with a fundamental focus on raising awareness about behaviours that maintain their health in optimal conditions, not only physical health, but also mental and nutritional health, in addition to the care of their organs and their functions.

Health Education as a Strategy to Prevent Alcoholism

Health education is defined as the discipline responsible for guiding and organizing educational processes with the purpose of positively influencing the knowledge, practices, and customs of individuals and communities in relation to their health [13].

To avoid the early onset of alcohol consumption, it is important to identify and provide information to the vulnerable population, habitual or regular in alcohol consumption.

What to do to understand the problem of alcoholism? That the individual knows the problem based on elements that accompany educational actions such as:

- Definition of alcoholism, alcohol addiction.
- Family history of alcohol consumption.
- Reasons or factors that could induce alcohol consumption.
- Symptoms, such as reservation or refusal to accept consistent alcohol consumption.
- Signs: physical effects of alcohol on health.
- Social impact.

Therefore, education in the field of health, aimed at the population with some type of risk, aims to positively and advantageously influence the knowledge, practices, and customs of the individual, family, and an entire community, as an active response to disease prevention and health promotion. This training also seeks to promote self-care dynamics, so that the individual achieves autonomy, capacity for responsibility, and management of conflicts regarding their own health. Appropriate educational strategies can ensure that the patient discards the idea that health personnel are solely responsible for the maintenance and care of each individual's health. Education against alcoholism is probably one of the least applied population actions.

Role of Health Professionals in Educating Alcohol Consumers

The Nursing professional is the key person in the prevention of consumption and the promotion of healthy lifestyles, given that their main function is to care for the health of individuals. Being present at all three levels of care, it plays a fundamental role in people's health throughout their lives [14].

It is evident that the doctor and nurses are in constant interaction with the individual, family, and community, which makes it possible for them to play an important role in positively influencing changes in favourable lifestyles, both in the patient and in their environment, family and social.

According to Amezcua et al. [13], to educate consumers about their health habits, it is necessary to identify key influencers. Health professionals, especially doctors, nurses, and community pharmacists, are the health educators par excellence. Closeness, trust, and accessibility support such a condition [15].

Proposal for Multidisciplinary Action from the Health Professional

For all that has been said, we propose:

- *Work coordination*: Coordinated work between institutions (schools, universities), health professionals, educators, community, and individuals.
- *Recruitment of risk groups*: Detect risk groups for alcohol addiction and recruit them to carry out educational work among them.
- *Early diagnosis*: Identify and perform early diagnosis and timely care.
- *Information*: Develop information plans. Basic information about alcoholism should be exchanged with the general population.
- *Self-esteem*: Provide motivational educational talks to raise the personal self-esteem of potential patients.
- *Sports*: Promote sports activities.
- *Healthy environments and values*: Create healthy environments that favour the formation of values.
- *Family promotion*: Promote rapprochement and understanding between parents and children. Raise parents' awareness about the need to establish communication, control measures, surveillance, and care for adolescents and young people and other family components.
- *Health programs*: Develop health education programs, focused on the prevention of alcohol consumption. Guide towards self-care and autonomy with responsibility towards your health.

Evaluation of Previous Proposals

Alcohol consumption varies widely in the general population of the Americas, with prevalence varying from 9.5% in El Salvador to 52% in Argentina and Uruguay. We also found consumption rates of more than 50% in both North and South America [15]. This indicates the convenience of a strategy of prioritizing preventive measures on our continent.

Given the fact that alcohol health education is a relevant strategy for preventing addictions, it is important to consider how it is carried out. It is recommended that when applied in regions, adaptation to local values, beliefs, and practices should be sought. It is recommended to implement public health promotion policies that are properly focused on local communities. Strategies linked to the arts have been recommended in order to achieve greater adherence and effectiveness [16].

In a review dedicated to the identification, efficiency study, and economic evaluations of prevention, treatment, and rehabilitation programs aimed at people with alcohol use disorders, it was observed that brief interventions are effective. Random blood alcohol measurement is surpassed in efficiency by other alternatives. Tax increases, advertising control, legal drinking age, and mass media campaigns are considered good strategies [17].

In a study conducted to evaluate prevention and treatment of harmful alcohol use, motivational interviewing and cognitive behavioural therapy were found to have a small effect. On the contrary, mentoring demonstrated a significant effect. This effect was lasting in the long term. In treatment, it was observed that the best results are obtained by combining pharmacological and psychosocial interventions [18].

A meta-analysis compared the effectiveness of in-person interventions carried out by professionals to those carried out digitally. The goal in both cases was the reduction of harmful alcohol consumption. Differences were found. Face-to-face interviews surpassed digital ones at 1 month and at 6 months, while both were equal at 12 months [19].

Conclusion

We may conclude that various forms of intervention are appropriate for the purpose of health education, particularly in the field of harmful alcohol consumption. In-person action shows differences in the short term with digital interventions, and mentoring has a good response in the long term. Early interventions are therefore recommended to achieve a good result in the field of health promotion education.

References

1. Redacción BBC News Mundo. 6 shocking facts about alcohol consumption in the world (including which Latin American countries consume the most). [6 datos impactantes sobre el consumo de alcohol en el mundo (incluido en qué países de América Latina se consume más)]. Septiembre 2018. https://www.bbc.com/mundo/noticias-45626675
2. Martínez González MA, Guillén Grima F, Robledo de Dios T. Alcohol and public health. [Alcohol y Salud Pública]. In: Martínez González MA, Sánchez Villegas A, editors. Life styles and public health. [Estilos de vida y salud pública]. Universidad de la Rioja; 2004. p. 225–243.
3. Martínez-Montilla JM, et al. Family coping strategies and repercussions on family health: a review of the literature. [Estrategias de afrontamiento familiar y repercusiones en la salud familiar: Una revisión de la literatura]. Enfermería Global. 2017;16(3):576–604. https://doi.org/10.6018/eglobal.16.3.255721.
4. Santo-Domingo J. The personal development of young people and alcohol. [El desarrollo personal del joven y el alcohol]. Trastornos Adictivos. 2002;4(4):223–32.
5. Gómez-Talegón MT, Álvarez González FJ. Work–related problems among alcohol-dependent patients: development a year of alcohol treatment. [Problemas laborales en pacientes dependientes del alcohol: Evolución en un año de tratamiento]. Med Segur Trab. 2009;55(216):20–5.
6. Tristán C, Llorens N, Brime B, León L, López M, García N, Molina M. Monografía alcohol 2021. Consumo y consecuencias. [Alcohol monograph 2021. Consumption and consequences]. Observatorio Español de las Drogas y las Adicciones (OEDA). Ministerio de Sanidad. Delegación del Gobierno para el Plan Nacional sobre Drogas (DGPNSD). [Spanish Observatory of Drugs and Addictions. Ministry of Health. Government Delegation for the National Drug Plan]. Madrid; 2021. p. 109.
7. Barrero Aguilar ME, Pérez Almeida MA. Evaluation of the risk of alcoholism in students of Vicente Quesada urban secondary school. Bayamo. [Evaluación del riesgo de alcoholismo en estudiantes de la secundaria básica Vicente Quesada. Bayamo]. Multimed Revista Médica Granma. 2018;22(4):761–76.
8. Pan American Health Organization. World Health Organization 51st Directing Council. 63rd Session of the regional committee. [Organización Panamericana de la Salud. Organización mundial de la salud 51° Consejo Directivo. 63ª Sesión del comité regional]. Washington, D.C. 2011. https://www.paho.org/es/temas/alcohol
9. Bolet Astoviza M, Socarras Suárez MM. Alcoholism, consequences and prevention. [El alcoholismo, consecuencias y prevención]. *Rev Cubana Invest Bioméd.* 2003; 22: n.1. http://scielo.sld.cu/scielo.php?script=sci_arttext&pid=S0864-03002003000100004&lng=es&nrm=iso
10. Public Health in the Americas. New Concepts, Performance Analysis and Basis for Action. [Organización Panamericana de la Salud (OPS). La Salud Pública en las Américas. Nuevos Conceptos, Análisis del Desempeño y Bases para la Acción].

Washington, D.C. OPS. Publicación Científica y Técnica No. 589. ISBN: 9275 31 589 2. 2002. https://www.binasss.sa.cr/opac-ms/media/digitales/La%20salud%20p%C3%BAblica%20en%20las%20Am%C3%A9ricas.%20Nuevos%20conceptos,%20an%C3%A1lisis%20del%20desempe%C3%B1o%20y%20bases%20para%20la%20acci%C3%B3n.pdf

11. Hernández-Sarmiento JM, Jaramillo-Jaramillo LI, Villegas-Alzate JD, Álvarez-Hernández LF, Roldan-Tabares MD, Ruiz-Mejía C, Calle-Estrada MC, Ospina-Jiménez MC, Martínez-Sánchez LM. Health education as an important promotion and prevention strategy. [La educación en salud como una importante estrategia de promoción y prevención]. Archivos de Medicina (Col). 2020;20(2):490–508. Universidad de Manizales, Colombia. https://www.redalyc.org/articulo.oa?id=273863770021
12. Ahumada-Cortez JG, Gámez-Medina ME, Valdez-Montero C. Alcohol consumption as a public health problema. [El consumo de alcohol como problema de salud pública]. Ra Ximhai. 2017;13(2):13–24. Universidad Autónoma Indígena de México El Fuerte, México
13. Amezcua M, García Pedregal E, Jordana J, Llisterri JL, Rodríguez Sampedro A, Villarino A. Education facing risk consumption of alcoholic beverages-A proposal for multidisciplinary action from the health care professionals. [La educación ante el consumo de riesgo de bebidas alcohólicas: propuesta de actuación multidisciplinar desde el profesional de la salud]. Nutr Hosp. 2020;37(3):609–15. https://doi.org/10.20960/nh.02930.
14. Herrera Molina AS, Machado Herrera PM, Tierra VR, Coro Tierra EM, Remache Ati KA. The nursing professional in health promotion at the second level of care. [El profesional de enfermería en la promoción de salud en el segundo nivel de atención]. Revista Eugenio Espejo. 2022;16(1):98–111. Universidad Nacional de Chimborazo
15. Organization of American States (OAS). Washington DC. 2019. Inter-American Commission for the Control of Drug Abuse (CICAD). Organization of American States (OAS). Report on Drug Use in the Americas 2019. [Organización de los Estados Americanos (OEA). Washington DC. 2019. Comisión Interamericana para el Control del Abuso de Drogas (CICAD). Organización de los Estados Americanos (OEA). Informe sobre el Consumo de Drogas en las Américas 2019]. Washington, D.C. 2019.
16. Araujo da Rocha R, Santana MAO. The use of health education strategies and art in rural health prevention focusing on alcohol abuse/addiction and other drugs. Rural Remote Health. 2023;23(1):8116. https://doi.org/10.22605/RRH8116.
17. Trapero-Bertran M, Gil-Doménech D, Vargas-Martínez AM. Economic evaluations of interventions aimed at the prevention, treatment and/or rehabilitation of alcohol-related disorders: a systematic review. Adicciones. 2023;35(3):325–48. https://doi.org/10.20882/adicciones.1649.
18. Botwright S, Sutawong J, Kingkaew P, Anothaisintawee T, Dabak SV, Suwanpanich C, Promchit N, Kampang R, Isaranuwatchai W. Which interventions for alcohol use should be included in a universal healthcare benefit package? An umbrella review of targeted interventions to address harmful drinking and dependence. BMC Public Health. 2023;23(1):382. https://doi.org/10.1186/s12889-023-15152-6.
19. Beyer FR, Kenny RPW, Johnson E, Caldwell DM, Garnett C, Rice S, Simpson J, Angus C, Craig D, Hickman M, Michie S, Kaner EFS. Practitioner and digitally delivered interventions for reducing hazardous and harmful alcohol consumption in people not seeking alcohol treatment: a systematic review and network meta-analysis. Addiction. 2023;118(1):17–29. https://doi.org/10.1111/add.15999.

Fetal Alcohol Spectrum Disorders

35

Virginia Leonor Herbas Pacheco, Pascual Jiménez Aguilar, Ana María Arias, Ruth Ávila Herbas, Virginia Ramos Chuquimia, Nicole Caldichoury, Juan Carlos Coronado, Marcos Constantino Josué Gargiulo, Mercedes María Lucrecia Gargiulo, Augusto Pascual Ítalo Gargiulo, Ángel José Martín Gargiulo, Ana Paula Colombini, Esteban Alejandro Romanowicz, Iker Barrutieta Arberas, Manuel Alejandro Guevara, Adriana Inés Landa de Gargiulo, Luis Echarte Alonso, José Vicente Lafuente, and Pascual Ángel Gargiulo

V. L. Herbas Pacheco · P. Jiménez Aguilar · A. M. Arias · R. Ávila Herbas · V. Ramos Chuquimia
Carrera de Enfermería. Facultad Ciencias de la Salud, Universidad Técnica de Oruro (UTO), Oruro, Bolivia

N. Caldichoury
Departamento de Ciencias Sociales, Universidad de Los Lagos, Los Lagos, Chile
e-mail: andrea.caldichoury@ulagos.cl

J. C. Coronado
Facultad de Ciencias de la Salud, Universidad Católica de Temuco, Araucanía, Chile
e-mail: jcoronado@uct.cl

M. C. J. Gargiulo · M. M. L. Gargiulo · A. P. Í. Gargiulo · Á. J. M. Gargiulo · A. P. Colombini
Laboratorio de Neurociencias y Psicología Experimental. Fundación Corporación Tecnológica Latinoamericana (FUCOTEL). Cátedra de Psicopatología. Facultad de Humanidades y Ciencias Económicas. Universidad Católica Argentina (UCA). Área de Farmacología. Facultad de Ciencias Médicas, Universidad Nacional de Cuyo (UNCuyo). Consejo Nacional de Investigaciones Científicas y Técnicas (CONICET), Mendoza, Argentina

Centro Integral de Salud Mental Argentino (CISMA), Buenos Aires, Argentina

E. A. Romanowicz · M. A. Guevara · A. I. Landa de Gargiulo
Laboratorio de Neurociencias y Psicología Experimental. Fundación Corporación Tecnológica Latinoamericana (FUCOTEL). Cátedra de Psicopatología. Facultad de Humanidades y Ciencias Económicas. Universidad Católica Argentina (UCA). Área de Farmacología. Facultad de Ciencias Médicas, Universidad Nacional de Cuyo (UNCuyo). Consejo Nacional de Investigaciones Científicas y Técnicas (CONICET), Mendoza, Argentina

P. Á. Gargiulo (✉)
Laboratory of Neurosciences and Experimental Psychology, Latin American Technological Corporation Foundation (FUCOTEL), Cathedra of Psychopathology, Catholic University of Argentina, Area of Pharmacology, Department of Pathology, National University of Cuyo, CONICET, Guaymallén, Mendoza, Argentina

I. Barrutieta Arberas · J. V. Lafuente
LaNCE-Neuropharm Research Group, Facultad de Medicina y Enfermería, Department of Neurosciences, University of the Basque Country (UPV-EHU), Leioa, Spain
e-mail: onplasav@lg.ehu.es; josevicente.lafuente@ehu.eus

L. Echarte Alonso
Humanities and Medical Ethics Unit, School of Medicine, University of Navarra, Pamplona, Spain
e-mail: lecharte@unav.es

P. Á. Gargiulo, H. L. Mesones-Arroyo (eds.), *Psychiatry and Neuroscience Update – Vol. V*,
https://doi.org/10.1007/978-3-031-72219-6_35

Introduction

Generally speaking, people drink to socialize, celebrate, and relax, despite the negative health effects of alcohol consumption. It has been pointed out that three periods of dynamic brain changes are particularly sensitive to the harmful effects of alcohol. They are: gestation (from conception to birth), late adolescence (15–19 years), and older adulthood (over 65 years) [1]. Unfortunately, alcohol consumption is common in many women during pregnancy. Studies by different authors reveal the significance of alcohol consumption in women of childbearing age and its repercussions on their pregnancies. We will show below some of the most important ones.

The term Foetal Alcohol Spectrum Syndrome refers to a large set of clinical features present in the foetus that are produced by the mother's alcohol consumption during pregnancy. This foetal alcohol spectrum disorder (FASD) is defined by its history and morphological manifestations. Among the antecedents, maternal alcohol consumption during pregnancy stands out. The physical attributes of the new-born are associated with this [2]. Foetal alcohol spectrum disorder (FASD) is suspected in new-borns based on a maternal history of alcohol consumption during pregnancy and the physical attributes present in the child at birth [3].

These foetal alcohol spectrum disorders (FASD) also present physical, mental, and behavioural disabilities caused by the harmful effect of alcohol during pregnancy or prenatal alcohol exposure (PAE). FASD is considered one of the leading preventable causes of developmental delay with an estimated 119,000 children born with this foetal alcohol syndrome (FAS) each year worldwide. Despite its prevalence, FASD is often misdiagnosed or underdiagnosed, making intervention difficult. This topic constitutes an area of relevance for doctors, nurses, psychologists, and other health professionals [2].

Various factors can converge in these disorders. This is the case of smoking, other drugs, and genetic and nutritional factors, both of the mother and of the child [4]. Given the known adverse effects of alcohol exposure in prenatal stages, and that these constitute a continuum of disabilities known as FASD, interest in specific diagnostic criteria has been of great interest. This has been the subject of numerous studies to establish reliable diagnoses [5–7].

There are rigorous literature search studies showing frequency and pointing to the need for more demanding prevention strategies against the problem of alcohol consumption during pregnancy and the detection of its consequences. Some of these studies included random effects meta-analyses for each country [6, 7]. A study realized in 76 countries considered a prevalence around >1%. This proportion would be higher in people excluded from home or included in mental health and justice systems [6]. From these studies, a global prevalence of prenatal alcohol consumption was estimated at 9.8%. A prevalence of FAS in the general population was also estimated at 14.6 per 10,000 people. It is estimated that one in every 67 women with prenatal alcohol consumption would conceive a child with FAS. In a global estimate, it has been argued that 119,000 children would be born with FAS in the world per year [6]. In the United States, FAS is more common than other congenital syndromes, such as spina bifida and Down syndrome [8]. Foetal alcohol spectrum disorder (FASD) is considered to be a very common cause of disability, with a prevalence of 1–6% of all births in the world. It highlights the fact that sensory processing deficits and consequent cognitive problems have been considered as an important characteristic of this condition [9].

Foetal alcohol disorder presents prenatal and/or postnatal growth retardation, facial dysmorphology, dysfunctional disorders of the central nervous system, and behavioural disabilities of neurological origin. The term "spectrum" is used when it refers to cases of people affected by maternal prenatal alcohol consumption, but who do not present all of the aforementioned criteria [10].

It has been proposed that the length of the right palpebral fissure, midfacial length, and width of the nose, together with machine learning methods, would be an efficient method for acceptable detection of patients with APS. This would allow objective and reliable detection of these patients [11]. In a first and recent systematic review, the variety and frequency of ocular anomalies reported in prenatal alcohol exposure (PAE) and Foetal alcohol Syndrome Disorder (FASD) were reported. These abnormalities include, among others, optic nerve hypoplasia with small optic discs and retinal tortuosity [12].

Objectives and Method

The aim of the present chapter is reviewing consequences on neurocognitive and behavioural profiles of foetal alcohol exposition. These consequences are defined today as foetal alcohol spectrum disorders. Here we analyse neuropsychological disorders of FASD, FASD and autism, alcohol as a teratogen, cause of FAS, animal models of FAS, potential complementary diagnostic methods, preventive care procedures, and suggested therapeutic approaches. The method used was a bibliographic research of last years and classical publications, consulting mainly PubMed and Scielo papers.

Neurocognitive and Behavioural Profile of Foetal Alcohol Spectrum Disorder

Current studies indicate that neurocognitive disorders are increasing in developed countries, citing different industrial toxins capable of causing brain damage. However, they also point out that, despite the aforementioned toxins, alcohol is one of the most teratogenic substances known and the main identifiable and preventable cause of congenital malformations and cognitive deficits. It additionally may cause collateral damage related to alcohol-dependent conditions. The mother and her social situation here are very important, such as, for example, the abandonment of children who suffer from this disorder.

Prenatal alcohol exposure is the leading preventable cause of cognitive deficits in developed countries and can lead to foetal alcohol spectrum disorder (FASD). This term encompasses a wide variety of physical, mental, behavioural, and cognitive effects that derive from the damage caused by exposure to alcohol during intrauterine life. The consumption of this substance among the general population is frequent in Eastern European countries and especially among women at risk of social exclusion, who are the most affected in processes of losing or renouncing custody of their children. This is the case of a high number of these children who are adopted in Spain. Many of them present neurocognitive and behavioural alterations, making FASD a public health problem. In many cases, this clinical condition is underdiagnosed due to the overlap of neuropsychological symptoms caused by abandonment and lack of attachment. To date, a specific neurocognitive and behavioural profile of FASD has not been described and many of the symptoms are common to other aetiologies [13].

Likewise, it highlights the fact that in the pathophysiology of damage caused by prenatal exposure to alcohol, the brain is the main target due to its greater metabolic demand and production of ROS (Acetaldehyde and reactive oxygen species). Likewise, the fact that ethanol crosses the placenta stands out. Additionally, although its levels in amniotic fluid are 40% of those in maternal blood, its slow clearance means prolonged foetal exposure. Apart from being teratogenic, alcohol decreases placental flow causing ischemia, infarctions, and thinning of the placenta. This enables intrauterine growth retardation and other anomalies [13]. Consequently, there is no safe consumption threshold during pregnancy, although the impact basically depends on the dose, time, consumption pattern, and individual genetic susceptibility. Alcohol can have deleterious effects at any time during pregnancy and all are avoided with abstinence. Stopping intake at any time improves the prognosis. This often occurs in the critical period of organogenesis, when pregnancy is unknown. The amount of alcohol that reaches the foetus varies depending on the time and intensity of consumption and maternal and foetal genetics [2, 13].

Neuropsychological Disorders of FASD

There is a set of functional, behavioural, or neuropsychological elements present in FASD. These have been described as linked to cognitive development, executive functions, motor functions, inattention and hyperactivity disorders, social skills, and other manifestations of the condition [13, 14].

In cognitive development, the presence of specific learning difficulties (mathematics, visual-spatial capacity deficits, etc.) has been described. Another characteristic feature is an uneven profile of cognitive abilities. Likewise, there is usually lower than expected academic performance. A discrepancy between verbal and non-verbal skills has been described. There are difficulties in processing information and it usually coexists with borderline intellectual functioning [13].

Executive functions may be altered. Difficulties are usually observed in the ability to organize and/or plan. They may coexist with difficulties in concrete thinking. As in all disorders of executive functions, there may be difficulties in behavioural inhibition and following instructions. There are often difficulties in understanding cause-effect logic and developing strategies. Judgment ability may be very poor. There are usually difficulties in generalizing and understanding abstract concepts [13]. Motor functions present disorders. There is delay in the development of motor skills. There are usually difficulties with fine motor skills, manifested in writing and/or drawing. There is a general lack of dexterity in motor skills. They may coexist with balance difficulties and tremors. In this disorder, there may also be attention deficit hyperactivity disorder. This will be characterized by inattention and an exaggerated degree of distractibility. There may be difficulty in driving calmly. There are usually difficulties with changes and completing tasks [13].

For all of the above, an evident decrease in social skills is common. They tend to behave recklessly and naively, thus being easily manipulated. All of this results in difficulties in social interactions, difficulties in social understanding, with immaturity and, consequently, with preferences in treatment for people of younger age. There may be difficulties understanding facial expressions. All of this leads to difficulties in developing skills relevant to daily life. There may be inappropriate sexual behaviour. Other elements may appear coexisting with the previous ones. There may be hypersensitivity or hyposensitivity, both to noise and pain. They may present memory deficits, often consecutive to attention disorders. They tend to respond poorly to behavioural strategies, such as punishment and positive reinforcement [13].

FASD and Autism

Foetal alcohol spectrum disorders (FASD) are a group of conditions associated with the effects of prenatal alcohol exposure and characterized by somatic and neuropsychological alterations. On the other hand, autism spectrum disorder (ASD) is characterized by a multifaceted neurobehavioural syndrome. Since alcohol can affect all stages of brain development, some authors hypothesized that alcohol exposure in utero could be related to an increased risk of ASD in genetically vulnerable subjects [15].

It is considered that ASD (Autism Spectrum Disorders) is caused by a functional alteration of the cerebral cortex, which leads to structural abnormalities in the brain. The role of immunological mechanisms linked to prenatal alcohol exposure has been proposed [16]. Possible relationships between FAS and autism spectrum disorder have been raised. The results are controversial. These two disorders are underdiagnosed or cause misdiagnoses. This suggests the need to continue these correlation studies by expanding the number and perspectives, that is, considering subsyndromal features and milder forms [17].

Alcohol as a Teratogen

The literature indicates that alcohol consumption during the perinatal stage is considered adverse, due to the risks it silently brings with it. For this reason, this substance is considered another drug, with depressant characteristics of the central nervous system. The ingestion of this toxin presumes teratogenicity because it passes the transplacental barrier.

Alcohol is a well-established teratogen that can cause variable physical and behavioural effects on the foetus. Likewise, it has been mentioned that differences in maternal and foetal enzymes, in terms of abundance and effectiveness, as well as reduced elimination, allow alcohol to have a prolonged effect on the foetus. This may act as a teratogen through numerous pathways, including reactive oxygen species, reduced levels of endogenous antioxidants, and inhibition of cofactors. Other risk factors have been mentioned. They include genetic factors, lower socioeconomic levels, and smoking [18].

Alcohol is the most important teratogen that causes APS, and there is no safe trimester for drinking alcohol or known safe amount of alcohol consumption during pregnancy. Therefore, clinicians should carefully evaluate women's alcohol consumption patterns and provide FAS education to women by understanding its pathophysiology. Likewise, they report that foetal alcohol syndrome (FAS) is a congenital and developmental disorder characterized by neurocognitive impairment, structural defects, and growth restriction due to prenatal exposure to alcohol [19].

The physical clinical characteristics of FAS include facial abnormalities, short stature, low body weight, and evidence of structural and/or functional damage to the central nervous system (CNS) [8, 20]. The prevalence of APS carriers worldwide is about 15 per 10,000 live births (around 119,000 children with APS born per year). Epidemiological data in the US show that the incidence of FAS exceeds other congenital syndromes such as Down syndrome and spina bifida [8]. The global prevalence of FAS is estimated in 2–5% in Europe and North America. It denotes the relevance of an early diagnosis and treatment [20].

The harmful effects of ethanol appear in different regions of the brain. These vary depending on the dose and the period of neural development when the embryo was exposed [8]. These harmful effects include:

1. Microcephaly.
2. Anomalies in cortical development, with a significant decrease in gyrification.
3. Agenesis or hypoplasia of the corpus callosum.
4. Cognitive and behavioural deficits (such as memory and learning impairment, speech difficulties, and hyperactivity).

There are countries, such as Korea, in which alcohol consumption during pregnancy has increased, particularly in childbearing age [19]. This consumption would reach 9.8% of pregnant women worldwide. It is estimated that the prevalence of alcohol foetal exposition in the general population would be 14.6 per 10,000 people. In Korea, women of childbearing age have increased alcohol consumption. During pregnancy, this reaches 16%. This has caused the prevalence of alcohol foetal exposition to range between 18 and 51 per 10,000 women. These numbers far exceed the global prevalence. As a consequence, this places a burden on society and increases medical expenses.

Foetal alcohol syndrome is considered to belong to a spectrum of disorders grouped under the general term foetal alcohol spectrum disorder (FASD). There is a total of five disorders that comprise foetal alcohol spectrum disorders [21].

1. Foetal alcohol syndrome (FAS).
2. Partial foetal alcohol syndrome (pFAS).
3. Alcohol-related neurodevelopmental disorder (ARND).
4. Neurobehavioural disorder associated with prenatal alcohol exposure (ND-PAE).
5. Alcohol-related birth defects (ARBD).

All of these FASDs are used to classify the broad physical and neurological effects that prenatal alcohol exposure can cause on the foetus.

The severity of the affectation depends on the interrelation of 5 factors: dose, consumption pattern, gestation phase, maternal nutrition, and genetics. They also point out that the therapeutic work of early care programs and psycho-pedagogical support at school age is often discouraging and must be accompanied by intense social work. In conclusion, the role of prevention is fundamental, but advice to pregnant women, motivational interviews, posters, etc. do not seem effective if transversal campaigns are not also undertaken with measures to control the accessibility of such a ubiquitous drug, which generates such a level of business profits and which is so socially rooted [22].

Causes of Foetal Alcohol Syndrome

The difference between the quantity and efficiency of maternal and foetal enzymes prolongs the duration of the presence of alcohol in the foetus. Alcohol acts as a teratogen through numerous described processes. These include, among others, reactive oxygen species and a decrease in the levels of endogenous antioxidants. Mitochondrial damage and lipid peroxidation have also been involved. This has led to the postulation of antioxidant agents. Prenatal administration of dietary supplements with antioxidants, folic acid, choline, neuroactive peptides, and neurotrophic growth factors has been mentioned [18]. Alcohol exposure also affects the foetal Blood Brain Barrier (BBB) [8].

The effects of maternal stress and associated mood dysregulation and its relationship with alcohol exposure during foetal development have been studied both clinically and in animal experiments. In this context, the role of the placenta has also been highlighted [23].

Various genetic studies suggest that different genetic factors, verifiable in both the mother and the foetus, influence the configuration of the final phenotype of these children. It is expected that these studies will provide additional data on the physiopathogenesis of alcohol teratogenicity and its intervention in the level of risk of negative effects of this order. This would allow for earlier detection of risks and could lead to earlier interventions [24].

Animal Models of FASD

Animal models have been used to make translational approaches to FASD. The intention has been to demonstrate the teratogenic effects of alcohol, its specificity, and what underlying changes alcohol induces in the central nervous system (CNS). More recently, efforts have been made to act therapeutically on the effects of alcohol. Particular attention has been paid to the impact of behaviour and social context on the effects of alcohol exposure during development. In this sense, animal models have been considered as useful instruments or approaches to study how the social context impacts the effect of alcohol throughout development [25].

Given the ethical and practical difficulties in studying the causes of birth defects in human beings, the contribution of animal models is very important. In this sense, animal models provide a large amount of resources. This makes it possible to identify causes of birth defects. This is particularly important in prenatal alcohol exposure, both to study interactions between genes and alcohol and the genetics of disorders linked to interaction with the environment [26].

This has led to the study of both the effects of maternal stress and the mood dysregulation, thus induced through stress and its relationship with alcohol exposure. These studies have been carried out both clinically and translationally. This has also led to studies of the effects of these variables on the placenta [23].

Behavioural touch screen tasks have been experimentally used in animals in order to observe the integration of dural recordings of electroencephalographic (EEG) activity in awake rodents. Translational generalization models are thus attempted. With this experimental scheme, it has been noted that with 5-choice continuous performance tasks [touchscreen 5-Choice Continuous Performance Task, 5C-CPT], cognitive control is affected. In this test, there are options with objectives to perceive and stimuli to reject. In an extension of this study, simultaneous EEG dural recordings were performed in the medial prefrontal cortex (mPFC) and posterior parietal cortex (PPC). More false alarm responses were observed in animals exposed to prenatal alcohol than controls, with a significant decrease in sensitivity index [27]. The translational use of these models would be a matter of interest aiming to relate cognitive parameters to brain electrical activity.

Complementary Diagnostic Methods

It has been postulated that screening may facilitate the early identification of foetal alcohol spectrum disorder (FASD) and the estimation of the prevalence of FASD for timely planning of prevention, diagnosis, and management. However, little is known about FASD screening tools [28]. Some research lines are today in development.

It has been sought to relate brain activity to the effect of alcohol on the developing brain. This would allow establishing relationships between brain dysfunctions and behavioural or functional disorders present in foetal alcohol syndrome. Initially, the brains of patients have been studied comparing them to normal individuals using Magnetic Resonance Imaging (MRI), Electroencephalography (EEG), Positron Emission Tomography (PET), and Single Photon Emission Computed Tomography (SPECT). Although these studies have provided some evidence, the set of findings is still very preliminary and not very systematized. There would be, in principle, some findings compatible with processing deficits [29].

Abnormalities of the corpus callosum and decreased size of basal ganglia and thalamic structures have been reported on MRI [14]. The cerebellum has been recently implicated also in this pathology [30]. In a broad review that involved various species, the presence of cerebellar dysfunctions was observed in several neurophysiological deficits associated with these symptoms of prenatal alcoholic damage. This highlights the importance of considering and weighing the structure and function of the cerebellum in this disorder and of considering these findings in its diagnosis. Additionally, this may lead to new therapeutic strategies to mitigate cerebellar damage resulting from alcohol exposure during pregnancy [30].

Recently, some findings have been reported with the use of analysis of specific frequency bands in computerized EEG. Thus, there would be a frontotemporal alpha predominance compared to controls in children with FAS. An increased theta/beta ratio was also observed in patients with FAS [31]. While these are preliminary findings, they are promising research lines.

As previously stated, there are preclinical translational models in rodents that tend to establish electroencephalographic and cognitive correlations in these disorders [27]. The continuation of these lines in humans could provide new evidence regarding cognitive disorders in FAS.

Preventive Care Procedures

Given that alcohol-induced disorders are stable and only partially modifiable with stimulation, the role of prevention is essential here. A series of desirable objectives have been proposed in the prevention and treatment of FASD. They would improve the quality of life of these people and prevent its presentation in future generations. In this sense, it has been suggested to provide them with equitable access to health systems and promote knowledge of the disorder to prevent its presentation in future generations [7].

Most intellectual disorders are diagnosed during or after school. It is vitally important to know the diagnostic criteria of both entities, identify the key clinical data that allow patients to be referred to the appropriate specialists, and perform an efficient evaluation.

The consequences related to the use of alcohol during pregnancy have no remission. This fact is valid for both physical and behavioural disorders. This is a valid reason to properly treat these conditions emphasizing prevention.

In order to carry out these purposes, the following is suggested:

- Early identification and treatment. It may contribute to mitigate secondary neurodevelopmental symptoms.
- Specialized maternal medical and health teams and specialized child care units. They may be preferentially in a strategic area of the institutions. It may allow to effective care and services.
- Attracting the attention and consults of mothers at risk. It may be also important to offer them prenatal care services.
- Facilitate extensive information about the problems and consequences of alcohol toxicity during pregnancy. Giving information about foetal alcohol spectrum disorders is here very important.
- Monitoring of children during the first 5 years of life evaluating their growth and development.
- The formation of a multidisciplinary team with family, social, and legal projection is strategic.
- Development of educational programs focusing on children with FASD and related disorders must be also considered.
- Early detection of suspected cases, including experts in foetal alcohol syndrome for evaluation and treatment, is also very relevant.

With the fulfilment of these objectives, a significant decrease in the presentation of this disorder can be expected.

Therapeutic Approaches

It has been suggested that early intervention services can reduce some of the secondary disabilities and mental and neurological problems. These may include: a special education trainer, a speech therapist, an occupational therapist, a physical therapist, and a psychologist [3]. The aim should be to support motor skills, social skills, and any other area that has a delay in development (Table 35.1).

Table 35.1 Intervention services

Services	Interventions
A special education trainer	Supports with social skills, walking, and other delays the child may be showing
A speech therapist	Supports with speaking skills
A physical and occupational therapist and a psychologist	Supports with learning and behaviour problems.

Source: Own elaboration with data from Patel et al. [3]

As it may be seen, multidisciplinary approach is suggested for its treatment. This scheme includes the treatment of comorbid conditions, such as nutrition, school, and psychological help for children with this problem, and education for parents. In this last point, total abstinence from alcohol should be advised, given the difficulty in verifying the amount of intake [10].

For the treatment of this condition, the use of anti-inflammatories and nutraceuticals in its acute aspect has been recently proposed [32]. The use of antioxidant agents was previously mentioned. It has led to prenatal administration of dietary supplements such as antioxidants, folic acid, choline, and other compounds [18].

However, when the lesions are installed, an effective treatment for alcohol sequelae is not present and, since there is here a brain damage, it cannot be expected that a specific pharmacological treatment will appear. Symptomatic treatments would be useful aiming to manage symptoms and comorbidities, but not as aetiological solutions.

Based on the fact that children with foetal alcohol spectrum disorder (FASD) present auditory, motor, and executive deficits, music training has been proposed for them as a way to compensate for their deficiencies. This therapy seems to act on these domains, modifying them positively. To this end, short-term music training was performed in children with FASD due to prenatal alcohol exposure. It was proposed that this could improve brain function. Results compatible with an improvement in attention were reported in these children [33].

Conclusion

Social awareness of foetal alcohol spectrum syndrome is important, as is the formation of consumption habits that exclude alcoholic beverages. In this task of raising awareness, health personnel with their entire multidisciplinary team is crucial, and also in establishing early diagnoses. Recognition of the mildest signs is extremely important to stop behaviours that, in the end, will be harmful. In this article, we have suggested a series of comprehensive interventions in women that complement alcohol awareness and avoidance strategies.

References

1. Pop-Jordanova N, Demerdzieva A. How alcohol damages brain development in children. Pril (Makedon Akad Nauk Umet Odd Med Nauki). 2022;43(3):29–42. https://doi.org/10.2478/prilozi-2022-0034.
2. Pan American Health Organization (PAHO). Washington DC. 2020. ISBN: 978-92-75-12224-2. E-ISBN: 978-92-75-12225-9. https://doi.org/10.37774/9789275122242.
3. Patel T, Narula S, Naderzad E, Early D, Nandhagopal T. Fetal alcohol spectrum disorder in a newborn. Cureus. 2022;14(9):e28836. https://doi.org/10.7759/cureus.28836.
4. Poskitt EM. Foetal alcohol syndrome. Alcohol. 1984;19(2):159–65.
5. Hoyme HE, Kalberg WO, Elliott AJ, Blankenship J, Buckley D, Marais AS, Manning MA, Robinson LK, Adam MP, Abdul-Rahman O, Jewett T, Coles CD, Chambers C, Jones KL, Adnams CM, Shah PE, Riley EP, Charness ME, Warren KR, May PA. Updated clinical guidelines for diagnosing fetal alcohol spectrum disorders. Pediatrics. 2016;138(2)
6. Popova S, Lange S, Probst C, Gmel G, Rehm J. Estimation of national, regional, and global prevalence of alcohol use during pregnancy and fetal alcohol syndrome: a systematic review and meta-analysis. Lancet Glob Health. 2017;5(3):e290–9. https://doi.org/10.1016/S2214-109X(17)30021-9.
7. Popova S, Charness ME, Burd L, Crawford A, Hoyme HE, Mukherjee RAS, Riley EP, Elliott EJ. Fetal alcohol spectrum disorders. Nat Rev Dis Primers. 2023;9(1):11. https://doi.org/10.1038/s41572-023-00420-x.
8. Siqueira M, Stipursky J. Blood brain barrier as an interface for alcohol induced neurotoxicity during development. Neurotoxicology. 2022;90 https://doi.org/10.1016/.neuro.2022.03.009.
9. Keum D, Pultorak K, Meredith MA, Medina AE. Effects of developmental alcohol exposure on cortical multisensory integration. Eur J Neurosci. 2023;57(5):784–95. https://doi.org/10.1111/ejn.15907.
10. Denny L, Coles S, Blitz R. Fetal alcohol syndrome and fetal alcohol spectrum disorders. Am Fam Physician. 2017;96(8):515–22.
11. Blanck-Lubarsch M, Dirksen D, Feldmann R, Bormann E, Hohoff A. Simplifying diagnosis of fetal alcohol syndrome using machine learning methods. Front Pediatr. 2022;9:707566.
12. Tsang TW, Finlay-Jones A, Perry K, Grigg JR, Popova S, Cheung MMY, Bower C, Tam P, Jamieson RV, Elliott EJ. Eye abnormalities in children with fetal alcohol spectrum disorders: a systematic review. Ophthalmic Epidemiol. 2023;30(4):340–51. https://doi.org/10.1080/09286586.2022.2123004.
13. Maya-Enero S, Ramis-Fernández SM, Astals-Vizcaino M, García-Algar Ó. Neurocognitive and behavioral profile of fetal alcohol spectrum disorder. An Pediatr (Engl Ed). 2021;95(3):208.e1–9. https://doi.org/10.1016/j.anpede.2020.12.012.
14. Mattson SN, Riley EP, Jernigan TL, Ehlers CL, Delis DC, Jones KL, Stern C, Johnson KA, Hesselink JR, Bellugi U. Fetal alcohol syndrome: a case report of neuropsychological, MRI and EEG assessment of two children. Alcohol Clin Exp Res. 1992;16(5):1001–3. https://doi.org/10.1111/j.1530-0277.1992.tb01909.x.
15. Charness ME. Fetal alcohol spectrum disorders: awareness to insight in just 50 years. Alcohol Res. 2022;42(1):05.
16. Bodnar TS, Raineki C, Wertelecki W, Yevtushok L, Plotka L, Granovska I, Zymak-Zakutnya N, Pashtepa A, Wells A, Honerkamp-Smith G, Coles CD, Kable JA, Chambers CD, Weinberg J, the CIFASD. Immune network dysregulation associated with child neurodevelopmental delay: modulatory role of prenatal alcohol exposure. J Neuroinflammation. 2020;17(1):39. https://doi.org/10.1186/s12974-020-1717-8.
17. Carpita B, Migli L, Chiarantini I, Battaglini S, Montalbano C, Carmassi C, Cremone IM, Dell'Osso L. Autism spectrum disorder and fetal alcohol spectrum disorder: a literature review. Brain Sci. 2022;12(6):792.
18. Gupta KK, Gupta VK, Shirasaka T. An update on fetal alcohol syndrome-pathogenesis, risks, and treatment. Alcohol Clin Exp Res. 2016;40(8):1594–602.
19. Hur YM, Choi J, Park S, Oh SS, Kim YJ. Prenatal maternal alcohol exposure: diagnosis and prevention of fetal alcohol syndrome. Obstet Gynecol Sci. 2022;65(5):385–94. https://doi.org/10.5468/ogs.22123.
20. Wozniak JR, Riley EP, Charness ME. Clinical presentation, diagnosis, and management of fetal alcohol spectrum disorder. Lancet Neurol. 2019;18(8):760–70. https://doi.org/10.1016/S1474-4422(19)30150-4.
21. Vorgias D, Bynum FD, Bernstein B. Fetal alcohol syndrome. 2023 May 27. In: StatPearls [Internet]. Treasure Island (FL): StatPearls Publishing; 2023.

22. García Algar O, Mendoza Berjano R. Consumo de alcohol en el embarazo. Prevención, diagnós-tico y atención temprana de los Trastornos del Espectro Alcohólico Fetal (TEAF). Madrid: Ediciones Díaz de Santos; 2021.
23. Ruffaner-Hanson C, Noor S, Sun MS, Solomon E, Marquez LE, Rodriguez DE, Allan AM, Caldwell KK, Bakhireva LN, Milligan ED. The maternal-placental-fetal interface: adaptations of the HPA axis and immune mediators following maternal stress and prenatal alcohol exposure. Exp Neurol. 2022;355:114121. https://doi.org/10.1016/j.expneurol.2022.114121.
24. Sambo D, Goldman D. Genetic influences on fetal alcohol spectrum disorder. Genes (Basel). 2023;14(1):195. https://doi.org/10.3390/genes14010195.
25. Kelly SJ, Goodlett CR, Hannigan JH. Animal models of fetal alcohol spectrum disorders: impact of the social environment. Dev Disabil Res Rev. 2009;15(3):200–8. https://doi.org/10.1002/ddrr.69.
26. Lovely CB. Animal models of gene-alcohol interactions. Birth Defects Res. 2020;112(4):367–79. https://doi.org/10.1002/bdr2.1623.
27. Olguin SL, Cavanagh JF, Young JW, Brigman JL. Impaired cognitive control after moderate prenatal alcohol exposure corresponds to altered EEG power during a rodent touchscreen continuous performance task. Neuropharmacology. 2023;236:109599. https://doi.org/10.1016/j.neuropharm.2023.109599.
28. Lim YH, Watkins RE, Jones H, Kippin NR, Finlay-Jones A. Fetal alcohol spectrum disorders screening tools: a systematic review. Res Dev Disabil. 2022;122:104168. https://doi.org/10.1016/j.ridd.2021.104168.
29. Coles CD, Li Z. Functional neuroimaging in the examination of effects of prenatal alcohol exposure. Neuropsychol Rev. 2011;21(2):119–32. https://doi.org/10.1007/s11065-011-9165-y.
30. Leung ECH, Jain P, Michealson MA, Choi H, Ellsworth-Kopkowski A, Valenzuela CF. Recent breakthroughs in understanding the cerebellum's role in fetal alcohol spectrum disorder: a systematic review. Alcohol. 2023;S0741-8329(23):00343–9. https://doi.org/10.1016/j.alcohol.2023.12.003.
31. Bauer W, Dylag KA, Lysiak A, Wieczorek-Stawinska W, Pelc M, Szmajda M, Martinek R, Zygarlicki J, Bańdo B, Stomal-Slowinska M, Kawala-Sterniuk A. Initial study on quantitative electroencephalographic analysis of bioelectrical activity of the brain of children with fetal alcohol spectrum disorders (FASD) without epilepsy. Sci Rep. 2023;13(1):109. https://doi.org/10.1038/s41598-022-26590-4.
32. Padilla-Valdez MM, Díaz-Iñiguez MI, Ortuño-Sahagún D, Rojas-Mayorquín AE. Neuroinflammation in fetal alcohol spectrum disorders and related novel therapeutic approaches. Biochim Biophys Acta Mol basis Dis. 2024;1870(1):166854. https://doi.org/10.1016/j.bbadis.2023.166854.
33. Gleichmann DC, Pinner JFL, Garcia C, Hakeem JH, Kodituwakku P, Stephen JM. A pilot study examining the effects of music training on attention in children with fetal alcohol spectrum disorders (FASD). Sensors (Basel). 2022;22(15):5642. https://doi.org/10.3390/s22155642.

Part IV

Explaining Human Pathological Behaviors. From Brain Disorders to Psychopathology

36 Values in Alcohol Use Disorders

Maria Julia Francischetto Ribeiro Soares
and Guilherme Peres Messas

Introduction

This chapter aims at:

A. Introducing the concept of values.
B. Explaining how this concept is related to clinical practice.
C. Explaining how it can be applied through value-based practice.
D. Explaining the reasons why it is important to work with values within the alcohol use disorder.
E. Relating the psychopathological changes of substance abuse and value-centered treatment.

What Are Values?

A value is a particular property of something, like a predicate. It is a kind of judgment, opinion or disposition, and as a disposition, it is linked to human actions, like an action guide [1]. It is about preferences, desires, and everything that people evaluate positively or negatively [2]. And to this, judgment of values is attributed to a social function of incorporating to the behavior guilt or the merit of a compliment [1]. Therefore, the operational concept of values is "values are attitudes or dispositions that are guides-actions subject to praise or guilt" [1, 3].

Although values determine principles, they are not generated by rational interpretations of experiences, but by the emotions experienced, being values and emotions connected by essence [3]. Responding to these concepts, Stanghellini [3] proposed the following aspects:

1. Values are beliefs, but not cold beliefs: they are not logical abstractions, but are original and intrinsically tied to emotions.
2. Values are motivational emotions: they refer to the desirable/undesirable goals that people strive to achieve or avoid.
3. Values are common attitudes that transcend particular actions and situations. This distinguishes values from norms that refer to specific actions and situations.
4. Values serve (often in an implicit and pre-reflective form) as criteria for emotional preference (reflective rather than rational choices): they guide the evolution of actions, people (including the self) and events.
5. Values form a structure rooted in the ontological constitution of the person: they compose an order not very coherent, but organized enough for personal emotions [3].

Maria Julia Francischetto Ribeiro Soares (✉) ·
G. P. Messas
Faculdade de Ciências Médicas da Santa Casa de São Paulo, Hospital do Servidor Público Estadual de São Paulo, São Paulo, Brazil
e-mail: guilherme.messas@fcmsantacasasp.edu.br

P. Á. Gargiulo, H. L. Mesones-Arroyo (eds.), *Psychiatry and Neuroscience Update – Vol. V*,
https://doi.org/10.1007/978-3-031-72219-6_36

Being ontological values, there are different values in different individuals, which are distant in different historical and cultural contexts [2]. There is the possibility of dividing values into personal valuations, which justify the actions of each individual in their life and cultural values, which justify collective actions [4].

How Do Values Present Themselves in Medical Practice?

Traditionally, the values recognized in medical practice are the ethical values [2]. The group's ethics code together with a series of values shared among professionals, such as autonomy of patients, confidentiality, and the goal of acting for the good of the patient, and these values help to guide decisions taken in daily life.

As we have seen before, values are not limited only to cultural values, as collective values. Individual values also determine actions, desires, and assessments of each person individually and during medical practice, and there are times when different individual values end up in conflict and may become complex [2].

Complex situations may appear in the interpretation of ethical values such as acting for the good of the patient. They can involve different moral judgments, for personal values, in the same situation. Conflicting values can arise in situations where we deal with the doubt of maintaining the autonomy of the patient and continue acting for his well-being, or even maintain confidentiality in cases of risk of life. That is, in different clinical contexts, we are faced with situations involving complex and conflicting values in which collective values are insufficient for decision-making [2].

Confronted with this insufficiency, Fulford [2] proposed the value-based practice (VBP) for situations involving conflicting and complex values, promoting the development of clinical skills [2, 5].

What Is Value-Based Practice?

VBP is a new and emerging way of working with conflicting and complex values in healthcare [2]. It is based on the development of certain clinical skills aimed at raising awareness about the individual values of patients in order to include them in clinical decisions. This is intended to improve the decision-making process [2].

PBV is organized into four levels, in 10 key elements. The first level is that of clinical skills, which constitute the first four key elements such as perception, reasoning, knowledge, and communication [2].

The second level is the model of application of services, marked by elements five and six, and emphasize the application of person-centered treatment and multidisciplinary practice, respectively [6].

The third level deals with the relationship of PBV with the scientific evidence, discriminating the elements seven, eight, and nine, respectively, the principle of "two supports," the principle of "creaking gear" and the principle of "scientific drive" [6].

The last level is also the last key element of PBV, the partnership, which consists of making it explicit that the decision must be shared between the healthcare team, the patient, and the people who provide support [6].

Why Work with Values in the Treatment of Alcohol Use Disorders? The Current Challenges of This Management

The World Health Organization (WHO) considers the consumption of alcohol as the largest single factor of increased morbidity and mortality in the world [7]. It is associated with more than 200 diseases reported in the International Classification of Diseases (ICD) [8], and individuals diagnosed with Alcohol Use Disorder (AUD) are involved in about half of the problems reported in association with the use of this substance [9].

This diagnosis is considered as one of the most subtracted mental disorders, less than 15% of individuals suffering from this disease receive treatment [9]. Furthermore, the time between the beginning of the development of the disorder and the first treatment is on average 30 years [9].

The treatment of AUD involves complex and conflicting decisions. The main therapeutic options present similar efficacy, both in the choice of medications to control the use of alcohol [10] and in the indication of therapies [11]. In order to direct therapy, guidelines for the management of this disorder are proposed, guided by the results of empirical research. However, there is evidence that the application of such guidelines in psychiatric practice in general does not achieve research effectiveness [12].

It is important to emphasize that besides the low effectiveness of these guidelines, most choose not to direct how to make important decisions for the management of AUD. The American Psychiatric Association (APA) does not guide, for example, how to choose the objective of treatment. The only suggestion is that the choice between abstinence from alcohol use, reduction or moderation of alcohol use or other elements of harm reduction be made between the clinician and the patient, and that it be documented [13, 14].

Therefore, when the objective is the accomplishment of an effective clinical practice, it is not enough just to mechanically reproduce the researches, ignoring nonideal situations, such as nonadherence. It is suggested that treatments guided by individual values in AUD present a higher adherence index [12]. This incorporation has the potential to increase the effectiveness of decision-making in medical care [2, 15].

By uniting this reasoning the current trend of increasing studies on substance use disorders involving shared decisions between health providers and users [16], it is proposed that treatment be centered on the values of individuals who are responsible for making clinical decisions.

The Psychopathology of Chemical Dependency and the Influence on Value-Based Treatment

Substance abuse emerges from a complex set of psychopathological experiences, personal choices, specific psychological vulnerabilities, personality types, and cultural values, and although it has different perspectives that influence research and clinical practice, there is no consensus on the central characteristic that makes substance use understandable as pathological or problematic [17].

Because of the difficulty in finding a comprehensive, unified, and convincing model, and the ineffectiveness of person-centered management therapeutic models, it presents itself as the best option [17]. This brings the importance of recognizing the psychopathological changes of substance users for understanding how they may influence complaints and treatment goals for each patient's decision-making.

Studies in phenomenological psychopathology aim at understanding the alterations experienced in substance abuse and, for a better understanding, the temporal and spatial alteration of alcohol abuse will be studied, respectively, hyperpresentification and fullness [17, 18]. Hyperpresentification is the experience of the present dominating the consciousness, with a proportional reduction of the past and the future at the moment of the experience, which makes the consciousness unstable, which can justify sudden changes in mood, risky behavior, and the difficulty of the individual to make plans [17]. Completeness is for spatiality, as hyperpresentification is for temporality. It is intoxication producing an effect of completeness in the abuser, the experience is homogeneous and all heterogeneity is expelled [17].

Faced with these alterations, the clinician to conduct the decision-making has an arduous work of helping the patient to balance the alterations, mainly in respect to the capacity to move towards the future [17]. To increase the patient's past and future experience, an important tool is the involvement of the family in treatment [17]. Together with the clinician, family members make up the group of stakeholders, which is fundamental for shared decision-making [17]. And if the patient decides to act according to free choice, he must be able to see the options he has to decide and to be able to consider his values at the time of choice [17]. For the decision to have the expression of the patient's values, he needs to be able to experience reality with fluid temporality and space with complexity, and be responsible for the choices and decisions shared and conducted by the clinician and the therapeutic alliance with stakeholders, despite the psychopathological changes [17].

Conclusion

The understanding of the values of patients diagnosed with AUD and their relationship with psychopathology is a subject little explored in the literature. It is believed that the need to listen to these individuals to demonstrate how the relationships between the pathology and its values emerge in the clinic. A study aiming at the relationship between the pathology and the values of the individuals has already been performed for patients with schizophrenia [3] and with the diagnosis of borderline disorder [19].

The proposal of studying these relationships can be enriching for the clinic, improving the decision-making process, and proposing a more effective treatment for these individuals, focused on their values.

Bibliography

1. Sadler JZ. Values in psychiactric diagnosis and classification. In: Fulford KWM, Davies M, Gipps RGT, Graham G, Sadler JZ, Stanghellini G, Thorton T, editors. The Oxford handbook of philosophy and psychiatry. Oxford: Oxford University Press; 2013. p. 753–79.
2. Fulford KWM. The value of evidence and evidence of values: bringing together values-based and evidence-based practice in policy and service development in mental health. J Eval Clin Pract. 2011;17(5):976–87. https://doi.org/10.1111/j.1365-2753.2011.01732.x.
3. Stanghellini G, Ballerini M. Values in persons with schizophrenia. Schizophr Bull. 2007;33(1):131–41. https://doi.org/10.1093/schbul/sbl036.
4. Sagiv L, Roccas S, Cieciuch J, et al. Personal values in human life. Nat Hum Behav. 2017;1:630–9. https://doi.org/10.1038/s41562-017-0185-3.
5. Fulford KWM. Values-based practice: a new partner to evidence-based practice and a first for psychiatry? Mens Sana Monogr. 2008;6(1):10–21.
6. Fulford KWM, Stanghellini G, Broome M. What can philosophy do for psychiatry? World Psychiatry. 2004;3(3):130–5.
7. World Health Organization. Global status report on alcohol and health 2018. Geneva: World Health Organization; 2018.
8. Nutt DJ, Gual A, Anderson P. Why less is always more in the treatment of alcohol use disorders. JAMA Psychiatry. 2019;76(4):359–60. https://doi.org/10.1001/jamapsychiatry.2018.2807.
9. Connor JP, Haber PS, Hall W. Alcohol use disorders. Lancet. 2016;387(10022):988–98. https://doi.org/10.1016/s0140-6736(15)00122-1.
10. Palpacuer C, et al. Pharmacologically controlled drinking in the treatment of alcohol dependence or alcohol use disorders: a systematic review with direct and network meta-analyses on nalmefene, naltrexone, acamprosate, baclofen and topiramate. Addiction. 2018;113(2):220–37. https://doi.org/10.1111/add.13974.
11. Gual A, Miquel L. New perspectives for the treatment of alcoholism. Med Clin (Barc). 2015;144(1):24–5.
12. Girlanda F, Fiedler I, Becker T, Barbui C, Koesters M. The evidence–practice gap in specialist mental healthcare: systematic review and meta-analysis of guideline implementation studies. Br J Psychiatry. 2017;210(01):24–30. https://doi.org/10.1192/bjp.bp.115.179093.
13. Reus VI, Fochtmann LJ, Bukstein O, Evan Eyler A, Hilty DM, Horvitz-Lennon M, Mahoney J, Pasic J, Weaver M, Wills CD, McIntyre J, Kidd J, Yager J, Hong SH. The American Psychiatric Association practice guideline for the pharmacological treatment of patients with alcohol use disorder. Am J Psychiatry. 2018;175(1):86–90. https://doi.org/10.1176/appi.ajp.2017.1750101.
14. Lieberman DZ, Cioletti A, Massey SH, Collantes RS, Moore BB. Treatment preferences among problem drinkers in primary care. Int J Psychiatry Med. 2014;47(3):231–40. https://doi.org/10.2190/pm.47.3.d.
15. Sackett DL, Straus SE, Richardson WS, Rosenberg W, Haynes RB. Evidence-based medicine: how to practice and teach EBM. 2nd ed. Edinburgh; London: Churchill Livingstone; 2000.
16. Joosten EAG, De Jong CAJ, de Weert-van Oene GH, Sensky T, Van der Staak CPF. Shared decision-making reduces drug use and psychiatric severity in substance-dependent patients. Psychother Psychosom. 2009;78:245–53. https://doi.org/10.1159/000219524.
17. Messas GP, Fukuda L, Pienkos E. A phenomenological contribution to substance misuse treatment: principles for person-Centered care. Psychopathology. 2019;52:85–93. https://doi.org/10.1159/000501509.
18. Messas GP. On the essence of drunkenness and the pathway to addiction: a phenomenological contribution. J Addict Behav Ther Rehabil. 2014;3:2. https://doi.org/10.4172/2324-9005.1000121.
19. Mancini M, Stanghellini G. Values in persons with borderline personality disorder: their relevance for the therapeutic interview. Res Psycho: Psychopathol Process Outcome. 2020;23(1):48–55. https://doi.org/10.4081/ripppo.2020.449.

37 Neuropsychological Instruments for the Evaluation of Alcohol Abuse Disorders

Jorge Herrera, Norman López, Carol Saldías Solís, Daniela Ripoll, Andrés Ledezma, Yuliana Flórez, Breiner Morales, and Pascual Ángel Gargiulo

Introduction

Some public health problems are very relevant for his psychosocial and interpersonal disturbances. It is the case for alcohol abuse disorder (AAD). It generates various medical illnesses and personal costs [1, 2]. One of the main problems is the consequences that AAD produces on the brain and, consequently, at the mental level. In this sense, AAD in the forms of alcohol excess and abuse affects higher functions. It implies effects on cognitive and adaptive functioning. The present chapter has been written in order to provide practical references for neuropsychologists and doctors in his field. Information was selected in order to provide them with actualized evaluation instruments in order to study patients with a history of AAD using specific batteries. The intention is to provide information on neuropsychological tools used to assess individuals with this condition. The tools are Repeatable Battery for the Assessment of Neuropsychological Status (RBANS), Mini-Mental State Examination (MMSE), Rey Auditory Verbal Learning Test (RAVLT), Controlled Oral Word Test, Controlled Oral Word Association Test (COWAT),

J. Herrera
College of Medicine Florida International University, University Park, FL, USA

N. López
Escuela de Kinesiología, Facultad de Salud, Universidad Santo Tomás, Temuco, Chile

Centro de Investigación en Gerontología Aplicada (CIGAP), Universidad Santo Tomas, Temuco, Chile
e-mail: normanlopezve@santotomas.cl

C. Saldías Solís
Escuela de Kinesiología, Facultad de Salud, Universidad Santo Tomás, Temuco, Chile
e-mail: carolsaldiasso@santotomas.cl

D. Ripoll · Y. Flórez · B. Morales
Departamento de Ciencias Sociales, Universidad de La Costa, Barranquilla, Colombia
e-mail: dripoll@cuc.edu.co; yflorez1@cuc.edu.co; bmorales3@cuc.edu.co

A. Ledezma
Centro de Investigación en Gerontología Aplicada (CIGAP), Facultad de Salud, Universidad Santo Tomas, Antofagasta, Chile

Escuela de Kinesiología, Facultad de Salud, Universidad Santo Tomás, Antofagasta, Chile
e-mail: aledezma@santotomas.cl

B. Morales
Departamento de Ciencias Sociales, Universidad de Los Lagos, Osorno, Chile
e-mail: bmorales3@cuc.edu.co

P. Á. Gargiulo (✉)
Laboratory of Neurosciences and Experimental Psychology, Latin American Technological Corporation Foundation (FUCOTEL), Cathedra of Psychopathology, Catholic University of Argentina, Area of Pharmacology, Department of Pathology, National University of Cuyo, CONICET, Guaymallén, Mendoza, Argentina

P. Á. Gargiulo, H. L. Mesones-Arroyo (eds.), *Psychiatry and Neuroscience Update – Vol. V*,
https://doi.org/10.1007/978-3-031-72219-6_37

Wisconsin Card Sorting Test (WCST), Test of Words and Colors (STROOP), Rey Osterrieth Complex Figure Test (ROCFT), Revised Benton Visual Retention Test (RBVRT), Symbols and Digits Test (SDMT), and the Halstead-Reitan Trail Making Test (TMT). A brief commentary describing the main uses and characteristics of these instruments is followed by a mention of recent studies that have applied these instruments in research studies to demonstrate the effects of alcoholism on specific cognitive functions, reviewing the current state of clinical application.

Repeatable Battery for Assessment of Neuropsychological Status (RBANS)

The RBANS [3, 4] is composed of 12 subtests, which are organized as follows within its five component indexes: (1) Immediate Memory Index (Word Learning and Story Memory), (2) Visual-Spatial/Constructive Index (Figure Copying and Line Orientation), (3) Language Index (Picture Naming and Semantic Fluency), (4) Attention Index (Digit Repetition and Number Key), and (5) Delayed Memory Index (List Recall, Word Recognition, Story Recall, and Figure Recall) [5].

The RBANS produces a standard score that describes the patient's overall neurocognitive function [6]. It consists of five indexes identifying deficits in specific areas and intact functions. The Immediate Memory Index assesses the patient's ability to recall information immediately after presentation. The Visual-Spatial/Constructive Index assesses the patient's ability to perceive spatial relationships and produce accurate copies. The RBANS Language Index evaluates the patient's verbal response ability through naming or recalling previously learned verbal material. The Attention Index evaluates the patient's capacity to process and remember information presented visually or orally in a short-term memory context. The Delayed Memory Index is useful for evaluating the patient's ability to form new memories [7].

Review of the Current State of Knowledge

A study conducted in the United States by Hart et al. [8] examined the impact of alcohol consumption on neurocognitive function in patients with end-stage liver disease. The study included 108 patients (70.4% male) awaiting liver transplantation. The sample had the following liver disease diagnoses: hepatitis (40.7%), alcoholic cirrhosis (25%), and other conditions, such as cryptogenic sarcoidosis and biliary cirrhosis (34.3%). Out of the entire sample, 62 patients reported alcohol abuse or dependence. When RBANS was administered, the patients with alcohol abuse or dependence had a lower, not significant mean total score.

On the RBANS Immediate Memory Index, the sample with alcohol abuse or dependence obtained a very lower mean score when compared with the sample without alcohol abuse or dependence ($p < 0.01$).

When Visual-Spatial/Constructive Index (Figure Copying and Line Orientation) was considered, a difference was observed, but it was not statistically significant. The RBANS Language Index scores for patients with and without alcohol abuse or dependence were different, but the difference between these means was not significant. Considering Attention Index, patients with alcohol abuse or dependence had a lower mean standard score when compared to patients without alcohol abuse or dependence. There was no significant difference between the means. Patients who reported alcohol abuse or dependence had a lower mean standard score on the RBANS Delayed Memory Index, compared with patients who did not report alcohol abuse or dependence ($p < 0.05$). A review of these findings revealed that patients with end-stage liver disease scored low on all RBANS indices. Regarding alcohol abuse or dependence, deficits in both immediate and delayed memory processes were observed.

In a study conducted in the United Kingdom [4], Brow et al. [9] investigated the usefulness of RBANS in detecting alcohol-related brain injury, studying two groups, aging 45–57 years. The first group (AL) consisted of 30 alcohol-dependent patients (19 women and 11 men) with a mean age of 46.1 years and a median year of drinking of 16 years. The second group consisted of 28 patients (18 men and 10 women) with a history of alcohol use and symptoms of alcohol-related brain damage (ADBD), with a mean age of 56.29 years. The median duration of alcohol consumption was 20 years. The sample included 11 patients with Korsakoff's syndrome and 17 patients with alcohol-related brain damage. The AL sample exhibited higher scores on total standard score, Attention Index, Immediate Memory Index, Visual-Spatial/Constructive Index, Linguistic Index ABD Delayed Memory Index. The discrepancies in the RBANS total standard score and the five indices between the two samples were highly significant.

The study's findings are significant. They demonstrate how heavy drinking causes brain damage that impairs several higher brain functions, including attention, immediate memory, delayed memory, *language*, and visual constructive praxis. The results also show that the RBANS is an effective neuropsychological instrument for identifying brain damage caused by heavy drinking.

Mini-Mental State Examination (MMSE)

The authors proposed this as a quick measure of cognitive functioning, which is particularly important for patients with poor stamina or perseveration due to their condition. This includes primarily the elderly, as well as other patients experiencing symptoms of dementia or cognitive impairment [10–12].

The instrument was also suggested as a standardized procedure that can be used multiple times to assess cognitive impairment. The Mini-Mental State Examination (MMSE) was initially validated by Folstein, Folstein, and McHugh [12] in three patient samples: those with dementia, depression with cognitive impairment, and depression. They established a cut-off score 20 between patients and healthy elderly controls from a sample of 137 patients and 63 controls. The MMSE consists of 11 items, with a maximum score of 30 points [13]. This instrument assesses cognitive functioning in orientation, memory, attention, language, and constructive visual praxis [14].

The MMSE is widely used in the brain-behavioral assessment [15]. However, specific bibliographic references on this instrument are not standard in the literature, particularly regarding its behavior in relation to different types of dementias or neurological conditions. The MMSE was previously in the public domain, but its copyright has recently been asserted. It is now available in English from Psychological Assessment Resources in Florida. The Spanish version can be purchased from *TEA Ediciones* in Madrid, Spain.

Review of the Current State of Knowledge

Ros-Cucurull et al. [16] conducted a study in Spain in which they examined the relationship between neurocognitive status and alcohol consumption in a sample of older participants. They selected a sample of 33 participants who were identified as "hazardous drinkers." The sample included 21 men and 12 women with an average age of 71. A total of 20 people in this sample had 10 or more years of education, and 13 had 10 or fewer years of education. In addition, 31 healthy controls (20 men and 11 women) with a mean age of 72.9 years participated. Twenty-two participants had 10 years or more of formal education, and 9 had 10 years or less. All participants were administered a comprehensive battery of neuropsychological tests, including the MMSE. The mean total score for the sample of patients with "hazardous drinking habits" was 26.62, with a corresponding score of 28.39 for the sample of healthy controls. The difference between these means was significant ($p < 0.05$). The results of this study further support the presence of changes in higher brain functions associated with increased alcohol consumption [17].

Wang et al. [18] investigated the effect of alcohol use disorder on functional connectivity of multisensory brain regions. Participants in this study, conducted in China, included 21 male patients diagnosed with alcohol use disorder (AUD) and 21 healthy male controls. They were in the range of 45–48 years old, with equivalent educational levels. The MMSE was administered to both samples, and significant differences were obtained ($p = 0.003$), with lower scores for AUD group. This study confirmed that excessive alcohol consumption has a deleterious effect on neurocognitive function and that the MMSE can reflect this effect [19].

Rey Auditory Verbal Learning Test (RAVLT)

The roots of the RAVLT [20–22] can be traced back to the original work of the physician and educator Edouard Claparède [23], who developed a memory assessment instrument in which patients listened to a list of 15 words and had to reproduce them in writing. From its beginnings in neuropsychology, the RAVLT proved its usefulness in differentiating neurological from non-neurological patient groups, including patients with severe psychiatric disorders [24].

By the 1980s, this instrument had already established its usefulness in assessing memory impairment associated with conditions such as human immunodeficiency virus (HIV) [25] and traumatic brain injury [26], among others. The RAVLT is currently one of the most widely used measures of auditory speech-mediated auditory memory in clinical and neuropsychological research [27]. It is widely used in the psychiatric and neurological literature and the assessment of neurocognitive status in patients with a variety of medical conditions [28, 29].

Review of the Current State of Knowledge

Moritz et al. [30] conducted a study in Germany in which they compared the neurocognitive profile of a sample of patients with alcohol use disorder (AUD) with that of a sample of healthy controls (HC) with no history of alcohol abuse. Participants in this study were 15 patients and 20 healthy controls. Age and education level were equivalent. A battery of neuropsychological instruments, including the German version of the RAVLT, was administered to both groups. The mean of the total number of words recalled in the sum of the first five administrations of List A of the RAVLT obtained from the sample of AUD patients was 43.13, while the corresponding value obtained from the sample of healthy controls was 56.95 ($p = 0.001$). The mean number of words recalled by the sample of patients with alcohol use disorder in the delayed recall of RAVLT List A was 8.73, while the corresponding value for the sample of healthy controls was 12.10 ($p = 0.006$).

The results of this study indicate the presence of impairments in auditory verbal episodic memory functions as assessed by the RAVLT in patients with alcohol use disorder [31].

In a study conducted in Italy, Ioime et al. [32] investigated the effects of heavy alcohol consumption on neuropsychological performance. These two samples had no significant differences in age, educational level, or gender composition.

The RAVLT, as part of the neuropsychological battery used by the authors of this study, was administered to both samples' participants. Scores obtained by the healthy controls was clearly higher than patients with alcohol abuse on the sum of the first five presentations of List A of the RAVLT ($p < 0.01$). In the delayed recall condition of the administration of these instruments, this difference between groups was also observed ($p < 0.01$). Once again, these results reflect and confirm the detrimental effect of excessive alcohol consumption on the auditory verbal episodic memory functions assessed by this instrument.

Controlled Oral Word Association Test (COWAT)

This test was originally called the TEST OF CONTROLLED VERBAL FLUENCY. However, when it was incorporated into the Multilingual Aphasia Examination [33, 34], the name was changed to the TEST OF CONTROLLED ORAL WORD ASSOCIATION. As a neuropsychological instrument, the COWAT is perhaps the most widely used in brain-behavioral studies [35–37]. The literature that has used is vast, in terms of the number of syndromes and conditions studied and the number of countries in which it has been used [38, 39].

Review of the Current State of Knowledge

Brand et al. [40] investigated the ability of alcoholics with Korsakoff's syndrome to make appropriate emotional and cognitive judgments. For this purpose, these authors studied a sample of 41 patients diagnosed with Korsakoff's syndrome of alcoholic origin together with a sample of healthy controls with no history of psychiatric or neurological disorders. The age and educational level of the sample of healthy controls was the same as that of the patient's sample. Alcoholic patients with Korsakoff's syndrome showed a lower score ($p < 0.01$).

Based on the results obtained by Brand et al. [40] in this study, it is clear that the verbal fluency process assessed by the COWAT is seriously affected by the effect of alcohol on brain tissue. These results also suggest that patients with Korsakoff's syndrome have memory deficits, as reported in the scientific literature, but also executive function deficits associated with the frontal lobes. In a study conducted in Spain, Asencio et al. [41] investigated the presence of damage in the brain structure of patients with alcohol abuse and its relationship to poor impulse control.

Using the COWAT, patients diagnosed with AAD scored significantly lower than controls ($p = 0.04$). Although the patients who participated in this study did not have a long history of alcohol abuse, i.e., 4–5 years, the adverse effects of heavy alcohol consumption on verbal fluency processes as assessed by the COWAT are beginning to show.

In a study conducted in South Korea, Lee et al. [42] compared the neurocognitive profile of 37 patients (19 men and 18 women) diagnosed with cirrhosis of viral origin, with a sample of 43 persons diagnosed with cirrhosis of the liver caused by excessive alcohol consumption. There were no significant differences between these two samples in the variables of age, gender composition, or educational level. A comparison was also realized between both groups and a normative sample of 1000 participants of the similar age and educational level. Both groups differed from the normative sample in the tests of memory, executive function and Korea-Mini Mental Status Examination. When both experimental groups were compared, lower memory scores were observed in alcoholic cirrhosis, specifically in the Verbal Learning Test, the visuospatial function (Ray-Complex Figure Copy Test), the frontal/executive function (Controlled Oral Ward Association), and the Korea-Mini-Mental Status Examination.

There is no doubt that both samples of patients with liver cirrhosis showed a lower verbal fluency ability than the normative sample. However, those with liver cirrhosis caused by excessive alcohol consumption obtained the worst results on these instruments.

Wisconsin Card Sorting Test (WCST)

The WCST was initially developed as a more valid and reliable assessment of organicity in psychiatric and neurological patients [43, 44]. The authors of this instrument intended to create a procedure that would be sensitive to the impairments in abstraction and cognitive flexibility often observed in organic patients [45].

Different versions of this instrument were used over the years until Heaton standardized it [46] and later revised by Heaton et al. [47]. It is used worldwide, and the number of research studies in which it is included is enormous. The WCST is considered one of the gold standards for assessing executive functions mediated primarily by the frontal lobes and identifying organicity [48, 49].

Review of the Current State of Knowledge

Martinez and Manoiloff [50] conducted a study in Argentina examining the executive functions of adolescents with different patterns of alcohol use. Participants in this study included 133 adolescents with a mean age of 21.26 years who were or had been university students. All participants were free of any medical or psychiatric conditions that might interfere with their participation in this study.

The sample was divided into three groups according to their reported drinking patterns: the first group consisted of light drinkers, the second group of moderate drinkers, and the third group of binge drinkers. Several neuropsychological instruments were administered, including the WCST. None of the differences between the means of the three groups were statistically significant.

According to these authors, the literature generally shows that executive functions are impaired in heavy drinkers. However, this was different in this study. The authors suggest two interesting possibilities to explain these findings. On the one hand, the drinking criteria they used to classify the participants in this study differed from those used in other studies. On the other hand, they also suggested that the adolescent brain has a higher degree of plasticity and, therefore, more compensatory capacity.

In general, the literature has reported that executive functions are impaired in heavy alcohol users. Therefore, the authors propose two possibilities that could explain their findings. The criteria used to classify the participants were different from those used in other studies, and the brains of adolescents have a greater degree of plasticity and therefore more compensatory capacity [51–53].

Dos Santos Rigoni et al. [54] conducted a study in Brazil in which they examined the neuropsychological functioning of alcoholics undergoing treatment. Two groups aging between 41 and 43 years and equivalent mean education level were compared. The first group was integrated by 101 alcoholic patients with a history of daily alcohol consumption. The second group was integrated by 41 healthy controls. None of the participants in the control sample reported daily alcohol consumption. Weekend drinking was reported by 19.5%, 34.1% reported occasional drinking, and 43.9% reported no drinking. The median number of categories achieved on the WCST was 2 for the alcoholic patients, with values ranging from 0 to 6 categories. Controls achieved a median of 6 categories, with scores ranging from 0 to 6. The difference between these scores was significant ($p \leq 0.001$).

A significant difference was observed in the median perseverative error, showing higher scores for the patients ($p = 0.004$). Significant differences were also observed in the nonperseverative errors, the number of trials completing the first category, and the failure to maintain the set. Based on these results, there is no doubt that excessive alcohol consumption has a detrimental effect on frontal lobe-mediated executive functions as assessed by the WCST.

Word and Color Test (STROOP)

In its different versions, it has a solid presence in the neuropsychological literature and has been and continues to be a very useful tool in neuropsychology [55–57]. It is based on the Stroop effect [58]. As a young experimental psychologist writing his doctoral dissertation, J.R. Stroop discovered that identifying the color in which a word is written, which is the name of another color, is particularly difficult, even for people with no clinical or neurological condition. This process requires executive functions and inhibitory control since the predominant behavior would be "reading" the word rather than saying the color in which it is written.

Review of the Current State of Knowledge

Connor et al. [59] investigated the direct and indirect effects of prenatal alcohol consumption on executive functions. Three groups of 20–25-year-old patients participated: 15 with fetal alcohol syndrome (**FAS**), 15 with the effects of fetal alcoholism (Fetal Alcohol Effects, FAE), and a third group of 15 healthy controls. The comparisons made between these groups were supplemented by values obtained in a sample of 219 participants, in whom there were reports of alcohol consumption by their mothers. The first two groups scored under controls on the word and color conditions of the instrument. Normative database showed similar scores than controls. The same was observed on the color-word condition.

The Stroop effect was clearly observed in the scores obtained by all samples in this study. That is, always, word reading showed higher scores, color reading intermediate scores, whereas in a task that required naming the color in which the word was written rather than naming the color it represented, the scores obtained were significantly much lower.

In terms of the clinical implications of this research, it is evident that both participants with and without fetal alcohol syndrome had impaired ability in the attentional and inhibitory control functions measured by the STROOP.

In a study of the ability of alcoholic patients with Korsakoff's syndrome to use frontal lobe-mediated executive functions, Brand et al. [40] administered a German-developed version of the STROOP to a sample of 41 patients diagnosed with Korsakoff's syndrome and another sample of 39 healthy controls with no history of neurological or psychiatric disorders. Both groups presented equivalent age and education level.

Based on the results obtained in this study, the word administration condition could not significantly discriminate between patients with Korsakoff's syndrome and those belonging to the healthy control sample, whereas the color or interference word administration condition was able to discriminate them. Although it is unlikely that clinicians reading this information will use the same version of the STROOP as used in this research, it is essential to appreciate the effect of Korsakoff's syndrome on the higher brain functions assessed by this type of instrument.

King Osterrieth Complex Figure Test (ROCFT)

This test is typically administered as a measure of visual construction practice, in which patients are asked to copy the figure, and as a measure of visual-spatial memory, in which patients are asked to reproduce the figure from memory at various intervals [60–62].

Review of the Current State of Knowledge

In a research study in which they developed a profile of neuropsychological deficits in female alcoholics, Sullivan et al. [63] examined the performance of 43 alcoholic women with an average age of 42 years, recruited from inpatient and outpatient programs at a U.S. veterans' hospital. Participants were also recruited from community-based treatment programs. The BECK DEPRESSION INVENTORY II (BDI II) was also administered [64] with a mean score of 10.2.

The performance of this sample of patients on the ROCFT was compared with that of a sample of 47 controls without a diagnosis of alcohol use disorder. While the means of the variables age and educational level did not differ significantly between alcoholic patients and healthy controls, they differed significantly in the mean scores of the BDI-II. No differences were observed between groups in the ROCFT.

Interestingly, although the difference in performance on the ROCFT administration copy condition was not markedly different between alcoholic patients and healthy controls, the difference in scores obtained on the BDI-II was. In this regard, it should be noted that in the presence of a marked difference in the level of depression, no marked difference in ROCFT performance was observed. Therefore, it can be concluded that the visual construction skills involved in the ROCFT are not affected by depression.

The presence of memory impairment in Korsakoff's syndrome caused by chronic alcohol use has been widely documented in the scientific literature [65–67]. However, other aspects, both cognitive and emotional judgment, are also negatively affected by this condition [68, 69].

To this end, Brand et al. [40] compared the performance of a sample of 41 patients with alcohol-associated Korsakoff's syndrome with that of a sample of 39 healthy controls using the

ROCFT. Both groups had equivalent age and education levels. Alcoholic patients reached significantly lower scores than healthy controls ($p = 0.003$).

In the delayed recall condition, i.e., 30 min after the initial presentation of the complex figure, patients with Korsakoff's syndrome obtained a very low mean score vs. controls. As with the Complex Figure Administration copy condition, this difference was highly significant ($p < 0.001$). The results of this study confirmed that in Korsakoff's syndrome caused by chronic alcohol consumption, memory processes are not the unique negatively affected parameter. Visual constructional practice functions necessary for the performance of the ROCFT copy administration is affected, as well as visual-spatial memory processes.

In a study conducted in Brazil, dos Santos Rigoni et al. [54] examined the neuropsychological performance of a sample of alcoholics in treatment. They included 101 alcoholic patients with a mean age of 43 and 31 years. Both groups were equivalent in age and educational levels.

In the sample of 101 alcoholic patients, 92 reported daily alcohol consumption. A battery of neuropsychological tests was administered to all participants, including a copy of the ROCFT. The scores were lower in the alcoholic patient's group. These results suggest that frequent and perhaps excessive alcohol consumption has a negative impact on the planning and visual-constructive practice processes assessed by administering copies of the ROCFT.

In another study conducted in the United States, Fama et al. [70] examined the neurological, nutritional, and alcohol consumption factors that lead to cognitive and motor deficits in chronic alcoholism. This study included a sample of 96 alcoholic patients and 41 healthy controls, aging 45–50 years and with an equivalent education. Significant differences were observed in the copy of complex figure in the ROCFT ($p = 0.022$) and the condition of complex figure reproduction from immediate memory ($p = 0.001$). In the delayed recall complex figure reproduction at 30 min after the initial presentation, a significant difference was also observed ($p = 0.008$).

The results of this study undoubtedly reflect the deleterious effects of chronic heavy alcohol use on visual construction practice and visual-spatial memory and the ability of the ROCFT to demonstrate this.

Revised Benton Visual Retention Test (RBVRT)

This instrument represents one of the Arthur L. Benton's most important contributions to neuropsychology and the study of the brain-behavior relationships [71–73]. This instrument is sensitive to sustained attention, perseverative endurance, immediate visual-spatial memory, and visual constructive praxis. Two different types of scores are usually derived from the RBVRT. The first is the number of errors in reproducing geometric drawings presented to the patient. The second type of score is derived from the number of correct reproductions of the 10 different sheets of drawings presented to patients.

Review of the Current State of Knowledge

In a study conducted in the United States, Goldstein et al. [74] examined the severity of neuropsychological alterations in cocaine and alcohol abusers and their relationship to frontal lobe metabolism. A sample of 72 healthy controls, 42 male cocaine addicts, and 40 alcoholics aging 35–40 years old, and with equivalent education was studied. Alcoholics exhibited a mean length of alcohol dependence in this sample was 23.8 years.

All study participants were administered a battery of neuropsychological instruments, including the RBVRT. The number of errors was used as one of the scores on this instrument. The mean number of errors made by the sample of healthy controls was 3.4, that of the cocaine abusers was 4.8, and the value for the sample of alcoholics was 6.2. The number of correctly reproduced drawings was also used as a score for the RBVRT. The mean number for the healthy controls was 7.7, for the cocaine abusers 6.5, and for the alcoholics 6.1.

The review of these results revealed a worse performance in this task by the alcoholic sample, certainly compared to the healthy controls, but also compared to the cocaine addict sample, both in terms of the number of errors made and in terms of the number of drawings correctly reproduced. Based on these results, there is no doubt that chronic and abusive alcohol consumption has a deleterious effect on attention and visual construction practice as assessed by the RBVRT.

Symbol and Digit Test (SDMT)

The SDMT [75–77] is among the most helpful and widely used neuropsychological instruments in the medical and scientific literature. The SDMT has been shown to contribute significantly to the identification of organicity in both psychiatric and neurological patients. This instrument has two forms of administration such as written and oral. The written administration of this instrument is sensitive to visual association processes, visuomotor processing speed and incidental memory. The oral administration is also sensitive to incidental memory and language naming function. Both administrations reflect the attentional processes of concentration and efficient execution.

Review of the Current State of Knowledge

In the study conducted by Goldstein et al. [74] and reported in the previous section of this chapter, the written administration of the SDMT was also included in the battery of neuropsychological instruments administered to the three samples of participants in that study: healthy controls, cocaine abusers, and alcoholics. The results obtained by these three samples on the SDMT were as follows. The mean score obtained by the sample of healthy controls was 54.3, the score obtained by the sample of cocaine addicts was 47.7, and the score obtained by the sample of alcoholics was 46.5.

Although no significant difference was observed between the two samples of substance abusers, both were significantly different from the mean score obtained from the sample of healthy controls. These results clearly indicate that both cocaine addiction and alcoholism negatively affect the attentional functions of processing speed and incidental memory as assessed by the SDMT.

Rothlind et al. [78] investigated the effect of alcohol consumption on neurocognitive function in patients with human immunodeficiency virus (HIV). Authors conclude that active heavy alcohol use may have additive adverse effects on NP function with HIV infection. These synergistic effects may be observed in cases of very heavy active alcohol use. Additionally, these authors postulate, starting from these results, that heavy drinking, associated with executive functioning, may be mediating abnormal behaviours observed in HIV disease.

Halstead-Retain Trail Making Test (TMT)

The TMT [79, 80] is one of the most widely used neuropsychological tests. As part of the HALSTEAD REITAN NEUROPSYCHOLOGICAL TEST BATTERY [80], it has been included as an instrument in hundreds of research studies. Within the flexible approach to neuropsychological assessment, this instrument has become one of the most widely used today in assessing the brain-behavior relationship [81–83].

Review of the Current State of Knowledge

The differential diagnosis of different types of dementia has been the subject of attention by many authors in the field of neuropsychology [84–86]. In this regard, Munro, Saxton, and Butters [87] studied the TMT performance of three samples of patients with dementia. They studied 11 patients with Alzheimer's disease (AD), 10 patients with dementia caused by alcohol abuse (DA), 29 patients with a history of alcohol abuse but without symptoms of dementia (AA), and 20 healthy controls (HC). The patients were 65–70 years old, with equivalent educational levels.

The results for each of the samples on the TMT were as follows. In Part A of this instrument, Sample AD completed the task in a mean of 74.9 s (sd = 32.09), while Sample DA completed this procedure in 45.7 s (sd = 9.70). Sample AA completed Part A of the TMT in a mean of 44.38 s (sd = 24.05); finally, sample HC completed this task in 32.15 s (sd = 8.95). The results obtained by the different groups of patients and participants in Part A of the TMT indicated that there was a marked difference between patients with Alzheimer's disease and the other samples. Furthermore, according to the authors of this study, the difference obtained between the alcohol-related dementia group and the control sample was also significant.

It is important to note that the standard deviation of the sample of patients with a history of alcohol abuse without the presence of dementia is much larger than that of the sample of patients in whom the etiology of their dementia is a product of alcohol abuse. However, the means do not differ much. The results of this study indicate that patients with Alzheimer's dementia have a much greater degree of dysfunction in visual perception and attention, as measured by Part A of the TMT, which is markedly different from that of patients with other types of dementia or those with severe alcohol abuse without dementia.

In Part B of the TMT, the mean time for the AD sample was 183.86 s (sd = 114.96). The DA sample's mean time to complete this task was 158 s (sd = 88.34). The AA sample was 120 s, while the HC sample completed Part B of the TMT in a mean of 91.15 s (sd = 26.79).

Although there were no statistically significant differences between these groups, it was observed that both samples of patients with dementia performed this task much slower than nondemented patients.

In this sense, the sequencing, inhibitory control, and learning of new series functions required by Part B of the TMT are more dysfunctional in patients with dementia than in those who have not been diagnosed with dementia, even in the presence of a history of alcohol abuse.

The TMT was also used by Goldstein et al. [74] in their study of neuropsychological functioning in cocaine abusers and alcoholics reported earlier in this chapter. According to the results, it is observed that the alcoholic sample performed this task much slower than the control sample and even more than the cocaine-dependent sample. The healthy control sample took a lower time to complete Part B of the TMT. Members of the cocaine-dependent sample and the alcoholic sample completed it in a higher time. These results indicate that both cocaine dependence and alcoholism negatively affect executive function, as assessed by Part B of the TMT.

Day et al. [88] examined the effects of acute and chronic alcohol use on TMT performance in a sample of underage alcohol consumers. This study involved a sample of 56 male alcohol consumers with a mean age of 19.39 years. The mean age of onset of alcohol use was 15.16 years, and the mean duration of alcohol use was 4.23 years. Another sample of 35 women who were also alcohol consumers participated in this study. This sample had a mean age of 19.34 years, and their mean age of onset of alcohol use was 15.46 years. The mean duration of alcohol use for this sample was 3.89 years. As with the male sample, these women began drinking before the age of majority.

The TMT was administered to both samples of participants. No differences were observed in completing neither Part A nor Part B of this instrument between males and females. No differences were observed in the difference of time completing Part B minus time completing Part A.

However, the scores obtained by these samples on the TMT correlated significantly with the number of years of alcohol consumption, with the breath alcohol concentration, and with a measure of the level of alcohol consumption.

Conclusions

Based on the results of the research studies reviewed in this chapter, there is no doubt that alcohol abuse has a detrimental effect on brain function. The higher brain functions adversely affected by this deleterious effect are attention, verbal and spatial memory processes, immediate and delayed memory, visual construction practice, verbal fluency, and executive functions. Conducting a neuropsychological evaluation of any patient with AAD is an essential component of a comprehensive clinical evaluation.

References

1. Nehring SM, Chen RJ, Freeman AM. Alcohol use disorder [Internet]. StatPearls; 2024. Available from: http://www.ncbi.nlm.nih.gov/pubmed/30439814
2. Mercer M, Stimpfel AW, Dickson VV. Psychosocial factors associated with alcohol use among nurses: an integrative review. J Nurs Regul. 2023;13(4):5–20.
3. Randolph C. RBANS repeatable battery for the assessment of neuropsychological status. San Antonio: PsyCorp; 1998.
4. Randolph C. RBANS UPDATE repeatable battery for the assessment of neuropsychological status. San Antonio: PsyCorp; 2012.
5. Kelley BJ, Bratt R, Lobue C. Using RBANS to characterize cognitive treatment response in autoimmune encephalopathy. Clin Neurol Neurosurg [Internet]. 2022;222:107438. Available from: https://linkinghub.elsevier.com/retrieve/pii/S0303846722003195
6. Duff K, Suhrie KR, Hammers DB, Dixon AM, King JB, Koppelmans V, et al. Repeatable battery for the assessment of neuropsychological status and its relationship to biomarkers of Alzheimer's disease. Clin Neuropsychol [Internet]. 2023;37(1):157–73. Available from: https://www.tandfonline.com/doi/full/10.1080/13854046.2021.1995050
7. Shura RD, Brearly TW, Rowland JA, Martindale SL, Miskey HM, Duff K. RBANS validity indices: a systematic review and meta-analysis. Neuropsychol Rev [Internet]. 2018;28(3):269–84. Available from: http://link.springer.com/10.1007/s11065-018-9377-5
8. Hart RP, Gibson DP, Bean MK, Fisher RA. Effects of illness severity and alcohol use on cognition in end stage liver disease after controlling for general intelligence and mood-cognition in end stage liver disease. Int J Clin Med [Internet]. 2012;03(02):125–31. Available from: http://www.scirp.org/journal/doi.aspx?DOI=10.4236/ijcm.2012.32025
9. Brown P, Heirene RM, Gareth-Roderique-Davies JB, Evans JJ. Applicability of the ACE-III and RBANS cognitive tests for the detection of alcohol-related brain damage. Front Psychol [Internet]. 2019;10. Available from: https://www.frontiersin.org/article/10.3389/fpsyg.2019.02636/full
10. Folstein MF, Folstein SE, McHugh PR, Fangiang G. MMSE Examen Cognoscitivo Mini-Mental. Madrid. TEA Ediciones, S.A; 2002.
11. Folstein MF, Folstein SE, McHugh PR, Fanjiang G. Mini-mental status examination. Odessa: Psychological Assessment Resources; 2001.
12. Folstein MF, Folstein SE, McHugh PR. Mini-mental state. J Psychiatr Res [Internet]. 1975;12(3):189–98. Available from: https://linkinghub.elsevier.com/retrieve/pii/0022395675900266
13. Ismail Z, Rajji TK, Shulman KI. Brief cognitive screening instruments: an update. Int J Geriatr Psychiatry [Internet]. 2010;25(2):111–20. Available from: https://onlinelibrary.wiley.com/doi/10.1002/gps.2306
14. Arevalo-Rodriguez I, Smailagic N, Roqué-Figuls M, Ciapponi A, Sanchez-Perez E, Giannakou A, et al. Mini-mental state examination (MMSE) for the early detection of dementia in people with mild cognitive impairment (MCI). Cochrane Database Syst Rev [Internet]. 2021;2021(7) Available from: http://doi.wiley.com/10.1002/14651858.CD010783.pub3
15. Santiago-Bravo G, Sudo FK, Assunção N, Drummond C, Mattos P. Dementia screening in Brazil: a systematic review of normative data for the mini-mental state examination. Clinics [Internet]. 2019;74:e971. Available from: https://linkinghub.elsevier.com/retrieve/pii/S1807593222006925
16. Ros-Cucurull E, Palma-Álvarez RF, Cardona-Rubira C, García-Raboso E, Jacas C, Grau-López L, et al. Alcohol use disorder and cognitive impairment in old age patients: a 6 months follow-up study in an outpatient unit in Barcelona. Psychiatry Res [Internet]. 2018;261:361–6. Available from: https://linkinghub.elsevier.com/retrieve/pii/S0165178117315548
17. Verdejo-Garcia A, Rezapour T, Giddens E, Khojasteh Zonoozi A, Rafei P, Berry J, et al. Cognitive training and remediation interventions for substance use disorders: a Delphi consensus study. Addiction [Internet]. 2023;118(5):935–51. Available from: https://onlinelibrary.wiley.com/doi/10.1111/add.16109
18. Wang Y, Zhao Y, Nie H, Liu C, Chen J. Disrupted brain network efficiency and decreased functional connectivity in multi-sensory modality regions in male patients with alcohol use disorder. Front Hum Neurosci [Internet]. 2018;12. Available from: https://www.frontiersin.org/article/10.3389/fnhum.2018.00513/full
19. Wang G, Li DY, Vance DE, Li W. Alcohol use disorder as a risk factor for cognitive impairment. J Alzheimer's Dis [Internet]. 2023;94(3):899–907. Available from: https://www.medra.org/servlet/aliasResolver?alias=iospress&doi=10.3233/JAD-230181
20. Rey A. L'examen clinique en psychologie. París: Presses Universitaires de France; 1964.
21. Schmidt M. Rey auditory verbal learning test: a handbook. Los Angeles: Western Psychological Service; 1996.
22. Strauss E, Sherman EMS, Spreen O. A compendium of neuropsychological tests. 3rd ed. New York: Oxford University Press; 2006.
23. Boake C. Édouard Claparède and the auditory verbal learning test. J Clin Exp Neuropsychol [Internet]. 2000;22(2):286–92. Available from: https://www.tandfonline.com/doi/full/10.1076/1380-3395%28200004%2922%3A2%3B1-1%3BFT286

24. Frydecka D, Beszłej JA, Gościmski P, Kiejna A, Misiak B. Profiling cognitive impairment in treatment-resistant schizophrenia patients. Psychiatry Res [Internet]. 2016;235:133–8. Available from: https://linkinghub.elsevier.com/retrieve/pii/S0165178115306958
25. Gibbs A, Andrewes DG, Szmukler G, Mulhall B, Bowden SC. Early HIV-related neuropsychological impairment: relationship to stage of viral infection. J Clin Exp Neuropsychol [Internet]. 1990;12(5):766–80. Available from: https://www.tandfonline.com/doi/full/10.1080/01688639008401018
26. Callahan CD, Johnstone B. The clinical utility of the Rey auditory-verbal learning test in medical rehabilitation. J Clin Psychol Med Settings [Internet]. 1994;1(3):261–8. Available from: http://link.springer.com/10.1007/BF01989627
27. Dawidowicz L, Ash E, Korczyn AD, Andelman F, Levy S, Elkana O. Can the RAVLT predict deterioration from MCI to dementia? Data from long term follow up. Exp Aging Res. 2021;47(4):347–56.
28. Moradi E, Hallikainen I, Hänninen T, Tohka J. Rey's auditory verbal learning test scores can be predicted from whole brain MRI in Alzheimer's disease. Neuroimage Clin. 2017;13:415–27.
29. Hammers DB, Spencer RJ, Apostolova LG. Validation of and demographically adjusted normative data for the learning ratio derived from the RAVLT in robustly intact older adults. Arch Clin Neuropsychol [Internet]. 2022;37(5):981–93. Available from: https://academic.oup.com/acn/article/37/5/981/6529048
30. Moritz S, Irshaid S, Lüdtke T, Schäfer I, Hauschildt M, Lipp M. Neurocognitive functioning in alcohol use disorder: cognitive test results do not tell the whole story. Eur Addict Res [Internet]. 2018;24(5):217–25. Available from: https://www.karger.com/Article/FullText/492160
31. Carbia C, Cadaveira F, Caamaño-Isorna F, Rodríguez-Holguín S, Corral M. Binge drinking during adolescence and young adulthood is associated with deficits in verbal episodic memory. Ryabinin AE, editor. PLoS One [Internet]. 2017;12(2):e0171393. Available from: https://dx.plos.org/10.1371/journal.pone.0171393
32. Ioime L, Guglielmo R, Affini GF, Quatrale M, Martinotti G, Callea A, et al. Neuropsychological performance in alcohol dependent patients: a one-year longitudinal study. Psychiatry Investig. 2018;15(5):505–13.
33. Benton AL, Hamnsher K dS. Multilingual aphasia examination. lowa City: AJA Associates; 1978.
34. Benton AL, Hamsher K dS, Rey HJ, Sivan AB. Multilingual aphasia examination. 3rd ed. Iowa City: AJA Associates; 1994.
35. Gamvrouli M, Gamvrouli I, Triantafyllou C. Evaluation tools of the characteristics of attention deficit and hyperactivity disorder (ADHD) in children and adolescents: A literature review. Psychiatriki [Internet]. 2021; Available from: https://www.psychiatriki-journal.gr/index.php?option=com_content&view=article&id=1700&lang=en
36. Kwak EH, Wi S, Kim M, Pyo S, Shin YK, Oh KJ, et al. Factors affecting cognition and emotion in patients with traumatic brain injury. NeuroRehabilitation [Internet]. 2020;46(3):369–79. Available from: https://www.medra.org/servlet/aliasResolver?alias=iospress&doi=10.3233/NRE-192893
37. Blume AW, Schmaling KB, Marlatt GA. Memory, executive cognitive function, and readiness to change drinking behavior. Addict Behav [Internet]. 2005;30(2):301–14. Available from: https://linkinghub.elsevier.com/retrieve/pii/S0306460304001911
38. Lim K, Kim J, Lee H, Yoo J, Kim HS, Kim C, et al. COWAT performance of persons with Alzheimer dementia, vascular dementia, and Parkinson disease dementia according to stage of cognitive impairment. PM&R [Internet]. 2019;11(7):737–44. Available from: https://onlinelibrary.wiley.com/doi/10.1002/pmrj.12125
39. Bauer K, Malek-Ahmadi M. Meta-analysis of Controlled Oral Word Association Test (COWAT) FAS performance in amnestic mild cognitive impairment and cognitively unimpaired older adults. Appl Neuropsychol Adult [Internet]. 2023;30(4):424–30. Available from: https://www.tandfonline.com/doi/full/10.1080/23279095.2021.1952590
40. Brand M, Kalbe E, Fujiwara E, Huber M, Markowitsch HJ. Cognitive estimation in patients with probable Alzheimer's disease and alcoholic Korsakoff patients. Neuropsychologia [Internet]. 2003;41(5):575–84. Available from: https://linkinghub.elsevier.com/retrieve/pii/S0028393202001835
41. Asensio S, Morales JL, Senabre I, Romero MJ, Beltran MA, Flores-Bellver M, et al. Magnetic resonance imaging structural alterations in brain of alcohol abusers and its association with impulsivity. Addict Biol [Internet]. 2016;21(4):962–71. Available from: https://onlinelibrary.wiley.com/doi/10.1111/adb.12257
42. Lee Y, Kim C, Suk KT, Choi HC, Bang CS, Yoon JH, et al. Differences in cognitive function between patients with viral and alcoholic compensated liver cirrhosis. Metab Brain Dis. 2016;31(2):369–76.
43. Berg EA. A simple objective technique for measuring flexibility in thinking. J Gen Psychol [Internet]. 1948;39(1):15–22. Available from: http://www.tandfonline.com/doi/abs/10.1080/00221309.1948.9918159
44. Grant DA, Berg E. A behavioral analysis of degree of reinforcement and ease of shifting to new responses in a Weigl-type card-sorting problem. J Exp Psychol [Internet]. 1948;38(4):404–11. Available from: http://doi.apa.org/getdoi.cfm?doi=10.1037/h0059831
45. Walsh K, Darby D. Neuropsychology: a clinical approach. 4th ed. Edinburg: Churchill Livingstone; 1999.
46. Heaton RK. Wisconsin card sorting test manual. Odessa: Psychological Assessment Resources; 1991.

47. Heaton RK, Chelune GJ, Talley JL, Kay GG, Curtiss G. Wisconsin Card Sorting Test manual. Revised and expanded. Odessa: Psychological Assessment Resources; 1993.
48. Steinke A, Kopp B. Toward a computational neuropsychology of cognitive flexibility. Brain Sci [Internet]. 2020;10(12):1000. Available from: https://www.mdpi.com/2076-3425/10/12/1000
49. Kopp B, Lange F, Steinke A. The reliability of the Wisconsin Card Sorting Test in clinical practice. Assessment [Internet]. 2021;28(1):248–63. Available from: http://journals.sagepub.com/doi/10.1177/1073191119866257
50. Martínez MV, Manoiloff LV. Evaluación europsicológica de la Función Ejecutiva en Adolescentes con Diferentes Patrones de Consumo de Alcohol. Rev Argent Cienc Comport [Internet] 2010;2:14–23. Available from: www.psyche.unc.edu.ar/racc
51. Maharjan S, Amjad Z, Abaza A, Vasavada AM, Sadhu A, Valencia C, et al. Executive dysfunction in patients with alcohol use disorder: a systematic review. Cureus [Internet]. 2022; Available from: https://www.cureus.com/articles/109740-executive-dysfunction-in-patients-with-alcohol-use-disorder-a-systematic-review
52. Powell A, Sumnall H, Kullu C, Owens L, Montgomery C. Subjective executive function deficits in hazardous alcohol drinkers. J Psychopharmacol [Internet]. 2021;35(11):1375–85. Available from: http://journals.sagepub.com/doi/10.1177/02698811211032605
53. Lees B, Meredith LR, Kirkland AE, Bryant BE, Squeglia LM. Effect of alcohol use on the adolescent brain and behavior. Pharmacol Biochem Behav [Internet]. 2020;192:172906. Available from: https://linkinghub.elsevier.com/retrieve/pii/S0091305719306021
54. dos Santos Rigoni M, Quarti Irigaray T, Duarte de Moraes JF, Ferrao Y, da Silva Oliveira M. Desempeño neuropsicológico y características sociodemográficas en pacientes alcohólicos en tratamiento. Adicciones [Internet]. 2014;26(3):221–9. Available from: https://www.redalyc.org/articulo.oa?id=289132251003
55. Golden CJ. STROOP: Test de Colores y Palabras. Madrid: TEA Ediciones, S.A; 2001.
56. Golden CJ, Freshwater SM. The Stroop Color and Word Test: a manual for clinical and experimental uses. Chicago: Stoelting Co; 2002.
57. Golden CJ. STROOP. Test de Colores y Palabras-Edición Revisada (B. Ruiz-Fernández, T. Luque y F. Sánchez-Sánchez, adaptadores). Madrid: TEA Ediciones; 2020.
58. Stroop JR. Studies of interference in serial verbal reactions. J Exp Psychol. 1935;18(6):643–62.
59. Connor PD, Sampson PD, Bookstein FL, Barr HM, Streissguth AP. Direct and indirect effects of prenatal alcohol damage on executive function. Dev Neuropsychol [Internet]. 2000;18(3):331–54. Available from: http://www.tandfonline.com/doi/abs/10.1207/S1532694204Connor
60. Rey A. Test de Copie et de Reproduction de Memoire de Figures Géometriques Complexes. París: Les Edicions du Centre de Psysichologie Appliquée; 1959.
61. Rey A. Test de Copia y Reproducción de Memoria de Figuras Complejas (8ª Edición). Madrid: TEA Ediciones, S.A.; 2003.
62. Meyers JE, Meyers KR. Rey complex figure test and recognition trial. Odessa: Psychological Assessment Resources; 1995.
63. Sullivan EV, Fama R, Rosenbloom MJ, Pfefferbaum A. A profile of neuropsychological deficits in alcoholic women. Neuropsychology [Internet]. 2002;16(1):74–83. Available from: http://doi.apa.org/getdoi.cfm?doi=10.1037/0894-4105.16.1.74
64. Beck AT, Steer RA. Beck depression Inventory manual. San Antonio: Psychological Corporation; 1993.
65. Mistarz N, Andersen K, Nielsen AS, Goudriaan AE, Michel TM, Skøt L, et al. Pharmacological enhancing agents targeting cognition in patients with alcohol-induced neurocognitive disorders: a systematic review. Neurosci Biobehav Rev [Internet]. 2021;125:608–26. Available from: https://linkinghub.elsevier.com/retrieve/pii/S0149763421000981
66. Maillard A, Laniepce A, Cabé N, Boudehent C, Chételat G, Urso L, et al. Temporal cognitive and brain changes in Korsakoff syndrome. Neurol Int. 2021;96(15) Available from: https://www.neurology.org/doi/10.1212/WNL.0000000000011749
67. van Dongen LCM, Wingbermühle E, van der Veld WM, Vermeulen K, Bos-Roubos AG, Ockeloen CW, et al. Exploring the behavioral and cognitive phenotype of KBG syndrome. Genes Brain Behav [Internet]. 2019;18(4) Available from: https://onlinelibrary.wiley.com/doi/10.1111/gbb.12553
68. El Haj M, Ndobo A, Moustafa AA, Allain P. "What did I tell this sad person?": Memory for emotional destinations in Korsakoff's syndrome. J Clin Med [Internet]. 2023;12(5):1919. Available from: https://www.mdpi.com/2077-0383/12/5/1919
69. Oey MJ, Brouwer VHEW, Buijs MJ, Wijnia JW, Postma A, Oudman E. Unraveling apathy in Korsakoff syndrome patients receiving long-term care with and without cerebrovascular comorbidity. Alcohol Clin Exp Res [Internet]. 2021;45(1):131–9. Available from: https://onlinelibrary.wiley.com/doi/10.1111/acer.14513
70. Fama R, Le Berre A, Hardcastle C, Sassoon SA, Pfefferbaum A, Sullivan EV, et al. Neurological, nutritional and alcohol consumption factors underlie cognitive and motor deficits in chronic alcoholism. Addict Biol [Internet]. 2019;24(2):290–302. Available from: https://onlinelibrary.wiley.com/doi/10.1111/adb.12584
71. Benton AL. Revised visual retention test. 4th ed. New York: The Psychological Corporation; 1974.
72. Benton AL. Test de Retención Visual de Benton: Manual (5ª Edición Revisada). Madrid: TEA Ediciones, S.A.; 2002.

73. Sivan AB. Benton visual retention test. 5th ed. San Antonio: The Psychological Corporation; 1992.
74. Goldstein RZ, Leskovjan AC, Hoff AL, Hitzemann R, Bashan F, Khalsa SS, et al. Severity of neuropsychological impairment in cocaine and alcohol addiction: association with metabolism in the prefrontal cortex. Neuropsychologia [Internet]. 2004;42(11):1447–58. Available from: https://linkinghub.elsevier.com/retrieve/pii/S0028393204000715
75. Smith A. Symbol digit modalities test. Los Angeles: Western Psycho-logical Services; 1973.
76. Smith A. Symbol digit modalities test. Los Angeles: Western Psycho-logical Services; 1982.
77. Smith A. SDMT: Test de Símbolos y Dígitos. Madrid: TEA Ediciones, S.A; 2002.
78. Rothlind JC, Greenfield TM, Bruce AV, Meyerhoff DJ, Flenniken DL, Lindgren JA, et al. Heavy alcohol consumption in individuals with HIV infection: effects on neuropsychological performance. J Int Neuropsychol Soc [Internet]. 2005;11(1):70–83. Available from: https://www.cambridge.org/core/product/identifier/S1355617705050095/type/journal_article
79. Reitan RM. Validity of the trail making test as an indicator of organic brain damage. Percept Mot Skills [Internet]. 1958;8(3):271–6. Available from: http://journals.sagepub.com/doi/10.2466/pms.1958.8.3.271
80. Reitan RM, Wolfson D. The Halstead-Reitan neuropsychological test battery: theory and clinical interpretation. 2nd ed. Tucson: Neuropsychology Press; 1993.
81. Guo Y. A selective review of the ability for variants of the Trail Making Test to assess cognitive impairment. Appl Neuropsychol Adult [Internet]. 2022;29(6):1634–45. Available from: https://www.tandfonline.com/doi/full/10.1080/23279095.2021.1887870
82. Simfukwe C, Youn YC, Kim SY, An SS. Digital trail making test-black and white: Normal vs MCI. Appl Neuropsychol Adult [Internet]. 2022;29(6):1296–303. Available from: https://www.tandfonline.com/doi/full/10.1080/23279095.2021.1871615
83. Llinàs-Reglà J, Vilalta-Franch J, López-Pousa S, Calvó-Perxas L, Torrents Rodas D, Garre-Olmo J. The trail making test: association with other neuropsychological measures and normative values for adults aged 55 years and older from a Spanish-speaking population-based sample. Assessment [Internet]. 2017;24(2):183–96. Available from: http://journals.sagepub.com/doi/10.1177/1073191115602552
84. Sokolovič L, Hofmann MJ, Mohammad N, Kukolja J. Neuropsychological differential diagnosis of Alzheimer's disease and vascular dementia: a systematic review with meta-regressions. Front Aging Neurosci [Internet]. 2023;15. Available from: https://www.frontiersin.org/articles/10.3389/fnagi.2023.1267434/full
85. Weintraub S. Neuropsychological assessment in dementia diagnosis. CONTINUUM [Internet]. 2022;28(3):781–99. Available from: https://journals.lww.com/10.1212/CON.0000000000001135
86. Chan CC, Fage BA, Burton JK, Smailagic N, Gill SS, Herrmann N, et al. Mini-Cog for the diagnosis of Alzheimer's disease dementia and other dementias within a secondary care setting. Cochrane Database Syst Rev [Internet]. 2019; Available from: https://doi.wiley.com/10.1002/14651858.CD011414.pub2
87. Munro C, Saxton J, Butters MA. Alcohol dementia: "cortical" or "subcortical" dementia? Arch Clin Neuropsychol [Internet]. 2001;16(6):523–33. Available from: http://linkinghub.elsevier.com/retrieve/pii/S0887617700000639
88. Day AM, Celio MA, Lisman SA, Johansen GE, Spear LP. Acute and chronic effects of alcohol on trail making test performance among underage drinkers in a field setting. J Stud Alcohol Drugs [Internet]. 2013;74(4):635–41. Available from: https://www.jsad.com/doi/10.15288/jsad.2013.74.635

38 Neurocognitive Effects of Substance Abuse and Their Measurement with Neuropsychological Tests

Norman López, Jorge Herrera, Yuliana Flórez, Cesar Castellanos, and Pascual Ángel Gargiulo

Introduction

The use of psychoactive substances (PAS) has been a complex public health problem for years [1] due to the high mortality risk and the increase in the prevalence of use in the population in recent years [2–4]. In this regard, the consensus of institutions such as the World Health Organization (WHO), the OCP, medical associations and scientific evidence point in an irrefutable direction regarding the harmful effects on the physical and mental health of regular drug use, and especially, more seriously, of PAS [5–9]. Cardiovascular diseases, liver diseases, and cancer [10–12], as well as various mood and personality disorders, constitute a set of clinical conditions that claim human lives every year, affect the quality of life and generate high costs for health systems [13].

The use of opioids, cocaine, amphetamines, and cannabis is included in PAS [4]. Recently, with globalization, the use of new psychoactive substances and illicit drugs (NPS) has increased [14, 15]. As a result of PAS, hallucinogenic effects that alter perception [16, 17] can be generated due to the action of receptor agonists, 5-HT2A of the cerebral cortex, which generates an imbalance at the level of the prefrontal cortex. So, it is expected to find alterations of reality that end up translating into illusions and hallucinations, which later end up affecting the capacity of judgment, reasoning, and distancing the patient from reality [18, 19]. Similarly, PAS can affect the normal functioning of the limbic system, so it is common to find changes in the subjects' mood, behavior, and emotional response [20]. Clinical manifestations have been widely described in the literature [21–25].

N. López
Escuela de Kinesiología, Facultad de Salud, Universidad Santo Tomás, Temuco, Chile

Centro de Investigación en Gerontología Aplicada (CIGAP), Universidad Santo Tomas, Temuco, Chile
e-mail: normanlopezve@santotomas.cl

J. Herrera
College of Medicine Florida International University, University Park, FL, USA

Y. Flórez
Departamento de Ciencias Sociales, Universidad de La Costa, Barranquilla, Colombia
e-mail: yflorez1@cuc.edu.co

C. Castellanos
Instituto Dominicano para el Estudio de la Salud Integral y la Psicología Aplicada (IDESIP), Santo Domingo, República Dominicana

P. Á. Gargiulo (✉)
Laboratory of Neurosciences and Experimental Psychology, Latin American Technological Corporation Foundation (FUCOTEL), Cathedra of Psychopathology, Catholic University of Argentina, Area of Pharmacology, Department of Pathology, National University of Cuyo, CONICET, Guaymallén, Mendoza, Argentina

P. Á. Gargiulo, H. L. Mesones-Arroyo (eds.), *Psychiatry and Neuroscience Update – Vol. V*,
https://doi.org/10.1007/978-3-031-72219-6_38

On the other hand, there are the neurocognitive effects of prolonged and chronic use of licit drugs, such as alcohol or psychoactive substances, which also ultimately produce changes in the nervous system that affect the normal functioning of a range of cognitive processes and human behavior [25]. Therefore, a group of neurocognitive effects associated with substance use will be discussed below, with particular emphasis on illicit substances.

First and foremost are amphetamine stimulants (ATS), which have the potential to produce significant changes in the responsiveness of the brain's cognitive processes, affecting the level of arousal, alertness, and attentional capacity [26, 27]. These are followed by problems with blood circulation and perfusion, which usually increase with the use of amphetamines. They produce an increase in blood pressure, bronchodilation, and abrupt changes in the heart rate [28]. Therefore, it is common that when people consume amphetamines, they end up suffering from cardiovascular and cerebrovascular diseases, coronary difficulties, hyperthermia, and hyperreflexia [29], among others, such as renal and hepatic failure and arrhythmias [30].

Second, there are methamphetamines, one of the most widely used illicit substances in the world [31]. Its use can have structural effects on the amygdala, prefrontal cortex, insula, orbitofrontal cingulate, striatum, and neurochemical substances in the brain that interfere with cognitive functions [32]. Some studies show a weakening of the prefrontal regions, resulting in problems with impulse control, memory deficits due to impaired dopaminergic activity, as well as poor performance in inhibitory control, social cognition, speed of execution, and information processing [33–35].

Another drug with the highest rate of use worldwide is cocaine [36]. Evidence shows that its use can affect the glutamatergic N-methyl-D-aspartate (NMDA) receptors, adrenergic receptors, and opioid receptors. This interferes with information between neurons with the dopaminergic receptor in the nucleus accumbens, the ventral tegmental area, and the prefrontal cortex [37]. Likewise, cocaine use can cause convulsions due to increased serotonergic activity, hallucinations, changes in perception, and changes in judgment [38, 39].

Heroin use has the potential to induce generalized cortical atrophy. Therefore, heroin users, regardless of age, are at an increased risk for generalized brain damage and cognitive impairment [40]. In this regard, Ghosh et al. [41] described persistent deficits in verbal and visual episodic memory in two groups of patients who used heroin intravenously and by inhalation, respectively. Both groups showed changes characteristic of amnestic syndromes, like older adults with dementia. In contrast, healthy controls with the same demographic characteristics showed a good general cognitive status.

Cannabis is perhaps one of the most widely consumed substances in the world [42]. It is composed of several chemicals, including cannabinoids, terpenoids, flavonoids, and alkaloids [43]. However, its use can cause problems with episodic memory, impairing information processing, decision-making, executive function, and performance of various tasks [44]. Duperrouzel et al. [45] reported that subjects who used cannabis had a higher risk of neurocognitive problems and brain-level changes compared to nonusers. In adolescents, cannabis use is associated with increased psychiatric comorbidity and deficits in working memory [46]. Neuroimaging studies show impairments in various prefrontal, limbic, and reward regions due to the dense concentration of cannabinoid receptors [47].

The truth is that the prolonged consumption of cannabinoids and synthetic cannabinoids (SC) can generate various health problems [48] and likewise deteriorate the normal functioning of executive functions and social cognition [49]. In this sense, Elrassas et al., [50] demonstrated the deterioration of several executive functions, such as processing speed, cognitive flexibility and working memory, in synthetic cannabinoid users; all these cognitive capacities are fundamental for the correct adaptive functioning of a person.

Another group of substances that affect brain function and cognitive processes would be integrated by inhalants that generate an effect on neurotransmitters and brain receptors, in particular, gamma-aminobutyric acid (GABA) [39]. As a result, essential changes in brain function occur; some are described as states of euphoria, delirium, tonic-clonic convulsions, memory loss, and sleep disturbances [51–53].

In the same vein, there are synthetic drugs such as lysergic acid diethylamide (LSD) [54]. At the same time, it is true that these psychedelic drugs have emerged as candidates for the treatment of various psychiatric disorders, such as major depression [55] and anxiety disorders [56]. It is a hallucinogenic substance with the potential to be addictive and disrupt brain function [57]. Recently, Bedford et al. [58] examined the effects of LSD on the functional connectivity patterns of a group of users and healthy controls using functional magnetic resonance imaging. The results suggest alterations in the general balance of cortical activity in LSD users, followed by difficulties in the visual connectivity network, supporting the presence of hallucinations and sensory-perceptual problems in this type of patients.

On the other hand, there is a group of substances present in the daily medication of several psychiatric and neurological disorders whose inappropriate or chronic use can cause severe neuropsychological problems. Benzodiazepines in this list, which, when used irresponsibly or chronically, can cause problems with speech, visual-motor coordination, lethargy, induce coma states, cardiorespiratory problems, and even sudden death [59].

Ketamine is another substance that has been used to treat psychiatric disorders, particularly depressive disorders [60]. Recently, its self-prescribed use has skyrocketed due to its hallucinogenic and dissociative properties [61], with severe contraindications for health, functionality, and cognitive performance [62]. In this regard, Zhang et al. [63] conducted a cross-sectional study in patients with depression treated with ketamine, demonstrating a significant pharmacological dependence and cognitive deterioration in patients with depression treated with this drug.

Finally, the use of opioids (OUD) has also skyrocketed in recent years [64] due to their highly addictive properties. Their use can affect several complex cognitive functions, interfering with decision-making, reasoning, and behavioral regulation [65, 66]. A recent study [67] analyzed the neuropsychological performance of a group of subjects, opioid users, patients who had recently completed the rehabilitation process for this substance, and healthy controls. The results were conclusive, showing a more significant deterioration in attention and executive processes and greater cognitive and motor impulsivity in the users, followed to a lesser extent by the recently referred patients, showing differences with the healthy controls. These results point in the direction of greater deterioration in executive functioning and cognitive sequelae in opiate users. It is, therefore, important to stop substance use quickly, as there is a high risk of addiction and neurocognitive effects that may persist over time [68] despite recovery or rehabilitation [69].

A major challenge in substance use clinics has been the objective measurement of effects on cognition. Over the past 20 years, lesional neuroimaging techniques and a variety of tests have been used to demonstrate the interrelationships between different cognitive processes and their neuroanatomical and neurophysiological correlates [70, 71]. As a result, several neuropsychological instruments were initially developed to detect cognitive deficits present in various disorders and diseases [72, 73], and they have demonstrated diagnostic utility in detecting neurocognitive alterations related to substance abuse and substance use disorders [74]. Therefore, the most used instruments are listed below, along with the supporting evidence. Details of the studies in which they have been used, along with the results obtained, are provided to objectify neuropsychological alterations in patients with substance use disorders.

Benton Revised Visual Retention Test (RBVRT)

Developed by A.L. Benton [75, 76], it is a neuropsychological test that assesses visuospatial processing, visual memory, visuoconstructive abilities, and visual and verbal conceptualization. It is useful for assessing sustained attention, perseverative endurance, immediate visual-spatial memory, and visual constructional practice [76, 77]. Two different types of scores are typically derived from the RBVRT. The first is the number of errors in reproducing geometric drawings presented to the patient. The second type of score is derived from the number of correct reproductions of the 10 different drawing sheets presented to patients [76, 78].

In a study conducted in the United States, Goldstein et al. [79] examined the severity of neuropsychological disturbances in cocaine and alcohol abusers and their relationship to frontal lobe metabolism. This study included 42 cocaine abusers, 40 alcoholics, and 72 healthy controls with a mean age of 40.7 years. The mean duration of addiction in this sample was 10.5 years (sd = 5.6). A review of these results showed that the alcoholic sample performed worse on this task than the healthy controls. Chronic and abusive alcohol consumption showed a detrimental effect on the attentional practice and visuoconstructive tasks of the RBVRT.

On the other hand, Ekanand and Ezhil Rajan [80] in India conducted a study in which they examined the inhibitory capacity to cognitive interference in cannabis users and healthy subjects aged 12–21 years. Both groups administered the Stroop test [81] and the RBVRT [77]. Lower inhibition and visual retention were observed in the cannabis users. Other studies have used the Benton Visual Retention Test, demonstrating its ability to detect neurocognitive changes due to substance use [79, 82–84].

Mini-Mental State Examination (MMSE)

The MMSE is a neuropsychological screening test originally developed by Dr. Folstein [85] to assess the mental status of psychiatric patients and the effectiveness of pharmacological treatment. Subsequently, it was recognized as a practical screening test to assess different cognitive domains involved in cognitive impairment and dementia. The MMSE takes utmost 10 min to administer. The original version consists of 30 questions divided into 10 sections that assess spatial and temporal orientation, attention, concentration, memory, abstraction, language, visuospatial perception, and ability to follow instructions. It is the most widely used screening instrument in the world to assess mental status [86]. Several cut-off scores have been proposed in the literature to detect cognitive impairment, but one of the most widely accepted is ≤24 points [87, 88].

Recently, the MMSE was used to assess cognitive performance in Brazilian adults with alcohol, crack, and polydrug use disorders [89]. It was found that those who consumed alcohol and also had a low level of education scored low on the instrument. In addition, they had a higher risk of suffering from cognitive impairment. Similarly, Shakeri et al. [90] used the MMSE to study a group of 202 cases and controls between the ages of 20 and 50. Opiate and methamphetamine users had low scores on the Orientation, Attention, and Altered Mental State subscales compared to healthy controls.

On the other hand, in Spain, Ros-Cucurull et al. [91] used the MMSE to evaluate the mental state of a sample of cases and controls, alcohol consumers over 70 years of age with the same level of education. The results were conclusive, showing that older alcoholics had a worse general mental state. This picture has been confirmed in other studies [92–96].

The Frontal Assessment Battery (FAB)

The FAB [97], developed by B. Dubois, is a neurocognitive test that evaluates executive functions. It is useful for detecting disexecutive changes associated with frontal lobe dysfunction as well as frontotemporal dementia. It includes six subtests to evaluate cognitive domains: (a) similarities (conceptualization); (b) lexical fluency (mental flexibility); (c) motor series (Luria test); (d) contradictory instructions; (e) GO-NO-GO; and (f) grasping behavior. The FAB is scored on a scale of 0 to 3, with a maximum score of 18. In its original version, the test was designed to detect frontotemporal dementia. However, it has been used in cases of frontal lobe dysfunction, executive dysfunction, and cognitive dysfunction [97, 98].

Fontes et al. [99] used the FAB to assess cognitive function in 107 abstinent cannabis users in Brazil compared with a group of 44 healthy subjects. The mean age of the users was 29.88 years. They found poor performance on the FAB, together with alterations in executive function in the group of users. Another study [100] analyzed the effectiveness of the FAB in detecting cognitive changes in a group of drug-dependent individuals during the abstinence period compared to healthy individuals with similar demographic characteristics. Low test performance was observed in the case group. Therefore, the FAB is another useful neuropsychological tool for the detection of general or specific cognitive changes in subjects who consume alcohol or other substances [99–101].

The Montreal Cognitive Assessment (MoCA)

After the MMSE, the MoCA became one of the world's best-known and most widely used mental status tests [102–104]. It is a screening test used in outpatient general neurology and neuropsychology consultations; it consists of seven cognitive domains: executive function, visuospatial ability, attention, concentration, working memory, language, abstract reasoning, memory, and orientation. It was developed by Ziad S. Nasreddine et al. It takes approximately 10 min to complete. It is scored out of a maximum of 30 points, adjusting +1 point if the participant has less than 13 years of education. A score ≤25 would indicate mild cognitive impairment [102].

Brujinen et al. [105] used the MoCA to assess the prevalence of cognitive impairment in a group of 656 middle-aged (40 years) patients using alcohol, cannabis, stimulants, and opioids in the Netherlands. Alcohol and cannabis were the most used substances. A prevalence of cognitive impairment of 31% was found in the studied population. Lower values were found in those who used cannabis. In Norway, Sømhovd et al. [106] used the MoCA to assess cognitive function and adherence to treatment in 132 substance users with an average age of 32 years. The results were striking, as they found a significant percentage of executive changes, and a higher risk of treatment discontinuation was observed in those who scored below the cut-off of the test compared with users who scored above the cut-off of the MoCA.

The fact is that there is a growing body of evidence in favor of MoCA for the assessment of cognitive performance in drug and alcohol users [93, 107–110].

The Neuropsychological Assessment Battery-Screening Module (S-NAB)

It is a screening battery used by clinicians and researchers to assess adults between 18 and 97, designed by Robert A. Stern and Travis White. It has an average administration time of 35 and 5 min for scoring. It provides information on cognitive domains such as attention, memory (immediate verbal and visual memory), visuospatial, language, and executive functions [111].

The S-NAB test differs from the original version, the Neuropsychological Assessment Battery (NAB), in duration and administration. In addition to being shorter to administer, it allows for a broad and comprehensive assessment of cognitive function [111]. A similar battery is the MicroCog Short Form [112], which assesses the same cognitive domains. However, this test is computerized, self-administered, and can take up to 1 h to complete [112, 113].

Cannizarro et al. [114] evaluated the clinical utility of the S-NAB to identify cognitive changes in cocaine users in New York City. However, 145 adults aged 45 years with a mean age of first cocaine use of 21.6 years were assessed. Forty-four percent of the subjects performed poorly on the test and met clinical criteria for substance use-related neurocognitive disorders [115].

In the same city, 10 years ago, Grohman and Fals-Stewart [116] analyzed the effectiveness of an adapted version of the instrument. They used the Neuropsychological Assessment Battery-Screening Module (NAB-SM) to detect cognitive impairment in young adults (30 years old), substance abusers in detoxification, and detoxified subjects. Both groups underwent 6 months of rehabilitation treatment. The levels of agreement and diagnostic efficiency of the battery were high, demonstrating that the NAB-SM can discriminate the cognitive status of substance abusers from that of recovering people with an addiction.

The Stroop Color and Word Test (STROOP)

Created by John Ridley Stroop [117], it is a test that assesses the ability to resist distraction or inhibitory control. It consists of three tasks: reading a set of words; then, identifying and reading some colors; finally, reading the color of some words printed in different colors, where the subject must read aloud the color of each word, avoiding reading the word. For example, the word "red" is written in blue ink. This last test is used to determine the degree of cognitive impairment. The Stroop test has been shown to be useful in assessing selective attention, inhibitory control, and processing speed [81, 118, 119].

In Saudi Arabia, Zahrani and Elsayed [120] applied the Stroop test to 154 young adults who were opioid, amphetamine, and alcohol users to determine the relationship between executive functions, mainly inhibitory control, and substance use disorders. It was demonstrated that the group of drug addicts had a greater and significant tendency to act impulsively without considering the consequences, with poor cognitive and behavioral control, compared to the healthy control group. In addition, this poor cognitive performance was found to be associated with substance use.

In another study focusing on patients with Korsakoff's syndrome due to chronic alcohol use, Brand et al. [121] used an adapted version of the Stroop for the German population. In a case-control study, they evaluated 41 patients diagnosed with Korsakoff's syndrome and 39 healthy controls with no history of neurological or psychiatric involvement. The subjects were between 50 and 59 years old and highly educated. The Stroop interference task, also known as the word color task, could identify and discriminate the neurocognitive changes associated with the frontal lobe atrophies described in the clinical case group. In the same vein, the available evidence suggests that [122–127].

Repeatable Battery for Assessment of Neuropsychological Status (RBANS)

The RBANS is used to assess the neuropsychological status of patients; it was designed by Chris Randolph to be administered individually to adults between the ages of 20 and 89. It is a rapid test that takes no more than 30 min to administer and includes 12 subtests: List Learning, Story Memory, Picture Copying, Line Orientation, Digit Span, Encoding, Picture Naming, Semantic Fluency, List Recall, List Recognition, Story Recall, and Picture Recall [128]. This instrument is widely used to detect dementia and neurocognitive changes and to monitor various disorders; it has also shown great utility in detecting cognitive changes in substance abusers [129–131].

In this regard, Hart et al. [132] analyzed the RBANS in a sample of North American patients with end-stage liver disease associated with a history of alcohol use. They included 108 subjects awaiting liver transplantation for diagnoses such as hepatitis, alcoholic cirrhosis, cryptogenic sarcoidosis, and biliary cirrhosis. The mean age of the patients with alcohol abuse was 81.2 years. The results showed that patients with end-stage liver disease scored low on all RBANS indices. Specific deficits were observed in the test's immediate and delayed memory processes.

In the United Kingdom, Brow et al. [133] investigated the usefulness of the RBANS for the detection of alcohol-induced brain damage. They assessed 30 subjects aged 46 years who were occasional drinkers and 28 with a history of chronic alcohol use. The latter showed symptoms of alcohol-related brain damage, with a mean age of 56.29 years. The differences between the two samples in the RBANS total standard score and the five indices were highly significant in favor of the occasional drinker group. In this regard, the available evidence has established a direct relationship between brain damage caused by excessive alcohol consumption [134], causing impairment in several higher brain functions, such as attention, immediate and delayed memory, language, and spatial and constructional orientation capacity. In addition, the ability of the RBANS as a neuropsychological tool to detect brain damage caused by excessive alcohol consumption has been highlighted.

Rey Auditory Verbal Learning Test (RAVLT)

It is an instrument for assessing auditory memory and learning ability. It was created by André Rey [135] and consists of a list of 15 words that the subjects must listen to and then recall from memory 5 times. It is accompanied by a list of interfering words and then recall the previous list of words. This instrument is handy for discriminating between groups of neurological and nonneurological patients, including patients with severe psychiatric disorders [136].

In Germany, Moritz et al. [137] compared the neurocognitive profile of a sample of patients with alcohol use disorder (AUD) to healthy controls (HC) with no history of alcohol abuse. They included 15 patients diagnosed with AUD with a mean age of 52.33 years and a mean education of 9.54 years versus 20 healthy controls with a mean age of 47.55 years and a mean education of 11.15 years. The results of this study indicate the presence of alterations in auditory verbal episodic memory functions assessed by the RAVLT in patients with alcohol use disorder [138].

Solowij et al. [139] investigated the long-term effects of cannabis and alcohol use on memory using the RAVLT. They studied 181 adolescents and young adults and found worse memory performance in the cannabis group, followed by the alcohol group. Of course, the healthy controls had better scores on the test. In addition, they described the degree of memory impairment, finding a solid association between cannabis and alcohol users from an early age, compromising functional autonomy and memory. In this vein, Goldstein et al. [79] examined the severity of neuropsychological alterations in cocaine and alcohol abusers and their relationship to frontal lobe metabolism. They studied a large sample of middle-aged Americans (40–45 years). They found that chronic and abusive use of alcohol and cocaine, in addition to accelerated cortical atrophy, was manifested by problem-solving the RAVLT test.

Rey–Osterrieth Complex Figure Test (ROCFT)

This instrument was created by André Rey. It consists of reproducing a drawing, observing the original image, and reproducing it from memory. The ROCFT is commonly used to assess visual construction practice when patients are asked to copy the figure and as a measure of visual-spatial memory when they are asked to reproduce it from memory at different time intervals [135, 140]. In addition, it is a useful tool for measuring several cognitive domains, such as attention, visuospatial memory and visuoconstructive abilities, planning, and organization [141]. It has been widely recognized as a test sensitive to right frontotemporal brain lesions associated with coordinating and managing visual, spatial, and constructional information [142–144].

In Brazil, dos Santos Rigoni et al. [145] studied the neuropsychological performance of this test in a sample of alcoholics undergoing treatment. They included 101 cases and 31 healthy controls of middle age (43 years) and education (13 years). The patients reported their daily alcohol consumption. The results of the study showed serious difficulties in the planning and execution of the ROCFT copying and memory task.

In the same vein, Brand et al. [121] compared the performance of a sample of patients with Korsakoff's syndrome associated with alcohol consumption with that of a sample of healthy controls using the ROCFT. The results of this study confirmed that not only the memory processes are negatively affected by Korsakoff's syndrome caused by chronic alcohol consumption, but also the visual constructional practice functions necessary for the performance of the ROCFT copy administration, as well as visual-spatial memory processes.

Mohamed and Elsayed [120] analyzed the relationship between substance use disorders and executive functions. They evaluated 154 patients in three consumption groups: opioids, amphetamines, and alcohol. They found neurological deficits at the level of the dorsolateral and anterior prefrontal cortex, together with poor test performance in alcoholics and, to a greater extent, in substance users.

Symbol Digit Modalities Test (SDMT)

The SDMT [146, 147] is one of the most useful and widely used neuropsychological instruments in the scientific literature. Aaron Smith had developed it, which has been shown to contribute significantly to identifying organicity in psychiatric and neurological patients. This instrument has two forms of administration: written and oral. The written administration of this instrument is typically used to assess visual association processes, visuomotor processing speed, and incidental memory. In contrast, the oral administration measures incidental memory and nominative language function. Both versions of the same test provide insight into the state of attentional processes of concentration and efficient execution [148, 149].

Rothlind et al. [150] investigated the effect of alcohol consumption on neurocognitive function in patients with human immunodeficiency virus (HIV). However, 270 subjects were assessed with the SDMT, divided into four groups: a first group of 72 HIV-positive patients with low alcohol consumption; a second group of 70 HIV-negative patients with high alcohol consumption, 70 HIV-positive patients with low alcohol consumption and 56 subjects with high alcohol consumption. On average, the participants were between 40 and 44 years old and had 15 years of education. The results showed that the combination of seropositivity and high alcohol consumption produced the lowest score, even compared to the sample of seropositive subjects with low alcohol consumption.

Trail Making Test Halstead-Reitan (TMT)

Developed by Ralph Reitan [151, 152], the TMT consists structurally of two elements: Part A, in which the subject must connect 25 dots in numerical order in the shortest possible time, and Part B, in which the subject must sequence numbers and letters (1-A-2-B...) without lifting the pencil and in the shortest possible time. The average test time is 35 s per item, and the total time to complete the TMT is between 5 and 30 min. The TMT is one of the most widely used neuropsychological tests in the world and has been used extensively in many studies where it is needed to assess visual attention, cognitive flexibility, task switching, and other executive functioning abilities [153, 154].

Roberts and Macneill Horton [155] in the United States used the TMT to analyze the neurocognitive effects of drug abuse in a group of patients in a rehabilitation program. They included 8.521 subjects of legal age. The results showed performance below the population average. These results suggest that the TMT is proper as a screening measure to detect dysexecutive disturbances in individuals with substance use disorders who are in treatment [156, 157].

Munro, Saxton, and Butters [158] examined TMT performance in three samples of older adults with and without dementia. They studied 11 patients with Alzheimer's disease, 10 patients with dementia caused by alcohol abuse, and 29 patients with a history of alcohol abuse but without symptoms of dementia, and healthy controls. The results were very striking since the impairment of executive functions was found to be worse in patients with Alzheimer's disease, followed by subjects with dementia related to chronic alcohol consumption, which was much higher compared to healthy controls but not so much compared to participants with a history of alcohol consumption but without dementia.

Wisconsin Card Sorting Test (WCST)

The WCST, originally developed by David A. Grant and Esta A. Berg, is a neuropsychological test that measures cognitive flexibility. It was originally developed as a more valid and reliable assessment of organicity in psychiatric and neurological patients [159, 160]. It consists of a series of colored and shaped cards that the subject must classify according to a criterion set by the examiner, which changes without warning as the test progresses [161].

Faustino et al. [162] evaluated the sensitivity and specificity of the WCST in 587 participants, including subjects with substance disorders and cognitive deficits and a group of subjects without cognitive impairment. They were divided into four groups: opioid users on methadone maintenance, opioid users in treatment, alcohol users in a therapeutic community, and a group of healthy subjects. The results showed adequate discriminant validity, suggesting that frontal lobe function and cognitive flexibility may be impaired by alcohol and drug use [163, 164].

On the other hand, Woicik et al. [165] analyzed perseverative behavior in substance users and nonusers using the WCST. In addition, relationships between perseveration and factors such as drug use, verbal learning, memory, trait inhibitory control, motivational state, and urinary status were examined. And 107 healthy subjects and 107 cocaine users were included. The results showed a more significant deterioration of cognitive functions in the latter group. In this regard, the available evidence points in the same direction as the results [166–169].

Conclusion

We may conclude that there is a wide repertoire of tests and batteries to be used in PAS use and abuse. Each test allows to identify specific dysfunctions induced by different agents. These procedures make possible an objective measure of brain functional problems. Its use should be generalized not only for research but also for everyday clinical activity.

References

1. Krendl AC, Perry BL. Stigma toward substance dependence: causes, consequences, and potential interventions. Psychol Sci Public Interest. 2023;24(2):90–126. https://doi.org/10.1177/15291006231198193.
2. Peacock A, Hall W, Degenhardt L. Epidemiology of substance use internationally. Cham: Springer; 2019. p. 19–36. https://doi.org/10.1007/978-3-030-00627-3_2.
3. Domingues LP, Bedendo A, Opaleye ES, Noto AR. Drug use and substance use disorders in Brazil and the world: epidemiological data. In: Drugs and human behavior: biopsychosocial aspects of psychotropic substances use. Springer; 2021. p. 27–38. https://doi.org/10.1007/978-3-030-62855-0_2/COVER.
4. Shen J, Hua G, Li C, Liu S, Liu L, Jiao J. Prevalence, incidence, deaths, and disability-adjusted life-years of drug use disorders for 204 countries and territories during the past 30 years. Asian J Psychiatr. 2023;86:103677. https://doi.org/10.1016/j.ajp.2023.103677.
5. Volkow ND, Blanco C. Substance use disorders: a comprehensive update of classification, epidemiology, neurobiology, clinical aspects, treatment and prevention. World Psychiatry. 2023;22(2):203–29. https://doi.org/10.1002/wps.21073.
6. Hefner K, Valentine G, Sofuoglu M. Electronic cigarettes and mental illness: reviewing the evidence for help and harm among those with psychiatric and substance use disorders. Am J Addict. 2017;26(4):306–15. https://doi.org/10.1111/ajad.12504.
7. Brady KT, Sinha R. Co-occurring mental and substance use disorders: the neurobiological effects of chronic stress. Am J Psychiatry. 2005;162(8):1483–93. https://doi.org/10.1176/appi.ajp.162.8.1483.
8. Pan American Health Organization [PAHO]. [Internet]. Substance use. Available from: https://www.paho.org/en/topics/substance-use

9. World Health Organization. Drug use epidemiology in Latin America and the Caribbean: a public health approach. Washington, DC: Pan American Health Organization; 2009.
10. Stein MD. Medical consequences of substance abuse. Psychiatr Clin N Am. 1999;22(2):351–70. https://doi.org/10.1016/S0193-953X(05)70081-2.
11. Rehm J. The risks associated with alcohol use and alcoholism. Alcohol Res Health. 2011;34(2):135–43.
12. Furlanello F, Serdoz LV, De Ambroggi L, Cappato R. Drug abuse in cardiovascular diseases. In: Drug abuse and addiction in medical illness. Springer: New York; 2012. https://doi.org/10.1007/978-1-4614-3375-0_32.
13. Martini F, Fregna L, Bosia M, Perrozzi G, Cavallaro R. Substance-related disorders. In: Fundamentals of psychiatry for health care professionals. Cham: Springer; 2022. https://doi.org/10.1007/978-3-031-07715-9_9.
14. Onaolapo OJ, Olofinnade AT, Ojo FO, Adeleye O, Falade J, Onaolapo AY. Substance use and substance use disorders in Africa: an epidemiological approach to the review of existing literature. World J Psychiatry. 2022;12(10):1268–86. https://doi.org/10.5498/wjp.v12.i10.1268.
15. Mohr ALA, Logan BK, Fogarty MF, Krotulski AJ, Papsun DM, Kacinko SL, et al. Reports of adverse events associated with use of novel psychoactive substances, 2017–2020: A review. J Anal Toxicol. 2022;46(6):e116–85. https://doi.org/10.1093/jat/bkac023.
16. Raj P, Rauniyar S, Sapkale B. Psychedelic drugs or hallucinogens: exploring their medicinal potential. Cureus. 2023;15(11):e48719. https://doi.org/10.7759/cureus.48719.
17. Martinotti G, Santacroce R, Pettorruso M, Montemitro C, Spano MC, Lorusso M, et al. Hallucinogen persisting perception disorder: etiology, clinical features, and therapeutic perspectives. Brain Sci. 2018;8(3). https://doi.org/10.3390/brainsci8030047.
18. Fiorentini A, Cantù F, Crisanti C, Cereda G, Oldani L, Brambilla P. Substance-induced psychoses: an updated literature review. Front Psychiatry. 2021:12. https://doi.org/10.3389/fpsyt.2021.694863.
19. Murray BP, Kiernan EA. Physiologic effects of substance use. Emerg Med Clin North Am. 2024;42(1):69–91. https://doi.org/10.1016/j.emc.2023.06.022.
20. Jones SA, Del Giacco AC, Barnes SJ, Nagel BJ. Adolescent substance use is associated with altered brain response during processing of negative emotional stimuli. J Stud Alcohol Drugs. 2022; https://doi.org/10.15288/jsad.22-00143.
21. Hansell S, White HR. Adolescent drug use, psychological distress, and physical symptoms. J Health Soc Behav. 1991;32(3):288. https://doi.org/10.2307/2136809.
22. Tschann JM, Adler NE, Irwin CE, Millstein SG, Turner RA, Kegeles SM. Initiation of substance use in early adolescence: the roles of pubertal timing and emotional distress. Health Psychol. 1994;13(4):326–33. https://doi.org/10.1037/0278-6133.13.4.326.
23. Otto MW, Powers MB, Fischmann D. Emotional exposure in the treatment of substance use disorders: conceptual model, evidence, and future directions. Clin Psychol Rev. 2005;25(6):824–39. https://doi.org/10.1016/j.cpr.2005.05.002.
24. Schweinhart A, Aramburú C, Bauer R, Simons-Rudolph A, Atwood K, Luseno WK. Changes in mental health, emotional distress, and substance use affecting women experiencing violence and their service providers during COVID-19 in a U.S. southern state. Int J Environ Res Public Health. 2023;20(4):2896. https://doi.org/10.3390/ijerph20042896.
25. Fosnocht AQ, Briand LA. Substance use modulates stress reactivity: behavioral and physiological outcomes. Physiol Behav. 2016;166:32–42. https://doi.org/10.1016/j.physbeh.2016.02.024.
26. Berman S, O'Neill J, Fears S, Bartzokis G, London ED. Abuse of amphetamines and structural abnormalities in the brain. Ann N Y Acad Sci. 2008;1141(1):195–220. https://doi.org/10.1196/annals.1441.031.
27. Salo R, Nordahl TE, Natsuaki Y, Leamon MH, Galloway GP, Waters C, et al. Attentional control and brain metabolite levels in methamphetamine abusers. Biol Psychiatry. 2007;61(11):1272–80. https://doi.org/10.1016/j.biopsych.2006.07.031.
28. Ciccarone D, Shoptaw S. Understanding stimulant use and use disorders in a new era. Med Clin North Am. 2022;106(1):81–97. https://doi.org/10.1016/j.mcna.2021.08.010.
29. Schep LJ, Slaughter RJ, Beasley DMG. The clinical toxicology of metamfetamine. Clin Toxicol. 2010;48(7):675–94. https://doi.org/10.3109/15563650.2010.516752.
30. Kevil CG, Goeders NE, Woolard MD, Bhuiyan MS, Dominic P, Kolluru GK, et al. Methamphetamine use and cardiovascular disease. Arterioscler Thromb Vasc Biol. 2019;39(9):1739–46. https://doi.org/10.1161/ATVBAHA.119.312461.
31. St. Peters MM, CHJ P, Turner A, Guerin AA, Kim JH. Past and current drug repurposing clinical trials to treat cognition in methamphetamine use: a scoping review of pharmacotherapy candidates. Addict Neurosci. 2023;5:100064. https://doi.org/10.1016/j.addicn.2023.100064.
32. Zhou Y, Yang WFZ, Wu Q, Ma Y, Zhou J, Ren H, et al. Altered spontaneous neurological activity in methamphetamine use disorders and its association with cognitive function. Asian J Psychiatr. 2024;94:103936. https://doi.org/10.1016/j.ajp.2024.103936.
33. Bari A, Robbins TW. Inhibition and impulsivity: behavioral and neural basis of response control. Prog Neurobiol. 2013;108:44–79. https://doi.org/10.1016/j.pneurobio.2013.06.005.

34. Serra M, Simola N, Pollack AE, Costa G. Brain dysfunctions and neurotoxicity induced by psychostimulants in experimental models and humans: an overview of recent findings. Neural Regen Res. 2024;19(9):1908–18. https://doi.org/10.4103/1673-5374.390971.
35. Fernández Ruiz PA, Cruz-Zúñiga N, Hernández Vergara CI, Martínez Alvarado JR, Chávez Flores YV, Magallanes-Rodríguez AG. Desempeño cognitivo durante la abstinencia de metanfetaminas. Horizon Interdiscipl J. 2023;1(2):42–57. https://doi.org/10.56935/hij.v1i2.18.
36. Stephenson RJ, Toth I. Anti-cocaine vaccine development: where are we now and where are we going? J Med Chem. 2023;66(11):7086–100. https://doi.org/10.1021/acs.jmedchem.3c00366.
37. Roque Bravo R, Faria AC, Brito-da-Costa AM, Carmo H, Mladěnka P, Dias da Silva D, et al. Cocaine: an updated overview on chemistry, detection, biokinetics, and pharmacotoxicological aspects including abuse pattern. Toxins (Basel). 2022;14(4):278. https://doi.org/10.3390/toxins14040278.
38. Pacifici R, Pichini S, Pellegrini M, Berretta P. Pharmacotoxicology of substances of abuse. In: Clinical and laboratory medicine textbook. Cham: Springer; 2023. https://doi.org/10.1007/978-3-031-24958-7_53.
39. Ciucă Anghel D-M, Nițescu GV, Tiron A-T, Guțu CM, Baconi DL. Understanding the mechanisms of action and effects of drugs of abuse. Molecules. 2023;28(13):4969. https://doi.org/10.3390/molecules28134969.
40. Tolomeo S, Steele JD, Ekhtiari H, Baldacchino A. Chronic heroin use disorder and the brain: current evidence and future implications. Prog Neuro-Psychopharmacol Biol Psychiatry. 2021;111:110148. https://doi.org/10.1016/j.pnpbp.2020.110148.
41. Ghosh A, Peyot M-L, Leung YH, Ravenelle F, Madiraju SRM, Prentki M. A peripherally restricted cannabinoid-1 receptor inverse agonist promotes insulin secretion and protects from cytokine toxicity in human pancreatic islets. Eur J Pharmacol. 2023;944:175589. https://doi.org/10.1016/j.ejphar.2023.175589.
42. Langa S, Magwaza LS, Mditshwa A, Tesfay SZ. Characterization of cannabis varieties and the intrinsic and extrinsic factors affecting cannabis germination and seedling establishment: A descriptive review. Ind Crop Prod. 2024;208:117861. https://doi.org/10.1016/j.indcrop.2023.117861.
43. Figueiredo PR, Tolomeo S, Steele JD, Baldacchino A. Neurocognitive consequences of chronic cannabis use: a systematic review and meta-analysis. Neurosci Biobehav Rev. 2020;108:358–69. https://doi.org/10.1016/j.neubiorev.2019.10.014.
44. Selamoglu A, Langley C, Crean R, Savulich G, Cormack F, Sahakian BJ, et al. Neuropsychological performance in young adults with cannabis use disorder. J Psychopharmacol. 2021;35(11):1349–55. https://doi.org/10.1177/02698811211050548.
45. Duperrouzel JC, Granja K, Pacheco-Colón I, Gonzalez R. Adverse effects of cannabis use on neurocognitive functioning: A systematic review of meta- analytic studies. J Dual Diagn. 2020;16(1):43–57. https://doi.org/10.1080/15504263.2019.1626030.
46. Sultan AA, Mio M, Dimick MK, Zou Y, Karthikeyan S, Kolla N, et al. Association of cannabis use with neurocognition in adolescents with bipolar disorder. J Psychopharmacol. 2023;37(9):920–7. https://doi.org/10.1177/02698811231187128.
47. Crane NA, Wade NE. Cannabis and neuropsychology. In: APA handbook of neuropsychology, Volume 1: neurobehavioral disorders and conditions: accepted science and open questions, vol. 1. Washington, DC: American Psychological Association; 2023. https://doi.org/10.1037/0000307-029.
48. Roque-Bravo R, Silva RS, Malheiro RF, Carmo H, Carvalho F, da Silva DD, et al. Synthetic cannabinoids: A pharmacological and toxicological overview. Annu Rev Pharmacol Toxicol. 2023;63(1):187–209. https://doi.org/10.1146/annurev-pharmtox-031122-113758.
49. Sainz-Cort A, Jimenez-Garrido D, Muñoz-Marron E, Viejo-Sobera R, Heeroma J, Bouso JC. The effects of cannabidiol and δ-9-tetrahydrocannabinol in social cognition: A naturalistic controlled study. Cannabis Cannabinoid Res. 2024;9(1):230–40. https://doi.org/10.1089/can.2022.0037.
50. Elrassas HH, Elsayed YAR, Abdeen MS, Mohamed AT, El Nagar ZM. Synthetic cannabinoids impact on cognitive functions. Egypt J Neurol Psychiatr Neurosurg. 2023;59(1):151. https://doi.org/10.1186/s41983-023-00756-x.
51. Salloum IM, Stewart CM, Abou-Saleh MT. Disorders due to substance use: inhalants. In: Tasman's psychiatry. Cham: Springer; 2023. https://doi.org/10.1007/978-3-030-42825-9_162-1.
52. Goodwin GJ, Gates-Woodyatt JJ, Salva CE, Allen DN. Substance use and impulse control disorders. In: Clinical neuropsychology: A pocket handbook for assessment. 4th ed. Washington: American Psychological Association; 2024. https://doi.org/10.1037/0000383-023.
53. Radparvar S. The clinical assessment and treatment of inhalant abuse. Perm J. 2023;27(2):99–109. https://doi.org/10.7812/TPP/22.164.
54. Correia B, Fernandes J, Botica MJ, Ferreira C, Quintas A. Novel psychoactive substances: the Razor's edge between Therapeutical potential and psychoactive recreational misuse. Medicines. 2022;9(3):19. https://doi.org/10.3390/medicines9030019.
55. Goodwin GM, Aaronson ST, Alvarez O, Arden PC, Baker A, Bennett JC, et al. Single-dose psilocybin for a treatment-resistant episode of major depression. N Engl J Med. 2022;387(18):1637–48. https://doi.org/10.1056/NEJMoa2206443.

56. Nutt D, Carhart-Harris R. The current status of psychedelics in psychiatry. JAMA Psychiatry. 2021;78(2):121. https://doi.org/10.1001/jamapsychiatry.2020.2171.
57. American Addiction Centers. [Internet]. What are synthetic drugs? Chemical research drugs. Available from: https://americanaddictioncenters.org/synthetic-drugs (2024)
58. Bedford P, Hauke DJ, Wang Z, Roth V, Nagy-Huber M, Holze F, et al. The effect of lysergic acid diethylamide (LSD) on whole-brain functional and effective connectivity. Neuropsychopharmacology. 2023;48(8):1175–83. https://doi.org/10.1038/s41386-023-01574-8.
59. Robertson S, Peacock EE, Scott R. Benzodiazepine use disorder: common questions and answers. Am Fam Physician. 2023;108(3):260–6.
60. Edinoff AN, Sall S, Koontz CB, Williams AK, Drumgo D, Mouhaffel A, et al. Ketamine evolving clinical roles and potential effects with cognitive, Motor and driving ability. Neurol Int. 2023;15(1):352–61. https://doi.org/10.3390/neurolint15010023.
61. Savić Vujović K, Jotić A, Medić B, Srebro D, Vujović A, Žujović J, et al. Ketamine, an old–new drug: uses and abuses. Pharmaceuticals. 2023;17(1):16. https://doi.org/10.3390/ph17010016.
62. Rybakowski JK, Permoda-Osip A, Bartkowska-Sniatkowska A. Ketamine: its safety, tolerability, and impact on neurocognition. In: Ketamine for treatment-resistant depression. Cham: Springer; 2016. https://doi.org/10.1007/978-3-319-42925-0_5.
63. Zhang C, Zhang B, Xu Y, Hao W, Tang WK. The impact of depressive symptoms on cognitive impairments in chronic ketamine users. Compr Psychiatry. 2024;129:152448. https://doi.org/10.1016/j.comppsych.2023.152448.
64. Castaldelli-Maia JM, Wang Y-P, Brunoni AR, Faro A, Guimarães RA, Lucchetti G, et al. Burden of disease due to amphetamines, cannabis, cocaine, and opioid use disorders in South America, 1990–2019: a systematic analysis of the Global Burden of Disease Study 2019. Lancet Psychiatry. 2023;10(2):85–97. https://doi.org/10.1016/S2215-0366(22)00339-X.
65. Brand M, Rothbauer M, Driessen M, Markowitsch H. Executive functions and risky decision-making in patients with opiate dependence. Drug Alcohol Depend. 2008;97(1–2):64–72. https://doi.org/10.1016/j.drugalcdep.2008.03.017.
66. van Steenbergen H, Eikemo M, Leknes S. The role of the opioid system in decision making and cognitive control: A review. Cogn Affect Behav Neurosci. 2019;19(3):435–58. https://doi.org/10.3758/s13415-019-00710-6.
67. Keleş DB, Bilici R, Ayık B, Kılıç MK, Kliewer W. Comparing attention, impulsivity, and executive functions between patients with opiate use disorder: buprenorphine maintenance treatment versus active users, in comparison with healthy controls. Indian J Psychiatry. 2024;66(1):90–7. https://doi.org/10.4103/indianjpsychiatry.indianjpsychiatry_520_23.
68. Lauvsnes ADF, Hansen TI, Håberg AK, Gråwe RW, Langaas M. Poor response inhibition and symptoms of inattentiveness are core characteristics of lifetime illicit substance use among young adults in the general Norwegian population: the HUNT study. Subst Use Misuse. 2022;57(9):1462–9. https://doi.org/10.1080/10826084.2022.2091788.
69. Cadet JL, Bisagno V. Neuropsychological consequences of chronic drug use: relevance to treatment approaches. Front Psychiatry. 2016:6. https://doi.org/10.3389/fpsyt.2015.00189.
70. Eslinger PJ, Flaherty-Craig CV, Benton AL. Developmental outcomes after early prefrontal cortex damage. Brain Cogn. 2004;55(1):84–103. https://doi.org/10.1016/S0278-2626(03)00281-1.
71. Szameitat AJ, Schubert T, Müller K, von Cramon DY. Localization of executive functions in dual-task performance with fMRI. J Cogn Neurosci. 2002;14(8):1184–99. https://doi.org/10.1162/089892902760807195.
72. López N, Allegri R, Soto-Añari M. Capacidad Diagnóstica y Validación Preliminar del Test del Reloj, Versión de Cacho a la Orden, para Enfermedad de Alzheimer de Grado Leve en Población Chilena. Revista Ecuatoriana de Neurología [Internet]. 2014 [cited 2024 Feb 25];23(3):1–3. Available from: https://revecuatneurol.com/magazine_issue_article/capacidad-diagnostica-validacion-preliminar-test-reloj-alzheimer-poblacion-chilena/
73. Lopez N, Russo M, Véliz A, Martella D, Carnero Pardo C, Allegri RF. Diagnostic accuracy of the phototest for cognitive impairment and dementia in Chile. J Neurol Sci. 2015;357:e230. https://doi.org/10.1016/j.jns.2015.08.791.
74. Stephan RA, Alhassoon OM, Allen KE, Wollman SC, Hall M, Thomas WJ, et al. Meta-analyses of clinical neuropsychological tests of executive dysfunction and impulsivity in alcohol use disorder. Am J Drug Alcohol Abuse. 2017;43(1):24–43. https://doi.org/10.1080/00952990.2016.1206113.
75. Sánchez González JL, Calvo Arenillas JI, Sánchez Rodríguez JL. Efectos del ejercicio físico moderado sobre la cognición en adultos mayores de 60 años. Rev Neurol. 2018;66(07):230. https://doi.org/10.33588/rn.6607.2017449.
76. Benton AL. Test de Retención Visual de Benton: Manual (5ª Edición Revisada). Madrid: TEA Ediciones, S.A.; 2002.
77. Benton AL. Revised visual retention test. 4th ed. New York: The Psychological Corporation; 1974.
78. Sivan AB. Benton visual retention test. 5th ed. San Antonio: The Psychological Corporation; 1992.
79. Goldstein RZ, Leskovjan AC, Hoff AL, Hitzemann R, Bashan F, Khalsa SS, et al. Severity of neuropsychological impairment in cocaine and alcohol addiction: association with metabolism in the prefrontal cortex. Neuropsychologia. 2004;42(11):1447–58. https://doi.org/10.1016/j.neuropsychologia.2004.04.002.

80. Ekanand D, Rajan JE. Visual retention and inhibition of cognitive interference among adolescents with cannabis use. Int J Indian Psychol. 2020;8(1). https://doi.org/10.25215/0801.023.
81. Golden CJ. STROOP: Test de Colores y Palabras. Madrid: TEA Ediciones, S.A; 2001.
82. Amir T, Bahri T. Effect of substance abuse on visuographic function. Percept Mot Skills. 1994;78(1):235–41. https://doi.org/10.2466/pms.1994.78.1.235.
83. Wegner A-J, Fahle M. Alcohol and visual performance. Prog Neuro-Psychopharmacol Biol Psychiatry. 1999;23(3):465–82. https://doi.org/10.1016/S0278-5846(99)00009-3.
84. Penk WE, Roberts WR, Dolan MP, Atkins HG, Robinowitz R, Brown AS. Visual memory of Black and White male heroin and nonheroin drug users. J Abnorm Psychol. 1981;90(5):486–9. https://doi.org/10.1037/0021-843X.90.5.486.
85. Folstein MF, Folstein SE, McHugh PR. "Mini-mental state". A practical method for grading the cognitive state of patients for the clinician. J Psychiatr Res. 1975;12(3):189–98. https://doi.org/10.1016/0022-3956(75)90026-6.
86. Gallegos M, Morgan ML, Cervigni M, Martino P, Murray J, Calandra M, et al. 45 years of the mini-mental state examination (MMSE): A perspective from ibero-america. Dement Neuropsychol. 2022;16(4):384–7. https://doi.org/10.1590/1980-5764-dn-2021-0097.
87. Folstein MF, Folstein SE, McHugh PR, Fangiang G. MMSE Examen Cognoscitivo Mini-Mental. Madrid. TEA Ediciones, S.A. 2002.
88. Folstein MF, Folstein SE, McHugh PR, Fanjiang G. Mini-mental status examination. Odessa: Psychological Assessment Resources; 2001.
89. Schuch JB, Becker N, Rabelo-da-Ponte FD, Ornell F, Freitas HJM, Rebelatto FP, et al. Assessment of cognitive functioning using the mini mental state examination in men with alcohol and crack cocaine use disorder. Trends Psychiatry Psychother. 2023. https://doi.org/10.47626/2237-6089-2022-0567.
90. Shakeri J, Farnia V, Golshani S, Rahami B, Salemi S, Hookari S, et al. Mini mental state examination (MMSE) in substance users and non substance users: A comparison study. J Subst Use. 2021;26(1):67–72. https://doi.org/10.1080/14659891.2020.1779360.
91. Ros-Cucurull E, Palma-Álvarez RF, Cardona-Rubira C, García-Raboso E, Jacas C, Grau-López L, et al. Alcohol use disorder and cognitive impairment in old age patients: a 6 months follow-up study in an outpatient unit in Barcelona. Psychiatry Res. 2018;261:361–6. https://doi.org/10.1016/j.psychres.2017.12.069.
92. Fals-Stewart W. Detection of neuropsychological impairment among substance-abusing patients: accuracy of the neurobehavioral cognitive status examination. Exp Clin Psychopharmacol. 1997;5(3):269–76. https://doi.org/10.1037/1064-1297.5.3.269.
93. Ridley N, Batchelor J, Draper B, Demirkol A, Lintzeris N, Withall A. Cognitive screening in substance users: diagnostic accuracies of the mini-mental state examination, Addenbrooke's cognitive examination–revised, and Montreal cognitive assessment. J Clin Exp Neuropsychol. 2018;40(2):107–22. https://doi.org/10.1080/13803395.2017.1316970.
94. Toledo-Fernández A, Villalobos-Gallegos L, Marín-Navarrete R. Is the mini-mental state examination (MMSE) useful for eligibility screening of research participants with substance use disorder? Rev Int Investig Adicc. 2016;2(1):39–44. https://doi.org/10.28931/riiad.2016.1.06.
95. Manning V, Gomez B, Guo S, Eng Wong K, Assam PN, Shih-Yen Chan E. Senior Research Fellow, National Addictions Management Service, Institute of Mental Health, Singapore; Turning Point 2016;54.
96. Smith KL, Horton NJ, Saitz R, Samet JH. The use of the mini-mental state examination in recruitment for substance abuse research studies. Drug Alcohol Depend. 2006;82(3):231–7. https://doi.org/10.1016/j.drugalcdep.2005.09.012.
97. Dubois B, Slachevsky A, Litvan I, Pillon B. The FAB. A frontal assessment battery at bedside. Neurology. 2000;55(11):1621–6. https://doi.org/10.1212/WNL.55.11.1621.
98. Appollonio I, Leone M, Isella V, Piamarta F, Consoli T, Villa ML, et al. The frontal assessment battery (FAB): normative values in an Italian population sample. Neurol Sci. 2005;26(2):108–16. https://doi.org/10.1007/s10072-005-0443-4.
99. Fontes MA, Bolla KI, Cunha PJ, Almeida PP, Jungerman F, Laranjeira RR, et al. Frontal assessment battery (FAB) is a simple tool for detecting executive deficits in chronic cannabis users. J Clin Exp Neuropsychol. 2011;33(5):523–31. https://doi.org/10.1080/13803395.2010.535505.
100. Cunha PJ, Nicastri S, de Andrade AG, Bolla KI. The frontal assessment battery (FAB) reveals neurocognitive dysfunction in substance-dependent individuals in distinct executive domains: abstract reasoning, motor programming, and cognitive flexibility. Addict Behav. 2010;35(10):875–81. https://doi.org/10.1016/j.addbeh.2010.05.005.
101. Cunha PJ, Novaes MA. Avaliação neurocognitiva no abuso e dependência do álcool: implicações para o tratamento. Rev Bras Psiquiatr. 2004;26(suppl 1):23–7. https://doi.org/10.1590/S1516-44462004000500007.
102. Nasreddine ZS, Phillips NA, Bédirian V, Charbonneau S, Whitehead V, Collin I, et al. The Montreal cognitive assessment, MoCA: A brief screening tool for mild cognitive impairment. J Am Geriatr Soc. 2005;53(4):695–9. https://doi.org/10.1111/j.1532-5415.2005.53221.x.
103. Correa-Naranjo MI, Camargo-Camargo L, Acosta-Camargo L, Ramos-Clason EC, López-Velásquez N. MoCA-T como herramienta de evaluación remota para precisar deterioro cognitivo en paci-

entes con SAHOS moderado a severo. Neurol Argent. 2023;15(1):15–9. https://doi.org/10.1016/j.neuarg.2022.12.001.

104. Montaño-Lozada JM, López N, Espejo-Zapata LM, Soto-Añari M, Ramos-Henderson M, Caldichoury-Obando N, et al. Cognitive changes in patients with epilepsy identified through the MoCA test during neurology outpatient consultation. Epilepsy Behav. 2021;122:108158. https://doi.org/10.1016/j.yebeh.2021.108158.
105. Bruijnen CJWH, Dijkstra BAG, Walvoort SJW, Markus W, VanDerNagel JEL, Kessels RPC, et al. Prevalence of cognitive impairment in patients with substance use disorder. Drug Alcohol Rev. 2019;38(4):435–42. https://doi.org/10.1111/dar.12922.
106. Sømhovd M, Hagen E, Bergly T, Arnevik EA. The Montreal cognitive assessment as a predictor of dropout from residential substance use disorder treatment. Heliyon. 2019;5(3):e01282. https://doi.org/10.1016/j.heliyon.2019.e01282.
107. Copersino ML, Schretlen DJ, Fitzmaurice GM, Lukas SE, Faberman J, Sokoloff J, et al. Effects of cognitive impairment on substance abuse treatment attendance: predictive validation of a brief cognitive screening measure. Am J Drug Alcohol Abuse. 2012;38(3):246–50. https://doi.org/10.3109/00952990.2012.670866.
108. Zaheer R, Ghazal P. Cognitive screening of Pakistani substance-dependent male patients using Montreal cognitive assessment score (MoCA). J Addict Sci. 2020;6(2):37–42. https://doi.org/10.17756/jas.2020-048.
109. Copersino ML, Fals-Stewart W, Fitzmaurice G, Schretlen DJ, Sokoloff J, Weiss RD. Rapid cognitive screening of patients with substance use disorders. Exp Clin Psychopharmacol. 2009;17(5):337–44. https://doi.org/10.1037/a0017260.
110. Marceau EM, Lunn J, Berry J, Kelly PJ, Solowij N. The Montreal cognitive assessment (MoCA) is sensitive to head injury and cognitive impairment in a residential alcohol and other drug therapeutic community. J Subst Abus Treat. 2016;66:30–6. https://doi.org/10.1016/j.jsat.2016.03.002.
111. Stern RA, White T, Lutz FL. Neuropsychological assessment battery: administration, scoring, and interpretation manual. Odessa: Psychological Assessment Resources; 2003.
112. Powell DH, Kaplan EF, Whitla D, Weintraub S, Catlin R, Funkenstein HH. The psychological corporation, editor. Microcog: Assessment of cognitive functioning (Version 2.1). [Computer software]. San Antonio; 1993.
113. Aharonovich E, Hasin DS, Brooks AC, Liu X, Bisaga A, Nunes EV. Cognitive deficits predict low treatment retention in cocaine dependent patients. Drug Alcohol Depend. 2006;81(3):313–22. https://doi.org/10.1016/j.drugalcdep.2005.08.003.
114. Cannizzaro DL, Elliott JC, Stohl M, Hasin DS, Aharonovich E. Neuropsychological assessment battery-screening module (S-NAB): performance in treatment-seeking cocaine users. Am J Drug Alcohol Abuse. 2014;40(6):476–83. https://doi.org/10.3109/00952990.2014.916718.
115. American Psychiatric Association. Diagnostic and statistical manual of mental disorders. American Psychiatric Association; 2013. https://doi.org/10.1176/appi.books.9780890425596.
116. Grohman K, Fals-Stewart W. The detection of cognitive impairment among substance-abusing patients: the accuracy of the neuropsychological assessment battery-screening module. Exp Clin Psychopharmacol. 2004;12(3):200–7. https://doi.org/10.1037/1064-1297.12.3.200.
117. Stroop JR. Studies of interference in serial verbal reactions. J Exp Psychol. 1935;18(6):643–62. https://doi.org/10.1037/h0054651.
118. Golden CJ, Freshwater SM. The Stroop color and word test: A manual for clinical and experimental uses. Chicago: Stoelting Co; 2002.
119. Golden CJ. STROOP. Test de Colores y Palabras-Edición Revisada (B. Ruiz-Fernández, T. Luque y F. Sánchez-Sánchez, adaptadores). Madrid: TEA Ediciones; 2020.
120. Al-Zahrani MA, Elsayed YA. The impacts of substance abuse and dependence on neuropsychological functions in a sample of patients from Saudi Arabia. Behav Brain Funct. 2009;5(1):48. https://doi.org/10.1186/1744-9081-5-48.
121. Brand M, Kalbe E, Fujiwara E, Huber M, Markowitsch HJ. Cognitive estimation in patients with probable Alzheimer's disease and alcoholic Korsakoff patients. Neuropsychologia. 2003;41(5):575–84. https://doi.org/10.1016/S0028-3932(02)00183-5.
122. Connor PD, Sampson PD, Bookstein FL, Barr HM, Streissguth AP. Direct and indirect effects of prenatal alcohol damage on executive function. Dev Neuropsychol. 2000;18(3):331–54. https://doi.org/10.1207/S1532694204Connor.
123. Streeter CC, Terhune DB, Whitfield TH, Gruber S, Sarid-Segal O, Silveri MM, et al. Performance on the Stroop predicts treatment compliance in cocaine-dependent individuals. Neuropsychopharmacology. 2008;33(4):827–36. https://doi.org/10.1038/sj.npp.1301465.
124. Brewer JA, Worhunsky PD, Carroll KM, Rounsaville BJ, Potenza MN. Pretreatment brain activation during Stroop task is associated with outcomes in cocaine-dependent patients. Biol Psychiatry. 2008;64(11):998–1004. https://doi.org/10.1016/j.biopsych.2008.05.024.
125. Silveri MM, Rogowska J, McCaffrey A, Yurgelun-Todd DA. Adolescents at risk for alcohol abuse demonstrate altered frontal lobe activation during Stroop performance. Alcohol Clin Exp Res. 2011;35(2):218–28. https://doi.org/10.1111/j.1530-0277.2010.01337.x.
126. Carpenter KM, Schreiber E, Church S, McDowell D. Drug Stroop performance: relationships with pri-

mary substance of use and treatment outcome in a drug-dependent outpatient sample. Addict Behav. 2006;31(1):174–81. https://doi.org/10.1016/j.addbeh.2005.04.012.
127. Banich MT, Crowley TJ, Thompson LL, Jacobson BL, Liu X, Raymond KM, et al. Brain activation during the Stroop task in adolescents with severe substance and conduct problems: A pilot study. Drug Alcohol Depend. 2007;90(2–3):175–82. https://doi.org/10.1016/j.drugalcdep.2007.03.009.
128. Randolph C, Tierney MC, Mohr E, Chase TN. The repeatable battery for the assessment of neuropsychological status (RBANS): preliminary clinical validity. J Clin Exp Neuropsychol. 1998;20(3):310–9. https://doi.org/10.1076/jcen.20.3.310.823.
129. Zhang XY, Tan Y-L, Chen D-C, Tan S-P, Yang F-D, Zunta-Soares GB, et al. Effects of cigarette smoking and alcohol use on neurocognition and BDNF levels in a Chinese population. Psychopharmacology. 2016;233(3):435–45. https://doi.org/10.1007/s00213-015-4124-6.
130. Cao H, Hou C, Huang S, Zhou X, Yang J, Bin XJ, et al. The evaluation of cognitive impairment in alcohol-dependent patients through RBANS combined with ERPs. Front Psychiatry. 2021:11. https://doi.org/10.3389/fpsyt.2020.598835.
131. Green A, Garrick T, Sheedy D, Blake H, Shores EA, Harper C. The effect of moderate to heavy alcohol consumption on neuropsychological performance as measured by the repeatable battery for the assessment of neuropsychological status. Alcohol Clin Exp Res. 2010;34(3):443–50. https://doi.org/10.1111/j.1530-0277.2009.01108.x.
132. Hart RP, Gibson DP, Bean MK, Fisher RA. Effects of illness severity and alcohol use on cognition in end stage liver disease after controlling for general intelligence and mood-cognition in end stage liver disease. Int J Clin Med. 2012;03(02):125–31. https://doi.org/10.4236/ijcm.2012.32025.
133. Brown P, Heirene RM, Gareth-Roderique-Davies JB, Evans JJ. Applicability of the ACE-III and RBANS cognitive tests for the detection of alcohol-related brain damage. Front Psychol. 2019:10. https://doi.org/10.3389/fpsyg.2019.02636.
134. Wei J, Qin L, Fu Y, Dai Y, Wen Y, Xu S. Long-term consumption of alcohol exacerbates neural lesions by destroying the functional integrity of the blood–brain barrier. Drug Chem Toxicol. 2022;45(1):231–8. https://doi.org/10.1080/01480545.2019.1681444.
135. Rey A. Test de Copie et de Reproduction de Memoire de Figures Géometriques Complexes. París: Les Edicions du Centre de Psysichologie Appliquée; 1959.
136. Frydecka D, Beszłej JA, Gościmski P, Kiejna A, Misiak B. Profiling cognitive impairment in treatment-resistant schizophrenia patients. Psychiatry Res. 2016;235:133–8. https://doi.org/10.1016/j.psychres.2015.11.028.
137. Moritz S, Irshaid S, Lüdtke T, Schäfer I, Hauschildt M, Lipp M. Neurocognitive functioning in alcohol use disorder: cognitive test results do not tell the whole story. Eur Addict Res. 2018;24(5):217–25. https://doi.org/10.1159/000492160.
138. Carbia C, Cadaveira F, Caamaño-Isorna F, Rodríguez-Holguín S, Corral M. Ryabinin AE, editor. Binge drinking during adolescence and young adulthood is associated with deficits in verbal episodic memory. PLoS One. 2017;12(2):e0171393. https://doi.org/10.1371/journal.pone.0171393.
139. Solowij N, Jones KA, Rozman ME, Davis SM, Ciarrochi J, Heaven PCL, et al. Verbal learning and memory in adolescent cannabis users, alcohol users and non-users. Psychopharmacology. 2011;216(1):131–44. https://doi.org/10.1007/s00213-011-2203-x.
140. Rey A. Test de Copia y Reproducción de Memoria de Figuras Complejas. (8ª Edición). Madrid: TEA Ediciones, S.A.; 2003.
141. Meyers JE, Meyers KR. Rey complex figure test and recognition trial. Odessa: Psychological Assessment Resources; 1995.
142. Gainotti G, Ferraccioli M, Quaranta D, Marra C. Cross-modal recognition disorders for persons and other unique entities in a patient with right fronto-temporal degeneration. Cortex. 2008;44(3):238–48. https://doi.org/10.1016/j.cortex.2006.09.001.
143. Sedda A, Passoni S, Bottini G. Perseverations and non-verbal confabulations on the Rey–Osterrieth Complex Figure Test in a fronto-temporal dementia single case study. Neurocase. 2012;18(5):366–76. https://doi.org/10.1080/13554794.2011.608368.
144. Chen H, Pan X, Lau JKL, Bickerton W-L, Pradeep B, Taheri M, et al. Lesion-symptom mapping of a complex figure copy task: A large-scale PCA study of the BCoS trial. Neuroimage Clin. 2016;11:622–34. https://doi.org/10.1016/j.nicl.2016.04.007.
145. dos Santos RM, Quarti Irigaray T, Duarte de Moraes JF, Ferrao Y, da Silva Oliveira M. Desempeño neuropsicológico y características sociodemográficas en pacientes alcohólicos en tratamiento. Adicciones [Internet]. 2014;26(3):221–9. Available from: https://www.redalyc.org/articulo.oa?id=289132251003
146. Smith A. Symbol digit modalities test. Los Angeles: Western Psycho-logical Services; 1982.
147. Smith A. SDMT: Test de Símbolos y Dígitos. Madrid: TEA Ediciones, S.A; 2002.
148. Silva PHR, Spedo CT, Baldassarini CR, Benini CD, Ferreira DA, Barreira AA, et al. Brain functional and effective connectivity underlying the information processing speed assessed by the symbol digit modalities test. NeuroImage. 2019;184:761–70. https://doi.org/10.1016/j.neuroimage.2018.09.080.
149. Sheridan L, Fitzgerald H, Adams K, Nigg J, Martel M, Puttler L, et al. Normative symbol digit modalities test performance in a community-based sample. Arch Clin Neuropsychol. 2006;21(1):23–8. https://doi.org/10.1016/j.acn.2005.07.003.
150. Rothlind JC, Greenfield TM, Bruce AV, Meyerhoff DJ, Flenniken DL, Lindgren JA, et al. Heavy alcohol consumption in individuals with HIV infection:

effects on neuropsychological performance. J Int Neuropsychol Soc. 2005;11(1):70–83. https://doi.org/10.1017/S1355617705050095.
151. Reitan RM. Validity of the trail making test as an indicator of organic brain damage. Percept Mot Skills. 1958;8(3):271–6. https://doi.org/10.2466/pms.1958.8.3.271.
152. Reitan RM, Wolfson D. The Halstead-Reitan neuropsychological test battery: theory and clinical interpretation. 2nd ed. Tucson: Neuropsychology Press; 1993.
153. Waggestad TH, Kirsebom BE, Strobel C, Wallin A, Eckerström M, Fladby T, et al. Improving validity of the trail making test with alphabet support. Front Psychol. 2023:14. https://doi.org/10.3389/fpsyg.2023.1227578.
154. Soukup VM, Ingram F, Grady JJ, Schiess MC. Trail making test: issues in normative data selection. Appl Neuropsychol. 1998;5(2):65–73. https://doi.org/10.1207/s15324826an0502_2.
155. Roberts C, Horton AM. Using the trail making test to screen for cognitive impairment in a drug abuse treatment sample. Int J Neurosci. 2001;109(3–4):273–80. https://doi.org/10.3109/00207450108986538.
156. Eno Lawani R, Tomar S. Executive dysfunction in drug-induced psychosis. Niger J Psychol Res [Internet]. 2022 [cited 2024 Feb 18];18(1):41–8. Available from: https://njpsyresearch.com/ojs3/index.php/njopr/article/view/136
157. Clergue-Duval V, Barré T, Cognat E, Brichet A-L, Géraud C, Azuar J, et al. Patients with severe alcohol-related cognitive impairment improve in flexibility when abstinence is maintained: A comparative study with Alzheimer's disease. Front Psychol. 2022:13. https://doi.org/10.3389/fpsyg.2022.936639.
158. Munro C, Saxton J, Butters MA. Alcohol dementia: "cortical" or "subcortical" dementia? Arch Clin Neuropsychol. 2001;16(6):523–33. https://doi.org/10.1016/S0887-6177(00)00063-9.
159. Berg EA. A simple objective technique for measuring flexibility in thinking. J Gen Psychol. 1948;39(1):15–22. https://doi.org/10.1080/00221309.1948.9918159.
160. Grant DA, Berg E. A behavioral analysis of degree of reinforcement and ease of shifting to new responses in a Weigl-type card-sorting problem. J Exp Psychol. 1948;38(4):404–11. https://doi.org/10.1037/h0059831.
161. Walsh K, Darby D. Neuropsychology: a clinical approach. 4th ed. Edinburg: Churchill Livingstone; 1999.
162. Faustino B, Oliveira J, Lopes P. Diagnostic precision of the Wisconsin card sorting test in assessing cognitive deficits in substance use disorders. Appl Neuropsychol Adult. 2021;28(2):165–72. https://doi.org/10.1080/23279095.2019.1607737.
163. Abdulaal A, El Tantawy A, Ibrahim O, Elbadry H, Hassan H. Cognitive dysfunction in adolescents with substance use disorder. Middle East Curr Psychiatry. 2023;30(1):13. https://doi.org/10.1186/s43045-023-00291-8.
164. Formiga MB, Galdino MKC, Vasconcelos SC, Neves JWJS, da Costa Lima MD. Executive functions and emotion regulation in substance use disorder. J Bras Psiquiatr. 2021;70(3):236–44. https://doi.org/10.1590/0047-2085000000331.
165. Woicik PA, Urban C, Alia-Klein N, Henry A, Maloney T, Telang F, et al. A pattern of perseveration in cocaine addiction may reveal neurocognitive processes implicit in the Wisconsin card sorting test. Neuropsychologia. 2011;49(7):1660–9. https://doi.org/10.1016/j.neuropsychologia.2011.02.037.
166. Grant S, Contoreggi C, London ED. Drug abusers show impaired performance in a laboratory test of decision making. Neuropsychologia. 2000;38(8):1180–7. https://doi.org/10.1016/S0028-3932(99)00158-X.
167. Verdejo-García A, Pérez-García M. Ecological assessment of executive functions in substance dependent individuals. Drug Alcohol Depend. 2007;90(1):48–55. https://doi.org/10.1016/j.drugalcdep.2007.02.010.
168. Dolan SL, Bechara A, Nathan PE. Executive dysfunction as a risk marker for substance abuse: the role of impulsive personality traits. Behav Sci Law. 2008;26(6):799–822. https://doi.org/10.1002/bsl.845.
169. Sullivan EV, Mathalon DH, Zipursky RB, Kersteen-Tucker Z, Knight RT, Pfefferbaum A. Factors of the Wisconsin card sorting test as measures of frontal-lobe function in schizophrenia and in chronic alcoholism. Psychiatry Res. 1993;46(2):175–99. https://doi.org/10.1016/0165-1781(93)90019-D.

Cognitive Dysfunction in Addictions

39

Marcela Waisman Campos and Pablo M. Bagnati

Introduction

A substance use disorder (SUD) is a maladaptive pattern of drug use, involving poor control over consumption activities, social impairment, risk-taking behavior, and pharmacological indicators such as tolerance and withdrawal [1].

This chapter aims to provide a brief review of recent evidence on cognitive factors related to addiction. Clinical observations, conventional wisdom, and well-reasoned theoretical mechanisms, all suggest acute and chronic use of psychoactive substances impair individual cognitive functioning. Neurocognitive assessment of addiction should be employed in daily practice. Early interventions aim to detect prodromal symptoms and provide prompt response to initial stages, as well as adequate adaptation of treatments to cognitive status, given the impact on suboptimal decision-making, poor executive function, and inadequate prioritization of daily goals.

M. Waisman Campos (✉) · P. M. Bagnati
Department of Cognitive Neurology, Neuropsychiatry and Neuropsychology, Instituto de Investigaciones Neurológicas "Raúl Carrea", Fundación para la Lucha contra las Enfermedades Neurológicas de la Infancia (FLENI), Buenos Aires, Argentina
e-mail: pbagnati@fleni.org.ar

The relationship between substance use and cognitive functioning has been known for many years in the case of alcohol, and this last decade has added to our understanding of the cognitive impact for other psychoactive substances. The impact will differ, given the influence of premorbid intellectual functioning, variable consumption patterns, polyconsumption, neuropsychiatric comorbidities, sleep dysfunction, and other pharmacological treatments.

Variations in cognitive development between individuals ultimately affect cognitive reserve and in the face of brain damage or insult, such as that caused by a psychoactive substance, clinical involvement will therefore be variable [2]. Most current research on drug users shows that cognitive changes are observed mainly in attention, memory, and executive functions [3].

Cognition is probably one of the first functions affected in users of psychoactive substances during intoxication. Because effects are reversible, they are often minimized, but later they can persist in early and late abstinence. We know that it is an important predictor of the level of autonomy, adaptation to academic, work and social environments as well as to treatment programs.

Cognitive screening is recommended for all individuals with a SUD. Statements such as "I've drawn a blank," "I don't remember," and "I can't concentrate" represent reversible cognitive states

P. Á. Gargiulo, H. L. Mesones-Arroyo (eds.), *Psychiatry and Neuroscience Update – Vol. V*,
https://doi.org/10.1007/978-3-031-72219-6_39

and are perhaps minimized in degree of severity, but continue to appear depending on level of intoxication, abstinence, single or sustained use (impact depending on accumulation of damage).

In adult rodents, acute administration of alcohol, nicotine, or marijuana alters aspects of learning and memory associated with the frontal cortex and hippocampus [4, 5], indicating that mechanisms responsible for learning and memory are sensitive to these substances. Other animal models confirm that rats show impaired reverse learning after exposure to methamphetamine [6], cocaine [7], alcohol [8], and nicotine [9], indicating decreased cognitive flexibility. Even after prolonged self-administration of cocaine or amphetamines, rats will continue to administer cocaine, even in the presence of a fearful stimulus, indicating abnormal response inhibition [10].

Polysubstance use is most common currently, i.e., combined use of depressants (alcohol, marijuana, benzodiazepines, and opiates) and stimulants (tobacco, cocaine, etc.), in an attempt to recover the physiological brain balance, lost from the beginning of psychoactive substance intake.

Patients start use at crucial stages of development and ensuing cognitive changes may often affect their adaptation to school, to academic and work environments, as well as to treatment programs. The impact is both direct due to neurotoxicity, and also secondary to progressive biopsychosocial decline, with loss of motivations and interests, early dropout from academic and sports-related activities, loss of social contacts as well as increased rates of accidents or injuries, all of which directly impact individual quality of life.

Including a neurocognitive assessment, with the analysis of cognitive phenotype, could be a valuable tool for diagnosis and for patient empowerment of motivation for change [11]. Also, adaptation of program contents to patient cognitive status can improve treatment adherence and efficacy [12].

Cognitive assessment objectives in addictions include the following aspects [13]:

- Identifying preserved functions and specific deficits.
- Determining patient's ability to care for themselves, manage their finances, and assist them in planning their return to work or study.
- Legal medical assessments.
- Selecting and adapting the most appropriate treatment program.
- Objective method to evaluate efficacy of treatments and patient situation, with the aim of preventing relapses.

Good practice recommendations suggest early neuropsychological evaluation in order to characterize drug-induced cognitive phenotypes. It is widely accepted that over 80% of subjects with addictions drop-out of treatment programs in the clinical setting. This may be due to a pattern of anosognosia, or lack of insight, regarding the severity of their own disorder. These aspects of denial are believed to be related to psychological mechanisms as well as to cognitive dysfunction in relation to insight and self-consciousness [14].

Quality of life, as defined by the World Health Organization, is both a subjective and a dynamic concept including physical, cognitive, psychological, social, and spiritual aspects, resulting from the interaction between expectations and current experience, conditioned in turn when starting and persisting in the use of psychoactive substances.

Assessment of Cognitive Functions in Patients with Substance Use Disorders

Neuropsychological assessment in addictions should include two components [15]:

(a) Evaluation of cognitive functioning through a neurocognitive assessment.
(b) Impact of cognitive deficits on daily personal functioning.

One of the issues to be further defined in the coming years is timing of cognitive screening, how long into abstinence should it be performed (to avoid residual effects of intoxication or of drugs used for detox). Options range from 1 week [16], to at least 6 weeks [17]. The general recommendation is to wait at least 30 days, ideally 60 days without substance use to perform the evaluation [13–18].

It is possible that the type of substance is selected with a certain objective in mind: to achieve greater efficiency and/or with less effort; improve social interactions; facilitate sexual behavior; facilitate stress management, self-medication for neuropsychiatric disorders; and/or improve cognitive performance.

Several psychoactive drugs are specifically engineered to enhance cognitive performance. Long-term regular use may induce tolerance for the cognitive effects and even lead to cognitive deficits [19].

Therefore, we may find patients with cognitive dysfunction prior to substance use (attention deficit disorder or mood disorders), or as a result of intoxication, withdrawal syndromes, chronic persistence of consumption, or irreversible damage.

The initial evaluation of a psychoactive substance user should include:

- Clinical neuropsychiatric evaluation, including age at onset, increased intensity, and frequency of use for each substance.
- Neuropsychiatric and neurocognitive battery.
- General clinical evaluation.

Regarding the neurocognitive battery, the Mini-Mental State Examination (MMSE) has been the standard tool used for screening, but it has been found to miss the subtler changes. Therefore, the Addenbrooke's assessment (ACE-R) and/or the Montreal Cognitive Assessment (MoCA) would be more indicated [20], both validated for use in cognitive impairment associated with substance abuse [16].

We still need to advance further in designing a specific battery for cognitive assessment in addictions, to better select useful tests for clinical practice, evaluating the cognitive domains referred to, as well as subprocesses typically altered in addictions.

Some examples include:

- *Processing speed*:
  - Processing speed Index (PVI) Wechsler Adult Intelligence Scale (WAIS-III) [21], consisting in digit-symbol coding and symbol search subtests: measures ability to process visual information rapidly.
  - Execution time for Trail Making Test Form A [22].
  - Alternating verbal fluency task for 1 min, in which the patient is asked to alternately produce a word (not a proper noun) beginning with "p" and with "m" [23].
- *Divided attention*:
  - Trail Making Test B.
  - Stroop test [21].
- *Sustained attention*:
- It refers to the ability to focus on what is relevant while ignoring what is irrelevant, maintaining attentional focus over time. Failures in this domain are demonstrated in lack of concentration, distractions and errors due to inattention, all described in addictions [24].
  - d2 Test. A test used to measure selective attention and concentration, requiring 10 min to complete. It evaluates processing speed, following instructions and execution of a task on discrimination of similar visual stimuli [25].
  - Digit Span Score.
  - Wechsler Adult Intelligence Scale (WAIS IV).
- *Attentional span and central executive function framed in what is called Working Memory.*
  - Reverse order digits and digit sequencing.
  - Wechsler Adult Intelligence Scale (WAIS IV): performance on this test is sensitive to "phonological loop" and "central executive" functioning working memory model [21].
  - Cognitive flexibility and verbal/semantic fluency.
  - Phonological verbal fluency (ability to generate words from a phonological cue: words beginning with a given letter) depends directly on cognitive flexibility.
  - Wisconsin Card Sorting Test (WCST) to assess cognitive flexibility.
  - For the assessment of semantic fluency, the subject can be asked to recall as many animals as possible in 1 min, and for phonological fluency, any words beginning with the letter "p" in 1 min [26].

  - Paced Auditory Serial Addition Test (PASAT) evaluates auditory information processing speed and cognitive flexibility, as well as calculation skills.
- *Decision-making.*
  - Iowa Gambling Task [27].
- *Inhibitory control.*
  - Stroop interference.
  - Five-digit test (5DT): also based on the Stroop interference paradigm, is a test of selective attention and response inhibition. Developed as an alternative to the Stroop test minimizing implications of schooling level in test performance, significantly correlating with equivalent sections [28].
  - Go/no go task, in which the subject must respond by hitting the table once or twice according to conflicting instructions requiring inhibition of motor responses [29].
- *Memory* [30].
  - Immediate and delayed reproduction of Rey Complex Figure Test.
  - WMS-III, logical memory subtest (verbal memory).
  - Rey-Auditory Verbal Learning Test.
- *Theory of Mind.*
  - "The Faux Pas Recognition Test" (version for adults) [31].
  - "Reading the Mind in the Eyes Test" [32].

Classification of Cognitive Impairment Related to Psychoactive Substances Use

Cognitive impairment goes through different stages ranging from normality to varying degrees of reversible and irreversible dementia, and it is common in many neurological and psychiatric pathologies, due to a variety of aetiologies, all of which need to be ruled out.

In DSM-V, 2013, a specific chapter was added on this topic of mild or major neurocognitive disorders due to substance use. In major neurocognitive disorders, there must be evidence of cognitive decline from a previous level in one or more cognitive domains, reported by the patient or informant, preferably documented by standardized neurocognitive tests.

Deficits interfere with independence in activities of daily living (paying bills or treatment adherence). Prior behavioral disturbances need to be specified, and whether current severity is mild, moderate or severe.

In mild neurocognitive impairment, there is evidence of decline in one or more domains, although this does not interfere with independence in daily activities, even when there may be need for greater effort, or for restoring to compensatory or adaptive techniques.

We must rule out that cognitive deficits are not better explained by another mental disorder.

Effects of Psychoactive Substances with Impact on Cognitive Function

Cognitive impact during acute consumption must be differentiated from effects in early and late abstinence, or in chronic consumers. In the last group, there is a window before deficits occur, and in others, possible tolerance develops. We will analyze the main findings for each substance.

Tobacco

In acute consumption, nicotine improves hippocampal-dependent learning [33]. It also appears to improve attention, verbal memory, working memory, and executive function in nonsmokers. These effects are mediated by activation of the cholinergic system, and subsequent effects on dopamine and serotonin release.

The adolescent brain, specifically the hippocampus and the frontal cortex, respond differently to nicotine exposure than the adult brain, generating a persistent attention deficit, a finding supported by findings in rodent animal models. Furthermore, hippocampal-based learning and memory are altered after exposure to nicotine in adolescents long after cessation of drug exposure. Chronic use alters learning when tolerance to nicotine has developed in smokers [34, 35].

Hypothesis of mechanisms involved:

1. Direct cerebral neurotoxicity: tobacco smoke (toxic substances produced) may cause brain toxicity [36].
2. Changes in cerebral blood flow: increases carbon monoxide concentration (combustion gas, cigarettes 2%, pipe 1–3%, and cigar 6%) altering oxygen levels [37–39].
3. Risk of cardiovascular and of chronic obstructive pulmonary disease (COPD): both affecting cognitive function. Smoking has been linked to accelerated brain atrophy, increased white matter lesions and brain hypoperfusion, as well as decreased cortical grey matter density.
4. Even in middle-aged adults, smoking has been linked to cognitive deficit, including reduced psychomotor processing speed and loss of cognitive flexibility [40].
5. Vascular endothelial damage: acting synergistically with increased arterial systolic blood pressure [36–41], doubling the risk of stroke and of haemorrhagic cerebral infarct, increases four-fold in moderate smokers and nine-fold in individuals consuming over 25 cigarettes a day [42].
6. Decreases neurogenesis and increments cell damage. Studies show that exposure to tobacco decreases neurogenesis and promotes glycogenesis in the dentate gyrus of adolescent rats. These effects may play a role in the increased risk for depression and cognitive impairment in adolescent smokers [43].
7. Oxidative stress: tobacco smoke contains large amounts of free radicals and prooxidants, causing oxidative damage to biological macromolecules [38, 44, 45].

Other situations with cognitive impact include passive smoking. In a study that used cotinine as a biomarker, authors showed a significant association with cognitive performance [46], and prenatal exposure to tobacco affects brain development, and can cause cell apoptosis and mitochondrial abnormalities [47].

Alcohol

Alcohol-related brain damage occurs through several pathophysiological processes: direct effects of neuroinflammation, neurodegeneration and oxidative stress, nutritional deficit such as lack of thiamine, along with damage from associated conditions such as liver disease, injury and trauma, and repeated periods of abstinence and intoxication [48].

The impact on intoxication would be related to:

- Inhibition of NMDA-activated ionic currents in the hippocampus [49].
- Inhibition of hippocampal long-term potentiation (LTP) [50].
- Decrease in hippocampal glutamate levels with acute alcohol concentration [51].
- Significant decrease in hippocampal theta rhythm [52].
- Decreased hippocampal expression of immediate early genes such as c-fos after acute intoxication [53].
- In the amygdala, it affects conditioned and emotional memories of fear [54–56]. It produces retrograde facilitation and anterograde impairment of emotional memories. Alcohol facilitates emotional recall of events occurring before intoxication [57]. In other words, it would not be convenient to "drink to forget" as the little prince once said [58].

In vivo and in vitro research in the rodent hippocampus has shown that exposure to ethanol 20 min prior to stimulation completely inhibits or reduces ability to induce long-term potentiation (LTP) [59].

Different studies find impairment in 50–70% of alcohol dependents in the following cognitive functions: visuospatial processing, problem solving, memory and learning ability, and executive function [60, 61]. Deficits tend to improve with sustained abstinence within 3–6 weeks, although certain patients do not experience deficit reversal, but consolidate chronic pathology [62].

Alcoholic dementia is a persistent and progressive disorder, which causes memory impairment and one or more cognitive impairments, such as aphasia, apraxia, agnosia, impaired performance (planning, organization, sequencing, and abstraction), and significant impairment of occupational or social activity. Specific alcohol-derived effects include Wernicke's encephalopathy, Korsakoff's syndrome, Marchiafava-Bignami disease, centropontine myelinolysis, hepatic encephalopathy, and cerebellar atrophy [63].

The association of alcohol use with other disorders remains a problem and is especially important in those with early-onset dementia, for which alcohol is a risk factor in men [64]. Alcohol is the second leading cause of adult dementia in the West, accounting for 10% of cases [65]. In the evaluation of the difference between AUD (alcohol use disorder) with and without Korsakoff, we observed that when Korsakoff is absent, for example, temporospatial orientation and gnosia is preserved, anosognosia is not present and symptoms improve with alcohol cessation [66].

Marihuana

Acute and chronic cannabis use impairs psychomotor function, memory, and attention, often in a dose-dependent manner [67, 68]. Variations in deficits between studies relate to age at onset, number of puffs per cigarette, and inspiration time, which modifies concentration achieved, e.g., different test, different cannabinoid composition, different resilient equipment, etc.

Studies in pubescent rats treated with a cannabinoid agonist showed persistent deficits in performing object recognition tasks, while adult rats did not [69]. Earlier age at onset of cannabis use in humans is associated with greater neuropsychological impairment [70]. The most sensitive periods of development according to preclinical models would be during gestation (dysfunction in excitatory/inhibitory balance, dysregulation of monoaminergic pathway, abnormal stress response) and in adolescence, (where in addition to the above, changes in glial cell activation, desynchronization of prefrontal neuronal cortex networks and excessive synaptic pruning are also added) [71].

Cannabis-induced cognitive deficits emerge from different processes acting together. These processes mainly involve: (i) increased glutamate release in the hippocampus, due to the preferential activation of CB1 receptors on GABAergic interneurons and astrocytes, in turn inducing LTD (long-term depression); (ii) interaction with other neurotransmitter systems involved in the modulation of memory, such as acetylcholine, adenosine, and serotonin; and (iii) decrease in neuronal respiration induced by activation of mitochondrial CB1 receptors, which, in turn, may also affect the previously described pathways. Repeated exposure to cannabis, especially at vulnerable ages, may magnify these effects, eventually leading to decreased LTP, reduction in dendritic spines and efficiency of the neural network circuits in the brain [72].

The development of tolerance to sustained cannabis use might explain why people with a history of heavy cannabis use showed less cognitive impairment after acute challenge with Δ9-THC in some [73] but not all studies [74]. In particular, the degree of tolerance manifested may vary depending on the domain investigated. Therefore, it is likely that tolerance to the effects of cannabis intoxication does not develop uniformly across different domains [75, 76].

Cocaine

Studies on cocaine users direct their interest towards neuronal loss, rate of gray matter loss over the years compared to normal aging, and the subsequent cognitive expression of defects [77]. Accumulation of minor vascular episodes, secondary to either vasospasm or hypertension may also impact neuropsychological findings.

Acute administration of cocaine in users appears to enhance response inhibition as well as the speed component of psychomotor tasks, but only when administered intranasally [78].

Cocaine, amphetamines, nicotine, or opiates can all induce and/or modulate forms of synaptic plasticity, such as LTP and LTD (long-term potentiation and depression) in brain regions known to be involved in addiction, learning, and memory, including the hippocampus, ventral tegmental area (VTA), nucleus accumbens, and the amygdala [79–83].

In a meta-analysis of 46 studies analysing 1452 chronic cocaine users and 1411 controls, findings indicated cocaine users evidenced deficits related to attention, episodic memory, and working memory, with effects of moderate to greater magnitude [84]. Other studies also found deficits in executive functioning, visuoperception, psychomotor speed, and manual dexterity [85, 86].

Another way to look at cognitive impact is through epidemiological studies. These have shown cocaine can increase the risk of being involved in driving accidents [87, 88].

In a metaanalysis by Elvik et al. in 2013, the best estimate of the relative risk of accidental cocaine involvement was 2.96 (95% CI 1.18–7.38) for fatal accidents, 1.66 (95% CI 0.91–3.02) for injury accidents, and 1.44 (95% CI 0.93–2.23) for accidents resulting in property damage [89].

A metaanalytic review indicated that cognitive impairment only improves after 5 months of sustained abstinence [84].

Treatment

Treatment should be based on discontinuation of consumption, to slow down disease progression and give time for altered cognitive function recovery, especially when the patient is young and is in crucial stages of development, such as finishing high school or starting a university career. Benefits of assessing and halting cognitive impairment progression and allowing recovery will impact the future of the individual, as well as of his or her family and environment. Although evidence is limited, provision for cognitive rehabilitation ideally through specialized inpatient services when the addiction is severe and the cognitive impact more significant has been shown to have positive effects on cognitive functioning.

Recommendations for adequate cognitive rehabilitation as part of a comprehensive treatment program can include:

1. Adaptive recommendations: keeping a diary which acts as a cue to memory and can guide future treatment planning; delaying some aspects of treatment until cognitive recovery; simplifying information given at the outset, etc.
2. Choose to withdraw or change medications that also alter cognitive functioning, considering the risk/benefit ratio.

   For example: sodium valproate use could be related to dose-dependent attentional deficits and memory impairment and/or delayed decision-making; topiramate to possible impairment (not clearly dose-related) in global cognitive functioning; benzodiazepines to possible impairment in attention, verbal and nonverbal memory, motor speed, reaction time, and anterograde amnesia [90, 91].
3. Improve patient nutritional status.
4. Starting a physical exercise program. Studies have shown that this increases BDNF: brain-derived neurotrophic factor [92]. For years, studies in patients with alcohol disorders showed that exercise was associated with both cognitive and functional benefits [93].
5. Cognitive rehabilitation: structured sessions with a neuropsychologist or in day hospital or therapeutic community models [94].
6. Psycho-education programs should be included for patients with mental illness before they initiate consumption as well as in special populations [11].
7. Specific procognitive drugs: Pharmacotherapies target cognitive impairments associated with executive control and include cholinesterase inhibitors (e.g., galantamine, rivastigmine) and monoamine transporter inhibitors, e.g., for cocaine addiction (modafinil, methylphenidate). Cognitive behavioral therapy and cognitive rehabilitation also improve executive control, while cognitive bias modification targets impairments associated with automatic processes [95].

Pharmacological treatments that improve cognitive symptoms demonstrate greater efficacy. For example, studies in smokers showed that varenicline was effective in the treatment of cognitive withdrawal symptoms [96]. In another study [97], bupropion, after withdrawal, improved correct response times for working memory and for a measure of sustained attention (numbers, but not letters; $p < 0.05$) compared with placebo. Future studies could examine whether this effect of bupropion contributes to its efficacy for long-term smoking cessation, and develop drugs that facilitate recovery.

8. To have drug treatment in place that improves all aspects related to the perpetuation of active disease, in its three stages such as intoxication, withdrawal, and craving stage [95].

Among the drugs under investigation are:

- For use during the intoxication stage: NK1 antagonists, oxytocin, gabapentin, topiramate, and vaccines.
- For the withdrawal and stress response recovery stage: e KOR antagonists, lofexidine, gabapentin, n-acetylcysteine, topiramate, and vaccines.
- For the preoccupation/anticipation stage, to restore executive control: NK1 antagonists, n-acetylcysteine, modafinil, transcranial magnetic stimulation, and deep brain stimulation [98].

Conclusions

The early approach to them allows an adequate evaluation and collaborates for a better perception of the initial stages—more silent or hidden regarding symptoms—but not from the perspective of progressive signs of disease. Most current research in drug users shows that cognitive changes are observed mainly in attention, memory, and executive function. The cognitive status assessment will enhance effectiveness and decrease bio-psycho-social impact, since it is an important predictor of the level of autonomy and adaptation to academic, work and social environments, as well as to treatment programs. We should increase the assessment of cognitive impact in this mostly young population and adapt treatment models administered to promote adherence, with a more precise knowledge of the real possibilities of these patients.

Both abstinence and treatment should be prolonged, to sustain the cognitive changes achieved and allow rehabilitation and adequate social reintegration.

The cognitive impact of psychotropic drugs to be used should be taken into consideration, although continued use of psychoactive substances will cause deficits to persist and progress, so a risk-benefit analysis needs to be made.

Our study highlights the importance of cognitive assessment in SUD. Impaired patients may not recognize the condition (anosognosia) or minimize it. Inclusion of cognitive evaluation in clinical practice is a tool that not only measures global functioning in patients with SUD, but also may help tailor treatments based on cognitive functioning. For example, high-intensity interval training could be used to reduce illicit drug cravings in individuals with methamphetamine dependence. It can also have a positive effect on cognitive functions, such as memory and executive functions.

Although the study of cognitive phenotypes will lead to better select diagnostic tools in the coming years, a specific cognitive evaluation for SUD patients is still missing. It will also be of interest to determine the functional consequences (social and occupational) of long-term abuse.

Careful review of metaanalyses on psychoactive substance dependence and cognition suggests a number of methodological limitations mostly related to abstinence duration that were present in the majority of studies, which would affect cognitive performances of abusers in the clinical trials.

Assessment of cognitive deficits, as well as the clinical approach to them, is relevant during phases of addiction, treatment, and follow-up, in order to improve clinical outcomes and early referral to a rehabilitation program.

Further research should address identification of specific diagnostic tools suitable for use in clinical practice for individuals SUD, above all for adolescents, in order to tailor early interventions based on cognitive remediation and functional rehabilitation.

References

1. American Psychiatric Association. Diagnostic and statistical manual, DSM V. Washington, DC: American Psychiatric Association Press; 2013.
2. Waisman Campos M, Ale L. Cap 5: Repercusiones cognitivas en usuarios de alcohol. In: Serebrisky D, editor. Trastornos por sustancias. Buenos Aires: Editorial Sciens; 2014.
3. Yucel M, Oldenhof E, Ahmed S et al. Addiction. 2018;114(6):1095–1109.
4. Semenova S, Stolerman IP, Markou A. Chronic nicotine administration improves attention while nicotine withdrawal induces performance deficits in the 5-choice serial reaction time task in rats. Pharmacol Biochem Behav. 2007;87:360–8.
5. Portugal GS, Wilkinson DS, Turner JR, Blendy JA, Gould TJ. Developmental effects of acute, chronic, and withdrawal from chronic nicotine on fear conditioning. Neurobiol Learn Mem. 2012;97: 482–94.
6. Izquierdo A, Belcher AM, Scott L, Cazares VA, Chen J, O'Dell SJ, Malvaez M, et al. Reversal-specific learning impairments after a binge regimen of methamphetamine in rats: possible involvement of striatal dopamine. Neuropsychopharmacology. 2010;35:505–14.
7. Calu DJ, Stalnaker TA, Franz TM, Singh T, Shaham Y, Schoenbaum G. Withdrawal from cocaine self-administration produces long-lasting deficits in orbitofrontal-dependent reversal learning in rats. Learn Mem. 2007;14:325–8.
8. McMurray MS, Amodeo LR, Roitman JD. Effects of voluntary alcohol intake on risk preference and behavioral flexibility during rat adolescence. PLoS One. 2014;9:e100697.
9. Ortega LA, Tracy BA, Gould TJ, Parikh V. Effects of chronic low- and high-dose nicotine on cognitive flexibility in C57BL/6J mice. Behav Brain Res. 2013;238:134–45.
10. Tse MT, Cantor A, Floresco SB. Repeated amphetamine exposure disrupts dopaminergic modulation of amygdala-prefrontal circuitry and cognitive/emotional functioning. J Neurosci. 2011;31:11282–94.
11. Waisman Campos M, Fonseca F. Cap: Trastorno esquizoafectivo y consumo de sustancias. In: Trastorno esquizoafectivo de Benabarre A. Madrid: Ed Panamericana; 2014.
12. Aharonovich E, Hasin DS, Brooks AC, Liu X, Bisaga A, Nunes EV. Cognitive deficits predict low treatment retention in cocaine dependent patients. Drug Alcohol Depend. 2006;81:313–22. https://doi.org/10.1016/j.drugalcdep.2005.08.003.
13. Waisman Campos M. Benabarre A. Adicciones. Madrid: Editorial Panamericana; 2017.
14. Goldstein RZ, Craig ADB, Bechara A, et al. The neurocircuitry of impaired insight in drug addiction. Trends Cogn Sci. 2009;13:372–80.
15. Bagnati P, Allegri R, Kremer J, et al. La evaluación neuropsiquiátrica. In: Semiología neuropsiquiátrica. Buenos Aires: Polemos; 2013. p. 25–32.
16. Copersino ML, Fals-Stewart W, Fitzmaurice G, Schretlen DJ, Sokoloff J, Weiss RD. Rapid cognitive screening of patients with substance use disorders. Exp Clin Psychopharmacol. 2009;17(5):337–44.
17. Walvoort SJ, Wester AJ, Egger JI. The neuropsychology of cognitive functions in alcohol abstinence. Tijdschr Psychiatr. 2013;55(2):101–11.
18. Oslin D, Atkinson RM, Smith DM, Hendrie H. Alcohol related dementia: proposed clinical criteria. Int J Geriatr Psychiatry. 1998;13(4):203–12.
19. Ahmed SH, Badiani A, Miczek KA, Müller CP. Non-pharmacological factors that determine drug use and addiction. Neurosci Biobehav Rev. 2020;110:3–27. https://doi.org/10.1016/j.neubiorev.2018.08.015.
20. Nasreddine ZS, Phillips NA, Bedirian V, et al. The Montreal Cognitive Assessment, MoCA: a brief screening tool for mild cognitive impairment. J Am Geriatr. 2005;53(4):695–9.
21. Wechsler D. WAIS-III. Escala de inteligencia de Wechsler para adultos-III. Madrid: TEA (Edición original); 1997. p. 1999.
22. Lezak MD, Howieson DB, Loring DW, et al. Neuropsychological assessment. 4th ed. New York: Oxford University Press; 2004.
23. Sánchez R, de León JM, Pedrero Pérez EJ, Rojo Mota G, et al. Propuesta de un protocolo para la evaluación neuropsicológica de las adicciones. Rev Neurol. 2011;53:483.
24. Goldstein RZ, Leskovjan AC, Hoff AL, et al. Severity of neuropsychological impairment in cocaine and alcohol addiction: association with metabolism in the prefrontal cortex. Neuropsychologia. 2004;42:1447–58.
25. Brickenkamp R, Zillmer E. The d2 test of attention. Seattle: Hogrefe & Hubber; 1998.
26. Butman J, Allegri R, Harris P, et al. Fluencia verbal en español datos normativos en Argentina. Med B Aires. 2000;60:561–4.
27. Bull PN, Tippett LJ, Addis DR. Decision making in healthy participants on the Iowa Gambling Task: new insights from an operant approach. Front Psychol. 2015;6:391.
28. de Castro Paiva GC, Fialho MB, de Souza Costa D, et al. Ecological validity of the five digit test and the oral trails test. Arq Neuropsiquiatr. 2015;74:29–34.

29. Ruiz Sánchez de León JM, Pedrero Pérez EJ, Rojo Mota G, et al. Propuesta de un protocolo para la evaluación neuropsicológica de las adicciones. Rev Neurol. 2011;53:483.
30. Tang WK, Lau CG, Ungvari GS, et al. Recovery of cognitive functioning following abstinence from ketamine. Addict Behav. 2019;99:106081.
31. Stone VE, Baron-Cohen S, Knight RT. Frontal lobe contributions to theory of mind. J Cogn Neurosci. 1998;10:640–56.
32. Baron-Cohen S, Ring HA, Wheelwright S, et al. Social intelligence in the normal and autistic brain: an fMRI study. Eur J Neurosci. 1999;11:1891–8.
33. Kutlu MG, Gould TJ. Nicotinic receptors, memory, and hippocampus. Curr Top Behav Neurosci. 2015;23:137–63.
34. Mooney-Leber S, Gould T. Review: the long-term cognitive consequences of adolescent exposure to recreational drugs of abuse. Rev Learn Mem. 2018;25(9):481–91. https://doi.org/10.1101/lm.046672.117.
35. Waisman Campos M, Serebrisky D, Mauricio Castaldelli-Maia J. Smoking and cognition. Curr Drug Abuse Rev. 2016;9:76–9.
36. Okusaga O, Stewart MC, Butcher I, Deary I, Fowkes FG, Pirce JF. Smoking, hypercholesterolemia and hypertension as risk factor for cognitive impairment in older adults. Age Ageing. 2013;42(3):306–1.
37. Dolan MC. El envenenamiento por monóxido de carbono. CMAJ. 1985;133(5):392–9.
38. Lorenzo P, Ladero JM, Leza JC, Lizasoain I. Drogodependencias. 3ª edición. Madrid: Ed Panamericana; 2009.
39. DeLorenze GN, Kharrazi M, Kaufman FL, Eskenazi B, Bernert JT. Exposure to environmental tobacco smoke in pregnant women: the association between self-report and serum cotinine. Environ Res. 2002;90(1):21–32.
40. Kalmijn S, et al. Cigarette smoking and alcohol consumption in relation to cognitive performance in middle age. Am J Epidemiol. 2002;156(10):936–44.
41. Shinton R, Beevers G. Meta-analysis of relation between cigarette smoking and stroke. BMJ. 1989;298(6676):789–94. PMID:2496858
42. Wolf PA, D'Agostino RB, Kannel WB, Bonita R, Belanger AJ. Cigarette smoking as a risk factor for stroke. The Framingham study. JAMA. 1988;259(7):1025–9. PMID:3339799
43. Bruijnzeel AW, Bauzo RM, Munikoti V, Rodrick GB, Yamada H, Fornal CA, Ormerod BK, Jacobs BL. Tobacco smoke diminishes neurogenesis and promotes gliogenesis in the dentate gyrus of adolescent rats. Brain Res. 2011;1413:32–42.
44. Pryor WA, Stone K. Oxidants in cigarette smoke. Radicals, hydrogen peroxide, peroxynitrate, and peroxynitrite. Ann N Y Acad Sci. 1993;686:12–27.
45. Waisman Campos M. Cap 6: alteraciones cognitivas en usuarios de tabaco. In: Serebrinsky D, editor. Trastornos por sustancias: tabaco. Madrid: Ed Sciens; 2015.
46. Llewllyn DJ, Lang IA, Langa KM, et al. Exposure to secondhand smoke and cognitive impairment in non-smokers: national cross sectional study with cotinine measurement. BMJ. 2009;338:b462.
47. Cornelius MD, Day NL. The effects of tobacco use during and after pregnancy on exposed children. Alcohol Res Health. 2000;24(4):242–9.
48. Hayes V, Demirkol A, Ridley N, Withall A, Draper B. Alcohol-related cognitive impairment: current trends and future perspectives. Neurodegener Dis Manag. 2016;6(6):509–23.
49. Lovinger DM, White G, Weight FF. NMDA receptor-mediated synaptic excitation selectively inhibited by ethanol in hippocampal slice from adult rat. J Neurosci. 1990;10:1372–9.
50. Zorumski CF, Mennerick S, Izumi Y. Acute and chronic effects of ethanol on learning-related synaptic plasticity. Alcohol. 2014;48:1–17.
51. Shimizu K, Matsubara K, Uezono T, Kimura K, Shiono H. Reduced dorsal hippocampal glutamate release significantly correlates with the spatial memory deficits produced by benzodiazepines and ethanol. Neuroscience. 1998;83:701–6.
52. Zhang Y, Yu H, Li W, Yang Y, Wang X, Qian Z. Effect of acute ethanol administration on the hippocampal region neural activity using a microelectrode array. Alcohol Clin Exp Res. 2016;2016(40):1857–64.
53. Ryabinin AE, Melia KR, Cole M, Bloom FE, Wilson MC. Alcohol selectively attenuates stress-induced c-fos expression in rat hippocampus. J Neurosci. 1995;15:721–30.
54. Gould TJ. Ethanol disrupts fear conditioning in C57BL/6 mice. J Psychopharmacol. 2003;2003(17):77–81.
55. Knowles SK, Duka T. Does alcohol affect memory for emotional and non-emotional experiences in different ways? Behav Pharmacol. 2004;15:111–21.
56. Gulick D, Gould TJ. Interactive effects of ethanol and nicotine on learning in C57BL/6J mice depend on both dose and duration of treatment. Psychopharmacology. 2008;2008(196):483–95.
57. Van Skike CE, Goodlett C, Matthews DB. Acute alcohol and cognition: remembering what it causes us to forget. Alcohol. 2019;2019(79):105–25.
58. Jacob A, Wang P. Alcohol intoxication and cognition: implications on mechanisms and therapeutic strategies. Front Neurosci. 2020;14:102.
59. Ramachandran B, Ahmed S, Zafar N, Dean C. Ethanol inhibits long-term potentiation in hippocampal CA1 neurons, irrespective of lamina and stimulus strength, through neurosteroidogenesis. Hippocampus. 2015;25:106–18.
60. Giancola PR, Moss HB. Executive cognitive functioning in alcohol use disorders. Recent Dev Alcohol. 1998;14:227–51.
61. Smith DM, Atkinson RM. Alcoholism and dementia. Int J Addict. 1995;30:1843–69.
62. Ryan P, Vetreno J, Hall J, Savage L. Alcohol-related amnesia and dementia: animal models have revealed the contributions of different etiological factors

on neuropathology, neurochemical dysfunction and cognitive impairment. Neurobiol Learn Mem. 2011;96(4):596–608.
63. Waisman Campos M. Cap 14 Deterioro cognitivo asociado al consumo de alcohol. In: Alcoholopatias de Sackmann. Ed corpus, Argentina; 2012.
64. Nordstrom P, Nordstrom A, Eriksson M, Wahlund LO, Gustafson Y. Risk factors in late adolescence for young-onset dementia in men: a nationwide cohort study. JAMA Intern Med. 2013;173:1612–8.
65. Luchsinger JA, Tang MX, Siddiqui M, Shea S, Mayeux R. Alcohol intake and risk of dementia. J Am Geriatr Soc. 2004;52:540–6.
66. Alonso M, Stern R. The Oxford handbook of adult cognitive disorders. New York: Oxford University Press; 2019.
67. Broyd SJ, van Hell HH, Beale C, Yücel M, Solowij N. Acute and chronic effects of cannabinoids on human cognition – a systematic review. Biol Psychiatry. 2016;79:557–67.
68. Ramaekers JG, Kauert G, Van Ruitenbeek P, Theunissen EL, Schneider E, Moeller MR. High-potency marijuana impairs executive function and inhibitory motor control. Neuropsychopharmacology. 2006;31:2296–303.
69. Schneider M, Schömig E, Leweke FM. Acute and chronic cannabinoid treatment differentially affects recognition memory and social behavior in pubertal and adult rats. Addict Biol. 2008;13(3–4):3453–7.
70. Fontes MA, Bolla KI, Cunha PJ, et al. Cannabis use before age 15 and subsequent executive functioning. Br J Psychiatry. 2011;198(6):442–7.
71. Testai F, Gorelick MD, Aparicio H, et al. Use of marijuana: effect on brain health: a scientific statement from the American Heart Association. Stroke. 2022;53(4):e176–87.
72. Prini P, Zamberletti E, Manenti D, et al. Neurobiological mechanisms underlying cannabis-induced memory impairment. Eur Neuropsychopharmacol. 2020;6:181–90.
73. Metrik J, Kahler CW, Reynolds B, McGeary JE, Monti PM, Haney M, de Wit H, Rohsenow DJ. Balanced placebo design with marijuana: pharmacological and expectancy effects on impulsivity and risk taking. Psychopharmacol. 2012;223:489–99.
74. Hart CL, Van Gorp W, Haney M, Foltin RW, Fischman MW. Effects of acute smoked marijuana on complex cognitive performance. Neuropsychopharmacology. 2001;25:757–65.
75. Colizzi M, Bhattacharyya S. Neurocognitive effects of cannabis: lessons learned from human experimental studies. Prog Brain Res. 2018;242:179–216.
76. Scott EP, Brennan E, Benitez A. A systematic review of the neurocognitive effects of cannabis use in older adults. Curr Addict Rep. 2019;6:443–55.
77. Ersche KD, Jones PS, Williams GB, Robbins TW, Bullmore ET. Cocaine dependence: a fast-track for brain aging? Mol Psychiatry. 2013;18:134–5.
78. Fillmore MT, Rush CR, Hays L. Acute effects of oral cocaine on inhibitory control of behavior in humans. Drug Alcohol Depend. 2002;67:157–67.
79. Bao G, Kang L, Li H, Li Y, Pu L, Xia P, Ma L, Pei G. Morphine and heroin differentially modulate in vivo hippocampal LTP in opiate-dependent rat. Neuropsychopharmacology. 2007;32:1738–49.
80. Goussakov I, Chartoff EH, Tsvetkov E, Gerety LP, Meloni EG, Carlezon WA Jr, Bolshakov VY. LTP in the lateral amygdala during cocaine withdrawal. Eur J Neurosci. 2006;23:239–50.
81. Grueter BA, McElligott ZA, Robison AJ, Mathews GC, Winder DG. In vivo metabotropic glutamate receptor 5 (mGluR5) antagonism prevents cocaine-induced disruption of postsynaptically maintained mGluR5-dependent long-term depression. J Neurosci. 2008;28:9261–927.
82. Nugent FS, Penick EC, Kauer JA. Opioids block long-term potentiation of inhibitory synapses. Nature. 2007;446:1086–90.
83. Yin HH, Park BS, Adermark L, Lovinger DM. Ethanol reverses the direction of long-term synaptic plasticity in the dorsomedial striatum. Eur J Neurosci. 2007;25:3226–32.
84. Potvin S, Stavro K, Rizkallah E, Pelletier J. Cocaine and cognition: a systematic quantitative review. J Addict Med. 2014;8(5):368–76.
85. Cadet JL, Bisagno V. Neuropsychological consequences of chronic drug use: relevance to treatment approaches. Front Psych. 2016;2016(6):189.
86. Winhusen T, Lewis D, Adinoff B, Brigham G, Kropp F, Donovan DM. Impulsivity is associated with treatment non-completion in cocaine- and methamphetamine-dependent patients but differs in nature as a function of stimulant-dependence diagnosis. J Subst Abus Treat. 2013;44:541–7.
87. Hels T, Bernhoft IM, Lyckegaard A, Houwing S, Hagenzieker M, Legrand SA, Isalberti C, van der Linden T, Verstraete A. Risk of injury by driving with alcohol and other drugs. DRUID (Driving under the Influence of Drugs, Alcohol and Medicines). 6th Framework programme; 2011.
88. Stoduto G, Mann RE, Ialomiteanu A, Wickens CM, Brands B. Examining the link between collision involvement and cocaine use. Drug Alcohol Depend. 2012;123:260–3.
89. Elvik R. Risk of road accident associated with the use of drugs: a systematic review and meta-analysis of evidence from epidemiological studies. Accid Anal Prev. 2013;60:254–67.
90. Goldberg J, Ernst C. Managing the side effects of psychotropic medications. Washington, DC: American Psychiatric Association; 2012.
91. Campos J, Waisman Campos M. Cap: Alteraciones cognitivas en usuarios de benzodiacepinas. In: de Sanchez Toranzo A, Hansen F, editors. Trastornos por sustancias. Psicofármacos. Madrid: Ed Sciens; 2015.

92. Hillman CH, Erickson KI, Kramer AF. Be smart, exercise your heart: exercise effects on brain and cognition. Nat Rev Neurosci. 2008;9:58–65.
93. Brown RA, Abrantes AM, Read JP, Marcus BH, Jakicic J, Strong DR. Aerobic exercise for alcohol recovery: rationale, program description, and preliminary findings. Behav Modif. 2009;33:220–49.
94. Nixon S, Lewis B. Cognitive training as a component of treatment of alcohol use disorder: a review. Rev Neuropsychol. 2019;33(6):822–41.
95. Carroll KM, Nich C, DeVito EE, Shi JM, Sofuoglu M. Galantamine and computerized cognitive behavioral therapy for cocaine dependence: a randomized clinical trial. J Clin Psychiatry. 2018;2018:79.
96. Rhodes JD, Hawk LW Jr, Ashare RL, Schlienz NJ, Mahoney MC. The effects of varenicline on attention and inhibitory control among treatment-seeking smokers. Psychopharmacology. 2012;223(2):131–8.
97. Perkins KA, Karelitz JL, Jao NC, et al. Effects of bupropion on cognitive performance during initial tobacco abstinence. Drug Alcohol Depend. 2013;133(1):283–6.
98. Volkow N. Adicciones. Presentation at the American Psychiatric Association. New York: EEUU; 2014.

Face Recognition as a Tool in Neuropsychiatric Studies

40

Maria Clotilde H. Tavares, Carlos Tomaz, and Jéssica Mendes de Souza

Introduction

Faces are complex visual stimuli that carry accurate information about the behavior in terms of the identity, age, and gender of the individuals with whom they live socially, but also about their attractiveness, emotional state, and intentions for each other [1] based on a context in which the behavior occurs. Details present in facial stimuli provide an idea of the level of involvement or the object of attention of the individual to the environment and information about their changing mental states, such as social attention, humor [2], and the attention to such details allows us to infer about character attributes such as reliability [3], among others. Thus, facial recognition confers an important social ability to the extent that it allows to identify aspects of the processes of the individual's thoughts and predict their behavior [4].

For human and nonhuman primates, facial expressions are considered important emotional manifestations, and the ability to recognize faces is essential for maintaining their social organization. In both, face processing and recognition have anatomical and functional homologies and similarities and share an extensive network of widely distributed neurons that operate in an integrated manner. In the next section, we will cover the evolutionary importance of facial recognition. We will be able to understand its relevance to nonhuman primates and how facial recognition developed through humans.

M. C. H. Tavares (✉) · J. Mendes de Souza
Laboratory of Neuroscience and Behavior, Institute of Biology, University of Brasília, Brasília, DF, Brazil

C. Tomaz
Laboratory of Neuroscience and Behavior and Graduate Program in Environment, University CEUMA, São Luís, MA, Brazil
e-mail: ctomaz@ceuma.br

Historical Perspective: Evolutionary Importance of Face Recognition

In social animals, communication through the expression of gestures and emotions represented mainly in the faces (in addition to body postures, and vocalizations, among others) emerged as an addition to vocal communication. The facial expressions acquired a role of great adaptive importance, as they expanded the form of interaction between the members of the same community [4]. Charles Darwin [5] was the first researcher to address the study of animal emotions in his classic book entitled *The Expression of Emotions in Men and Animals.* He argued that the facial expressions displayed by humans share several characteristics with the facial expressions displayed by other animals, including the same facial muscles, which are somewhat more intelligible if we believe in their descent from a common ancestor.

P. Á. Gargiulo, H. L. Mesones-Arroyo (eds.), *Psychiatry and Neuroscience Update – Vol. V*,
https://doi.org/10.1007/978-3-031-72219-6_40

Darwin's hypothesis that facial expressions were innate and universal and capable of reproducing human emotions came to be confirmed almost a century later after Paul Ekman's [6] remarkable work, in which he demonstrated that human emotions share universal facial expressions, not only transcultural but also shared with other animal species. The development of the first tool to measure objectively, in humans, facials movements [7], which received a review in 2002 with Hagar [8] was also an important mark. The *Facial Action Coding System (FACS)* remains the gold standard for identifying any action expressed by human faces. In 2007, Vick, Waller, Parr, Smith-Pasqualini, & Bard developed the *ChimpFACS—The Chimpanzee Facial Action Coding System* [9], a standardized system of the taxonomy of facial expressions in chimpanzees following the same methodological procedure of FACS. This shows the pattern of innervation of the facial musculature that humans, nonhuman primates, and other mammals share, which allowed the researchers to suggest a homology between some of their facial expressions. Thus, people of different ethnicities and ages presented very similar facial movements to the same state of mind [10], which would be consistent with the popular notion that specific expressions can be signs or symbols of feelings and intentions [11].

Face perception is a relevant ability among species, with ecological and evolutionary importance [12, 13]. Face processing and recognition are some of the most important social abilities in primates, which allow individuals to access a range of information associated with facial stimuli. This information allows them to establish interindividual and long-term relationships with several members of a group [14]. Facial expressions are usually coordinated with the emission of vocalizations, giving such facial expressions relevant meanings for the social group, as demonstrated in chimpanzees [4] which most likely occurs in other species of primates.

Although the similarity between some forms of expression of monkeys and men, the lack of experience with these animals makes it impossible to discern affiliative or agonistic meanings to the facial expressions exhibited by them, which can generate misinterpretations about some of their facial expressions. An example is the expression of pleasure described by Darwin [5] for the species *Cynopithecus niger*. The feeling of contentment exhibited by this primate causes the corners of the mouth to pull back and forth, revealing the teeth, and the long tuft present on the forehead is lowered with the skin of the head pulled. His eyebrows rise briefly, and his eyes are wide open [5] (Fig. 40.1). As a rule, for an unknown,

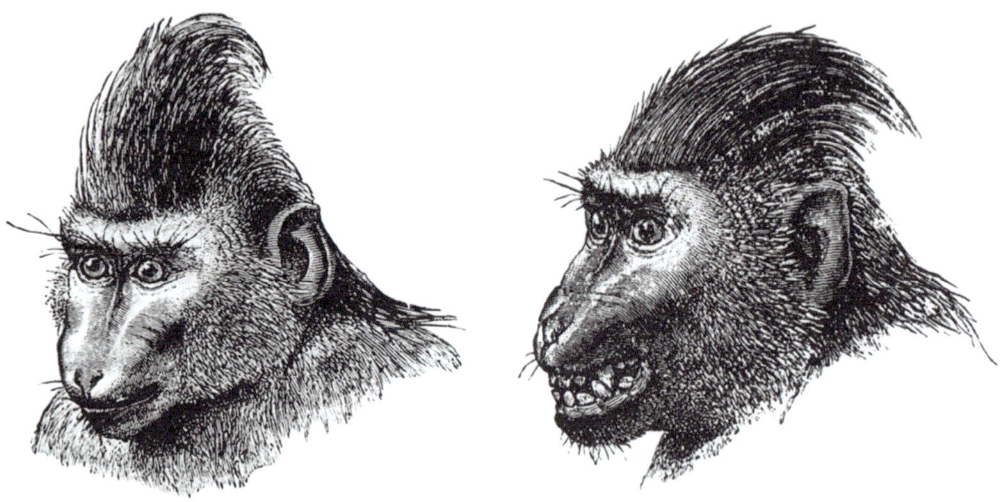

Fig. 40.1 *Cynopithecus niger* with a placid expression on the left. The same monkey, happy to be petted on the right. (Figure adapted from Darwin [5])

that facial expression would never be recognized as an expression associated with pleasure.

Humans, in turn, are considered experts in conspecific face recognition, due to a differentiated way of processing facial stimuli. They can identify, differentiate, and recall with greater precision countless faces throughout life in different contexts [15]. This ability allows them to organize their social world according to the information obtained through the faces, as these are used as a label of visual identification and as a source of information, mainly related to emotional state [16].

Like humans, primates benefit from the ability to recognize individuals through their faces. This ability allows them to remember those with whom they interacted since their social groups consist of individuals of different ages, genders, hierarchy status, and degrees of kinship [16]. They have an extensive repertoire of facial expressions to communicate their emotional states, followed by postures and vocalizations [17] within a context. From this perspective, faces are relevant stimuli whose recognition ensures individual identification within the group [18]. This ability has been successfully demonstrated in several primate species [16, 19–21].

Darwin's investigations on facial expressions show how animals perceive and what social information they took from it in a specific social context. Darwin [5] suggested that, as most expressive movements must have been obtained gradually and later became innate, we might suppose—a priori—that the recognition of emotions had also become innate [5]. If this hypothesis is the closest to what we can find in nature, we could assume that we were born ready for the processing and recognition of faces. In this sense, this ability would be restricted to species that present some socioecological demand. Additionally, if the ability to recognize faces is a skill only acquired through learning, a wide variety of species would be able to present this ability [15]. Therefore, the study of facial perception within a comparative and evolutionary context is necessary to understand how and when the main characteristics related to facial recognition emerged during the course of evolution, which requires a high level of social cognition [22].

Within the group of nonhuman primates, the main species studied are chimpanzees and monkeys of the genus *Macaca*. These species share several characteristics related to facial processing with humans, for example, the same patterns of responses of face-selective cells. It suggests that spontaneity in the perception of facial stimuli may have arisen similarly in the most recent common ancestor of this group of primates that lived more than 20 million years ago [4].

Although there are few behavioral studies on facial processing performed in New World monkeys, with a small number of species investigated, their results suggest that these animals also have sophisticated processing mechanisms for face perception [21, 23]. And concerning neural specialization for facial recognition in these animals, the origin of complex facial processing by primates may arise with the first anthropoids dating back more than 40 million years [24].

Neurobiological Basis of Facial Recognition and Holistic Processing

In recent decades, the identification of a system dedicated to processing faces in the brain of primates (genus *Macaca*) has been the result of research efforts using different investigation methods [12]. This effort demonstrated that the brain has specialized machinery for face recognition and, therefore, several of its regions respond more intensely to facial stimuli contrasted to stimuli such as objects or scenes [25]. It is believed that the remaining mechanisms of this system: (1) are present in today's nonhuman primates [25, 26]; (2) have functional similarities in their areas (which indicates that they are homologous) [12]; and (3) depend on a distributed neural network composed of areas and selective neurons for face processing [12] that establish selective connections over long distances [27] and operate in an integrated manner according to organizational principles [28]. Anatomically, this system is divided into a ventral and a dorsal portion organized into selective cortical areas for faces in spatial arrangements and functional specializations that simultaneously indicate a mode of operation that includes hierarchical and parallel information processing [25].

Multiple brain areas spatially dedicated to faces have been identified in human temporal and frontal lobes (see Duchaine & Yovel [29] for review). This specialization appears to occur early in development with subsequent refinement throughout growth [30]. As in monkeys, areas of the human ventral face are adjacent to selective body areas [31, 32] and are similarly accompanied, ventrally, by regions responsible for color processing [33]. In humans and monkeys, the total number of brain areas for the face is similar. Its spatial arrangement in the temporal lobe occurs in two occipitotemporal regions, one in the ventral temporal cortex and the other dorsally located in the superior temporal sulcus [25]. Other similarities between the organization of brain areas in humans and monkeys concern the functional specializations along the ventral region of the face areas that follow a similar progression, suggesting a hierarchical organization. In this sense, in the occipitotemporal direction, the selectivity of neurons for faces increases [34], the position dependence decreases [35], a mirrored symmetric confusion emerges from the views of faces in profile [36, 37], and finally, the selectivity of the facial identity is strengthened [38]. Likewise, for both, the response to faces is increased in the presence of an anatomically placed body in a correct position (relative to the face), and this increase in specific response to faces grows more strongly from the posterior to the anterior areas [39–41]. Furthermore, selectivity for facial movements is highly pronounced in dorsal areas but not in the ventral areas [42, 43]. Similarly, to that observed in monkeys, in humans, the ventral areas for the processing of faces seem to be interconnected, but aspects related to connectivity between the ventral and dorsal regions are not well established yet [44, 45].

The similarities between the systems extend beyond the temporal lobe, as the homology between the face-processing systems in humans and apes follows the criteria of anatomical location and functional specialization [12]. Neurons and selective areas for faces have been found in monkeys in the three principal regions of the prefrontal cortex [46–48] and, subsequently, studies using functional magnetic resonance imaging (fMRI), have confirmed the presence of selective areas for faces in the human prefrontal cortex [36, 43, 49].

In 1986, Bruce & Young [1] proposed a facial recognition model by indicating the presence of distinct functional pathways for facial identity and facial expression. Almost 20 years later, Haxby et al. [2] mapped the regions involved in visual processing for face perception and proposed a model compatible with two functionally and neurologically distinct pathways for the visual analysis of faces [50]. The first route of facial perception would be related to the regions of the inferior occipital gyrus and the superior temporal sulcus (STS), they would be responsible for the analysis of the variable or dynamic facial properties, that is, the movements related to the direction of the gaze, the lip movement during speech, and the identification of expressions. The second pathway of facial perception would comprehend the regions of the lateral fusiform gyrus (fusiform face area—FFA) and inferior occipital gyrus (GOI) [50]. These regions would have an independent functionality, as it would be related to the invariable properties of the faces that allow determining identity, for instance, the shape of the eyes, mouth, and nose and their relative spatial configuration.

Thus, the following regions stand out as the main ones involved in human facial processing: the fusiform face area, inferior occipital gyrus, superior temporal sulcus [25], and amygdala [51]. Together with the amygdala, the regions of the insula lobe and ventral striatum, which correspond to an extension of the areas proposed by Haxby et al. [2], play a significant role in helping to interpret facial emotions. The current view found in the literature is that facial processing does not depend on a single and independent neuroanatomical system [50] but, the ventral network related to facial processing is incorporated into the visual system more generally. Visual regions outside the facial process network and their interaction with it—for example, through long-range white matter connections—is significant and contribute to the efficiency of facial processing, as proposed by Grill-Spector and collaborators [52].

Also noteworthy is the selectivity of cells present in the areas related to facial processing [53] that have different characteristics. Thus, primates and humans have cells tuned to the orientation of the head or gaze [54–56], which suggests their involvement in the direction of social care; cells tuned to facial expressions [57, 58], and cells associated with physical features of the face that are involved in the analysis of facial features and identity [59, 60]. Mechanisms for processing facial expressions and identity may overlap in mutual neural systems [39, 50] and neural population codes that reflect another social quality, in this case, familiarity [60, 61]. In this sense, it is plausible to conclude the existence of neural mechanisms that support the processing of different social dimensions of facial recognition.

Theoretical and experimental models using monkeys and humans have demonstrated two distinct pathways involved in facial perception, one of which is related to holistic face processing. The *face-specific perceptual development theory* proposes that the development of facial perception continues to develop throughout childhood and adolescence due to the extensive experience with faces, which directly contributes to increasing the ability of holistic processing of faces [62], which is associated with the perception of facial identity.

The processing of dynamic or variable characteristics of the faces (e.g., emotional expressions) occurs in the previously mentioned regions that include the amygdala, insula, and ventral striatum. Even though these are not regions specialized in interpreting emotions from facial signals per se, they are essential to help in this interpretation [50]. In addition, facial expressions are not processed by a single system. There is a differentiation in brain regions that allows the recognition of different emotional expressions, such as fear, disgust, and anger [50]. This suggests the importance of developing these regions throughout childhood to increase the specialization in the perception of facial stimuli, especially concerning the interpretation of emotions.

Recent studies based on the functional magnetic resonance imaging (fMRI) technique in monkeys have found six brain regions for faces. These are regions referring to the posterior, medial, and anterior portions that cover the entire temporal lobe, and each one of them has different functions in facial processing [63]. These regions have a hierarchical functionality in facial processing, mainly related to the first- and second-order processing of facial elements fundamental for the holistic processing of faces. In Old World primate species (*Macaca fascicularis* and *Macaca mulatta*), studies using fMRI indicate consistency of association of these temporal lobe regions for facial perception [12, 63].

Despite the emphasis of these studies on the *Macaca* genus, possible homologies with humans are still carried out with caution due to the difference in absolute brain size between them and the variation in the number of cortical fields related to facial recognition [25]. Few studies used other primates from the Old World and, fewer used species from the New World. Only one behavioral study was carried out with a neotropical species, the *Ateles geoffroyi* (spider monkey), and the results indicated the possible presence of holistic processing for conspecific and human faces (due to familiarity), using the paradigm of Composition Face Effect [64].

Another gap in this area concerns the need to develop behavioral studies with primates [25, 59]. Although studies from single-cell recording and neuroimaging studies can provide important information about the brain circuitry and its functioning, in the absence of a verbal report, as occurs for humans, only a behavioral measure can provide information about the perception of faces by animals. Limitations are also related to the difficulty of establishing differentiation in multiple branches of the order of primates, given the insufficient number of species used [25]. Additionally, it is necessary to evaluate the *Own-age effect theory* in humans and other aspects that may influence face processing. The human visual system presents sensitivity to recognizing individual faces, related to the frequency with which this type of face is encountered in everyday situations. Studies investigating the own-age effect suggest that individuals usually have more contact and experience with individuals with age equivalent to their own. Thus, this contact would facilitate the development of expertise in this face recognition of greater coexistence compared to faces of other ages [65]. These investigations are relevant to elucidate the mechanisms of face recognition, brain organization principles, and social perceptual skills' evolution. When we better understand the homologies between systems using different primate species, it will be possible to apply this knowledge of one species to understand another.

Facial Recognition vs. Facial Discrimination

Humans and other primates evolved to high levels of social cognition and developed a variety of behaviors related to their social communication as they faced the challenges of living in society [22]. Even though facial stimuli have several components that allow perception and carry a variety of social information [4], the principal element of facial perception is identification. Determining an individual's identity is the central aspect of facial recognition [66]. However, facial discrimination does not indicate recognition [16]. Recognition involves specific neurological bases, mainly related to the perception of the invariant characteristics of the faces, which we will address in the next topic.

Human beings have a specialized facial processing system to determine facial identity, using the configurational information present on the faces, that is, the relationships between the individual features of the face. Thus, in humans, faces are not easily recognized when their elements are separated into parts [67], which suggests they are processed holistically. Familiar and unfamiliar faces are discriminated differently by humans. Face recognition of familiar faces is increased due to perceptual, semantic, emotional, and social information that it is possible to extract from it. In addition, individuals can perceive changes in face positioning and sudden expression changes during the recognition of these stimuli, which is not possible for unfamiliar faces [68]. These characteristics reflect the main objective of facial recognition in primates, which is the recognition of familiar individuals in social contexts [12]. Due to the lesser influence of these components, unfamiliar faces are ideal for isolating aspects involved in facial perception. Thus, facial recognition of unknown individuals in a social context becomes a challenge due to the limited amount of information available, as there are no clues or elements that facilitate their discrimination [12].

Nonhuman primates can recognize and discriminate members of their species more easily than other species [4] and have advantages for facial discrimination with which they are very familiar [16], which is biologically adaptive. This ability can be associated with the *Other-race effect*, also verified in humans, where the faces belonging to the same ethnicity as the individual are more easily recognized compared to the faces of other ethnicities [69, 70]. Unlike facial discrimination, recognition refers to the ability to associate a face as belonging to an individual. It is believed that this ability would only be present in humans; however, studies have shown that rhesus monkeys (*Macaca mulatta*) can emit socially adequate responses to images of conspecific faces, such as lip-smacking, threatening the image, or avoiding looking [71], showing that they can associate a facial representation to real individuals that are familiar to them, just as we humans know whom we see in a photograph [18]. Further evidence of this ability was presented in a study where chimpanzees' heart rates were measured as they looked at images of conspecific faces and humans. It was found that this frequency varied depending on the quality of the subject's relationship with the observed individual, that is, they are associated the images with real individuals present in their environment [72].

Capuchin monkeys (*Sapajus* sp.) also demonstrate the ability of individual identification. They can detect differences between the images of conspecific faces, recognize individuals, and extract the identity that the individual represents even when presented from different points of view. They can even perform better in discriminating against unfamiliar individuals compared to family members. It is believed that this occurs as a result of the attention given to this new group and that the face of these individuals could provide additional social information to the study subjects [16].

Configurational Analysis—Holistic Face Processing

Facial perception depends on the interrelationships between the salient features of the face [73], and, at the individual level, it involves the configurational processing of the elements present at the facial stimuli. The configurational processing presents two types of information: (1) the configurations of the first-order that refer to the basic configuration of the features of a face and that all faces share (a standard appearance consisting of the presence of two eyes above the nose and the nose above a mouth), and (2) the configurations of second-order that refer to variations between spaces and positioning of facial features. In this case, individuals are differentiated due to subtle variations in this facial pattern, and such characteristics help discriminate individual faces [73].

Holistic processing involves a configurational analysis of facial aspects within a gestalt, which allows the face to be perceived as a whole that represents more than the sum of its parts, as pointed out by *Gestalt Theory* [74]. That is a very complex type of processing, as it takes place in a fraction of a second during the microgenesis of perception [75]. The holistic perception precedes the analysis of individual characteristics [76], making this phenomenon very particular because it considers not only the presence of global aspects of the face (first-order configurations) but also the spatial organization of these elements that become integrated (second-order configurations) within a total perception [77]. Thus, all facial aspects are included (shape, color, and distance between features) and simultaneously perceived during holistic processing. The perception of these facial components occurs through a hierarchical organization [68].

Paradigms Used to Investigate Holistic Processing

There are several paradigms used in the study of holistic processing in monkeys and humans, among which three stand out: Thatcher's Illusion and/or Face Inversion Effect [78, 79]; Part-whole effect [80]; and the Composition Face Effect [81]. These paradigms reveal that alterations in a small region of a face can critically modify the perception of other regions of the face, as well as the entire face. This shows that holistic processing is a type of perceptual processing, as it does not consider decision-making or the influence of attentional aspects [82].

The Face Inversion Effect refers to the difficulty in recognizing faces and objects when they are presented rotated 180°. This effect only allows an indirect measure of holistic processing to be obtained, as it occurs disproportionately between facial stimuli and objects, which prevents the assessment of qualitative differences in the processing of these stimuli [73]. When faces are in an inverted position, there is a change in the first-order configuration of the facial elements, so their detection is impaired. The face inversion also causes a change in sensitivity for the perception of the second-order configuration. Thus, the spatial organization between the common aspects of the faces is reduced [68]. This also occurs in the Thatcher illusion, in which the facial stimulus is also rotated 180°, and some internal elements of the face, such as the mouth and eyes, also undergo this modification. The curious thing about this illusion is that the alterations of the internal elements, despite the great modification, are not easily perceived. Individuals can notice small changes, but these only become grotesquely visible when the face returns to its original position (Fig. 40.2). The use of this paradigm was a relevant demonstration of the possible presence of specific mechanisms for processing the information present on faces. If facial processing occurs analytically, the change

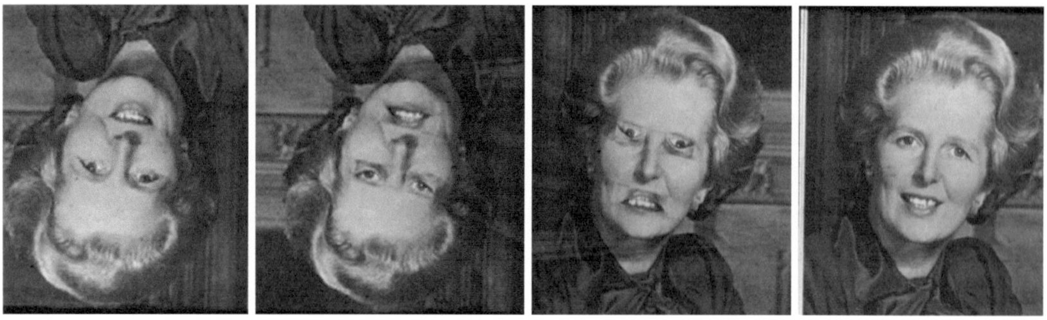

Fig. 40.2 Examples of stimuli used in the investigation of the Thatcher Illusion [78]. (Figure adapted from Thompson [78]. http://www-users.york.ac.uk/~pt2/html/research.html)

in facial characteristics, as performed in Thatcher's Illusion test, would be readily coded, as we would realize a separate analysis of each of these elements. However, as we perform a holistic analysis of faces, these changes become less visible, as we do not only consider the presence of facial elements, but also the positioning, distances, and integration between them.

The second paradigm consists of two images where the only difference is the orientation of a component, such as a mouth. When the mouth's position is changed on vertical faces, an illusion is created that the entire facial region has been modified, compromising even the recognition of identity. This illusory effect is not identified on inverted faces. Furthermore, when studying the memorization of specific components, the perception of these components is more accurate when they are presented within the entire face compared to the isolated form [82] (Fig. 40.3).

The third paradigm is a unique processing style for faces [64] that consists of deconstructing images of human faces into two halves, superior (forehead) and inferior (mouth-chin), followed by recombination of the same upper half with different lower halves, to build the test stimuli. The images used to compose the facial stimuli consisted of celebrities' faces, due to the familiarity of the faces and thus the possible ease of being named by the subjects. The stimuli were presented in two configurations (Fig. 40.4), wherein the first, the two halves of the face would be aligned and in the second, the two halves would be misaligned.

Holistic processing of these stimuli creates difficulty in recognizing the superior half of the face, even when individuals are instructed to ignore information from the lower half of the stimulus [83]. The combination of the two halves is perceived together, that is, as a gestalt. Thus, it becomes difficult to correctly judge the upper half of the stimuli alone, as we perceive the stimulus as a new face. On the other hand, in the misaligned form, there is a disruption in the processing, and it becomes easier to identify who belongs to the upper half of the image [84]. This advantage of recognizing the upper half of misaligned faces compared to aligned faces was seen as strong evidence that humans perceive and recognize faces as a whole and not as a collection (sum) of independent aspects [64].

Inability with holistic processing has been pointed out by many researchers for populations of people whose perception of faces is impaired to the extent that it interferes with their social functioning [85–87]. Although for most people this perception can be performed without effort and in an automatic way, others cannot do it. Such groups include those who are face blindness (prosopagnosia) that can't make use of the global, holistic, or configurational information that is of crucial importance in successful face perception but also includes people with autism and schizophrenia which is described a local bias in sensory processing and face recognition difficulties [88]. Since a global or holistic processing strategy is known to be important when recognizing emotional faces, and emotions are affected in these

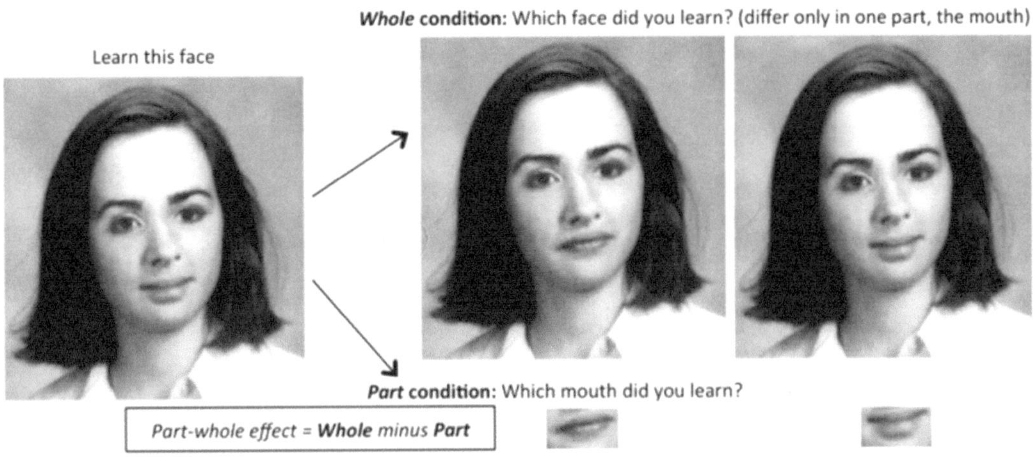

Fig. 40.3 Test used to test the memorization of specific face components. In the upper right there are the images where the component is integrated into the face and in the lower right the test of the isolated form [82]. (Figure adapted from McKone et al. [82])

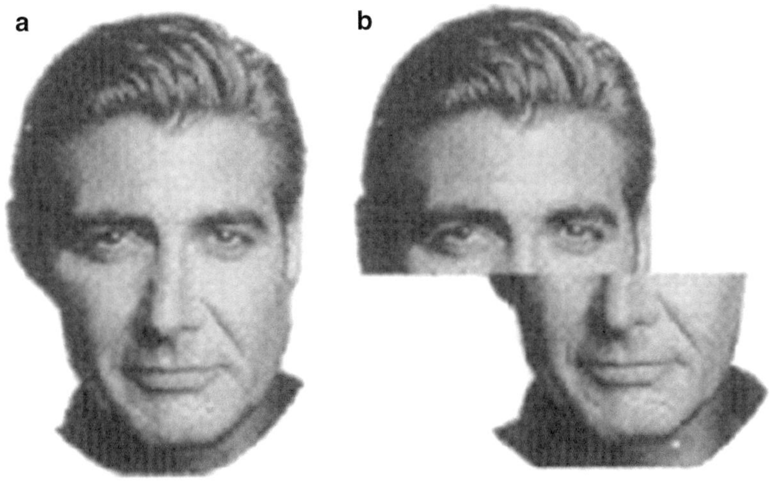

Fig. 40.4 Examples of stimuli used in the Face Composition Effect test [81]. The faces of the famous have been rearranged to form (**a**) aligned or (**b**) misaligned where the upper half of the face (George Clooney) and the lower half (Harrison Ford) belong to different individuals. (Figure adapted from Parr [14])

disorders, schizophrenic patients exhibit a strong deficit in face processing and cannot extract facial information that allows for efficient processing [87].

Is There Impairment of Holistic Processing in Patients with Schizophrenia?

A global or holistic processing strategy is known to be important when recognizing faces [88], as well as face recognition, relies on emotional, and nonemotional information. The distinction between these two facial aspects follows the dominant model for face perception [1, 2]. They are related to the processing of invariant and changeable features found in facial stimuli that are crucial to the social interaction between individuals [85]. However, some individuals cannot perform this effortless and automatic perception and cannot recognize their relatives or even their faces in a mirror. These people usually have impaired face recognition or prosopagnosia that directly interferes with their social lives [86]. Face recognition deficits can occur mainly due to neuropsychological disorders, like autism and Turner's syndrome in children or schizophrenia, Alzheimer's disease, and Parkinson's disease in adults [86].

Prosopagnosia, specifically, refers to selective visual agnosia characterized by the inability to recognize the identity of faces [86]. This face blindness can be either acquired or developmental. The first seems to have a genetic basis, a relatively common disorder in 2.5% of the population. The developmental prosopagnosia impairs face recognition besides the accurate visual and memory and no lesions brain on the patients [86]. On the other hand, acquired prosopagnosia is rare and usually results from brain injury. Although this visual agnosia is related to the identification of a person through their faces, it can also impair the processing of additional information associated with the face stimuli (e.g., familiarity, memory, semantics, and voice) since the model for face perception [1, 2] is a multistage model involved in different cognitive levels.

However, these impairments occur primarily for the most basic nonemotional facial information (e.g., identity and gender) and affect the holistic or configurational face processing. It is well known the high deficit in face processing by schizophrenic patients has been more pronounced for facial emotion recognition. But researchers also mention impairment in other perceptual aspects, like holistic/configurational face processing. This strategy represents "a rapid, involuntary face-specific perceptual process that integrates information across the face as a whole" [85]. Baudouin and collaborators [87] investigated the information related to the second-order relational face information in 28 patients with schizophrenia, who were asked whether the space between the eyes was the same in two side-by-side faces [87]. The results show that patients needed a space that was twice as great as controls to see a difference. They believe that this difficulty was related to a reduced perceptual sensitivity acquired from an abnormal visual scanning of faces [87]. This lack of appropriate scanning could explain a global impairment in face processing by schizophrenic patients. However, the investigation did not consider the holistic processing itself and proposed a new paradigm based on the part-whole effect paradigm. That way is hard to evaluate possible dysfunction in holistic face recognition by patients with schizophrenia.

Reviews conducted by Darke and collaborators [85] and Watson [88] clarify this possible impairment of holistic processing in patients with schizophrenia. These patients seem to have reduced face detection and discrimination ability; however, they do not lack holistic/configuration face processing. Although holistic processing is a very complex type of processing, it seems to be the central strategy for face recognition that is necessary even in individuals with impaired face recognition, such as patients with schizophrenia and autism [88]. Nevertheless, holistic/configuration face processing does not seem to be a sufficient strategy for optimal face recognition. The information extracted from faces requires a more general perceptual process besides the face-specific process. It suggests an investigation through the visual and attentional function related to face recognition that can somehow explain the deficits that patients with schizophrenia present.

On the other hand, it is well known that patients with schizophrenia have difficulties judging other people's emotions and intentions. This inability to recognize the emotional intent of faces is also one of the reasons for the psychotic symptoms of these individuals that can lead to social dysfunction (e.g., aggressive behavior) [89]. A review conducted by Gao et al. [89] analyzed 47 studies that investigate, to some extent, the cognitive impairment in facial emotion recognition in schizophrenia. These studies show deficits primarily manifested through face recognition of negative emotions (sadness, fear, and anger). Furthermore, the clinical characteristics of schizophrenic patients tend to influence the impairment of facial emotion recognition, becoming worst as the disease progresses [89].

To conclude, there are many questions about the deficits in face recognition in patients with schizophrenia and others with neuropsychological disorders. One of them is to establish the importance of holistic face processing for optimal face recognition and its influence on perceptual nonemotional and emotional information from a face.

Conclusion

The complex ability to recognize and discriminate faces from specialized neural systems and mechanisms present in the nervous system for millions of years is required in interactions between social individuals such as primates. In humans, the relevance of this skill is essential in multiple aspects of everyday life, for example, in different contexts verified in socialization or its impairment by neurological and mental disorders (e.g., autism, prosopagnosia, and schizophrenia), in diagnostic identification for various purposes such as criminal identification, fraud detection, court decisions, the digital use of face recognition in electoral processes, among many others. Therefore, the more we understand the neural bases of these processes in different species, the better we will be able to understand the complex challenge of recognizing faces.

Acknowledgments This work was supported by CNPq (National Council for Scientific and Technological Development)—Research Productivity Scholarship—PQ 2 (311582/2015-0) for MCHT and a postgraduate scholarship to JMS. We are also grateful for the financial support of the Institute of Biological Sciences of the University of Brasília to the Primate Center of the University of Brasília.

References

1. Bruce V, Young AW. Understanding face recognition. Br J Psychol. 1986;77:305–27.
2. Haxby JV, Hoffman EA, Gobbini MI. The distributed human neural system for face perception. Trends Cogn Sci. 2000;4:223–33.
3. Todorov A. Evaluating faces on trustworthiness: an extension of systems for recognition of emotions signaling approach/avoidance behaviors. Ann N Y Acad Sci. 2008;1124:208–24.
4. Leopold DA, Rhodes G. A comparative view of face perception. J Comp Psychol. 2010;124(3):233–51.
5. Darwin CR. A expressão das emoções no homem e nos animais (LSL. Garcia, trans). São Paulo: Companhia das Letras; 2009.
6. Ekman P. Facial expressions of emotion: an old controversy and new findings. In: Bruce V, Cowey A, Ellis AW, Perrett DI, editors. Processing the facial image. New York: Clarendon Press/Oxford University Press; 1992.
7. Ekman P, Friesen WV. The facial action coding system: a technique for the measurement of facial movement. Palo Alto: Consulting Psychologist Press; 1978.
8. Ekman P, Friesen WV, Hager JC. Facial action coding system. Salt Lake City: Research Nexus; 2002.
9. Parr LA, Waller BM, Vick SJ, Bard KA. Classifying chimpanzee facial expressions using muscle action. Emotion. 2007;7(1):172–81.
10. Chevalier-Skolnikoff S. Facial expression of emotion in nonhuman primates. In: Ekman P, editor. Darwin and facial expression: a century of research in review. New York: Academic Press; 1973.
11. Izard CE. Innate and universal facial expressions: evidence from developmental and cross-cultural research. Psychol Bull. 1994;115(2):288–99.
12. Freiwald WA, Duchaine B, Yovel G. Face processing systems: from neurons to real-world social perception. Ann Rev Neurosci. 2016;39:325–46.
13. Weiner KS, Grill-Spector K. The evolution of face processing networks. Trends Cogn Sci. 2015;19(5):240–1.
14. Parr LA. The evolution of face processing in primates. Philos Trans R Soc B Biol Sci. 2011;12:1764–77.
15. Taubert J. Evidence of human-like holistic face processing in spider monkey (*Ateles geoffroyi*). J Comp Psychol. 2010;124:57–65.
16. Pokorny JJ, de Waal FB. Face recognition in capuchin monkeys (*Cebus apella*). J Comp Psychol. 2009;123(2):151–60.
17. Seyfarth RM, Cheney DL. Signalers and receivers in animal communication. Annu Rev Psychol. 2003;54:145–73.
18. Pokorny JJ, de Waal FBM. Monkeys recognize the faces of group mates in photographs. PNAS. 2009;106(51):21539–43.
19. Parr LA, Heintz M, Akamagwuna U. Three studies on configural face processing by chimpanzees. Brain Cogn. 2006;62(1):30–42.
20. Bovet D, Washburn DA. Rhesus macaques (*Macaca mulatta*) categorize unknown conspecifics according to their dominance relations. J Comp Psychol. 2003;117(4):400–5.
21. Dufour V, Pascalis O, Petit O. Face processing limitation to own species in primates: a comparative study in brown capuchins, tonkean macaques and humans. Behav Process. 2006;73:107–13.
22. Calcutt SE, Rubin TL, Pokorny JJ, de Waal FBM. Discrimination of emotional facial expressions by tufted capuchin monkeys (*Sapajus apella*). J Comp Psychol. 2017;131(1):40–9.
23. Phelps MT, Roberts WA. Memory for pictures of upright and inverted primate faces in humans (*Homo sapiens*), squirrel monkeys (*Saimiri sciureus*), and pigeons (*Columba livia*). J Comp Psychol. 1994;108(2):114–25.
24. Janecka JE, Miller W, Pringle TH, Wiens F, Zitzmann A, Helgen KM, Springer MS, Murphy WJ. Molecular

and genomic data identify the closest living relative of primates. Science. 2007;318(5851):792–4. https://doi.org/10.1126/science.1147555.
25. Yovel G, Freiwald WA. Face recognition systems in monkey and human: are they the same thing? F1000Prime Rep. 2013;5(10):1–8.
26. Hung CC, Yen CC, Ciuchta JL, Papoti D, Bock NA, Leopold DA, Silva AC. Functional mapping of face-selective regions in the extrastriate visual cortex of the marmoset. J Neurosci. 2015;35(3):1160–72.
27. Moeller S, Freiwald WA, Tsao DY. Patches with links: a unified system for processing faces in the macaque temporal lobe. Science. 2008;320:1355–9.
28. Freiwald WA, Tsao DY. Functional compartmentalization and viewpoint generalization within the macaque face-processing system. Science. 2010;330:845–51.
29. Duchaine B, Yovel G. A revised neural framework for face processing. Ann Rev Vis Sci. 2015;1:293–416.
30. Deen B, Richardson H, Dilks DD, Takahashi A, Keil B, Wald LL, Kanwisher N, Saxe R. Organization of high-level visual cortex in human infants. Nat Commun. 2017;8(13995):1–10.
31. Peelen MV, Downing PE. Selectivity for the human body in the fusiform gyrus. J Neurophysiol. 2005;93:603–8.
32. Schwarzlose RF, Baker CI, Kanwisher N. Separate face and body selectivity on the fusiform gyrus. J Neurosci. 2005;25:11055–9.
33. Lafer-Sousa R, Conway BR, Kanwisher NG. Color-biased regions of the ventral visual pathway lie between face- and place-selective regions in humans, as in macaques. J Neurosci. 2016;36:1682–97.
34. Bell AH, Hadj-Bouziane F, Frihauf JB, Tootell RB, Ungerleider LG. Object representations in the temporal cortex of monkeys and humans as revealed by functional magnetic resonance imaging. J Neurophysiol. 2009;101:688–700.
35. Hemond CC, Kanwisher NG, Op de Beeck HP. A preference for contralateral stimuli in human object and face-selective cortex. PLoS One. 2007;2:e574.
36. Axelrod V, Yovel G. The challenge of localizing the anterior temporal face area: a possible solution. NeuroImage. 2013;81:371–80.
37. Kietzmann TC, Swisher JD, Konig P, Tong F. Prevalence of selectivity for mirror symmetric views of faces in the ventral and dorsal visual pathways. J Neurosci. 2012;32:11763–72.
38. Yang H, Susilo T, Duchaine B. The anterior temporal face area contains invariant representations of face identity that can persist despite the loss of right FFA and OFA. Cereb Cortex. 2016;26:1096–107.
39. Bernstein M, Oron J, Sadeh B, Yovel G. An integrated face-body representation in the fusiform gyrus but not the lateral occipital cortex. J Cogn Neurosci. 2014;26:2469–78.
40. Fisher C, Freiwald WA. Whole-agent selectivity within the macaque face-processing system. PNAS. 2015;112:14717–22.
41. Song Y, Luo YL, Li X, Xu M, Liu J. Representation of contextually related multiple objects in the human ventral visual pathway. J Cogn Neurosci. 2013;25:1261–9.
42. Fox CJ, Moon SY, Iaria G, Barton JJ. The correlates of subjective perception of identity and expression in the face network: an fMRI adaptation study. NeuroImage. 2009;44:569–80.
43. Pitcher D, Dilks DD, Saxe RR, Triantafyllou C, Kanwisher N. Differential selectivity for dynamic versus static information in face-selective cortical regions. NeuroImage. 2011;56:2356–63.
44. Gschwind M, Pourtois G, Schwartz S, Van De Ville D, Vuilleumier P. White-matter connectivity between face-responsive regions in the human brain. Cereb Cortex. 2012;22:1564–76.
45. Yeatman JD, Weiner KS, Pestilli F, Rokem A, Mezer A, Wandell BA. The vertical occipital fasciculus: a century of controversy resolved by in vivo measurements. PNAS. 2014;111:E5214–23.
46. O Scalaidhe SP, Wilson FAW, Goldman-Rakic PS. Areal segregation of face-processing neurons in prefrontal cortex. Science. 1997;278:1135–8.
47. Rolls ET, Critchley HD, Browning AS, Inoue K. Face-selective and auditory neurons in the primate orbitofrontal cortex. Exp Brain Res. 2006;170:74–87.
48. Tsao DY, Schweers N, Moeller S, Freiwald WA. Patches of face-selective cortex in the macaque frontal lobe. Nat Neurosci. 2008;11:877–9.
49. Chan AW, Downing PE. Faces and eyes in human lateral prefrontal cortex. Front Hum Neurosci. 2011;5(51):1–10.
50. Calder AJ, Young AW. Understanding the recognition of facial identity and facial expression. Neuroscience. 2005;6:641–51.
51. Hoffman KL, Gauthier I. Evolutionary specializations for processing faces and objects. In: Kaas JH, editor. Evolution of nervous systems. Amsterdam: Elsevier; 2010.
52. Grill-Spector K, Weiner KS, Kay K, Gomez J. The functional neuroanatomy of human face perception. Ann Rev Vis Sci. 2017;3:167–96.
53. Carlin JD, Calder AJ, Kriegeskorte N, Nili H, Rowe JB. A head view-invariant representation of gaze direction in anterior superior temporal sulcus. Curr Biol. 2011;21(21):1817–21.
54. De Souza WC, Eifuku S, Tamura R, Nishijo H, Ono T. Differential characteristics of face neuron responses within the anterior superior temporal sulcus of macaques. J Neurophysiol. 2005;94(2):1252–66.
55. Desimone R, Albright TD, Gross CG, Bruce C. Stimulus-selective properties of inferior temporal neurons in the macaque. J Neurosci. 1984;4(8):2051–62.
56. Perrett DI, Smith PAJ, Potter DD, Mistlin AJ, Head AS, Milner AD, Jeeves MA. Visual cells in the temporal cortex sensitive to face view and gaze direction. Proc R Soc B. 1985;223:293–317.
57. Gothard KM, Battaglia FP, Erickson CA, Spitler KM, Amaral DG. Neural responses to facial expression and face identity in the monkey amygdala. J Neurophysiol. 2007;97(2):1671–83.

58. Sugase Y, Yamane S, Ueno S, Kawano K. Global and fine information coded by single neurons in the temporal visual cortex. Nature. 1999;400(6747):869–73.
59. Cole MW, Yeung N, Freiwald W, Botvinick M. Cingulate cortex: diverging data from humans and monkeys. Trends Neurosci. 2009;32(11):566–74.
60. Young MP, Yamane S. Sparse population coding of faces in the inferotemporal cortex. Science. 1992;256(5061):1327–31.
61. Eifuku S, De Souza WC, Nakata R, Ono T, Tamura R. Neural representations of personally familiar and unfamiliar faces in the anterior inferior temporal cortex of monkeys. PLoS One. 2011;6(4):e18913.
62. Crookes K, McKone E. Early maturity of face recognition: no childhood development of holistic processing, novel face encoding, or face-space. Cognition. 2009;111:219–47.
63. Farzmahdi A, Rajaei K, Ghodrati M, Ebrahimpour R, Khaligh-Razavi SM. A specialized face-processing model inspired by the organization of monkey face patches explains several face-specific phenomena observed in humans. Sci Rep. 2016;6:25025.
64. Taubert J, Qureshi AA, Parr LA. The composite face effect in chimpanzees (*Pan troglodytes*) and rhesus monkeys (*Macaca mulatta*). J Comp Psychol. 2012;126:339–46.
65. Burton AM. Why has research in face recognition progressed so slowly? The importance of variability. Q J Exp Psychol. 2013;66(8):1467–85.
66. Rhodes MG, Anastasi JS. The own-age bias in face recognition: a meta-analytic and theoretical review. Psychol Bull. 2012;138(1):146–74.
67. Carey S, Diamond R. From piecemeal to configurational representation of faces. Science. 1977;195(4275):312–4.
68. Taubert J, Apthorp D, Aagten-Murphy D, Alais D. The role of holistic processing in face perception: evidence from the face inversion effect. Vis Res. 2011;51:1273–8.
69. Malpass RS, Kravitz J. Recognition for faces of own and other race. J Pers Soc Psychol. 1969;13(4):330–4.
70. Meissner CA, Brigham JC. Thirty years of investigating the own-race bias in memory for faces: a meta-analytic review. Psychol Public Policy Law. 2001;7(1):3–35.
71. Sackett GP. Responses of rhesus monkeys to social stimulation presented by means of colored slides. Percept Mot Skills. 1965;20:1027–8.
72. Boysen ST, Berntson GG. Conspecific recognition in the chimpanzee (*Pan troglodytes*): cardiac responses to significant others. J Comp Psychol. 1989;103:215–20.
73. Piepers DW, Robbins RA. A review and clarification of the terms "holistic," "configural," and "relational" in the face perception literature. Front Psychol. 2012;3(559):1–11.
74. Wagemans J, Feldman J, Gepshtein S, Kimchi R, Pomerantz JR, van der Helm PA, van Leeuwen C. A century of gestalt psychology in visual perception II. Conceptual and theoretical foundations. Psychol Bull. 2012;138:1218–52.
75. Sergent J. Microgenesis of face perception. In: Ellis H, Jeeves MA, Newcombe F, Young AW, editors. Aspects of face processing. Dordrecht: InDordrecht; 1986.
76. Schiltz C, Rossion B. Faces are represented holistically in the human occipito-temporal cortex. NeuroImage. 2006;32(3):1385–94.
77. Farah MJ, Wilson KD, Drain M, Tanaka JN. What is "special" about face perception? Psychol Rev. 1998;105(3):482–98.
78. Thompson P. Margaret Thatcher: a new illusion. Perception. 1980;9(4):483–4.
79. Maurer D, Le Grand R, Mondloch CJ. The many faces of configural processing. Trends Cogn Sci. 2002;6:255–60.
80. Tanaka JW, Farah MJ. Parts and wholes in face recognition. Q J Exp Psychol Sect A. 1993;46(2):225–45.
81. Young AW, Hellawell D, Hay DC. Configural information in face perception. Perception. 1987;16:747–59.
82. McKone E, Davies AA, Darke H, Crookes K, Wickramariyaratne T, Zappia S, Fiorentini C, Favelle S, Broughton M, Fernando F. Importance of the inverted control in measuring holistic face processing with the composite effect and part-whole effect. Front Psychol. 2013;4(33):1–21.
83. Garcia-Marques T, Fernandes A, Fonseca R, Prada M. Social presence and the composite face effect. Acta Psychol. 2015;158:61–6.
84. Wiese H, Komes J, Schweinberger SR. Daily-life contact affects the own-age bias and neural correlates of face memory in elderly participants. Neuropsychologia. 2012;50(14):3496–508.
85. Darke H, Peterman J, Park S, Sundram S, Carter O. Are patients with schizophrenia impaired in processing non-emotional features of human faces? Front Psychol. 2013;4(529):1–8.
86. Corrow SL, Dalrymple KA, Barton JJ. Prosopagnosia: current perspectives. Eye Brain. 2016;8:165–75. https://doi.org/10.2147/EB.S92838.
87. Baudouin JY, Vernet M, Franck N. Second-order facial information processing in schizophrenia. Neuropsychology. 2008;22(3):313–20. https://doi.org/10.1037/0894-4105.22.3.313.
88. Watson TL. Implications of holistic face processing in autism and schizophrenia. Front Psychol. 2013;4:414. https://doi.org/10.3389/fpsyg.2013.00414.
89. Kohler CG, Turner TH, Bilker WB, Brensinger CM, Siegel SJ, Kanes SJ, Gur RE, Gur RC. Facial emotion recognition in schizophrenia: intensity effects and error pattern. Am J Psychiatry. 2003;160(10):1768–74. https://doi.org/10.1176/appi.ajp.160.10.1768.

41

Alcohol Binge Drinking in Adolescence: The Who, the How, and the Why

Luis Fernando Antón-Toro,
Alberto del Cerro León, Danylyna Shpakivska,
Ángeles Correas, Marcos Uceta, Fernando Maestú,
and Luis Miguel García-Moreno

Introduction

Alcohol is a psychoactive substance that depresses the central nervous system with variable effects depending on the dose ingested, genetic factors, and the previous drinking experiences. Globally, alcohol is the most harmful substance in society (in the social, economic, and health fields). Traditionally, many cultures have used alcohol as part of their habits and customs. Nowadays, its consumption has become normalized despite its potential for dependence and its serious health consequences [1]. However, alcohol intake can have different effects depending on the amount of alcohol ingested and the speed of the consumption. In this context, during the last decades, a new pattern of intensive consumption, called binge drinking (BD), has emerged among young people. The BD pattern is characterized by an intense alcohol consumption in short periods of time separated by periods of abstinence [2]. The National Institute on Alcohol Abuse and Alcoholism (NIAAA) has defined BD as a consumption pattern that brings blood alcohol concentration to 0.08 grams per deciliter (0.08%) or higher. This typically occurs after the intake of 4 units of alcohol standard unit (SAU; 10 ml of pure ethanol) for women and 5 for men in a 2-h time frame [3].

Concerning the prevalence of alcohol consumption, the latest data from the World Health Organization (WHO) show that, in 2016, 43% of the world population over 15 years old have consumed alcohol during the last 12 months. Remarkably, geographic regions with more incomes, as Europe (59.9%), USA (54.1%), and

L. F. Antón-Toro (✉) · A. del Cerro León
D. Shpakivska
Department of Experimental Psychology, Complutense University of Madrid (UCM), Madrid, Spain

Center for Cognitive and Computational Neuroscience (C3N), University Complutense of Madrid (UCM), Madrid, Spain
e-mail: lfanton@ucm.es; Aldelcer@ucm.es; danyshpa@ucm.es;

Á. Correas · F. Maestú
Department of Experimental Psychology, Complutense University of Madrid (UCM), Madrid, Spain
e-mail: macorr112@ucm.es; fmaestuu@ucm.es

M. Uceta
Department of Experimental Psychology, Complutense University of Madrid (UCM), Madrid, Spain

Department of Cell Biology, Faculty of Biological Sciences, Complutense University of Madrid (UCM), Madrid, Spain
e-mail: muceta@ucm.es

L. M. García-Moreno
Department of Psychobiology and Methodology in Behavioral Sciences, Complutense University of Madrid (UCM), Madrid, Spain
e-mail: luismgm@ucm.es

P. Á. Gargiulo, H. L. Mesones-Arroyo (eds.), *Psychiatry and Neuroscience Update – Vol. V*,
https://doi.org/10.1007/978-3-031-72219-6_41

the Western Pacific region (53.8%) had greater prevalence of alcohol use (see Fig. 41.1). On the other hand, since 2000, the percentage of drinkers has decreased by 5%, whereas the total alcohol per capita among drinkers have risen from 11.5 liters in 2005 to 15.1 liters in 2016, representing a global increase, except from the European region where there was a decrease of 0.9 liters. These data represent a decrease in the number of drinkers but an increase in the amount of individual alcohol consumption. In turn, this also represent a problematic use of alcohol in which 39.5% of drinkers acknowledge having practiced BD patterns. However, these reports become worrying when we focus on the adolescent population between 15 and 19 years old, which reflect similar patterns of consumption. Regarding the drinking episodes in the last 12 months, young people show high prevalence of alcohol intake in European region (43.8%), USA (38.2%), and the Western Pacific region (37.9%). Moreover, apart from the high rates of consumption, the statistics depict a scenario where almost half of the young and teenage drinkers admit to practicing BD (see Fig. 41.2) [1].

However, this type of consumption does not appear sporadically, but rather the onset of alcohol consumption and its subsequent evolution usually follows a gradual pattern. Commonly, the onset of alcohol consumption occurs during early adolescence (12–14 years) and, over the years, there is an increase for alcohol consumed per episode until frequent episodes of drunkenness during adolescence (16–18 years old). This consumption results in many social and health problems such as traffic accidents, risky sexual behavior, poor academic performance, injuries, criminal problems, and health issues (intoxications, ethyl coma, etc.). It is important to note that adolescence is a period of multiple biological, psychological, and social changes. In this context, adolescence is a critical window of vulnerability in which excessive alcohol consump-

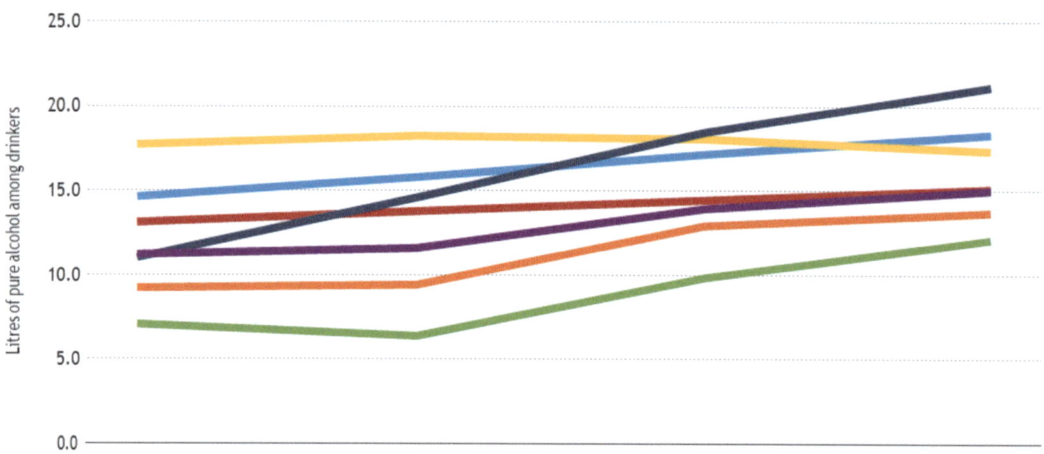

	2000	2005	2010	2016
AFR	14.5	15.7	17.2	18.4
AMR	13.1	13.7	14.5	15.1
EMR	10.9	14.5	18.5	21.2
EUR	17.6	18.3	18.0	17.2
SEAR	7.0	6.3	9.8	12.1
WPR	9.2	9.3	12.9	13.8
World	11.1	11.5	14.0	15.1

Fig. 41.1 Global trends in alcohol consumption
Note. Trends in total alcohol consumption per capita (in liters of alcohol) over 15 years old. Provided by WHO (Global status report on alcohol and health 2018. Geneva: World Health Organization; 2018. Licence: CC BY-NC-SA 3.0 IGO)

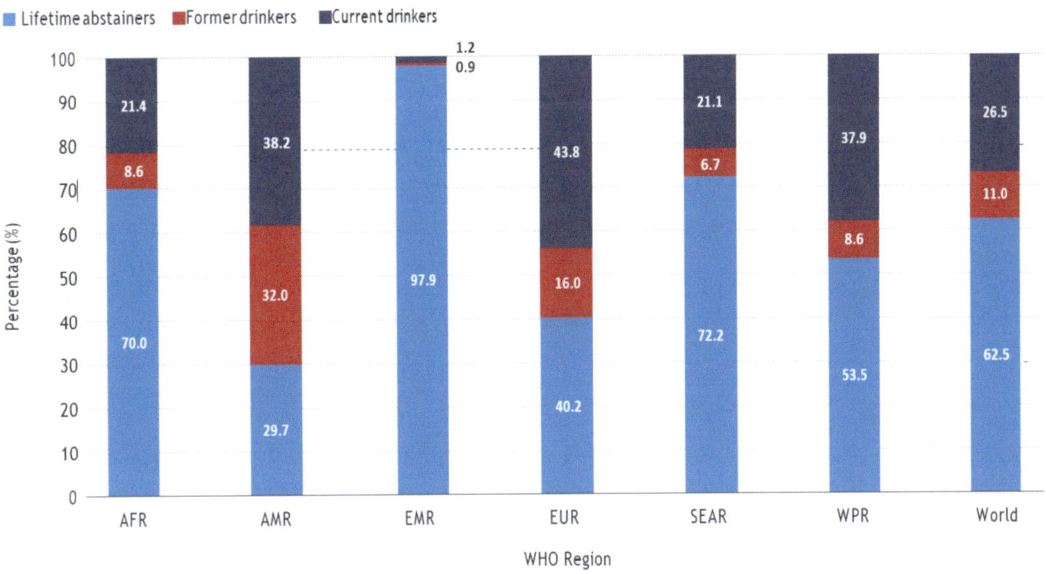

Fig. 41.2 Percentage of drinkers among adolescents Note. Percentage of current drinkers, former drinkers, and lifetime abstainers among total population (**15–1**9 years), provided by WHO (Global status report on alcohol and health 2018. Geneva: World Health Organization; 2018. Licence: CC BY-NC-SA 3.0 IGO)

tion acquires serious emerging side effects leading to lasting consequences [3].

Adolescent Development and Alcohol Intake

As previously stated, adolescence is a period of biological, cognitive, and social changes, partly as a consequence of significant brain' maturation at several levels such as molecular, neuronal, structural, and functional domains. This section will describe the principal neurodevelopmental milestones through this period, in order to understand the implication of alcohol drinking over adolescent brain.

At the neuronal level, changes in the soma, dendrites, and axonal projections will occur throughout adolescence. Just as the sensory and motor brain regions become fully myelinated during the first years of life, the oligodendrocytes of the frontal cortex continue to form myelin bands in adolescence. These changes translate into an increase of the transmission speed of neural information, improving neural computation in the adolescent brain [4]. On the other hand, postnatal development is characterized by a process of synaptic proliferation, up to several months; followed by an experienced-dependent process of synaptic pruning, which occurs over a period of years. Though, there are studies that evidence a second wave of synaptogenesis and synaptic pruning during puberty in several regions involved in high-level processing and behavioral control as prefrontal cortex (PFC), anterior cingulate cortex (ACC), temporal gyrus, insula, amygdala, hippocampus, and subcortical structures related to the mesocortical and reward system [5, 6]. These changes, far from affecting only the pyramidal cells of the cortex, restructure several of the most important neurotransmitter systems of the central nervous system, such as GABAergic, dopaminergic, and serotonergic. Specifically, one of the most important modifications occurs in the GABAergic neurons of the PFC. During adolescence, dopaminergic inputs to inhibitory cells are increased, improving inhibitory tone within this region, which leads to a decrease in the noisy activity of pyramidal cells, adjusting the dynamic activation of cortical networks, including the coordination of oscillatory activity [7]. On the other hand, the refinement of dopaminergic (DA) neurotransmitter pathways will be of relevance during this stage. DA innervation of the PFC through mesocortical pathways appears late in development, being among the last neurotransmitter systems to fully mature [8, 9].

At the structural level, there are many maturational events essential in the adolescent neurodevelopment. Thus, axonal myelination is reflected in a linear increase in global white matter tracts, whereas the change in synaptogenesis and synaptic pruning triggers a nonlinear decrease in gray matter, especially in the dorsal prefrontal and parietal cortexes throughout adolescence. Reductions of gray matter on those cortical regions continues after adolescence, accelerating between the childhood and adolescence in the dorsal PFC and the parietal cortex whereas the rest of the frontal lobe decrease its gray matter during the adolescent-adult transition [6, 10]. By contrast, subcortical regions as ventral tegmental area (VTA), nucleus accumbens (NAcc) or amygdala, which regulate reward-based behaviors, mature earlier than the PFC, and likely contributing to many of youth's risky behaviors such as substances use [11]. Interestingly, the regions that exhibit the most robust decrease in gray matter density also develop the strongest postpubertal increase in white matter [6, 12].

Together with those macrostructural maturations observed during the neurodevelopment of adolescents, myelination processes among high-order brain structures contribute to the maturation of improved neural interconnections leading to changes in the behavior and brain functioning. For instance, sensation-seeking behaviors, defined as the need to live new, exciting, and intense experiences, show a peak at the time of pubertal maturation. In the same way, early adolescence is characterized by an increased impulsivity. Such psychological traits negatively impair the behavioral outcomes during adolescence, leading to an increase of risky and potentially harmful behaviors such as drug use [11]. Parallelly, executive functions (defined as high-order control cognitive skills) improve gradually during this period because of the neurodevelopment of prefrontal and parietal regions. These changes contribute to the development of cognitive control processes like working memory, inhibitory control (IC), cognitive flexibility, and performance monitoring [6]. At a neurofunctional level, functional magnetic resonance imaging (fMRI) shows a peak of brain activations in regions involved in the brain reward system, including the ventral and dorsal striatum, insula, and the NAcc [5]. Additionally, neural activations in regions directly associated with specific cognitive skills generally trend to decrease (considering exceptions) as consequence of neural circuitry and cognitive optimization (Fig. 41.3).

In addition to the study of local activation in specific regions, more holistic paradigms such as functional connectivity studies provide a perspective of the brain functioning as a complex and changing network, essential to understand adolescent's development. Techniques such as fMRI, electroencephalography (EEG), and magnetoencephalography (MEG) allow to describe

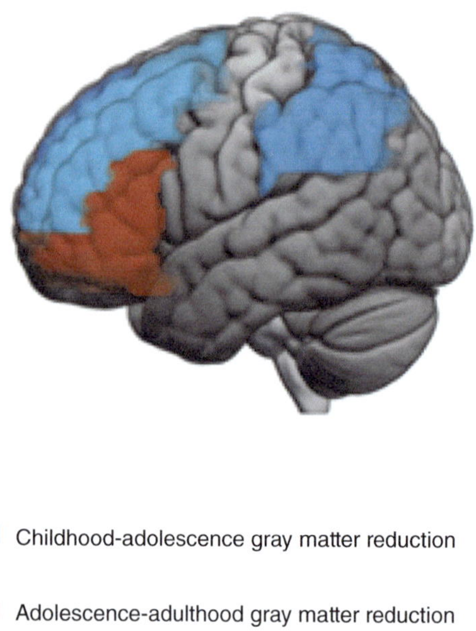

Fig. 41.3 Cortical gray matter maturation during adolescence
Note. Changes in the cortical gray matter during the child-adolescent transition that includes regions such as the dorsal PFC and the parietal cortex (blue). Changes in the cortical gray matter during the adolescent-adult transition that includes the rest of the PFC (red)

the connectivity patterns of the brain based on the statistical dependence of neurophysiological signals from different regions of the brain [13]. Within this framework, a resting-state paradigm evaluates the intrinsic connectivity of spontaneous brain activity, allowing to study the synchronization of different regions in the formation of several neural networks. Among others, default mode network (DMN) and the executive control network (ECN) are relevant, which are predominantly active during introspective thought and cognitive control respectively [14]. Throughout adolescence, brain synchronization tends to change from a predominantly local intraarea connectivity (more connections within a singular brain area), to an enhancement of interregions connectivity pattern (more connections between distant regions). This allows a more efficient transmission of information between neural cores, optimizing brain communication, and in turn, improving behavioral and cognitive outcomes [15]. In general terms, along with adolescence tends to improve the connectivity within neural networks (increased connectivity between regions forming a network) and decrease between the network and external regions. In other words, as neuromaturation progress neural networks become more refined, decreasing the number of inefficient or unnecessary connections.

Taken together, all these modifications show that the adolescent's brain undergoes several important changes for its adaptation to adult life. In this context, alcohol toxicity supposes an increased risk by interfering with these neurodevelopmental mechanisms. The special neurobiology of adolescent's brains makes them especially "blind" to the aversive aspects of alcohol abuse, such as the acute withdrawal. Moreover, during adolescence, we find a developing and inefficient cognitive and behavioral control system, together with an exacerbated rewarding and hedonic value of drug-related stimuli. These facts joint to a social environment which promotes alcohol consumption as the prevalent leisure choice, makes adolescence a critical period to initiates in alcohol intake. More importantly, the same developmental mechanisms that bring adolescents closer to substance abuse make their brains especially vulnerable to its effects and lasting consequences [3, 16]. Through the following sections, cognitive, structural, and functional deficits associated with BD will be detailed.

Neurocognitive Consequences

Neuropsychological and behavioral deficits related to BD could be some of the emerging consequences which characterize BD's cognitive functioning. These neurocognitive dysfunctions would be in tight relationship with underlying neurobiological deficiencies elicited by alcohol consumption. In this sense, neuropsychological impairments would represent just one of the last links, in a chain of neurochemical, subcellular, neuroanatomical, and functional disturbances on brain maturation, related to heavy drinking during adolescent stages.

A recent systematic review of 27 studies concluded that BD is associated with several cognitive deficits [17]. Studies which explored verbal memory performance suggest that Binge drinkers (BDs) have poorer strategy use and impaired free immediate and delayed recall, added to more susceptibility to interference. Respecting to visuospatial memory, BDs appear to display difficulties in visuospatial tasks with a high degree of interference, due to limited ability to inhibit task-induced information. Regarding executive functioning, it includes constructs as working memory, inhibition, cognitive flexibility, and planning. This cognitive domain is one of the main milestones in cognitive development during adolescence, and its impairments have been associated to a wide variety of alcohol use disorders (AUD). Related to working memory, BDs show deficits on monitoring of information and executive strategies to complement storage limits, when assessed with demanding self-ordered search tasks. IC is the most affected capacity by BD, decreasing the ability to suppress prepotent or contextually inappropriate responses, domineer impulsive reactions and regulate behavior. This deficit is consistent on different forms of IC, as response inhibition (go/no-go and stop signal tasks), interference control (Stroop), and self-control (premature responding tasks). Impairment of the IC has been proposed to play a dual role in BD: a preceding characteristic, making some individual prone to engage in problematic behaviors, as well as an effect caused by heavy alcohol consumption. Moreover, acute effects of alcohol on IC could promote a continuous autoadministration of the substance which leads to binge drinking thresholds, contributing to a further deterioration of the IC system. In addition, deficient IC is also linked to increased *impulsivity* during this period, which may enhance behaviors that are risky, poorly planned, and that entail undesirable or negative consequence [18]. Another crucial cognitive skill is the decision-making processes, defined as the ability to assess and choose among different alternatives, based on intrinsic and extrinsic factors. In this regard, BD population exhibits poorer decision-making abilities measured by Iowa Gambling task; it means, lower capacity of choosing from advantageous decks that yield long-term gains, because of their hypersensitivity to reward. Disadvantageous decision-making, added to a low executive control, contributes to perpetuating the BD pattern in a vicious circle [19]. Finally, BDs seem to show worse performance on focalized attentional and sustained tasks [20], as well as faster reaction times on sustained attention, selective attention, and processing speed, reflecting a greater impulsivity. Besides, even when neurocognitive performance is found unaltered, ecological and self-reported executive functioning questionnaires show that BD could exhibit everyday life dysexecutive behaviors related to prefrontal symptomatology [21] (Fig. 41.4).

In summary, psychological and neuropsychological impairments cited above seems an undoubtable consequence of BD consumption. Several of these neurocognitive deficits, particularly those related with executive control, could at the same time sustain hazardous intake habits, increasing the negative outcomes. As BD intake remains along adolescence, brain's integrity will suffer from a progressive degeneration, leading to more severe AUD. However, nowadays, there are some evidences pointing that neurocognitive deficits could not be purely be a cause of alcohol intake, with potential dysfunctions taking place before BD initiation. Even when neurocognitive deficits associated with BD has been strongly supported by the literature, some recent studies challenge this idea [22]. Testing the evidence for the *causal relationship* between alcohol use and cognitive functioning, the observational study included 3155 adolescents and their parents (fully adjusted models) from the Avon Longitudinal Study of Parents and Children (ALSPAC). Their findings suggest that binge drinking in adolescence and early adulthood may

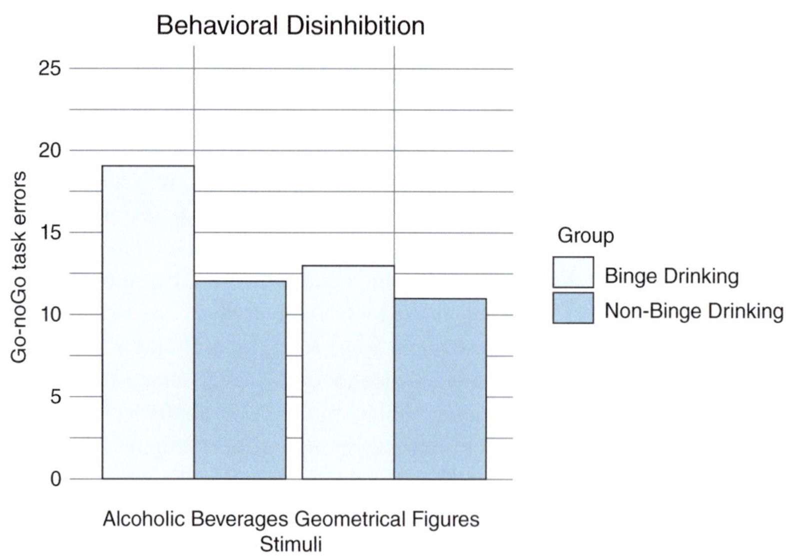

Fig. 41.4 Inhibitory performance of binge drinkers
Note. Performance of go/no-go task with alcoholic and nonalcoholic stimulus. BD adolescents shows higher rate of error in the inhibition (no-go) of alcoholic beverage stimuli

not be causally related to deficiencies in working memory, response inhibition or emotion recognition in youths. Previous studies as those conducted by Boelema and colleagues [23] support this line if thinking.

In the next sections, neuroanatomical and neurofunctional consequences in which these cognitive deficits rely, will be discussed, as well as the implication of differences predating BD onset which may play an important role in the development of such behaviors.

Neuroanatomical Consequences

Several studies have shown that repetitive consumption of alcohol during adolescence have an impact on neuroanatomical maturation. In general, BD is associated with an excessive synaptic pruning, myelin damage, and/or neuronal death, causing different alterations in specific brain regions. Such alterations contribute to disturb normal maturational courses, accelerating the decreases in gray matter, and/or delaying developmental increases in white matter maturation [24, 25]. Along this section, we will analyze some of the most prevalent neuroanatomical alterations (volumetric and structural connectivity) and its macrocharacteristics associated with BD.

Volumetric Studies

Magnetic resonance imaging (MRI) studies have been used to examine the effects of binge drinking during the ongoing brain maturation through young adulthood. Several cross-sectional studies have examined brain structure abnormalities in BDs, with unconclusive evidence. However, although there is no clear consensus on the direction of the results, the majority have reported that binge drinking produces a reduction in gray matter, with the strongest effects in the prefrontal areas [26]. These studies have found smaller volumes or thinner gray matter across neocortical structures, such as the ACC, orbitofrontal cortex (OFC), or the insular cortex [24, 27], as well as in areas related to the Visual Network (VN), the sensorimotor cortex network (SMN), and the ventral attention network (VAN) [28]. Parallel to these results, volumetric differences have also been described in subcortical regions such as the hippocampus [29], the brain stem [30], or the cerebellum [31]. They are characterized by an accelerated decline in the anterior lobules and the vermis, and an accelerated expansion of the vermian white matter and the cerebrospinal fluids in the anterior lobules [32]. Conversely, two studies have reported increased volume of gray matter in BDs compared to controls in the dorsolateral prefrontal cortex [33] and middle frontal gyrus [34]. Also, some studies reported a wider surface area of the left insula in BD teenagers, correlated positively with the number of drinks per BD episode [35]. Within this research line, Sousa and colleagues [36] evidenced that BD adolescents had greater volume in the NAcc, while studies performed by Pérez-García and colleagues [35] showed that the maturation speed for NAcc in BD teenagers was significantly higher (Fig. 41.5).

Structural Connectivity

Diffusion tensor imaging (DTI) is an MRI technique that measures water molecule diffusion and its directionality in the white matter tissue of the brain. The most used outcome measures are fractional anisotropy (FA), mean diffusivity (MD) and axial diffusivity (AD). Following this procedure, different studies have used DTI to examine brain connectivity differences between BDs and moderate/light drinkers. Nevertheless, the results of the different studies that analyze the structural connectivity in BDs do not converge in the same direction.

On one hand, Kashfi and colleagues found increased connectivity of the BD brain in the right corona radiata, right external capsule, and both the right and left cingulum. Also, FA and AD values of these regions correlated with alcohol drinking behaviors of the BDs. In this sense, these authors proposed that increased connectivity in the BDs may produce difficulties with regulatory control, contributing to their propen-

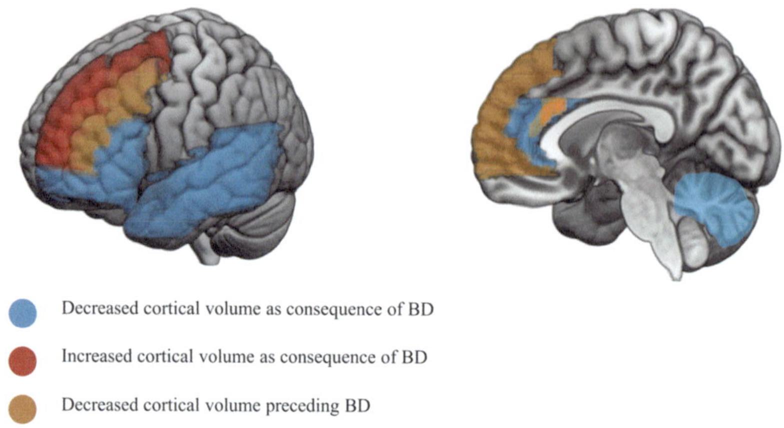

Fig. 41.5 Cortical volume changes after binge drinking
Note. Cortical regions with gray matter differences as consequence and/or preceding BD

sity to binge drinking [37]. On the other hand, it has been also found lower white matter integrity in BDs than in nondrinkers. A longitudinal study using DTI technique investigated the relationship between BD, structural connectivity, and cognitive performance in two sessions 1 year apart. They found lower FA for BDs than for men controls but this did not hold true for women. In the same way, lower FA was associated with higher BD score and worse spatial working memory in men and women [38]. In other study where the goal was to examine white matter integrity in adolescents with histories of BD and marihuana use, they found that FA was lower for BDs in superior corona radiata, inferior longitudinal fasciculus, inferior frontoccipital fasciculus, and superior longitudinal fasciculus. Interestingly, in four of these same tracts, BDs who are also heavy marihuana users had higher FA than BDs who did not use marijuana [39]. Finally, new studies performed by Qingyu Zhao and colleagues [40] showed how there was a FA reduction in the genu and body of the corpus callosum in BD groups, correlating the amount episodes of drinking.

On the contrary, two independent studies that analyzed the structural connectivity in the resting-state network and in the ECN have found no significant differences in white matter integrity between BDs and nondrinkers [41, 42]. This inconsistency highlights the need for new metadata studies or research with larger samples aiming to clarify the conclusions. Taken together, these findings indicate that repeated exposure to alcohol throughout adolescence is linked with structural abnormalities at both cortical and subcortical levels in white and gray matter. However, to discern between abnormal traits associated with binge drinking during adolescence, it is necessary to carry on longitudinal studies capable of differentiating risk traits from the effects of consumption on binge drinking.

Neurofunctional Consequences

As discussed in the previous section, BD consumption has several consequences over the structural integrity of the adolescent's brain. These differences embrace both cortical gray matter, disturbing regional neural processing in a greater or lesser degree, and whiter matter tracts, affecting the interregional connectivity, which will impact on brain's network functionality. Throughout the following section, some of the most relevant neurofunctional consequences of BD will be depicted. This topic will be addressed from the point of view of resting state (RS) and executive task-based activity, supported by both BOLD fMRI and neurophysiological MEG-EEG studies. With the purpose of offer a wider scope, evidence from local brain activity and functional networks interactions will be discussed. As different techniques and methodologies may report incommensurable results, it would be important to extract common conclusions in order to understand the big picture of this complex phenomenon.

Resting-State Studies

RS studies are based on the measure of spontaneous oscillatory or hemodynamic activity which emerge while participants are not engaged in any specific task. This paradigm has proved to be an excellent approach in the depiction of brain activity associated with plenty of neurological and neuropsychiatric states [43–45]. In this regard, some studies have used RS measurements in order to address the BD-related neurofunctional outcomes. When exploring the brain's electrophysiological properties of BD population compared with non-BD or light-drinkers (LD) groups, majority of works reach similar and consistent conclusions. BD eye-closed RS tend to be characterized by power increases of posterior theta band (4–8 Hz) and alpha band (8–12 Hz) reductions, while eye-open exhibit increased theta band power in frontal areas and beta band power (12–30 Hz) in temporal regions [46–48] (Fig. 41.6). As previously seen, as healthy neurodevelopmental progress, the cortical electrophysiological activity tends to be characterized by progressive power decrement of several frequency bands. However, those increments of activity power found in diverse studies may be supporting the idea of neurodevelopmental delays or disruptions among BD adolescents as a consequence of continuous drinking episodes. Additional source of evidence comes from the FC studies which explore the functional interactions between several brain regions. This approach has become a crucial tool in the understanding of brain functional dynamics. The RS spontaneous activity is known to reflect regional synchronization. These synchronized activities bound in several brain functional networks, so called *Resting-State Networks* (RSN), in which the majority of cognitive processing underlie [49]. Several works have successfully applied this methodology, delivering interesting results about how BD intake affects the integrity of different neural networks. For instance, the DMN includes brain regions such as the precuneus, posterior and anterior cingulate, middle prefrontal cortex, and the inferior parietal cortex. It is highly active when the brain is not involved in an externally imposed goal-directed activity, and it deactivates during task performance. It has commonly been associated (among others) with introspective though and the formation episodic memories. This network has been shown to be hyperconnected in BD college students than in their CN counterparts in recent neurophysiological studies. Specifically, adolescent BD presents a pattern of hypersynchrony among several regions of the DMN (frontal medial cortex, inferior parietal cortex, and precuneus) for delta, theta, and beta frequency bands [41]. Interestingly, this pattern of hypersynchronization increased after 2 years of regular BD intake, while not drinkers' adolescents show the opposite trend (Fig. 41.7).

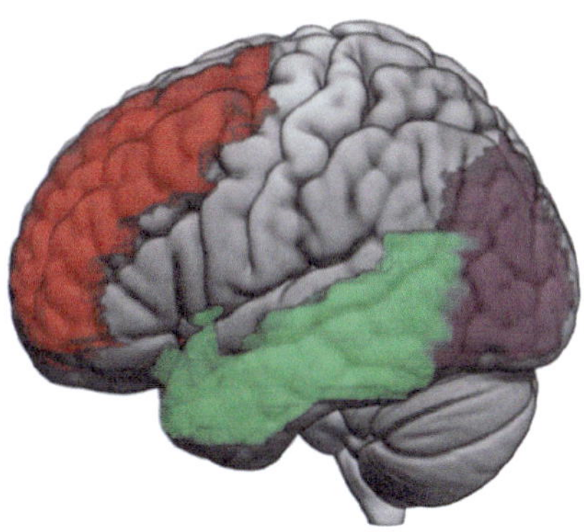

Increased theta and decreased alpha band power

Increased theta band power

Increased beta band power

Fig. 41.6 Electrophysiological changes in resting-state after binge drinking
Note. Regions with differences in electrophysiological activity during resting state in binge drinkers

In a similar way, fMRI studies have found synchronization differences in the ECN related to BD consumption. ECN is a front-parietal network which includes regions such as dorsolateral prefrontal cortex (DLPFC) and the lateral parietal cortex, being engaged in high-order cogni-

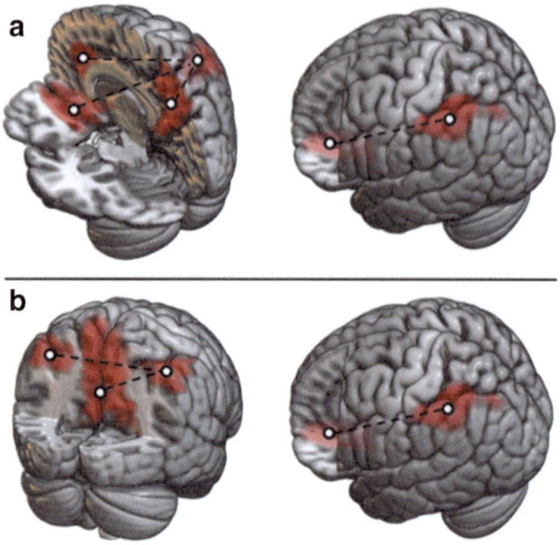

Fig. 41.7 Functional connectivity differences in resting state after binge drinking
Note. Regions of the DMN which shows differences in functional connectivity (red regions linked). BD adolescents exhibit increases FC in theta band (a) and beta band (b) in EC resting state. (Adapted from Ref. [41])

tive functions such as working memory, cognitive control, and goal-directed behavior. In this sense, those who engage in BD behaviors exhibit a higher synchronization in the left part of the ECN (left middle frontal gyrus) compared with CN individuals [42]. Accordingly, the increase in FC along adolescence observed in BD youths may be a representative of a disrupted neurodevelopmental trajectory, being related with several of the cognitive and behavioral deficits usually associated with BD population [50]. Moreover, the FC between regions directly implicated in the regulation of addictive-like behaviors, appears to be altered among BD population. Crucial regions in the behavioral and cognitive control such as the OFC present a higher connectivity with reward striatal areas and the ACC, together with lower connectivity with the amygdala [51, 52]. In this sense, dysregulations of neural networks bounded to reward and behavioral control systems may underline many of BD-related traits and behaviors such as lesser risk perception, higher alcohol-motivated appetitive habits, and greater sensation seeking. However, nowadays, it is not totally clear whether behind these differential patterns of functional activity could exist early neurobiological deviations which made some individuals prone to engage in risky behaviors such as alcohol consumption. Undoubtedly, more longitudinal research are necessary to clarify the complex relationship between early neurobiological predispositions and behavioral outcomes. Altogether, RS studies seem to deliver a clear state of harmful consequences of intensive drinking over neurodevelopmental course and adolescent brain integrity. In the following section, neurofunctional consequences in the performance of executive cognitive tasks will be mentioned in detail.

Task-Based Studies

In the above section, BD consequences over several neural systems and network dynamics in RS periods were exposed. However, it becomes necessary to explore the brain's neurofunctional differences associated with a wide repertoire of high-order cognitive processes. As AUD has been proposed to be tightly bound to deficiencies in executive control, with particular impairments in skills such as IC or working memory (WM) [18, 53], several studies have investigated the influence of BD over those cognitive skills. As general trend, a few longitudinal fMRI studies have revealed a neurofunctional "shift" between a predate reduced activation of task-relevant regions in youths which will transit into future BD and an extensive increase in the activation once intensive consumption takes place. Regarding specific cognitive skills, in the first term, IC is a crucial component of human behavior, involved in a wide range of executive control processes. Generally, it is defined as the ability to suppress or withhold an inconvenient response, and its impairment has been associated with several neuropsychiatric conditions, including AUD. In this vein, adolescents BD tend to exhibit greater activation in the right inferior frontal cortices (and left in a lesser magnitude) during the performing of successful inhibitions of classical inhibitory tasks (go/no-go, stop-signal task) compared with nondrinkers counterparts [54–56]. Another study based on EEG FC revealed that BDs exhibit increased beta and theta band FC in a right frontoparietal network during the inhibition of responses in face of stimuli with alcoholic contents [57]. Besides IC, several fMRI works have observed abnormal brain responses in a wide variety of cognitive task. For instance, WM studies have reported greater activation of task-related regions (superior and inferior frontal, and inferior parietal cortices) together with increased recruitment of regions which usually are not engaged in the performance of such cognitive process [58–60]. However, these effects may be sex-dependent, presenting opposite patterns of neural activation in females (reduced activation) and males (increased activation) [61]. Similar results are obtained during verbal-encoding task, where heavy drinkers adolescents exhibit higher activation in the superior frontal gyrus and parietal regions, joint to a reduced activity of left hippocampal areas [62]. This pattern of hyperactivity in BD adolescents, common across different cognitive tasks, appears even when no task performance differences are detected. In this sense, some authors have proposed the hypothesis of compensatory mechanisms whereby BD overactivate and/or recruit additional brain structures in order to maintain an optimal level of performance despite its dysregulated neural circuitry. Regarding decision-making ability, crucial in substance abuse habits and addictive disorders, some studies found alterations in BD population. They are characterized by a poorer development and assumption of greater risks in the performance classical decision tasks. This poorer ability to choose optimal decisions was associated with a greater activation of motivational/reward system structures such as NAcc and bilateral insula, joint to a less activation of the orbital frontal cortex [63, 64]. By contrast, a study of 1041 young adults and 74 young adult rats based on an ERP auditory oddball paradigm revealed a significantly lower phase-locking between frontal and parietal cortices in the theta frequencies in both the humans and the rats with a history of adolescent alcohol exposure as compared to their controls [65].

Finally, recent studies using alcohol cued reactivity task were able to detect FC differences in BDs population to the viewing of alcohol-related stimuli. This experimental paradigm consists in the presentation of pictures with or without alcoholic content, while the participants only have to look at the pictures, without requiring a response. In this kind of task, BDs adolescents show greater beta band FC in a right fronto-parieto-occipital network when processing alcoholic cues, while they show reduced theta band left frontooccipital FC in the face of nonalcoholic cues [66].

Altogether, evidence provided by diverse studies supports the idea of neurodevelopmental deviation among BD adolescents. As previously seen, healthy neurodevelopmental course is characterized by decreases in the neural activity as a result of circuitry refining and optimization. However, BD adolescents tend to reflect a common state of cortical hyperexcitability, both in local activity as in FC, which increase as alcohol intake episodes are sustained in time. This general pattern of hyperactivation may come about by disruptions in neuroreceptors functioning, such as N-methyl D-aspartate (NMDA) and gamma-aminobutyric acid-A (GABA-A), known to be particularly affected by ethanol neurotoxicity. Accordingly, as detailed in above sections, BDs are also characterized by higher cortical volumes, likely indicative of deficit in neural pruning, contributing to the increased neural activation and excitability reported by neurofunctional research.

Predisposition Profiles Towards BD Initiation

As discussed in the previous sections, BD is a pattern of alcohol consumption widespread among adolescent population, which cause several cognitive, structural, and functional harmful consequences. These disturbances over brain's integrity have been widely described in plenty of cross-sectional studies, stating the aversive outcomes of the intermittent but intensive alcohol intake. However, it is important to note that the cross-sectional nature of these type of studies on BDs makes it impossible to infer a conclusion about whether the neurocognitive impairment of

BDs is just due to alcohol consumption or if there exist prior abnormal brain condition which make some individuals prone to initiate in substances use. In this sense, some authors have proposed the presence of abnormal neurocognitive and neurological developments, mainly in brain systems associated with executive control and impulsivity traits, years before their first drinking episode. These profiles could represent a vulnerability factor that increases the probability of engaging in BD or developing any risk-taking behavior [18, 67]. Accordingly, recent reviews of longitudinal studies with a prospective experimental design [68, 69] detail several functional and anatomical disparities manifest in young subjects that engage in alcohol use few years later. A recent review in the same line of thinking points those developmental deviations in the frontal region, which plays a critical role in executive functions, appeared to be a key risk factor for the onset of binge drinking in adolescents and young adults. Young people who displayed structural, functional, and cognitive deviations from the expected developmental trajectory were more likely to initiate binge drinking [70]. At the date, there is a scarce of works which shed light over this matter; however, the current evidence allows to outline a preliminary "predisposition" profile towards BD engagement.

From a systemic perspective, adolescents prone to BD would be characterized by an impaired or dysfunctional ability in executive functions domains, particularly those related with behavioral control. These abnormalities would embrace aspects as a reduced IC, worse working memory, and/or maladaptive decision-making. Some psychological traits seem also associated with BD predisposition, such as higher impulsivity, sensation seeking, extraversion, and lower sensitivity to punishment, all intimately related with motivational and reward-directed behaviors. Regarding brain' integrity evidence, the general trend in longitudinal fMRI studies is to find a reduced BOLD activity in regions associated with the regulation of these cognitive processes (predominantly prefrontal, temporal and parietal areas), as well as differences in brain cortical volumes and white matter tracts [71, 72] Concerning FC studies, adolescents prone to BD exhibit reduced fMRI connectivity between prefrontal cortices (ventromedial and orbital prefrontal cortex), and subcortical regions such as nucleus accumbens and the amygdala, all involved in the mesocortical circuit implicated in the motivated and reward-directed behavior [52, 64]. In general terms, the evidence suggests that future BDs have smaller brain volume in frontal regions, less cerebellar white matter, smaller prefrontal surface area, less brain activation in frontoparietal regions during inhibition, and working memory tasks [70].

Complementarily, a few MEG FC studies have depicted the electrophysiological FC signatures of predisposition to BD. They are characterized by an increased beta band FC between frontal and temporal cortices during the performance of IC processes [73] and increased gamma band FC in the resting-state activity [74]. Interestingly, these hyperconnectivity patterns were associated with dysexecutive behavior and sensation seeking traits.

Further evidence in support of the existence of predisposition profiles comes from studies with alcoholic patients' offspring. Adolescents with family history (FH+) of AUDs used to exhibit brain differences even in lack of personal alcohol intake episodes. FH+ adolescents use to present a blunted brain response under several experimental conditions as risky decision-making, IC, and emotional tasks among frontoparietal regions and prefrontal-subcortical FC. In a similar way, they tend to show differences in volumes (but not consistently) of structures such as amygdala, Nacc, hippocampus, and decreased white matter tracts in prefrontal-parietal [69]. The nature of these works allows to consider the importance of genotypical differences, besides learning' experiential history, in the modulation of the neurobiological factors which conform predisposition states of vulnerability.

The knowledge of brain and psychological preconsumption states has become an essential cornerstone in the understanding of neurobiological and cognitive mechanisms which govern BD hazardous behaviors. Moreover, longitudinal studies are required in order to enhance early detection of adolescents at risk of engage in substances misuse, allowing professionals to launch preventive programs. Neuropsychological and neuroimaging works would provide relevant and helpful biomarkers in the task of prevent and reduce the nefarious effects of alcohol consumption in this vulnerable population.

Conclusions

All through this chapter, a wide description of binge drinking consumption pattern and its several consequences were depicted. As could be seen, this mode of intensive alcohol intake, while intermittent, it is not free of deleterious outcomes for the adolescent developing brain. Due to the stronger necessity of this youth population to engage in new sensations and behaviors, there is an inherent risk of getting involved in hazardous activities such as alcohol drinking. Adolescents are particularly vulnerable against negative consequences of BD engagement due to their developing brain. Ethanol neurotoxicity is especially harmful for its integrity, causing remarkable disturbances as were stated above. Moreover, in the last decade, there is a growing body of evidence alerting about potential neurobiological differences taking placed before BD initiation, making certain individuals even more prone to engage in risky behaviors, such as substances abuse. This fact calls the imperative necessity of developing more longitudinal studies, in order to deeply understand these predisposing factors. Building up precise "profiles of vulnerability" would allow professional to design optimal prevention and intervention programs, helping to reduce the notorious harmful consequences of BD in adolescent health and society.

References

1. Hammer JH, Parent MC, Spiker DA, World Health Organization. Global status report on alcohol and health 2018, vol. 65. Global status report on alcohol; 2018. 74–85p
2. Courtney KE, Polich J. Binge drinking in young adults: data, definitions, and determinants. Psychol Bull. 2009;135(1):142–56. https://doi.org/10.1037/a0014414. PMID: 19210057; PMCID: PMC2748736
3. Cronce J, Toomey T, Lenk K, Nelson T, Kilmer J, Larimer M. NIAAA's college alcohol intervention matrix: CollegeAIM. Alcohol Res. 2018;39(1):43.
4. Guerri C, Pascual M. Mechanisms involved in the neurotoxic, cognitive, and neurobehavioral effects of alcohol consumption during adolescence. Alcohol [Internet]. 2010;44(1):15–26. Available from: https://linkinghub.elsevier.com/retrieve/pii/S0741832909001712
5. Vijayakumar N, Op de Macks Z, Shirtcliff EA, Pfeifer JH. Puberty and the human brain: insights into adolescent development. Neurosci Biobehav Rev. 2018;92:417–36.
6. Blakemore S-J, Choudhury S. Development of the adolescent brain: implications for executive function and social cognition. J Child Psychol Psychiatry [Internet]. 2006; [cited 2019 Jul 10];47(3–4):296–312. Available from: http://www.ncbi.nlm.nih.gov/pubmed/16492261
7. Tseng KY, O'Donnell P. Dopamine modulation of prefrontal cortical interneurons changes during adolescence. Cereb Cortex. 2007;17(5):1235–40.
8. Caballero A, Granberg R, Tseng K. Mechanisms contributing to prefrontal cortex maturation during adolescence. Neurosci Biobehav Rev. 2016;70:4–12.
9. Hoops D, Flores C. Making dopamine connections in adolescence. Trends Neurosci. 2017;40(12):709–19.
10. Tamnes CK, Østby Y, Fjell AM, Westlye LT, Due-Tønnessen P, Walhovd KB. Brain maturation in adolescence and young adulthood: regional age-related changes in cortical thickness and white matter volume and microstructure. Cereb Cortex [Internet]. 2010;20(3):534–48. Available from: https://academic.oup.com/cercor/article-lookup/doi/10.1093/cercor/bhp118
11. Mills KL, Goddings AL, Clasen LS, Giedd JN, Blakemore SJ. The developmental mismatch in structural brain maturation during adolescence. Dev Neurosci. 2014;36(3–4):147–60.
12. Pfefferbaum A, Rohlfing T, Pohl KM, Lane B, Chu W, Kwon D, et al. Adolescent development of cortical and white matter structure in the NCANDA sample: role of sex, ethnicity, puberty, and alcohol drinking. Cereb Cortex. 2016;26(10):4101–21.
13. Friston KJ. Functional and effective connectivity in neuroimaging: a synthesis. Hum Brain Mapp. 1994;2(1–2):56–78.
14. Krmpotich TD, Tregellas JR, Thompson LL, Banich MT, Klenk AM, Tanabe JL. Resting-state activity in the left executive control network is associated with behavioral approach and is increased in substance dependence. Drug Alcohol Depend [Internet]. 2013;129(1–2):1–7. https://doi.org/10.1016/j.drugalcdep.2013.01.021.
15. Stevens MC, Pearlson GD, Calhoun VD. Changes in the interaction of resting-state neural networks from adolescence to adulthood. Hum Brain Mapp. 2009;30(8):2356–66.

16. Herman AM, Duka T. Facets of impulsivity and alcohol use: what role do emotions play? Neurosci Biobehav Rev [Internet]. 2019;106(January):202–16. https://doi.org/10.1016/j.neubiorev.2018.08.011.
17. Carbia C, López-Caneda E, Corral M, Cadaveira F. A systematic review of neuropsychological studies involving young binge drinkers. Neurosci Biobehav Rev [Internet]. 2018; [cited 2020 Jun 6]; 90:332–49. Available from: https://linkinghub.elsevier.com/retrieve/pii/S0149763417303846
18. López-Caneda E, Rodríguez Holguín S, Cadaveira F, Corral M, Doallo S. Impact of alcohol use on inhibitory control (and vice versa) during adolescence and young adulthood: a review. Alcohol. 2013.
19. van Hemel-Ruiter ME, de Jong PJ, Ostafin BD, Wiers RW. Reward sensitivity, attentional bias, and executive control in early adolescent alcohol use. Addict Behav [Internet]. 2015;40:84–90. Available from: https://linkinghub.elsevier.com/retrieve/pii/S0306460314002950
20. Crego A, Holguín SR, Parada M, Mota N, Corral M, Cadaveira F. Binge drinking affects attentional and visual working memory processing in young university students. Alcohol Clin Exp Res [Internet]. 2009;33(11):1870–9. Available from: http://doi.wiley.com/10.1111/j.1530-0277.2009.01025.x
21. Gil-Hernandez S, Garcia-Moreno LM. Executive performance and dysexecutive symptoms in binge drinking adolescents. Alcohol [Internet]. 2016;51:79–87. https://doi.org/10.1016/j.alcohol.2016.01.003.
22. Mahedy L, Suddell S, Skirrow C, Fernandes G, Field M, Heron J, Hickman M, Wootton R, Munafo M. Alcohol use and cognitive functioning in young adults: improving causal inference. Addiction. 2021;116(2):292–302.
23. Boelema S, Harakeh Z, Van Zandvoort M, Reijneveld S, Verhulst F, Ormel J, Vollebergh W. Adolescent heavy drinking does not affect maturation of basic executive functioning: longitudinal findings from the TRAILS study. PLoS One. 2015;10(10):e0139186.
24. Mashhoon Y, Czerkawski C, Crowley DJ, Cohen-Gilbert JE, Sneider JT, Silveri MM. Binge Alcohol consumption in emerging adults: anterior cingulate cortical "thinness" is associated with Alcohol use patterns. Alcohol Clin Exp Res [Internet]. 2014;38(7):1955–64. [cited 2020 May 13]. Available from: http://doi.wiley.com/10.1111/acer.12475
25. Bava S, Tapert SF. Adolescent brain development and the risk for alcohol and other drug problems. Neuropsychol Rev. 2010;20(4):398–413.
26. Infante M, Eberson S, Zhang Y, Brumback T, Brown S, Colrain I, Baker F, Clark D, De Bellis M, Goldston D, et al. Adolescent binge drinking is associated with accelerated decline of gray matter volume. Cereb Cortex. 2022;32(12):2611–20.
27. Heikkinen N, Niskanen E, Könönen M, Tolmunen T, Kekkonen V, Kivimäki P, et al. Alcohol consumption during adolescence is associated with reduced grey matter volumes. Addiction. 2017;112(4):604–13.
28. Guo X, Yan T, Chen M, Ma X, Li R, Li B, Yang A, Chen Y, Fang T, Yu H, et al. Differential effects of alcohol-drinking patterns on the structure and function of the brain and cognitive performance in young adult drinkers: a pilot study. Brain Behav. 2022;12(1):e2427.
29. Medina KL, Schweinsburg AD, Cohen-Zion M, Nagel BJ, Tapert SF. Effects of alcohol and combined marijuana and alcohol use during adolescence on hippocampal volume and asymmetry. Neurotoxicol Teratol. 2007;29(1):141–52.
30. Squeglia LM, Rinker DA, Bartsch H, Castro N, Chung Y, Dale AM, et al. Brain volume reductions in adolescent heavy drinkers. Dev Cogn Neurosci [Internet]. 2014;9:117–25. https://doi.org/10.1016/j.dcn.2014.02.005.
31. Lisdahl KM, Thayer R, Squeglia LM, McQueeny TM, Tapert SF. Recent binge drinking predicts smaller cerebellar volumes in adolescents. Psychiatry Res Neuroimag. 2013;211(1):17–23.
32. Sullivan E, Brumback T, Tapert S, Brown S, Baker F, Colrain I, Prouty D, De Bellis M, Clark D, Nagel B, et al. Disturbed cerebellar growth trajectories in adolescents who initiate alcohol drinking. Biol Psychiatry. 2020;87(7):632–44.
33. Doallo S, Cadaveira F, Corral M, Mota N, López-Caneda E, Rodríguez HS. Larger mid-dorsolateral prefrontal gray matter volume in young binge drinkers revealed by voxel-based morphometry. PLoS One. 2014;9(5):e96380.
34. Sousa SS, Sampaio A, Marques P, Gonçalves ÓF, Crego A. Gray matter abnormalities in the inhibitory circuitry of young binge drinkers: a voxel-based morphometry study. Front Psychol. 2017;8(SEP):Article 1567.
35. Perez-Garcia J, Cadaveira F, Canales-Rodriguez E, Suarez-Suarez S, Holguin S, Corral M, Blanco-Ramos J, Doallo S. Effects of persistent binge drinking on brain structure in emerging adults: a longitudinal study. Front Psych. 2022;13:935043.
36. Sousa S, Sampaio A, Lopez-Caneda E, Bec C, Gonçalves, Crego A. Increased nucleus accumbens volume in college binge drinkers-preliminary evidence from manually segmented MRI analysis. Front Psychiatry. 2020;10:1005.
37. Kashfi K, Al-Khalil K, Hou J, Fang D, Anderson R, Rajmohan R, et al. Hyper-brain connectivity in binge drinking college students: a diffusion tensor imaging study. Neurocase. 2017;23(3–4):179–86.
38. Smith KW, Gierski F, Andre J, Dowell NG, Cercignani M, Naassila M, et al. Altered white matter integrity in whole brain and segments of corpus callosum, in young social drinkers with binge drinking pattern. Addict Biol. 2017;22(2):490–501.
39. Jacobus J, McQueeny T, Bava S, Schweinsburg BC, Frank LR, Yang TT, et al. White matter integrity in adolescents with histories of marijuana use and binge drinking. Neurotoxicol Teratol. 2009 Nov;31(6):349–55.

40. Zhao Q, Sullivan E, Honnorat N, Adeli E, Podhajsky S, De Bellis M, Voyvodic J, Nooner K, Baker F, Colrain I, et al. Association of heavy drinking with deviant fiber tract development in frontal brain systems in adolescents. JAMA Psychiatry. 2021;78(4):407–15.
41. Correas A, Cuesta P, López-Caneda E, Rodríguez Holguín S, García-Moreno LM, Pineda-Pardo JA, et al. Functional and structural brain connectivity of young binge drinkers: a follow-up study. Sci Rep [Internet]. 2016; https://doi.org/10.1038/srep31293.
42. Sousa SS, Sampaio A, Marques P, López-Caneda E, Gonçalves ÓF, Crego A. Functional and structural connectivity of the executive control network in college binge drinkers. Addict Behav. 2019 Dec;1:99.
43. Deco G, Jirsa VK, McIntosh AR. Emerging concepts for the dynamical organization of resting-state activity in the brain, vol. 12. Nature Reviews Neuroscience. Nature Publishing Group; 2011. p. 43–56.
44. Raichle ME, Raichle ME. Searching for a baseline: functional imaging and the resting human brain. Nat Rev Neurosci. 2001;2(10):685–94.
45. Baillet S. Magnetoencephalography for brain electrophysiology and imaging. Nat Neurosci. 2017;20(3):327–39.
46. Correas A, Rodriguez Holguín S, Cuesta P, López-Caneda E, García-Moreno LM, Cadaveira F, et al. Exploratory analysis of power Spectrum and functional connectivity during resting state in young binge drinkers: a MEG study. Int J Neural Syst [Internet]. 2015;25(03):1550008. Available from: http://www.worldscientific.com/doi/abs/10.1142/S0129065715500082
47. López-Caneda E, Cadaveira F, Correas A, Crego A, Maestú F, Rodríguez Holguín S. The brain of binge drinkers at rest: alterations in theta and beta oscillations in first-year college students with a binge drinking pattern. Front Behav Neurosci [Internet]. 2017;11. [cited 2020 Apr 6]. Available from: http://journal.frontiersin.org/article/10.3389/fnbeh.2017.00168/full
48. Affan RO, Huang S, Cruz SM, Holcomb LA, Nguyen E, Marinkovic K. High-intensity binge drinking is associated with alterations in spontaneous neural oscillations in young adults. Alcohol. 2018;70:51–60.
49. Brookes MJ, Woolrich M, Luckhoo H, Price D, Hale JR, Stephenson MC, et al. Investigating the electrophysiological basis of resting state networks using magnetoencephalography. Proc Natl Acad Sci [Internet]. 2011;108(40):16783–8. Available from: http://www.pnas.org/cgi/doi/10.1073/pnas.1112685108
50. Ruan H, Zhou Y, Luo Q, Robert GH, Desrivières S, Quinlan EB, et al. Adolescent binge drinking disrupts normal trajectories of brain functional organization and personality maturation. NeuroImage Clin. 2019 Jan;1:22.
51. Arienzo D, Happer JP, Molnar SM, Alderson-Myers A, Marinkovic K. Binge drinking is associated with altered resting state functional connectivity of reward-salience and top down control networks. Brain Imaging Behav. 2019.
52. Crane NA, Gorka SM, Phan KL, Childs E. Amygdala-orbitofrontal functional connectivity mediates the relationship between sensation seeking and alcohol use among binge-drinking adults. Drug Alcohol Depend. 2018;192:208–14.
53. Kamarajan C, Porjesz B, Jones KA, Choi K, Chorlian DB, Padmanabhapillai A, et al. Alcoholism is a disinhibitory disorder: neurophysiological evidence from a go/no-go task. Biol Psychol. 2013;69(3):353–73.
54. López-Caneda E, Rodríguez Holguín S, Corral M, Doallo S, Cadaveira F. Evolution of the binge drinking pattern in college students: neurophysiological correlates. Alcohol. 2014;48(5):407–18.
55. Wetherill RR, Squeglia LM, Yang TT, Tapert SF. A longitudinal examination of adolescent response inhibition: neural differences before and after the initiation of heavy drinking. Psychopharmacology. 2013;230(4):663–71.
56. López-Caneda E, Cadaveira F, Crego A, Gómez-Suárez A, Corral M, Parada M, et al. Hyperactivation of right inferior frontal cortex in young binge drinkers during response inhibition: A follow-up study. Addiction. 2012;107(10):1796–808.
57. Blanco-Ramos J, Anton-Toro L, Cadaveira F, Doallo S, Suarez-Suarez S, Rodriguez Holguin S. Alcohol-related stimuli modulate functional connectivity during response inhibition in young binge drinkers. Addict Biol. 2022;27(2):e13141.
58. Squeglia LM, Pulido C, Wetherill RR, Jacobus J, Brown GG, Tapert SF. Brain response to working memory over three years of adolescence: influence of initiating heavy drinking. J Stud Alcohol Drugs. 2012;73(5):749–60.
59. Feldstein Ewing SW, Sakhardande A, Blakemore SJ. The effect of alcohol consumption on the adolescent brain: A systematic review of MRI and fMRI studies of alcohol-using youth. NeuroImage Clin. 2014;5:420–37.
60. Jacobus J, Tapert SF. Neurotoxic effects of alcohol in adolescence. Annu Rev Clin Psychol [Internet]. 2013;9(1):703–21. Available from: http://www.annualreviews.org/doi/10.1146/annurev-clinpsy-050212-185610
61. Squeglia LM, Schweinsburg AD, Pulido C, Tapert SF. Adolescent binge drinking linked to abnormal spatial working memory brain activation: differential gender effects. Alcohol Clin Exp Res [Internet]. 2011;35(10):1831–41. [cited 2020 Jun 12]. Available from: http://doi.wiley.com/10.1111/j.1530-0277.2011.01527.x
62. Schweinsburg AD, McQueeny T, Nagel BJ, Eyler LT, Tapert SF. A preliminary study of functional magnetic resonance imaging response during verbal encoding among adolescent binge drinkers. Alcohol. 2010;44(1):111–7.
63. Xiao L, Bechara A, Gong Q, Huang X, Li X, Xue G, et al. Abnormal affective decision making revealed in adolescent binge drinkers using a functional magnetic resonance imaging study. Psychol Addict Behav [Internet]. 2013;27(2):443–54. [cited 2020

Jun 9]. Available from: http://doi.apa.org/getdoi.cfm?doi=10.1037/a0027892
64. Morales AM, Jones SA, Harman G, Patching-Bunch J, Nagel BJ. Associations between nucleus accumbens structural connectivity, brain function, and initiation of binge drinking. Addict Biol. 2020;25(3):e12767.
65. Ehlers C, Phillips E, Wills D, Benedict J, Sanchez-Alavez M. Phase locking of event-related oscillations is decreased in both young adult humans and rats with a history of adolescent alcohol exposure. Addict Biol. 2020;25(2):e12732.
66. Almeida-Antunes N, Anton-Toro L, Crego A, Rodrigues R, Sampaio A, Lopez-Caneda E. "It's a beer!": brain functional hyperconnectivity during processing of alcohol-related images in young binge drinkers. Addict Biol. 2022;27(2):e13152.
67. Verdejo-García A, Lawrence AJ, Clark L. Impulsivity as a vulnerability marker for substance-use disorders: review of findings from high-risk research, problem gamblers and genetic association studies. Neurosci Biobehav Rev. 2008;32(4):777–810.
68. O'Halloran L, Nymberg C, Jollans L, Garavan H, Whelan R. The potential of neuroimaging for identifying predictors of adolescent alcohol use initiation and misuse. Addiction. 2017;112(4):719–26.
69. Spear LP. Effects of adolescent alcohol consumption on the brain and behaviour, vol. 19. Nature Reviews Neuroscience. Nature Publishing Group; 2018. p. 197–214.
70. Lees B, Mewton L, Stapinski L, Squeglia L, Rae C, Teesson M. Neurobiological and cognitive profile of young binge drinkers: a systematic review and meta-analysis. Neuropsychol Rev. 2019;29(3):357–85.
71. Cheetham A, Allen NB, Whittle S, Simmons J, Yücel M, Lubman DI. Volumetric differences in the anterior cingulate cortex prospectively predict alcohol-related problems in adolescence. Psychopharmacology. 2014;231(8):1731–42.
72. Squeglia LM, Ball TM, Jacobus J, Brumback T, McKenna BS, Nguyen-Louie TT, et al. Neural predictors of initiating alcohol use during adolescence. Am J Psychiatry. 2017;174(2):172–85.
73. Anton-Toro L, Bruna R, Suarez-Mendez I, Correas A, Garcia-Moreno L, Maestu F. Abnormal organization of inhibitory control functional networks in future binge drinkers. Drug Alcohol Depend. 2021;218:108401.
74. Anton-Toro L, Bruna R, Del Cerro-Leon A, Shpakivska D, Mateos-Gordo P, Porras-Truque C, Garcia-Gomez R, Maestu F, Garcia-Moreno L. Electrophysiological resting-state hyperconnectivity and poorer behavioural regulation as predisposing profiles of adolescent binge drinking. Addict Biol. 2022;27(4):e13199.

42 M/EEG Hallmarks of Healthy and Pathological Aging

Brenda Chino, Jaisalmer de Frutos Lucas, Luis Fernando Antón-Toro, Gianluca Susi, Guiomar Niso, and Fernando Maestú

Electrophysiological Basis of M/EEG Signal

Neuronal communication in the brain is associated with small electrical currents, which give rise to measurable voltage differences on the scalp, and magnetic fields outside the head. Electroencephalography (EEG) and magnetoencephalography (MEG) are neurophysiological techniques that allow us to map the brain electrical and magnetic activity in a noninvasive manner. EEG and MEG reflect in essence the same elementary neuronal phenomena: the postsynaptic activity of synchronously activated neurons [1].

Each neuron—which typically has thousands of synapses with other neurons

B. Chino (✉)
Center for Cognitive and Computational Neuroscience (C3N), Complutense University of Madrid, Madrid, Spain

Institute of Neuroscience, Autonomous University of Barcelona (UAB), Barcelona, Spain

Achucarro Basque Center for Neuroscience, Leioa, Spain
e-mail: brenda.chino@achucarro.org

J. de Frutos Lucas
Center for Cognitive and Computational Neuroscience (C3N), Complutense University of Madrid, Madrid, Spain

Department of Experimental Psychology, Complutense University of Madrid, Madrid, Spain

Centre for Precision Health, Edith Cowan University, Joondalup, WA, Australia
e-mail: jaidefru@ucm.es

L. F. Antón-Toro
Center for Cognitive and Computational Neuroscience (C3N), Complutense University of Madrid, Madrid, Spain

Department of Psychology, Faculty of health, University Camilo José Cela (UCJC), Madrid, Spain
e-mail: lfanton@ucm.es

G. Susi
Center for Cognitive and Computational Neuroscience (C3N), Complutense University of Madrid, Madrid, Spain

Department of Structure of Matter, Thermal Physics and Electronics. School of Physics, Complutense University of Madrid, Madrid, Spain
e-mail: gsusi@ucm.es

G. Niso
Psychological & Brain Sciences, Indiana University, Bloomington, IN, USA

Universidad Politécnica de Madrid, Madrid, Spain
e-mail: guiomar.niso@ctb.upm.es

F. Maestú
Center for Cognitive and Computational Neuroscience (C3N), Complutense University of Madrid, Madrid, Spain

Department of Experimental Psychology, Complutense University of Madrid, Madrid, Spain

Instituto de Investigación Sanitaria San Carlos (IdISSC), Madrid, Spain
e-mail: fmaestuu@psi.ucm.es

P. Á. Gargiulo, H. L. Mesones-Arroyo (eds.), *Psychiatry and Neuroscience Update – Vol. V*,
https://doi.org/10.1007/978-3-031-72219-6_42

[2]—continuously integrates postsynaptic potentials (PSP), caused in turns by the action potentials (AP) of presynaptic afferent neurons. Although AP and PSP are part of the same process, they represent different underlying mechanisms, which attribute them different features: the AP is characterized by a considerable amplitude (~100 mV) and a small duration (~1 ms), whereas the PSP presents a smaller amplitude (~10 mV) but a larger duration (10 ms), important factors which at the scale of cell assemblies translate to a more likely overlap in time for PSPs (Fig. 42.1).

Among the different existing types of neurons, pyramidal neurons—which approximately constitute two-thirds of the neurons present in the cerebral cortex—possess geometrical properties that are able to foster the detection of postsynaptic activity at a certain distance from the neuronal sources when activated with a sufficient degree of synchrony [1, 3].

Indeed, pyramidal neurons present an elongated shape which constrains the circulation of the intracellular current along the somatodendritic axis [4], which can be modeled with a current dipole (that is, a popular source model used to approximate the flow of current in a small area [2]). Furthermore, they are arranged in the form of a palisade, with their main axes parallel to each other and perpendicular to the cortical surface, and the apical dendrites oriented toward the pial surface of the cortex [5]. Such features are ideal for the generation of coherent electric and magnetic fields.

The intracellular (primary) current generates a magnetic field around it, following the right-hand rule of the electromagnetism (Fig. 42.2a). Such current is compensated by extracellular (volume, or secondary) currents that circulate in the opposite direction elsewhere along the membrane, completing the loop of ionic flow in the surrounding medium (Fig. 42.2b), and able to induce voltage differences on the scalp.

This is the reason why the EEG (which measures voltage differences) reflects mainly the extracellular currents, while the MEG (which measures *magnetic fields*) is more sensitive to the intracellular currents [1]. Due to the approximately spherical shape of the head, and since magnetic fields generated by pyramidal neurons in the cortex are radial to their axis, intracellular currents that have a component oriented tangentially to the skull (e.g., those generated by pyramidal neurons in sulcal walls) will produce stronger contributions to MEG signal than currents generated from radial sources (e.g., pyramidal neurons in gyral crowns) [4–6]. Differently, those intracellular currents that are oriented radially to the skull do not generate a magnetic field outside the head but contribute to the EEG [7] (Fig. 42.2c).

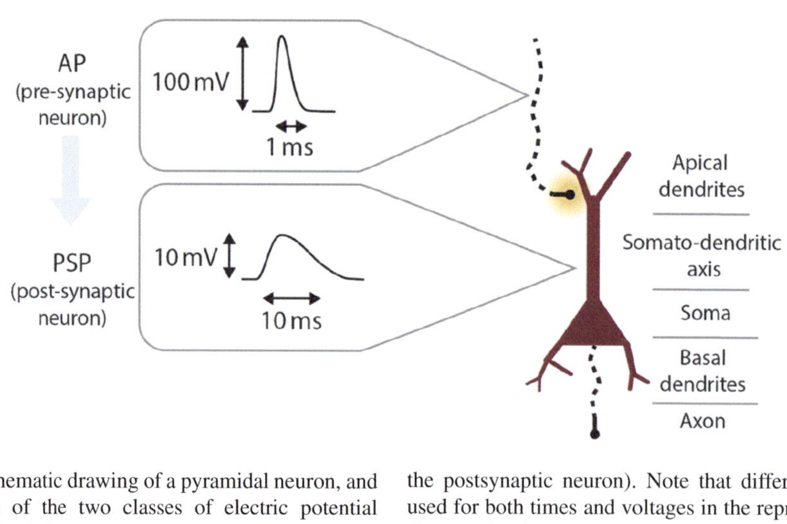

Fig. 42.1 Schematic drawing of a pyramidal neuron, and representation of the two classes of electric potential involved in the information signaling process between neurons: AP (from the presynaptic neuron) and PSP (on the postsynaptic neuron). Note that different scales are used for both times and voltages in the representations of the two signals

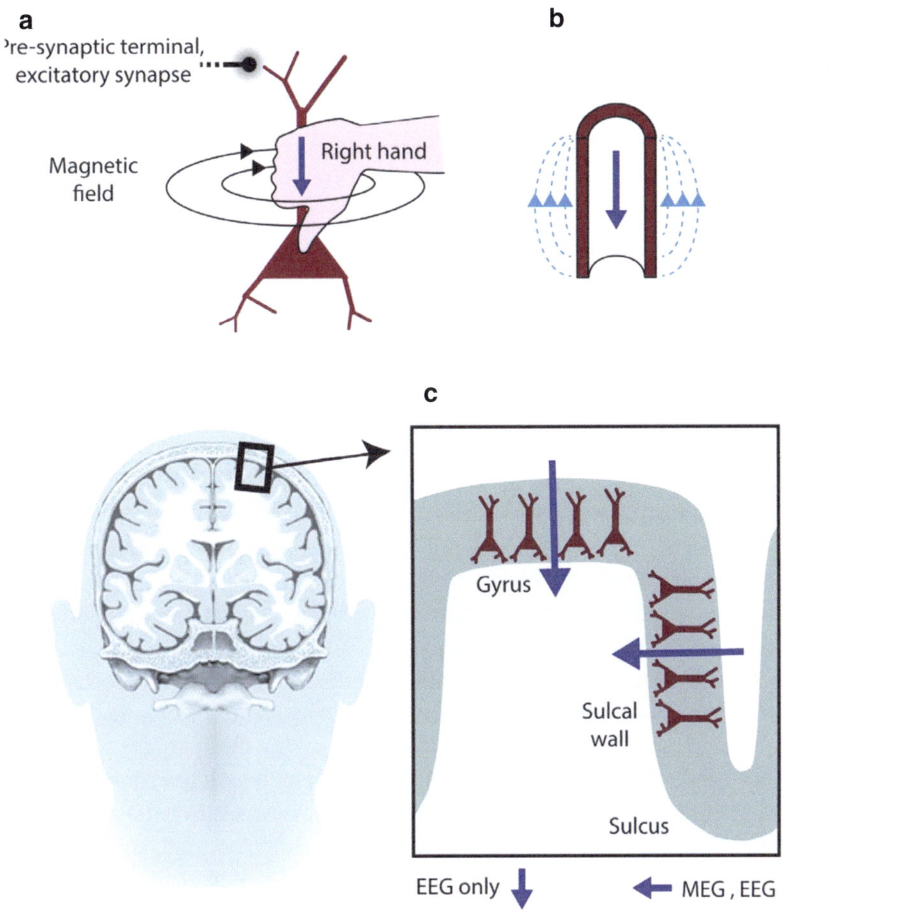

Fig. 42.2 (**a**) An excitatory synaptic stimulation at the level of the apical dendrites is associated with a magnetic field generated around the somatodendritic axis, in accordance with the right-hand rule of electromagnetism. Note that, an inhibitory synapse at the level of the soma will produce the same effect whereas an inhibitory (excitatory) synapse at the level of apical dendrites (soma) will produce an intracellular current upward. This process causes (**b**) the flow of intracellular (primary) current (solid blue arrow) along the somatodendritic axis and related extracellular (volume or secondary) currents in the surrounding medium (dashed blue arrows). (**c**) Scheme of pyramidal neuron disposition in the cortex (*palisade*). Since the primary currents flow roughly perpendicular to the cortex, MEG is much less sensitive to neural currents with a radial orientation with respect to the scalp

In addition to the study of the signal measured at the level of the sensors (sensor space), MEG and EEG allow the scientist to obtain the signals at the level of neural sources (source space). The inference of the position of the current sources from external sensors (known as the inverse problem) can be achieved by combining the signal acquired from the sensors with the structural MRI of the subject, or by using proper existing structural templates.

Since EEG and MEG are sensitive to different aspects of these sources, the combined EEG/MEG source analysis can yield more accurate results than using either method alone [8].

EEG and MEG are particularly appropriate for the study of neurocognitive processes because: (1) they directly measure neural activity, not relying on vascular responses differently to other in-vivo functional neuroimaging techniques (e.g., functional magnetic resonance imaging [fMRI]); (2) they are able to capture cognitive dynamics with high-temporal-resolution (i.e., 1 ms), that is, an appropriate time frame for cognition processes. In addition, MEG presents a good spatial resolution (up to 2–5 mm) and lacks interaction with biologic tissues, avoiding smearing and distortion outside of the scalp [4].

The characteristics of MEG and EEG allow us to study brain activity during the execution of cognitive tasks. Many studies have highlighted the potential of M/EEG as a tool for understanding the resting brain and the nature of connectivity that binds network nodes. Such techniques represent a useful tool to unveil neurobiological mechanisms related to the functional modifications observed during aging.

Brain Oscillations Captured by M/EEG

M/EEG systems are able to capture brain signals containing rhythmic activity. This rhythmic activity is directly linked to neural oscillations in the cortex produced by fluctuations in the excitation/inhibition of underlying populations of neurons. There are three main features that characterize any oscillation: its power (i.e., the amount of energy per unit time), its frequency (i.e., the number of cycles per second), and its phase (i.e., the position along the cosine wave). Some oscillations could be modified by tasks or events, while some others seem to remain unchanged for longer periods of time.

In the brain, oscillations of multiple frequencies coexist simultaneously. These frequencies have been historically grouped into bands, which include delta (2–4 Hz), theta (4–8 Hz), alpha (8–12 Hz), beta (15–30 Hz), low gamma (30–80 Hz), and high gamma (80–150 Hz). These bands are not unique, but the most typically related to cognitive processes in the literature, and their boundaries could slightly vary between studies [6].

The field of spectral analysis enables studying the frequency content of brain signals. By means of the power spectral density (PSD) (also referred as *power spectrum* or *power density spectrum*), one can analyze how the signal power is distributed over the different frequency components. Several studies show that individual differences in peak frequencies have been linked to a number of individual characteristics, highlighting their potential as biomarkers for specific diseases [9]. In the last decades, studying dynamically the frequency content of brain signals has drawn interest revealing promising results in the field of aging [7–10].

Analyzing the oscillatory components of brain signals is considered a key step to further study the "interaction" between brain regions (i.e., in terms of functional connectivity, FC).

M/EEG Instrumentation

Both EEG and MEG techniques allow us to measure a large frequency range (up to 1000 Hz), although bands of interest span typically across 1–80 Hz.

While the detection of surface potentials can be made through small electrodes attached to the scalp, without particular constraints, the sensing of tiny magnetic fields implies a more complex system. To this purpose, classical MEG equipment employs superconducting quantum interference devices (SQUIDs), i.e., particular sensors (magnetometers and gradiometers) made up of superconducting material and based on the so-called Josephson effect. To maintain superconductivity, the entire device needs to operate within a few degrees of absolute zero and cooled with liquid helium. This need reflects on a much more complex system, sketched in Fig. 42.3.

The unit of measurement of EEG is the *volt* (typically, microvolts or μV) while the unit of MEG is the *tesla* (typically, femtotesla or fT). Differently to MEG, for EEG, the measured values are relative with respect to a reference, e.g., an electrode placed somewhere else on the head, such as the ear lobe.

The fact that MEG does not require a reference electrode greatly simplifies the data interpretation. In addition, the possibility of performing continuous head monitoring for subsequent movement compensation ensures versatility in relation to specific types of subjects, such as infants, or patients with movement disorders. On the other hand, MEG technology imposes substantial capital and operating costs.

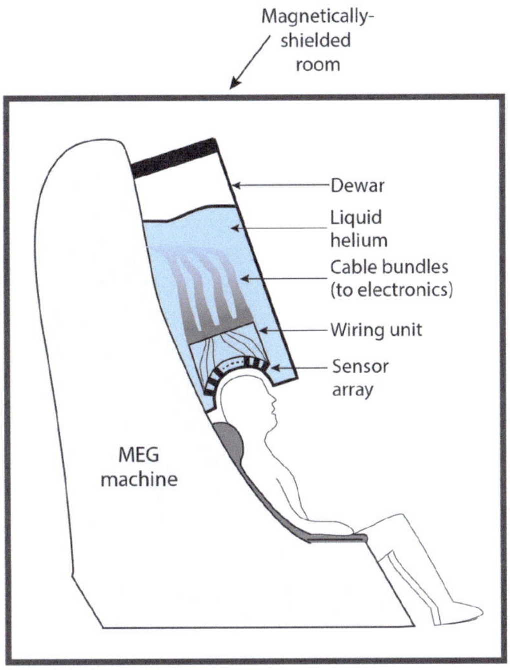

Fig. 42.3 Schematic drawing of an MEG machine

Fortunately, cost-effective solutions are being increasingly used, as onsite helium recycling or helium-free alternatives to SQUID-based technology (i.e., optically pumped magnetometers) [11].

Aging in Figures: A Current Epidemiological Overview

There are 7.7 billion people in the world, and 12.3% are over 60 years old [12]. In 2018, for the first time in history, people over the age of 65 outnumbered children under the age of five. It is estimated, also, that by 2050, one in six will be elderly which implies a radical increase in the ratio of old to young [13]. Demographic aging is a natural process associated with a series of biological changes that include the gradual decrease in physical and mental capacities, increased risk of disease and death [14]. This increase in demand can be particularly significant in developing countries, where population aging occurs at a faster rate than in developed countries. For example, in 2010, the global population of people aged 60 and over residing in developing countries was 65%, and this figure is projected to increase to 80% by 2050 [13]. The pace reached by aging is attributed to two aspects: first, to the increase in life expectancy, which in 2019 was 72.6 years; second, to the decrease in fertility rates, less than 3.2 births per woman reached in 1990 (2.5 in 2019) [13].

Latin America and the Caribbean still cannot have an aging region. According to the United Nations data, adults over 65 years represent 15.2% of its population concerning people between 20 and 64 years. This value is lower than that observed in Europe, North America, Oceania, Asia, and Africa, where we found figures like 32%, 28.5%, 22.6%, 14.8%, and 7.7%, respectively [15]. However, regional data hide strong heterogeneities. Any other way, countries such as Belize, Bolivia, Guatemala, Guyana, and Haiti will be as China is today, with around 15% of the population over 60 years of age. Else, Bahamas, Barbados, Brazil, Chile, Colombia, Costa Rica, Jamaica, Trinidad and Tobago, and Uruguay can be compared to Germany, Finland, and even Japan, with a proportion of older adults close to 30% [12].

This panorama has also led to a growth in the prevalence of various diseases such as dementia. These clinical characteristics directly affected the independence and quality of life of the elderly [16, 17].

In a systematic review of the data obtained in 195 countries from 1990 to 2016 published by the Global Burden of Disease Study, an analysis of mortality, prevalence, and incidence of cases with this pathology concluding that in 2016, the global number of people living with the disease was 43.8 million. This figure increased to 20.2 million compared to 1990 [18]. In the same way, the latest report from Alzheimer's disease International (2018) indicates there are 50 million people worldwide who live with dementia [19]. It implies that there is a new diagnosis of dementia somewhere in the world every 3 s. This figure will more than triple to reach 152 million by 2050. Dementias are a pressing problem for global public health, with costs that exceed $160 billion annually [20]; being, even more, pressing in low–/middle-income countries [21, 22].

In Latin America, in a study by Nitrini et al. [23], the prevalence of dementia in older adults (≥65 years) was determined to be 7.1%, a score similar to that of developed countries. Among dementias, Alzheimer's disease was the most frequent cause, reaching 49.9% in Maracaibo, Venezuela, up to 84.5% in Concepción, Chile. Vascular dementia was the second most prevalent disease, reaching 8.7% in Lima, Peru, up to 26.5% in Maracaibo, Venezuela. Similarly, a high prevalence of dementia is evident in relatively young individuals among older people (65–69 years of age), significantly high compared to that seen in developed countries [23]. In the Andean region alone, there are an estimated 250,000 people with dementia [24].

In recent years, many investigations of Alzheimer's dementia (AD) concluded that interventions must be started in the early stages of AD [25–27], before that the neurodegeneration destroys regions of the brain [28, 29]. In addition, this intervention will be making it possible to reduce the costs of institutionalization, time of care, and medication that in Peru, for example, exceeds up to 2.5 times the assigned minimum wage [30].

Thus, the call to combat dementia has become global [31] and implies the need to transform health systems to provide timely care with affordable diagnostic tools to the general population, which favors the identification of case principles and promotes a preventive approach to the risk associated with the disease.

Cognitive Changes Associated with Healthy Aging

Aging is a natural process that involves the progressive accumulation of physiological changes over time [32]. The physiological decline is accompanied by a slowdown in cognitive processes, which begins shortly after individuals reach maturity [33, 34].

The findings indicate that complex processes are more vulnerable to aging. Between 61 and 96 years old, there would be a decline of −0.04 to −0.05 standard deviations (SD) per year, much more pronounced than that found in people younger than 60 years (− 0.02 to −0.03 SD per year) in the general performance [35].

However, not all aspects of cognitive functioning exhibit early age-related declines. Based on accumulated knowledge, crystallized skills such as vocabulary and general knowledge remain stable or gradually improve at a rate of 0.02–0.03 SD per year during the sixth and seventh decades of life [14, 35, 36]. For example, when comparing their performance to that of people between 20 and 40 years, older people aged between 70 and 80 years old obtained higher vocabulary scores [14, 36].

In contrast, fluent intelligence, referred to skills that involve problem-solving and reasoning about things that are less familiar and independent of learning, declines with the age. Psychomotor ability and processing speed are including in this category, and peaks in the third decade of life and then decreases at an estimated rate of −0.02 standard deviations per year [14, 35, 37]. The last one usually appears as an early sign of normal aging [33] and its slowdown negatively impacts performance in many specific neuropsychological tests to measure other cognitive domains (for example, working memory) [38].

Attention resources decrease with age, specifically in activities that depend on more complex levels of care [39], for example, when engaging in conversation in a noisy environment (selective attention) or cooking while talking on the phone (divided attention). However, the simple listening attention evaluates, classically, with the repetition of a string of digits, shows only a slight decline in late life [14].

The typical memory decline is usually a common complaint in the elderly. However, it remains stable until before the 60 s, and then decreases with age [36]. The alteration of the memory is characterized by difficulties in the free acquisition and/or recovery of the information but not in consolidation [33, 37]. For example, in free recall tests, the support provided by the task is minimal and the demand for self-initiated processes is maximum. On the other hand, in the recognition task, the elderly receives greater environmental support and less need for self-initiated processing, decreasing differences by age [39].

Moreover, research has determined that executive function (EF) could also be altered. Components of the EF like concept formation, abstraction, and flexibility which usually decrease after the 70 s [14]. Other types of executive functions, such as the ability to identify similarities, describe the meaning of proverbs, and reason about familiar material remain stable throughout life.

These findings have practical implications. Age-adjusted cognitive data and longitudinal assessments are essential to define impairment and detect deviations in the clinic that may herald the presence of neuropathology.

What Can Neuroimaging Techniques (EEG/MEG) Tell Us About the Aging Process?

The aging is accompanied by changes in spectral power and topographic distribution of the brain signal. The recent literature describes EEG/MEG as an ideal tool for evaluating the progressive loss of efficiency of the neuronal networks in normal aging and the dysfunctions at the synaptic level that occur at early stages of pathological aging [40–42]. The study of these changes can be addressed from two perspectives: resting state paradigms, where participants do not have to engage in any particular cognitive activity, and task paradigms, where participants have to perform a specific perceptual or cognitive task. Both approaches are alternative ways to study power spectrum and neurophysiological FC networks, and the differences associated with a healthy aging course.

Power in Healthy Aging Using EEG/ MEG

Resting State

EEG studies show a decrease in delta and theta waves overage and an increase in beta compared to younger subjects. Duffy et al. [43] noted the existence of a negative correlation between age and delta and theta waves, indicating that the amount of slow activity on the quantitative EEG does not increase with age in the context of a good state of health. Also, a nonsignificant slowdown of alpha waves is observed in aging but evident between 60 and 80 years. Their results are similar to those found by Pollock et al. [44]; however, the latter also indicates a decrease in the power of beta. Ponomareva et al. [45] found the same results in subjects between 20 and 87 years old, which relates the increase in power in beta with subjects at risk of developing Alzheimer's disease.

Years later, Babiloni et al. [46], in a study carried out on a sample of 215 subjects between 18 and 85 years of age, adds evidence to the decrease in delta band power, specifically the reduction of the magnitude of the delta sources in the occipital. Keeping in mind these data, a tentative explanation of the present findings might be that a significant magnitude increase of low-band EEG sources is not a marker of physiological aging. Rather, it may be a marker of subclinical cognitive deterioration in physiological aging. Besides, there is a decrease in alpha sources in the parietal, occipital, temporal, and limbic areas, related to age. Similarly, Ponomareva et al. [47] indicate a decrease in alpha 3 power in the occipital area, and Reichert et al. [48] indicate a decrease in alpha 2 power in the parietal area, reduced with age.

In the same manner, Dias et al. [49] found an inverse correlation between alpha and theta power during the baseline and age. Theta showed modulations with age mainly in front-central regions while the young sample (22–33 years old) have a greater increase in power than the 40-year-old sample. For some authors, like Arakaki et al. [50], frontal abnormalities in the power spectrum act like first signs of the presymptomatic AD and they can be visible by a simple task. In contrast, only one study has shown that relatively high resting theta power correlates with healthy cognitive aging in subjects between the ages of 56 and 70 years old [51]. Theta power could be a marker of healthy cognitive aging, at least in those without significant cognitive decline, such as MCI, according to the author.

On the other hand, MEG studies about healthy aging in resting state indicate a general shift from low- to high-frequency bands of the PSD distribution until the end of middle age, followed by an opposite behavior for subsequent age stages [52]. In addition, a widespread reduction of low-frequency relative power (delta and theta bands) with increasing age is reported until the end of the middle age. For elder adults, some authors report a perpetuated and linear relative power decrease (e.g., Vlahou et al. [53]), while an increase is highlighted in other studies involving a greater number of subjects (e.g., Gómez et al. [52]), individuating a quadratic trend across the lifespan (discrepancies among the findings may be due to the different power normalization methods used). Relative power of higher frequency bands (alpha and beta) follows an opposite trend with respect to that of low frequency bands [52]. Vlahou et al. [53] highlighted that for older adults, but not for younger participants, higher delta and theta relative power in central and temporal regions is associated with improved cognitive performances (separately assessed with cognitive tests). With regard to task execution studies, the common trait seems to be the greater beta power required by older adults with respect to younger participants during the early/preparatory phase of the task, but these results cannot be generalized due to the limited number of comparative studies and the differences between the experimental designs.

Tasks Paradigms

Regarding the effects of aging on task-related power measurements, there are not as many studies as for resting state, and the results are less convergent, as was to be expected, given the greater variability among the experiment designs. With regard to EEG, as early as 2001 McEvoy et al., [54], the effects on EEG power arising from a spatial working memory task were analyzed, finding decreases of the alpha power with age attributable to the fact that more neurons become involved in task-related processing. By increasing the difficulty of the task, older people showed decreased alpha power over both frontal and parietal regions, while young adults showed a decrease in alpha power over parietal regions only. This suggests that normal aging may be associated with changes in the frontoparietal networks involved with spatial working memory processes. Cummings and Finnigan [55] observed a significantly lower theta power in older adults during both the retention and recognition intervals of a modified version of the Sternberg test. This difference was greatest at the frontocentral midline. Interestingly, Ho et al. [56] measured the EEG power in response to a recognition task based on auditory stimuli, finding for elderly participants a decreased power in the alpha bands and an increased power in the delta band. The power increases in anterior areas where it decreases in the posterior area.

Regarding the MEG technique, among the most emblematic works, Proskovec et al. [57] studied the MEG power in relation to a modified Sternberg working memory task. They reported that older people show an increased alpha/beta power during the *early encoding* phase in the right hemispheric homologue of Wernicke's area, whereas in the right hemispheric homologue of Broca's area, the same effect has been noted during the subsequent period, persisting throughout the *memory maintenance* phase. In addition, a stronger alpha activity is detected during the maintenance phase, involving occipital areas and more cortical tissue. Rondina et al. [10] characterized the power with regard to a visuospatial memory task, observing that during the prestimulus activity, older present significantly lower theta and greater beta power with respect to younger, across all brain areas. In this study, older adults showed an increase in theta power from prestimulus to poststimulus phase in medial temporal channels, as well as a decrease in alpha power from prestimulus to poststimulus phases in occipitotemporal regions.

Taken together, the results emerging from MEG studies seem to highlight a common trait: with respect to younger participants, older adults show greater activation power in the beta band during the early phase of the task. Regarding the age-related modification in EEG power under task execution, the findings indicate a reorganization of frontoparietal networks, as well as a power decrease in the alpha band, attributable to the fact that more neurons become involved in task-related processing.

Nevertheless, these results cannot be generalized due to the limited number of comparative studies and the differences between the experimental designs.

Functional Connectivity in Healthy Aging Using EEG/MEG

Several studies have explored differences in FC networks associated with aging. These works, despite applying different metrics in order to depict the synchronized activation of brain regions, claim to reflect the FC changes related to nonpathologic physiological aging. The study of these changes can be addressed from two perspectives: resting state paradigms and task paradigms.

Resting State (RS)

The study of RS FC networks aims to depict the functional interactions of spontaneous brain oscillations. Some researchers have evidenced that nonpathological aging is associated with changes in these functional networks. For instance, Duffy et al. [58], evaluated 371 healthy adults, from 20 to 80 years old (171 males and 200 females) with EEG RS recordings. They found age-related reductions in EEG interhemispheric coherence. These changes were located in temporal lobes, particularly in theta, alpha, and beta bands. Comparable results in alpha band were reported by Shinosaki et al. [59]. In an EEG study over 38 elder subjects (50–89 years old) and a control group formed by 22 individuals (20–29 years old), they calculated FC patterns using relative power contribution analysis. They reported a decreased left temporooccipital functional interdependence in ages from 50 to 80 years old, and additional reductions of alpha interdependence in right inferior frontal areas for ages from 70 to 80 years old, indicating a progressive alteration of alpha FC as normal aging advance.

In the same line, Schlee et al. [60], using MEG RS recordings with 53 (18–89 years old), found FC several age-related changes. These changes were characterized by a lower FC inflow in posterior cingulum and precuneus, together with and increased FC within temporal lobes. This last one was found to be inversely correlated with cognitive performance.

In other study, Balsters et al. [61], combined fMRI and EEG recordings in order to explore age-related differences in the FC of diverse resting state networks (RSn). They compared a group of 15 young adults (age 18–28) with a group of 27 older adults (age 65–78). Some of the more robust differences in older adults were a reduction in beta band connectivity between the default mode network (DMN) (particularly, the anterior part) and hippocampus, and between the DMN and the SMA. In another MEEG study with 48 EEGs (age 18–72 years old) and 31 MEGs (age 20–75 years old), information process and sharing among brain regions were analyzed by transfer entropy methods.

McIntosh et al. [62], reported an age-related reduction of distributed entropy across hemispheres. Additionally, they found a reduced high-alpha activity within the left frontoparietal network. In another study carried out by Vysata et al. [63], a large sample of healthy adults (17722) by EEG coherence method was analyzed. They reported reductions in global theta and alpha bands coherence, accompanied by an increase in the coherence of beta band. Conversely, Nakamura et al. [64] found increased FC in low frequency bands between precuneus and the bilateral inferior parietal lobules in healthy aging, correlating with amyloid-β deposition.

A complementary line of research is the novel machine learning methodology, which allows us to identify the common features that define a particular brain state. Using these machine learning classification methods, as a minimum spanning tree, Escudero et al. [65] identified FC features as potential classifiers of old-age adults brain networks. In a sample of 1500 healthy participants, from 7 to 71 years old, they found in the >50 years old range, a decrease in the alpha band FC calculated by PLI metric. These reductions were observed specially in frontoparietal regions (bihemispheric) and interhemispheric connections.

In a similar way, Moezzi et al. [66] employed a different machine learning classifier (support vector machine) to sort the FC features, measured with imaginary coherence method, of a group of young adults (19–37 years old) and a group of older adults (63–85 years old). They found that older adults group presented decreased FC particularly in the alpha band, involving frontal, temporal, and parietal electrodes. These findings were interpreted as reduced connectivity in the networks which govern attention and awareness. In contrast, increased beta FC was reported for the older group in sensorimotor functional networks. EEG FC of older adults has been also related with differences in the "individual alpha peak frequency" (IAPF) by Scally et al. [67]. In this work, the authors found a lower alpha band FC in the old adult's group (N = 32; mean age 69) compared with younger adults (N = 37; mean age = 20). However, an important finding of this study was the absence of differences in terms of FC when groups were compared, adapting the results to each individual IAPF. An additional line of RS works focused on depicting FC changes regarding healthy aging by means of sleep stages analysis. In this line, recent research carried out by Ujma et al. [68] studied the age-related EEG FC (wPLI) characteristics during sleep. A large cohort of 172 individuals (from 17 to 69 years old) was evaluated by EEG recordings during NREM and REM sleep stages. Healthy aging was characterized by a steady decrease of NREM sigma (11.5–15.5 Hz) band among frontal, parietal, and occipital electrodes, joint to stage-independent increased in theta, in frontal electrodes and beta FC in frontooccipital electrodes. Similar findings were reported by Bouchard et al. [69] in a quite similar work. They analyzed the FC differences (imaginary coherence) between a group of 30 individuals (20–30 years old) and a group of older participants (50–70 years old) during a NREM and REM sleep episodes. Main findings pointed to a reduced FC of older-age group in sleep stage N2 for high-delta, theta, and sigma bands, but higher in N3 and REM stages in lower frequency bands, delta, and theta, compared with the younger group. These results were interpreted by the authors as a reduced ability of older brains to "disconnect" active networks in comparison with young brains.

Altogether, the study of RS networks variations with healthy aging seem to shed consistent evidence: age-related changes are generally characterized by a reduction in the synchronization of spontaneous brain activity among diverse cortical areas. This reduced FC is particularly seen in slow frequency bands, joint to increases of beta band synchronization within sensorimotor networks. However, different methodologies employed in the measurement of FC patterns must be borne in mind when drawing conclusions.

Cognitive and Perceptual Tasks

Traditionally, M/EEG task paradigms are employed to study the brain functional activity associated with diverse cognitive "states." By means of the FC analysis, these kinds of paradigms allow investigators to depict the functional brain regions interactions in order to accomplish specific cognitive processes. The functional dynamics engaged in these processes may be affected by multiple factors, among which, aging, is a crucial one. In the following section, we will provide further information regarding how healthy aging alters task-related functional networks.

Some researchers have put their efforts in characterizing the old-ages electrophysiological connectivity which emerge as a consequence of relatively simple cognitive process, such as visual-stimuli discrimination or auditory oddball detection. For instance, Maurits et al. [70], investigated the EEG coherence differences between a group of 11 young adults (mean age = 27.8) and 10 older adults (mean age = 61.3) while performing an auditory oddball task. This task aims to study the electrophysiological response to the detection of a "deviant" stimuli within a relatively stable sequence of "standard" stimuli. The authors found a higher interhemispheric EEG coherence in the delta band and higher intrahemispheric coherence for theta and alpha bands for older adults. In another study using a similar paradigm, Muller et al. [71] reported an age-related increase of phase coherence in older-ages for delta, theta, and alpha bands, measured as mean global connectivity of Cz electrode in deviant condition. Moreover, the level of FC in older-ages correlated negatively with measures of perceptual speed.

A different line of works employed a visual perceptual task in order to analyses FC patterns of older ages during the encoding of visual stimulus. Werkle-Bergner et al. [72] evaluated age-related FC differences due effect of stimulus size in three groups: 17 children (10–12 years old), 16 young adults (20–26 years old), and 17 old adults (70–76 years old). Main results reported an increased gamma band synchronization in older ages for smaller stimulus, but a less increment of FC for higher stimulus size. Similar pattern of FC changes was reported by Wang et al. [73] during an audiovisual integration task. In this work, a group of 12 young adults (22–28 years old) and a group of 12 older adults (60–78 years old) were evaluated, finding that old adults presented higher FC in beta band among temporal and central electrodes. A complementary line of task studies is related to the sensorimotor activity in older ages. A recent study conducted by Ferreri et al. [74], found that older adults exhibit a higher functional coupling between M1 cortices with homolateral PFC after TMS stimulation.

Regarding age-related changes involving high-order cognitive processes, several works have found interesting results pointing to differences in the way how brain networks synchronize to support them. For instance, Tóth et al. [75] evaluated age-related changes in the frontal midline (FM) theta synchronization during delayed math-to-sample WM task. They compared a group of 20 young adults (18–22 years old) and 16 older adults (60–71 years old), revealing that the last, presented reduced theta FC strength in the FM with temporal areas, being related with worse WM performance. In a similar way, an MEG study of participants performing an interference-based working memory task showed that older adults require higher alpha synchronization between cortical brain regions in order to achieve a successful recognition. In this scenario, the main differences between age groups arose during the interference window, where older participants had a reduced ability to reorganize their brain functional network [76]. In a similar work, by means of WM interference-task, Arnau et al. [77], evaluated the theta FM connectivity changes between 18 young (19–29 years old) and 18 old adults (62–71 years old). Using an Fz electrode as seed for FM, they reported that older adults were characterized by increased theta FC in right parietooccipital areas during primary task response and reduced theta FC in centrooccipital areas for upcoming interference signaling. In another study, Hou et al. [78] measured the PLI FC networks during a N-back cognitive task in a group of 15 young adults (mean age = 23) and 13 old adults (mean age = 64). In the condition of high cognitive load, 2-back, older adults showed in this case, a reduced FC in alpha band among frontoparietal electrodes and an enhancement of theta band connectivity among prefrontal electrodes.

In general, most of the studies regarding age-related differences in simple cognitive processes seem to report similar patterns in their results. These findings in healthy aging changes are commonly characterized by an increased synchronization among diverse brain areas. Moreover, these changes seem to engage particularly slow frequency bands for perceptual discrimination tasks, such as oddball paradigm, and fast frequency bands for perceptual integration paradigms (i.e., audio-visual) and motor tasks. Conversely, the works which focus on FC age-related differences related with high cognitive processes deliver less cohesive findings. For instance, works which evaluated FC in WM delayed-match-to-sample performance paradigms showed divergent results; while some studies reported reduced frontal-midline theta synchronization in the maintenance state, others showed an increased connectivity in this frequency band and just a reduced synchronization as response to interference conditions. Additionally, other works reported widespread higher alpha connectivity in WM interference states as a neurophysiological compensatory mechanism of the brain to accomplish successful performances. Divergently, reduced frontoparietal alpha band and enhanced prefrontal theta band synchronization were reported in the performance of N-back task. Nevertheless, variations in the experimental paradigms and FC analysis methodologies would be an important bias towards coming up with similar results. This fact shed light to the necessity of carrying on additional research to enhance the growing body of evidence regarding this important matter. Even then, despite discrepant evidence, there is a strong consensus regarding the existence of age-related changes in brain functional networks involved in a wide variety of high-order cognitive processes.

How Does Pathology Modify the Electrophysiological Footprints of the Aging Brain?

The Alzheimer's Disease Continuum

One of the most relevant age-related disorders affecting the brain is Alzheimer's disease (AD), which is a neurodegenerative disease that is characterized by progressive and fatal cognitive impairment as a result of the abnormal accumulation of proteins in the brain parenchyma, which causes the loss of neurons and brain atrophy. There is strong evidence to affirm that AD pathology starts to accumulate in the brain up to 20 years before the earliest clinical manifestations. This process is usually referred to as the AD continuum, which includes preclinical, prodromal, and dementia stages. The first of these is known as subjective cognitive decline (SCD) [79, 80] which is followed by mild cognitive impairment (MCI) [81]. There is a high rate of progression from this state to AD [82, 83], while a significant percentage is not progressing into dementia at all [82, 83]. After this long process, the final stage will be reached, accompanied by a formal diagnosis of AD.

M/EEG studies build upon our knowledge on how the electrophysiological properties of the aging brain are affected by AD neuropathology. Taking a power spectrum characterization approach has yielded highly consistent outcomes, where a general slowing of background activity characterizes the AD continuum, including prodromal and preclinical stages of the disease [84–86].

This profile features an increase in power in low frequencies (delta band) together with a decrease in power decrease in higher frequency bands (alpha and beta bands) (Verdoorn et al., 2011) [86–90]. According to de Waal et al. [91], it is possible to observe an increase in delta and theta power in the temporal, parietal, and/or occipital region in patients with AD even after a 3-year follow-up. These changes can be observed even in the early stages of the disease for both hemispheres and the anterior and posterior areas [88, 92]. Some studies also indicate an alteration of the gamma power; however, the results are still contradictory. McBride et al. [93] point, for example, to a decrease in gamma in the right frontal and left temporal regions, while Sarma et al. [94] indicated a high-power gamma in AD.

Probably, the best described feature of the aforementioned slowing and also the one that has raised greatest interest in the scientific community is reduction in alpha power, which makes this the most robust finding in neurophysiological research on AD. This reduction in alpha power is associated with worse cognitive functioning in AD patients [95]. Such slowing is even more exacerbated among multidomain MCI patients (MCI cases showing alterations in more than one cognitive domain) compared to single-domain MCI patients. Moreover, the latter groups present an association between such slowing and worse cognitive outcomes [86]. Similarly, in an EEG study, Van der Hiele et al. [89] described an increase in theta relative power and a decrease in alpha reactivity in AD patients, which indicated worse performance in several cognitive domains.

In the case of MCI, the findings are controversial. According to Hsiao et al. [96], the cortical activity of resting-state oscillations is altered during the transition from MCI to AD. However, 1 year later, the same authors concluded that there is no significant difference between AD and

MCI in spectral power, but that averaged power values in AD were larger for theta and delta bands and smaller alpha and beta bands [97]. On the other hand, longitudinal studies on MCI, such as the ones by Rossini et al. [40, 98] and Musaeus et al. [99], point out to a decrease in power in the alpha and beta band in temporal and frontal areas both in AD and MCI. Moreover, progressive MCI was characterized by decreased beta power in parietal, temporal, and central regions, a feature that could be considered as a good classifier to distinguish between MCI progressive and MCI stable at 2-years follow-up. Additionally, high spectral power of the slower rhythms (delta and theta) in frontotemporal areas also warns of "conversion from MCI to AD" [100] and could be considered as a biomarker of the disease [101]. Altogether, the reported evidence indicates that an early increase in theta power and a decrease in beta power, followed by a subsequent decrease in alpha power and later a decrease in delta power would be the process of conversion of normal adults to AD [102].

Conversely, brain connectivity alterations play a fundamental role in the study of the mechanisms underlying disturbances in cognition. AD has often been defined as a disconnection syndrome [103]. Abnormal interactions between brain areas in AD could be linked to early neuropathological changes, which degenerate white matter tracts and synaptic transmission, even decades before the first clinical symptoms appear [104, 105]. Therefore, brain functional connectivity alterations could be detectable in early stages of the disease, such as in SCD and MCI using in-vivo FC and SC methods. Hypersynchronization has been suggested as an AD biomarker of synaptic dysfunction, showing abnormal excitation/inhibition levels in the brain [106–109].

In the continuum of the disease, it has been found that people with SCD and MCI, in comparison to HCs, present a hypersynchronization in the anterior network and a hyposynchronization in posterior regions in the resting state, the latter being significantly lower in MCI as compared to SCD subjects [110–114]. This hyposynchronization between different areas is often interpreted as a disruption and a loss of the network communication, while the hypersynchronization is often attributed to a compensatory recruitment of brain areas due to the progressive loss of cognitive function. At the same time, network-based studies in MCI have revealed that these changes of connectivity occur often more randomly and inefficiently. These disruptions are also present in SCD subjects, but to a lesser degree [113, 115].

In AD, MEG papers report a decrease in FC [106–108]. This decreased synchronization seems to affect especially to higher frequency bands (e.g., [107, 116–118]), which may reflect local connectivity changes [84]. Some studies have also found an increased connectivity in slow frequencies (3–7 Hz), particularly in posterior regions, but these have been less reported (e.g., [116, 118, 119]). Connectivity between long-range regions was reported diminished in the left hemisphere, involving main frontal, temporal, and parietal regions, while the connectivity within a region was primarily decreased in the right hemisphere frontal and parietal areas (for a review, see [42, 84, 108]). The findings from studies using network analysis confirm some previous results reported in AD. A lower and more vulnerable concentration is observed [120], weaker connections between modules [121, 122], and a more random configuration in several bands [109, 117, 123]. These findings allowed evaluating the risk of conversion from MCI to AD in a longitudinal study. This was done by comparing the resting-state MEG networks of FC from patients with MCI, who remained "stable" after several months of evaluation, and patients with MCI, who converted to AD at the same time later. Two characteristic networks were identified in the theta and beta bands, involving frontotemporal and frontooccipital connections, with reduced FC levels in the progressive MCI group. However, at baseline, patients with progressive MCI presented higher synchronization than patients with stable MCI, while in the postcondition, this pattern was reversed. These results suggest an "X" form model where the hypersynchrony predicts conversion, leading subsequently to a network breakdown in progressive MCI [109].

Despite their different measure approaches to FC and cognitive function frequently used, cognitive impairment correlates with modification of functional connectivity (e.g., [107, 112, 116, 120]). This is in line with previous findings from other neuroimaging techniques [124] and with neuropathological studies that found that synapses disturbances lead to connection impairment [125], supporting the notion of AD as a disconnection syndrome.

In summary, different reports of FC in the AD continuum using MEG confirm the existence of an anteroposterior dual pattern along the network failures that occur in predementia and AD stages. There seems to be an early loss of synchronization in posterior regions but increased in anterior regions, when the cognitive impairment is still not perceptible by neuropsychological assessments, followed by a similar pattern but with a more decreased synchrony in posterior networks at the MCI phase, and a final network desynchronization when the patient is diagnosed as AD. However, still more research on other neurodegenerative diseases than AD is necessary to unravel the pattern of network disturbances that occur in dementia.

Influence of Lifestyle on Electrophysiological Measures

Lifestyle and Healthy Aging

Based on this knowledge about the neurophysiological footprints of aging, different studies have explored the potential of lifestyle modifications to promote healthy brain aging. One of these factors is physical activity. Exercise has been found to exert a positive response in the brain, promoting neurogenesis, synaptogenesis, angiogenesis, and myelin remodeling [126, 127]. In this line, it has been found that the individual alpha frequency peak was higher among highly active older adults, compared to moderately and low active older adults [128]. A different study on healthy aging observed that incidental physical activity (activity associated with unstructured daily activities) was related to slower activity in frontal, central, and temporal regions across different frequency bands [129]. At the network level, an objectively measured physical activity was also found to be associated with reduced left-temporal hypersynchrony in older adults. Moreover, cardiovascular fitness has been associated with increased intermodular connectivity and reduced within-modules connectivity [130].

Other authors have analyzed the effect on factors that contribute to cognitive reserve could have on neurophysiological measures. For example, an MEG study showed that that older woman who had learnt to read after the age of 50 presented reduced functional asymmetry during the execution of a language recognition test than those who had attended school for at least 10 years [131]. This was interpreted as a sign of compensation, so that both groups performed similarly at the behavioral level, yet ex-illiterate women required greater neural resources. In a different MEG study, healthy older adults scoring higher in cognitive reserve (using a composite measure combining educational attainment and occupation) showed lower functional connectivity across several frequency bands than those with lower cognitive reserve [86]. This was again interpreted as a sign of compensation. Finally, in a recent resting state MEG study bilingualism was associated with greater parieto-occipital functional connectivity [132].

Last but not least, diet could also contribute to foster brain health, which could be tracked using neurophysiological devices. In particular, diet patterns rather than specific nutrients are nowadays the focus of interventional studies within this field. In this sense, Mediterranean diet is linked to slower cognitive impairment and greater grey matter volumes among older adults. In this line, a preliminary MEG study shows that higher adherence to Mediterranean diet seems to be associated with increased functional connectivity between the anterior and posterior DMN in healthy older adults [132]. One controversial element associated with diet is alcohol consumption. Moderate wine consumption has traditionally been part of Mediterranean diet. However, there is a growing body of evidence that suggests that no dose of alcohol intake can be attributed health benefits [133]. Although there is a lack of electrophysiological studies looking at the effect of alcohol consumption on brain aging, there is some evidence that both acute and chronic alcohol consumption induce changes. For example, both moderate and heavy regular alcohol consumption has been found to alter alpha and beta synchronization during a mental rehearsal of pictures task [134]. In social drinkers, acute alcohol intake induces an increase in functional connectivity at rest, which has been suggested to exert the opposite effect long-term [135]. Additionally, alcohol consumption has been found to impair neuroplasticity (defined as theta-gamma coupling potentiation) in the dorsolateral prefrontal cortex [136]. Acute consumption of low doses of ethanol has also been found to induce a lowering in peak power in the fast-alpha range [137].

Neurophysiological tools, being completely non-invasive, could play a key role in the study of how lifestyle modifications promote healthy aging. However, very few studies have been conducted under this framework and even less have taken a longitudinal approach. Future studies looking at the effect of lifestyle interventions on the brain, as well as longitudinal observational studies following a cohort for several years and also studies combining several lifestyle factors, are needed in order to determine which lifestyle elements are the most effective to preserve brain health.

Lifestyle and Dementia

Despite the efforts of hundreds of scientists globally, no cure has yet been found for Alzheimer's disease. This is partly explained by the fact that Alzheimer's neuropathology begins decades before the very first clinical symptoms arise [104, 138]. For this reason, attention has shifted towards disease prevention. Education, diet, or exercise are some of the lifestyle variables that could aid to delay AD onset and reduce its symptoms. In other words, lifestyle changes could provide individuals at greater risk of AD, as well as patients, with greater quality of life for longer periods. Electrophysiological techniques are excellent tools to monitor the effect that lifestyle changes could exert on the brain, since it is safe to repeat the procedure as many times as needed.

One of its most relevant lifestyle factors is physical activity. Physical exercise has been proposed to delay the onset of AD and enhance cognition. Electrophysiological studies can foster our understanding of how physical activity affects the brain. For example, a few studies have looked at the effect of physical activity in healthy older adults at increased genetic risk for AD. MEG data provided evidence of an association between greater spontaneous physical activity and higher individual alpha peak frequencies [128]. However, such association only remained significant among those who did not carry genetic risk factors for AD. Conversely, in another MEG study, during a working memory task, physically active older adults at increased genetic risk for AD presented higher right temporal lobe activation in matching probe trials than their sedentary counterparts [139]. Noncarriers of that genetic risk factor did not show such association. In this line, a recent MEG study found that the physical activity was associated with left temporal hyposynchronization in slow wave bands during rest [132]. Interestingly, this association remained significant in both carriers and noncarriers of genetic risk factors for AD. However, while in carriers, this neurophysiological profile was associated with better preserved gray and white matter structure, as well as reduced anxiety, in noncarriers, this profile was associated with improved cognition.

Additional studies have been carried out looking specifically at the effect that the physical activity has in pathological conditions. For example, in an EEG study [140], it was found that after an exercise-based rehabilitation program, the alpha wave was reduced in dementia patients, paired with an improvement in cognition and daily activities performance. Another study observed that, after an intervention program using whole-body vibration, women with senile dementia showed greater EEG activation [140]. Moreover, in line with the idea that, evolutionary, locomotion would signal the brain the presence of a cognitive challenge [141, 142], a few studies have combined physical and cognitive training programs. This way, in a sample of MCI seniors, Styliadis et al. [143] observed that the precuneus/posterior cingulate cortex activity across several frequency bands increased with training, but only after a combined intervention program. Such increase, once again, correlates with enhanced cognitive function. Similarly, an EEG study looking at the network level showed that in MCI patients, a combined intervention resulted in network reorganization in the beta band, mainly not only in the dorsal but also in the ventral streams [144].

Beyond the physical activity, several proxies of cognitive reserve have also been studied as candidates to contribute to the delay of AD onset. Cognitive reserve could be described as interindividual differences in the ability of the brain to preserve its functioning despite the presence of underpinning neuropathology [145]. Factors such as educational attainment or bilingualism do not counteract pathological processes at the cellular and molecular levels, but they seem to be able to delay the emergence of clinical and cognitive alterations. For example, in an EEG study with MCI , patients [146] observed that greater cognitive reserve was paired with higher neural efficiency. MCI patients, compared to healthy controls, showed reduced P300 amplitudes, but cognitive reserve modulated this relationship.

Finally, one additional lifestyle factor that could contribute to delay AD and ameliorate its symptoms is nutrition. A diet rich in antioxidants, paired with high consumption of monounsaturated and polyunsaturated fat acids and low levels of saturated fat acids seems to protect against dementia and cognitive decline (see Solfrizzi et al., [147] for an in-depth review). A decade ago, MEG was already proposed as a useful tool to assess nutritional interventions in AD [148, 149]. Unfortunately, just a few studies have been developed with this purpose. For example, the efficacy of Suvenaid, a medical food designed to counteract synaptical loss in AD, was tested in an EEG study with mild AD patients. After a 24-week intervention, it was found that the experimental group presented enhanced memory, reduced slowing of the peak frequency and differential mean PLI trajectories in the delta band [150]. The experimental group also seemed more resilient to network disruption in the beta band [150]. However, in a later MEG study, these results could not be replicated, most likely due to the smaller sample size [151].

As this section highlights, electrophysiological techniques could play a key role in the study of lifestyle interventions to prevent AD. The studies presented above show that EEG and MEG are able to measure even subtle differences in brain function across individuals who engage in healthy lifestyles at varying levels. However, very few studies have taken this approach so far. Given that AD progression employing EEG and MEG has been thoroughly described, it is high time to evaluate ways to alter the trajectory of the disease by implementing healthier daily habits.

Conclusions

Brain nonpathological aging involves several neurobiological changes which in turn affect neurophysiological functioning. As above exposed, the consequences of these changes can be explored under the framework of brain power spectrum and regional synchronizations.

Resting state EEG / MEG studies on healthy aging coincide in pointing out a generalized reduction of the relative power of low frequency (delta and theta bands) with increasing age until the end of the mature age. The relative power of the higher-frequency bands (alpha and beta) follows an opposite trend to low-frequency bands.

On the other hand, electrophysiological studies on AD also find an exacerbated slowing of background activity, where the alterations within the alpha band, especially the alpha peak have been widely studied. Power spectrum studies have also identified valuable features to distinguish stable and progressive MCI.

On the other hand, FC analysis methodologies applied to M/EEG recordings have proved to be a useful and reliable tool in the identification of age-related variations. FC differences along healthy aging are evidenced in several studies, using different paradigms, and employing different analysis approaches. In general, RS studies reported slow frequency bands (delta, theta, and alpha) reduced synchronization, together with increased sensorimotor beta-band synchronization. Such alterations have been proposed to be associated with the loss of white matter tract integrity and nonpathological processes of neural degeneration. Similarly, task-induced functional networks appear sensitive to age-related changes, revealing a wider variety of FC differences across regions and frequency bands. Both FC increases in some networks and reductions in others were reported by several works. Some authors have proposed different models of "compensatory mechanisms" as a potential explanation for the increases of FC usually observed in older adults. The brain would engage additional neural resources to successfully develop a particular cognitive task. However, considering the relatively scarce number of works addressing this topic as well as the variety of paradigms employed, drawing firm conclusions becomes challenging.

Moreover, FC alterations along the AD continuum have also been addressed in M/EEG studies. SCD and MCI individuals, as opposed to HCs, present anterior hypersynchronization and posterior hyposynchronization during resting state, where the latter is more intense in MCI. At the end of the spectrum, AD could be considered a disconnection syndrome, where widespread decreased FC is the most remarkable feature.

Finally, a few studies have applied electrophysiological approaches to the study of how lifestyle could exert a beneficial effect in the brain to minimize the alterations that are associated with healthy and pathological aging. They are excellent tools for this aim, since they are completely noninvasive, and it is safe to reapply them in longitudinal and interventional designs. However, although results so far are promising, more research is needed in this field to provide robust evidence upon which to determine future lifestyle guidelines.

Acknowledgements BChV appreciates the financial support of the National Council for Science, Technology and Technological Innovation (CONCYTEC, Peru) through the National Fund for Scientific and Technological Development (FONDECYT, Peru) by fund 235-2018-FONDECYT. Additionally, JdFL was supported through a scholarship by the School of Medical and Health Sciences from Edith Cowan University (Australia). GN received financial support through a postdoctoral fellowship from the AXA Research Fund. GN and FM acknowledge the Community of Madrid through the project Madrid Neurocenter (B2017/BMD-3760).

References

1. Lopes da Silva F. EEG and MEG: relevance to neuroscience. Neuron. 2013;80(5):1112–28.
2. Hämäläinen M, Hari R, Ilmoniemi RJ, Knuutila J, Lounasmaa OV. Magnetoencephalography—theory, instrumentation, and applications to noninvasive studies of the working human brain. Rev Mod Phys. 1993;65(2):413–97.
3. Buzsáki G, Anastassiou CA, Koch C. The origin of extracellular fields and currents—EEG, ECoG, LFP and spikes. Nat Rev Neurosci. 2012;13(6):407–20.
4. Baillet S. Magnetoencephalography for brain electrophysiology and imaging. Nat Neurosci. 2017;20(3):327–39.
5. Hansen P, Kringelbach M, Salmelin R, editors. MEG: an introduction to methods [Internet]. New York: Oxford University Press; 2010. 448 p
6. Lopes da Silva F. Neural mechanisms underlying brain waves: from neural membranes to networks. Electroencephalogr Clin Neurophysiol. 1991;79(2):81–93.
7. Fernández A, Hornero R, Mayo A, Poza J, Gil-Gregorio P, Ortiz T. MEG spectral profile in Alzheimer's disease and mild cognitive impairment. J Int Fed Clin Neurophysiol. 2006;117(2):306–14.
8. Aydin Ü, Vorwerk J, Dümpelmann M, Küpper P, Kugel H, Heers M, et al. Combined EEG/MEG can outperform single modality EEG or MEG source reconstruction in Presurgical epilepsy diagnosis. PLoS One. 2015;10(3):e0118753.
9. Başar E, Başar-Eroğlu C, Güntekin B, Yener GG. Brain's alpha, beta, gamma, delta, and theta oscillations in neuropsychiatric diseases: proposal for biomarker strategies. In: Başar E, Başar-Eroĝlu C, Özerdem A, Rossini PM, Yener GG, editors. Supplements to clinical neurophysiology, vol. 62. Elsevier; 2013. p. 19–54.
10. Rondina R, Olsen RK, McQuiggan DA, Fatima Z, Li L, Oziel E, et al. Age-related changes to oscillatory dynamics in hippocampal and neocortical networks. Neurobiol Learn Mem. 2016;134 Pt A:15–30.
11. Tierney TM, Holmes N, Mellor S, López JD, Roberts G, Hill RM, et al. Optically pumped magnetometers: from quantum origins to multi-channel magnetoencephalography. NeuroImage. 2019;199:598–608.
12. Aranco N, Stampini M, Ibarrarán P, Medellín N. Panorama de envejecimiento y dependencia en América Latina y el Caribe. Inter-American Development Bank; 2018.
13. United Nations, editor. Department of economic and social affairs. World population prospects 2019—

volume II: demographic profiles. United Nations; 2020. 1237 p
14. Harada CN, Natelson Love MC, Triebel K. Normal cognitive aging. Clin Geriatr Med. 2013;29(4):737–52.
15. World Population Prospects 2019 Volume II: Demographic Profiles | Population Division.
16. Sperling RA, Aisen PS, Beckett LA, Bennett DA, Craft S, Fagan AM, et al. Toward defining the preclinical stages of Alzheimer's disease: recommendations from the National Institute on Aging-Alzheimer's association workgroups on diagnostic guidelines for Alzheimer's disease. Alzheimers Dement J Alzheimers Assoc. 2011;7(3):280–92.
17. Mukadam N, Sommerlad A, Huntley J, Livingston G. Population attributable fractions for risk factors for dementia in low-income and middle-income countries: an analysis using cross-sectional survey data. Lancet Glob Health. 2019;7(5):e596–603.
18. GBD 2016 Dementia Collaborators. Global, regional, and national burden of Alzheimer's disease and other dementias, 1990–2016: a systematic analysis for the Global Burden of Disease Study 2016. Lancet Neurol. 2019;18(1):88–106.
19. World Alzheimer Report. The state of the art of dementia research: new frontiers. New Front. 2018; 48.
20. Prince M, Acosta D, Ferri CP, Guerra M, Huang Y, Llibre Rodriguez JJ, et al. Dementia incidence and mortality in middle-income countries, and associations with indicators of cognitive reserve: a 10/66 dementia research group population-based cohort study. Lancet Lond Engl. 2012;380(9836):50–8.
21. Wimo A, Guerchet M, Ali GC, Wu YT, Prina AM, Winblad B, et al. The worldwide costs of dementia 2015 and comparisons with 2010. Alzheimers Dement J Alzheimers Assoc. 2017;13(1):1–7.
22. Xu J, Zhang Y, Qiu C, Cheng F. Global and regional economic costs of dementia: a systematic review. Lancet. 2017;390:S47.
23. Nitrini R, Bottino CMC, Albala C, Custodio Capuñay NS, Ketzoian C, Llibre Rodriguez JJ, et al. Prevalence of dementia in Latin America: a collaborative study of population-based cohorts. Int Psychogeriatr. 2009;21(4):622–30.
24. Custodio N, Lira D, Herrera-Pérez E, Del Prado LN, Parodi J, Guevara-Silva E, et al. Cost-of-illness study in a retrospective cohort of patients with dementia in Lima. Peru Dement Neuropsychol. 2015;9(1):32–41.
25. Contador I, Fernández-Calvo B, Ramos F, Tapias-Merino E, Bermejo-Pareja F. El cribado de la demencia en atención primaria. Rev Neurol. 2010;51(11):677–86.
26. Gomez RG, White DA. Using verbal fluency to detect very mild dementia of the Alzheimer type. Arch Clin Neuropsychol. 2006;21(8):771–5.
27. Olazarán J, Hoyos-Alonso MC, del Ser T, Garrido Barral A, Conde-Sala JL, Bermejo-Pareja F, et al. Aplicación práctica de los test cognitivos breves. Neurologia. 2016;31(3):183–94.
28. Silverberg NB, Ryan LM, Carrillo MC, Sperling R, Petersen RC, Posner HB, et al. Assessment of cognition in early dementia. Alzheimers Dement J Alzheimers Assoc. 2011;7(3):e60–76.
29. Skoog J, Backman K, Ribbe M, Falk H, Gudmundsson P, Thorvaldsson V, et al. A longitudinal study of the mini-mental state examination in late nonagenarians and its relationship with dementia, mortality, and education. J Am Geriatr Soc. 2017;65(6):1296–300.
30. Rojas G, Bartoloni L, Dillon C, Serrano CM, Iturry M, Allegri RF. Clinical and economic characteristics associated with direct costs of Alzheimer's, frontotemporal and vascular dementia in Argentina. Int Psychogeriatr. 2011;23(4):554–61.
31. Parra MA, Baez S, Allegri R, Nitrini R, Lopera F, Slachevsky A, et al. Dementia in Latin America: assessing the present and envisioning the future. Neurology. 2018;90(5):222–31.
32. Carmona JJ, Michan S. Biology of healthy aging and longevity. Rev Investig Clin Organo Hosp Enfermedades Nutr. 2016;68(1):7–16.
33. Ferreira D, Correia R, Nieto A, Machado A, Molina Y, Barroso J. Cognitive decline before the age of 50 can be detected with sensitive cognitive measures. Psicothema. 2015;27(3):216–22.
34. Nikolai T, Stepankova H, Kopecek M, Sulc Z, Vyhnalek M, Bezdicek O. The uniform data set, Czech version: normative data in older adults from an international perspective. J Alzheimers Dis JAD. 2018;61(3):1233–40.
35. Salthouse TA. When does age-related cognitive decline begin? Neurobiol Aging. 2009;30(4):507.
36. Salthouse TA. Trajectories of normal cognitive aging. Psychol Aging. 2019;34(1):17–24.
37. Salthouse T. Consequences of age-related cognitive declines. Annu Rev Psychol. 2012;63:201–26.
38. Laurence BD, Michel L. The fall in older adults: physical and cognitive problems. Curr Aging Sci. 2017;10(3):185–200.
39. Luo L, Craik FIM. Aging and memory: a cognitive approach. Can J Psychiatry Rev Can Psychiatr. 2008;53(6):346–53.
40. Rossini PM, Del Percio C, Pasqualetti P, Cassetta E, Binetti G, Dal Forno G, et al. Conversion from mild cognitive impairment to Alzheimer's disease is predicted by sources and coherence of brain electroencephalography rhythms. Neuroscience. 2006;143(3):793–803.
41. Mufson EJ, Binder L, Counts SE, DeKosky ST, deTolledo-Morrell L, Ginsberg SD, et al. Mild cognitive impairment: pathology and mechanisms. Acta Neuropathol. 2012;123(1):13–30.
42. Maestú F, Solesio-Jofre E, Bajo R. Towards the understanding of healthy and pathological aging through MEG. In: Supek S, Aine CJ, editors. Magnetoencephalography: from signals to dynamic

cortical networks [Internet]. Cham: Springer; 2019. p. 817–51.
43. Duffy FH, Albert MS, McAnulty G, Garvey AJ. Age-related differences in brain electrical activity of healthy subjects. Ann Neurol. 1984;16(4):430–8.
44. Pollock VE, Schneider LS, Lyness SA. EEG amplitudes in healthy, late-middle-aged and elderly adults: normality of the distributions and correlations with age. Electroencephalogr Clin Neurophysiol. 1990;75(4):276–88.
45. Ponomareva NV, Andreeva TV, Protasova MS, Shagam LI, Malina DD, Goltsov AY, et al. Quantitative EEG during normal aging: association with the Alzheimer's disease genetic risk variant in PICALM gene. Neurobiol Aging. 2017;51:177.e1–8.
46. Babiloni C, Binetti G, Cassarino A, Dal Forno G, Del Percio C, Ferreri F, et al. Sources of cortical rhythms in adults during physiological aging: a multicentric EEG study. Hum Brain Mapp. 2006;27(2):162–72.
47. Ponomareva N, Andreeva T, Protasova M, Shagam L, Malina D, Goltsov A, et al. Age-dependent effect of Alzheimer's risk variant of CLU on EEG alpha rhythm in non-demented adults. Front Aging Neurosci [Internet]. 2013.
48. Reichert JL, Kober SE, Witte M, Neuper C, Wood G. Age-related effects on verbal and visuospatial memory are mediated by theta and alpha II rhythms. Int J Psychophysiol. 2016 Jan;1(99):67–78.
49. Dias NS, Ferreira D, Reis J, Jacinto LR, Fernandes L, Pinho F, et al. Age effects on EEG correlates of the Wisconsin card sorting test. Physiol Rep. 2015;3(7):e12390.
50. Arakaki X, Lee R, King KS, Fonteh AN, Harrington MG. Alpha desynchronization during simple working memory unmasks pathological aging in cognitively healthy individuals. PLoS One. 2019;14(1):e0208517.
51. Finnigan S, Robertson IH. Resting EEG theta power correlates with cognitive performance in healthy older adults. Psychophysiology. 2011;48(8):1083–7.
52. Gómez C, Pérez-Macías JM, Poza J, Fernández A, Hornero R. Spectral changes in spontaneous MEG activity across the lifespan. J Neural Eng. 2013;10(6):066006.
53. Vlahou EL, Thurm F, Kolassa IT, Schlee W. Resting-state slow wave power, healthy aging and cognitive performance. Sci Rep. 2014;4:5101.
54. McEvoy LK, Pellouchoud E, Smith ME, Gevins A. Neurophysiological signals of working memory in normal aging. Brain Res Cogn Brain Res. 2001;11(3):363–76.
55. Cummins TDR, Finnigan S. Theta power is reduced in healthy cognitive aging. Int J Psychophysiol. 2007;66(1):10–7.
56. Ho MC, Huang CF, Chou CY, Lin YT, Shih CS, Wu MT, et al. Task-related brain oscillations in normal aging. Health (N Y). 2012;4(9):762–8.
57. Proskovec AL, Heinrichs-Graham E, Wilson TW. Aging modulates the oscillatory dynamics underlying successful working memory encoding and maintenance. Hum Brain Mapp. 2016;37(6):2348–61.
58. Duffy FH, Mcanulty GB, Albert MS. Effects of age upon interhemispheric EEG coherence in normal adults. Neurobiol Aging. 1996;17(4):587–99.
59. Shinosaki K, Ishii R, Ukai S, Mizuno-Matsumoto Y, Inouye T, Tutiyama M, et al. Effect of normal aging on functional connectivity of the brain: an EEG study. Psychogeriatrics. 2003;3(2):49–53.
60. Schlee W, Leirer V, Kolassa IT, Weisz N, Elbert T. Age-related changes in neural functional connectivity and its behavioral relevance. BMC Neurosci. 2012 Feb;14(13):16.
61. Balsters JH, O'Connell RG, Galli A, Nolan H, Greco E, Kilcullen SM, et al. Changes in resting connectivity with age: a simultaneous electroencephalogram and functional magnetic resonance imaging investigation. Neurobiol Aging. 2013;34(9):2194–207.
62. McIntosh AR, Vakorin V, Kovacevic N, Wang H, Diaconescu A, Protzner AB. Spatiotemporal dependency of age-related changes in brain signal variability. Cereb Cortex. 2014;24(7):1806–17.
63. Vysata O, Kukal J, Prochazka A, Pazdera L, Simko J, Valis M. Age-related changes in EEG coherence. Neurol Neurochir Pol. 2014;48(1):35–8.
64. Nakamura A, Cuesta P, Kato T, Arahata Y, Iwata K, Yamagishi M, et al. Early functional network alterations in asymptomatic elders at risk for Alzheimer's disease. Sci Rep. 2017;7:6517.
65. Escudero J, Smith K, Azami H, Abasolo D. Inspection of short-time resting-state electroencephalogram functional networks in Alzheimer's disease. Annu Int Conf IEEE Eng Med Biol Soc. 2016;2016:2810–3.
66. Moezzi B, Pratti LM, Hordacre B, Graetz L, Berryman C, Lavrencic LM, et al. Characterization of young and old adult brains: an EEG functional connectivity analysis. Neuroscience. 2019;422:230–9.
67. Scally B, Burke MR, Bunce D, Delvenne JF. Resting-state EEG power and connectivity are associated with alpha peak frequency slowing in healthy aging. Neurobiol Aging. 2018;71:149–55.
68. Ujma PP, Konrad BN, Simor P, Gombos F, Körmendi J, Steiger A, et al. Sleep EEG functional connectivity varies with age and sex, but not general intelligence. Neurobiol Aging. 2019;78:87–97.
69. Bouchard M, Lina JM, Gaudreault PO, Dube J, Gosselin N, Carrier J. EEG connectivity across sleep cycles and age. Sleep. 2020;43(3):zsz236.
70. Maurits NM, Scheeringa R, van der Hoeven JH, de Jong R. EEG coherence obtained from an auditory oddball task increases with age. J Clin Neurophysiol. 2006;23(5):395–403.
71. Müller V, Gruber W, Klimesch W, Lindenberger U. Lifespan differences in cortical dynamics of auditory perception. Dev Sci. 2009;12(6):839–53.
72. Werkle-Bergner M, Shing YL, Müller V, Li SC, Lindenberger U. EEG gamma-band synchronization in visual coding from childhood to old age: evidence

from evoked power and inter-trial phase locking. Clin Neurophysiol. 2009;120(7):1291–302.

73. Wang J, Fang Y, Wang X, Yang H, Yu X, Wang H. Enhanced gamma activity and cross-frequency interaction of resting-state electroencephalographic oscillations in patients with Alzheimer's disease. Front Aging Neurosci. 2017;9:243.
74. Ferreri F, Vecchio F, Guerra A, Miraglia F, Ponzo D, Vollero L, et al. Age related differences in functional synchronization of EEG activity as evaluated by means of TMS-EEG coregistrations. Neurosci Lett. 2017;647:141–6.
75. Tóth B, Kardos Z, File B, Boha R, Stam CJ, Molnár M. Frontal midline theta connectivity is related to efficiency of WM maintenance and is affected by aging. Neurobiol Learn Mem. 2014;114:58–69.
76. Ariza P, Solesio-Jofre E, Martínez JH, Pineda-Pardo JA, Niso G, Maestú F, et al. Evaluating the effect of aging on interference resolution with time-varying complex networks analysis. Front Hum Neurosci. 2015.
77. Arnau S, Wascher E, Küper K. Age-related differences in reallocating cognitive resources when dealing with interruptions. NeuroImage. 2019;191:292–302.
78. Hou F, Liu C, Yu Z, Xu X, Zhang J, Peng CK, et al. Age-related alterations in electroencephalography connectivity and network topology during n-Back working memory task. Front Hum Neurosci. 2018;12:484.
79. Riedel-Heller SG, Matschinger H, Schork A, Angermeyer MC. Do memory complaints indicate the presence of cognitive impairment? Results of a field study. Eur Arch Psychiatry Clin Neurosci. 1999;249(4):197–204.
80. Roberts JL, Clare L, Woods RT. Subjective memory complaints and awareness of memory functioning in mild cognitive impairment: a systematic review. Dement Geriatr Cogn Disord. 2009;28(2):95–109.
81. Albert MS, DeKosky ST, Dickson D, Dubois B, Feldman HH, Fox NC, et al. The diagnosis of mild cognitive impairment due to Alzheimer's disease: recommendations from the National Institute on Aging-Alzheimer's association workgroups on diagnostic guidelines for Alzheimer's disease. Alzheimers Dement J Alzheimers Assoc. 2011;7(3):270–9.
82. Petersen RC. Mild cognitive impairment as a diagnostic entity. J Intern Med. 2004;256(3):183–94.
83. Petersen RC, Caracciolo B, Brayne C, Gauthier S, Jelic V, Fratiglioni L. Mild cognitive impairment: a concept in evolution. J Intern Med. 2014;275(3):214–28.
84. Engels MMA, van der Flier WM, Stam CJ, Hillebrand A, Scheltens P, van Straaten ECW. Alzheimer's disease: the state of the art in resting-state magnetoencephalography. Clin Neurophysiol. 2017;128(8):1426–37.
85. Poza J, Hornero R, Abásolo D, Fernández A, García M. Extraction of spectral based measures from MEG background oscillations in Alzheimer's disease. Med Eng Phys. 2007;29(10):1073–83.
86. López ME, Aurtenetxe S, Pereda E, Cuesta P, Castellanos NP, Bruña R, et al. Cognitive reserve is associated with the functional organization of the brain in healthy aging: a MEG study. Front Aging Neurosci. 2014.
87. Besthorn C, Zerfass R, Geiger-Kabisch C, Sattel H, Daniel S, Schreiter-Gasser U, et al. Discrimination of Alzheimer's disease and normal aging by EEG data. Electroencephalogr Clin Neurophysiol. 1997;103(2):241–8.
88. Moretti DV, Babiloni C, Binetti G, Cassetta E, Dal Forno G, Ferreric F, et al. Individual analysis of EEG frequency and band power in mild Alzheimer's disease. Clin Neurophysiol. 2004;115(2):299–308.
89. van der Hiele K, Vein AA, Reijntjes RHAM, Westendorp RGJ, Bollen ELEM, van Buchem MA, et al. EEG correlates in the spectrum of cognitive decline. Clin Neurophysiol. 2007;118(9):1931–9.
90. Mizuno T, Takahashi T, Cho RY, Kikuchi M, Murata T, Takahashi K, et al. Assessment of EEG dynamical complexity in Alzheimer's disease using multiscale entropy. Clin Neurophysiol. 2010;121(9):1438–46.
91. de Waal H, Stam CJ, de Haan W, van Straaten ECW, Blankenstein MA, Scheltens P, et al. Alzheimer's disease patients not carrying the apolipoprotein E ε4 allele show more severe slowing of oscillatory brain activity. Neurobiol Aging. 2013;34(9):2158–63.
92. Czigler B, Csikós D, Hidasi Z, Anna Gaál Z, Csibri E, Kiss E, et al. Quantitative EEG in early Alzheimer's disease patients—power spectrum and complexity features. Int J Psychophysiol. 2008;68(1):75–80.
93. McBride JC, Zhao X, Munro NB, Smith CD, Jicha GA, Hively L, et al. Spectral and complexity analysis of scalp EEG characteristics for mild cognitive impairment and early Alzheimer's disease. Comput Methods Prog Biomed. 2014;114(2):153–63.
94. Sharma N, Kolekar MH, Jha K, Kumar Y. EEG and cognitive biomarkers based mild cognitive impairment diagnosis. IRBM. 2019;40(2):113–21.
95. de Haan W, Stam CJ, Jones BF, Zuiderwijk IM, van Dijk BW, Scheltens P. Resting-state oscillatory brain dynamics in Alzheimer disease. J Clin Neurophysiol. 2008;25(4):187–93.
96. Hsiao FJ, Wang YJ, Yan SH, Chen WT, Lin YY. Altered oscillation and synchronization of default-mode network activity in mild Alzheimer's disease compared to mild cognitive impairment: an electrophysiological study. PLoS ONE. 2013;8(7).
97. Hsiao FJ, Chen WT, Wang YJ, Yan SH, Lin YY. Altered source-based EEG coherence of resting-state sensorimotor network in early-stage Alzheimer's disease compared to mild cognitive impairment. Neurosci Lett. 2014;13(558):47–52.
98. Rossini PM, Buscema M, Capriotti M, Grossi E, Rodriguez G, Del Percio C, et al. Is it possible to automatically distinguish resting EEG data of normal elderly vs. mild cognitive impairment subjects

with high degree of accuracy? Clin Neurophysiol. 2008;119(7):1534–45.
99. Musaeus CS, Nielsen MS, Osterbye NN, Hogh P. Decreased parietal Beta power as a sign of disease progression in patients with mild cognitive impairment. J Alzheimers Dis. 2018;65(2):475–87.
100. Jiang Z, yan. Study on EEG power and coherence in patients with mild cognitive impairment during working memory task. J Zhejiang Univ Sci B. 2005;6(12):1213–9.
101. Dimpfel W. Neurophysiological biomarker of mild cognitive impairment. Adv Alzheimers Dis. 2014;3(2):64–77.
102. Smailovic U, Koenig T, Kåreholt I, Andersson T, Kramberger MG, Winblad B, et al. Quantitative EEG power and synchronization correlate with Alzheimer's disease CSF biomarkers. Neurobiol Aging. 2018;63:88–95.
103. Delbeuck X, Van der Linden M, Collette F. Alzheimer's disease as a disconnection syndrome? Neuropsychol Rev. 2003;13(2):79–92.
104. Braak H, Braak E. Neuropathological stageing of Alzheimer-related changes. Acta Neuropathol (Berl). 1991;82(4):239–59.
105. Villemagne VL, Burnham S, Bourgeat P, Brown B, Ellis KA, Salvado O, et al. Amyloid β deposition, neurodegeneration, and cognitive decline in sporadic Alzheimer's disease: a prospective cohort study. Lancet Neurol. 2013;12(4):357–67.
106. Berendse HW, Verbunt JPA, Scheltens P, van Dijk BW, Jonkman EJ. Magnetoencephalographic analysis of cortical activity in Alzheimer's disease: a pilot study. Clin Neurophysiol. 2000;111(4):604–12.
107. Stam CJ, van Walsum AMC, Pijnenburg YAL, Berendse HW, de Munck JC, Scheltens P, et al. Generalized synchronization of MEG recordings in Alzheimer's disease: evidence for involvement of the gamma band. J Clin Neurophysiol. 2002;19(6):562–74.
108. Stam CJ. Use of magnetoencephalography (MEG) to study functional brain networks in neurodegenerative disorders. J Neurol Sci. 2010;289(1):128–34.
109. Pusil S, Eugenia Lopez M, Cuesta P, Bruna R, Pereda E, Maestu F. Hypersynchronization in mild cognitive impairment: the "X" model. Brain. 2019;142:3936–50.
110. Bajo R, Maestú F, Nevado A, Sancho M, Gutiérrez R, Campo P, et al. Functional connectivity in mild cognitive impairment during a memory task: implications for the disconnection hypothesis. J Alzheimers Dis. 2010;22(1):183–93.
111. Bajo R, Castellanos NP, Cuesta P, Aurtenetxe S, Garcia-Prieto J, Gil-Gregorio P, et al. Differential patterns of connectivity in progressive mild cognitive impairment. Brain Connect. 2012;2(1):21–4.
112. Lopez-Sanz D, Bruna R, Garces P, Carmen Martin-Buro M, Walter S, Luisa Delgado M, et al. Functional connectivity disruption in subjective cognitive decline and mild cognitive impairment: a common pattern of alterations. Front Aging Neurosci. 2017;21(9):109.
113. Lopez-Sanz D, Garces P, Alvarez B, Luisa Delgado-Losada M, Lopez-Higes R, Maestu F. Network disruption in the preclinical stages of Alzheimer's disease: from subjective cognitive decline to mild cognitive impairment. Int J Neural Syst. 2017;27(8):1750041.
114. Bajo R, Castellanos NP, López ME, Ruiz JM, Montejo P, Montenegro M, et al. Early dysfunction of functional connectivity in healthy elderly with subjective memory complaints. Age. 2012;34(2):497–506.
115. Stam CJ. Functional connectivity patterns of human magnetoencephalographic recordings: a "small-world" network? Neurosci Lett. 2004;355(1–2):25–8.
116. Stam CJ, Jones BF, Manshanden I, van Walsum AMC, Montez T, JPA V, et al. Magnetoencephalographic evaluation of resting-state functional connectivity in Alzheimer's disease. NeuroImage. 2006;32(3):1335–44.
117. Stam CJ, De Haan W, Daffertshofer A, Jones BF, Manshanden I, van Walsum AMC, et al. Graph theoretical analysis of magnetoencephalographic functional connectivity in Alzheimer's disease. Brain. 2009;132(1):213–24.
118. Alonso JF, Poza J, Mañanas MA, Romero S, Fernández A, Hornero R. MEG connectivity analysis in patients with Alzheimer's disease using cross mutual information and spectral coherence. Ann Biomed Eng. 2011 Jan;39(1):524–36.
119. Escudero J, Sanei S, Jarchi D, Abásolo D, Hornero R. Regional coherence evaluation in mild cognitive impairment and Alzheimer's disease based on adaptively extracted magnetoencephalogram rhythms. Physiol Meas. 2011 Aug;32(8):1163–80.
120. Yu M, Engels MMA, Hillebrand A, van Straaten ECW, Gouw AA, Teunissen C, et al. Selective impairment of hippocampus and posterior hub areas in Alzheimer's disease: an MEG-based multiplex network study. Brain. 2017;140:1466–85.
121. de Haan W, van der Flier WM, Wang H, Van Mieghem PFA, Scheltens P, Stam CJ. Disruption of functional brain networks in Alzheimer's disease: what can we learn from graph spectral analysis of resting-state magnetoencephalography? Brain Connect. 2012;2(2):45–55.
122. De Haan W, Van der Flier WM, Koene T, Smits LL, Scheltens P, Stam CJ. Disrupted modular brain dynamics reflect cognitive dysfunction in Alzheimer's disease. NeuroImage. 2012;59(4):3085–93.
123. Franciotti R, Iacono D, Della Penna S, Pizzella V, Torquati K, Onofrj M, et al. Cortical rhythms reactivity in AD, LBD and normal subjects: a quantitative MEG study. Neurobiol Aging. 2006 Aug;27(8):1100–9.
124. Teipel S, Grothe MJ, Zhou J, Sepulcre J, Dyrba M, Sorg C, et al. Measuring cortical connectivity in Alzheimer's disease as a brain neural net-

work pathology: toward clinical applications. J Int Neuropsychol Soc. 2016;22(2):138–63.

125. Coleman P, Federoff H, Kurlan R. A focus on the synapse for neuroprotection in Alzheimer disease and other dementias. Neurology. 2004;63(7):1155–62.
126. Phillips C, Baktir MA, Srivatsan M, Salehi A. Neuroprotective effects of physical activity on the brain: a closer look at trophic factor signaling. Front Cell Neurosci. 2014;8.
127. Kennedy G, Hardman RJ, Macpherson H, Scholey AB, Pipingas A. How does exercise reduce the rate of age-associated cognitive decline? A review of potential mechanisms. J Alzheimers Dis JAD. 2017;55(1):1–18.
128. de Frutos-Lucas J, López-Sanz D, Zuluaga P, Rodríguez-Rojo IC, Luna R, López ME, et al. Physical activity effects on the individual alpha peak frequency of older adults with and without genetic risk factors for Alzheimer's disease: a MEG study. Clin Neurophysiol. 2018;129(9):1981–9.
129. Sanchez-Lopez J, Silva-Pereyra J, Fernández T, Alatorre-Cruz GC, Castro-Chavira SA, González-López M, et al. High levels of incidental physical activity are positively associated with cognition and EEG activity in aging. PLoS One. 2018;13(1):e0191561.
130. Douw L, Nieboer D, van Dijk BW, Stam CJ, Twisk JWR. A healthy brain in a healthy body: brain network correlates of physical and mental fitness. PLoS One. 2014;9(2):e88202.
131. Nunes MVS, Castro-Caldas A, Rio DD, Maestú F, Ortiz T. The ex-illiterate brain: the critical period, cognitive reserve and HAROLD model. Dement Neuropsychol. 2009;3(3):222.
132. de Frutos-Lucas J, Lopez-Sanz D, Cuesta P, Bruna R, de la Fuente S, Serrano N, et al. Enhancement of posterior brain functional networks in bilingual older adults. Biling-Lang Cogn. 2020;23(2):387–400.
133. Burton R, Sheron N. No level of alcohol consumption improves health. Lancet. 2018;392(10152):987–8.
134. de Bruin EA, Stam CJ, Bijl S, Verbaten MN, Kenemans JL. Moderate-to-heavy alcohol intake is associated with differences in synchronization of brain activity during rest and mental rehearsal. Int J Psychophysiol Off J Int Organ Psychophysiol. 2006;60(3):304–14.
135. Lithari C, Klados MA, Pappas C, Albani M, Kapoukranidou D, Kovatsi L, et al. Alcohol affects the Brain's resting-state network in social drinkers. PLoS One. 2012;7(10):e48641.
136. Loheswaran G, Barr MS, Zomorrodi R, Rajji TK, Blumberger DM, Foll BL, et al. Impairment of neuroplasticity in the dorsolateral prefrontal cortex by alcohol. Sci Rep. 2017;7(1):5276.
137. Ehlers CL, Wall TL, Schuckit MA. EEG spectral characteristics following ethanol administration in young men. Electroencephalogr Clin Neurophysiol. 1989;73(3):179–87.
138. Jack CR, Wiste HJ, Weigand SD, Rocca WA, Knopman DS, Mielke MM, et al. Age-specific population frequencies of cerebral β-amyloidosis and neurodegeneration among people with normal cognitive function aged 50-89 years: a cross-sectional study. Lancet Neurol. 2014;13(10):997–1005.
139. Deeny SP, Poeppel D, Zimmerman JB, Roth SM, Brandauer J, Witkowski S, et al. Exercise, APOE, and working memory: MEG and behavioral evidence for benefit of exercise in epsilon4 carriers. Biol Psychol. 2008;78(2):179–87.
140. Choi MR, Kim JY, Yi ES. Development and validation of exercise rehabilitation program for cognitive function and activity of daily living improvement in mild dementia elderly. J Exerc Rehabil. 2018;14(2):207–12.
141. Raichlen DA, Alexander GE. Adaptive capacity: an evolutionary-neuroscience model linking exercise, cognition, and brain health. Trends Neurosci. 2017;40(7):408–21.
142. Kempermann G, Fabel K, Ehninger D, Babu H, Leal-Galicia P, Garthe A, et al. Why and how physical activity promotes experience-induced brain plasticity. Front Neurosci. 2010;4:189.
143. Styliadis C, Kartsidis P, Paraskevopoulos E, Ioannides AA, Bamidis PD. Neuroplastic effects of combined computerized physical and cognitive training in elderly individuals at risk for dementia: an eLORETA controlled study on resting states. Neural Plast. 2015;2015:172192.
144. Klados MA, Styliadis C, Frantzidis CA, Paraskevopoulos E, Bamidis PD. Beta-band functional connectivity is reorganized in mild cognitive impairment after combined computerized physical and cognitive training. Front Neurosci. 2016;10:55.
145. Steffener J, Stern Y. Exploring the neural basis of cognitive reserve in aging. Biochim Biophys Acta. 2012;1822(3):467–73.
146. Gu L, Chen J, Gao L, Shu H, Wang Z, Liu D, et al. Cognitive reserve modulates attention processes in healthy elderly and amnestic mild cognitive impairment: an event-related potential study. Clin Neurophysiol. 2018;129(1):198–207.
147. Solfrizzi V, Custodero C, Lozupone M, Imbimbo BP, Valiani V, Agosti P, et al. Relationships of dietary patterns, foods, and micro- and macronutrients with Alzheimer's disease and late-life cognitive disorders: a systematic review. J Alzheimers Dis. 2017;59(3):815–49.
148. Sizonenko SV, Babiloni C, de Bruin EA, Isaacs EB, Jönsson LS, Kennedy DO, et al. Brain imaging and human nutrition: which measures to use in intervention studies? Br J Nutr. 2013;110(Suppl 1):S1–30.
149. de Wilde MC, Kamphuis PJGH, Sijben JWC, Scheltens P. Utility of imaging for nutritional intervention studies in Alzheimer's disease. Eur J Pharmacol. 2011;668(Suppl 1):S59–69.

150. Scheltens P, Twisk JWR, Blesa R, Scarpini E, von Arnim CAF, Bongers A, et al. Efficacy of Souvenaid in mild Alzheimer's disease: results from a randomized, controlled trial. J Alzheimers Dis. 2012;31(1):225–36.
151. van Straaten ECW, de Waal H, Lansbergen MM, Scheltens P, Maestu F, Nowak R, et al. Magnetoencephalography for the detection of intervention effects of a specific nutrient combination in patients with mild Alzheimer's disease: results from an exploratory double-blind, randomized, controlled study. Front Neurol. 2016;7:161.

43 Brain Imaging: From Ramón Y Cajal Epoch to Our Days

Nicolás Fayed, Humberto Morales, and Alicia Fayed

Introduction

Santiago Ramón y Cajal: The Neuron

Cajal graduated from the Zaragoza Faculty of Medicine (Spain). He refined the technique of silver staining, previously established by Golgi (Cajal ended up sharing the Novel Prize with him on 1906). This technique improved the visualization of the nervous system components, allowing him to posit, the now well-known, description of the neurons, as independent elements with a separation between them, called synapsis. His scientific papers describing his theories were multiple, one of the most important papers is "Histology of the Nervous System in Human and Vertebrates," published between 1897 and 1904 [1].

He realized that a neuronal system had greater capacity of processing information, and generate intelligent decisions, than any other networking or tissue system. Moreover, he foresaw how the neurons send and receive the information they process.

He envisioned that the connecting space (synapsis) could somehow be filled with chemical substances, which would activate or deactivate the receptive neuron. This neuron could modify the information received from other neurons, forming complicated neural circuits. The human mind, the creation of emotions, and the human thought and perceptions, would be possible, thanks to this complex neuronal activity. Cajal thought that the dendritic spines were plastic structures, which could contain the memory and also participate in our intelligence. Thus, the intellect would relate not only to the number and size of neurons but also to the connections between them. These dendritic spines would be necessary to form connections when we learn or perform an intellectual task.

Cajal also thought that the glial cells participate in mental processes. Interestedly, this is something that we are starting to understand. In 1913, Cajal developed a method, based on sublaminated gold, to stain the neuroglia. He described the neuroglia as a cell with prolongations, calling it astrocyte; at the same time, he described a third adendritic element. Years after, Pio del Rio Ortega showed that the third element was constituted by oligodendrocytes and the microglia [2]. These discoveries by the Spanish school have been of transcendental importance and they have allowed the development of the neuroanatomy and neurophysiology of our days.

N. Fayed (✉)
Department of Radiology, Section of Neuroradiology, Quirónsalud Hospital, Zaragoza, Spain

H. Morales
Department of Radiology, Division of Diagnostic and Interventional Neuroradiology, University of Kentucky, Lexington, KY, USA
e-mail: humberto.morales@uky.edu

A. Fayed
Department of Hematology, Hospital Miguel Servet, Zaragoza, Spain

P. Á. Gargiulo, H. L. Mesones-Arroyo (eds.), *Psychiatry and Neuroscience Update – Vol. V*,
https://doi.org/10.1007/978-3-031-72219-6_43

In 1944, Rafael Lorente de No (Cajal's disciple) published a paper that described multiple circuits in the brain where the neurons would interconnect in a reciprocal way [3].

Later, Donald Hebb, a Canadian scientist, postulated an associative plasticity. This plasticity allowed the neurons, according to their activity, to modify their morphology and metabolism, with subsequent potentiation of their efficacy. In 1973, Terje Lomo and Timothy Bliss were able to prove this theory. They stimulated hippocampal neurons with weak high frequency electric currents, which resulted in a potentiated effect that lasted for weeks [4].

Eric Kandel proved that the learning process improved the neurons response and their interconnections, resulting in precise chemical changes within the cells [5].

In 1999, the journal *Nature* confirmed Cajal's theory [6], with state-of-the-art microscopy showed the sprout of new spines in stimulated hippocampal neurons. However, as the spines can grow or increase their number, they can also diminish their number or disappear. These findings could be related to our capacity of forget. It is also believed to be related to pathologic mental states such as autism or mental retardation, where the dendritic spines have a form deviated from normal or are more elongated and immature.

In 2005, it was demonstrated that the synapsis is not the only form of communication between the neurons, but there is also discharge of neurotransmitter outside the synapsis. This phenomenon has been called ectopic neurotransmission [7]. They concluded that "the combination of mathematic models with physiologic, anatomical, and behavioral data is the future of the neurobiology."

Angelo Mosso: The Blood Flow

The correct function of the brain is reflected, among other aspects, by its perfusion, i.e., the amount of oxygen and nutrients being supplied to the brain tissue. Some pathologic states such as cerebrovascular diseases, brain tumors, or Alzheimer disease can be diagnosed by the quantification of some perfusion parameters, such as the cerebral blood volume and cerebral blood flow, the mean transit time or the capillary permeability.

Angelo Mosso, a nineteenth-century Italian physiologist and pharmacologist, invented the first technique of neuroimaging. It was called "human circulation balance" [8], and it predeceases recent techniques such as functional magnetic resonance imaging (fMRI) and positron emission tomography (PET). He invented multiple instruments to measure the pulse and wrote about the variation in the volume of the pulse during sleep, mental activity, or emotions.

In 1884, he was convinced that his bascule would show the relation between brain blood flow and cognitive performance. He designed a table, where a person could lie still until the balance reached an equilibrium. Then, he asked the person to read a philosophic statement; thus, the body would increase the blood to the brain. This minimum change in the blood flow triggered a change in the dispositive around the head, turning it down. Currently, all the experiments of mental activation are based on the primordial idea from Mosso: the cognitive tasks are related to the blood flow to the brain. In recent times, we rely on fMRI to visualize the areas of the brain that are activated with certain cognitive tasks, although it is not possible yet to relate the exact changes in the volume of blood flowing through these areas of activation.

Korbinian Brodmann: Brain Cartography

Ramon y Cajal's discovery of multiple types of neurons lead to a classification methodology and to subsequent studies of structural similarities, which allowed to define specific zones in the cerebral cortex. Von Economo and Koskinas, Brodmann, Campbell, and many others followed on Cajal's footsteps.

Von Economo and Koskinas brilliantly divided the cerebral cortex into five types, with a differentiate structure and composition. Brodmann, during the same epoch, performed a study about the effects of structural maturation of the distinct areas of the human brain cortex. He numbered these areas from number 1 to 48. Today, we are still using this mapping to localize, precisely, brain lesions [9]. During the first half of the twentieth century, and thanks to advances in the electrophysiology and neurosurgery, Foester was able to describe a new electrophysiological classification. His classification defined concrete functional areas and stemmed from Brodmann mapping.

Neuroimaging

Current neuroimaging techniques allow to observe the brain with amazing detail. Our brain, with more than 100,000 million of neurons and billions of synapsis, is able to develop networks of exquisite complexity. Through deep knowledge of magnetism and physics, scientists have been able to image the brain with significant structural and functional detail.

Magnetic Resonance Diffusion-Weighted Imaging

Diffusion is defined as the random movement of the water molecules at a temperature superior to −273 °C (0 Kelvin). This movement is related to different properties of the medium such as temperature and viscosity. In biologic tissues, there are different types of barriers, such as the cell membrane, that limits the free motion of water. In 1965, an MRI sequence sensitive to the motion of the water molecules was introduced [10].

Diffusion-weighted images can show areas of hyperintensity related to restriction of the free movement of water. Objective measurements of the apparent diffusion coefficient (ADC) can also be performed. The ADC represents the magnitude of the water motion in a tissue volume, although is not able to represent the heterogeneity of the lesions. Today, it is considered the more sensitive method to diagnose ischemic brain lesions. It is also helpful in the diagnosis of central nervous system (CNS) infections, brain tumors, acute demyelination, epilepsy, metabolic alterations, neurodegenerative processes, and traumatic brain injuries.

Diffusion Tensor Imaging

Diffusion tensor imaging (DTI) has revolutionized our understanding of the CNS. The technique is based on the principle of anisotropic diffusion and allow a qualitative and quantitative assessment of the white matter tracts and their integrity and relations to different types of brain lesions. Fractional anisotropy (FA) measures the dominant direction of the movement of the water molecules.

Median diffusivity is derived from the diffusion tensor and is the average of apparent diffusion coefficients in different directions. Thus, it is a more accurate apparent diffusion coefficient. FA is another parameter derived from the diffusion tensor and measures the degree of deviation from isotropic water motion. Hence, FA is a reflection of the alignment of the cell structures and tissue coherency. FA varies from 0, which reflects equal movement of water in all directions (isotropy); to 1, which reflects a dominant single direction of movement (anisotropy). DTI is a technique based on the anisotropy of diffusion, reflecting the structure of a tissue. In the brain, the myelin sheaths limit the free motion of water; herein, DTI reflects the structure of the white matter. These natural microstructural barriers lead to an anisotropic water diffusion, with a dominant direction between axons. Thus, although in an indirect way, DTI allows the assessment of the integrity of the white matter tracts.

FA appears increased in tubular structures such as the white matte tracts. On the other hand, FA appears decreased in spherical structures such as the gray matter cells.

Current computer software is capable to find a high value of FA and follow the longitudinal axis of the diffusion tensor. The representation stops when FA values are significantly low and similar than the gray matter. Then, the software finds another voxel with high FA and start tracking again.

A Magnetic Resonance Imaging (MRI) machine is capable of tracing the water motion in thousands of points within the brain, revealing the presence of fibers or tracts. We are able to see multiple lines of different colors, each color representing a direction, reflecting thousands of millions of axons. With this technique, we can see impressive 3D models of fiber tracts in the brain. Studies have shown that children with delay in reading can have decreased FA in language areas of the brain [11]. Similarly, schizophrenic patients have shown decreased FA in frontal areas responsible of cognition [12].

DTI is used with increased frequency in psychology research. Studies have shown that FA is related to the development of cognitive capacities, and in early infancy, the FA values have shown to increase as the corpus callosum and anterior aspect of the frontal lobe [13] (prefrontal cortex, which participates in the working memory and control of behavior and attention) are developed.

Moreover, diffusion tensor imaging contributes in the research of personality disorders, providing clues on their neurologic bases. In 2009, a study was able to associate the creativity of a group of persons with the integrity of white matter in certain brain regions: anterior frontal lobe, basal ganglia, and transition zones of the temporal and parietal lobes [14].

Magnetic Resonance Angiography

Egas Moniz, neurosurgeon and psychiatrist, invented the cerebral angiography in the 1930s. Currently, less invasive techniques can also be used for the visualization of the cerebral vessels, such as computed tomography and magnetic resonance angiography.

Brain Perfusion

Blood perfusion is defined as the supply of blood to a specific tissue. Nutrients and oxygen are supplied by this mechanism [15]. Magnetic Resonance Imaging (MRI) is a powerful tool for evaluation of the brain anatomy. Advances on MRI technology allow the evaluation of the brain function and its metabolism. One of these parameters is the brain perfusion. MRI perfusion evaluates the blood passing through a vascular network in the brain. Multiple noninvasive hemodynamic parameters and measures are retrieved by MRI perfusion [16].

Unfortunately, this technique is only able to obtain relative measurements. This limitation precludes a direct comparison between subjects and sometimes within the same subject. Multiple publications suggest that magnetic resonance perfusion in combination with diffusion-weighted imaging (DWI) is able to determine viable ischemic tissue in cases of stroke, or ischemic penumbra [17]. In theory, the mismatch between perfusion and diffusion represents the ischemic tissue able to recover [18].

Magnetic resonance perfusion has been used in the diagnosis of neurodegenerative and psychiatric diseases. Harris et al. found that the ratios of cerebral blood volume (rCBV) in relation to the cerebellum, in the temporoparietal cortex, were 20% decreased in patients with Alzheimer, with a 95% sensitivity in cases of moderate disease and 88% sensitivity in mild cases. Specificity was 96%, and MR perfusion showed improved sensitivity as compared with SPECT perfusion [19].

Other study showed decreased ratios of cerebral blood volume rCBV in the temporoparietal cortex of patients with Alzheimer disease, with sensitivity and specificity of 91% and 90%, respectively. Lower values were obtained in the sensory-motor cortex and the hippocampus [20]. Johnson et al. [21] found that there was hypoperfusion in the right inferior parietal cortex, bilateral posterior cingulate gyri, bilateral superior and middle frontal gyri, and less frequent in the left inferior parietal region. Callen et al. showed that patients with Alzheimer had a significant decreased perfusion in the limbic structures. Perfusion values in the cingulate discriminated between control and Alzheimer patients with accuracy of 93% (sensitivity of 95% and specificity of 88%) [22].

Alzheimer disease should be discriminated from major depression. Perfusion studies have also shown utility to differentiate these two entities. There was decreased flow in the lateral parietal, lateral temporal, precuneus, and posterior cingulate in patient with Alzheimer as compared with patients with major depression. On the other hand, there was decreased flow in the lateral frontal region, left thalamus, and middle frontal region in patients with major depression as compared with Alzheimer patients [23].

Magnetic resonance perfusion can improve the sensitivity and specificity in the diagnosis of some CNS pathologies. It can improve the prediction of histologic findings as well as the evaluation of disease progression and therapeutic response. In the near future, perfusion studies should evaluate in a quantitive way the cerebral blood volume and flow, improving the postprocessing of images and decreasing artifacts secondary to blood brain barrier rupture and recirculation [24].

Functional Magnetic Resonance Imaging

The ability to observe the brain thoughts has been an old dream of scientist. During recent years, this dream is becoming true, thanks to modern techniques such as fMRI. This technique is able to demonstrate what is happening in our brains as we see, hear, talk, feel, or think.

Recent advances in neuroimaging allowed us to improve the subjective parcellation of histologic sections. Nowadays, the investigation is centered in the variability between subjects, the recollection of cytoarchitectonic data in a common space, the connectivity, and molecular and functional aspects of the brain. High-field MRI allows the visualization of some in-vivo microstructures of human brains.

This is the first step towards an individual cartography of the brain. In the future, in combination with fMRI, it will be possible to associate specific areas of the brain with concrete functions.

It will be a milestone to map the microstructure of the brain cortex and overly this information with functional activity. We would be able to observe whether a single area of the cortex is activated with a motor, sensorial or cognitive task, or there are actually simultaneous activation of other brain regions.

High field MRI (7 Tesla) is able to delineate the thickness of the myelin sheaths, through T1 relaxation. In zones of high density of myelin (primary motor cortex, somatosensory cortex, auditory or visual cortex), a specific relaxation change is observed.

Recently, a method that compares T1 maps of myelin from in-vivo brains with postmortem histology has allowed specific delineation of some brain regions. First, a bloc tissue from the central sulcus is retrieved from a postmortem brain [25]. Then, it is imaged by high-field MRI for a period of hours. Thus, obtaining an exact T1 map. Differences on T1 contrast correlate with the myelin architecture, and is also capable to stablish the limits between the area 4 (primary motor cortex) and area 3 (somatosensorial cortex). Subsequently, microslices of the tissue bloc are staining, and histologic correlation of the brain cortex is performed with the T1 maps [26].

The year 2009 marked the 100th anniversary of the historic publication of the Brodmann maps of the brain. One day in the near future, personal microanatomical maps would be associated with the brain function, in-vivo, without a need for median values from a larger group of persons.

Functional Connectivity

However, fMRI has the capacity of measuring the functional activity of the brain through a signal derived from the changes in the oxygen level of the blood oxygen level dependent (BOLD contrast). Because of this, fMRI has become a powerful tool in neuroscience. The development of these imaging techniques had modified the way we examine the functional cartography of the brain. Our brain is made up of multiple regions distributed in the space, but functionally connected, sharing information in a constant manner.

Thus, the recent advances have catalyzed the exploration of the functional connectivity of the human brain.

Functional connectivy can be analyzed by fMRI related to a task or in resting-state. Functional connectivity is defined as the temporal dependence of multiple regions of the brain that are anatomically separated. Recently, an increasing number of studies are evaluating this connectivity by multiple temporal series of fMRI in the resting-state. Some areas share a common path to complete a task, despite the fact they are not always connected by white matter fibers. The areas can also be activated when the brain is resting.

In 1995 [27], a group of researchers found that the same group of motor and supplementary areas could be activated in resting-state as well as during the movement of hand fingers. Since the recognition of this phenomenon, multiple studies have been able to validate the existence of well-defined brain circuits. Resting-state fMRI is becoming an accepted tool for neuroscientific research [28]. For instance, fMRI studies can predict the age of a brain. The color of a sphere correlates with a function, the size is correlated with a predictive power and the thick of a line that link all the interaction zones correlates with the strength of this connection, finally predicting a patient's age [29, 30].

Work performed at the Allen Institute has established, for the first time, a map of neuronal networks in the mouse brain. Before this, there were only partial maps of different connections in the brain, but this is the first "connectome" of a complete brain from a mammal. A quarter of century ago, a complete connectome of the warm C. elegans, which brain contains only 302 neurons, was deciphered. However, the mouse brain contains 75 millions of neurons, which are organized in a similar way than the human brain.

The cartography of the human connectome, i.e., the complete neurons connections between different brain areas, as well as the investigation of the relation between the connectome, behavior and genetic maps were performed between 2010 and 2015, with more than 1200 healthy patients. The group used functional MRI, looking for any correlation in time between different activity measures and different regions of the brain. Then, they elaborated patterns that described the connections that were formed and the intensity of them. Later, they look for any unique identifier, like a fingerprint, and found until 99% of certainty in two partial networks in the frontal, temporal, and parietal lobes [31]. Finally, they tried to identify any correlation between the connections and fluid intelligence with a model to predict the intensity of the connections and the intelligence quotient. They found that there are individual differences in the functional connectivity and that this connectivy was heterogeneous in the brain cortex [32, 33].

Artificial Neuronal Networks

The study of the brain is not exclusive to biologist or physicians, as physics, mathematicians and engineers have been investigating mathematical and electronic models of artificial neurons for years. The artificial neuronal networks (ANN) are processing structures inspired by the structure of the neurons in the brain. They are capable of learning from examples and are capable of executing some intelligent tasks. Thus, ANNs can facilitate the life of disable or elderly persons, they can identify emotions and mood, and they can predict responses or help with decision-making processes.

There is a new three-dimensional (3D) imaging technique capable to resolve individual neurons, intracellular organelles, and also able to trace the connections between them. This technique has been developed in the Massachusetts Institute of Technology (MIT, Cambridge, MA-USA), the University of California at Berkeley and the Howard Hughes Medical Institute (HHMI, Ashburn, VA-USA) among other institutions. The technique uses both the expansion as well as the optical microscopy and is able to obtain images of the proteins of the brain at a nanometric scale. In one study, the researchers imaged the brain of the Drosophila fly, including the synaptic proteins in the dendritic spines, the myelin in the axons and the presynaptic junctions of the dopaminergic neurons in each brain region. They were able to calculate the thickness of the myelin covering different axons and to calculate the gaps between myelin segments. The technology was also able to visualize intracellular organelles such as mitochondrias and lysosomes [34].

Joining the optical microscope and the expansion microscopy is essential to improve the sensitivity, resolution, and scalability of imaging. With this technique, it is possible to analyze millions of synapsis in just some days. It is possible to count conglomerates of postsynaptic markers in the cortex, and also observe the differences of synaptic density in distinct layers of the cortex. Using electronic microscopy, this type of study would have taken years.

This technique allows the researchers to map great number of circuits within the brain, and at the same time, it offers a unique perspective about the function of individual neurons. Using grid-enhanced optical microscopy along with expansion microscopy, we are able to obtain images with high resolution without losing the nanoscale configuration of the biomolecules.

The expansion microscopy works with a thin preserved sample of tissue. The sample is infused with an absorbent polymer, which allows the tissue to expand at least four time its volume. Through this process, the sample becomes more transparent, which is an advantage for the grid-enhanced optical microscope. The microscope sends the light from one side and take images from the other side. According to the researchers, this technology should allow the study of neural development, sexual dimorphism, stereotyping, and structural correlations of the neural activity with a significant statistical power. All of this, thanks to molecular contrast.

Brain Fluorescence

The Brainbow technique is improving our understanding of the function and development of neuronal circuits. In 2007, a group of researchers [35] described a technique where genes from bacteria, corals, or squids were inserted in nervous cells of mouses to codify three fluorescent proteins. They created neurons that expressed a random combinations of proteins. These combinations illuminated cells with more than 90 colors, offering a detailed view of the function of specific neurons and their variations according to specific behaviors. The daughter cells inherited the same color of the mother cells, which allows to study the development of specific cellular groups [36].

Genetic Atlas

The German scientist Korbinian Brodmann, during the early twentieth century, divided the brain cortex in dozens of regions, and slowly noticed that each region was responsible of a concrete brain function. This parceling model have acquired renewed attention, thanks to the fMRI technique, which is being used to build maps in relation to human behavior.

In 2003, our DNA was sequenced, it is comprised of about 20,000 genes. A decade later, a three-dimensional atlas was created mapping genes and their function in normal brains. These discoveries will certainly accelerate the progress of neurosciences [37].

The idea that the left hemisphere specializes in certain functions such as mathematics and language, and the right hemisphere in other functions such as the artistic and creative thinking is generally accepted. However, there is no prove of such differences in the genetic activity. Most genes are active in each of the largest regions of the brain, contributing to particular functions. However, 97% of the time, when there is a significant amount of RNA from certain gene in one part of the brain, the same quantity is observed in the brain of other individuals. Moreover, the brain and cerebellar cortices (which have comparatively more recent evolutionary development) present a homogeneous genetic activity. Their function seems to be related more with neurons connection than with the genetic variations from one Brodmann area to other.

Cartography of Gene Expression

Researchers from 11 institutions are working to diagram the neural circuit of extensive areas of the brain, combining four imaging techniques, to include MRI. The project allows the combined diagram of white matter fibers, histologic findings, and genetic expression.

Scientists from the Allen Institute for the Brain Science (owned by the Microsoft co-founder, Paul Allen) have revealed an atlas of the human brain, which is the first guide that relates the anatomy with the active genes in the brain.

This map is considered important because it is able to combine multiple imaging techniques in a single three-dimensional file, detailing at the same time, the anatomy, the nervous and cells structures, and the genetic activity of the brain. The atlas is a catalog of 1000 anatomic points of two donated normal brains. It links the brain tissue to thousands of genes. The atlas is grouping more than 100 million data points, measuring the strength or weakness of distinct genes in each region of the brain.

The atlas offers a complete visualization, during the embryologic development, of each active gene in a concrete region of the brain and with each cell type. This improves our understanding of the normal development of the brain and offers a powerful tool to investigate the abnormalities behind different diseases.

The authors highlight the importance of this atlas, which contributes to the understanding of pathologies such as autism, that seems to originate during embryologic stages. "Pathologies such as autism o schizophrenia demonstrate subtle alterations in the brain architecture, due to the expression of different types of genes" [38].

Optogenetics

Optogenetics covers the development of light-sensitive proteins (natural or chemically modified), strategies to introduce the genes that encode these proteins into target cells or tissues and, finally, the generation of systems for detecting behavioral changes produced in said cells and tissues.

Optogenetic methods are based on the introduction of exogenous genes that encode light-sensitive proteins into certain cells. These proteins allow behavior to be modified at the cellular level through the presence or absence of light. The key idea is the fusion in a protein of light-absorbing domains with effector domains, capable of a function. Thus, light-sensitive variants of effector proteins fused with photosensitive proteins have been created [39].

The use of opsins from microorganisms (bacteria) and their adaptation for use as cellular switches has allowed an important advance in these technologies. These opsins combine a light-sensitive domain and an ion channel in the same protein. The procedure begins by placing opsins in one type of neurons. Opsins are a group of light-sensitive proteins. This is the "genetic" part. The "Opto" component consists of applying light shots on these opsins, so that they stimulate the neurons on which they were "placed."

Scientists have designed particles capable of transforming infrared light into visible radiation. This allows us to manipulate neuronal activity in deep areas of the brain.

Conclusion

Since the second half of the twentieth century, the investigation of the brain has been characterized by a multidisciplinary approach, combining distinct methods, practices and concepts, and giving birth to new scientific communities, in conjunction denominated as neurosciences.

Neuroscience is a malleable activity that explores the brain from different fields and with different methods. Today, the scientific community discusses about the most important problems and the way of solving them.

The current imaging techniques can improve our understanding of an individual brain, beyond the need to understand a significant group of individuals. It seems better to investigate an individual brain in a normal or unsettled state, so in the future, this information can be used to give a treatment that fits a specific person.

Neuroscience might be able to explain distinct human phenomena, such as psychopatological changes, which as we know are characterized by a significant complexity.

Neuroscience is in a very important moment, due to the different methods able to register simultaneously the action potential of thousands of neurons and generate huge data points. The optogenetic, which allows to activate or deactivate selective neurons in the cortex, will be able to decipher the way the signals from neurons can control our behavior, and unlock the secret code that the brain uses to communicate with itself. In the future, we should be able to build machines that imitate the function of this wonderful organ. Hopefully, the understating of the brain through the genetic map is helpful. Thanks to the connectome project, in a near future, we will be able to map the distinct connections in our brain. Another challenge is the development of software that can use at a maximum the potential of supercomputers. Finally, neuroscientists need more research about imaging formation with more sophisticated machines, and there is a need for consensus and validation of the distinct imaging techniques.

References

1. Annex Volume II-1st part of the Histology of the Nervous System of Man and the Vertebrates of Cajal, 2009). September 2018.
2. Pérez-Cerdá F, Sánchez-Gómez MV, Matute C. Pío del Río Hortega and the discovery of the oligodendrocytes. Front Neuroanat. 2015;9:92.
3. Rafael Lorente de Nó. A Study of Nerve Physiology, Volúmenes 131–132 de Rockefeller University, New York. StudiesStudies from The Rockefeller Institute for Medical Research, Rockefeller Institute for Medical Research.
4. Bliss TVP, Lomo T. Long-lasting potentiation of synaptic transmission in the dentate area of the anaesthetized rabbit following stimulation of the perorant path. J Physiol. 1973;232:331–56.
5. Kandel ER, Schwartz JH, Jessell TM, Siegelbaum SA, Hudspeth AJ. Principles of neural science. 5th ed. McGraw Hill Professional; 2012.
6. Bonhoeffer T, Caroni P. Chapter 19. In: Stuart G, Spruston N, Häusser M, editors. Structural plasticity in dendrites and spines. Oxford University Press; 1999.
7. Coggan JS, Bartol TM, Esquenazi E, Stiles JR, Lamont S, Martone ME, Berg DK, Ellisman MH, Sejnowski TJ. Evidence for ectopic neurotransmission at a neuronal synapse. Science. 2005;309:446–51.
8. Sandrone S. Weighing brain activity with the balance: Angelo Mosso's original manuscripts come to light. Brain. 2014;137:621–33.
9. Brodmann K. Ergleichende Lokalisationlehre der Grosshiernrinde in ihren prinzipien dargestellt auf grund des zellenbaues. Leipzig: J.A. Barth; 1909.
10. Geyer S, Weiss M, Reimann K, Lohmann G, Turner R. Microstructural Parcellation of the human cerebral cortex—from Brodmann's post-mortem map to *in vivo* mapping with high-field magnetic resonance imaging. Front Hum Neurosci. 2011;5:19.
11. S. Geyer y R. Turner. Microstructural parcellation of the human cerebral cortex. Berlin/Heidelberg: Springer; 2013.
12. Stejskal E. 6 Tanner JE. Spin diffusion measurements: spin echoes in the presence of time-dependent field gradient. J Chem Phys. 1965;42:288–92.
13. Rimrodt SL, Peterson DJ, Denckla MB, Kaufmann WE, Cutting LE. White matter microstructural differences linked to left perisylvian language network in children with dyslexia. Cortex. 2010;46:739–49.
14. Yang X, Cao D, Liang X, Zhao J. Schizophrenia symptomatic associations with diffusion tensor imaging measured fractionalanisotropy of brain: a meta-analysis. Neuroradiology. 2017;59:699–708.
15. Barnea-Goraly N, Menon V, Eckert M, Tamm L, Bammer R, Karchemskiy A, et al. White matter development during childhood and adolescence: a cross-sectional diffusion tensor imaging study. Cereb Cortex. 2005;15:1848–54.
16. Takeuchi H, Taki Y, Sassa Y, Hashizume H, Sekiguchi A, Fukushima A, et al. Whitte matter structures associated with creativity: evidence from diffusion tensor imaging. NeuroImage. 2010;51:11–8.
17. Alsop DC. Imagen de RM de perfusion. In: Scott W, editor. Atlas. Magnetic resonance imaging of the brain and spine (3rd Spanish ed.). Madrid: Marban; 2004. p. 215–37.
18. Gili J. Tecnicas especiales en IRM. In: Introduccion biofísica a la resonancia magnetica en neuroimagen. Barcelona: Centre Diagnostic Pedralbes; 1993. p. 21–8.
19. Sorensen AG, Buonanno FS, Gonzalez RG, Schwamm LH, Lev MH, Huang-Hellinger FR, et al. Hyperacute stroke: evaluation with combined multisection diffusion-weighted and hemodynamically weighted echo-planar MR imaging. Radiology. 1996;199:391–401.
20. Kidwell CS, Saver JL, Starkman S, Duckwiler G, Jahan R, Vespa P, et al. Late secondary ischemic injury in patients receiving intraarterial thrombolysis. Ann Neurol. 2002;52:698–703.

21. Harris GJ, Lewis RF, Satlin A, English CD, Scott TM, Yurgelun-Todd DA, et al. Dynamic susceptibility contrast MR imaging of regional cerebral blood volume in Alzheimer disease: a promising alternative to nuclear medicine. AJNR Am J Neuroradiol. 1998;19:1727–32.
22. Bozzao A, Floris R, Baviera ME, Apruzzese A, Simonetti G. Diffusion and perfusion MR imaging in cases of Alzheimer's disease: correlations with cortical atrophy and lesion load. AJNR Am J Neuroradiol. 2001;22:1030–6.
23. Johnson NA, Jahng GH, Weiner MW, Miller BL, Chui HC, Jagust WJ, et al. Pattern of cerebral hypoperfusion in Alzheimer disease and mild cognitive impairment measured with arterial spin-labeling MR imaging: initial experience. Radiology. 2005;234:851–9.
24. Callen DJ, Black SE, Caldwell CB. Limbic system perfusion in Alzheimer's disease measured by MRI-coregistered HMPAO SPECT. Eur J Nucl Med Mol Imaging. 2002;29:899–906.
25. Hanada K, Hosono M, Kudo T, Hitomi Y, Yagyu Y, Kirime E, et al. Regional cerebral blood flow in the assessment of major depression and Alzheimer's disease in the early elderly. Nucl Med Commun. 2006;27:535–41.
26. Fayed-Miguel N, Castillo-Blandino J, Medrano-Lin J. Perfusión por resonancia magnética: bases físicas y aplicación clínica. Rev Neurol. 2010;50:23–32.
27. Biswal BB, Van Kylen J, Hyde JS. Simultaneous assessment of flow and BOLD signals in resting-state functional connectivity maps. NMR Biomed. 1997;10:165–70.
28. Lowe M. A historical perspective on the evolution of resting-state functional connectivity with MRI. MAGMA. 2010;
29. Greicius M, Srivastava G, Reiss A, Menon V. Default-mode network activity distinguishes Alzheimer's disease from healthy aging: evidence from functional MRI. Proc Natl Acad Sci USA. 2004;101:4637–42.
30. Wang K, Liang M, Wang L, Tian L, Zhang X, Li K, et al. Altered functional connectivity in early Alzheimer's disease: a resting-state fMRI study. Hum Brain Mapp. 2007;28:967–78.
31. Finn ES, Shen X, Scheinost D, Rosenberg MD, Huang J, Chun MM, et al. Functional connectome fingerprinting: identifying individuals using patterns of brain connectivity. Nat Neurosci. 2015;18:1664–71.
32. Mueller S, Wang D, Fox MD, Yeo BT, Sepulcre J, Sabuncu MR, et al. Individual variability in functional connectivity architecture of the human brain. Neuron. 2013;77:586–95.
33. Shen X, Finn ES, Scheinost D, Rosenberg MD, Chun MM, Papademetris X, et al. Using connectome-based predictive modeling to predict individual behavior from brain connectivity. Nat Protoc. 2017;12:506–18.
34. Gao R, Asano SM, Upadhyayula S, Pisarev I, Milki DE, Liu T-L, et al. Cortical column and whole-brain imaging with molecular contrast and nanoscale resolution. Science. 2019;18:363(6424).
35. Livet J, Weissman TA, Kang H, Draft RW, Lu J, Bennis RA, et al. Transgenic strategies for combinatorial expression of fluorescent proteins in the nervous system. Nature. 2007;450:56–62.
36. Weissman TA, Pan YA. Brainbow: new resources and emerging biological applications for multicolor genetic labeling and analysis. Genetics. 2015;199:293–306.
37. Hawrylycz MJ, Lein ES, Guillozet-Bongaarts AL, Shen EH, Ng L, Miller JA, et al. An anatomically comprehensive atlas of the adult human brain transcriptome. Nature. 2012;489:391–9.
38. Thompson CL, Ng L, Vilas M, Martinez S, Lee CK, Glattfelder K, et al. A high-resolution spatiotemporal atlas of gene expression of the developing mouse brain. Neuron. 2014;83:309–23.
39. Bamberg E, Gärtner W, y Trauner, D. Introduction: optogenetics and photopharmacology. Chem Rev. 2018;118(21):10627–8. https://doi.org/10.1021/acs.chemrev.8b00483.

Neuroimaging in Drug and Substance Abuse

44

Humberto Morales, Nicolás Fayed, and Alicia Fayed

Introduction

Psychostimulants are the most used psychotropic substances over the world. A "psychostimulant" can be defined as a psychotropic substance with the capacity to stimulate the central nervous system (CNS). It causes excitation and elevated mood, as well as increased alertness and arousal. Its global effect is to speed up signals into the brain. A psychostimulant can also be negatively defined as a substance other than a depressant or a hallucinogenic substance. In many cases, its use is purely recreational, at risk of abusive consumption, suffering intoxication and generating with its withdrawal a syndrome in which effects contrary to those generated by intoxication appear. As the main components of this category, we find cocaine, amphetamines, xanthines, and nicotine.

For its euphoric effects, heroin is used as a semisynthetic recreational drug. Derived from morphine and originated from poppy, the plant from which opium is extracted, its frequent and regular administration is associated with tolerance and strong physical dependence.

They will often be the neuroimaging findings that raise the possibility of consumption, and even, in the face of characteristic patterns, suggest the specific type of drug.

In this chapter, we will take a tour of drugs with the greatest neurological impact (cocaine, amphetamines, heroin, alcohol, and cannabis), as well as describing CNS acute and complications using conventional and functional magnetic resonance imaging (fMRI), positron emission tomography (PET), emission tomography of single photon (SPECT), and magnetic resonance imaging (MRI) perfusion.

Marijuana-Cannabis

Cannabis is by far the most commonly used drug of abuse. Worldwide, there were an estimated 192 million users of cannabis in 2018, corresponding to 3.9% of the global population aged 15–64. Israel reported the largest prevalence of cannabis use in the world with 27% in 2016, followed by USA with 19.4% in 2018 [1]. Over the past decade, there has been a significant increase in the consumption of the drug, in part due to legalization in multiple countries and multiple states in the USA (either for medical and/or recreational use) as well as a change in sociopolitical perceptions towards the use of cannabis. In

H. Morales
Department of Radiology, University of Kentuchy, Lexington, KY, USA
e-mail: humberto.morales@uky.edu

N. Fayed (✉)
Department of Radiology, Quironsalud Hospital, Zaragoza, Spain

A. Fayed
Department of Hematology, Miguel Servet Hospital, Zaragoza, Spain

P. Á. Gargiulo, H. L. Mesones-Arroyo (eds.), *Psychiatry and Neuroscience Update – Vol. V*, https://doi.org/10.1007/978-3-031-72219-6_44

terms of clinical implications, cannabis now accounts for around half of all first-time entrants to specialist drug treatment worldwide [2] and has now superseded opiates as the primary reason for first-time treatment entry of all illicit drugs in Europe [3]. One possible contributor to the increase in cannabis-related treatment admissions may be the increase potency of cannabis products, resulting in a higher dose of Δ9-tetrahydrocannabinol (THC) and greater harm to users [4].

The main psychoactive component of cannabis, Δ9-tetrahydrocannabinol (THC), and other cannabinoids interact with specific receptors. There are two known cannabinoid receptor subtypes such as CB1 and CB2. CB1 are G-protein-coupled receptors and are present in many presynaptic neurons, mainly located on GABAergic axon terminals, and one of their main functions is inhibiting the release of excitatory and inhibitory neurotransmitters [5]. The CB1 receptors exist abundantly in the prefrontal cortex, hippocampus, amygdala, basal ganglia, and cerebellum [6]. The CB2 receptors are expressed in the peripheral tissues of the nervous system, gastrointestinal system, and immune system. The psychoactive effects of cannabis are mainly linked to CB1 receptors. Thus, CB1 stimulation leads to diverse neuronal and cellular alterations and the modulation of dopaminergic, serotonergic, glutamatergic, and opioid neurotransmission in a wide range of neuronal networks [5].

Medical uses of cannabis include the treatment of nausea and vomiting due to chemotherapy, seizures control, neuropathic, and chronic pain; and antispastic properties in stroke and multiple sclerosis. However, the drug is not innocuous. The detrimental effects in the brain can be divided into cerebrovascular and neurological/psychological.

There is cumulative evidence of cannabis-related cerebrovascular events. Although the exact mechanism is not elucidated yet, a reversible vasoconstriction syndrome (RCVS) seems to be the most plausible pathologic association (see Figs. 44.1 and 44.2). Recent reviews of the published literature have found more than 100 cases of cerebrovascular events related to marijuana consumption since 1967 [7, 8], with ischemic strokes reported in more than 80% of cases. Rarely, hemorrhagic strokes or other intracranial hemorrhagic changes have been reported. From the published data, it is evident that young people are severely affected by neurovascular diseases as they consume cannabis in higher amount compared to older people [7]. Moreover, it can also be noted that the occurrence of cerebrovascular insults such as stroke has drastically increased after 2010. Legalization and increased availabil-

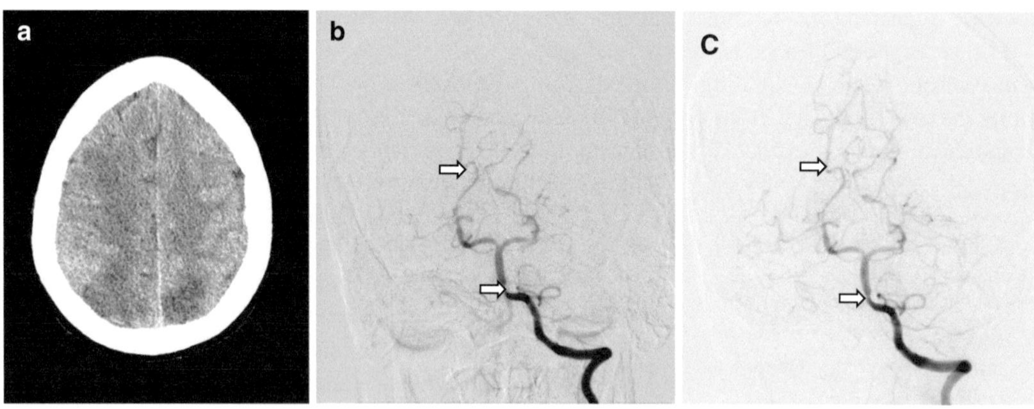

Fig. 44.1 Ischemic stroke and reversible cerebral vasoconstriction syndrome (RCVS). (**a**) CT showing symmetric areas of low attenuation in the bilateral parietal lobes, (**b**) angiogram of the posterior circulation pre-verapamil, and (**c**) angiogram post-verapamil infusion. There are multiple areas of vasoconstriction, more conspicuous in the proximal basilar artery and the distal posterior cerebral arteries that improve after verapamil infusion (arrows). Patient with a history of heavy use of marijuana before admission

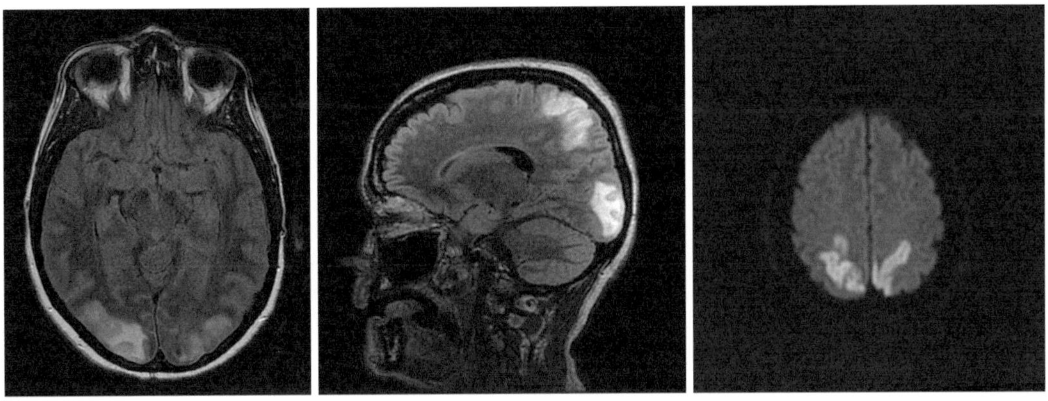

Fig. 44.2 Reversible cerebral vasoconstriction syndrome (RCVS) and marijuana. Similar pattern of involvement than patient in Fig. 44.1, in this case with bilateral infarcts in the parietal lobes and occipital lobes. Angiogram (not shown) also demonstrated vasoconstriction phenomenon

ity of the drug across the world may be the underlying reasons for this.

The detrimental neurologic/psychological effects can be acute or chronic, including hyperemesis syndrome, impaired coordination, anxiety, psychotic symptoms, cognitive dysfunction, memory and attention deficiency. The high density of CB1 receptors in regions associated with memory, perception, and motor control explain the neurologic effects, whereas the low density in the brain stem might explain the overall lack of lethality of cannabis.

Cannabis use disorder (CUD) is a clinical diagnosis that a substantial number of people currently meet criteria or at risk of developing. Similarly to other substance use disorder (SUD), a diagnosis of CUD is characterized by problematic use, including escalation with loss of control over use, repeated failures to reduce or quit, and continued use despite of negative consequences [9]. Consistent with the characteristics of a complex psychiatric disorder, environmental as well as genetic factors mediate vulnerability to CUD. Irrespective of other factors, age of onset is a strong predictive variable, with significant correlations between younger age of initiation and CUD liability. Thus, the risk for CUD onset normally peaks in late adolescence, when the brain has not achieved full adult maturity and it is more vulnerable to psychiatric disorders [10].

The acute alterations that cannabis produces in the cerebral blood flow (CBF) and metabolism have been studied by imaging. Nearly every study using H2 [15O]- positron emission tomography (PET) found Δ9-tetrahydrocannabinol (THC)-induced increases in the cerebral blood flow in the frontal cortex, insula, and cingulate gyrus [4, 11, 12]. Subsequently, magnetic resonance imaging (MRI) measures of cerebral blood flow with arterial spin labelling (ASL) have corroborated the PET findings [13]. In terms of metabolism, using [18F]-deoxyglucose (FDG) PET, Volkow et al. [14] demonstrated that acute Δ9-tetrahydrocannabinol (THC) increased metabolism in the basal ganglia and the orbitofrontal cortex (OFC) and prefrontal cortex (PFC). Collectively, these studies show that acute cannabis exposure causes region-specific increases in cerebral blood flow and metabolism, particularly in frontal regions [4].

Despite some contradictory findings, most human structural magnetic resonance imaging (MRI) studies document brain architectural alterations particularly in the cortico-limbic structures such as the prefrontal cortex (PFC), hippocampus and amygdala with CUD. The orbitofrontal cortex (OFC; located within the PFC), which contributes to cognition and valuation and decision-making, is commonly damaged in SUD. Overall, greater disease severity is associated with reduced volume of the medial OFC [10,

15, 16]. Decreased OFC volume in young teens predicts initiation of cannabis later in life, suggesting a preexisting neurobiological risk factor. Similarly, in the hippocampus (related to learning and memory), reduced gray matter is associated with increased consume of cannabis. The latter emphasizes the direct contribution of CB1 receptors stimulation. Overall, the deficits in gray matter volume observed in CUD are similar than in many other SUD. One particular difference is the cerebellum, which show increased gray matter in subjects with CUD [15, 17]. In contrast to consistent cerebellar findings, the striatum (critical to reward and habit formation) shows no clear pattern of structural alterations in CUD [10].

Multiple diffusion tensor imaging (DTI) studies have found evidence of structural dysconnectivity in cannabis users, in the form of reduced mean diffusivity in the corpus callosum (prefrontal section and splenium), fornix, and commissural fibers [4, 18, 19]. Other studies have found effects on orbitofrontal connectivity [20]. There is also longitudinal evidence of cannabis effects on white matter (WM). Two studies [21, 22] found that greater cannabis consumption was associated with reduced connectivity in several key pathways including the inferior longitudinal fasciculus.

In addition to morphologic changes, various fMRI studies have shown specific brain activity signatures with cannabis use, both during resting conditions and when specific tasks are given. One of the most common patterns of resting stage activity identified is similar than in other SUD, with increased connectivity associated with the default mode network (DMN) (a collection of brain regions involved in self-referential cognitive tasks: posterior cingulate cortex, adjacent medial prefrontal cortex (PFC) and portions of the parietal cortex, the precuneus and angular gyri) and insular networks [23, 24]. During neurocognitive tasks, for example, with cost-benefit decision-making conditions, there is reduced activity of the OFC and dorsolateral PFC, but also increased cerebellar activity, in heavy cannabis users. An effect is related with impaired choose outcome [25]. There is converging evidence that cannabis use is associated with working memory impairments due to the hyperactivation and hyperconnectivity of working memory circuits particularly in the PFC [4]. These effects have been associated with total cannabis exposure [26] which may be mediated by CB1 receptors genotype [27].

The important question whether cannabis can cause irreversible brain damage is still a matter of debate. Particularly, because some of the changes described by structural and functional MRI in the brain appear to reverse once the consumption ceases. Nevertheless, there is mounting evidence about the association of cannabis and cerebrovascular injuries, particularly ischemic stroke related to reversible cerebral vasoconstriction syndrome (RCVS). The perception of a harmless drug might be due to the unawareness of complications. In the current context, every young patient with stroke or symptoms related to reversible cerebral vasoconstriction syndrome, such as thunderclap headaches, should be asked and actively screened for the use of drugs such as cannabis. The same could be extrapolated to neurological and psychiatric symptoms such as psychosis.

Opiates and Derivatives (Heroin)

Opiates are drugs derived from the opium poppy plant, and they are naturally occurring peptide compounds such as morphine and codeine. Opioid is a term used to describe any nonpeptide compound, synthetic or partly synthetic, that can also bind at the opiate receptor site [28]. Opioids include heroine, hydrocodone, oxycodone, fentanyl, meperidine, and methadone.

Opiates and opioids constitute the second most common illicit drug of abuse after cannabis [1]. However, they are the predominant substance that cause death in drug abusers [29]. In 2018, 57.8 million people globally were estimated to have used opioids in the past year. The use of opioids is higher than the global average in North America, Australia and New Zealand, the Near and Middle East, and Asia [1]. There is a well-known epidemic of opioid addiction and abuse in the United States, and unfortunately, drug dealers looking for ways to increase their profits have begun to mix heroin with highly potent fentanyl, even worsening their fatal effect [30].

Opiates offer beneficial analgesic properties, but many of the compounds are some of the most addictive substance in the world, leading to tolerance, withdrawal, and relapse. Opiates have their biochemical and physiological effects via stimulation of three types of opiate receptors that are the μ, κ, and δ opioid receptors [28]. These receptors are coupled to G1 proteins and act by regulating calcium channels and rectifying potassium channels. This results in hyperpolarization and reduction in neuronal excitability. The drugs also decrease intracellular cyclic adenosine monophosphate (cAMP) which modulates the release of nociceptive neurotransmitters. Stimulation of the μ opioid receptor will result in analgesic effects, euphoria, respiratory depression, and miosis, while stimulation of the κ and δ opioid receptors causes analgesic, dysphoric, and psychotomimetic effects [31, 32]. Morphine and all of the clinically significant opiates exert their primary effect at the μ receptor. The μ-receptors are mainly located in the periaqueductal gray region of the brain. High densities of μ-receptors are also found in the nucleus accumbens (an area deeply implicated in the process of addiction), the amygdala, some portions of the cerebral cortex, the cerebellum, and the superficial dorsal horn of the spinal cord [28, 33].

Heroin is the most common drug of abuse within opiates [34]. The drug is taken orally, via inhalation, and/or by intravenous injections. Acute and chronic effects of heroin include cerebrovascular disorders, leuko-encephalopathy, and atrophy [35]. Heroin users show several cognitive deficits in neuropsychological tests. These deficits include visual memory, working memory, processing speed, and executive function [36, 37].

Ischemic stroke is the most common acute cerebrovascular complication caused by heroin [32]. Although the prevalence of a cerebrovascular injury associated with heroin is not as high as the neurovascular complications associated with cocaine, the proposed mechanisms are similar: (1) direct effects of the heroin with reversible vasospasm from stimulation of the vascular smooth muscles by the μ opioid receptors or (2) embolic events from crystalline impure additives [38]. A drug-associated vasculitis has also been proposed but the evidence of this phenomenon is poor. Ischemia is more often encountered following intravenous injection compared with other routes. The globus pallidus is the most commonly involved location, and infarcts in this location are present in approximately 5–10% of chronic heroin abusers [39] (see Fig. 44.3). Hypoxic-ischemic injury occurs most commonly in the setting of drug overdose, secondary to a heroin-induced respiratory depression with subsequent

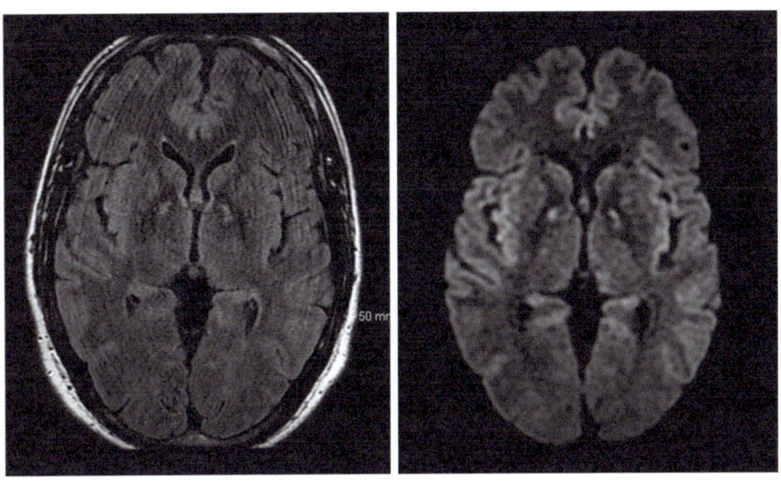

Fig. 44.3 Globus pallidi infarction associated with heroin abuse. Note the symmetric hyperintensity in the bilateral globus pallidi

Fig. 44.4 Hypoxic ischemic injury and heroin overdose. Diffuse loss of the gray-white matter differentiation and effacement of the cerebral sulci consistent with diffuse edema

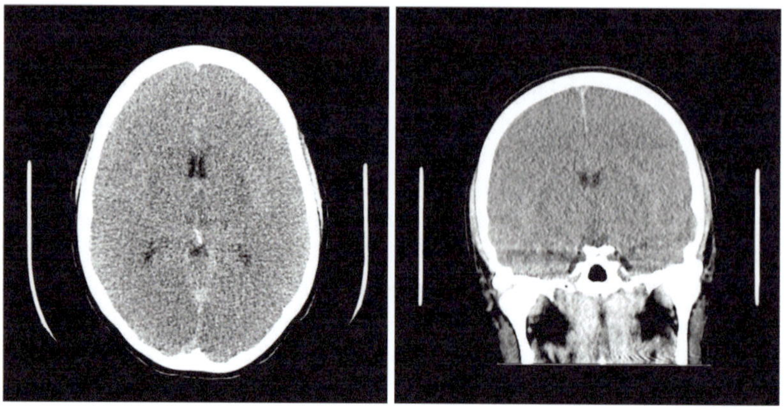

hypoxia and in some cases hypotension [40] (see Fig. 44.4).

Toxic leukoencephalopathy is a unique and rare disorder in heroin abusers. The route of administration and the time of onset after the acute heroin intoxication appear to correlate with distinct patterns of toxic leukoencephalopathy on MR imaging and also with distinct clinical prognosis [41]. An acute or delayed-onset leukoencephalopathy has been identified after IV-injection of heroin, and is characterized by diffuse involvement of the brain WM on MRI, to include the subcortical U-fibers (see Fig. 44.5). On the other hand, a progressive pattern of leukoencephalopathy has been identified in inhalation-users, and is characterized by involvement of the posterior more than anterior brain WM, including the posterior limb of the internal capsule and cerebellum. The latter has been called "Chasing the Dragon" pattern and corresponds to a spongiform leukoencephalopathy. On neuropathologic examination, there is a diffuse spongiform and vacuolar white-matter degeneration with loss of oligodendrocytes, axonal reduction, astrogliosis, and subcortical U fiber sparing [40, 42].

Recently, a cluster of patients was identified with acute hippocampal injury and amnesia, most likely associated with opioid use, particularly fentanyl [43]. On MRI, the patients present well defined restricted diffusion (see Fig. 44.6). In rats, fentanyl has been shown to cause acute neuronal injury in the hippocampus, limbic structures, and areas of association [44]. Thus, the hippocampus might be the structure most sensitive to the neurotoxic effects (possibly hypermetabolism and excitotoxicity) of fentanyl and related agents [43].

Structural MRI studies often find reduced gray matter in the prefrontal cortex, anterior cingulate, insula, and temporal cortex of opiate/heroin abusers [45–47]. The duration of heroin use appears to negatively correlate with gray matter density in many of these brain regions [47]. Thus, continued and prolonged use of opiates may lead to neuronal damage or death [35]. Opioids are known to decrease dendritic spine density, and this decrease could explain the smaller volumes [48]. Reduced gray matter density in the prefrontal cortex is consistent with MRI studies reporting cerebral blood flow changes to the prefrontal cortex [49]. The nucleus accumbens [50] and amygdale [51], important regions in reward processing, also show smaller volumes.

WM abnormalities have been reported using DTI in opiate users. These studies find diminished WM integrity in frontal, temporal, and parietal regions [45, 52–54]. Associations between duration of use and fractional anisotropy (FA) in these WM regions have been observed such that the longer the duration of opioid abuse, the more the damage to the tissue. Additionally, decreased fractional anisotropy in opiate abusers has been observed in the stria terminalis, amygdalofugal fibers, and uncinate fasciculus that connect the amygdala with other subcortical and cortical structures, including the nucleus accumbens and

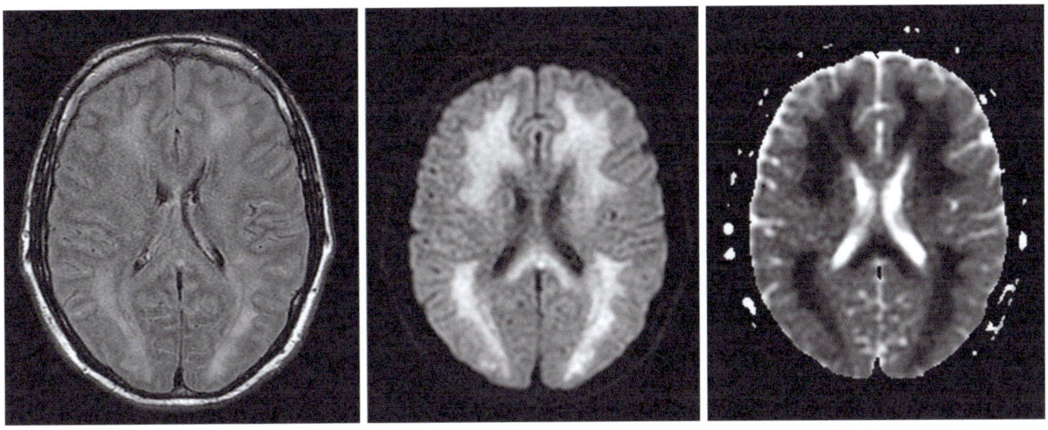

Fig. 44.5 Toxic leukoencephalopathy and heroin overdose. There is extensive white matter signal alteration in this MRI from a patient who was found down and with known heroin use

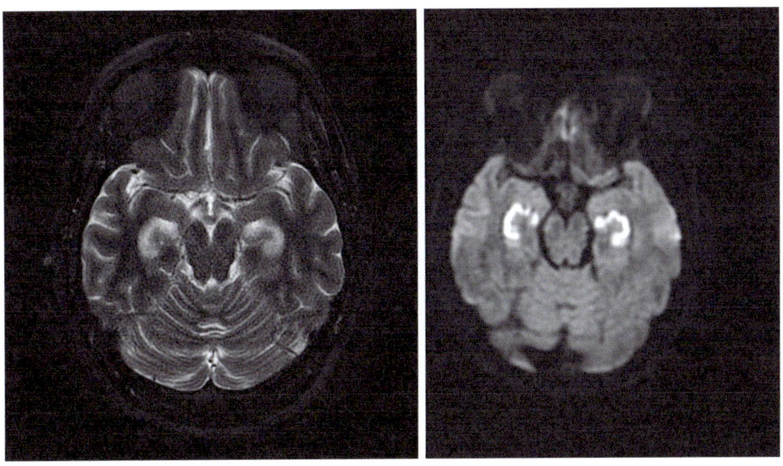

Fig. 44.6 Hippocampal injury and fentanyl. Note the symmetric hyperintensity in the bilateral hippocampi in this patient with antegrade amnesia who was found unresponsive at initial presentation

insula [51]. Overall, structural MRI studies have found alterations to gray and WM within the frontal-subcortical networks underlying the rewards system.

Regarding brain function, studies have shown that heroin users are at increased risk for long-term deficits in their decision-making capacity when compared to healthy controls [55–57]. Evidence of abnormal function has also been obtained by fMRI. Using the resting-stage fMRI, heroin use has been associated with dysfunction of the DMN [58–60]. Disturbance within the DMN appeared to worsen as heroin use duration increased and was positively correlated with poor performance on gambling and impulsiveness tests.

Other fMRI studies have shown that the brain circuits responsible for exerting executive control over areas associated with self-control were weakened in heroin users compared to healthy individuals [60–62]. Specific areas related to significant functional changes are the left prefrontal cortex (PFC), bilateral orbital frontal cortices (OFC), left anterior cingulate gyrus, and limbic regions (amygdala and hippocampus). Existing research also showed that the brain circuits associated with primary drives, motives, and memory are strengthened in heroin users compared to healthy individuals [60]. Collectively, the studies suggest that the abnormal brain connectivity in heroin users contribute to decreased self-control, impaired inhibitory functions, and deficits in stress regulation.

Cocaine

This psychostimulant obtained from the plant Erythroxylum coca is one of the most well-known and dangerous plant-based excitatory substances, as well as being among the most addictive drugs. It is consumed by an estimation of 19 million people worldwide, 0.4% of the global population aged 15 to 64 years [1].

There are two forms of presentation such as hydrochlorin (fine powder) and the alkaloid (also known as crack) [63].

The effect of cocaine is mediated through enhancement of the monoamine neurotransmitter activity in the central and peripheral nervous system. Cocaine blocks the reuptake of dopamine, norepinephrine, and to a lesser degree serotonin [64, 65], increasing their extracellular concentrations, especially in the nucleus accumbens [66].

The onset of action is very fast for the smoked or injected form (within seconds) and a couple of minute for the snorted form. The oral form, rarely observed, would take about 20–30 min to produce effects. The action lasts typically 15–30 min for the smoked or injected form, about 1 h for the snorted form, and 2–3 h for the ingested one.

The amount of cocaine taken has also been linked to the risk of addiction. In general, the addictive potential is high, and community-based interview surveys show that up to one in six persons who use cocaine will become dependent [67]. With increasing dose and duration of use, the incidence of unintended adverse effect increases. They include dysphoric mood, panic attack, paranoid reactions, impaired judgment, and psychotic symptom as delusions and hallucinations.

The physical harms are mainly related to cardiovascular accidents and consequences of injection and sharing equipment (e.g., blood borne viruses, abscess, and endocarditis). Increased cardiac oxygen demand, vasoconstriction, and platelets activation are synergic in causing acute coronary syndromes [68] cerebral strokes [69], or toxic leucoencephalopathy [70, 71], even in young healthy individuals.

The cerebrovascular bed is also concerned: a US study found a 14-fold increase in the risk of ischemic or hemorrhagic stroke among cocaine users compared with matched controls (and a fourfold increased risk for methamphetamine) (see Fig. 44.7) [72]. Other neurologic acute events concerns seizures that can happen even at the first time of use and without prior history of seizure [73].

The main brain complications arising from cocaine abuse are vascular, mainly bleeding subarachnoid and intraparenchymatous hemorrhage. The bleeding events are, on the whole, twice as frequent as ischemic heart attacks [32] (see Fig. 44.7). However, the shape of the drug and the absorption pathway influence the type of

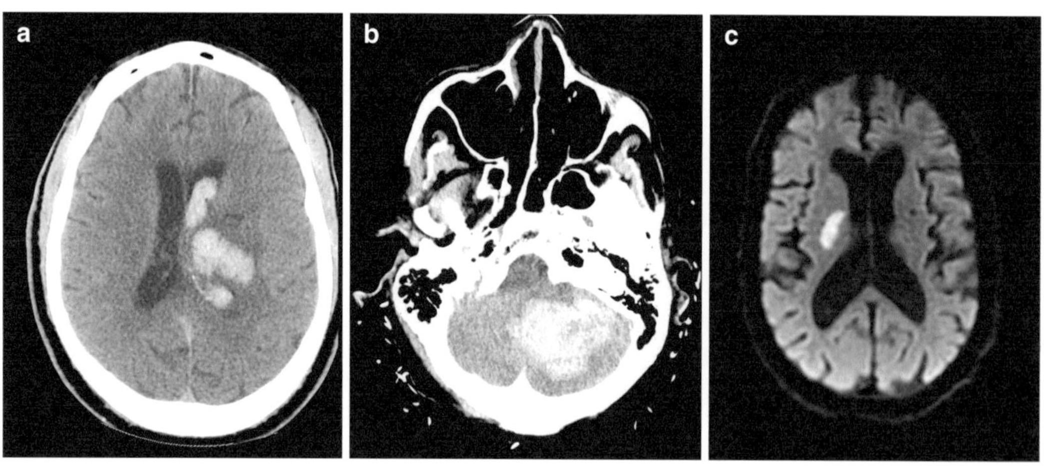

Fig. 44.7 Hemorrhagic and ischemic cerebrovascular complications of cocaine abuse. (**a**) There is a left thalamic hemorrhage with associated intraventricular extension. (**b**) There is a prominent left cerebellar hemorrhage. (**c**) There is a small area of restricted diffusion on the right corona radiata (ischemic event)

adverse event. When cocaine is smoked in the form of crack, the incidence of bleeding events is higher, while there are no significant differences between ischemic and hemorrhagic events when the drug snorts [74, 75].

Recent cocaine ingestion is associated with hemorrhages that occur more frequently in subcortical locations, have a higher risk of intraventricular hemorrhage (see Fig. 44.7), and have a poor prognosis compared to patients with cocaine-negative, spontaneous intracerebral hemorrhage [76]. Up to 50% of patients with hemorrhagic complications of cocaine have underlying vascular pathology, like aneurysms and vascular malformations [63]. A sudden rise in systemic arterial pressure may cause hemorrhages, sometimes in association with an underlying aneurysm or arteriovenous malformation (AVM).

Chronic cocaine use appears to predispose patients who harbor incidental neurovascular anomalies to present at an earlier point in their natural history than similar noncocaine users. Cocaine use has been temporally associated with neurovascular complications, including the rupture of intracerebral aneurysms. Joint cocaine and ethanol abuse are not uncommon, which synergistically increases the likelihood of bleeding subarachnoid [75].

One study has shown that users of cocaine with subarachnoid hemorrhage (SAH) had smaller aneurysms at a younger age than a noncocaine user control group with SAH and that mortality was 27.3% for patients who presented with neurovascular sequelae of their cocaine use, with 77.8% of deaths occurring in patients who presented with SAH [77].

Ischemic heart attacks often affect territories of the middle and posterior cerebral arteries, border territories, the inner capsule, and the hippocampus, without a specific pattern of affectation [74]. The mesencephalic infarction has been associated with simultaneous use cocaine and amphetamines [78].

Vasospasm [79], arteritis [80, 81], myocardial infarction with cardiac arrhythmias, and increased platelet aggregation may provoke infarcts [82].

Chronic cocaine snoring can cause the classic nasal septum perforation, oropharyngeal ulcers, and osteolytic sinusitis [83]. More important are the neuropsychiatric long-term consequences. Cocaine has been shown to be neurotoxic for the dopamine neurons, especially in the midbrain [84].

Chronic addicts feature characteristically atrophy in the insular, orbitofrontal, cingulate, and temporal cortices [32, 85] and a decrease in metabolic activity in PET studies with 18-fluorodeoxyglucose [86]. Infusion studies with single photon emission computed tomography (SPECT) have shown a 30% generally reduced blood flow which has a specific decrease in relative cerebral blood flow in the prefrontal cortex, anterior cingulate gyrus, thalamus, basal ganglia, occipital cortex, and cerebellum [87]. Using nuclear-medicine imaging (PET/SPECT) provides evidence that there are ongoing changes in the dopaminergic system associated with the use of stimulants. The striatal dopamine transporter (DAT) availability was significantly increased in cocaine users [88].

The brain structure was examined in a mega-analysis of previously published data pooled from 23 laboratories, including 3240 individuals, 2140 of whom had substance dependence on one of five substances: alcohol, nicotine, cocaine, methamphetamine, or cannabis. Lower volume or thickness was observed in many brain regions in individuals with substance dependence. A set of affected regions related to dependence in general, regardless of the substance, included the insula and the medial orbitofrontal cortex [89].

The majority of studies reported statistically significant differences between cocaine users and non-drug-using controls in brain structures, blood-oxygen-level dependent signals, and brain metabolism. However, the current evidence does not support the view that chronic cocaine use is associated with broad cognitive deficits. The view that cocaine users have broad cognitive deficits is inaccurate based upon current evidence, and the perpetuation of this view may have negative implications for treatment programs and development of public policies [90].

Dorsal medial prefrontal cortex alterations may not be substance-specific, but rather related to the number of substances used, whereas ventrolateral prefrontal cortex pathology is specifically associated with cocaine use [91]. Studies have determined that it is possible to decrease frontal and striatal reactivity to drug signals in cocaine users through continuous stimulation of the theta burst (cTBS) to the left ventromedial prefrontal cortex (VMPFC) [92].

The orbitofrontal cortex and the anterior cingulate gyrus, which are regions neuroanatomically connected with limbic structures, are the frontal cortical areas most frequently implicated in drug addiction. They are activated in addicted subjects during intoxication, craving, and bingeing, and they are deactivated during withdrawal. These regions are also involved in higher-order cognitive and motivational functions, such as the ability to track, update, and modulate the salience of a reinforcer as a function of context and expectation and the ability to control and inhibit prepotent responses [93]. The latter study noted negative correlations between normalized prefrontal volumes and years of either cocaine or heroin use, implying a cumulative effect of substance abuse on frontal volumes. Additional support is provided by studies done in rats. For example, it has been recently shown that self-administration of cocaine, but not food, results in morphological changes in dendrites and dendritic spines in the prefrontal cortex and nucleus accumbens [94].

Another line of evidence supporting the role of the frontal cortex in craving derives from studies conducted shortly after the subjects last drug use. For example, it has been shown a higher regional brain glucose metabolism, including in the orbitofrontal cortex and striatum, in cocaine abusers tested during early withdrawal (<1 week since last cocaine use) than in normal comparison subjects [86].

Cocaine withdrawal syndrome is a situation of considerable importance that often causes both physical and psychic disorders and often lead to the compulsive need to continue consuming. Abnormalities in the human cortex associated with withdrawal from cocaine in regular cocaine abusers were documented as early as 1988 [95, 96]. This group showed that the relative CBF values for the prefrontal cortex and the left lateral frontal cortex were significantly lower in the cocaine users than in the normal comparison subjects. A follow-up study in active cocaine abusers demonstrated differences in regional brain glucose metabolism between cocaine abusers tested within 1 week of last cocaine use and cocaine abusers tested 2–4 weeks after last cocaine use [86]. During more protracted withdrawal (1–6 weeks since last use), brain metabolism was found to be lower in cocaine abusers than in normal comparison subjects, an effect that was most accentuated in the frontal cortex [97].

Other neuroimaging studies found cerebral gray matter atrophy, small cerebral perfusion defects, and decreased D2 dopamine receptors in the striatum [74] and especially in the nucleus accumbens, which is attributed to an important role in pleasure, so it is involved in the reward-reward circuit [98]. Voxel-based morphometry of long-term abstinent former regular users of cocaine has shown that abstinence duration positively correlated with volume in both subcortical regions (particularly the nucleus accumbens) and prefrontal regions [99].

Functional MRI studies at rest have been conducted on hospitalized crack-cocaine users who had been abstinent for at least 4 weeks and age-matching drug nonuse checks, and the results suggest that selective extrinsic network connectivity of the DMN related to motor and executive function is impaired during crack-cocaine addiction [100].

Research of dopaminergic deficits has focused on the ventral striatum with many studies elucidating altered resting-state functional connectivity in cocaine-dependent individuals, and findings suggesting a different pattern of subregional functional connectivity of the ventral striatum in altered resting state in cocaine dependence.

The findings can provide a new view of ventral striatum circuit deficits in cocaine dependence and provide an alternative analytical framework for addressing functional disconnectivity in other mental illnesses [101].

Brain imaging studies indicate that chronic cocaine users display altered functional connectivity between prefrontal cortical, thalamic, striatal, and limbic regions. However, the use of cross-sectional designs in these studies precludes measuring baseline brain activity prior to cocaine use. Thus, fMRI studies have been conducted in private cocaine rats, and the results suggest that cocaine and sucrose can change the arrangement of functional connectivity of brain regions involved in cognition and emotion, but that these changes dissipate across the early stages of abstinence [102].

Recently, using an advanced imaging method called magnetic field correlation imaging, it has been observed that individuals with cocaine use disorder have excess iron in the globus pallidus internal segment, as indexed by magnetic field correlation, and lack the age-related gradual iron deposition seen in normal aging. Because the globus pallidus is critical for the transition of goal-directed behavior to compulsive behavior, significantly elevated iron in the globus pallidus internal segment may contribute to the persistence of cocaine use disorder, and support pursuing this new line of research [103].

It has also been observed by MRI studies with diffusion tensor imaging (DTI) in cocaine users, alterations in the white substance, and in particular, users tended to exhibit differences in the microstructure of major fiber pathways, such as the corpus callosum, though it is unclear to what extent such alterations are permanent [104]. Converging lines of evidence from diffusion tensor imaging (DTI) studies reveal significant alterations in the WM microstructure in the prefrontal cortex of chronic stimulant users compared to controls, suggesting compromised axonal microstructure and/or myelin [105]. Furthermore, no significant differences were found between cocaine and methamphetamine-based groups [106].

Human neuroimaging studies indicate that the amygdala plays a key role in cocaine addiction. It has been suggested that compulsive use of drugs of abuse is, at least in part, mediated by structural and functional changes in the amygdala, an area that signals negative emotional states [107]. For instance, amygdala volume is reduced in cocaine addicts [108, 109], but the amygdala-striatum connectivity is increased in cocaine addicts in response to losing outcomes [110]. Cocaine users show amygdala hyperresponsiveness during fear conditioning and in response to angry and fearful facial expressions.

Amphetamine and Derivatives

These substances are designer drugs that are classified as psychostimulants and hallucinogens. Nevertheless, methylenedioxymethamphetamine's (MDMA, ecstasy) hallucinogenic properties are light and normally limited to visual disturbances [111]. MDMA is one of the most commonly used synthetic drugs today.

Ecstasy is mainly sold in the form of pills or tablets, but may be found in powder that can be snorted or smoked. The drug has central stimulant and psychedelic effects mediated by serotonin (5-HT), and to a lesser proportion by dopamine [112, 113].

The intraneuronal 5-HT stores are depleted, and the 5-HT concentration in the synaptic cleft is increased. The effect typically begins within the first hour, and lasts for 3–6 h [114]. Other chemically close substances can be found mixed with MDMA in the preparations. These include MDA (methylenedioxyamphetamine), known as "love pill" because of intense euphoria and entactogen effect, MDEA (methylenedioxyethamphetamine) a substance very similar to MDMA, and PMA (paramethoxyamphetamine), suspected to be more toxic that MDMA. The clinical effects of MDMA include a feeling of euphoria together with relaxation, empathy, and energy. Sexual desire and satisfaction are enhanced. The effects may include impulsive or paranoid reactions. The sense of appetite and the need to sleep are suppressed; still, the feeling of thirst can sometimes be enhanced even without a water deficit after MDMA use. This can lead to absorption of large quantities of water, leading to hyponatremia, cerebral edema, and even death [115].

In the week following use of MDMA, depression and low concentration and/or memory problems are reported by users as being relatively common. The risk of development of more severe psychopathological problems exists, with 31 cases of psychiatric complications described in the medical literature comprising episodes of depression, panic attacks, "flashbacks," and delusion. This can occur even after one single take of MDMA [116].

The street names of methamphetamine are "Meth," "Crystal Meth," "Speed," or "Ice." It can be easily manufactured from widely available pseudoephedrine, with a risk of explosion and burns for careless producers. The substance can be taken orally, smoked, snored, injected, or inserted rectally. Its effect and high addictive potential can largely be compared to cocaine, but its half-life is longer and about 12 h. It produces a rapid and pleasurable rush related to the release of dopamine, norepinephrine, and serotonin, followed by euphoria, heightened level of alertness, and increased energy. Increased libido and enhanced sexual pleasure also occur, followed by increased sexual activity with high risk behavior.

The main acute side effects seem to be cardiovascular (myocardial infarction, stroke). The other adverse events are those of the others amphetamine derivatives (hyperthermia, rhabdomyolysis, acute renal failure, and seizures) [117].

Psychiatric acute reactions include anxiety, insomnia, paranoia, and psychosis. Chronic use of methamphetamine can cause important neurological and psychiatric problems caused by dopamine depletion (anxiety, motor slowing, and psychosis), as well as serotonin depletion.

Although the biochemical mechanism of amphetamines produces long-term ischemia, the most common urgent complications are bleeding caused by increased blood pressure. As with cocaine use (see Fig. 44.7), increased blood pressure conditions an increased risk of ruptured malformations arteriovenous and preexisting aneurysms. Vasoconstriction in brain microcirculation produces ultimately necrosis of irrigated tissue. The areas most frequently affected by this ischemia are the globus pallidi -as with heroin-, (see Fig. 44.3) and the occipital cortex, where the highest concentration of 5-hydroxytryptamine receptors (called 5HT 2A) are found [32]. In fact, the most common finding in autopsies is globus pallidus necrosis [118].

Mephedrone, also known as 4-methyl methcathinone (4-MMC) or 4-methyl ephedrone, is a synthetic stimulant drug of the amphetamine and cathinone classes. It comes in the form of tablets or a powder, which users can swallow, snort, or inject, producing similar effects to ecstasy, amphetamines, and cocaine. While posterior reversible encephalopathy syndrome (PRES) has been rarely associated with cocaine ingestion, it can also be associated with mephedrone [119]. Posterior reversible encephalopathy syndrome has been associated with hypertension, preeclampsia, cancer chemotherapy, and drugs of abuse, such as amphetamine and methamphetamine. CT and MRI showed extensive WM changes consistent with edema in the posterior regions of both cerebral hemispheres (see Fig. 44.8). Although the pathogenesis of PRES is not fully understood, abnormal cerebral blood flow regulation likely contributes to its development [120]. As the arterial blood pressure rises, this pressure change could cause blood-brain barrier disruption and extravasation of fluid into the

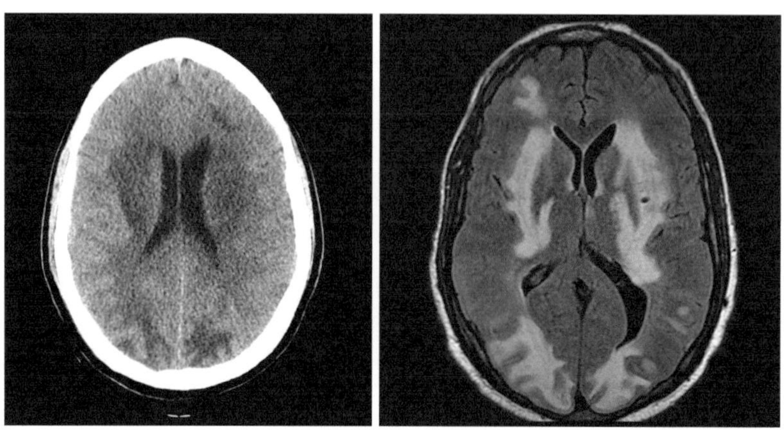

Fig. 44.8 Posterior reversible encephalopathy syndrome (PRES) with drug overdose. Diffuse areas of abnormality are demonstrated in the white matter consistent with vasogenic edema in this patient with known heroin overdose and associated hypertension

brain parenchyma, producing vasogenic edema [121].

With PET, a selective damage is observed in the serotonin neurons and a decrease in their conveyors [122]. Using positron emission tomography to identify binding of translocator protein (TSPO), which is upregulated in reactive glial cells and activated microglia during pathological states, high TSPO levels have been shown in methamphetamine use but exhibits variable patterns in cocaine use [123].

As for the infusion measured with SPECT, a relative decrease in blood flow has been found in the visual cortex, caudate, upper parietal lobe, and the dorsolateral region of the frontal lobe, related to ecstasy induced vasoconstriction [124]. MR perfusion has shown a decrease in relative cerebral blood volume of that dorsolateral region of the frontal cortex as the first functional manifestation after the first contacts with ecstasy (MDMA) in young subjects [125].

There are studies indicating that individuals with a history of chronic methamphetamine abuse often display several signs of corticostriatal dysfunction, including abnormal gray- and white-matter integrity, monoamine neurotransmitter system deficiencies, neuroinflammation, poor neuronal integrity, and aberrant patterns of brain connectivity and function, both when engaged in cognitive tasks and at rest. More importantly, many of these neural abnormalities were found to be linked with certain addiction-related phenotypes that may influence treatment response (e.g., poor self-control, cognitive inflexibility, and maladaptive decision-making), raising the possibility that they may represent novel therapeutic targets [126].

Methamphetamine dependence can lead to psychotic symptoms which may be mediated by frontal, striatal, limbic, and thalamic regions. Furthermore, they indicate that glucose metabolism and cerebral perfusion in these regions are disrupted in methamphetamine dependent individuals with psychotic symptoms. Methamphetamine dependent with psychotic symptoms had: (1) decreased glucose metabolism in the left precentral gyrus and the left inferior frontal gyrus and (2) increased glucose metabolism in the putamen and pallidum. Methamphetamine dependent with psychotic symptoms participants also had increased cerebral perfusion in the right putamen and right pallidum compared to methamphetamine dependent [127].

Structural brain abnormalities are associated with abuse of amphetamines. A brief history of amphetamine use/abuse and evidence for toxicity is followed by a summary of findings from structural magnetic resonance imaging (MRI) studies of human subjects who had abused amphetamines and children who were exposed to amphetamines in utero. These included lower cortical gray matter volume and higher striatal volume than control subjects. High striatal volumes might reflect compensation for toxicity in the dopamine-rich basal ganglia. Prenatal exposure was associated with striatal volume that was below control values, suggesting that such compensation might not occur in utero. Several forms of WM abnormality are also common and may involve gliosis. In relation to long-term effects, it has been shown selective atrophy in the occipital and frontal cortex, the left temporal lobe and brain stem compared to users who abuse other drugs exclusively or together [128].

Using diffusion tensor imaging in methamphetamine users with 3T magnetic resonance imaging, it has been shown that the striato-thalamo-orbitofrontal circuit has reduced microstructural integrity in methamphetamine users, and the microstructural changes in the thalamus may compensate for dysfunction in functionally connected cortices. The methamphetamine group had significant fractional anisotropy reduction in the bilateral nucleus accumbens, orbitofrontal cortex, and right thalamus. Lower left orbitofrontal cortex fractional anisotropy and right nucleus accumbens fractional anisotropy/axial diffusion were associated with longer duration of methamphetamine use. Lower right orbitofrontal cortex fractional anisotropy was associated with younger age at first methamphetamine use. Higher fractional anisotropy and lower mean diffusivity/radial diffusion in the thalamus, as well as higher left orbitofrontal cortex radial diffusion, were associated with increased psychiatric symptoms [129]. Compared with healthy control subjects, methamphetamine users showed lower fractional anisotropy in right frontal WM and higher apparent diffusion coefficient in left caudate and bilateral putamen. Higher left putamen apparent diffusion coefficient was associated with earlier initiation of methamphetamine use, greater daily amounts, and a higher cumulative lifetime dose. Similarly, higher right putamen apparent diffusion coefficient was associated with greater daily amounts and a higher cumulative lifetime dose. The lower fractional anisotropy in the right frontal WM suggests axonal injury in these methamphetamine users. The higher apparent diffusion coefficient in the basal ganglia suggests greater inflammation or less myelination in these brain regions of those with younger age of first methamphetamine use and greater methamphetamine usage [130].

It has been demonstrated, in a chronic methamphetamine administration model, that discontinuation of drug for more than a week produces much larger changes in overall meth-induced brain connectivity and cerebral blood volume (CBV) response than changes that occur immediately following meth administration. Areas showing the largest changes were hippocampal, limbic striatum, and sensorimotor cortical regions as well as brain stem areas including the pedunculopontine tegmentum (PPTg) and pontine nuclei—regions known to be important in mediating reinstatement of drug-taking after abstinence. These changes occur concomitantly with behavioral sensitization and appear to be mediated through increases in dopamine D1 and D3 and decreases in D2 receptor protein and mRNA expression [131].

There are studies that show improvement in behavior and cognitive function after long-term abstinence, although the patients still show an abnormal brain structure [132].

Alcohol

Alcohol in the form of ethanol that is probably the most common recreational drug in the world [133]. It is estimated that approximately 90% of people consume it at some stage [134]. Alcohol consumption in moderation can have beneficial effects [135, 136]. Problems arise when it is abused. Alcohol use disorder (AUD) is one of the most common psychiatric disorders in first world countries and affects millions around the globe [137, 138]. It is estimated that AUD accounts for 4% of the global disease burden [139]. In the United States, 36% of the male and 23% of the female population met Diagnostic and Statistical Manual of Mental Disorders (DSM5) criteria for AUD at least once during their lifetime [140].

The consideration of alcohol as an addictive drug is more complicated than the consideration of other addictive substances because alcohol (ethanol) is also a source of calories through its metabolism, and can be considered a food [141]. The subject of alcohol metabolism by brain remains controversial to this day [142]. However, many years of investigation to elucidate the molecular site of ethanol action in the CNS has shed some light into the mystery. Ethanol interacts with certain protein subunits of the γ-aminobutyric acid (GABA-A) receptor and the glutamate neurotransmitter systems (N-methyl-D-aspartate—NMDA receptors). These are currently considered the primary pathways for ethanol-induced intoxication as well as the addicting effects. Similarities between the behavioral effects of benzodiazepines, which are known to act through sites on GABA-A receptors, and ethanol's actions are quite obvious (reduce anxiety, produce sedation, anticonvulsant actions, and produce tolerance/addiction) [142]. In animals, a relatively large body of the literature demonstrates that acute ethanol, at concentrations associated with intoxication, potentiates GABA-A receptor function and GABA release [143, 144] while inhibiting glutamate NMDA receptors [145, 146].

Overall, the effects of AUD in the brain can be classified as indirect (mediated by nutritional deficits or electrolytes imbalances) or direct effects (toxic effects). From the indirect effects, Wernicke encephalopathy (WE) is one of the most common pathologies affecting the brain of chronic alcohol users. It is due to thiamine (vitamin B1) deficiency. The classic triad of WE includes ataxia, global confusion, and ophthalmoplegia. On MRI, WE typically affects medial thalami, mamillary bodies, the tectal plate, and periaqueductal gray matter in a symmetric fashion [147] (see Fig. 44.9). Marchiafava-Bignami disease (MBD) is a rare entity characterized by acute demyelination of the corpus callosum, also associated with alcohol abuse. On MRI, patients with MBD show areas of high signal intensity on T2 images in the body of the corpus callosum, genu, splenium, and adjacent WM [148]. During the acute phase, the lesions may show peripheral contrast enhancement. As the disease progresses, residual atrophy of the involved structure is usually observed. Osmotic demyelination syndromes are seen in the setting of altered plasma osmolarity that is associated with alcohol abuse. The syndromes can present in the way of central pontine (CPM) or extrapontine myelinolysis (EPM). In acute CPM, MRI shows signal alteration in the central pons with sparing of the tegmentum, ventrolateral pons, and corticospinal tracts [149]. In EPM, symmetric signal alterations can be seen in the basal ganglia, thalami, lateral geniculate body, cerebellum, and cerebral cortex [150].

Direct brain damage produced by excessive consumption of alcohol has been well documented, primarily as regional brain atrophy in both gray matter and WM structures. The production of toxic ethanol metabolites and damage of cellular proteins is one of the proposed mechanisms for neuronal damage [151–153]. The first toxic metabolite of ethanol, acetaldehyde, can form adducts with the e-amino group of lysine residues. These covalent modifications can disrupt the function of proteins resulting in cellular injury [154]. One of the major targets of acetaldehyde-mediated adduction is a-tubulin, which can influence microtubule polymerization [155]. Although the nature of alcohol-related WM loss has not yet been elucidated, it is likely that the disruption involves changes in both myelination and axonal integrity [156, 157]. Nevertheless, there is evidence in animals (ethanol-fed rats) that acetaldehyde-protein adducts are present within the WM, frontal cortex, midbrain, dentate gyrus, and cerebellum. The same adducts are present in the frontal cortex and midbrain of an alcoholic [153].

Alcoholics have a reduced brain weight compared to controls and the degree of brain atrophy has been shown to correlate with the rate and amount of alcohol consumed over a lifetime [158]. Neuronal loss has been documented in specific regions of the cerebral cortex (superior frontal association cortex), hypothalamus, and cerebellum in alcoholics [159]. Atrophy of the cerebellum is commonly associated with alcoholism. Imaging [160] and examination of the cerebellum at autopsy reveal shrinkage of the anterior superior cerebellar vermis (see Fig. 44.10). Quantitative pathological studies have shown that there is a loss of Purkinje cells in the vermis (reduced on average by 43%) that correlates with clinical ataxia/unsteadiness [159]. These are permanent changes reported in the brain and cerebellum. However, some longitudinal structural MRI studies demonstrate that some morphologi-

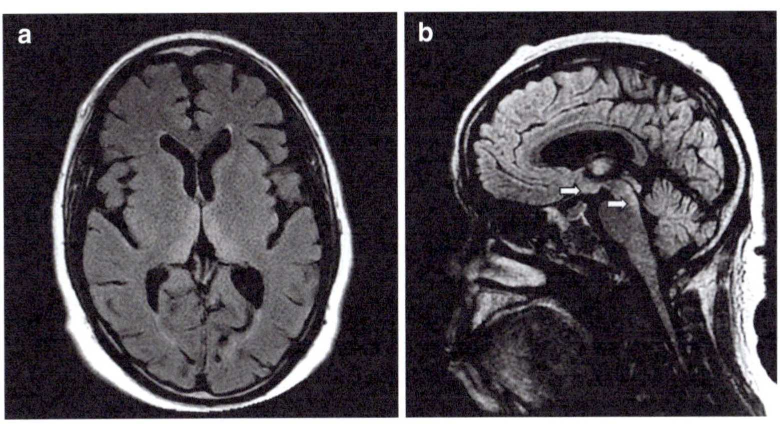

Fig. 44.9 Wernicke's encephalopathy. Abnormal signal is seen in a symmetric way in (**a**) the medial thalamic regions and also (**b**) (arrows) in the periaqueductal gray matter and mammillary bodies

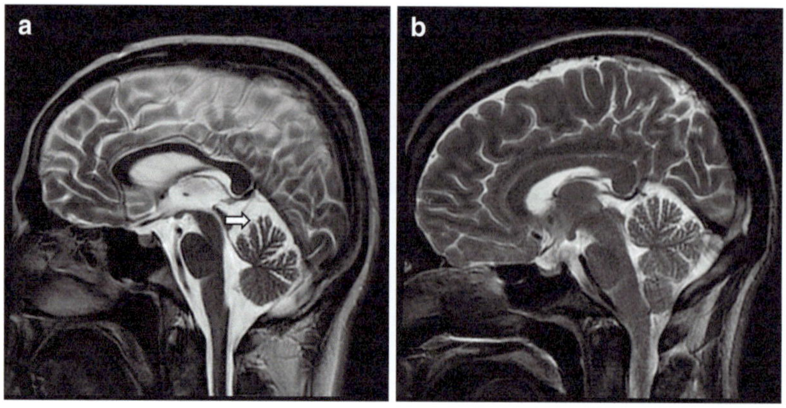

Fig. 44.10 Cerebellar atrophy associated with alcohol abuse. Compare the volume loss of the superior vermis on (**a**) (arrow) with the appearance of a control subject on (**b**)

cal changes are reversible upon discontinuation of alcohol consumption [138]. After periods of abstinence, previously enlarged ventricles decrease in size [161] and a number of brain areas increase in volume including the temporal, insular, and anterior cingulate cortices; amygdala, thalamus, hippocampus, brainstem, and cerebellar cortex [162–164]. Thus, alcoholic brain pathology may have two components, one reflecting permanent change and the other transient change.

Many other specific regions of the brain of uncomplicated alcoholics have shown reduced volume on MRI in comparison with control subjects, for example, frontal cortex, thalamus, mammillary bodies, corpus callosum, and pons [165–168]. Basal ganglia structures are affected and include the caudate, putamen, amygdala, and nucleus accumbens [169, 170]. Such changes of the basal ganglia may contribute to the gradual progression of AUD, as these structures are involved in habit formation and reward evaluation. It is interesting to notice that some of the specific regional changes in volume are not only affected in uncomplicated alcoholism but also in patients with known pathologic entities such as WE or MBD, which suggest that these entities might occur on a continuum during the dynamic course of alcoholism [138].

Diffusion tensor imaging can detect WM abnormalities in alcoholics without quantifiable WM volume loss [171]. Significant abnormalities (reduced fractional anisotropy and increased mean diffusivity) have been detected in the corpus callosum, frontal forceps, internal and external capsules, fornix, superior cingulate, and longitudinal fasciculi of alcoholics relative to control group [172]. Quantitative diffusion tensor imaging investigations have reported microstructural compromise of WM tracts between midbrain and pons, and in fronto-limbic, fronto-parietal, and fronto-occipital fiber tracts [173, 174]. Moreover, WM deficits may be more pronounced in alcoholic women, despite a lower quantity of lifetime alcohol consumed [175, 176]. As with other modalities, diffusion tensor imaging studies support brain recovery with abstinence.

Functional MRI has also been used in the investigation of AUD. For example, many studies have shown an alcohol cue induced attentional bias in alcoholics compared to control group [177, 178]. However, fMRI investigations have linked visual alcohol cues to a hemodynamic response in the brain regions related to the reward circuitry including the anterior cingulate cortex, medial prefrontal cortex, ventral striatum, and insula [179]. Other studies have shown functional changes in brain areas related to self-control, memory, and reflective thinking [180], indicating significant changes in the decision-making circuitry. During resting-state fMRI, uncomplicated alcoholics change the DMN from connectivity between posterior cingulate cortex and middle cingulate cortex (MCC) toward increased connectivity between midbrain and MCC. These results indicate a compromised executive control [181].

Conclusions

Imaging plays a significant role in the acute and chronic evaluation of neurologic complications in drug abuse patients. Moreover, advanced imaging techniques have a preeminent role in the current understanding of the neurobiology involved in drug abuse. There is a consistent pattern in functional imaging studies with disruption of connectivity and impaired function in areas related to reward circuitry, decision-making, and self-control. For instance, the prefrontal cortex, specifically the orbitofrontal cortex, appears consistently abnormal regardless of the drug of abuse. There is also evidence by imaging that changes in volume can precede a pattern of abuse in some patients, favoring a predisposition in certain individuals and strengthening the role of genetics. Imaging also demonstrates that some structural changes in the brain are reversible after periods of abstinence, giving an important role to neural plasticity.

References

1. World Drug Report 2020—Booklet 2. United Nations publication, Sales No. E.20.XI.6. Available from: https://wdr.unodc.org/wdr2020/field/WDR20_Booklet_2.pdf
2. World Drugs Report. United Nations Office on drugs and crime (UNODC). Vienna: United Nations Publications; 2018.
3. European Drug Report. Trends and developments. Luxembourg: Publications Office of the European Union: European Monitoring Centre for Drugs and Drug Addiction (EMCDDA); 2018.
4. Bloomfield MAP, Hindocha C, Green SF, Wall MB, Lees R, Petrilli K, et al. The neuropsychopharmacology of cannabis: a review of human imaging studies. Pharmacol Therap. 2019;195:132–61. Epub 2018/10/23. PubMed PMID: 30347211; PubMed Central PMCID: PMCPMC6416743. https://doi.org/10.1016/j.pharmthera.2018.10.006.
5. Cohen K, Weizman A, Weinstein A. Modulatory effects of cannabinoids on brain neurotransmission. Eur J Neurosci. 2019;50(3):2322–45. Epub 2019/03/19. https://doi.org/10.1111/ejn.14407.
6. Herkenham M, Lynn AB, Johnson MR, Melvin LS, de Costa BR, Rice KC. Characterization and localization of cannabinoid receptors in rat brain: a quantitative in vitro autoradiographic study. J Neurosci. 1991;11(2):563–83. Epub 1991/02/01. PubMed PMID: 1992016; PubMed Central PMCID: PMCPMC6575215. https://doi.org/10.1523/jneurosci.11-02-00563.1991.
7. Archie SR, Cucullo L. Harmful effects of smoking cannabis: a cerebrovascular and neurological perspective. Front Pharmacol. 2019;10:1481. Epub 2020/01/11. PubMed PMID: 31920665; PubMed Central PMCID: PMCPMC6915047. https://doi.org/10.3389/fphar.2019.01481.
8. Wolff V, Jouanjus E. Strokes are possible complications of cannabinoids use. Epilepsy Behav. 2017;70(Pt B):355–63. Epub 2017/02/27. https://doi.org/10.1016/j.yebeh.2017.01.031.
9. American Psychiatric Association. Diagnostic and statistical manual of mental disorders. 5th ed; 2013.
10. Ferland JN, Hurd YL. Deconstructing the neurobiology of cannabis use disorder. Nat Neurosci. 2020;23(5):600–10. Epub 2020/04/07. https://doi.org/10.1038/s41593-020-0611-0.
11. Mathew RJ, Wilson WH, Turkington TG, Hawk TC, Coleman RE, DeGrado TR, et al. Time course of tetrahydrocannabinol-induced changes in regional cerebral blood flow measured with positron emission tomography. Psychiatry Res. 2002;116(3):173–85. Epub 2002/12/13. https://doi.org/10.1016/s0925-4927(02)00069-0.
12. O'Leary DS, Block RI, Koeppel JA, Schultz SK, Magnotta VA, Ponto LB, et al. Effects of smoking marijuana on focal attention and brain blood flow. Hum Psychopharmacol. 2007;22(3):135–48. Epub 2007/04/03. https://doi.org/10.1002/hup.832.
13. van Hell HH, Bossong MG, Jager G, Kristo G, van Osch MJ, Zelaya F, et al. Evidence for involvement of the insula in the psychotropic effects of THC in humans: a double-blind, randomized pharmacological MRI study. Int J Neuropsychopharmacol. 2011;14(10):1377–88. Epub 2011/04/15. https://doi.org/10.1017/s1461145711000526.
14. Volkow ND, Gillespie H, Mullani N, Tancredi L, Grant C, Valentine A, et al. Brain glucose metabolism in chronic marijuana users at baseline and during marijuana intoxication. Psychiatry Res. 1996;67(1):29–38. Epub 1996/05/31. https://doi.org/10.1016/0925-4927(96)02817-x.
15. Battistella G, Fornari E, Annoni JM, Chtioui H, Dao K, Fabritius M, et al. Long-term effects of cannabis on brain structure. Neuropsychopharmacology. 2014;39(9):2041–8. Epub 2014/03/19. PubMed PMID: 24633558; PubMed Central PMCID: PMCPMC4104335. https://doi.org/10.1038/npp.2014.67.
16. Chye Y, Solowij N, Suo C, Batalla A, Cousijn J, Goudriaan AE, et al. Orbitofrontal and caudate volumes in cannabis users: a multi-site mega-analysis comparing dependent versus non-dependent users. Psychopharmacology. 2017;234(13):1985–95. Epub 2017/04/02. https://doi.org/10.1007/s00213-017-4606-9.
17. Cousijn J, Wiers RW, Ridderinkhof KR, van den Brink W, Veltman DJ, Goudriaan AE. Grey matter

alterations associated with cannabis use: results of a VBM study in heavy cannabis users and healthy controls. NeuroImage. 2012;59(4):3845–51. Epub 2011/10/11. https://doi.org/10.1016/j.neuroimage.2011.09.046.
18. Arnone D, Barrick TR, Chengappa S, Mackay CE, Clark CA, Abou-Saleh MT. Corpus callosum damage in heavy marijuana use: preliminary evidence from diffusion tensor tractography and tract-based spatial statistics. NeuroImage. 2008;41(3):1067–74. Epub 2008/04/22. https://doi.org/10.1016/j.neuroimage.2008.02.064.
19. Zalesky A, Solowij N, Yücel M, Lubman DI, Takagi M, Harding IH, et al. Effect of long-term cannabis use on axonal fibre connectivity. Brain: J Neurol. 2012;135(Pt 7):2245–55. Epub 2012/06/07. https://doi.org/10.1093/brain/aws136.
20. Filbey FM, Aslan S, Calhoun VD, Spence JS, Damaraju E, Caprihan A, et al. Long-term effects of marijuana use on the brain. Proc Natl Acad Sci U S A. 2014;111(47):16913–8. Epub 2014/11/12. PubMed PMID: 25385625; PubMed Central PMCID: PMCPMC4250161. https://doi.org/10.1073/pnas.1415297111.
21. Becker MP, Collins PF, Lim KO, Muetzel RL, Luciana M. Longitudinal changes in white matter microstructure after heavy cannabis use. Dev Cogn Neurosci. 2015;16:23–35. Epub 2015/11/26. PubMed PMID: 26602958; PubMed Central PMCID: PMCPMC4691379. https://doi.org/10.1016/j.dcn.2015.10.004.
22. Epstein KA, Kumra S. White matter fractional anisotropy over two time points in early onset schizophrenia and adolescent cannabis use disorder: a naturalistic diffusion tensor imaging study. Psychiatry Res. 2015;232(1):34–41. Epub 2015/03/18. https://doi.org/10.1016/j.pscychresns.2014.10.010.
23. Pujol J, Blanco-Hinojo L, Batalla A, López-Solà M, Harrison BJ, Soriano-Mas C, et al. Functional connectivity alterations in brain networks relevant to self-awareness in chronic cannabis users. J Psychiatr Res. 2014;51:68–78. Epub 2014/01/15. https://doi.org/10.1016/j.jpsychires.2013.12.008.
24. Wetherill RR, Fang Z, Jagannathan K, Childress AR, Rao H, Franklin TR. Cannabis, cigarettes, and their co-occurring use: disentangling differences in default mode network functional connectivity. Drug Alcohol Depend. 2015;153:116–23. Epub 2015/06/22. PubMed PMID: 26094186; PubMed Central PMCID: PMCPMC4509835. https://doi.org/10.1016/j.drugalcdep.2015.05.046.
25. Bolla KI, Eldreth DA, Matochik JA, Cadet JL. Neural substrates of faulty decision-making in abstinent marijuana users. NeuroImage. 2005;26(2):480–92. Epub 2005/05/24. https://doi.org/10.1016/j.neuroimage.2005.02.012.
26. Tervo-Clemmens B, Simmonds D, Calabro FJ, Day NL, Richardson GA, Luna B. Adolescent cannabis use and brain systems supporting adult working memory encoding, maintenance, and retrieval. NeuroImage. 2018;169:496–509. Epub 2017/12/19. PubMed PMID: 29253654; PubMed Central PMCID: PMCPMC6537905. https://doi.org/10.1016/j.neuroimage.2017.12.041.
27. Colizzi M, Fazio L, Ferranti L, Porcelli A, Masellis R, Marvulli D, et al. Functional genetic variation of the cannabinoid receptor 1 and cannabis use interact on prefrontal connectivity and related working memory behavior. Neuropsychopharmacology. 2015;40(3):640–9. https://doi.org/10.1038/npp.2014.213. Epub 2014/08/21. PubMed PMID: 25139064; PubMed Central PMCID: PMCPMC4289952
28. Karch SB, Drummer OH. Chapter 5. Opiates and opioids. In: Karch's pathology of drug abuse. 5th ed. Boca Raton: CRC Press; 2016.
29. Büttner A. The neuropathology of drug abuse. Curr Opin Behav Sci. 2017;13:8–12.
30. Bates DDB, Gallagher K, Yu H, Uyeda J, Murakami AM, Setty BN, et al. Acute radiologic manifestations of America's opioid epidemic. Radiographics. 2018;38(1):109–23. Epub 2018/01/11. https://doi.org/10.1148/rg.2018170114.
31. Trescot AM, Datta S, Lee M, Hansen H. Opioid pharmacology. Pain Physician. 2008;11(2 Suppl):S133–53. Epub 2008/06/17
32. Geibprasert S, Gallucci M, Krings T. Addictive illegal drugs: structural neuroimaging. Am J Neuroradiol. 2010;31(5):803–8.
33. Herz A, Millan MJ. Opioids and opioid receptors mediating antinociception at various levels of the neuraxis. Physiol Bohemoslov. 1990;39(5):395–401. Epub 1990/01/01
34. Büttner A, Mall G, Penning R, Weis S. The neuropathology of heroin abuse. Forensic Sci Int. 2000;113(1-3):435–42. Epub 2000/09/09. https://doi.org/10.1016/s0379-0738(00)00204-8.
35. Büttner A. Review: the neuropathology of drug abuse. Neuropathol Appl Neurobiol. 2011;37(2):118–34. Epub 2010/10/16. https://doi.org/10.1111/j.1365-2990.2010.01131.x.
36. Gruber SA, Silveri MM, Yurgelun-Todd DA. Neuropsychological consequences of opiate use. Neuropsychol Rev. 2007;17(3):299–315. Epub 2007/08/11. https://doi.org/10.1007/s11065-007-9041-y.
37. Cadet JL, Bisagno V, Milroy CM. Neuropathology of substance use disorders. Acta Neuropathol. 2014;127(1):91–107. https://doi.org/10.1007/s00401-013-1221-7. Epub 2013/12/03. PubMed PMID: 24292887; PubMed Central PMCID: PMCPMC7453825
38. Brust JC, Richter RW. Stroke associated with addiction to heroin. J Neurol Neurosurg Psychiatry. 1976;39(2):194–9. https://doi.org/10.1136/jnnp.39.2.194. Epub 1976/02/01. PubMed PMID: 1262894; PubMed Central PMCID: PMCPMC492246
39. Andersen SN, Skullerud K. Hypoxic/ischaemic brain damage, especially pallidal lesions, in heroin

addicts. Forensic Sci Int. 1999;102(1):51–9. Epub 1999/07/29. https://doi.org/10.1016/s0379-0738(99)00040-7.
40. Weis S, Büttner A. Neurotoxicology and drug-related disorders. Handb Clin Neurol. 2017;145:181–92. Epub 2017/10/11. https://doi.org/10.1016/b978-0-12-802395-2.00014-6.
41. Cheng MY, Chin SC, Chang YC, Wu T, Lim SN, Hsieh HY, et al. Different routes of heroin intake cause various heroin-induced leukoencephalopathies. J Neurol. 2019;266(2):316–29. Epub 2018/11/28. https://doi.org/10.1007/s00415-018-9131-1.
42. Wolters EC, van Wijngaarden GK, Stam FC, Rengelink H, Lousberg RJ, Schipper ME, et al. Leucoencephalopathy after inhaling "heroin" pyrolysate. Lancet (London, England). 1982;2(8310):1233–7. Epub 1982/12/04. https://doi.org/10.1016/s0140-6736(82)90101-5.
43. Barash JA, Kofke WA. Connecting the dots: an association between opioids and acute hippocampal injury. Neurocase. 2018;24(2):124–31. Epub 2018/05/19. https://doi.org/10.1080/13554794.2018.1475572.
44. Kofke WA, Garman RH, Stiller RL, Rose ME, Garman R. Opioid neurotoxicity: fentanyl dose-response effects in rats. Anesth Analg. 1996;83(6):1298–306. Epub 1996/12/01. https://doi.org/10.1097/00000539-199612000-00029.
45. Brown GG, Jacobus J, McKenna B. Structural imaging for addiction medicine: From neurostructure to neuroplasticity. Progr Brain Res. 2016;224:105–27. Epub 2016/01/30. PubMed PMID: 26822356; PubMed Central PMCID: PMCPMC4856004. https://doi.org/10.1016/bs.pbr.2015.07.029.
46. Lyoo IK, Pollack MH, Silveri MM, Ahn KH, Diaz CI, Hwang J, et al. Prefrontal and temporal gray matter density decreases in opiate dependence. Psychopharmacology. 2006;184(2):139–44. Epub 2005/12/22. https://doi.org/10.1007/s00213-005-0198-x.
47. Yuan Y, Zhu Z, Shi J, Zou Z, Yuan F, Liu Y, et al. Gray matter density negatively correlates with duration of heroin use in young lifetime heroin-dependent individuals. Brain Cogn. 2009;71(3):223–8. Epub 2009/09/25. https://doi.org/10.1016/j.bandc.2009.08.014.
48. Liao D, Grigoriants OO, Wang W, Wiens K, Loh HH, Law PY. Distinct effects of individual opioids on the morphology of spines depend upon the internalization of mu opioid receptors. Mol Cell Neurosci. 2007;35(3):456–69. Epub 2007/05/22. PubMed PMID: 17513124; PubMed Central PMCID: PMCPMC1931568. https://doi.org/10.1016/j.mcn.2007.04.007.
49. Daglish MR, Weinstein A, Malizia AL, Wilson S, Melichar JK, Britten S, et al. Changes in regional cerebral blood flow elicited by craving memories in abstinent opiate-dependent subjects. Am J Psychiatry. 2001;158(10):1680–6. Epub 2001/10/02. https://doi.org/10.1176/appi.ajp.158.10.1680.
50. Seifert CL, Magon S, Sprenger T, Lang UE, Huber CG, Denier N, et al. Reduced volume of the nucleus accumbens in heroin addiction. Eur Arch Psychiatry Clin Neurosci. 2015;265(8):637–45. Epub 2014/12/04. https://doi.org/10.1007/s00406-014-0564-y.
51. Upadhyay J, Maleki N, Potter J, Elman I, Rudrauf D, Knudsen J, et al. Alterations in brain structure and functional connectivity in prescription opioid-dependent patients. Brain J Neurol. 2010;133(Pt 7):2098–114. Epub 2010/06/19. PubMed PMID: 20558415; PubMed Central PMCID: PMCPMC2912691. https://doi.org/10.1093/brain/awq138.
52. Qiu Y, Jiang G, Su H, Lv X, Zhang X, Tian J, et al. Progressive white matter microstructure damage in male chronic heroin dependent individuals: a DTI and TBSS study. PloS One. 2013;8(5):e63212. Epub 2013/05/08. PubMed PMID: 23650554; PubMed Central PMCID: PMCPMC3641135. https://doi.org/10.1371/journal.pone.0063212.
53. Bora E, Yücel M, Fornito A, Pantelis C, Harrison BJ, Cocchi L, et al. White matter microstructure in opiate addiction. Addict Biol. 2012;17(1):141–8. Epub 2010/11/13. https://doi.org/10.1111/j.1369-1600.2010.00266.x.
54. Liu H, Li L, Hao Y, Cao D, Xu L, Rohrbaugh R, et al. Disrupted white matter integrity in heroin dependence: a controlled study utilizing diffusion tensor imaging. Am J Drug Alcohol Abuse. 2008;34(5):562–75. Epub 2008/08/23. https://doi.org/10.1080/00952990802295238.
55. Pirastu R, Fais R, Messina M, Bini V, Spiga S, Falconieri D, et al. Impaired decision-making in opiate-dependent subjects: effect of pharmacological therapies. Drug Alcohol Depend. 2006;83(2):163–8. Epub 2005/12/14. https://doi.org/10.1016/j.drugalcdep.2005.11.008.
56. Kirby KN, Petry NM, Bickel WK. Heroin addicts have higher discount rates for delayed rewards than non-drug-using controls. J Exp Psychol Gen. 1999;128(1):78–87. Epub 1999/04/01. https://doi.org/10.1037//0096-3445.128.1.78
57. Madden GJ, Petry NM, Badger GJ, Bickel WK. Impulsive and self-control choices in opioid-dependent patients and non-drug-using control participants: drug and monetary rewards. Exp Clin Psychopharmacol. 1997;5(3):256–62. Epub 1997/08/01. https://doi.org/10.1037//1064-1297.5.3.256
58. Ma X, Qiu Y, Tian J, Wang J, Li S, Zhan W, et al. Aberrant default-mode functional and structural connectivity in heroin-dependent individuals. PloS One. 2015;10(4):e0120861. Epub 2015/04/11. PubMed PMID: 25859661; PubMed Central PMCID: PMCPMC4393019. https://doi.org/10.1371/journal.pone.0120861.
59. Wang L, Zou F, Zhai T, Lei Y, Tan S, Jin X, et al. Abnormal gray matter volume and resting-state functional connectivity in former heroin-dependent

individuals abstinent for multiple years. Addict Biol. 2016;21(3):646–56. Epub 2015/03/03. https://doi.org/10.1111/adb.12228.
60. Fareed A, Kim J, Ketchen B, Kwak WJ, Wang D, Shongo-Hiango H, et al. Effect of heroin use on changes of brain functions as measured by functional magnetic resonance imaging, a systematic review. J Addict Dis. 2017;36(2):105–16. Epub 2017/01/18. https://doi.org/10.1080/10550887.2017.1280898.
61. Liu J, Liang J, Qin W, Tian J, Yuan K, Bai L, et al. Dysfunctional connectivity patterns in chronic heroin users: an fMRI study. Neurosci Lett. 2009;460(1):72–7. Epub 2009/05/20. https://doi.org/10.1016/j.neulet.2009.05.038.
62. Ma N, Liu Y, Li N, Wang CX, Zhang H, Jiang XF, et al. Addiction related alteration in resting-state brain connectivity. NeuroImage. 2010;49(1):738–44. Epub 2009/08/26. PubMed PMID: 19703568; PubMed Central PMCID: PMCPMC2764798. https://doi.org/10.1016/j.neuroimage.2009.08.037.
63. Brown E, Prager J, Lee H, Ramsey R. CNS complications of cocaine abuse: prevalence, pathophysiology, and neuroradiology. AJR Am J Roentgenol. 1992;159(1):137–47.
64. Rothman RB, Baumann MH, Dersch CM, Romero DV, Rice KC, Carroll FI, et al. Amphetamine-type central nervous system stimulants release norepinephrine more potently than they release dopamine and serotonin. Synapse. 2001;39(1):32–41.
65. Howell LL, Kimmel HL. Monoamine transporters and psychostimulant addiction. Biochem Pharmacol. 2008;75(1):196–217.
66. Dackis CA, Dackis MAP, Martin D, Pottash A, Gold MS. Platelet serotonin transporter in cocaine patients. Problems Drug Depend. 1985;46:164.
67. Anthony JC, Warner LA, Kessler RC. Comparative epidemiology of dependence on tobacco, alcohol, controlled substances, and inhalants: basic findings from the National Comorbidity Survey. 1997.
68. Afonso L, Mohammad T, Thatai D. Crack whips the heart: a review of the cardiovascular toxicity of cocaine. Am J Cardiol. 2007;100(6):1040–3.
69. Neiman J, Haapaniemi H, Hillbom M. Neurological complications of drug abuse: pathophysiological mechanisms. Eur J Neurol. 2000;7(6):595–606.
70. Abdilla Y, Cauchi M, Vella N. Cocaine-induced toxic leucoencephalopathy with complete clinical recovery. BMJ Case Rep CP. 2019;12(7):e229134.
71. Mader EC Jr, Ramos AB, Cruz RA, Branch LA. Full recovery from cocaine-induced toxic leukoencephalopathy: emphasizing the role of neuroinflammation and brain edema. J Investig Med High Impact Case Rep. 2019;7:2324709619868266.
72. Petitti DB, Sidney S, Quesenberry C, Bernstein A. Stroke and cocaine or amphetamine use. Epidemiology. 1998:596–600.
73. Brust JC. Acute neurologic complications of drug and alcohol abuse. Neurol Clin. 1998;16(2):503–19.
74. Rojas R, Riascos R, Vargas D, Cuellar H, Borne J. Neuroimaging in drug and substance abuse part I: cocaine, cannabis, and ecstasy. Top Magn Reson Imaging. 2005;16(3):231–8.
75. Levine SR, Brust JC, Futrell N, Ho K-L, Blake D, Millikan CH, et al. Cerebrovascular complications of the use of the crack form of alkaloidal cocaine. N Engl J Med. 1990;323(11):699–704.
76. Martin-Schild S, Albright KC, Hallevi H, Barreto AD, Philip M, Misra V, et al. Intracerebral hemorrhage in cocaine users. Stroke. 2010;41(4):680–4.
77. Fessler RD, Esshaki CM, Stankewitz RC, Johnson RR, Diaz FG. The neurovascular complications of cocaine. Surg Neurol. 1997;4(47):339–45.
78. Kaufman MJ, Levin JM, Ross MH, Lange N, Rose SL, Kukes TJ, et al. Cocaine-induced cerebral vasoconstriction detected in humans with magnetic resonance angiography. JAMA. 1998;279(5):376–80.
79. Levine S, Brust J, Futrell N, Brass L, Blake D, Fayad P, et al. A comparative study of the cerebrovascular complications of cocaine: alkaloidal versus hydrochloride—a review. Neurology. 1991;41(8):1173.
80. Unger MD, Georges J, Shaikh HA, Kavi T. Moyamoya tipping point: fatal bilateral MCA territory infarction following cocaine abuse. Case Rep. 2018:bcr-2017-222883.
81. Storen EC, Wijdicks EF, Crum BA, Schultz G. Moyamoya-like vasculopathy from cocaine dependency. Am J Neuroradiol. 2000;21(6):1008–10.
82. Daras M, Tuchman A, Koppel B, Samkoff L, Weitzner I, Marc J. Neurovascular complications of cocaine. Acta Neurol Scand. 1994;90(2):124–9.
83. Boghdadi MS, Henning RJ. Cocaine: pathophysiology and clinical toxicology. Heart Lung. 1997;26(6):466–83.
84. Little KY, Ramssen E, Welchko R, Volberg V, Roland CJ, Cassin B. Decreased brain dopamine cell numbers in human cocaine users. Psychiatry Res. 2009;168(3):173–80.
85. Franklin TR, Acton PD, Maldjian JA, Gray JD, Croft JR, Dackis CA, et al. Decreased gray matter concentration in the insular, orbitofrontal, cingulate, and temporal cortices of cocaine patients. Biol Psychiatry. 2002;51(2):134–42.
86. Volkow ND, Fowler JS, Wolf AP, Hitzemann R, Dewey S, Bendriem B, et al. Changes in brain glucose metabolism in cocaine dependence and withdrawal. Am J Psychiatry. 1991;148(5):621–6.
87. Adinoff B, Devous MD Sr, Cooper DB, Best SE, Chandler P, Harris T, et al. Resting regional cerebral blood flow and gambling task performance in cocaine-dependent subjects and healthy comparison subjects. Am J Psychiatry. 2003;160(10):1892–4.
88. Proebstl L, Kamp F, Manz K, Krause D, Adorjan K, Pogarell O, et al. Effects of stimulant drug use on the dopaminergic system: a systematic review and meta-analysis of in vivo neuroimaging studies. Eur Psychiatry. 2019;59:15–24.
89. Mackey S, Allgaier N, Chaarani B, Spechler P, Orr C, Bunn J, et al. Mega-analysis of gray mat-

ter volume in substance dependence: general and substance-specific regional effects. Am J Psychiatry. 2019;176(2):119–28.

90. Frazer KM, Richards Q, Keith DR. The long-term effects of cocaine use on cognitive functioning: a systematic critical review. Behav Brain Res. 2018;348:241–62.
91. Kaag A, Schulte M, Jansen J, Van Wingen G, Homberg J, van den Brink W, et al. The relation between gray matter volume and the use of alcohol, tobacco, cocaine and cannabis in male polysubstance users. Drug Alcohol Depend. 2018;187:186–94.
92. Kearney-Ramos TE, Dowdle LT, Lench DH, Mithoefer OJ, Devries WH, George MS, et al. Transdiagnostic effects of ventromedial prefrontal cortex transcranial magnetic stimulation on cue reactivity. Biol Psychiatry Cogn Neurosci Neuroimag. 2018;3(7):599–609.
93. Goldstein RZ, Volkow ND. Drug addiction and its underlying neurobiological basis: neuroimaging evidence for the involvement of the frontal cortex. Am J Psychiatry. 2002;159(10):1642–52.
94. Robinson TE, Gorny G, Mitton E, Kolb B. Cocaine self-administration alters the morphology of dendrites and dendritic spines in the nucleus accumbens and neocortex. Synapse. 2001;39(3):257–66.
95. Volkow ND, Mullani N, Gould KL, Adler S, Krajewski K. Cerebral blood flow in chronic cocaine users: a study with positron emission tomography. Br J Psychiatry. 1988;152:641–8.
96. Volkow ND, Wang G-J, Fowler JS, Hitzemann R, Angrist B, Gatley SJ, et al. Association of methylphenidate-induced craving with changes in right striato-orbitofrontal metabolism in cocaine abusers: implications in addiction. Am J Psychiatry. 1999;156(1):19–26.
97. Volkow ND, Hitzemann R, Wang GJ, Fowler JS, Wolf AP, Dewey SL, et al. Long-term frontal brain metabolic changes in cocaine abusers. Synapse. 1992;11(3):184–90.
98. Montoya-Filardi A, Mazón M. The addicted brain: imaging neurological complications of recreational drug abuse. Radiología (English Edition). 2017;59(1):17–30.
99. Korponay C, Kosson DS, Decety J, Kiehl KA, Koenigs M. Brain volume correlates with duration of abstinence from substance abuse in a region-specific and substance-specific manner. Biol Psychiatry Cogn Neurosci Neuroimag. 2017;2(7):626–35.
100. Martins DLN, Valiatti TDS, D'Ávila J, Ferreira LF, Batista EK, Bazán PR, et al. Extrinsic functional connectivity of the default mode network in crack-cocaine users. Radiologia Brasileira. 2018;ahead:0.
101. Zhang S, Li C-SR. Ventral striatal dysfunction in cocaine dependence–difference mapping for subregional resting state functional connectivity. Transl Psychiatry. 2018;8(1):1–11.
102. Orsini CA, Colon-Perez LM, Heshmati SC, Setlow B, Febo M. Functional connectivity of chronic cocaine use reveals progressive neuroadaptations in neocortical, striatal, and limbic networks. eNeuro. 2018;5(4):ENEURO.0081-18.2018. https://doi.org/10.1523/ENEURO.0081-18.2018.
103. Adisetiyo V, McGill CE, DeVries WH, Jensen JH, Hanlon CA, Helpern JA. Elevated brain iron in cocaine use disorder as indexed by magnetic field correlation imaging. Biol Psychiatry Cogn Neurosci Neuroimag. 2019;4(6):579–88. Epub 2018/12/26. https://doi.org/10.1016/j.bpsc.2018.11.006.
104. Narayana PA, Ahobila-Vajjula P, Ramu J, Herrera J, Steinberg JL, Moeller FG. Diffusion tensor imaging of cocaine-treated rodents. Psychiatry Res. 2009;171(3):242–51. Epub 2009/02/17. PubMed PMID: 19217266; PubMed Central PMCID: PMCPMC2677684. https://doi.org/10.1016/j.pscychresns.2008.04.004.
105. Kaag AM, van Wingen GA, Caan MWA, Homberg JR, van den Brink W, Reneman L. White matter alterations in cocaine users are negatively related to the number of additionally (ab)used substances. Addict Biol. 2017;22(4):1048–56. Epub 2016/02/11. https://doi.org/10.1111/adb.12375.
106. Beard CL, Schmitz JM, Soder HE, Suchting R, Yoon JH, Hasan KM, et al. Regional differences in white matter integrity in stimulant use disorders: a meta-analysis of diffusion tensor imaging studies. Drug Alcohol Depend. 2019;201:29–37. Epub 2019/06/09. PubMed PMID: 31176066; PubMed Central PMCID: PMCPMC6660908. https://doi.org/10.1016/j.drugalcdep.2019.03.023.
107. Koob GF, Le Moal M. Review. Neurobiological mechanisms for opponent motivational processes in addiction. Philos Trans R Soc London Ser B Biol Sci. 2008, 363;(1507):3113–23. Epub 2008/07/26. PubMed PMID: 18653439; PubMed Central PMCID: PMCPMC2607326. https://doi.org/10.1098/rstb.2008.0094.
108. Makris N, Gasic GP, Seidman LJ, Goldstein JM, Gastfriend DR, Elman I, et al. Decreased absolute amygdala volume in cocaine addicts. Neuron. 2004;44(4):729–40. Epub 2004/11/16. https://doi.org/10.1016/j.neuron.2004.10.027.
109. Mei S, Xu J, Carroll KM, Potenza MN. Self-reported impulsivity is negatively correlated with amygdalar volumes in cocaine dependence. Psychiatry Res. 2015;233(2):212–7. https://doi.org/10.1016/j.pscychresns.2015.07.013. Epub 2015/07/19. PubMed PMID: 26187551; PubMed Central PMCID: PMCPMC4536101
110. Worhunsky PD, Potenza MN, Rogers RD. Alterations in functional brain networks associated with loss-chasing in gambling disorder and cocaine-use disorder. Drug Alcohol Depend. 2017;178:363–71. Epub 2017/07/12. PubMed PMID: 28697386; PubMed Central PMCID: PMCPMC5551408. https://doi.org/10.1016/j.drugalcdep.2017.05.025.
111. Beebe DK, Walley E. Substance abuse: the designer drugs. Am Fam Physician. 1991;43(5):1689–98. Epub 1991/05/01

112. Buchert R, Thomasius R, Nebeling B, Petersen K, Obrocki J, Jenicke L, et al. Long-term effects of "ecstasy" use on serotonin transporters of the brain investigated by PET. J Nucl Med. 2003;44(3):375–84. Epub 2003/03/07
113. Daws LC, Irvine RJ, Callaghan PD, Toop NP, White JM, Bochner F. Differential behavioural and neurochemical effects of Para-methoxyamphetamine and 3,4-methylenedioxymethamphetamine in the rat. Prog Neuro-Psychopharmacol Biol Psychiatry. 2000;24(6):955–77. Epub 2000/10/21. https://doi.org/10.1016/s0278-5846(00)00113-5.
114. Rattray M. Ecstasy: towards an understanding of the biochemical basis of the actions of MDMA. Essays Biochem. 1991;26:77–87. Epub 1991/01/01
115. Milroy CM, Clark JC, Forrest AR. Pathology of deaths associated with "ecstasy" and "eve" misuse. J Clin Pathol. 1996;49(2):149–53. Epub 1996/02/01. PubMed PMID: 8655682; PubMed Central PMCID: PMCPMC500349. https://doi.org/10.1136/jcp.49.2.149.
116. Cohen RS, Cocores J. Neuropsychiatric manifestations following the use of 3,4-methylene dioxymethamphetamine (MDMA: "ecstasy"). Prog Neuro-Psychopharmacol Biol Psychiatry. 1997;21(4):727–34. Epub 1997/05/01. https://doi.org/10.1016/s0278-5846(97)00045-6.
117. Kiyatkin EA, Sharma HS. Acute methamphetamine intoxication: brain hyperthermia, blood-brain barrier, brain edema, and morphological cell abnormalities. Int Rev Neurobiol. 2009;88:65–100. Epub 2009/11/10. PubMed PMID: 19897075; PubMed Central PMCID: PMCPMC3145326. https://doi.org/10.1016/s0074-7742(09)88004-5.
118. Reneman L, Habraken JB, Majoie CB, Booij J, den Heeten GJ. MDMA ("ecstasy") and its association with cerebrovascular accidents: preliminary findings. AJNR Am J Neuroradiol. 2000;21(6):1001–7. Epub 2000/06/28
119. Omer TA, Doherty C. Posterior reversible encephalopathy syndrome (PRES) complicating the 'legal high' mephedrone. BMJ Case Rep. 2011;2011. Epub 2011/01/01. PubMed PMID: 22689272; PubMed Central PMCID: PMCPMC3166585. https://doi.org/10.1136/bcr.02.2011.3904.
120. Hinchey J, Chaves C, Appignani B, Breen J, Pao L, Wang A, et al. A reversible posterior leukoencephalopathy syndrome. N Engl J Med. 1996;334(8):494–500. Epub 1996/02/22. https://doi.org/10.1056/nejm199602223340803.
121. Castillo A, Payne JD, Nugent K. Posterior reversible leukoencephalopathy syndrome after kratom ingestion. Proceedings (Baylor University Medical Center). 2017;30(3):355–7. Epub 2017/07/04. PubMed PMID: 28670086; PubMed Central PMCID: PMCPMC5468044. https://doi.org/10.1080/08998280.2017.11929647.
122. Mena JC, Cuellar H, Vargas D, Riascos R. PET and SPECT in drug and substance abuse. Topics Magn Resonan Imag. 2005;16(3):253–6. Epub 2005/12/13. https://doi.org/10.1097/01.rmr.0000192177.01789.c0.
123. Kohno M, Link J, Dennis LE, McCready H, Huckans M, Hoffman WF, et al. Neuroinflammation in addiction: a review of neuroimaging studies and potential immunotherapies. Pharmacol Biochem Behav. 2019;179:34–42. Epub 2019/01/30. PubMed PMID: 30695700; PubMed Central PMCID: PMCPMC6637953. https://doi.org/10.1016/j.pbb.2019.01.007.
124. Chang L, Grob CS, Ernst T, Itti L, Mishkin FS, Jose-Melchor R, et al. Effect of ecstasy [3,4-methy lenedioxymethamphetamine (MDMA)] on cerebral blood flow: a co-registered SPECT and MRI study. Psychiatry Res. 2000;98(1):15–28. Epub 2000/03/10. https://doi.org/10.1016/s0925-4927(99)00048-7.
125. de Win MM, Reneman L, Jager G, Vlieger EJ, Olabarriaga SD, Lavini C, et al. A prospective cohort study on sustained effects of low-dose ecstasy use on the brain in new ecstasy users. Neuropsychopharmacology. 2007;32(2):458–70. Epub 2006/11/02. https://doi.org/10.1038/sj.npp.1301225.
126. London ED, Kohno M, Morales AM, Ballard ME. Chronic methamphetamine abuse and corticostriatal deficits revealed by neuroimaging. Brain Res. 2015;1628(Pt A):174–85. Epub 2014/12/03. PubMed PMID: 25451127; PubMed Central PMCID: PMCPMC4418947. https://doi.org/10.1016/j.brainres.2014.10.044.
127. Vuletic D, Dupont P, Robertson F, Warwick J, Zeevaart JR, Stein DJ. Methamphetamine dependence with and without psychotic symptoms: a multi-modal brain imaging study. NeuroImage Clin. 2018;20:1157–62. Epub 2018/11/01. PubMed PMID: 30380522; PubMed Central PMCID: PMCPMC6205927. https://doi.org/10.1016/j.nicl.2018.10.023.
128. Berman S, O'Neill J, Fears S, Bartzokis G, London ED. Abuse of amphetamines and structural abnormalities in the brain. Ann N Y Acad Sci. 2008;1141:195–220. Epub 2008/11/11. PubMed PMID: 18991959; PubMed Central PMCID: PMCPMC2769923. https://doi.org/10.1196/annals.1441.031.
129. Li Y, Dong H, Li F, Wang G, Zhou W, Yu R, et al. Microstructures in striato-thalamo-orbitofrontal circuit in methamphetamine users. Acta Radiol (Stockholm, Sweden : 1987). 2017;58(11):1378–85. Epub 2017/02/10. https://doi.org/10.1177/0284185117692170.
130. Alicata D, Chang L, Cloak C, Abe K, Ernst T. Higher diffusion in striatum and lower fractional anisotropy in white matter of methamphetamine users. Psychiatry Res. 2009;174(1):1–8. Epub 2009/09/29. PubMed PMID: 19782540; PubMed Central PMCID: PMCPMC2925833. https://doi.org/10.1016/j.pscychresns.2009.03.011.
131. Choi JK, Lim G, Chen YI, Jenkins BG. Abstinence to chronic methamphetamine switches connectiv-

ity between striatal, hippocampal and sensorimotor regions and increases cerebral blood volume response. NeuroImage. 2018;174:364–79. Epub 2018/03/09. PubMed PMID: 29518566; PubMed Central PMCID: PMCPMC5949272. https://doi.org/10.1016/j.neuroimage.2018.02.059.

132. Zhang Z, Li P, Fan L, Tao F, Li Y, Jiang B, et al. Change of brain structure imaging of long-term withdrawal of methamphetamine-dependent patients. Zhong nan da xue xue bao Yi xue ban = J Centr South Univer Med Sci. 2018;43(1):41–8. https://doi.org/10.11817/j.issn.1672-7347.2018.01.007. Epub 2018/08/30

133. Alderazi Y, Brett F. Alcohol and the nervous system. Curr Diagn Pathol. 2007;13(3):203–9.

134. Sher L. Alcohol and suicide: neurobiological and clinical aspects. Sci World J. 2006;6:700–6. Epub 2006/06/27. PubMed PMID: 16799741; PubMed Central PMCID: PMCPMC5917128. https://doi.org/10.1100/tsw.2006.146.

135. Truelsen T, Thudium D, Grønbaek M. Amount and type of alcohol and risk of dementia: the Copenhagen City heart study. Neurology. 2002;59(9):1313–9. Epub 2002/11/13. https://doi.org/10.1212/01.wnl.0000031421.50369.e7.

136. Ganguli M, Vander Bilt J, Saxton JA, Shen C, Dodge HH. Alcohol consumption and cognitive function in late life: a longitudinal community study. Neurology. 2005;65(8):1210–7. Epub 2005/10/26. https://doi.org/10.1212/01.wnl.0000180520.35181.24.

137. Rehm J, Anderson P, Barry J, Dimitrov P, Elekes Z, Feijão F, et al. Prevalence of and potential influencing factors for alcohol dependence in Europe. Eur Addict Res. 2015;21(1):6–18. Epub 2014/10/25. https://doi.org/10.1159/000365284.

138. Fritz M, Klawonn AM, Zahr NM. Neuroimaging in alcohol use disorder: from mouse to man. J Neurosci Res. 2019; https://doi.org/10.1002/jnr.24423. Epub 2019/04/23. PubMed PMID: 31006907; PubMed Central PMCID: PMCPMC6810809.

139. Connor JP, Haber PS, Hall WD. Alcohol use disorders. Lancet (London, England). 2016;387(10022):988–98. Epub 2015/09/08. https://doi.org/10.1016/s0140-6736(15)00122-1.

140. Grant BF, Goldstein RB, Saha TD, Chou SP, Jung J, Zhang H, et al. Epidemiology of DSM-5 alcohol use disorder: results from the national epidemiologic survey on alcohol and related conditions III. JAMA Psychiatry. 2015;72(8):757–66. https://doi.org/10.1001/jamapsychiatry.2015.0584. Epub 2015/06/04. PubMed PMID: 26039070; PubMed Central PMCID: PMCPMC5240584

141. Yeomans MR. Alcohol, appetite and energy balance: is alcohol intake a risk factor for obesity? Physiol Behav. 2010;100(1):82–9. Epub 2010/01/26. https://doi.org/10.1016/j.physbeh.2010.01.012.

142. Tabakoff B, Hoffman PL. The neurobiology of alcohol consumption and alcoholism: an integrative history. Pharmacol Biochem Behav. 2013;113:20–37. https://doi.org/10.1016/j.pbb.2013.10.009. Epub 2013/10/22. PubMed PMID: 24141171; PubMed Central PMCID: PMCPMC3867277

143. Lobo IA, Harris RA. GABA(A) receptors and alcohol. Pharmacol Biochem Behav. 2008;90(1):90–4. https://doi.org/10.1016/j.pbb.2008.03.006. Epub 2008/04/22. PubMed PMID: 18423561; PubMed Central PMCID: PMCPMC2574824

144. Olsen RW, Hanchar HJ, Meera P, Wallner M. GABAA receptor subtypes: the "one glass of wine" receptors. Alcohol (Fayetteville, NY). 2007;41(3):201–9. https://doi.org/10.1016/j.alcohol.2007.04.006. Epub 2007/06/27. PubMed PMID: 17591543; PubMed Central PMCID: PMCPMC2852584

145. Criswell HE, Ming Z, Griffith BL, Breese GR. Comparison of effect of ethanol on N-methyl-D-aspartate- and GABA-gated currents from acutely dissociated neurons: absence of regional differences in sensitivity to ethanol. J Pharmacol Exp Ther. 2003;304(1):192–9. Epub 2002/12/20. https://doi.org/10.1124/jpet.102.041590.

146. Hoffman PL, Rabe CS, Moses F, Tabakoff B. N-methyl-D-aspartate receptors and ethanol: inhibition of calcium flux and cyclic GMP production. J Neurochem. 1989;52(6):1937–40. Epub 1989/06/01. https://doi.org/10.1111/j.1471-4159.1989.tb07280.x.

147. Zuccoli G, Pipitone N. Neuroimaging findings in acute Wernicke's encephalopathy: review of the literature. Am J Roentgenol. 2009;192(2):501–8.

148. Arbelaez A, Pajon A, Castillo M. Acute Marchiafava-Bignami disease: MR findings in two patients. AJNR Am J Neuroradiol. 2003;24(10):1955–7. Epub 2003/11/20

149. Thompson PD, Miller D, Gledhill RF, Rossor MN. Magnetic resonance imaging in central pontine myelinolysis. J Neurol Neurosurg Psychiatry. 1989;52(5):675–7. Epub 1989/05/01. PubMed PMID: 2732743; PubMed Central PMCID: PMCPMC1032189. https://doi.org/10.1136/jnnp.52.5.675.

150. Zuccoli G, Siddiqui N, Cravo I, Bailey A, Gallucci M, Harper CG. Neuroimaging findings in alcohol-related encephalopathies. AJR Am J Roentgenol. 2010;195(6):1378–84. Epub 2010/11/26. https://doi.org/10.2214/ajr.09.4130.

151. Erdozain AM, Morentin B, Bedford L, King E, Tooth D, Brewer C, et al. Alcohol-related brain damage in humans. PloS One. 2014;9(4):e93586. https://doi.org/10.1371/journal.pone.0093586. Epub 2014/04/05. PubMed PMID: 24699688; PubMed Central PMCID: PMCPMC3974765

152. Zahr NM, Kaufman KL, Harper CG. Clinical and pathological features of alcohol-related brain damage. Nat Rev Neurol. 2011;7(5):284–94. Epub 2011/04/14. https://doi.org/10.1038/nrneurol.2011.42.

153. Nakamura K, Iwahashi K, Furukawa A, Ameno K, Kinoshita H, Ijiri I, et al. Acetaldehyde adducts in the brain of alcoholics. Arch Toxicol.

2003;77(10):591–3. Epub 2003/10/24. https://doi.org/10.1007/s00204-003-0465-8.
154. Tuma DJ, Smith SL, Sorrell MF. Acetaldehyde and microtubules. Ann N Y Acad Sci. 1991;625:786–92. Epub 1991/01/01. https://doi.org/10.1111/j.1749-6632.1991.tb33920.x.
155. Smith SL, Jennett RB, Sorrell MF, Tuma DJ. Acetaldehyde substoichiometrically inhibits bovine neurotubulin polymerization. J Clin Investig. 1989;84(1):337–41. https://doi.org/10.1172/jci114159. Epub 1989/07/01. PubMed PMID: 2500458; PubMed Central PMCID: PMCPMC303987
156. Harper C, Matsumoto I. Ethanol and brain damage. Curr Opin Pharmacol. 2005;5(1):73–8. Epub 2005/01/22. https://doi.org/10.1016/j.coph.2004.06.011.
157. Pfefferbaum A, Sullivan EV. Disruption of brain white matter microstructure by excessive intracellular and extracellular fluid in alcoholism: evidence from diffusion tensor imaging. Neuropsychopharmacology. 2005;30(2):423–32. Epub 2004/11/25. https://doi.org/10.1038/sj.npp.1300623.
158. Harper C. The neuropathology of alcohol-related brain damage. Alcohol Alcoholism. 2009;44(2):136–40.
159. Baker KG, Harding AJ, Halliday GM, Kril JJ, Harper CG. Neuronal loss in functional zones of the cerebellum of chronic alcoholics with and without Wernicke's encephalopathy. Neuroscience. 1999;91(2):429–38. Epub 1999/06/12. https://doi.org/10.1016/s0306-4522(98)90664-9.
160. Sullivan EV, Deshmukh A, Desmond JE, Lim KO, Pfefferbaum A. Cerebellar volume decline in normal aging, alcoholism, and Korsakoff's syndrome: relation to ataxia. Neuropsychology. 2000;14(3):341–52. Epub 2000/08/06. https://doi.org/10.1037//0894-4105.14.3.341
161. Shear PK, Jernigan TL, Butters N. Volumetric magnetic resonance imaging quantification of longitudinal brain changes in abstinent alcoholics. Alcohol Clin Exp Res. 1994;18(1):172–6. Epub 1994/02/01. https://doi.org/10.1111/j.1530-0277.1994.tb00899.x.
162. Liu RS, Lemieux L, Shorvon SD, Sisodiya SM, Duncan JS. Association between brain size and abstinence from alcohol. Lancet (London, England). 2000;355(9219):1969–70. https://doi.org/10.1016/s0140-6736(00)02332-1. Epub 2000/06/20
163. van Eijk J, Demirakca T, Frischknecht U, Hermann D, Mann K, Ende G. Rapid partial regeneration of brain volume during the first 14 days of abstinence from alcohol. Alcohol Clin Exp Res. 2013;37(1):67–74. Epub 2012/10/18. https://doi.org/10.1111/j.1530-0277.2012.01853.x.
164. Demirakca T, Ende G, Kämmerer N, Welzel-Marquez H, Hermann D, Heinz A, et al. Effects of alcoholism and continued abstinence on brain volumes in both genders. Alcohol Clin Exp Res. 2011;35(9):1678–85. Epub 2011/05/24. https://doi.org/10.1111/j.1530-0277.2011.01514.x.
165. Zahr NM, Pfefferbaum A. Alcohol's effects on the brain: neuroimaging results in humans and animal models. Alcohol Res Curr Rev. 2017;38(2):183–206. Epub 2017/10/11. PubMed PMID: 28988573; PubMed Central PMCID: PMCPMC5513685
166. van Holst RJ, de Ruiter MB, van den Brink W, Veltman DJ, Goudriaan AE. A voxel-based morphometry study comparing problem gamblers, alcohol abusers, and healthy controls. Drug Alcohol Depend. 2012;124(1-2):142–8. Epub 2012/01/25. https://doi.org/10.1016/j.drugalcdep.2011.12.025.
167. Estruch R, Nicolás JM, Salamero M, Aragón C, Sacanella E, Fernández-Solà J, et al. Atrophy of the corpus callosum in chronic alcoholism. J Neurol Sci. 1997;146(2):145–51. Epub 1997/03/10. https://doi.org/10.1016/s0022-510x(96)00298-5.
168. Sullivan EV, Harding AJ, Pentney R, Dlugos C, Martin PR, Parks MH, et al. Disruption of frontocerebellar circuitry and function in alcoholism. Alcohol Clin Exp Res. 2003;27(2):301–9. Epub 2003/02/28. https://doi.org/10.1097/01.alc.0000052584.05305.98.
169. Durazzo TC, Tosun D, Buckley S, Gazdzinski S, Mon A, Fryer SL, et al. Cortical thickness, surface area, and volume of the brain reward system in alcohol dependence: relationships to relapse and extended abstinence. Alcohol Clin Exp Res. 2011;35(6):1187–200. https://doi.org/10.1111/j.1530-0277.2011.01452.x. Epub 2011/03/18. PubMed PMID: 21410483; PubMed Central PMCID: PMCPMC3097308
170. Sullivan EV, Deshmukh A, De Rosa E, Rosenbloom MJ, Pfefferbaum A. Striatal and forebrain nuclei volumes: contribution to motor function and working memory deficits in alcoholism. Biol Psychiatry. 2005;57(7):768–76. Epub 2005/04/12. https://doi.org/10.1016/j.biopsych.2004.12.012.
171. Pfefferbaum A, Sullivan EV, Hedehus M, Adalsteinsson E, Lim KO, Moseley M. In vivo detection and functional correlates of white matter microstructural disruption in chronic alcoholism. Alcohol Clin Exp Res. 2000;24(8):1214–21. Epub 2000/09/01
172. Fortier CB, Leritz EC, Salat DH, Lindemer E, Maksimovskiy AL, Shepel J, et al. Widespread effects of alcohol on white matter microstructure. Alcohol Clin Exp Res. 2014;38(12):2925–33. https://doi.org/10.1111/acer.12568. Epub 2014/11/20. PubMed PMID: 25406797; PubMed Central PMCID: PMCPMC4293208

173. Bagga D, Sharma A, Kumari A, Kaur P, Bhattacharya D, Garg ML, et al. Decreased white matter integrity in fronto-occipital fasciculus bundles: relation to visual information processing in alcohol-dependent subjects. Alcohol (Fayetteville, NY). 2014;48(1):43–53. https://doi.org/10.1016/j.alcohol.2013.10.009. Epub 2014/01/07
174. Maksimovskiy AL, McGlinchey RE, Fortier CB, Salat DH, Milberg WP, Oscar-Berman M. White matter and cognitive changes in veterans diagnosed with alcoholism and PTSD. J Alcohol Drug Depend. 2014;2(1):144. https://doi.org/10.4172/2329-6488.1000144. Epub 2014/05/24. PubMed PMID: 24855633; PubMed Central PMCID: PMCPMC4023485
175. Pfefferbaum A, Adalsteinsson E, Sullivan EV. Supratentorial profile of white matter microstructural integrity in recovering alcoholic men and women. Biol Psychiatry. 2006;59(4):364–72. Epub 2005/08/30. https://doi.org/10.1016/j.biopsych.2005.06.025.
176. Sasaki H, Abe O, Yamasue H, Fukuda R, Yamada H, Takei K, et al. Structural and diffusional brain abnormality related to relatively low level alcohol consumption. NeuroImage. 2009;46(2):505–10. Epub 2009/02/24. https://doi.org/10.1016/j.neuroimage.2009.02.007.
177. Schacht JP, Anton RF, Myrick H. Functional neuroimaging studies of alcohol cue reactivity: a quantitative meta-analysis and systematic review. Addict Biol. 2013;18(1):121–33. https://doi.org/10.1111/j.1369-1600.2012.00464.x. Epub 2012/05/12. PubMed PMID: 22574861; PubMed Central PMCID: PMCPMC3419322
178. Vollstädt-Klein S, Loeber S, Richter A, Kirsch M, Bach P, von der Goltz C, et al. Validating incentive salience with functional magnetic resonance imaging: association between mesolimbic cue reactivity and attentional bias in alcohol-dependent patients. Addict Biol. 2012;17(4):807–16. Epub 2011/07/28. https://doi.org/10.1111/j.1369-1600.2011.00352.x.
179. Ihssen N, Cox WM, Wiggett A, Fadardi JS, Linden DE. Differentiating heavy from light drinkers by neural responses to visual alcohol cues and other motivational stimuli. Cerebr Cortex (New York, NY : 1991). 2011;21(6):1408–15. https://doi.org/10.1093/cercor/bhq220. Epub 2010/11/04
180. Krienke UJ, Nikesch F, Spiegelhalder K, Hennig J, Olbrich HM, Langosch JM. Impact of alcohol-related video sequences on functional MRI in abstinent alcoholics. Eur Addict Res. 2014;20(1):33–40. Epub 2013/08/08. https://doi.org/10.1159/000349909.
181. Müller-Oehring EM, Jung YC, Pfefferbaum A, Sullivan EV, Schulte T. The resting brain of alcoholics. Cerebr Cortex (New York, NY : 1991). 2015;25(11):4155–68. Epub 2014/06/18. PubMed PMID: 24935777; PubMed Central PMCID: PMCPMC4816777. https://doi.org/10.1093/cercor/bhu134.

45 Drinking to Cope as a Vulnerability Factor for Alcohol Use Disorder: Evidence from Clinical and Preclinical Research

Ricardo Marcos Pautassi, Adrián J. Bravo, Agustín Salguero, and Angelina Pilatti

Abbreviations

DTC	drinking to cope
AUD	alcohol use disorder
PBS	protective behavioral strategies
ARC	alcohol-related consequences
EOD	early onset of drinking
EPM	elevated plus maze
LDB	light-dark box
MCSF	multivariate concentric square field
PAE	prenatal alcohol exposure
PDYN	prodynorphin
KOR	kappa-opioid receptor
mRNA	messenger ribonucleic acid
VTA	ventral tegmental area
P rats	alcohol-preferring rats
NP rats	alcohol nonpreferring (or low-preferring) rats
ADHI	adolescent high ethanol drinking rats
ADLO	adolescent low ethanol drinking rats
EMA	ecological momentary assessment

R. M. Pautassi (✉) · A. Salguero
Facultad de Psicología, Universidad Nacional de Córdoba (UNC), Córdoba, Argentina

Instituto de Investigación Médica M. y M. Ferreyra, INIMEC-CONICET-UNC, Córdoba, Argentina
e-mail: rpautassi@immf.uncor.edu; asalguero@immf.uncor.edu

A. J. Bravo
Department of Psychological Sciences, William & Mary, Williamsburg, VA, USA
e-mail: ajbravo@wm.edu

A. Pilatti
Facultad de Psicología, Universidad Nacional de Córdoba (UNC), Córdoba, Argentina

Instituto de Investigaciones Psicológicas, IIPsi-CONICET-UNC, Córdoba, Argentina
e-mail: apilatti@unc.edu.ar

Introduction

Alcohol use disorder (AUD) is a condition in which the individual keeps drinking despite recognizing a plethora of negative social, occupational, and health consequences. It is a chronic disorder in which alcohol-free periods are punctuated with periods of heavy drinking. Relapse is often triggered by stress exposure or by stimuli associated with the effects of the drug.

The harmful use of alcohol is a leading cause of premature death and disability among people between 15 and 49 years. Moreover, risky drinking patterns are associated with greater probability of having domestic injuries, car crashes, engaging in interpersonal violence, unsafe sexual practices, and reduced work or academic performance. Binge drinking [i.e., the ingestion of 4 or 5 (men/women, respectively) standard alcohol drinks in a single and short (usually 2 h or less) occasion] is one of those risky drinking patterns. Within the United States, a standard drink or alcohol unit contains about 14 grams of absolute alcohol, the quantity found in 350 ml of regular

P. Á. Gargiulo, H. L. Mesones-Arroyo (eds.), *Psychiatry and Neuroscience Update – Vol. V*,
https://doi.org/10.1007/978-3-031-72219-6_45

beer or in a typical serving of wine. Binge drinking is significantly more prevalent among adolescent and youth than in older individuals and increases the number and severity of negative consequences [1], including the likelihood of developing an alcohol use disorder [2].

Vulnerability Factors Associated with AUD and Risky Drinking: Mediation, Moderation, and Confounding Effects

AUD runs in the families, suggesting that at least part of the susceptibility to the condition is genetic. The initial studies on the topic conflated genetic and environmental exposure, yet later studies, for instance, those that measured risk of AUD in twins separated at birth, disaggregated risk of AUD attributable to genetic, environmental, and gene x environment interactions. In general, it has been shown that 40 to 60% of the risk for AUD can be attributed to our genetic makeup [3]. Finding a single gene responsible for the disease has proven elusive, yet variations in the enzymatic machinery that breaks down alcohol into acetaldehyde, and then the latter into acetate, significantly modulate alcohol use [4]. Heritability is but one of the factors collectively known as vulnerability factors that increase the likelihood associated with AUD. Another is exposure to aversive lifetime events, more commonly known as stress. These factors interact in increasingly complex ways. For instance, a vulnerability factor for AUD is being diagnosed with a psychiatric or psychological disorder. However, the latter are usually associated with greater likelihood of experiencing aversive lifetime events such as divorce or prolonged unemployment. Other factors deter (e.g., high levels of paternal monitoring, low levels of impulsivity-like personality traits) from risky drinking and AUD and are thus referred to as protective factors. Most of the factors we have described so far (e.g., personality traits, genetic risk) can be described as distal factors that ultimately affect drinking via the mediation of factors more proximal to the actual behavior of alcohol ingestion, such as drinking motives, greater perception of alcohol-related cues or greater sensitivity to ethanol's pharmacological effects. We will expand on the concept of mediation shortly.

Sometimes the risk associated with exposure to a vulnerability factor interacts with that of another factor. By interaction we indicate a synergistic mechanism by which apparently smaller risks add up geometrically to produce a large dose effect. For instance, a study showed little increase in risk effect (measured as the volume of alcohol drank per day) in those exhibiting an early age of drinking onset (i.e., having had the first drink at 14 or younger) or that had experience 6 or more stress events during the last year. Yet, the combination of both events was associated with a dramatic increase in the volume of alcohol consumed per day [5]. Other example of interaction is that in which the outcome of a treatment is affected by a given characteristics of the sample applied. For instance, aspirin may protect from heart attack in men, but can cause internal bleeding in women [6].

Sometimes, however, the relationship between two risk factors (e.g., A and B) is such that B serves as the mechanism by which A ultimately exerts its action. Such an interplay, referred to as mediation in the clinical literature, is illustrated by several behavioral alterations that provide risk for AUD, but are ultimately a consequence of genetic vulnerability for the disease. These traits have been also termed, particularly within the preclinical literature, as endophenotypes [7]: behavioral or neural traits with substantial degree of heritability that are significantly associated with (and temporally prior to the emergence of) AUD. Individuals with genetic risk for AUD have been shown, among several other features, to be more sensitive to the psychomotor stimulation induced by the acute alcohol intoxication, which can be assessed via hearth rate changes [8]. Similarly, rats and mice that spontaneously exhibit heightened alcohol intake are more prone to exhibit greater reactivity to novel environments, blunted responsiveness to ethanol-induced malaise and aversion, yet greater sensitivity to ethanol-induced reward [9].

An example of mediation can be found in the stress-hypertension literature. Chronic stress has been traditionally linked to cardiovascular diseases such as stroke, yet the specific underlying mechanisms remain elusive. Some studies indicate that stress increases hypertension via behavioral (i.e., favoring the acquisition of high-fat diets) or psychological (increasing rumination of previously experienced stress events) mediators [10]. In the clinical literature of risky drinking, in turn, some mediators extensively studied are drinking motives and protective behavioral strategies (PBS). PBS are behaviors that drinkers can execute during (e.g., keeping their alcohol drink within reach, refusing refilling or alternating alcoholic and nonalcoholic drinks) or even before (plan how many and what types of drinks to have) or after drinking (e.g., return home with a trusted person), to reduce their level of exposure to negative alcohol-related consequences (ARC). Use of alcohol PBS is associated with lower alcohol consumption and negative alcohol-related consequences [11, 12]. Further, PBS use has been shown to mediate the effects of known risk factors (i.e., sex, age of alcohol use onset, college alcohol use beliefs, and impulsivity-like traits) on alcohol outcomes (i.e., use and consequences [13–15]). Drinking motives are conscious or unconscious reasons that ignite the decision to drink, and include drinking to modulate negative or positive affect [16, 17] or better fit into a social group [18]. Drinking to reduce negative states, including anxiety and depression, is usually referred to as drinking to cope (DTC) and will be a main focus of the present chapter.

Summarizing the interplay, we have discussed up to this point, the variables linking distal antecedents (e.g., mental health status, personality dimensions) and alcohol-related outcomes (i.e., consumption and consequences) are usually referred to as mediators (also known as process variables) or moderators (also known as conditional variables). Mediation and moderation are traditionally measured via different statistical approaches (path analysis or SEM models and regression or analysis of variance, respectively) and have of course quite different implications for untangling causation phenomena. A third possibility of interplay between variables is, in turn, that of confounding. A confounder occurs when two variables of interest [namely, the association between an early onset of drinking (EOD) and later development of AUD] are in turn associated with a third variable that spuriously accentuates the relationship between them [19]. Usually, statistical adjustment for the confounder significantly decreases the strength of the relationship between the putative independent and dependent variables.

The previous reference to the association between EOD and the risk of being diagnosed with AUD or exhibiting risky drinking is meant to highlight the discussion on whether or not these two events are casually related. The phenomena are strongly correlated. We have found, for instance, that circa 80% of Argentinean college students that began drinking by age 14 or younger (the typical definition of EOD) reported binge drinking in the last 6 months, whereas the prevalence of that behavior was around 50% in those that began drinking after age 15 [20]. Moreover, the proposals grounded in the so-called gateway theories of addiction [21] suggest that the effect of EOD may be broader, affecting the likelihood of ingesting substances other than alcohol. Consistent with this, in Pilatti et al. [20] last-month prevalence of marijuana use was 30% in those with EOD, yet circa 13% in those that began drinking after the age of 15. This and other findings support the public health strategy of increasing efforts to prevent as much as possible the age of alcohol drinking onset. However, many have indicated that EOD may be a marker of genetic vulnerability or that its effect upon AUD is confounded by, and disappears when adjusted for, factors such as externalizing psychopathology or deviant behavior. Under this perspective, EOD would merely be an indicator of risk for AUD, not a causal influence [22].

Aim of the Chapter

Motivational models of alcohol use [16, 23] posit that drinking motives are one of the most proximal antecedent to alcohol use (i.e., the decision to drink), and different drinking motives are associated with different patterns of alcohol consumption. DTC motives are directly related to alcohol-related consequences [24] and have been shown to be associated with alcohol dependence. Since Kuntsche et al.'s review [24] (also see a later review by Cooper et al. [17]), several studies have examined the role of DTC motives as a mediator or moderator between distal antecedents (i.e., mental health and personality dimensions) and alcohol consumption or consequences.

In the chapter, we analyze the possibility that an anxiety-prone phenotype or the motivation of DTC with negative emotions is a common and proximal mediator or moderator of a wide range of vulnerability factors for AUD or risky drinking, ranging from personality traits to environmental exposure to aversive life events or early alcohol exposure. In the first section, we review preclinical studies indicating that rats or mice selectively bred for high alcohol drinking across several generations or exposed to ethanol during pregnancy or to varieties of experimental stress exhibit reduced exploration of brightly lit environments, greater shelter seeking or other anxiety-like behaviors, measured in tests such as the elevated plus maze (EPM), the light-dark box (LDB), or the multivariate concentric square field (MCSF) test. The second section, in turn, describes clinical work indicating that DTC motives are a primary mechanism through which personality or psychosocial constructs relate to problematic alcohol use. In this section, we summarize recent research examining DTC motives as a mediator or moderator between both personality dimensions and mental health on alcohol outcomes. Across the sections, we identify gaps in the literature and offer suggestions for future research that may be used to better inform and tailor interventions aimed reducing the impact of risky drinking on emerging adults, particularly college students.

Emerging adults, compared to any other developmental stage, exhibit the highest prevalence of binge drinking [25]. The transition from high school to college is a particularly risky period for increased alcohol use among emerging adults [26]. Therefore, most of the evidence presented in this review focuses on this developmental stage or in preclinical models that measure alcohol-related behaviors in adolescent or young adult subjects.

Anxiety as Measured in Preclinical Studies

Measuring "personality" traits in rats or mice can be daunting, yet researchers have designed tasks that take advantage of innate, species-specific, behavioral predispositions. Rats or mice tend to avoid brightly lit and open spaces and prefer to explore dark and enclosed areas. This is the basis of the LDB and EPM tests. The former is a cage with two compartments, one white and brightly illuminated, whereas the EPM is a cross-shaped maze with enclosed or open sections.

There is a great variability in the exploration of these devices, and thus, one can find subpopulations of rodents that, compared to their peers, exhibit heightened preference for these open, potentially risky, spaces, or that, vice versa, avoid these spaces more than the usual, and thus can be referred to as exhibiting spontaneous high anxiety response. In one of those studies, Acevedo et al. [27] found that adolescent female rats classified as high anxiety responders exhibited significantly more ethanol intake and ethanol preference than counterparts classified as low-anxiety responder (i.e., 5 g/kg/24 h vs 1.5 g/kg/24 h or 65% vs 25%, respectively). Another study [28] found similar results in adult rats and, intriguingly, was able to inhibit the exacerbated drinking of the high-anxiety responders by modulating the levels of neuropeptide Y in the amygdala. The central amygdala is the major output of the amygdala and is thought to integrate fear and anxiety-related signals and relay them to downstream effector regions. Another alternative, to test the association between anxiety and ethanol drinking in animals, is to use rats selectively bred for high or low anxiety, across several generations, and test ethanol intake in those populations. Using that approach, it has been shown that Floripa L rats drink more ethanol than their

Floripa H rats [29]. These strains were selected for exhibiting relatively low and high levels, respectively, of locomotion in the central, anxiety-inducing, section of an open field. Together, these studies indicate that inborn anxiety can promote ethanol intake in rodents, probably a self-medication behavior aimed at reducing this innate, trait-like, anxiety. Yet, these studies do not help decide if anxiety can mediate the effectiveness of other relevant risk factors for AUD. We will have to look elsewhere to find support for this possibility.

Prenatal alcohol exposure (PAE) is highly relevant across the Western world, with recent studies indicating that 20–30% of pregnant woman drink at least one glass of an alcoholic beverage during pregnancy and a sizeable proportion of them (e.g., 15% in Lopez et al. [30]) achieve binge drinking. PAE is associated with increased alcohol drinking at adolescence and young adulthood, both in clinical and preclinical studies. The classical studies by Baer et al. (e.g., [31]) reported that the association kept significant event after adjustment for or test of interaction with family history and other environmental covariates.

The mechanism underlying this promoting effect of PAE in later alcohol drinking is still elusive. Recently, Diaz et al. [32] gave pregnant rats a single exposure to ethanol on gestational day 12, consisting of two doses of 2.5 g/kg, separated by 2 h. The offspring subsequently exhibited greater ethanol drinking and, particularly in males, greater social anxiety. The latter was measured via a test in which the rats actively seek or avoid asocial interaction with a peer. Intriguingly, when the male rats were divided into high/medium/low anxiety responders, only high anxiety males that had been exposed to ethanol in-utero demonstrated heightened voluntary ethanol intake.

The study by Diaz et al. [32] is but one of the several reports of heightened anxiety after PAE. We have shown that PAE rats spent less time in the brightly lit areas of an LDB apparatus [33]. The LDB is a rather simple test, in which the rats are put into a white and brightly lit open area connected to a dark and enclosed chamber. It is a so-called binary task, which is surpassed in complexity by the MCSF test, in which the rats are introduced in an interconnected set of chambers, with varying degree with illumination and potential risk, from an enclosed and dark "shelter" to a central, open-field like, square to an elevated and illuminated "bridge" [34, 35]. Interestingly, time spent in the sheltered area was twofold greater in PAE than in control rats, and PAE rats also exhibited less propensity to explore the bridge, when compared to controls [33]. We have traced the anxiety-prone phenotype of PAE rats to changes in the functionality of the kappa opioid and nociceptive transmitter systems, within the mesocorticolimbic brain pathway [36]. Specifically, PAE rats exhibited enhanced prodynorphin (PDYN) and kappa-opioid receptor (KOR) mRNA levels in the ventral tegmental area (VTA) or in the prefrontal cortex. Upregulated PDYN/KOR functioning, which is likely to explain the anxiety and ethanol-drinking prone phenotype of PAE rats, was accompanied by reduced functioning of the nociceptin system. The latter is thought to counteract the aversive stimulation associated with KOR activity.

Another strategy to identify endophenotypes associated with risky drinking is selectively bred rats or mice, for high or low alcohol drinking across several generations. Usually, this involves the mating of male and female animals that drink relatively high levels of alcohol, as assessed in two-bottle choice tests. After several generations, the offspring of these rats will spontaneously drink more ethanol when compared to non-selected counterparts or when compared to rats derived from couples selected for exhibiting low intake and preference for ethanol [37]. The strategy also allows measuring behavioral or neural traits correlated, and perhaps casually related, to ethanol intake.

Alcohol-preferring rats (P rats, perhaps the most studied strain created by selecting high drinkers across generations) exhibit, when compared to their low-preferring (NP rats) counterparts, reduced sensitivity to the aversive motivational effects of ethanol [38]. Perhaps, more important for the purposes of the present chapter the P rats display [39], when compared with NP rats, (a) greater sensitivity to the suppressing effect exerted by foot shock (i.e., exteroceptive nociceptive stimulation) upon operant responding, (b) greater latency to access a chamber in which they had experienced foot shock and (c), similar to the PAE rats of [32] or [33], reduced exploration of open and brightly lit spaces [39]. These effects were normalized by the administration of ethanol in P but not in NP rats. Reduced time spent in the open spaces of the elevated plus maze and other signs of innate anxiety (e.g., reduced mobility in an open field test) are also observed in another strain selected for high alcohol drinking, the Sardinian alcohol-preferring rat [40–42].

The intriguing finding we have just reviewed suggest that an anxiety-prone phenotype may mediate the heightened levels of ethanol ingestion observed in the line selected for high ethanol consumption at adulthood. Recently, we applied selective breeding for high or low alcohol drinking, yet conducted the selection during adolescence, and thus produced two replicas of rat lines (high and low adolescent ethanol drinking, ADHI and ADLO lines, respectively) that significantly differ in ethanol drinking at adolescence [43, 44]. The phenotypic assessment of the lines revealed greater and reduced sensitivity to the appetitive and aversive motivational effects of ethanol in ADHI vs. ADLO rats, respectively. More intriguing the adolescent ADHI rats exhibited, when compared to their ADLO counterparts, several signs of inborn anxiety, including taste neophobia, reduced level of exploratory behavior in an open field and reduced propensity to spend time in the white section of the LDB test [43]. They also exhibited greater neural activity in brain areas responsible for the processing of fear and aversive stimuli (e.g., amygdala, [45]) and, when tested in the MSCF test the ADHI rats spent exhibited greater shelter seeking and reduced time exploring the attractive yet potentially dangerous area of the bridge. Responsivity to stress was also greater in ADHI than in ADLO or nonselected Wistars. Specifically, when tested at adulthood, these three groups of rats exhibited fairly similar ethanol intake and preference scores. Yet, exposure to psychological (i.e., 5 sessions of restraint, 2 h each) stress was associated with a significant increase in ethanol intake and preference in ADHI, but not in ADLO or nonselected Wistars [44]. This suggests a synergistic effect between experimental stress and some innate trait of the ADHI rats, probably their relatively high level of inborn anxiety.

Drinking to Cope as a Mediator or Moderator in Clinical Studies

Theoretical Models of Drinking to Cope

Stress-dampening [46] and tension-reduction models of alcohol use [47] posit that individuals dealing with high levels of stress may use alcohol as a mean to alleviate that stress. Social Learning Theory [48] and the Self-Medication Hypothesis [49, 50] posit that some individuals engage in DTC expecting that drinking provides immediate coping benefits by alleviating their negative affect [51]. Based on these models, DTC may serve as a mediator through which more distal antecedents (e.g., negative affect) may relate to more alcohol consumption and problematic drinking.

Conversely, the Attention-Allocation Model [52] posits that in the absence of distractors, alcohol-induced impairment facilitates individuals to allocate their attention on the most salient internal or external cues (e.g., focusing on their negative mood or thoughts), which may exacerbate their negative affect and lead to more problematic alcohol consumption [53]. Thus, individuals who engage in high levels of DTC motives (compared to low) may be more prone to problematic drinking as a result of refocusing their attention on their reasons (i.e., stressors) for using alcohol as a coping mechanism. Further, behavioral models of addiction (e.g., cognitive-behavioral model of relapse [54]) posit that engaging in an unhealthy coping response (i.e., DTC) when dealing with stressors (e.g., sadness and anxiety) leads to increased probability of consuming that desired substance [55]. Based on these models, DTC motives may serve as a moderator between distal antecedents (e.g., depression and anxiety) and alcohol-related outcomes.

Drinking to Cope and Personality Dimensions

Cross-sectional research has indicated that conscientiousness (i.e., the tendency to be organized, self-controlled, task-and goal-oriented, and to follow norms/rules) relates to both decreased alcohol consumption [56] and ARC [57] via decreased reports of DTC motives. Neuroticism (i.e., the disposition to experience negative affect, including anxiety, anger, irritability, emotional instability, and depression) relates to increased alcohol consumption and ARC via increased reports of DTC motives [57, 58]. Further, research suggests that DTC motives mediate the associations between impulsivity and ARC [59, 60]. One longitudinal study examined, in a sample of freshman college students, changes in drinking motives (i.e., coping and enhancement) as explanatory mechanisms by which changes in personality relate to changes in alcohol problems [61]. Individuals who declined in impulsivity and neuroticism over time had reductions in alcohol problems via decreased DTC motives over time.

Cross-sectional findings suggest that DTC motives may mediate the associations between negative urgency—another dimension of impulsivity—and both alcohol consumption [62] and ARC [59]. In a sample of college athletes, sports-related alcohol coping motives have been found to mediate the relationship between trait urgency and alcohol consumption [63]. A longitudinal study [64] examined drinking motives as explanatory mechanisms by which four distinct personality constructs (i.e., hopelessness, anxiety sensitivity, impulsivity, and sensation-seeking) were associated with increased alcohol-related outcomes in drinking college students. At the between-subjects level, the researchers found that DTC-depression motives, while controlling for other drinking motives, uniquely mediated the association between hopelessness and ARC as well as impulsivity and ARC. Higher hopelessness and higher impulsivity predicted higher DTC-depression motives, which in turn uniquely predicted increased ARC.

Rather than examining DTC motives as a mediator, Stojek and Fischer [65] examined coping and enhancement motives as moderators of the established relationships between impulsivity-related constructs (i.e., negative urgency, positive urgency, lack of deliberation, lack of persistence, and sensation seeking) and AUD over a 3-month period in a sample of female college student drinkers. When controlling for other personality traits and drinking motives, they found a synergistic interaction between DTC motives and negative urgency, such that the harmful effect of negative urgency at baseline on AUD symptoms 3 months later (i.e., positive relationship) was stronger among women with higher DTC motives at baseline.

Conclusion of Personality Factors DTC motives appear to be one explanatory mechanism through which personality factors (i.e., neuroticism, impulsivity, negative urgency, hopelessness, and anxiety sensitivity) are related to both elevated reports of alcohol consumption and ARC among college student drinkers. Conscientiousness appears to be one protective personality factor that is associated with lower levels of problematic alcohol consumption via decreased DTC motives. Longitudinal studies have found that DTC motives may explain how changes in specific personality dimensions (e.g., impulsivity) relate to changes in alcohol problems [61, 64]. Because personality-targeted interventions that target how to cope with certain high-risk personality traits are effective at improving alcohol-related outcomes among adolescents [66], clinicians, and researchers who implement college alcohol interventions should examine whether these same principles apply to college students with high levels of negative urgency, impulsivity, and neuroticism.

Mental Health

Depression Cross-sectional findings suggest that DTC is one mechanism through which depressive symptoms (including suicidal ideation) is associated with increased alcohol consumption [67] and ARC [14, 48, 68, 69]. In one such longitudinal study, Kenney and colleagues

[70] found that, for women, higher pre-college depressive symptoms predicted higher DTC motives during college, which in turn were associated with more ARC during college. However, the association between pre-college depressive symptoms and *alcohol consumption* during college was not mediated by DTC motives. Pedrelli et al. [71] also found gender-specific pathways linking DTC motives with alcohol use and ARC. Curiously, the results were somewhat in a different direction. Specifically, DTC motives significantly mediated the path from depressive symptoms to ARC in both, men and women. However, the double mediated path, via DTC motives and heavy drinking (DTC → Heavy Drinking → ARC), was significant among women but not among men. Moreover, Foster et al. [72] found that, among women, the association between DTC motives and ARC was stronger at lower levels of depressive symptoms but, among men, this association was stronger at higher levels of depressive symptoms. Other variables seem to also affect these associations. Illustrating this point, Kenney et al. [73] found that DTC motives significantly mediated the relationship between depressive symptoms and ARC in the subsample of college students. However, and despite exhibiting similar levels of DTC motives and similar drinking outcomes, the mediational role of DTC motives was not significant among non-college emerging adults.

Rather than examining DTC motives as a mediator, Kelley and colleagues [74] found a synergistic interaction, such that the harmful effect of depressive symptoms on ARC was relatively stronger among women with high levels of DTC motives (compared to average or low levels). However, there have been mixed findings when longitudinally examining DTC motives as a moderator between depression and alcohol outcomes. Hussong [75] used survival analyses (28 days of daily diary data, n = 85 college students) to examine whether DTC motives and alcohol-related consequences moderated the relationship between depressed mood (i.e., sadness) and alcohol consumption within a time-to-drink model. She found that men with higher DTC motives were more likely to drink during the days immediately following elevated sadness (compared to men with low DTC motives). Among women, greater DTC motives and alcohol-related consequences were related to earlier drinking days after peak days of sadness.

Comparably, using multilevel modeling within a prospective study (using both daily and aggregate daily data; n = 530 drinking college students), Armeli et al. [76] found that the individuals with stronger DTC motives showed decreased drinking frequency during periods of high depressed mood. Further, the relationship between daily depressed mood and alcohol consumption did not differ by levels of DTC motivation. A similar finding has been found within a more recent longitudinal study [77], suggesting that the relationship between daily depressed mood and alcohol consumption does not differ by levels of global DTC motivation.

Anxiety Researchers have found cross-sectional support that DTC is one mechanism through which global anxiety symptoms [1, 14, 78] and social anxiety symptoms [79] are associated with alcohol outcomes. Moreover, the findings for social anxiety have been replicated and shown to vary by gender [80] and clinical levels of social anxiety [81]. Although these cross-sectional studies support these mediated effects, caution must be taken until these findings are replicated longitudinally.

Similar to depression, there have been mixed findings when longitudinally examining DTC motives as a moderator between anxiety and alcohol outcomes. In one longitudinal study, Armeli et al. [82] examined whether DTC motives moderated the relationship between weekly anxiety levels and alcohol consumption within a time-to-drink model (n = 458 college students; 30 days of daily diary data). They found that individuals with higher DTC motives (compared to lower DTC motives) initiated drinking relatively earlier during high (compared to low) anxiety weeks. In another longitudinal study,

Armeli et al. [83] longitudinally examined DTC motives as a moderator of the established relationships between depressive and anxiety symptoms and alcohol outcomes (n = 844 first year college student drinkers). A three-way interaction suggested that the harmful effect of anxiety on ARC was stronger among those with higher DTC motives and increased alcohol consumption.

However, other longitudinal studies have found that the relationship between *daily* anxiety and alcohol consumption does not differ by levels of DTC motivation [61, 76, 77]. For example, Littlefield et al. [84] found that the relationship between daily anxiety and alcohol consumption did not differ by levels of global DTC motivation. One explanation for these inconsistent findings may be that increased construct specificity for assessing DTC motives (e.g., DTC-anxiety motives) can better explain the relationships between different daily moods and alcohol consumption [18]. Moreover, contexts of substance use seem to affect these associations. Buckner and Terlecki [85] found that the association between social anxiety and ARC was affected by drinking contexts. Specifically, those with greater social anxiety are more likely to engage in solitary drinking which in turn was associated to greater drinking frequency and more ARC.

Stress In support of the stress-dampening [46] and tension-reduction models of alcohol use [47], cross-sectional studies suggest that stress relates to increased alcohol consumption and ARC via increased reports of DTC motives [86, 87]. These findings have been shown to be stronger for women [87] and for those with low restraint coping [86].

Conclusion of Mental Health As posited by self-medication models of alcohol use [49, 50], there is strong support for the notion that poor mental health leads to more alcohol consumption [88] and ARC [89] via DTC motives. Specifically, DTC motives may explain and exacerbate (at high levels) the relationships between poor mental health and ARC among college students.

Discussion

The chapter described the relationships among personality facets, mental health, DTC motives, and alcohol outcomes among emerging adult drinkers (particularly, college students). It also described works that attempt to analyze, using preclinical models that carefully control for genetic background, rearing and dietary environment, if anxiety-like behaviors can predict predisposition for ethanol intake.

Globally, there is strong support for the notion that DTC motives may explain and exacerbate (at high levels) the relationships between poor mental health, distinct personality factors, and risk factors to alcohol use and misuse among college students. The chapter highlights the impact DTC motives have as a maladaptive coping strategy. Specifically, individuals with poor mental health, high levels of impulsivity, anxiety sensitivity, negative urgency, and neuroticism, may engage in high levels of DTC, which may lead to and exacerbate ARC. Noteworthy, the preclinical work pinpointed that exacerbated anxiety—likely leading the rats to drink to reduce negative affect—maybe likely mechanisms by which notorious vulnerability factors for AUD (namely, PAE) exert their effects. Thus, for clinicians and researchers who implement college alcohol interventions, more targeted interventions to reduce the urge to use alcohol as a coping mechanism are needed. Future research should also examine what factors may decouple the relationship between negative emotional states and DTC motives because those associations put emerging adults, and particularly college students, at a heightened risk for problematic drinking.

Gaps in Knowledge

Theoretical Comparisons and Crosstalk Between Clinical and Preclinical Research A majority of theoretical models (e.g., Social Learning Theory, Self-medication Hypothesis, and tension-reduction models) were generally supported within the present review. However, there is a lack of research testing "competing" alcohol models against each other among college populations. According to competitive hypothesis testing [90], we can move the field forward by viewing theoretical models as consisting of a set of separable predictions as opposed to an unbreakable whole. For example, researchers may be able to test distinct theoretical pathways (e.g., alcohol expectancies vs. avoidant coping strategies) in order to identify which factors more strongly lead individuals to use alcohol as a coping mechanism when dealing with stressors. More comparative theory research, especially longitudinal studies using competitive hypotheses testing, is needed to advance the field. Moreover, little interplay was detected between clinical and preclinical research. Clinical research would benefit from the identification of endophenotypes carefully laid out by pre-clinical research. A major roadblock in the interaction between clinical and preclinical research is the apparent incommensurability of tasks employed by each, yet there are some promising avenues. For instance, the Delay-discounting and the 5-choice serial reaction time tasks [91] offer alternatives to test impulsivity in rodents that are both analogous and homologous to those employed to measure such personality factor in humans.

Operationalization of DTC Motives The problem of how to operationalize some of the constructs discussed also arises in the clinical research. Although DTC motives are most commonly operationalized as a single construct [16], an increasing number of studies have distinguished between DTC-depression motives and DTC-anxiety motives [18]. Although some studies have attempted to validate distinguishing these motives [92], some have found a strong enough overlap between them to warrant combining them into a single index (e.g., $r = 0.76$ [93]). On the one hand, if there are differential effects on alcohol-related outcomes depending on the specific affect motivating DTC [57], examining DTC motives as a single construct may obscure the true relationships between DTC motives and alcohol-related outcomes. On the other hand, if there are significant recall biases into the retrospective recall of the specific affective states motivating DTC, differences found between specific types of DTC motives and alcohol-related outcomes may be little more than chance variation [14].

The current common operationalizations of drinking motives stem from the Cox-Klinger motivational model of alcohol use [23], which distinguishes between drinking to modulate positive vs. negative mood (i.e., enhancement vs. coping motives). However, more recent ecological momentary assessment (EMA) studies have been able to examine the near real-time associations between various specific affective states and alcohol-related outcomes beyond depression and anxiety (e.g., fear, guilt, hostility, and sadness [94]). Therefore, at least in the context of EMA studies, it may be prudent to further distinguish DTC motives by more specific affective states. Empirical work is needed to determine the degree to which DTC motives should be examined more generally (i.e., overall DTC motives) or specific to distinct affective states.

Assessment and Sex Bias Other primary issues are the reliance of using long-term retrospective self-report measures (i.e., past 30 days, past 90 days, etc.) in clinical studies, and the focus in males only, in preclinical studies. Recall bias for alcohol consumption is significant as evidenced by the declining accuracy of reports on consumption over just 1 week [95]. One way to overcome recall bias is using prospective studies using daily diary or ecological momentary assessment methods [65]. These approaches would conceptually provide more accurate accounts of how DTC motives, distal antecedents, and alcohol outcomes interrelate among college students. Importantly, some studies using these methods have found inconsistent results between how DTC motives, negative mood and alcohol outcomes interrelate over weekly [76] and daily assessments [88].

The use of only male rats or mice is, in turn, a major problem of preclinical research. This is a chronic problem, despite recommendations of funding agencies to include individuals of either sexes or the methodological reassurance that, if the designs are adequately powered, the variations in estrous cycle should not obscure the variability associated with the phenomena under analysis.

Future Directions

Given these gaps in the literature, future studies are needed to replicate many of the cross-sectional and experimental studies within the present chapter, to use new methods in assessing how DTC motives interrelate with personality dimensions, mental health, and alcohol outcomes, and to use methods that allow significant cross-talk between clinical and preclinical studies. Studies should focus on who is most susceptible to higher DTC motives, when individuals are more likely to engage in DTC motives, and what factors may reduce the role DTC motives has on the relationships between distal antecedents.

Who Identifying who is most susceptible to use alcohol as a coping mechanism would provide critical information for clinicians and researchers who implement brief interventions. Specifically, it would be useful to identify which college students are at a particular risk of escalated levels of DTC because DTC motives exacerbate the relationships between personality dimensions and alcohol outcomes, as well as mental health and alcohol outcomes. For example, numerous studies in the present review found that the relationships between both mental health and personality dimensions on alcohol outcomes through DTC motives was significant only among women [80, 87, 89]. Some studies have already examined the role that DTC motives have on specific subpopulations of college students, such as American students studying abroad [96] or student athletes [97]. However, these studies are not as prevalent. Similarly, preclinical studies should advance from describing how inborn anxiety is associated with greater ethanol intake to studies inquiring how double or triple-hits (i.e., ethanol drinking in rats exhibiting high or low innate anxiety exposed to paternal negligence followed by stress exposure) affect the outcome under analysis.

Further research is also needed to examine whether the associations between distal antecedents, DTC motives and alcohol outcomes are conditional upon subsamples of drinkers. For example, in one cross-sectional study, Goldsmith and colleagues [78] found that increased generalized anxiety is associated with increased negative-affect heavy drinking via subtypes of alcohol expectancies (i.e., tension-reduction and worry-reduction) and DTC motives. Further, invariance analyses across subsamples of non-hazardous and hazardous drinkers (identified by a cut-off score ≥ 8 on the Alcohol Use Disorders Identification Test) revealed that the indirect effects were stronger among hazardous drinkers compared to non-hazardous drinkers. Thus, future studies should attempt to implement multi-group analyses to examine whether their findings are noninvariant across not only gender, but also across other subsamples of college students, especially type of drinkers.

When Examining when individuals are more likely to engage in DTC might provide important information for future EMA intervention studies. For example, research using daily diary studies [83] revealed that individuals engaging in high DTC motive levels leads to drink larger amounts in risky drinking contexts (e.g., drinking alone). Further, research has shown that using hazard and survival analysis models trying to pinpoint when (e.g., time of day as well as day of the week) students engage in alcohol consumption [77] might be extended to determining when students are more likely to engage in DTC. Preclinical work has also shown that the drinking differences between adolescent and adults are exacerbated when testing takes place during the first hours of the dark cycle. For instance, Wille-Bille et al. [98] reported greater ethanol drinking in adult vs. adolescent Wistar rats, when tested in lengthy 18-h two bottle tests. Yet, ethanol drinking was dramatically greater in adolescent than in adults (3.0 g/kg vs 1.25 g/kg) when testing took place in the first 2 h of the dark cycle and a single bottle was provided [99]. These future studies would be beneficial for prevention or intervention studies, such that those interventions may give personalized feedback and/or alternative coping methods in the moment to deter students from using alcohol as a coping mechanism.

What Examining what factors may reduce the role DTC motives have on the relationships between distal antecedents, especially poor mental health and alcohol outcomes is especially needed. Behavioral models of addiction posit that engaging in an effective coping response instead of an ineffective coping response (i.e., DTC) leads to a decreased probability of consuming a desired substance [100]. Thus, research is needed to examine adaptive coping strategies that may decouple the associations between negative emotional states and DTC in order to reduce ARC among college students.

Concluding Remarks

The present chapter attempted to disentangle how distal antecedents (i.e., personality dimensions and mental health) relate to alcohol outcomes via DTC motives and why using alcohol as a coping mechanism places college student drinker at risk for heavier, more problematic drinking. Specifically, we examined recent literature summarizing the role of DTC motives as a process variable (i.e., mediator) or conditional variable (i.e., moderator) between both mental health and personality dimensions on alcohol-related outcomes. We also revised preclinical studies that assessed how innate differences in anxiety-like behaviors may serve as an endophenotype predicting exacerbated ethanol intake or how increased anxiety seems to be a common mediator or mechanisms by which genetic or environmental factors provide vulnerability for such exacerbated ethanol intake, with a focus in animal models of adolescence.

Among college students, the literature has found strong support for DTC motives as a primary mechanism through which psychosocial constructs relate to problematic alcohol use and problems. Moreover, longitudinal studies have supported the notion that engaging in high levels of DTC motives puts student drinkers at a heightened risk for ARC even when controlling for alcohol consumption. Given that "college years" are a critical development period and brief alcohol interventions have become popular to disseminate among college students, it is important for clinicians and researchers to focus on mechanisms to deter student drinkers from engaging in high levels of DTC motives because it is associated with more ARC and consumption. Overall, the present chapter should highlight that college student and young adult drinkers are a critical population that deserves special attention.

References

1. Bravo AJ, Pilatti A, Pearson MR, Read JP, Mezquita L, Ibáñez MI, et al. Cross-cultural examination of negative alcohol-related consequences: measurement invariance of the Young adult alcohol consequences questionnaire in Spain, Argentina, and USA. Psychol Assess. 2019;31(5):631–42.
2. Tavolacci MP, Berthon Q, Cerasuolo D, Dechelotte P, Ladner J, Baguet A. Does binge drinking between the age of 18 and 25 years predict alcohol dependence in adulthood? A retrospective case-control study in France. BMJ Open. 2019;9(5):e026375.
3. Ducci F, Goldman D. Genetic approaches to addiction: genes and alcohol. Addiction. 2008;103(9):1414–28.
4. Quertemont E. Genetic polymorphism in ethanol metabolism: acetaldehyde contribution to alcohol abuse and alcoholism. Mol Psychiatry. 2004;9(6):570–81.
5. Dawson DA, Grant BF, Li TK. Impact of age at first drink on stress-reactive drinking. Alcohol Clin Exp Res. 2007;31(1):69–77.
6. van Kruijsdijk RCM, Visseren FLJ, Ridker PM, Dorresteijn JAN, Buring JE, van der Graaf Y, et al. Individualised prediction of alternate-day aspirin treatment effects on the combined risk of cancer, cardiovascular disease and gastrointestinal bleeding in healthy women. Heart. 2015;101(5):369.
7. Mitchell SH. Linking delay discounting and substance use disorders: genotypes and phenotypes. Perspect Behav Sci. 2019;42(3):419–32.
8. Caneto F, Pautassi RM, Pilatti A. Ethanol-induced autonomic responses and risk taking increase in young adults with a positive family history of alcohol problems. Addict Behav. 2018;76:174–81.

9. Pautassi RM, Nizhnikov ME, Spear NE. Assessing appetitive, aversive, and negative ethanol-mediated reinforcement through an immature rat model. Neurosci Biobehav Rev. 2009;33(6):953–74.
10. William Gerin MJZ, Jos F. Brosschot, Julian F. Thayer, Nicholas J. S. Christenfeld, Tavis S. Campbell, Joshua M. Smyth. Rumination as a Mediator of Chronic Stress Effects on Hypertension: A Causal Model. International Journal of Hypertension. 2012;2012.
11. Pearson MR. Use of alcohol protective behavioral strategies among college students: a critical review. Clin Psychol Rev. 2013;33(8):1025–40.
12. Prince MA, Carey KB, Maisto SA. Protective behavioral strategies for reducing alcohol involvement: a review of the methodological issues. Addict Behav. 2013;38(7):2343–51.
13. Bravo AJ, Prince MA, Pearson MR. A multiple replication examination of distal antecedents to alcohol protective behavioral strategies. J Stud Alcohol Drugs. 2016;77(6):958–67.
14. Bravo AJ, Pearson MR. In the process of drinking to cope among college students: an examination of specific vs. global coping motives for depression and anxiety symptoms. Addict Behav. 2017;73:94–8.
15. Bravo AJ, Weinstein AP, Pearson MR. Protective strategies study T. The relationship between risk factors and alcohol and marijuana use outcomes among concurrent users: a comprehensive examination of protective behavioral strategies. J Stud Alcohol Drugs. 2019;80(1):102–8.
16. Cooper ML. Motivations for alcohol use among adolescents: development and validation of a four-factor model. Psychol Assess. 1994;6(2):117–28.
17. Cooper ML, Kuntsche E, Levitt A, Barber LL, Wolf S. Motivational models of substance use: a review of theory and research on motives for using alcohol, marijuana, and tobacco. The Oxford handbook of substance use and substance use disorders, Oxford library of psychology, vol. 1. New York: Oxford University Press; 2016. p. 375–421.
18. Grant VV, Stewart SH, O'Connor RM, Blackwell E, Conrod PJ. Psychometric evaluation of the five-factor modified drinking motives questionnaire—revised in undergraduates. Addict Behav. 2007;32(11):2611–32.
19. MacKinnon DP, Krull JL, Lockwood CM. Equivalence of the mediation, confounding and suppression effect. Prevent Sci. 2000;1(4):173–81.
20. Pilatti A, Read JP, Pautassi RM. ELSA 2016 cohort: alcohol, tobacco, and marijuana use and their association with age of drug use onset, risk perception, and social norms in Argentinean college freshmen. Front Psychol. 2017;8:1452.
21. Lynskey MT, Agrawal A. Denise Kandel's classic work on the gateway sequence of drug acquisition. Addiction. 2018;113(10):1927–32.
22. King KM, Chassin L. A prospective study of the effects of age of initiation of alcohol and drug use on young adult substance dependence. J Stud Alcohol Drugs. 2007;68(2):256–65.
23. Cox WM, Klinger E. A motivational model of alcohol use. J Abnorm Psychol. 1988;97(2):168–80.
24. Kuntsche E, Knibbe R, Gmel G, Engels R. Why do young people drink? A review of drinking motives. Clin Psychol Rev. 2005;25(7):841–61.
25. Patrick ME, Schulenberg JE, O'Malley PM. High school substance use as a predictor of college attendance, completion, and dropout: a National Multi-cohort Longitudinal Study. Youth Soc. 2016;48(3):425–47.
26. Riordan BC, Carey KB. Wonderland and the rabbit hole: a commentary on university students' alcohol use during first year and the early transition to university. Drug Alcohol Rev. 2019;38(1):34–41.
27. Acevedo MB, Fabio MC, Fernandez MS, Pautassi RM. Anxiety response and restraint-induced stress differentially affect ethanol intake in female adolescent rats. Neuroscience. 2016;334:259–74.
28. Primeaux SD, Wilson SP, Bray GA, York DA, Wilson MA. Overexpression of neuropeptide Y in the central nucleus of the amygdala decreases ethanol self-administration in "anxious" rats. Alcohol Clin Exp Res. 2006;30(5):791–801.
29. Izidio GS, Ramos A. Positive association between ethanol consumption and anxiety-related behaviors in two selected rat lines. Alcohol. 2007;41(7):517–24.
30. Lopez MB, Filippetti VA, Cremonte M. Alcohol consumption before and during pregnancy in Argentina: prevalence and risk factors. Revista panamericana de salud publica (Pan Am J Public Health). 2015;37(4–5):211–7.
31. Baer JS, Sampson PD, Barr HM, Connor PD, Streissguth AP. A 21-year longitudinal analysis of the effects of prenatal alcohol exposure on young adult drinking. Arch Gen Psychiatry. 2003;60(4):377–85.
32. Diaz MR, Johnson JM, Varlinskaya EI. Increased ethanol intake is associated with social anxiety in offspring exposed to ethanol on gestational day 12. Behav Brain Res. 2020;393:112766.
33. Wille-Bille A, Miranda-Morales RS, Pucci M, Bellia F, D'Addario C, Pautassi RM. Prenatal ethanol induces an anxiety phenotype and alters expression of dynorphin & nociceptin/orphanin FQ genes. Prog Neuro-Psychopharmacol Biol Psychiatry. 2018;85:77–88.
34. Roman E, Meyerson BJ, Hyytia P, Nylander I. The multivariate concentric square field test reveals different behavioural profiles in male AA and ANA rats with regard to risk taking and environmental reactivity. Behav Brain Res. 2007;183(2):195–205.
35. Meyerson BJ, Augustsson H, Berg M, Roman E. The Concentric Square field: a multivariate test arena for analysis of explorative strategies. Behav Brain Res. 2006;168(1):100–13.
36. Wille-Bille A, Bellia F, Jimenez Garcia AM, Miranda-Morales RS, D'Addario C, Pautassi RM. Early exposure to environmental enrichment

modulates the effects of prenatal ethanol exposure upon opioid gene expression and adolescent ethanol intake. Neuropharmacology. 2020;165:107917.

37. Bell RL, Sable HJ, Colombo G, Hyytia P, Rodd ZA, Lumeng L. Animal models for medications development targeting alcohol abuse using selectively bred rat lines: neurobiological and pharmacological validity. Pharmacol Biochem Behav. 2012;103(1):119–55.
38. Stewart RB, Murphy JM, McBride WJ, Lumeng L, Li TK. Place conditioning with alcohol in alcohol-preferring and -nonpreferring rats. Pharmacol Biochem Behav. 1996;53(3):487–91.
39. Stewart RB, Gatto GJ, Lumeng L, Li TK, Murphy JM. Comparison of alcohol-preferring (P) and nonpreferring (np) rats on tests of anxiety and for the anxiolytic effects of ethanol. Alcohol. 1993;10(1):1–10.
40. Richter RM, Zorrilla EP, Basso AM, Koob GF, Weiss F. Altered amygdalar CRF release and increased anxiety-like behavior in sardinian alcohol-preferring rats: a microdialysis and behavioral study. Alcohol Clin Exp Res. 2000;24(12):1765–72.
41. Colombo G, Lobina C, Carai MAM, Gessa GL. Phenotypic characterization of genetically selected Sardinian alcohol-preferring (sP) and -non-preferring (sNP) rats. Addict Biol. 2006;11(3/4):324–38.
42. Ciccocioppo R, Economidou D, Cippitelli A, Cucculelli M, Ubaldi M, Soverchia L, et al. Genetically selected Marchigian Sardinian alcohol-preferring (msP) rats: an animal model to study the neurobiology of alcoholism. Addict Biol. 2006;11(3/4):339–55.
43. Fernandez MS, Baez B, Bordon A, Espinosa L, Martinez E, Pautassi RM. Short-term selection for high and low ethanol intake yields differential sensitivity to ethanol's motivational effects and anxiety-like responses in adolescent Wistar rats. Progr Neuro Psychopharmacol Biol Psychiatry. 2017;79(Pt B):220–33.
44. Fernandez MS, Bellia F, Ferreyra A, Chiner F, Jimenez Garcia AM, D'Addario C, et al. Short-term selection for high and low ethanol intake during adolescence exerts lingering effects in stress-induced ethanol drinking and yields an anxiety-prone phenotype. Behav Brain Res. 2020;380:112445.
45. Fernandez MS, Ferreyra A, de Olmos S, Pautassi RM. The offspring of rats selected for high or low ethanol intake at adolescence exhibit differential ethanol-induced Fos immunoreactivity in the central amygdala and in nucleus accumbens core. Pharmacol Biochem Behav. 2019;176:6–15.
46. Sher KJ, Levenson RW. Risk for alcoholism and individual differences in the stress-response-dampening effect of alcohol. J Abnorm Psychol. 1982;91(5):350–67.
47. Greeley J, Oei T. Alcohol and tension reduction. Psychological theories of drinking and alcoholism, The Guilford substance abuse series. 2nd ed. New York: The Guilford Press; 1999. p. 14–53.
48. Maisto SA, Carey KB, Bradizza CM. Social learning theory. Psychological theories of drinking and alcoholism, The Guilford substance abuse series. 2nd ed. New York: The Guilford Press; 1999. p. 106–63.
49. Conger JJ. Alcoholism: theory, problem and challenge. II. Reinforcement theory and the dynamics of alcoholism. Q J Stud Alcohol. 1956;17(2):296–305.
50. Khantzian EJ. The self-medication hypothesis of substance use disorders: a reconsideration and recent applications. Harv Rev Psychiatry. 1997;4(5):231–44.
51. Cooper ML, Russell M, George WH. Coping, expectancies, and alcohol abuse: a test of social learning formulations. J Abnorm Psychol. 1988;97(2):218–30.
52. Steele CM, Josephs RA. Alcohol myopia. Its prized and dangerous effects. Am Psychol. 1990;45(8):921–33.
53. Merrill JE, Read JP. Motivational pathways to unique types of alcohol consequences. Psychol Addict Behav. 2010;24(4):705–11.
54. Larimer ME, Palmer RS, Marlatt GA. Relapse prevention. An overview of Marlatt's cognitive-behavioral model. Alcohol Res Health. 1999;23(2):151–60.
55. Bowen S, Chawla N, Collins SE, Witkiewitz K, Hsu S, Grow J, et al. Mindfulness-based relapse prevention for substance use disorders: a pilot efficacy trial. Subst Abus. 2009;30(4):295–305.
56. Kuntsche E, Stewart SH, Cooper ML. How stable is the motive-alcohol use link? A cross-national validation of the drinking motives questionnaire revised among adolescents from Switzerland, Canada, and the United States. J Stud Alcohol Drugs. 2008;69(3):388–96.
57. Mezquita L, Stewart SH, Ruipérez MÁ. Big-five personality domains predict internal drinking motives in young adults. Personal Individ Differ. 2010;49(3):240–5.
58. Mezquita L, Bravo AJ, Ortet G, Pilatti A, Pearson MR, Ibáñez MI. Cross-cultural examination of different personality pathways to alcohol use and misuse in emerging adulthood. Drug Alcohol Depend. 2018;192:193–200.
59. Adams ZW, Kaiser AJ, Lynam DR, Charnigo RJ, Milich R. Drinking motives as mediators of the impulsivity-substance use relation: pathways for negative urgency, lack of premeditation, and sensation seeking. Addict Behav. 2012;37(7):848–55.
60. Magid V, Maclean MG, Colder CR. Differentiating between sensation seeking and impulsivity through their mediated relations with alcohol use and problems. Addict Behav. 2007;32(10):2046–61.
61. Littlefield AK, Sher KJ, Wood PK. Do changes in drinking motives mediate the relation between personality change and "maturing out" of problem drinking? J Abnorm Psychol. 2010;119(1):93–105.

62. Coskunpinar A, Cyders MA. Mediation-moderation analysis of problematic alcohol use: the roles of urgency, drinking motives, and risk/benefit perception. Addict Behav. 2012;37(7):880–3.
63. Martens MP, Pedersen ER, Smith AE, Stewart SH, O'Brien K. Predictors of alcohol-related outcomes in college athletes: the roles of trait urgency and drinking motives. Addict Behav. 2011;36(5):456–64.
64. Mackinnon SP, Kehayes IL, Clark R, Sherry SB, Stewart SH. Testing the four-factor model of personality vulnerability to alcohol misuse: a three-wave, one-year longitudinal study. Psychol Addict Behav. 2014;28(4):1000–12.
65. Stojek M, Fischer S. Impulsivity and motivations to consume alcohol: a prospective study on risk of dependence in young adult women. Alcohol Clin Exp Res. 2013;37(2):292–9.
66. Conrod PJ, Castellanos-Ryan N, Mackie C. Long-term effects of a personality-targeted intervention to reduce alcohol use in adolescents. J Consult Clin Psychol. 2011;79(3):296–306.
67. Gonzalez VM, Bradizza CM, Collins RL. Drinking to cope as a statistical mediator in the relationship between suicidal ideation and alcohol outcomes among underage college drinkers. Psychol Addict Behav. 2009;23(3):443–51.
68. Bravo AJ, Pearson MR, Baumgardner SF. The relationship between negative affect and alcohol and marijuana use outcomes among dual users. Subst Use Misuse. 2020;55(4):658–65.
69. Gonzalez VM, Reynolds B, Skewes MC. Role of impulsivity in the relationship between depression and alcohol problems among emerging adult college drinkers. Exp Clin Psychopharmacol. 2011;19(4):303–13.
70. Kenney S, Jones RN, Barnett NP. Gender differences in the effect of depressive symptoms on prospective alcohol expectancies, coping motives, and alcohol outcomes in the first year of college. J Youth Adolesc. 2015;44(10):1884–97.
71. Pedrelli P, Collado A, Shapero BG, Brill C, MacPherson L. Different pathways explain alcohol-related problems in female and male college students. J Am Coll Health. 2016;64(7):535–44.
72. Foster DW, Young CM, Steers M, Quist MC, Bryan JL, Neighbors C. Tears in your beer: gender differences in coping drinking motives, depressive symptoms and drinking. Int J Ment Health Addict. 2014;12(6):730–46.
73. Kenney SR, Anderson BJ, Stein MD. Drinking to cope mediates the relationship between depression and alcohol risk: different pathways for college and non-college young adults. Addict Behav. 2018;80:116–23.
74. Kelley ML, Linden AN, Milletich RJ, Lau-Barraco C, Kurtz ED, D'Lima GM, et al. Self and partner alcohol-related problems among ACOAs and non-ACOAs: associations with depressive symptoms and motivations for alcohol use. Addict Behav. 2014;39(1):211–8.
75. Hussong AM. Predictors of drinking immediacy following daily sadness: an application of survival analysis to experience sampling data. Addict Behav. 2007;32(5):1054–65.
76. Armeli S, Conner TS, Cullum J, Tennen H. A longitudinal analysis of drinking motives moderating the negative affect-drinking association among college students. Psychol Addict Behav. 2010;24(1):38–47.
77. O'Hara RE, Armeli S, Tennen H. Drinking-to-cope motivation and negative mood-drinking contingencies in a daily diary study of college students. J Stud Alcohol Drugs. 2014;75(4):606–14.
78. Goldsmith AA, Tran GQ, Smith JP, Howe SR. Alcohol expectancies and drinking motives in college drinkers: mediating effects on the relationship between generalized anxiety and heavy drinking in negative-affect situations. Addict Behav. 2009;34(6):505–13.
79. Villarosa-Hurlocker MC, Bravo AJ, Pearson MR. The relationship between social anxiety and alcohol and marijuana use outcomes among concurrent users: a motivational model of substance use. Alcohol Clin Exp Res. 2019;43(4):732–40.
80. Norberg MM, Norton AR, Olivier J, Zvolensky MJ. Social anxiety, reasons for drinking, and college students. Behav Ther. 2010;41(4):555–66.
81. Terlecki MA, Buckner JD. Social anxiety and heavy situational drinking: coping and conformity motives as multiple mediators. Addict Behav. 2015;40:77–83.
82. Armeli S, Todd M, Conner TS, Tennen H. Drinking to cope with negative moods and the immediacy of drinking within the weekly cycle among college students. J Stud Alcohol Drugs. 2008;69(2):313–22.
83. Armeli S, O'Hara RE, Ehrenberg E, Sullivan TP, Tennen H. Episode-specific drinking-to-cope motivation, daily mood, and fatigue-related symptoms among college students. J Stud Alcohol Drugs. 2014;75(5):766–74.
84. Littlefield AK, Talley AE, Jackson KM. Coping motives, negative moods, and time-to-drink: exploring alternative analytic models of coping motives as a moderator of daily mood-drinking covariation. Addict Behav. 2012;37(12):1371–6.
85. Buckner JD, Terlecki MA. Social anxiety and alcohol-related impairment: the mediational impact of solitary drinking. Addict Behav. 2016;58:7–11.
86. Corbin WR, Farmer NM, Nolen-Hoekesma S. Relations among stress, coping strategies, coping motives, alcohol consumption and related problems: a mediated moderation model. Addict Behav. 2013;38(4):1912–9.
87. Rice KG, Van Arsdale AC. Perfectionism, perceived stress, drinking to cope, and alcohol-related problems among college students. J Couns Psychol. 2010;57(4):439–50.
88. Dvorak RD, Pearson MR, Day AM. Ecological momentary assessment of acute alcohol use disorder symptoms: associations with mood, motives, and use on planned drinking days. Exp Clin Psychopharmacol. 2014;22(4):285–97.

89. Kenney SR, Lac A, Labrie JW, Hummer JF, Pham A. Mental health, sleep quality, drinking motives, and alcohol-related consequences: a path-analytic model. J Stud Alcohol Drugs. 2013;74(6):841–51.
90. Brewer NT, Gilkey MB. Comparing theories of health behavior using data from longitudinal studies: a comment on Gerend and shepherd. Ann Behav Med. 2012;44(2):147–8.
91. Dalley JW, Mar AC, Economidou D, Robbins TW. Neurobehavioral mechanisms of impulsivity: fronto-striatal systems and functional neurochemistry. Pharmacol Biochem Behav. 2008;90(2):250–60.
92. Grant VV, Stewart SH, Mohr CD. Coping-anxiety and coping-depression motives predict different daily mood-drinking relationships. Psychol Addict Behav. 2009;23(2):226–37.
93. Roos CR, Pearson MR, Brown DB. Drinking motives mediate the negative associations between mindfulness facets and alcohol outcomes among college students. Psychol Addict Behav. 2015;29(1):176–83.
94. Hussong AM, Hicks RE, Levy SA, Curran PJ. Specifying the relations between affect and heavy alcohol use among young adults. J Abnorm Psychol. 2001;110(3):449–61.
95. Ekholm O. Influence of the recall period on self-reported alcohol intake. Eur J Clin Nutr. 2004;58(1):60–3.
96. Pedersen ER, Neighbors C, Lee CM, Larimer ME. Not all those who wander are lost: examining the impact of sojourner adjustment and drinking motives on alcohol consequences experienced by Americans studying in foreign countries. J Stud Alcohol Drugs. 2012;73(6):1005–15.
97. Doumas DM. Alcohol-related consequences among intercollegiate student athletes: the role of drinking motives. J Addict Offender Couns. 2013;34(1):51–64.
98. Wille-Bille A, de Olmos S, Marengo L, Chiner F, Pautassi RM. Long-term ethanol self-administration induces DeltaFosB in male and female adolescent, but not in adult, Wistar rats. Prog Neuro-Psychopharmacol Biol Psychiatry. 2017;74:15–30.
99. Salguero A, Suarez A, Luque M, Ruiz-Leyva L, Cendan CM, Moron I, et al. Binge-like, naloxone-sensitive, voluntary ethanol intake at adolescence is greater than at adulthood, but does not exacerbate subsequent two-bottle choice drinking. Front Behav Neurosci. 2020;14:50.
100. Grant S, Colaiaco B, Motala A, Shanman R, Booth M, Sorbero M, et al. Mindfulness-based relapse prevention for substance use disorders: a systematic review and meta-analysis. J Addict Med. 2017;11(5):386–96.

Exploring the Neurobiology of Ethanol Relapse and Its Prevention Using N-Acetylcysteine

46

Sandra Fernández-Rodríguez, M. José Cano-Cebrián, Ana Polache, and Teodoro Zornoza

Introduction

The latest World Health Organization report "Global Status Report on Alcohol and Health" stated that 5.1% of the adult population worldwide suffered from alcohol use disorder (AUD) and around 3 million persons had died in 2016 due to ethanol misuse [1]. Relapse is one of the most severe issues of this psychopathological condition. Repeated ethanol intake produces persistent neuroadaptations in key brain circuits that promote this susceptibility to return to drug use following abstinence. These neurobiological changes that persist over time lead patients to relapse in alcohol consumption even after several months or years of abstinence [2, 3]. Unfortunately, nowadays there are no completely successful pharmacotherapies available to prevent ethanol relapse or at least reduce alcohol intake. In fact, relapse rates remain high even for people receiving currently available treatments [4]. Although in the last decade, a large number of studies have investigated the neurobiological mechanisms involved in the various phases of AUD, there are still gaps lingering in the literature. Abstinence represents a critical period of vulnerability within the addiction cycle, and the consecutive alterations of chronic ethanol abstinence remain poorly understood. Recently, some authors have pointed out the need of unraveling molecular mechanisms linked to relapse in vulnerable individuals [5]. These findings would have the potential to improve AUD treatments. For this purpose, preclinical models focused on alcohol relapse are an invaluable tool, which will be presented and discussed herein. Subsequently, data derived from the application of the alcohol deprivation effect (ADE) model in our laboratory are presented. According to the obtained results, it was possible to distinguish two different subpopulations of rats based on their vulnerability against ethanol relapse behavior. Both subpopulations allowed us to differentially explore the molecular mechanisms associated to relapse vulnerability and its neurobiology.

Preclinical Models to Study Alcohol Relapse-Like Behavior

There are two groups of commonly accepted experimental models that allow the analysis of the efficacy of potential antirelapse pharmacotherapies: the so-called reinstatement models and the models that use the assessment of the phe-

S. Fernández-Rodríguez · M. J. Cano-Cebrián · A. Polache (✉) · T. Zornoza
Department of Pharmacy and Pharmaceutical Technology and Parasitology, Faculty of Pharmacy, University of Valencia, Valencia, Spain
e-mail: sanfero5@uv.es; Maria.Jose.Cano@uv.es; ana.polache@uv.es; teodoro.zornoza@uv.es

P. Á. Gargiulo, H. L. Mesones-Arroyo (eds.), *Psychiatry and Neuroscience Update – Vol. V*,
https://doi.org/10.1007/978-3-031-72219-6_46

nomenon so-called alcohol deprivation effect (ADE), in animals with long-term experience in ethanol consumption.

Reinstatement models are operant self-administration models in which the animal, during a first phase called *conditioning*, learns to perform a certain task, such as manipulating what is called an operand (for example, pressing a lever), in order to obtain the drug. In this learning or conditioning phase, the manipulation of the operand is associated with the obtaining of the drug, but is also often associated with the presentation of a visual stimulus (for example, a light) or sound (a certain sound of a specific frequency). After reaching stable ethanol consumption, due to the stable manipulation of the operand, animals are subjected to an *extinction phase*, in which the manipulation of the operand is no longer associated with drug availability and, consequently, the animal stops performing the task. After extinction, the experimenter places the animal in different situations and/or stimuli that had previously been paired with the drug experience during the conditioning phase. The researcher can evaluate whether the animal reinstates the operand manipulation response even without the presence of the drug: this is the so-called *reinstatement phase*. Three types of situations or stimuli are normally used to trigger drug-seeking behavior: cues or environmental stimuli (which had previously been associated with the reinforcing effects of the drug), the administration of a noncontingent small dose of the drug (priming effect) or situations of stress [6]. The advantage of these procedures is that the experimenter can vary the complexity of the response that the animal must perform in order to obtain the drug. Hence, in the context of ethanol research, the animal's degree of motivation to seek alcohol can be evaluated [7]. There are many authors who consider reinstatement patterns to be a good indicator of drug seeking and relapse to alcohol use [8, 9]. In this sense, the currently most widely used antirelapse drugs for the treatment of alcoholism, acamprosat and naltrexone are capable of suppressing reinstatement after an extinction phase [10, 11]. This fact justifies the predictive validity of this preclinical model.

However, relapse can be defined as a return to alcohol consumption after a period of abstinence. Therefore, other authors consider reinstatement a valid model for the study of drug-seeking behavior but not for the study of relapse, since: i) there is no period of withdrawal itself (the animal continues to perform the same tasks to obtain the drug, even if it does not succeed) and ii) the animal does not receive the drug during the reinstatement phase, so the psychoactive effects associated with its intake do not occur [6, 12]. For this reason, this type of model lacks of construct validity, i.e. its resemblance of human behavior is limited.

There is another preclinical model of alcohol relapse in which the ADE phenomenon is evaluated. ADE is a temporary increase in alcohol consumption that occurs after a period or periods of forced abstinence. It was first described in rats by Sinclair and Senter in 1967 [13]. Animals that had had voluntary access to ethanol for a prolonged period showed a significant and transient increase in drug intake after a period of forced deprivation. Since this study was published, ADE has been described not only in rats [14, 15] but also in mice [16], monkeys [17] and in humans [18]. The ADE phenomenon has been identified not only under non-operant continuous voluntary alcohol drinking procedures but also under intermittent procedures as well as under operant self-administration paradigms [19]. All in all, this ADE-based model is probably one of the most commonly used preclinical approaches to study the ethanol relapse-like drinking behavior, due to its face, predictive and ecological validity [20]. This animal model encompasses the entire range of the addiction cycle, including acquisition and maintenance of drug taking, withdrawal, and craving during periods of drug abstinence and ultimately relapse. These processes are repeated several times in this experimental model [21]. The predictive value of this experimental approach is best illustrated by the fact that the latest approved medications for alcohol relapse prevention -acamprosate and naltrexone- were developed by means of adequate animal models, more concretely this particular ADE model, and then translated into a clinical setting [20]. This pharmacological validation has provided predictive validity to the ADE model in relation to the search for new and better drugs in the treatment of ethanol intake relapse.

Nonetheless, it is necessary to take into consideration that this model differs in certain aspects from the usual situation in humans. For instance, one of the few limitations of this animal model could be that the abstinence is not freely chosen by the rat, i.e., the withdrawal period is not under the control of the animal. Hence, the model serves to characterize the return to alcohol consumption because of the reexposure to the drug, while the motivation that, in humans, precedes the drug seeking is not fully analyzed. Thus, recently new rat models of relapse after voluntary abstinence (achieved either by introducing adverse consequences to drug taking or seeking or by providing mutually exclusive choices between the self-administered drug and nondrug rewards) are being developed. Nevertheless, at present it is not known whether the use of these novel models will improve the predictive validity of classical relapse models as, to date, there are no published reports showing their postdictive validity using approved medications [22].

Despite the above-commented drawbacks, the ADE-based model has become a widely used paradigm for studying the efficacy of new drugs that could potentially be useful in the relapse treatment in alcohol consumption. Several reviews show that processes underlying the relapse phenomenon seem to include the same neuronal circuits in rodents and humans, making animal models an excellent basis for the development of new pharmacotherapies [20, 23]. Therefore, the results achieved in pre-clinical studies that use ADE evaluation provide a solid basis for the subsequent development of controlled clinical trials.

Identification of Two Subpopulations of Rats Depending on Their Alcohol-Relapse Drinking Behavior

It is well known that the alcoholic population is heterogeneous [24, 25]. In fact, AUDs can be considered the result of a complex interplay between polygenic, environmental, and neurobiological components leading to very heterogeneous patient [26]. Identifying specific behavioral and genetic traits that could predispose individuals to develop drug abuse is a major goal in the field of neurobiology of addiction [27, 28]. The reported data using the ADE model have revealed the existence of an enormous heterogeneity in the relapse behavior in nonselected rat lines that has been linked by many authors to a greater variability in the expression of several genes that may have a great importance in the functioning of critical brain areas [29].

In this context, using a heterogeneous and nonselected cohort of rats as well as the ADE model, we have been able to identify and categorize two different subpopulations of rats that showed specific behavioral endophenotypes related to their relapse-like drinking behavior. To do so, we evaluated the ADE phenomenon after three abstinence periods by comparing the average alcohol intake of the last three preabstinence days and the average ethanol intake of the 3 days following the reintroduction of the ethanol bottles (Fig. 46.1).

Based on the manifestation or not of the ADE phenomenon, we categorized our rats according to their relapse-like drinking behavior. We were able to differentiate them between two subpopulations named ADE or no-ADE (Fig. 46.2).

As can be observed in Fig. 46.2a, the average ethanol intake displayed by ADE rats increased significantly, with respect to the basal value, along the three consecutive deprivation periods assayed, thus confirming the deprivation effect in this group of animals. Contrarily, animals assigned to the no-ADE subgroup clearly showed a different relapse-like drinking behavior pattern. Another differential behavioral trait between

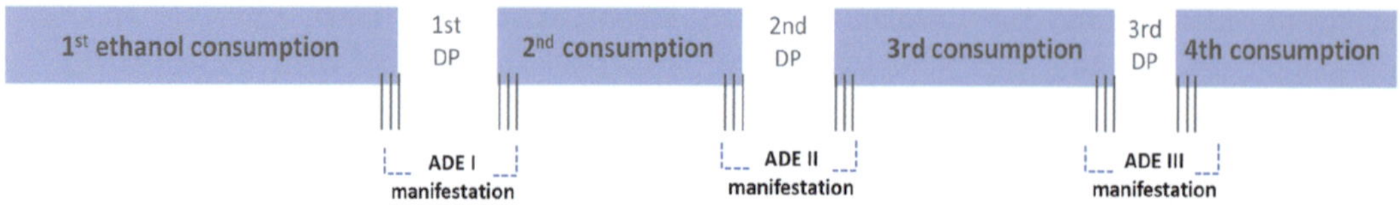

Fig. 46.1 Schematic representation of the ADE model performed in our laboratory. Rats were subjected to a long-term voluntary ethanol drinking procedure with repeated deprivation phases, which lasted for a total of 31–33 weeks. During the consumption period, animals were given continuous access to tap water and to 5%, 10% and 20% (v/v) ethanol solutions in their home cages. Rats were subjected to three random drinking (6 ± 2 weeks) and deprivation (2 ± 1 weeks) periods (DP). The duration of these periods was irregular in order to prevent behavioral adaptations. The blue rectangles represent the periods of free access to ethanol intake. The manifestation of the ADE phenomenon was determined by comparing the average alcohol intake of the last three pre-abstinence days and the average ethanol intake of the 3 days following the reintroduction of the ethanol bottles (represented by vertical lines)

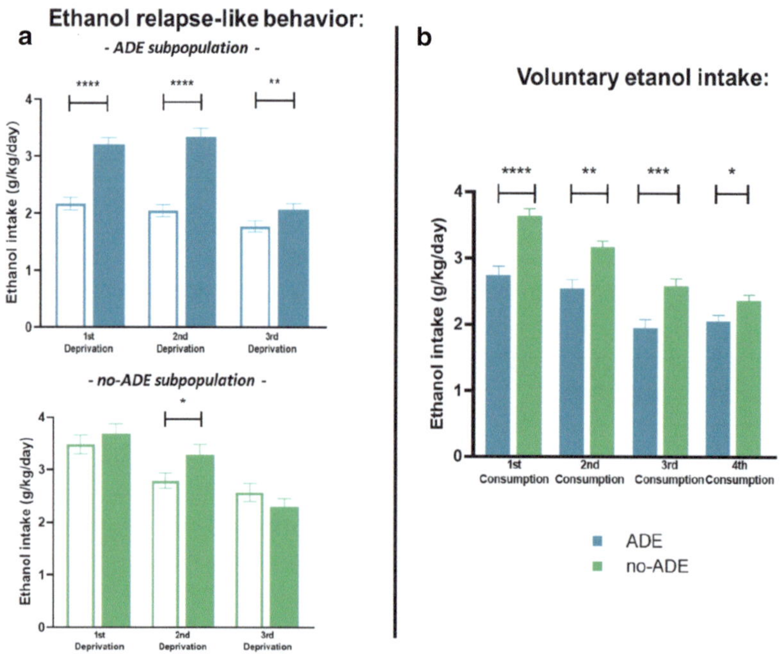

Fig. 46.2 (**a**) Identification of the ADE and no-ADE subpopulation of rats based on their ethanol relapse-like behavior. Framed bars indicate average basal ethanol consumption (expressed in g/kg/day) determined during the 3 days before the deprivation period, whereas solid bars indicate the mean daily ethanol consumption 3 days after ethanol reintroduction (ADE manifestation) during the three deprivation periods assayed. Paired Student t-test revealed statistical differences between pre- and postabstinence ethanol intake in the three deprivation periods of the ADE subpopulation. In contrast, animals assigned to the no-ADE subpopulation only displayed one slight ADE phenomenon during the second deprivation period. Data is represented as mean ± SEM. (Student test: $*p < 0.05$, $**p < 0.01$, $****p < 0.0001$)**.** (**b**) Compared average voluntary ethanol intake between ADE (blue solid bars) and NO-ADE (green solid bars) groups along the four ethanol-consumption periods assayed. Asterisks denote significant differences between ADE and NO-ADE groups. Data are represented as mean ± SEM. ($*p < 0.05$; $**p < 0.01$; $***p < 0.001$; $****p < 0.0001$)

these two subpopulations of rats is the voluntary alcohol intake displayed along time. As can be observed in Fig. 46.2b, ADE rats displayed a lower alcohol consumption than no-ADE animals since statistical differences in mean ethanol consumption were detected between both experimental groups in the four consecutive consumption periods compared.

Our results demonstrated that the relapse-like drinking behavior correlates with their pattern of voluntary alcohol-drinking. Specifically, animals with a high probability of displaying alcohol-relapse (called "ADE group") always showed lower alcohol intake rates than those observed in no-ADE animals. Similar results were obtained when total ethanol preference was analyzed. Again, a great difference between both groups was detected when the particular pattern of ethanol consumption was studied (data not shown; for extensive results see [30]). The identification of these two subpopulations provided us a suitable experimental substrate for studying molecular basis involved in alcohol relapse.

Potential Molecular Mechanisms Involved in Alcohol Relapse

Oxidative Stress

Brain functioning requires a considerably quantity of oxygen, whose metabolization produces high levels of reactive oxygen species (ROS). Together with the low prevalence of antioxidant enzymes and the presence of polyunsaturated lipids, the antioxidant defences are crucial to maintain redox homeostasis in the brain [31]. Particularly, antioxidants are quite important in brain areas innervated with dopamine, such as the nucleus accumbens or hippocampus, since dopamine metabolism results in ROS production as well [32]. The metabolism of ethanol also induces an imbalance in oxidative stress not only because ethanol is metabolized by alcohol dehydrogenase into acetaldehyde in a process that enhances ROS levels, but also because the accumulation of acetaldehyde is highly toxic and causes an augmentation of oxidative stress which damages cells and organelles [33]. Accumulating evidence from preclinical and clinical studies suggests that chronic alcohol consumption is associated with excessive oxidative damage and reduced levels of endogenous antioxidants, leading to excessive ROS production [34, 35]. These alterations in the oxidative stress status are not only restricted to the period of consumption itself but have also been linked to the early withdrawal phase. Thus, Huang et al. (2009) demonstrated the existence of alterations in the oxidative stress status only during early and prolonged alcohol withdrawal symptoms in alcoholic patients. In experimental animals, Jung et al. [37] clearly showed that oxidative stress is even more intense during early withdrawal than during previous ethanol exposure. Hence, according to the gaps detected in the literature, we explored whether the brain oxidative status was misbalanced after experiencing a protracted ethanol withdrawal period. If so, it could be linked to the vulnerability against ethanol relapse behavior, providing a plausible mechanism for the neurobiology of relapse. To this end, we used the male Wistar rats previously categorized as ADE or no-ADE subpopulations under the ADE preclinical model: the ADE group, including animals that repeatedly displayed a relapse-like drinking behavior and the no-ADE group, animals that did not tent to relapse. Our research focused particularly on the exploration of a crucial stage of the disease: the abstinence period which leads to the relapse phenomenon, and more specifically the long-lasting abstinence period (21 days, **abstinence group**). We also examined the effect of the alcohol reintroduction (**reintroduction group**) on brain oxidative stress in hippocampus since this brain area is highly affected by ethanol consumption [38]. To evaluate the oxidative stress status of the hippocampus, we measured the oxidized glutathione (GSSG)/reduced glutathione (GSH) ratio as it is one of the most common parameters to determine oxidative stress levels. In parallel, we measured the GSSG/GSH quotient in two additional groups: rats that were given continuous ad libitum access to tap water (**control group**) or tap water and 5%, 10%, and 20% alcohol dilutions (**alcohol group**) without any deprivation phase (Fig. 46.3a).

Even though ethanol-induced hippocampal oxidative damage has been well documented in rats [39–41], under our experimental conditions, the GSSG/GSH ratio was not modified by prolonged chronic ethanol consumption in the hippocampus (alcohol group, Fig. 46.3a). In previous papers in which significant effects

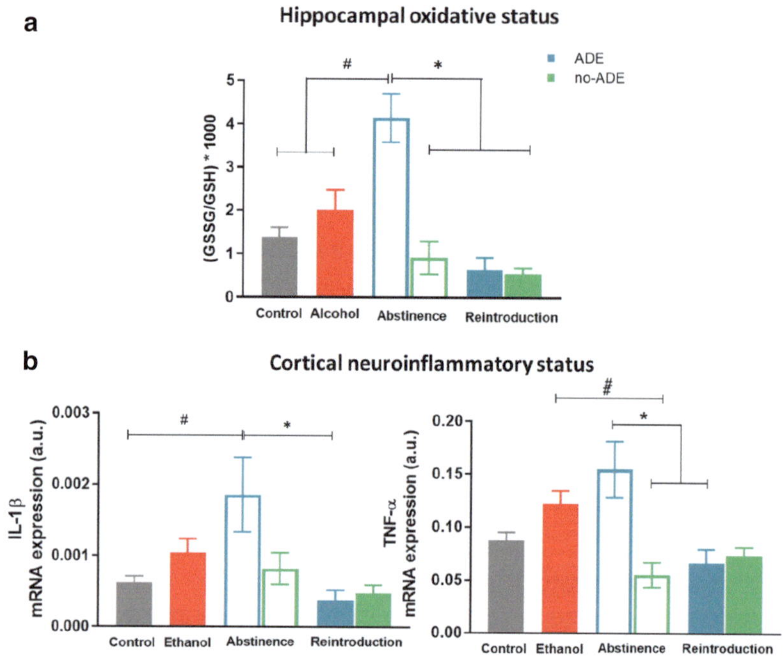

Fig. 46.3 (**a**) GSSH/GSH ratio determined after chronic ethanol intake, during the abstinence period or after ethanol reintroduction in the ADE and no-ADE subpopulation. Data are expressed as nmol/mg of protein. Each bar represents metabolite levels from rats under different conditions: animals exposed to water consumption (control) in grey; animals chronically exposed to ethanol consumption (ethanol) in red; animals under abstinence conditions (blue framed bar for ADE subpopulation and green framed bar for the no-ADE subpopulation), and after ethanol reintroduction (blue solid bar for the ADE subpopulation and green solid bar for the no-ADE subpopulation). (**b**) Levels of IL-1B (left) and TNFα (right) mRNA, expressed in arbitrary units, in the rat Prefrontal Cortex under the above-mentioned experimental conditions. The color legend is the same as the one described in Fig. 46.3a. For both panels, data is represented as mean ± SEM. For data analysis, one- or two-way ANOVA followed by Tukey's post hoc was applied. Asterisk (*) indicates significant differences among groups, and the hash symbol (#) indicates significant differences with respect to "water" or "ethanol" group

were reported, rats were exposed to the Lieber-deCarli alcohol liquid diet, that enhances the rate of alcohol consumed by the animal [39], or elevated ethanol doses (3 g/kg) were intraperitoneally administered [41]. Nonetheless, when a lower ethanol dose was administered, for example, by oral gavage (1.5 g/kg), no changes in GSH levels were observed in the frontal cortex, hippocampus, or striatum of male Sprague–Dawley [42]. Under the free-choice four-bottle paradigm used in our research, our male Wistar rats displayed a voluntary average ethanol intake of 2.21 ± 0.12 g/kg during 24 h, which is a low ethanol dosing rate compared to previous data reported. Probably, this low ethanol consumption was not enough to alter the GSSG/GSH ratio in the hippocampus.

However, the analysis of the hippocampal oxidative stress during protracted abstinence reported remarkable results. As can be seen in Fig. 46.3a, a striking difference was detected between the ADE and no-ADE groups in the GSSG/GSH ratio when animals were subjected to a 21-day deprivation period. In particular, rats belonging to the **ADE group** suffered a great increase in oxidative stress levels during abstinence (up to 300%) with regard to control animals, i.e., animals that were only exposed to water consumption, or with respect to ethanol group. These results suggest the critical role that oxidative stress might play in triggering alcohol craving and relapse. Our results correlate somewhat with clinical data according to which serum oxidative stress markers remain elevated after

1–2 weeks of alcohol detoxification [36]. Contrarily, the GSSG/GSH ratio in **no-ADE rats** (0.917 ± 0.382) remained invariable with respect to control group during the abstinence period.

Another interesting aspect that emerges from the results obtained is the role of alcohol when it is reintroduced. In particular, whereas high GSSG/GSH ratio levels were detected in ADE rats during abstinence, these levels were normalized after 24 h of ethanol reintroduction (Fig. 46.3a). Although alcohol is considered a prooxidant substance, our results evidence that it has different effects depending on the distinct endophenotypes displayed by the rats. In fact, when ethanol was reintroduced in ADE rats, it restored altered oxidative stress indicators, whereas it did not cause any change in the no-ADE GSSG/GSH ratio. This paradoxical result should be considered in future pharmacological research when an antirelapse drug is being evaluated and the action mechanism is being explored, as not only the drug but also the alcohol could have an effect on the obtained results.

Neuroinflammation

Oxidative stress and neuroinflammation are tightly connected and the existence of a drug-induced brain oxidative stress-neuroinflammation vicious cycle has been proposed. Augmented ROS levels activate astrocytes and microglia stimulating the release of proinflammatory factors that will, in turn, enhance oxidative stress [43]. Hence, it has been suggested that inflammatory factors also play a key role in the development of alcohol-related behavioral and mood disorders [44, 45]. In the case of AUDs, several animal and human studies have demonstrated the role of neuroinflammation in the pathophysiology of the disease [46]. The neuroinflammatory response has been observed at the mRNA and/or protein level when different cells or tissues are directly exposed to ethanol [47, 48]. Systemic administration of ethanol to experimental animals also induces neuroinflammation [49]. Thus, binge intoxication induces an inflammatory response in the brain of rats [35, 43] or mice [50, 51], as does chronic exposure to ethanol in mice [47, 52]. The inflammatory response has also been described after 24-hour ethanol withdrawal and a 15-day period of alcohol exposure. However, if the alteration of the neuroinflammatory markers appears in late withdrawal situations and whether these alterations can be correlated with relapse behavior in alcohol consumption has not been explored yet. Hence, we decided to study the neuroinflammatory status in the prefrontal cortex of animals from the two identified subpopulations, ADE and no-ADE, under protracted abstinence and after alcohol reintroduction conditions. To this aim, we evaluated the mRNA levels of two inflammatory mediators, IL-1B and TNFα (Fig. 46.3b) in these experimental groups, also including two groups of rats chronically exposed to water or chronic consumption named control and alcohol group, respectively.

Under our experimental conditions, prolonged chronic ethanol consumption did not alter any inflammatory mediator. However, several studies have demonstrated that after chronic ethanol exposure, rats show significantly elevated cytokine expression in the hippocampus and cortex. Yet, in those experiments, high ethanol doses were administered following a forced schedule (10 g/kg by oral gavage for 10 weeks), or animals were fed the Lieber-deCarli diet (5 months), respectively [53, 54]. Again, the moderate ethanol dosing rate displayed by our animals chronically exposed to voluntary ethanol consumption was insufficient to alter mRNA levels of IL-1B and TNFα in PFC.

As previously, the study of neuroinflammation during long-term abstinence yielded interesting results. After a 3-week period of ethanol withdrawal, ADE rats presented an increased IL-1B value up to 200% with regard to control conditions. Conversely, after prolonged abstinence, the mRNA levels of this cytokine in rats from the no-ADE group were not significantly modified in comparison to those determined in the control group (Fig. 46.3b). The same trend was observed in the case of TNFα mRNA expression (Fig. 46.3b). Our results are in accordance with previous reports, using procedures similar to ours, but under much shorter periods of abstinence (a maximum of 5 days) [55, 56]. In the clinical setting, Yen et al. [57] reported that alcohol-dependent patients, during early withdrawal, showed higher plasma cytokine levels than healthy controls for all cytokines analyzed, including IL-1β and TNF-α. However, after 4 weeks of alcohol abstinence, cytokine expression levels were significantly lower except for IL-1β and IL-5. In a study performed with 29 patients, after an average of 6 days of ethanol abstinence, increased serum levels of IL-6, IL-10, and IL-8 at the beginning of the abstinence period declined [58]. All in all, data evidence that the time course of each neuroinflammation mediator is different and depends on the brain nuclei considered. As can be observed, under our experimental conditions, only in ADE rats, but not in the no-ADE subpopulation, IL-1β and TNF-α mRNA levels remained altered after prolonged ethanol abstinence, suggesting that neuroinflammation could also play a role in the alcohol craving that will lead to relapse process.

Again, the effects of alcohol reintroduction on the gene expression levels of neuroinflammatory mediators in the prefrontal cortex were paradoxical. As previously, it can be observed that the presence of alcohol after a long period of abstinence, rapidly normalized IL-1B and TNFα mRNA expression in ADE rats. This evidences that the alcohol reintroduction differently affects ADE and no-ADE subpopulations and its impact in neuroinflammatory processes must be considered when performing antirelapse pharmacological experiments.

Glutamate Homeostasis

According to the literature, another potential mechanism that may underlie the neurobiological effects of ethanol could be related to the alteration of glutamate homeostasis, which is also relevant in drug relapse [59, 60]. Brain glutamate homeostasis is closely related to the oxidative stress status and inflammatory processes. High levels of extracellular glutamate cause the overactivation of postsynaptic neuron causing excitotoxicity. An immediate consequence of this effect is the increase in reactive oxygen species (ROS) previously reported. In the same way, there is also a crosstalk between glutamate and immunomodulatory signals. Concretely, changes in glutamate levels can cause the microglial liberation of proinflammatory factors. In parallel, immunomodulatory signals can alter synaptic transmission through their influence over astrocytes [5]. In this context, it is important to consider that, as in the case of oxidative stress and neuroinflammation, glutamate homeostasis may also play a role in triggering relapse behavior. In recent years, several researchers have suggested that the existence of neural mechanisms could explain relapse behavior to different drugs of abuse. This mechanism entails the glutamatergic projections from the PFC, hippocampus and amygdala to the nucleus accumbens. Concretely, it has been shown that astrocytic dysfunction in regulating both the basal glutamate levels as well as the clearance of synaptic glutamate in the nucleus accumbens is a primary mechanism whereby cues associated with drugs of abuse can drive relapse [59, 61]. Hence, numerous authors consider that glutamate homeostasis in the nucleus accumbens seems to be involved in the vulnerability to relapse [62]. Regarding AUD, it has been suggested that increased levels of glutamate in the mesocorticolimbic system during the abstinence period are involved in triggering cue-induced alcohol relapse [60]. Consequently, numerous studies have focused their efforts on unraveling the relationship between AUD and glutamate homeostasis with the purpose of finding new targets for addressing new pharmacoterapies. In this sense, the study of the effects of chronic alcohol consumption and abstinence on astroglial high affinity glutamate transporters and/or glutamatergic signaling machinery has been crucial. These studies have essentially focused on (i) the astrocytic excitatory amino acid transporter 2 (EAAT2, known as GLT1 in rodents) and EAAT1 (known as GLAST in rodents), which are mainly expressed in astrocytes, and clear synaptic glutamate preventing excitotoxicity [63], as well as (ii) the cystine/glutamate antiporter (xCT) which interchanges intracellular glutamate for extracellular cysteine in a 1:1 ratio [64] and works as the major extracellular glutamate supplier in many brain regions such as the nucleus accumbens, striatum, or hippocampus [65]. Furthermore, the results found in the literature are not fully coincident. The high variability and discrepancies reported are probably related to different variables such as rat strains, the use of ethanol preferent vs naïve animals and, particularly, the ethanol administration paradigm used [66]. Overall, an in-depth analysis of the data shows that chronic ethanol intake provokes a decrease or no alteration of expression levels of these Glu transporters [67, 68]. On the other hand, according to the literature focused on the glutamate homeostasis during the withdrawal period, the results are scarce and controversial. For instance, early abstinence conditions were reported not to affect GLT1 and GLAST expression in Nucleus accumbens [69, 70], but to downregulate xCT expression [71, 72]. Instead, the only study found analyzing the consequences of protracted abstinence showed no alteration in GLT1 and xCT protein expression, while GLAST levels were found to be diminished in Nucleus Accumbens of female P rats [73].

All in all, the effects of chronic alcohol consumption and, in particular, the effect of abstinence on astroglial high affinity glutamate transporters and/or the glutamatergic signaling machinery so far they have not been completely understood. It should be considered that abstinence represents a critical period of vulnerability within the addiction cycle, and the altered glutamatergic homeostasis sequelae of protracted ethanol abstinence remains poorly known [5]. To date, very few studies have examined how glutamate transporters are altered across a protracted period of abstinence compared to chronic ethanol exposure, and if such changes are causally linked to relapse-like drinking behavior [73].

In this context, some studies have suggested that pharmacological agents acting upstream of glutamate transport systems (e.g., GLT-1 or xCT) could influence broader aspects of the glial function and may also disrupt drug reinstatement and relapse [59, 74]. Thus, agents that have glutamatergic properties, such as N-acetylcysteine (NAC), are being assayed in the preclinical and clinical setting as a potential antirelapse pharmacotherapy for several substance use disorders (SUDs) [75].

N-acetylcysteine as a New Antirelapse Pharmacotherapy for AUD

NAC is a pleiotropic drug associated with antioxidant and antiinflammatory capabilities [43, 76]. Additionally, there is growing evidence showing that NAC also has glutamatergic properties. Concretely, as NAC is a cysteine prodrug, it has been hypothesized that it is able to increase the extrasynaptic glutamate levels in critical brain regions, such as the nucleus accumbens core, through the glial xCT, which exchanges extracellular cysteine for intracellular glutamate [59, 64]. Although preclinical and clinical research has increasingly explored the potential efficacy of NAC to regulate/modify drug-related behaviors [77, 78], the literature has shown mixed results, particularly depending on the drug of abuse considered. For instance, with respect to cocaine, NAC has been found to reduce cocaine-seeking behavior in rats [79–81], to prevent the escalation of drug intake [82], and to facilitate self-imposed abstinence after cocaine escalation [83]. Likewise, preliminary clinical data indicate that repeated administration of NAC to cocaine-dependent human subjects produced a significant reduction in craving [79]. The clinical trial conducted by La Rowe et al. [84] failed to demonstrate that NAC reduces cocaine use in actively using cocaine-dependent individuals, but they demonstrated its antirelapse effect in patients who had already achieved abstinence from this drug. Nicotine self-administration, extinction response, and cue-induced reinstatement have also been reduced in rats treated with NAC [40, 85]. Human smokers treated with NAC reported a reduction in cigarette smoking but without any effect on the assessment of withdrawal and craving symptoms [86]. Nevertheless, Froeliger et al. [87] reported that NAC was able to prevent nicotine craving. In a general sense, metaanalyses of

NAC trials support the use of NAC in ameliorating drug craving, although in some trials NAC failed to reduce craving [88]. In a preclinical setting, effects of NAC on heroin-seeking behavior have also been identified [89], and a potential role in the management of methamphetamine dependence has also been claimed [90]. Thus, there is currently sufficient evidence that points to the potential usefulness of NAC in the management of several SUDs. It is probably due to its capacity to restore drug-induced alterations in glutamate homeostasis, oxidative stress status, and/or the inflammatory process associated with the mesocorticolimbic system (for review, see [78, 91]).

In contrast, studies with ethanol evaluating the preclinical effectiveness of NAC are scarce and, moreover, show controversial results as well. For example, Weiland et al. [92] reported that NAC did not attenuate the cue-primed reinstatement of alcohol seeking in male Sprague–Dawley rats. Quintanilla et al. [93] demonstrated that NAC (30 or 60 mg/ kg, ip) was able to reduce voluntary drug intake during the maintenance phase, but not along the acquisition phase. Later, the same group also reported that oral NAC administration during a 14-day period reduced ethanol binge-like behavior [40]. Naassila and Vilpoux's group also showed that NAC, under different alcohol exposure protocols, was able to reduce ethanol-motivational properties, ethanol-seeking behavior, and reacquisition after abstinence in rats but it failed to limit reacquisition after extinction [72, 94]. Curiously, in all these latter experiments, only a single dose of the drug was intraperitoneally injected 60 min before the session. Thus, it seems difficult to attribute the restoration of systems disrupted in addiction to NAC, but rather to the acute effects of NAC. Finally, Garcia-Keller et al. [95] also demonstrated that subchronic NAC treatment, using several timing variations, is able to reduce conditioned stress reinstatement after cocaine or alcohol self-administration. It expands the potential use of this drug in the treatment of SUDs, given that, until now, NAC had principally been explored in preventing cue-induced or context-induced reinstatement.

Presently, the number of drugs marketed to relieve abstinence syndrome symptoms and prevent relapse in alcohol-addicted individuals is limited. This fact, together with the potential mechanism of action of NAC underlying the process of drug relapse prompted us to evaluate the efficacy of prolonged NAC treatment in the prevention of alcohol relapse using the preclinical model based on the ADE. We tested two different NAC doses (60 and 100 mg/kg) that were subcutaneously administered once a day for 13 days (9 days under abstinence conditions and 4 days during ethanol reintroduction) to rats that repeatedly displayed a relapse-like drinking behavior, i.e., the ADE subpopulation (Fig. 46.4a). Then, we evaluated the manifestation of the ADE phenomenon after the fourth abstinence period (Fig. 46.4b).

As expected, after ethanol reintroduction, vehicle-treated animals showed a significant increase in alcohol intake by up to 25% in comparison with that observed in the baseline period, confirming that vehicle-treated rats experienced the ADE phenomenon. Interestingly, NAC treatment was able to block the expression of the ADE phenomenon. Concretely, animals treated with the 60 mg/kg dose displayed a significant decrease (around −20%) in ethanol intake after the forced abstinence period, while the NAC 100 mg/kg treatment did not significantly change the amount of ethanol consumed before and after abstinence [96]. In order to rule out that a possible loss of interest in the consumption of liquids could have caused the observed reduction in ethanol intake displayed by the animals treated with NAC, total fluid intake was also evaluated. Total fluid intake was not significantly reduced during the postabstinence days in any of the experimental groups, suggesting that NAC might have a specific effect on the mechanisms that mediate relapse.

Under our experimental conditions, the antirelapse effect of NAC was more pronounced with 60 mg/kg/day NAC than 100 mg/kg/day. This observation might fit with an inverted U-shaped dose-effect curve. From a mechanistic point of view, this result could agree with data reported [81] using electrophysiological techniques (in

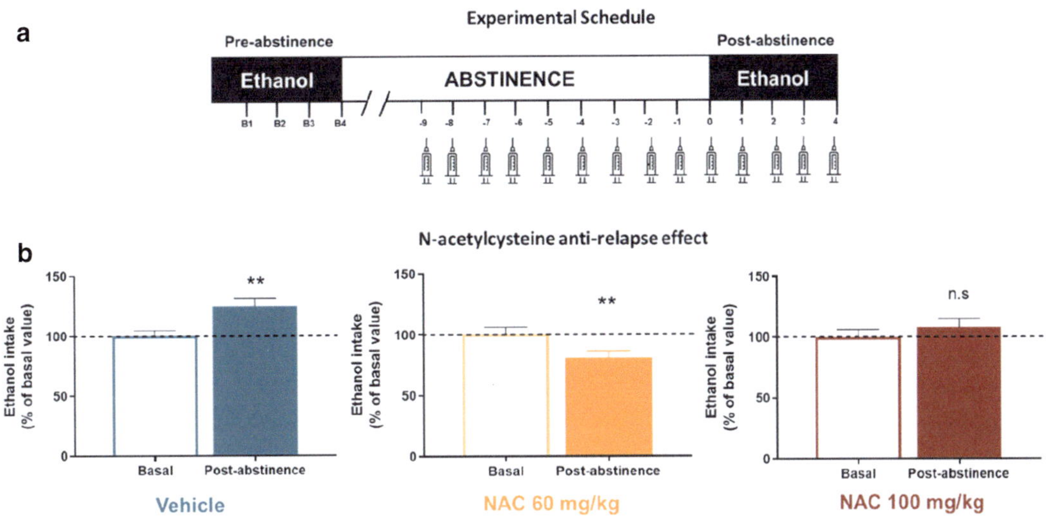

Fig. 46.4 (**a**) Schematic representation of the experimental procedure used in this study. B1, B2, B3, and B4 represent the baseline measurements taken throughout 4 days prior to the abstinence period. Hatch bars correspond to a 12-day period in both experiments, so that the total duration of the abstinence period was 21 days. (**b**) Effect of the subcutaneous injections once a day for 12 days of vehicle (blue pattern), NAC 60 mg/kg (yellow pattern) or NAC 100 mg/kg (pattern) on ethanol intake referred to % of basal value. Framed columns represent the mean daily ethanol intake determined during the 4 days before (baseline) under each experimental condition whereas solid columns represent mean daily ethanol intake after (post-abstinence) the imposed withdrawal period. The dashed line represents the mean baseline value. Paired Student t-test was performed at each experimental group. Asterisks denote statistically significant differences within groups (**$p < 0.01$). Data are presented as mean ± SEM

vitro whole cell recording). They demonstrate that low concentrations of NAC inhibit glutamate transmission into nucleus accumbens core spiny cells via activation of presynaptic mGluR2/3. However, higher concentrations of the drug counteract this effect by stimulating mGluR5 at the postsynaptic level. Along this line, they concluded that the effect of NAC on relapse to cocaine seeking depends on the balance between stimulating mGluR2/3 and mGluR5 in this brain region of the mesocorticolimbic system. In the same way, our group recently reported that a single 120 mg/kg NAC dose was able to activate glutamatergic transmission that lead to an increase in cFOS IR-cell expression in the nucleus accumbens, while a lower dose of NAC 30 mg/kg did not have any effect. Moreover, the negative allosteric modulator of mGLuR5 (MTEP) was able to abolish the activating effect of the higher dose of NAC assayed, suggesting that this effect could be mediated by mGluR5 [97]. All in all, we are aware that our preclinical conditions are far from those used in vitro by Kupchik and colleagues, but, generally, the results obtained point in the same direction and underline the importance of selecting the appropriate NAC dose.

Conclusions and Future Directions

The underlying mechanisms involved in various phases of the AUD development are not only multiple but also complex. The use of appropriate preclinical models is necessary to unravel these mechanisms. Using the preclinical model based on the ADE effect, we have demonstrated that after a prolonged ethanol withdrawal, brain redox, and neuroinflammation status remain altered, but only in animals that display ethanol-relapse behavior. It may be a plausible key in the induction of the craving that will lead to the relapse process. The next step in our research should be the elucidation of the underlying mechanisms (precise causes), probably from the genetic point of view, that would lead to the different redox/neuroinflammation status identified in the different individuals. These aspects could be considered a robust criterion for predicting the alcohol-addiction and nonaddiction vulnerability of individuals. Additionally, our results gather mechanistic evidence concerning the use of antioxidant, antiinflammatories, or combined therapies for preventing alcohol relapse, as currently being evaluated by different groups [43, 98]. In this context, we have evaluated the potential alcohol antirelapse effect of NAC. Our results have demonstrated the antirelapse efficacy of NAC 60 or 100 mg/kg treatment using a robust preclinical model such us the ADE model. However, the mechanisms by which NAC exerts its diverse effects are complex and still remain unclear. Moreover, several papers have recently reported gender differences in the psychopharmacological effects of NAC under different indications and experimental paradigms [99, 100]. Hence, following the pipeline to the clinical evaluation of its alcohol antirelapse effect, it would be highly recommended to elucidate the NAC molecular mechanism of action, considering the paradoxical effects induced by ethanol reintroduction. In other words, to assess the underlying mechanism of action of NAC in ethanol relapse, analyzing its neurobiological effects during the abstinence period, in absence of ethanol that potentially interferes in the altered neuroimmune and oxidative status and would mask NAC effects. Finally, it would be necessary to determine plasma NAC levels that correlate with their pharmacological response as well as to evaluate different NAC treatment regimens and doses focusing on the sex and gender differences previously reported for this drug.

References

1. World Health Organization. Global status report on alcohol and health 2018. World Health Organization; 2019.
2. Barrick C, Connors GJ. Relapse prevention and maintaining abstinence in older adults with alcohol-use disorders. Drugs Aging. 2002;19(8):583–94.
3. Weiss F, Ciccocioppo R, Parsons LH, Katner S, Liu XIU, Zorrilla EP, et al. Compulsive drug-seeking behavior and relapse: neuroadaptation, stress, and conditioning factors. Ann N Y Acad Sci. 2001;937(1):1–26.
4. National Institute on Alcohol Abuse and Alcoholism. Understanding alcohol use disorder; 2021. Available in: https://www.niaaa.nih.gov/publications/brochures-and-fact-sheets/understanding-alcohol-use-disorder
5. Namba M, Leyrer-Jackson JM, Nagy EK, Olive MF, Neisewander JL. Neuroimmune mechanisms as novel treatment targets for substance use disorders and associated comorbidities. Front Neurosci. 2021;15:650785.
6. Shaham Y, Shalev U, Lu L, de Wit H, Stewart J. The reinstatement model of drug relapse: history, methodology and major findings. Psychopharmacol (Berl). 2003;168(1–2):3–20.
7. Samson HH, Doyle TF. Oral ethanol self-administration in the rat: effect of naloxone. Pharmacol Biochem Behav. 1985;22(1):91–9.
8. Rodd ZA, Bell RL, Sable HJ, Murphy JM, McBride WJ. Recent advances in animal models of alcohol craving and relapse. Pharmacol Biochem Behav. 2004;79:439–50.
9. Spanagel R, Kiefer F. Drugs for relapse prevention of alcoholism: ten years of progress. Trend Pharm Sci. 2008;29:109–15.
10. Bachteler D, Economidou D, Danysz W, Ciccocioppo R, Spanagel R. The effects of acamprosate and neramexane on cue-induced reinstatement of ethanol-seeking behavior in rat. Neuropsychopharmacology. 2005;30(6):1104–10.
11. Katner SN, Magalong JG, Weiss F. Reinstatement of alcohol-seeking behavior by drug-associated discriminative stimuli after prolonged extinction in the rat. Neuropsychopharmacology. 1999;20(5):471–9.
12. Sanchis-Segura C, Spanage R. Behavioural assessment of drug reinforcement and addictive features in rodents: an overview. Addict Biol. 2006;11:38.
13. Sinclair JD, Senter RJ. Development of an alcohol-deprivation effect in rats. Q J Stud Alcohol. 1968;29(4):863–7.
14. Rodd-Henricks ZA, McKinzie DL, Shaikh SR, Murphy JM, McBride WJ, Lumeng L, Li TK. Alcohol deprivation effect is prolonged in the alcohol preferring (P) rat after repeated deprivations. Alcohol Clin Exp Res. 2000;24(1):8–16.
15. Sinclair JD, Tiihonen K. Lack of alcohol-deprivation effect in AA rats. Alcohol. 1988;5(1):85–7.
16. Salimov RM, Salimova NB. The alcohol-deprivation effect in hybrid mice. Drug Alcohol Depend. 1993;32(2):187–91.
17. Kornet M, Goosen C, Van Ree JM. Effect of naltrexone on alcohol consumption during chronic alcohol drinking and after a period of imposed abstinence in free-choice drinking rhesus monkeys. Psychopharmacol (Berl). 1991;104(3):367–76.

18. Burish TG, Maisto SA, Cooper AM, Sobell MB. Effects of voluntary short-term abstinence from alcohol on subsequent drinking patterns of college students. J Stud Alcohol. 1981;42(11):1013–20.
19. Martin-Fardon R, Weiss F. Modeling relapse in animals. Curr Top Behav Neurosci. 2013;13:403–32.
20. Spanagel R. Animal models of addiction. Dialog Clin Neurosci. 2017;19(3):247–58.
21. Leong KC, Cox S, King C, Becker H, Reichel CM. Oxytocin and rodent models of addiction. Int Rev Neurobiol. 2018;140:201–47.
22. Fredriksson I, Venniro M, Reiner DJ, Chow JJ, Bossert JM, Shaham Y. Animal models of drug relapse and craving after voluntary abstinence: a review. Pharmacol Rev. 2021;73(3):1050–83.
23. Bell RL, Hauser SR, Liang T, Sari Y, Maldonado-Devincci A, Rodd ZA. Rat animal models for screening medications to treat alcohol use disorders. Neuropharmacology. 2017;122:201–43.
24. Lesch OM, Walter H. Subtypes of alcoholism and their role in therapy. Alcohol. 1996;31:63–7.
25. Windle M, Scheidt DM. Alcoholic subtypes: are two sufficient? Addiction. 2004;99:1508–19.
26. Cannella N, Ubaldi M, Masi A, Bramucci M, Roberto M, Bifone A, Ciccocioppo R. Building better strategies to develop new medications in alcohol use disorder: learning from past success and failure to shape a brighter future. R Neurosci Biobehav Rev. 2019;103:384–98.
27. Reilly MT, Noronha A, Warren K. Perspectives on the neuroscience of alcohol from the National Institute on Alcohol Abuse and Alcoholism. Handb Clin Neurol. 2014;125:15–29.
28. Spanagel R, Vengeliene V. New pharmacological treatment strategies for relapse prevention. Curr Top Behav Neurosci. 2013;13:583–609.
29. Vengeliene V, Bilbao A, Spanagel R. The alcohol deprivation effect model for studying relapse behavior: a comparison between rats and mice. Alcohol. 2014;48(3):313–20.
30. Fernández-Rodríguez S, Cano-Cebrián MJ, Rius-Pérez S, Pérez S, Guerri C, Granero L, Zornoza T, Polache A. Different brain oxidative and neuroinflammation status in rats during prolonged abstinence depending on their ethanol relapse-like drinking behavior: effects of ethanol reintroduction. Drug Alcohol Depend. 2022;232:109284.
31. Dringen R. Metabolism and functions of glutathione in brain. Prog Neurobiol. 2000;62(6):649–71.
32. Womersley JS, Townsend DM, Kalivas PW, Uys JD. Targeting redox regulation to treat substance use disorder using N-acetylcysteine. Eur J Neurosci. 2019;50(3):2538–51.
33. Tapia-Rojas C, Pérez MJ, Jara C, Vergara EH, Quintanilla RA. Ethanol consumption affects neuronal function: role of the mitochondria. Mitochondrial Dis; 2017.
34. Das SK, Vasudevan DM. Alcohol-induced oxidative stress. Life Sci. 2007;81(3):177–87.
35. Crews F, Nixon K, Kim D, Joseph J, Shukitt-Hale B, Qin L, Zou J. BHT blocks NF-kappa B activation and ethanol-induced brain damage. Alcohol Clin Exp Res. 2006;30(11):1938–49.
36. Huang MC, Chen CH, Peng FC, Tang SH, Chen CC. Alterations in oxidative stress status during early alcohol withdrawal in alcoholic patients. J Formos Med Assoc. 2009;108(7):560–9.
37. Jung ME, Yan LJ, Forster MJ, Simpkins JW. Ethanol withdrawal provokes mitochondrial injury in an estrogen preventable manner. J Bioenerg Biomembr. 2008;40(1):35–44.
38. Elibol-Can B, Jakubowska-Dogru E, Severcan M, Severcan F. The effects of short-term chronic ethanol intoxication and ethanol withdrawal on the molecular composition of the rat hippocampus by FT-IR spectroscopy. Alcoholism: Clin Exp Res. 2011;35(11):2050–62.
39. Almansa I, Barcia JM, López-Pedrajas R, Muriach M, Miranda M, Romero FJ. Naltrexone reverses ethanol-induced rat hippocampal and serum oxidative damage. Oxidative Med Cell Longev. 2013;2013:296898.
40. Quintanilla ME, Morales P, Ezquer F, Ezquer M, Herrera-Marschitz M, Israel Y. Commonality of ethanol and nicotine reinforcement and relapse in Wistar-derived UChB rats: inhibition by N-acetylcysteine. Alcoholism: Clin Exp Res. 2018;42(10):1988–99.
41. Scolaro B, Delwing-de Lima D, da Cruz JG, Delwing-Dal Magro D. Mate tea prevents oxidative stress in the blood and hippocampus of rats with acute or chronic ethanol administration. Oxidative Med Cell Longev. 2012;2012:314758.
42. Sommavilla M, Sánchez-Villarejo MV, Almansa I, Sánchez-Vallejo V, Barcia JM, Romero FJ, Miranda M. The effects of acute ethanol exposure and ageing on rat brain glutathione metabolism. Free Radic Res. 2012;46(9):1076–81.
43. Berríos-Cárcamo P, Quezada M, Quintanilla ME, Morales P, Ezquer M, Herrera-Marschitz M, et al. Oxidative stress and neuroinflammation as a pivot in drug abuse. A focus on the therapeutic potential of antioxidant and anti-inflammatory agents and biomolecules. Antioxidants. 2020;9(9):830.
44. Kelley KW, Dantzer R. Alcoholism and inflammation: neuroimmunology of behavioral and mood disorders. Brain Behav Immun. 2011;25:S13–20.
45. Leclercq S, De Saeger C, Delzenne N, de Timar P, Stärkel P. Role of inflammatory pathways, blood mononuclear cells, and gut-derived bacterial products in alcohol dependence. Biol Psychiatry. 2014;76(9):725–33.
46. Robinson G, Most D, Ferguson LB, Mayfield J, Harris RA, Blednov YA. Neuroimmune pathways in alcohol consumption: evidence from behavioral and genetic studies in rodents and humans. Int Rev Neurobiol. 2014;118:13–39.
47. Alfonso-Loeches S, Pascual-Lucas M, Blanco AM, Sanchez-Vera I, Guerri C. Pivotal role of TLR4

receptors in alcohol-induced neuroinflammation and brain damage. J Neurosci. 2010;30(24):8285–95.
48. Alfonso-Loeches S, Ureña-Peralta JR, Morillo-Bargues M, Guerri C. Role of mitochondria ROS generation in ethanol-induced NLRP3 inflammasome activation and cell death in astroglial cells. Front Cel Neurosci. 2014;8:216.
49. Pascual M, Blanco AM, Cauli O, Miñarro J, Guerri C. Intermittent ethanol exposure induces inflammatory brain damage and causes long-term behavioural alterations in adolescent rats. Eur J Neurosci. 2007;25(2):541–50.
50. Kane CJ, Phelan KD, Douglas JC, Wagoner G, Johnson JW, Xu J, Phelan PS, Drew PD. Effects of ethanol on immune response in the brain: region-specific changes in adolescent versus adult mice. Alcohol Clin Exp Res. 2014;38(2):384–91.
51. Montesinos J, Pascual M, Rodríguez-Arias M, Miñarro J, Guerri C. Involvement of TLR4 in the long-term epigenetic changes, rewarding and anxiety effects induced by intermittent ethanol treatment in adolescence. Brain Behav Immun. 2016;53:159–71.
52. Whitman BA, Knapp DJ, Werner DF, Crews FT, Breese GR. The cytokine m RNA increase induced by withdrawal from chronic ethanol in the sterile environment of brain is mediated by CRF and HMGB 1 release. Alcoholism: Clin Exp Res. 2013;37(12):2086–97.
53. Tiwari V, Kuhad A, Chopra K. Suppression of neuro-inflammatory signaling cascade by tocotrienol can prevent chronic alcohol-induced cognitive dysfunction in rats. Behav Brain Res. 2009;203(2):296–303.
54. Vallés SL, Blanco AM, Pascual M, Guerri C. Chronic ethanol treatment enhances inflamamatory mediators and cell death in the brain and in astrocytes. Brain Pathol. 2004;14(4):365–71.
55. Knapp DJ, Harper KM, Whitman BA, Zimomra Z, Breese GR. Stress and withdrawal from chronic ethanol induce selective changes in neuroimmune mRNAs in differing brain sites. Brain Sci. 2016;6(3):25.
56. Schneider R Jr, Bandiera S, Souza DG, Bellaver B, Caletti G, Quincozes-Santos A, Elisabetsky E, Gomez R. N-acetylcysteine prevents alcohol related Neuroinflammation in rats. Neurochem Res. 2017;42(8):2135–41.
57. Yen CH, Ho PS, Yeh YW, Liang CS, Kuo SC, Huang CC, Chen CY, Shih MC, Ma KH, Sung YF, Lu RB, Huang SY. Differential cytokine levels between early withdrawal and remission states in patients with alcohol dependence. Psychoneuroendocrinol. 2017;76:183–91.
58. González-Quintela A, Dominguez-Santalla MJ, Pérez LF, Vidal C, Lojo S, Barrio E. Influence of acute alcohol intake and alcohol withdrawal on circulating levels of IL-6, IL-8, IL-10 and IL-12. Cytokine. 2000;12(9):1437–40.
59. Kalivas PW. The glutamate homeostasis hypothesis of addiction. Nat Rev Neurosci. 2009;10(8):561–72.
60. Alasmari F, Goodwani S, McCullumsmith RE, Sari Y. Role of glutamatergic system and mesocorticolimbic circuits in alcohol dependence. Prog Neurobiol. 2018;171:32–49.
61. Scofield MD, Heinsbroek JA, Gipson CD, Kupchik YM, Spencer S, Smith AC, Roberts-Wolfe D, Kalivas PW. The nucleus Accumbens: mechanisms of addiction across drug classes reflect the importance of glutamate homeostasis. Pharmacol Rev. 2016;68(3):816–71.
62. Kalivas PW, Volkow ND. The neural basis of addiction: a pathology of motivation and choice. Am J Psychiatry. 2005;162(8):1403–13.
63. Pajarillo E, Rizor A, Lee J, Aschner M, Lee E. The role of astrocytic glutamate transporters GLT-1 and GLAST in neurological disorders: potential targets for neurotherapeutics. Neuropharmacology. 2019;161:107559.
64. Massie A, Boillée S, Hewett S, Knackstedt L, Lewerenz J. Main path and byways: non-vesicular glutamate release by system xc(−) as an important modifier of glutamatergic neurotransmission. J Neurochem. 2015;135(6):1062–79.
65. Baker DA, Shen H, Kalivas PW. Cystine/glutamate exchange serves as the source for extracellular glutamate: modifications by repeated cocaine administration. Amino Acids. 2002;23(1–3):161–2.
66. Abulseoud OA, Camsari UM, Ruby CL, Kasasbeh A, Choi S, Choi DS. Attenuation of ethanol withdrawal by ceftriaxone-induced upregulation of glutamate transporter EAAT2. Neuropsychopharmacology. 2014;39(7):1674–84.
67. Hakami AY, Hammad AM, Sari Y. Effects of amoxicillin and augmentin on cystine-glutamate exchanger and glutamate transporter 1 isoforms as well as ethanol intake in alcohol-preferring rats. Front Neurosci. 2016;10:171.
68. Ezquer F, Quintanilla ME, Morales P, Santapau D, Munita JM, Moya-Flores F, Ezquer M, Herrera-Marschitz M, Israel Y. A dual treatment blocks alcohol binge-drinking relapse: Microbiota as a new player. Drug Alcohol Depend. 2022;236:109466.
69. Melendez RI, Hicks MP, Cagle SS, Kalivas PW. Ethanol exposure decreases glutamate uptake in the nucleus accumbens. Alcoholism: Clin and Exp Res. 2005;29(3):326–33.
70. Pati D, Kelly K, Stennett B, Frazier CJ, Knackstedt LA. Alcohol consumption increases basal extracellular glutamate in the nucleus accumbens core of S prague–D awley rats without increasing spontaneous glutamate release. Eur J Neurosci. 2016;44(2):1896–905.
71. Peana AT, Muggironi G, Bennardini F. Change of cystine/glutamate antiporter expression in ethanol-dependent rats. Front Neurosci. 2014;8:311.
72. Lebourgeois S, González-Marín MC, Antol J, Naassila M, Vilpoux C. Evaluation of N-acetylcysteine on ethanol self-administration in ethanol-dependent rats. Neuropharmacology. 2019;150:112–20.

73. Ding ZM, Rodd ZA, Engleman EA, Bailey JA, Lahiri DK, McBride WJ. Alcohol drinking and deprivation alter basal extracellular glutamate concentrations and clearance in the mesolimbic system of alcohol-preferring (P) rats. Addict Biol. 2013;18(2):297–306.
74. Sari Y, Sreemantula SN, Lee MR, Choi DS. Ceftriaxone treatment affects the levels of GLT1 and ENT1 as well as ethanol intake in alcohol-preferring rats. J Mol Neurosci. 2013;51(3):779–87.
75. Smaga I, Frankowska M, Filip M. N-acetylcysteine in substance use disorder: a lesson from preclinical and clinical research. Pharmacol Rep. 2021;73(5):1205–19.
76. Badisa RB, Goodman CB, Fitch-Pye CA. Attenuating effect of N-acetyl-L-cysteine against acute cocaine toxicity in rat C6 astroglial cells. Int J Mol Med. 2013;32(2):497–502.
77. Brown RM, Kupchik YM, Kalivas PW. The story of glutamate in drug addiction and of N-acetylcysteine as a potential pharmacotherapy. JAMA Psychiatry. 2013;70:895–7.
78. McClure EA, Gipson CD, Malcolm RJ, Kalivas PW, Gray KM. Potential role of N-acetylcysteine in the management of substance use disorders. CNS Drugs. 2014;28(2):95–106.
79. Amen SL, Piacentine LB, Ahmad ME, Li SJ, Mantsch JR, Risinger RC, Baker DA. Repeated N-acetyl cysteine reduces cocaine seeking in rodents and craving in cocaine-dependent humans. Neuropsychopharmacology. 2011;36:871–8.
80. Bake DA, McFarland K, Lake RW, Shen HUI, Toda S, Kalivas PW. N-acetyl cysteine-induced blockade of cocaine-induced reinstatement. Ann N Y Acad Sci. 2003;1003:349–51.
81. Kupchik YM, Moussawi K, Tang XC, Wang X, Kalivas BC, Kolokithas R, et al. The effect of N-acetylcysteine in the nucleus accumbens on neurotransmission and relapse to cocaine. Biol psy. 2012;71(11):978–86.
82. Madayag A, Lobner D, Kau KS, Mantsch JR, Abdulhameed O, Hearing M, Grier MD, Baker DA. Repeated N-acetylcysteine administration alters plasticity-dependent effect of cocaine. J Neurosci. 2007;27:13968–76.
83. Ducret E, Puaud M, Lacoste J, Belin-Rauscent A, Fouyssac M, Dugast E, Murray JE, Everitt BJ, Houeto J, Belin D. N-acetylcysteine facilitates self-imposed abstinence after escalation of cocaine intake. Biol Psyc. 2016;80:226–34.
84. LaRowe SD, Kalivas PW, Nicholas JS, Randall PK, Mardikian PN, Malcolm RJ. A double-blind placebo-controlled trial of N-acetylcysteine in the treatment of cocaine dependence. Am J Addict. 2013;22:443–52.
85. Moro F, Orrú A, Marzo CM, Di Clemente A, Cervo L. mGluR2/3 mediates short-term control of nicotine-seeking by acute systemic N-acetylcysteine. Addict Biol. 2018;23:28–40.
86. Knackstedt LA, Melendez RI, Kalivas PW. Ceftriaxone restores glutamate homeostasis and prevents relapse to cocaine seeking. Biol Psychiatry. 2010;67(1):81–4.
87. Froeliger B, McConnell PA, Stankeviciute N, McClure EA, Kalivas PW, Gray KM. The effects of N-acetylcysteine on frontostriatal resting-state functional connectivity, withdrawal symptoms and smoking abstinence: a double-blind, placebo-controlled fMRI pilot study. Drug Alcohol Depend. 2015;156:234–42.
88. Duailibi MS, Cordeiro Q, Brietzke E, Ribeiro M, LaRowe S, Berk M, Trevizol AP. N-acetylcysteine in the treatment of craving in substance use disorders: systematic review and meta-analysis. Am J Addict. 2017;26(7):660–6.
89. Hodebourg R, Murray JE, Fouyssac M, Puaud M, Everitt BJ, Belin D. Heroin seeking becomes dependent on dorsal striatal dopaminergic mechanisms and can be decreased by N-acetylcysteine. Eur J Neurosci. 2019;50(3):2036–44.
90. McKetin R, Dean OM, Baker AL, Carter G, Turner A, Kelly PJ, Berk M. A potential role for N-acetylcysteine in the management of methamphetamine dependence. Drug Alcohol Rev. 2017;36:153–9.
91. Morley KC, Baillie A, Van Den Brink W, Chitty KE, Brady K, Back SE, Seth D, Sutherland G, Leggio L, Haber PS. N-acetyl cysteine in the treatment of alcohol use disorder in patients with liver disease: rationale for further research. Expert Opin Investig Drugs. 2018;27:667–75.
92. Weiland A, Garcia S, Knackstedt LA. Ceftriaxone and cefazolin attenuate the cue-primed reinstatement of alcohol-seeking. Front Pharmacol. 2015;6:44.
93. Quintanilla ME, Rivera-Meza M, Berríos-Cárcamo P, Salinas-Luypaert C, Herrera-Marschitz M, Israel Y. Beyond the "first hit": marked inhibition by N-acetyl cysteine of chronic ethanol intake but not of early ethanol intake. Parallel effects on ethanol-induced saccharin motivation. Alcoholism: Clin Exp Res. 2016;40(5):1044–51.
94. Lebourgeois S, González-Marín MC, Jeanblanc J, Naassila M, Vilpoux C. Effect of N-acetylcysteine on motivation, seeking and relapse to ethanol self-administration. Addict Biol. 2018;23(2):643–52.
95. Garcia-Keller C, Smiley C, Monforton C, Melton S, Kalivas PW, Gass J. N-Acetylcysteine treatment during acute stress prevents stress-induced augmentation of addictive drug use and relapse. Addict Biol. 2019;25:e12798.
96. Cano-Cebrián MJ, Fernández-Rodríguez S, Hipólito L, Granero L, Polache A, Zornoza T. Efficacy of N-acetylcysteine in the prevention of alcohol relapse-like drinking: study in long-term ethanol-experienced male rats. J Neurosci Res. 2021;99(2):638–48.
97. Fernández-Rodríguez S, Esposito-Zapero C, Zornoza T, Polache A, Granero L, Cano-Cebrián MJ. The effects of N-Acetylcysteine on the rat

Mesocorticolimbic pathway: role of mGluR5 receptors and interaction with ethanol. Pharmaceuticals (Basel). 2021;14(6):593.
98. Quintanilla ME, Ezquer F, Morales P, Ezquer M, Olivares B, Santapau D, Herrera-Marschitz M, Israel Y. N-acetylcysteine and acetylsalicylic acid inhibit alcohol consumption by different mechanisms: combined protection. Front Behav Neurosci. 2020;14:122.
99. Goenaga J, Powell GL, Leyrer-Jackson JM, Piña J, Phan S, Prakapenka AV, Koebele SV, Namba MD, McClure EA, Bimonte-Nelson HA, Gipson CD. N-acetylcysteine yiels sex-specific efficacy for cue induced reinstatement of nicotine seeking. Addict Biol. 2020;25:e12711.
100. Monte AS, da Silva FER, Lima CNC, Vasconcelos GS, Gomes NS, Miyajima F, Vasconcelos SMM, Gama CS, Seeman MV, de Lucena DF, Maced DS. Sex influences in the preventive effects of N-acetylcysteine in a two-hit animal model of schizophrenia. J Psychopharmacol. 2020;34:125–36.

Effects of Psychoactive Drugs on the Brain

47

Raul Gagliardi

Introduction

Addictions are widespread, and many cases negatively affect addicts, their families, and society. In addition, some addictions, such as illegal psychoactive drugs, cause serious problems nationally and internationally.

One of the characteristics of addictions to drugs is that they develop in some individuals who use psychoactive substances, while other users do not develop addictions. Unfortunately, relatively little is known about the origin of these differences. Understanding why they exist can help to develop new therapies to help addicts overcome their addiction, in addition to the knowledge that can be provided in studying the mechanisms of the brain's functions [1].

For the treatment of addictions, it is also necessary to understand what effects they have on the physiology and the behavior of the addicts and how they dominate them. The appearance of new synthetic drugs, which are very addictive and can produce very adverse effects, determines the importance of linking investigations on their molecular and neuronal mechanisms and their effects on behavior.

Like all processes of transformation of an individual, the changes produced by psychoactive drugs are determined simultaneously by individual factors and social factors. In the individual factors, we can mention those that depend on the individual's will and behavior and genetic factors that can partly determine these behaviors. The social factors are mainly the characteristics of the addicts' families, their friends, and the social environment.

Addiction to psychoactive drugs is defined as chronic relapsing with three stages such as preoccupation/anticipation, binge/intoxication, and withdrawal/negative effects. These three stages occur as the person increases the frequency of use and the amount of the drug dose until reaching the pathological state that is addiction.

Addictions, including substance use disorders, require exposure to an addictive agent, meaning that addiction is not a spontaneous result of the brain activity but an interaction between the body and a specific agent, such as a psychoactive drug.

Addictions are considered as chronic diseases that modify the activities in some regions of the brain, including the nucleus accumbens, anterior cingulate cortex, basal forebrain, and amygdala. These modifications determine alterations in the addict's behavior, which replace self-care behaviors.

Addictions also affect interactions between the hippocampus and the cortical region and reward structures. These new interactions modify the memory of previous reward mechanisms, such as food, sex, alcohol, or other drugs, which in turn determines greater addiction to the drug [2].

R. Gagliardi (✉)
International Center for Migrations, Health, and Development, Geneva, Switzerland

P. Á. Gargiulo, H. L. Mesones-Arroyo (eds.), *Psychiatry and Neuroscience Update – Vol. V*,
https://doi.org/10.1007/978-3-031-72219-6_47

Kinds of Psychoactive Drugs

There are different psychoactive drugs: depressants of the central nervous system or psycholeptics, stimulants or psychoanaleptics, and hallucinogens or psycholeptics. Some drugs have a structure similar to certain neurotransmitters, activating the nerve cells to send abnormal messages. Other drugs can cause nerve cells to release excessively high amounts of natural neurotransmitters (mainly dopamine) or block the regular recycling of these chemicals in the brain. The result is that the brain is saturated with dopamine provoking pleasure feelings.

Depending on the effects on the central nervous system, drugs can be classified into the following categories:

Depressants of the central nervous or psycholeptics inhibit the functioning of the central nervous system, slowing down the nervous activity and the rhythm of bodily functions. The effects are relaxation, sedation, drowsiness, sleep, analgesia, and even coma. Examples of these substances would be alcohol, various types of opiates, such as heroin, morphine, and methadone, and drugs such as benzodiazepines or barbiturates.

Depressants have agonistic characteristics, activating the gamma-aminobutyric acid (GABA), an inhibitory neurotransmitter, and antagonistic ones imbibing glutamate, an excitatory neurotransmitter.

Stimulants or psychoanaleptics produce a general activation of the central nervous system, giving rise to an increase in bodily functions. A distinction is made between major stimulants (such as cocaine or amphetamines) and minor stimulants (such as nicotine or xanthines: caffeine, theine, or theobromine).

Amphetamines are dopamine agonists, inducing its production in the synaptic button and keeping it out in the synapsis longer than it usually would be allowed to stay. Amphetamines also act agonistically on norepinephrine, competing with it for postsynaptic receptors and turning those postsynaptic receptors on.

Cocaine blocks the reuptake of the neurotransmitters dopamine and serotonin.

Hallucinogens or psychodisleptics produce an altered state of consciousness, distort perception, and evoke sensory images without sensory input. These substances include LSD or some synthetic drugs, which, due to their effects, would be considered stimulant-hallucinogenic mixed substances. LSD antagonizes serotonin by blocking its release. The effect of psychotropic drugs on neurotransmitters is presented in Table 47.1.

Table 47.1 Effects of psychoactive drugs on neurotransmitters [3]

Neurotransmitter	What it does	What drugs affect it
Dopamine	Involved in regulation of movement, reward and punishment, pleasure, energy	Every drug that affects feelings of pleasure, including cocaine, amphetamine, opiates, marijuana, heroin, and PCP
Epinephrine (also called adrenaline)	Excitatory neurotransmitters involved in peripheral effects of arousal and alertness	Peripheral effects of stress response
Norepinephrine (also called Noradrenaline)	Involved in brain effects of arousal and alertness, energy, and feelings of pleasure	Stimulants
Serotonin	Involved in regulation of mood and impulsivity	Alcohol, hallucinogens, stimulants, antidepressants
Acetylcholine	Involved in the movement, memory function, motivation, and sleep	PCP and hallucinogens, marijuana, stimulants
GABA (Gamma-Aminobutyric Acid)	Inhibitory neurotransmitters involved in arousal, judgment, and impulsiveness	Depressant drugs, marijuana
Glutamate	Excitatory neurotransmitter	Main excitatory brain neurotransmitter. Cognitive processes
Endorphins	Substances involved in pain relief and reward/punishment	Opioids, opiates, and depressants

Different Addictions Are Related to Similar Brain Mechanisms

An addiction is considered as a chronic disease that can be difficulty to overcome. It includes effects on the brain's reward system and also acts on circuits related to memory and motivation [4].

Various investigations indicate that different addictions involve similar effects in the brain, in which the neurotransmitter dopamine acts on the "reward center," causing the motivation for the consumption of the psychoactive drug or the continuation of the addictive behavior. Addictions also involve the cancellation of synapses in the prefrontal cortex, causing the addict's attention to focus on continuing the addiction. These simultaneous effects of pleasure and attention orientation to the addiction cause the addict's brain to be dominated by the drug or the addictive behavior. These changes in brain function are reversible, although it is difficult to overcome addiction in many cases.

Psychoactive drugs have an immediate effect on the reward center. However, they can also have a long-term effect that produces addiction, that is, the persistence in the need to consume the drug, even after periods of abstinence. The difference between the immediate and long-term effects is the basis of psychological and social problems that the addict suffers. In the processes that lead to addiction, there are short-term effects of psychoactive drugs mediated by interactions between dopaminergic projections and reward circuits. There are also other projections that do not participate in the reward circuits but that collaborate in the addiction processes because they are related to pathological states that become stronger than the rewarding effects of psychoactive drugs.

In the long term, there are permanent epigenetic changes in the brain, due to the expression of genes related to addictions. Figure 47.1 shows these processes.

There may be a predisposition to addictions, such as a risk behavior during adolescence, a personal history that facilitates trying new substances, or a social environment that favors drugs. An addiction can also result from exposure to a drug for health reasons, such as using opiates for pain relief.

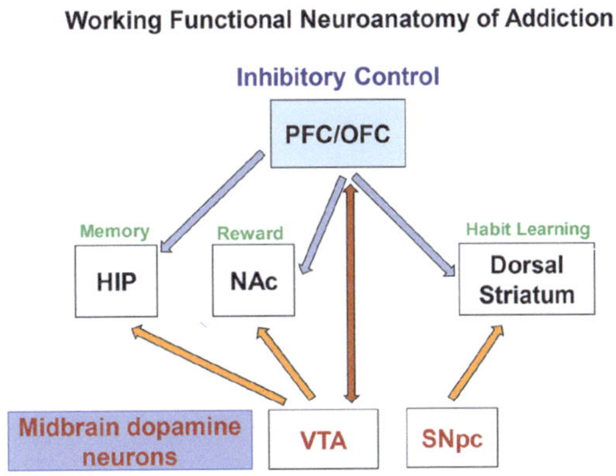

Fig. 47.1 Neuroanatomy of addictions [5]*VTA* Ventral Tegumentun, *HIP* Hippocampus, *NAC* Nucleus Accumbens, *SNpc* Substantia Nigra pars compacta Dopaminergic projections that participate in reward circuits related with the development and maintenance of addictive states

Effects of Psychoactive Drugs on the Reward System

Some psychoactive drugs are converted into metabolites that have psychotropic properties. However, most psychoactive drugs are probably not converted into molecules that exist in the body and interact with brain neuroreceptors. For example, morphine interacts with endorphin receptors.

One of the main effects of psychoactive drugs is to affect neurotransmission and the interactions between the reward structures of the brain, including the nucleus accumbens, anterior cingulate cortex, basal forebrain, and amygdala, altering the hierarchies related to motivation and causing a reduction in self-care behaviors. Addiction also affects neurotransmission and the interactions between cortical and hippocampal circuits with reward structures, which are responsible for the memory of other reward exposures, such as sex and food [2].

The psychoactive drugs infiltrate the brain's communication system, disrupting the sending, receiving, and standard processing of information between nerve cells. The two ways that drugs can do are by (1) mimicking the natural chemical messengers of the brain and (2) stimulating the brain's "reward circuit."

Some drugs like marijuana and heroin are similar to certain neurotransmitters, which the brain naturally produces. This resemblance allows drugs to "cheat" the brain's receptors and activate the nerve cells to send abnormal messages.

Other drugs, such as cocaine or methamphetamine, can cause nerve cells to release excessively high amounts of natural neurotransmitters (mainly dopamine), or they can block the regular recycling of these chemicals into the brain, which is necessary to cut the sending and receiving signals between neurons. The result is that the brain is saturated with dopamine.

Dopamine is a neurotransmitter in brain regions that controls movement, emotions, motivation, and pleasurable sensations. Usually, the gratification system responds to natural behaviors related to survival, such as eating or drinking. Alternatively, social are spending time with loved ones. When psychoactive drugs overstimulate, the reward system produces euphoric effects. This reaction initiates a vicious reinforcement cycle that "teaches" people to repeat the drug abuse behavior that caused the gratification.

When a person continues abusing drugs, the brain adapts to these overwhelming waves of dopamine by producing less dopamine or decreasing the number of dopamine receptors in the reward circuit. The result is a lower impact of dopamine on the gratification circuit, which limits the pleasure that the user can derive from drugs and events in his life that previously caused him pleasure. This decrease in pleasure forces the drug addict to continue abusing drugs to regain pleasure (maintaining the dopamine function). Besides, he frequently needs to consume a more considerable amount of the drug to elevate the dopamine function to its initial average level. This effect is known as tolerance.

Long-term abuse also causes changes in other systems and chemical circuits of the brain. For example, glutamate is a neurotransmitter that influences the gratification circuit and learning ability. When drug abuse alters the optimal concentration of glutamate, the brain tries to compensate for this imbalance, which can impair cognitive function. In addition, imaging studies of the brain of drug addicts show changes in areas of the brain essential for judgment, decision-making, learning, memory and behavior control. All these changes can make the drug addict seek and use drugs compulsively despite knowing his behavior's adverse and even devastating consequences.

There are many ways a drug can act to enhance (agonize) a given neurotransmitter or to be antagonistic to neurotransmitters.

An agonistic drug can increase the production of particular neurotransmitters. It can act on presynaptic receptors, and interferes with the release of neurotransmitters into the synapse. It can also interfere with the reuptake of neurotransmitters forcing them to remain in the synapse and interacting with receptors longer than usual. Another effect can bypass the neurotransmitter entirely and bind with and activate the neurotransmitter's receptors.

An antagonistic drug can displace the drug or agonist neurotransmitter from the receptor and thus nullify its effect on it. It can compete with the neurotransmitter for binding to its receptor without activating it and blocking the neurotransmitter receptors. An antagonistic drug can also cause neurotransmitters to leak out of their containers in the terminal button, making the neurotransmitter unavailable for release into the synapse.

Changes in the Brain Structure Provoked by Psychoactive Drugs

Some psychoactive drugs can produce structural changes in the brain. For example, cannabis use during adolescence is associated with altered neurodevelopment, particularly in cortices rich in cannabinoid receptors and undergoing the most remarkable age-related thickness change in middle to late adolescence [6].

Processes Associated with the Prefrontal Cortex that Are Disrupted in Addiction

Addictions are considered as chronic diseases that modify the activities in some regions of the brain, including the nucleus accumbens, anterior cingulate cortex, basal forebrain, and amygdala. These modifications determine alterations in the addict's behavior, which replace self-care behaviors.

Addictions also affect interactions between the hippocampus and the cortical region and reward structures. These new interactions modify the memory of previous reward mechanisms, such as food, sex, alcohol, or other drugs, which in turn determines greater addiction to the drug.

The loss of control over drug use in an addict results from changes at the central nervous system level. Initially, it was believed that the loss of control in drug addiction resulted from changes in the reward system's circuitry, which exists at the subcortical level.

Further investigations using neuroimaging indicated that the behavioral effects of psychoactive drug addiction are related to modifications of the prefrontal cortex. It exerts a regulation on limbic reward regions and controls on the brain's high-order executive functions, such as self-control, attention mechanisms (salience attribution), and the ability to understand.

Because addiction affects the brain's executive functions, centered in the prefrontal cortex, people who develop an addiction may not realize that their behavior is causing problems for themselves and others. Over time, pursuing the pleasurable effects of the substance or behavior can control an individual's activities.

The effects of a psychoactive drug on the central nervous system are multiple and can modify certain brain functions. One of these effects is to alter the inhibition responses, the coordination of behavior, the ability to predict errors, and the monitoring of the decisions taken. A psychoactive drug can modify the mechanisms of self-control and behavior monitoring. These transformations increase impulsivity and risk-taking and make behaviors more compulsive. They also make self-monitoring difficult, for example, in the automatic and habitual mechanisms of response to external stimuli. As a result, the addict who undergoes these transformations in his functions has less control over his actions and is more likely to make decisions that involve risks to his health or well-being or that may be related to crimes.

These alterations in executive functions explain the personality changes that can be observed in addicts of certain highly addictive drugs, who do not stop consuming even though their body is visibly destroying itself, as in the case of the drug called "crocodile" that causes severe ulcerations on the skin of addicts who consume it.

A change that an addict may suffer is reduction in the ability to understand the signals that the organism itself sends to the central nervous system (interoception). This reduced attention to internal cues can lead to neglection of health problems or denial of the need for medical treatment. In addition, the "fixation" on the drug causes less attention to other external stimuli, which increases the risks that the addict runs. Finally, attention deficits are also related to flexibility of thought.

Within the long list of phenomena related to the effects of psychoactive drugs, we must mention working memory problems or short-term memory oriented towards drug use and less efficient for other issues. For example, an investigation demonstrated in animal models that the administration of cocaine induces changes in dentate gyrus plasticity and hippocampal-dependent behavior [7].

The effects of psychoactive drugs on the control exerted by the prefrontal cortex over the reward system determine that the addict is more attentive to the pleasure obtained by consumption than to the rewards that can be obtained for other reasons unrelated to addiction. This situation can determine a lower learning capacity and a reduction in long-term memory, associated with a lower capacity for associations between stimuli and responses and difficulty in latent inhibition.

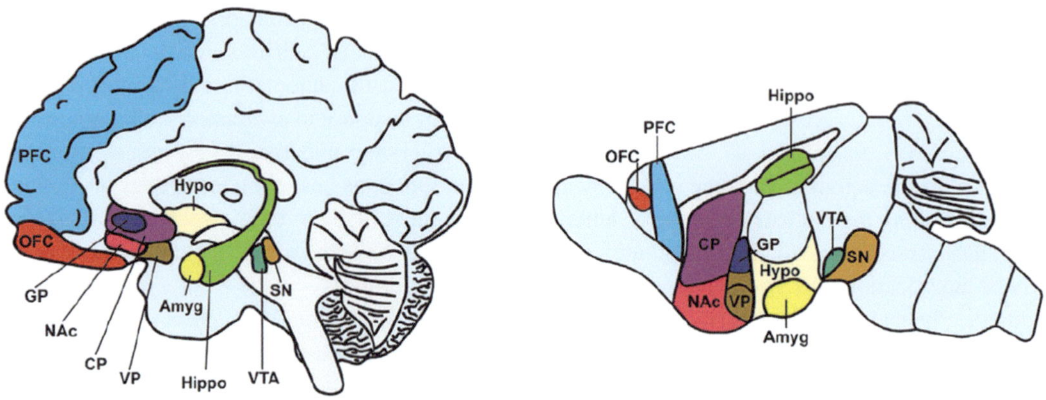

Fig. 47.2 Brain regions implicated in drug addiction [8]Left: Human brain. Right: Mouse brain*Amy* amygdala (yellow), *CP* caudate putamen (purple), *GP* globus pallidus (navy), *Hippo* hippocampus (light green), *Hypo* hypothalamus (ivory), *NAc* nucleus accumbens (pink), *OFC* orbitofrontal cortex (red), *PFC* prefrontal cortex (blue), *SN* substantia nigra (brown), *VP* ventral pallidum (dark brown), *VTA* ventral tegmental area (green)

Focusing on the consumption of a drug determines that the addict seeks the immediate pleasure determined by the consumption and is less critical to rewards in the medium and long term. Focusing on drug use also reduces the ability to plan and evaluate the future result of their actions. This situation can determine behavior that leads to difficult future situations. An addict "lives for the day" does not act beyond immediate consumption. Only same-day or next-day dose planning is expected. The addict is more attentive to the phenomena related to drug use than to other phenomena that tend to have less subjective importance. Different brain regions are implicated in drug addiction, as shown in Fig. 47.2.

A characteristic of addictions to psychoactive drugs is a fort reaction to stressful situations and a reduced ability to control the intensity of an emotion, for example, anxiety. The addict may have untimely emotional reactions to events that are relatively unimportant. He may also have a propensity to react with uncontrolled violence, which can lead to committing serious acts against him or others. These behavioral changes are also the result of changes in the central nervous system, particularly in the prefrontal cortex, that alter the regulation of emotions, that is, the cognitive or affective suppression of negative emotions.

One of the characteristics of the changes in behavior related to addictions is a motivation to obtain the drug, while the addict is less motivated for other goals, which can lead to losing their job, breaking relationships, or not taking enough care of their health. Addiction "focuses" the addict's mind on obtaining the drug. These behavioral changes are also related to the effects of psychoactive drugs on the prefrontal cortex.

Inductive Factors Related to Addictions

A critical question for understanding the addictions is why someone goes from a recreational behavior to a behavior that causes damage and cannot be abandoned.

Addiction to psychoactive drugs can be considered as a result of nonadaptive changes allowed by the plasticity of the central nervous system. The transition between using a psychoactive drug only on some occasions (recreational use) and having an addiction is possible, thanks to the plasticity of the central nervous system related to motivation, which responds to external and internal stimuli. Frequent drug use can lead to increased sensitivity to that drug in some individuals, greatly influencing behavior and causing a need for the drug, even after long-term abstinence.

The journey to addiction is determined by intrinsic factors specific to the addict, such as his personal history, genes, or culture. There are also extrinsic factors related to addictions, such as family characteristics or social environment.

These factors determine an addiction propensity, but it is always the personal decision that leads to the initiation of addictive behavior and the journey to the addiction, although once the addiction is installed, it is difficult for the addict to leave it and return to a life without addiction.

Among the intrinsic factors, we will see one of great theoretical and practical importances, the inheritance of the propensity to the addictions, whether directly through the individual's genes or the epigenetic inheritance, and to determine the inheritance of the modifications of the transcription systems of the genes.

Using a psychoactive drug or engaging in behavior that can be addictive does not necessarily lead to addiction. For this to happen, the intervention of several intrinsic factors is necessary, such as genotype, sex, age, the existence of a previous addictive disorder, or mental health problems. There are also extrinsic factors, such as access to drugs, the influence of peers, childhood problems, family characteristics, and socioeconomic status.

All these factors determine a propensity to addiction. However, it is always the personal decision that leads to the beginning of addictive behavior and the passage to addiction. While once the addiction is installed, it is difficult for the addict to get out of it.

The relative importance of these factors may vary according to age. In general, the influence of the family and peers is more important during adolescence. These factors are also crucial for the onset of consumption or addictive behavior. Genetic factors, epigenetics traits, and factors related to mental disorders influence the passage to systematic consumption and addiction [9].

The characteristics of the addictive agent are also a factor of great importance in developing an addiction. Certain substances are very addictive, and in a short time, their consumption leads to an addiction that is very difficult to overcome. An example is the opiates used in medicine, such as oxycodone, which causes addiction in just over a month of regular use. All addictive agents act on the same brain centers, but the addiction is determined by their pharmacological characteristics, psychoactive properties, and mode of administration [10–12].

Within the intrinsic factors, we will see one of the great theoretical and practical importances, the inheritance of the propensity to addictions, either directly by the genes of the individual or by epigenetic inheritance, that is, the inheritance of the modifications of the transcription systems of the genes.

The Role of Genetics and the Environment in the Development of an Addiction

In the medical/biological sciences and the social and psychological sciences, there is an old discussion about the determination of the characteristics of a person, if the genes determine them or if they are determined by the influences of the family and social environment.

Regarding a person's behavior, there are also old discussions about whether they are only the result of individual decisions or if they are the result of phenomena such as the morality to which they ascribe or the influences of the social environment to which they belong.

Transferred to the discussion on addictions, we can summarize that there are approaches that focus on individual responsibility, while other approaches give more importance to the circumstances of their lives, their social environment, or their genetics.

These discussions are not just theoretical. For example, when deciding the degree of responsibility of an addict for his actions in court, the verdicts will be different if they are based only on the idea that it was his will to take drugs; therefore, he is fully responsible for his actions, or if the addiction is the result of their genetics, the responsibility for their actions is less or null. These discussions are similar to when addiction is considered a disease that must be cured or when it is thought that the addict can stop using the drug when he decides.

An example allows us to clarify this situation: In the State of Florida (USA), there were cases of cannibalism associated with consuming a drug called cloud nine or flake. Once the addict who committed these acts has been arrested, the question arises: what should be done with him? Intern him as mentally ill or accuse him of the crime he committed? The answer is that he should be hospitalized and treated as mentally ill.

However, what should be done in cases of crimes committed by consumers of other drugs that promote violence, such as alcohol or cocaine? Determining the total or relative responsibility of the addict means, in the case of a trial, different verdicts. If it is thought that addiction is not only a disease but also that the propensity to addiction is inherited, the verdict will be closer to medical treatment than jail.

Different investigations have shown that certain addictions have a genetic basis. Others have shown that addictions result from epigenetic processes, that is, changes in gene expression due to the effect of psychoactive drugs. In some of these investigations, another element for discussion appears, some epigenetic modifications determined by drugs can be inherited in the first generations.

This information raises questions about an addict's responsibility if his parents were addicts and he inherited the propensity for addictions.

We do not claim to provide answers to these questions. However, we believe that research on the mechanisms of action of psychoactive drugs, and in particular, the epigenetic mechanisms and their possible inheritance can be helpful to help solve one of the world's most serious problems.

Genetics of Addictions

A hypothesis supported by investigations on the effect of psychoactive drugs is that the vulnerability to transform a recreational behavior into an addiction depends on genetic and nongenetic factors. The nongenetic factors are permanent environmental factors or random phenomena and can produce lasting changes in the individual.

The genetic memory of an individual, the set of genes that it possesses, translates into specific characteristics, a phenotype, based on the control of the expression of the genes. These genes are repressed and expressed, which determine the individual's development and characteristics. New research technologies have allowed the understanding of the relationship between addictions and an individual's genes.

One example is cannabis addiction. It is known that the risk of dependency on this drug has a genetic factor, a genetic locus located on chromosome 8 that controls the levels of expression of the CHRNA2 gene in the cerebrum and cerebellum. Low gene expression levels in the cerebellum are associated with cannabis addiction, including younger diagnoses and age. In addition, it was shown that genetic factors related to educational attainment are protective against cannabis addiction [13].

Two of the most frequently consumed psychoactive drugs which cause severe damage to health are nicotine and alcohol. Determining the genetic factors of addictions to those drugs was difficult. However, an investigation with a sample of 1.2 million people found that 566 genetic variants in 406 loci are associated with tobacco use in different stages. This research also showed the relationship between genes and alcohol consumption, with 150 loci showing a pleiotropic association. In addition, the research showed that, in nicotine and alcohol addiction, there are genes involved in nicotinic, dopaminergic, and glutamatergic neurotransmission [14].

Environmental and genetic factors related to addictions to psychoactive drugs act differently according to age. For nicotine, alcohol, and cannabis, family environmental factors are critical in early adolescence but are less important as age advances. In contrast, genetic factors are of little importance in early adolescence but gradually increase their effects with age. Substantial correlations were found between cannabis, nicotine, and alcohol consumption. A correlation was also found between the consumption of nicotine and caffeine [15].

Epigenetics Mechanism Related to Addictions

An individual's genetic makeup, its genotype, partly determines its characteristics, but development is not an exact result of genes. The interaction with the environment determines which genes are expressed and to what extent they do so. The characteristics of a person are not the result of genetics or the environment; they are the result of the interaction between them in the continuous processes of self-construction (autopoiesis).

In the case of psychoactive drugs, the influence of the family and social environment can play an essential role in determining whether or not a person will develop drug or other types of addictions. Studies conducted by the National Institute for Drug Abuse have shown that there is a reduced vulnerability to drug addictions in a community where there are healthy activities after study hours. Those data also show that physical exercise reduces drug-seeking behavior. This effect is more pronounced in men than in women.

How Psychoactive Drugs Can Provoke Epigenetic Effects

Epigenetic mechanisms transduce environmental stimuli in alterations of chromatin structure, which activate or repress gene expression. Proteins called histones surround the DNA and determine its compression. For RNA to be synthesized, histones must be uncoupled from DNA.

In the regions of DNA where the histones are connected, the DNA-to-RNA translation systems cannot act. The separation of histones from DNA releases these genes and allows their translation into RNA, which will then be translated into proteins and determine specific characteristics of the cell and the individual. Histone release is one of the mechanisms of genetic regulation or, in other words, one of the epigenetic mechanisms.

Different investigations have demonstrated the importance of epigenetic mechanisms in permanent changes in different tissues and organs, including the brain.

A characteristic of addictions to psychoactive drugs is the persistence of behavioral changes, that is, phenotypic changes produced by epigenetic mechanisms. The persistence of these changes suggests that there may be changes in the gene expression in some brain regions, particularly in the reward region. These changes result from the modulation of gene expression by environmental factors, in this case, by consuming psychoactive drugs. An example of the epigenetic effects of drugs is cocaine. When a person uses this drug, it can affect gene control by increasing the production of proteins related to addiction. In addition, animal research has shown increased levels of these proteins in animals with drug-seeking behaviors.

The behavioral changes related to the ingestion of psychoactive drugs and, in particular, the development of addictions, are related to brain plasticity, mediated by epigenetic mechanisms in the reward regions. The existence of three mechanisms of epigenetic regulation in the brain has been demonstrated: histone modifications such as acetylation and methylation, DNA methylation, and noncoding RNAs.

DNA methylation can be done by nucleotide or dinucleotide methylation. For example, a common process is the methylation of cytosine in which methyl groups are covalently linked at carbon 5. DNA methyltransferases 1, 3A, and 3B participate in these processes. Cytosine methylation occurs in cytosine-guanine dinucleotides and more frequently in dinucleotides with one of the other three nucleotides (adenine, thymine, and cytosine) [16–18].

Proteins and transcription factors sensitive to methyl groups can bind to methylated cytosine and interact with the repressor and chromatin, remodeling them and determining the expression of the corresponding genes [19, 20].

Methylated cytosine is stable but can be oxidized by methylcytosine dioxygenases, which convert it to hydroxymethylcytosine. This molecule can persist as a stable epigenetic modification or be subsequently oxidized by some methylxytosine dioxidase into formylcytosine and carboxylcytosine.

On DNA repair, mechanisms by demethylation formylcytosine and carboxylcytosine are excised and replaced with unmethylated cytosine.

The epigenetic mechanisms determined by psychoactive drugs include changes in gene expression in mature, postmitotic neurons without causing changes in DNA sequence. There is evidence that psychoactive drug-mediated chromatin remodeling associated with continued expression of addiction-associated genes includes enzymatic modifications of DNA and histones.

Addictions produce many epigenetic adaptations, changing the balance in the synthesis and destruction of enzymes in some specific loci of medium spiny neurons nucleus (MSN). Addictions also induce some transcription factors that mediate the transcription of genes that encode neurotransmitters receptors, cytoskeletal proteins, and ion channels. All these modifications alter the physiological functions of MSN and increase dendritic spine density [21]. The epigenetic modifications of the neurones of the MSN are presented in Fig. 47.3.

Epigenetic regulation produces changes in the regular expression of some genes or their "inducibility" that occurs throughout life in response to external or internal stimuli. These changes favor an individual's vulnerability to addictions.

Third, there is the possibility that drugs induce epigenetic changes in sperm or eggs, which means that offspring may be vulnerable to addictions (transgenerational epigenetic inheritance).

An example of epigenetic mechanisms terminated by psychoactive drugs is that of opioids. Scientific evidence indicates that these drugs act on brain reward circuits, increasing the acetylation levels of the histones that release genes (permissive histones) and lowering the methylation levels of the histones that prevent the expression of those genes (repressive histones). Opioids also alter the patterns of DNA methylation and noncoding RNA [22].

Epigenetic mechanisms, including histone modifications, noncoding RNA expression, and DNA methylation, may explain the relationship between the prenatal environment of a mother addicted to psychoactive drugs and the future health consequences she may suffer for the child during adolescence or as an adult [23].

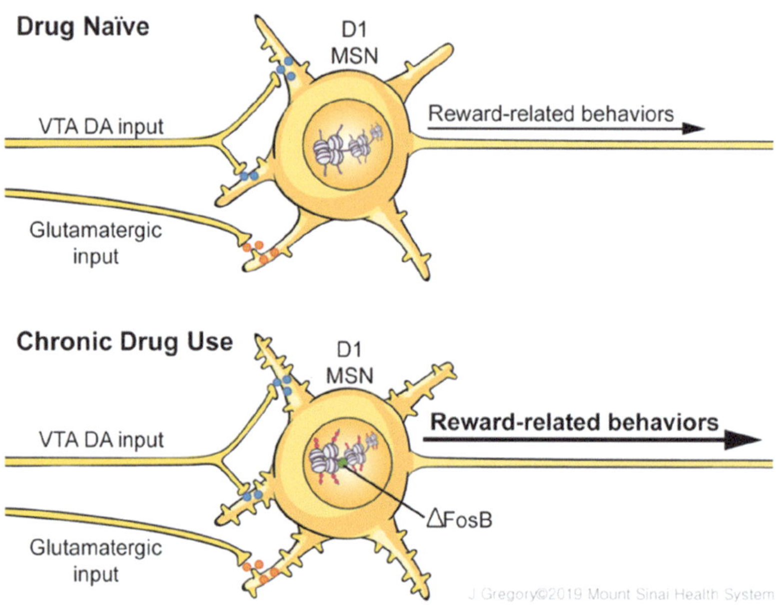

Fig. 47.3 Epigenetic modifications of neurons related to addictions *MSNs* medium spiny neurons, *Nac* nucleus accumbens, *VTA* ventral tegmental area

Epigenetic Heredity of Psychotropic Drug Abuse

An extensive review of the literature on the effects of drug use on subsequent generations indicates the existence of epigenetic inheritance of psychoactive drug addiction. The epigenetic modifications an addiction undergoes are transmitted to the embryo during fertilization and modify the expression of genetic and developmental programs. There are intergenerational mechanisms (transmission to the first generation) and transgenerational (that is, transmission to successive generations). In particular, alcohol, cocaine, nicotine, cannabinoids, and opiates are epigenetic inheritances [24].

Epigenetic inheritance can be intergenerational or transgenerational. Intergenerational inheritance occurs when males or females are subjected to an environmental stressor prior to mating, and their tissues, including their gametes, are directly exposed to the stressor. Therefore, their gametes will carry the epigenetic transformation expressed in the first generation. The gametes of the first generation were not subjected to the stressor, and therefore, the second generation will not have the epigenetic transformation. However, if the gametes of the first generation also carry the epigenetic modification, the second generation will also carry it. In this case, it is a transgenerational epigenetic inheritance. A particular case is when a pregnant female is exposed to an environmental stressor, the fetus is also subjected to that stressor, and the gametes of the fetus can also carry epigenetic modification, which produces a transgenerational inheritance. According to this information, epigenetic effects may be transmitted in successive generations.

Epigenetic inheritance can solve some of the problems of animal or plant evolution studies and open new theoretical and practical fields in biology. From the point of view of understanding the action of psychoactive drugs, the epigenetic inheritance would explain the addiction propensity of children of addicts.

Conclusion

Addictions to psychoactive drugs are related to modifications in the brain's reward systems that focus the addict's attention on drug consumption.

Various regions of the brain are related to the development of addictions.

Addiction to psychoactive drugs is related to processes of modification of the action of neurotransmitters, particularly dopamine. Various regions of the brain are involved in the development of addictions, including the frontal cortex.

The action of psychoactive drugs includes epigenetic mechanisms, in which certain genes are unlocked and promote addiction. Those epigenetic mechanisms can be passed on to the addict's offspring, which can increase the likelihood that those offspring will be addicted.

There are different psychoactive drugs such as depressants of the central nervous system or psycholeptics, stimulants or psychoanaleptics, and hallucinogens or psycholeptics. Some drugs have a structure similar to certain neurotransmitters, activating the nerve cells to send abnormal messages. Other drugs can cause nerve cells to release excessively high amounts of natural neurotransmitters (mainly dopamine) or block the regular recycling of these chemicals in the brain. The result is that the brain is saturated with dopamine provoking pleasure feelings.

References

1. Kaplan G, Xu H, Abreu K, Feng J. DNA epigenetics in addiction susceptibility. Front Genet. 2022;13.
2. Public policy statement: definition of addiction. American Society of Addiction Medicine; 2011.
3. How drugs affect the brain. MentalHealth.Net Online https://www.mentalhelp.net/substance-abuse/how-drugs-affect-the-brain/
4. Nora D, Volkow ND, Michaelides M, Baler R. The neuroscience of drug reward and addiction. Physiol Rev. 2019; Online https://journals.physiology.org/doi/full/10.1152/physrev.00014.2018
5. Cadet JL, Jayanthi S. Epigenetics of addiction. Neurochem Int. 2021.

6. Albaugh M, et al. Association of Cannabis use during adolescence with neurodevelopment. JAMA Psychiatry. 2021;78(9):1031.
7. Perez MF, Gabach LA, Almiron RS, Carlini VP, De Barioglio SR, Ramirez OA. Different chronic cocaine administration protocols induce changes in dentate gyrus plasticity and hippocampal dependent behavior. Synapse. 2010;64(10):742–53.
8. Kaplan G, Xu H, Abreu K, Feng J. opus cité.
9. Roberts AJ, Koob GF. The neurobiology of addiction: an overview. Lancet Psychiatry. 2016;3(8):760–73.
10. Reuter J, Raedler T, Rose M, et al. Pathological gambling is linked to reduced activation of the mesolimbic reward system. Nat Neurosci. 2005;8(2):147–8.
11. Ducci F, Goldman D. The genetic basis of addictive disorders. Psychiatry Clin North Am. 2012;35(2):495–519.
12. Merikangas KR, Avenevoli S. Implications of genetic epidemiology for preventing substance use disorders. Addict Behav. 2000;25(6):807–20.
13. Genetics and epigenetics of addiction drugfacts. National Institute of Drug Abuse. The USA. 2019.
14. Liu M, Jiang Y, Wedow R, et al. Association studies of up to 1.2 million individuals yield new insights into the genetic etiology of tobacco and alcohol use. Nat Genet. 2019;51:237–44.
15. Kendler KS, Schmitt E, Aggen SH, Carol A, Prescott CA. Genetic and environmental influences on alcohol, caffeine, cannabis, and nicotine use from early adolescence to middle adulthood. Arch Gen Psychiatry. 2008;65(6):674–82.
16. Xie W, Barr CL, Kim A, Yue F, Lee AY, Eubanks J, et al. Base-resolution analyses of sequence and parent-of-origin dependent DNA methylation in the mouse genome. Cell. 2012;148:816–31.
17. Jaenisch R, Bird A. Epigenetic regulation of gene expression: how the genome integrates intrinsic and environmental signals. Nat Genet. 2003;33(Suppl l):245–54.
18. Lister R, Mukamel EA, Nery JR, Urich M, Puddifoot CA, Johnson ND, et al. Global epigenomic reconfiguration during mammalian brain development. Science. 2013;341:1237905-1.
19. Clemens AW, Gabel HW. Emerging insights into the distinctive neuronal methylome. Trends Genet. 2020;36:816–32.
20. Skene PJ, Illingworth RS, Webb S, Kerr ARW, James KD, Turner DJ, et al. Neuronal MeCP2 is expressed at near histone-octamer levels and globally alters the chromatin state. Mol Cell. 2010;37:457–68.
21. Hamilton PJ, Nestler EJ. Epigenetics and addiction. Curr Opin Neurobiol. 2019;59:128.
22. Browne CJ, Godino A, Salary M, Nestler EJ. Epigenetic mechanisms of opioid. Addict Biol Psychiatry. 87(1):22–33.
23. Wanner NM, Colwell ML, Christopher Faulk C. The epigenetic legacy of illicit drugs: developmental exposures and late-life phenotypes. Environ Epigenet. 2019:1–10.
24. Baratta AM, Rathod RS, Plasil SL, Seth A, Homanics GE. Exposure to drugs of abuse induce effects that persist across generations. Int Rev Neurobiol. 2021;156:217–27.

48 Drugs Abuse by Adolescents

Raul Gagliardi

> We started knocking on doors to see how we could help the kids. So that they get out, not only from drugs but from the vulnerability they are in. That they stop to think, that they love each other, that they value themselves and that opportunities are given.[1]
>
> Misrepresented, misjudged, and mishandled. Addiction is a misunderstood tragedy, to often hushed up. Not anymore, my child is dying a slow death from the disease of addiction….We have the power to change the way addiction is perceived, we have the power to change the way addiction is believed. We have the power to change the way in which our beloved addicts are judged and treated. Our voices, together and unashamed, are fierce. We'll know we've succeeded once comfort is baked into bundt cakes—as it is for every other disease.[2]

Introduction

Writing a chapter of a book is usually a pleasant act. However, some themes produce sadness, leaving the feeling of something unfinished, with questions that the author does not know how to answer. The issue of adolescents and psychoactive drugs is one of these themes. When many children, adolescents, and young people worldwide destroy their lives—dying in many cases - due to drug abuse, and when gangs dominate cities and provinces, there are no clear solutions to avoid it.

In the street of many cities, children, adolescents, and young people move erratically, with lost eyes, begging. Many of them prostitute themselves. Others participate in the bloody struggles of drug gangs or are dealers. Each of them requires help to overcome the cause of these situations: psychoactive drug abuse.

Crack, cocaine, methamphetamine, heroin, fentanyl, and other opiates for legal or illegal sale, glues and alcohol are the various substances consumed that produce an immediate, pleasant, euphoric effect. Substances that calm hunger and anguish but destroy the future of the addicts and their families.

[1] Corvalan B. Madres Contra el Paco una Organizacion que lucha Dia a Dia. La Noticia Solidaria. Con la Gente Noticias. 2018. Online https://conlagentenoticias.com/madres-contra-el-paco-una-organizacion-que-lucha-dia-a-dia/

[2] Swenson S. When Your Child Is Addicted And hope hurts. 2017. The USA. Online. https://www.hazeldenbettyford.org/articles/child-addiction

R. Gagliardi (✉)
International Center for Migrations, Health, and Development, Vernier, Switzerland

P. Á. Gargiulo, H. L. Mesones-Arroyo (eds.), *Psychiatry and Neuroscience Update – Vol. V*, https://doi.org/10.1007/978-3-031-72219-6_48

One of the most severe and complex problems in modern society is drug abuse. The production, distribution, and sale of illegal drugs are significant challenges worldwide. Most countries must face the economic, political, and social power of drug trafficking and the psychological and other health problems related to the abuse of drugs.

Worldwide special police forces fight drug trafficking. Nevertheless, the main drug czars have enormous fortunes, and some of the gangs weigh the money because counting it would be much work. In some countries, drug traffickers dominate society and corrupt governments. Thousands of people die from gang violence.

Adolescents know the risk of being part of drug trafficking gangs. However, belonging to drug trafficking gangs is attractive to many young people who, in addition to the risk of prison, can die in struggles against the Police or other gangs.

Addiction is a phenomenon with significant effects on the family, the addict's environment and society. Millions of people worldwide are addicted to different substances or activities such as masturbation, gambling, the Internet, food, pornography, sex, sugar, technology, smartphone, social media, video games, shopping, physical exercise, and legal and illegal psychoactive drugs.[3]

The consumption of legal psychoactive drugs, such as opiates, used initially to reduce pain, is also a big problem, with hundreds of deaths and personal and family destruction, as has happened in the epidemic of opiates of legal sale in the USA.[4] and in some African countries.[5]

Some of the addictions, such as sugar, harm the health.[6] Others, such as gambling, provoke economic problems. The abuse of psychoactive drugs harms the health and the economy, provoking psychological problems, and promoting illegal activities.

Abuse of psychoactive drugs, including alcohol, can lead to death by provoking illnesses, accidents, unprotected sex, motor vehicle accidents, suicides, physical dependence, and psychological addiction. Moreover, the abuse of drugs jeopardizes the future of adolescents that start the consumption of drugs and become addicts. They can suffer physiological and psychological problems, changes in their sociocognitive niche and illegal activities. Adolescents who are drug abusers experience higher rates of physical and mental disorders and diminished well-being.

Effects of the Psychoactive Drugs on the Adolescent's Brain

The adolescent years are a crucial window for substance use and the development of substance use disorders. Brain systems governing emotion and reward-seeking are fully developed by this time, but circuits governing judgment and self-inhibition are still maturing, causing teenagers to act on impulse, seek new sensations, and be easily swayed by their peers—all of which may draw them to take risks such as trying psychoactive drugs. Moreover, because critical neural circuits are still forming, teens' brains are particularly susceptible to being modified by those substances in a lasting way—making developing a substance use disorder much more likely.

Autopoiesis, Homeostasis, and Homeorhesis

We can use different theories in the analysis of addictions. One of them, coming from biology, is that of autopoiesis. The basic concept is that an organism builds itself and determines the conditions that allow its construction. In other words, a living organism is a recurrent system that is con-

[3]Zaved A. Sugar Addiction: Causes, Dangers and Withdrawal Symptoms. Addiction Resource, 2021.

[4]Opioid Overdose Crisis, National Institute of Drugs Abuse. USA, 2021.

[5]Opioids in Africa: cheap and accessible. DW 2019.

[6]Avena N. M., Rada P., and Hoebel B. G. Evidence for sugar addiction: Behavioral and neurochemical effects of intermittent, excessive sugar intake. Neurosci Biobehav Rev. 2008; 32(1): 20–39.

structed and allows its construction by maintaining certain stable conditions in a changing environment.[7,8]

This concept can explain two phenomena characteristic of living organisms, which may appear contradictory, their stability in a changing environment and their ability to transform during their life in their development. In other words, stability keeps certain conditions constant and changes others in a programmed development answering simultaneously to environmental characteristics. The conditions of stability maintain homeostasis while the conditions that allow changes during development allow homeorhesis, that is, the maintenance of conditions that allow reaching a future state determined by genetic information. An embryonic organism or a young organism develops by homeostasis, and from its initial state, it has changes that lead it to the characteristics of the adult state.[9,10]

If we apply this idea to psychological phenomena, we can say that there are conditions of stability and conditions that allow developmental changes in the development of a child and a teenager.

The development of intelligence and personality can be interpreted according to the concepts mentioned above, the autopoiesis that determines the conditions of homeostasis (permanence of essential characteristics) and the conditions of homeorhesis that determines the arrival in an adult state in which there are changes in relationships with the younger states, and there are similar characteristics to them.

Addiction is a profound transformation of autopoiesis, homeostasis, and homeorhesis processes. The abuse of drugs alters the psychological mechanisms of self-building (autopoiesis) and changes stability (homeostasis) by guiding the behavior toward the search for the drug. It also influences homeorhesis by transforming physiological and psychological conditions.

The changes in adolescent physiology modify the developmental conditions and determine a different adult state from the one that would have been reached without drug use.

Hard and Soft Drugs

Psychoactive drugs that cause serious health problems and are highly addictive are called "hard drugs," for example, cocaine, morphine, heroin, and amphetamines. The psychoactive drugs that provoke more minor problems are called "soft drugs," such as marijuana. This distinction exists in both official discourse and informal speech.

There are campaigns to legalize soft drugs. Some countries allow the production and consumption of soft drugs, such as Uruguay and some states of the USA, where the production and sale of marihuana are allowed with controls, or in the Netherlands, where public consumption of cannabis is not penalized in certain bars that sell different forms of marijuana.

One of the arguments against the legalization of soft drugs is that they can facilitate the passage to hard drugs. Another argument is that consuming soft drugs can have long-term adverse effects. Also, it is necessary to consider the augment of the concentration of the psychoactive substance in the drug by the artificial selection made by the producers. For example, the concentration of tetra-hydro-cannabinol, the substance that produces the psychotropic effects of marijuana, in the drug consumed today is usually 10–20 times

---

[7] Maturana H, and Varela F. Autopoiesis and Cognition: The Realization of the Living. Dordecht: D. Reidel Publishing Co., 1980.

[8] Gagliardi R. Relationships between living organisms and environment. Thesis for the Grade of Doctor in Sciences. Faculty of Sciences. The University of Geneva. 1985.

[9] Munari A. Les concepts d'équilibration majorante et d'homéorhèse dans la psychogenèse du sujet individuel. Archives de psychologie (Genève). 1988, Vol 56, Num 219, pp. 271–28.

[10] Pereira A. Developing the Concepts of Homeostasis, Homeorhesis, Allostasis, Elasticity, Flexibility, and Plasticity of Brain Function. Neurosci, 2, 372–382. 2021.

higher than in the marijuana consumed 30 years ago.

The opioid epidemic in the USA, where hundreds of thousands of addicts died from an overdose, is another unfortunate example of the ease of going from a consumption determined by the need to calm the pain to an addiction that ruins lives.

An argument in favor of the decriminalization of the consumption of psychoactive drugs is that the prohibition determines the illegal production, drug trafficking, and the associated crimes, among them the search for money to buy the drug.

We believe that the legalization of soft drugs should be related to a vigorous campaign for educating the population, particularly children and adolescents, about the harmful effects of the drugs on health and quality of life, and the very negative impact on society of trafficking. It is also important to consider addiction as an illness and provide medical and psychological care to the addicts and not punish them only for consuming the drug.

"Responsible" Use of Psychoactive Substances

The concept of "responsible use of drugs" indicates that a person can use them by reducing or eliminating the risks of adversely affecting their own life or the lives of others. For example, some people argue that well-known artists or intellectuals use drugs to enhance their creativity. We believe this is an excuse for drug abuse because creativity is not the result of any substance but individual capacity.

Critics of the concept of responsible use of drugs say it is an escape from problems and that it can cause dangerous effects that are difficult to predict, including addiction. These critics point out that drug use affects the drug addict and the familiar and social environment. It can also have effects at a distance, such as the problems caused by drug trafficking. In addition, certain socially admitted drugs, such as tobacco and alcohol, provoke diseases that jeopardize the future of the addict.

A general rule is to "avoid the risks" of addiction and all its consequences, avoiding the initiation of consumption. This rule should apply to all cases where the social environment favors "testing drugs" (schoolmates or friends). The alleged reasonable use is nothing more than a false idea that only favors addiction.

Death by an Overdose of Psychoactive Drugs

The impact on the health of drug abuse is severe worldwide. More than 1.5% of the global disease burden in health results from illicit drug or alcohol addiction. In some countries, the burden is over 5%. Nearly 12 million people worldwide die from diseases provoked by alcohol and tobacco each year.

Death from overdoses is high around the world. With 245.8 overdoses by million inhabitants, the USA has the high rate. The second and third countries are Iceland with 221.2 and El Salvador with 160.1 overdoses by million inhabitants. Sweden, Australia, Ukraine, Canada, Estonia, Russia, and Seychelles are the next eight countries with higher frequency of overdoses.[11]

Between 1999 and 2019, one and a half million people died from overdoses in the USA.[12] Moreover, 96,779 people died from drug overdoses from March 2020 to March 2021. This figure is 36.1% higher than the previous annual high from December 2018 to December 2019 (71,130 deaths).[13]

The pandemic of COVID—19 provoked an augment in overdose deaths. In 2021, the number

[11] Highest Overdose & Drug Related Death Rates In The World. World Atlas. Online. https://www.worldatlas.com/articles/10-highest-overdose-and-drug-related-death-rates-in-the-world.html

[12] Drug Overdoses in Youth. National Institute on Drug Abuse. 2020.

[13] Drug Overdose Deaths. CDC, National Center for Health Statistics. 2020.

of deaths by overdose in the USA was higher than one hundred thousand.

Overdoses are a leading cause of death for adolescents and youngers. There is a constant growth of overdose deaths among 14–24 years old. In the USA, mainly caused by synthetic opioids (primarily illicitly manufactured fentanyl).

Frequently, overdoses are provoked by differences in the concentration of the psychoactive substance in the doses. For example, a more pure dose of the drug can provoke an overdose. Another frequent cause of overdose is the substance used to "cut" the drug. For example, the use of fentanyl for cutting cocaine or heroine in the dose can provoke the death of the addict. Every dealer who buys cocaine breaks it up. Some do it with nontoxic substances, such as starch. Others give it hallucinogens and if there is no type of control.[14]

Suicides are often related to drug use. Postmortem tests carried out on people who committed suicide are very significant. In 2013, 38.2% of those tests were positive for alcohol, 35.3% for antidepressants, 31.3% for benzodiazepines, 26.8% for opiates, and 16.6% for marijuana. Probably, the causes of suicide may be related to the psychological and social effects of drugs, or to the need to use drugs due to depression or other psychological conditions.[15]

In February of 2022 in Argentine, 24 persons died, and a hundred needed urgent treatment, including respirators, because of a high concentration of piperazine, a precursor of fentanyl, in the cocaine they consumed. The Police could confiscate 25,000 doses, and avoid a much larger quantity of deaths.[16,17]

Frequency of Addictions to Psychoactive Drugs by Adolescents

> (in the USA) By the time they are seniors, almost 70 percent of high school students will have tried alcohol, half will have taken an illegal drug, nearly 40 percent will have smoked a cigarette, and more than 20 percent will have used a prescription drug for a nonmedical purpose.[18]

Drug abuse is more common in men than in women. In addition, half of those who die from alcohol or drug overdoses are younger than 50.[19]

Addictions of psychoactive drugs are widespread in adolescents. An example is India, where 50% of male students have tried a drug gateway at least once.[20,21]

Alcohol is the most commonly abused substance among teens and young adults. The

[14] Berni: "Quienes compraron droga en estas últimas 24 horas tienen que descartarla". Infobae. 2022, Online. https://www.infobae.com/sociedad/policiales/2022/02/02/berni-quienes-compraron-droga-en-estas-ultimas-24-horas-tienen-que-descartarla/

[15] Drug Use Among Youth: Facts & Statistics. National Center for Drug Abuse Statistics. The USA. 2022. Online. https://drugabusestatistics.org/teen-drug-use/

[16] Tragedia en Argentina: al menos 20 muertos y más de 70 hospitalizados por consumir cocaína envenenada. El Pais. 2022. Online https://elpais.com/internacional/2022-02-02/tragedia-en-argentina-varios-muertos-y-decenas-de-hospitalizados-por-consumir-cocaina-envenenada.html#

[17] Narcotráfico en el conurbano: hay 20 muertos y aumentó a 84 el número de personas internadas. Infobae. 2022. Online https://www.infobae.com/sociedad/policiales/2022/02/02/cuatro-muertos-y-diez-internados-por-consumir-cocaina-adulterada-en-el-conurbano/

[18] Johnston, L.D.; O'Malley, P.M.; Bachman, J.G.; and Schulenberg, J.E. Monitoring the Future National Results on Adolescent Drug Use: Overview of Key Findings, National Institute on Drug Abuse, 2013.

[19] Ritchie H., and Roser M. Drug Use. Our World in Data, 2019.

[20] John R.C. Social and Cultural Aspects of Drug Abuse in Adolescents. Review, Delhi Psychiatry Journal Vol. 12 No.2, 2009.

[21] Kastner P. and Silbereisese RK. Drogengebrauch Jugendlicher auaentwicklungs psychologischer Sicht. In BildunUnd Erziehung, 1984; 37: 271–285. Cited in: Jiloha R.C. Social and Cultural Aspects of Drug Abuse in Adolescents. Review, Delhi Psychiatry Journal Vol. 12 No.2, 2009.

National Institute of Drug Abuse of the USA alerted that youth drug abuse is a high-profile public health concern. It informed that at least one-in-eight teenagers have used an illicit substance in the last year. By 12th grade, 62% of students have consumed alcohol in lifetime, and 16,8% did 5 or plus drinks in a row.

- Binge drinking is the most frequent mode of consuming alcohol, with a high risk of being drunk, 1.19 million of 12- to 17-year-olds and 11.72 million of 18- to 25-year-olds report binge drinking in the last month.[22]

In 2021, in the USA, 407,000 teenagers aged 12- to 17 years old met the criteria for Alcohol Use Disorder (AUD).

In the USA, 50% of teenagers have misused a drug at least once, 15% of high school students reported having ever used select illicit or injection drugs (i.e., cocaine, inhalants, heroin, methamphetamines, hallucinogens, or ecstasy), and 43% of college students use illicit drugs. In addition, 14% of students reported misusing prescription opioids, 86% of teenagers know someone who smokes, drinks or uses drugs during the school day, and drug use among 8th graders increased 61% between 2016 and 2020.[23,24,25,26,27] About half of the adolescents in the 12th grade consumed an illicit drug at least once. The most frequent is marijuana. Teens can also use drugs they find at home, such as prescription medications, glues, and aerosols. Each day, 15,000 teens use drugs for the first time.[28]

Surveys carried out in schools in the USA in 2023 indicate the high frequency of psychoactive drug use by students.[29] When asked what drugs had been used in the previous year, it was observed that alcohol was the most consumed drug, by 45.7% of 12th graders, 15.1% of 8th graders, and 30.6% of 10th graders. The consumption of illegal drugs was also very frequent, by 31.2% of 12th graders, 19.8% of 10th graders, and 10.9% of 8th graders. The most frequently consumed illegal drug was marijuana, by 29% of 12th graders, and 17.8% of 8th graders and 8.3% of 10th graders. Cigarette consumption was 15% in 12th graders, 9.4% in 10th graders, and 5.8% in 8th graders, vaping nicotine (e-cigarettes) was performed by 23.2% of 12th graders, 17.6% of 10th graders, and 11.4% of 8th grade.

Cocaine use in the USA decreased in the last 20 years, from 1 million in 2002 to 671,000 in 2019. People aged 18 and 25 were the largest group using cocaine (476,000). Among them, 59,000 were adolescents. These studies indicate that adolescents initiate cocaine use in college rather than high school. Those who start consumption in adolescence or youth become addicts more quickly than adults who start cocaine use.

In Nigeria, most drug addicts start smoking from a young age. Sixty-five percent of high school students used drugs to have a good time, 54% wanted to experiment to see what it is like, and 20–40% used it to alter their moods. Drug abuse results in gang formation, armed robbery, mental illness, and cultism.[30]

In Morocco, 16% of girls and 40% of boys reported alcohol, hashish, or psychotropic drugs at some point in their lifetime. Lower grades in

[22]Drug Use Among Youth: Facts & Statistics. talkheart-2heart.org. 2022, Online. https://talkheart2heart.org

[23]Drug Overdoses in Youth. National Institute on Drug Abuse. The USA. Op. cité.

[24]CDC. Youth Risk Behavior Surveillance, 2019. *MMWR Suppl* 2020;69(1):1–83. the USA.

[25]CDC, Division of Adolescent and School Health, National Center for HIV/AIDS, Viral Hepatitis, STD, and TB Prevention. *Youth Risk Behavior Survey Data Summary & Trends Report, 2009–2019* pdf icon[PDF – 31 MB]. Atlanta, GA: US Department of Health and Human Services, Centers for Disease Control and Prevention, Office of Infectious Diseases, NCHHSTP; 2020.

[26]Clayton, H.B, Lowry, R., August, E., & Jones, S.E. Nonmedical use of prescription drugs and sexual risk behaviors. *Pediatrics*.2016; 137 (1),e20152480.

[27]Clayton, H.B., Lowry, R, Basile, K.C., et al. Physical and Sexual Dating Violence and Nonmedical Use of Prescription Drugs. *Pediatrics*.2017; 140 (6): e20172289.

[28]Morin A. The Truth About Troubled Teens. VeryWellMind.com Online, 2021.

[29]Jones B. Teenage Drug Addiction: An Overview. Verywellhealth. 2023. Online https://www.verywell-health.com/teenage-drug-addiction-5213002

[30]Mamman H., Othman A. T., Lian L. H: Adolescents and Drugs Abuse in Nigeria. Journal of Biology, Agriculture and Healthcare Vol.4, No.1, 2014.

both genders were associated with using any substance in the last 30 days.[31]

A German study of 16-year-old middle-class students indicated that 6% of them used methamphetamine. The main factors associated with consumption were a single-parent family and having friends who used the drug.[32]

Factors Associated with Psychoactive Substance Abuse by Adolescents

Any exposure to psychoactive drugs is a challenge for many adolescents. Nevertheless, some become drug addicts while others do not.

There is no single factor determining whether someone will become a drug addict. Instead, the risk of developing drug addiction is influenced by the biological constitution, the social environment, and the age or stage of development. The more risk factors, the greater the likelihood that drug use will become an addiction.

In Morocco, 65% of high school students used drugs to have a good time, 54% wanted to experiment to see what it is like consuming a drug, and 20–40% used it to alter their moods.[33]

In Serbia, some of the factors that favor the consumption of psychoactive substances by adolescents are a low involvement of parents in the education of the sons and daughters, conflicts in the family, drug abuse by parents, neighbors, or friends, alcoholism of the parents, divorce of them, and death of one of the parents.[34]

[31]El Omari F., Salomonsen-Sautel S., Hoffenberg A., Anderson T., Hopfer Ch. Toufiq J. Prevalence of substance use among Moroccan adolescents and association with academic achievement. World J Psychiatr5(4): 425–431. 2015.

[32]Dhein S., Schmelmer K., Guenther J. and Salameh A. Aspects of Methamphetamine Abuse in Adolescents and Young Adults in a Thuringian County. Eur Addict Res. 24(2) 98–105. 2018.

[33]El Omari F. Opus cited.

[34]Janicijevic K. M., Kocic S. S., Radovic S. R, Jovanovic M. R., and Radovanovic S. M.: Socioeconomic Factors Associated with Psychoactive Substance Abuse by Adolescents in Serbia. Frontiers in Pharmacology. Volume 8, page 366. 2017.

Although there are common elements in the processes that lead to addiction and the effects that this produces, each case has particular characteristics, determined by the personal history, the environment, the conceptions, and the psychological problems of the addict. For this reason, actions adapted to each individual, each medium, and each culture are necessary for helping adolescents to stop drug abuse.

Genetic and environmental factors interact with the critical stages of development, affecting addiction susceptibility. In combination with the influences of the environment, the genes are responsible for half of the vulnerability to addiction. Genre, ethnicity, and mental disorders can also influence the risk of drug abuse and drug addiction.[35,36]

While drug use at any age can lead to addiction, the earlier the start of the consumption of drugs, the more likely the progress to abuse and addiction.

Adolescents are frequently motivated to seek pleasure rewards and avoid pain, but their judgment and decision-making skills remain limited, affecting their ability to weigh risks and make informed decisions, including drug use. In addition, the brain areas that govern decision-making, judgment, and self-control are still actively developing during adolescence; teenagers may be prone to risky behaviors, including drug experimentation.[37]

The beginning of drug use by adolescents is not a casual event. Familiar, cultural, and social factors may favor the abuse of drugs by teenagers. First-time drug use often occurs in social settings with easily accessible substances, such as alcohol and cigarettes. Very frequently, the abuse of drugs continues, and it is challenging for the addict to stop it. The majority of adults who meet the criteria for substance use disorder started using substances during their teen and young adult years.

[35]Nestler EJ, Malenka RC. The addicted brain. Scientific American. 2004 Mar;290:78–85.

[36]Teens: Alcohol And Other Drugs. American Association of Child and Adolescent Psychiatry. 2018.

[37]National Institute of Drug Abuse. 2014 Opus cité.

Each person's environment involves many factors, from family and friends to socioeconomic level and quality of life. However, certain factors, such as the social pressure of friends or colleagues for consuming drugs, physical or sexual abuse, stress, and the quality of parenting given to them, can significantly influence whether the person comes to use drugs and if this progresses to drug addiction.

Other motivations are boredom, looking for feel-good, the necessity to forget the problems, looking for relaxation, curiosity about the effects of the drugs easing pain, or showing independence from parents. Belonging to peer groups that consume drugs is also an essential motivation for abusing drugs.[38] Continued use might result from insecurities or a desire for social acceptance.

There is a clear relationship between adolescents' drug abuse and the pressures that they suffer. Frequently drug consumption means a deliberate violation of social norms, a test to verify if it is possible to behave like an adult, the desire to test one's limits, a lack of control related to underdevelopment, and the desire to integrate with delinquent or substance-using peers.

Other factors that favor adolescents' abuse of drugs are a family history of substance abuse, family rejection of sexual orientation or gender identity, favorable parental attitudes towards drug use, and poor parental monitoring. The absence of love and parental care in some families in which both parents work can be a factor that stimulates the consumption of drugs.[39]

Mental health issues can promote the beginning of drug use. Adolescent with depression, anxiety, low self-esteem, feelings of social rejection, impulsive or risk-taking behavior, or attention-deficit/hyperactivity disorder (ADHD) are more prone to consuming drugs. A history of traumatic events, such as suffering abuse or watching car accidents, are also elements that contribute to the abuse of drugs.[40] Lack of school connectedness and low academic achievement are also elements that stimulate drug use.

Some people mention that the decline in moral values can increase drug use among adolescents. Other factors are the decrease of social control due to the migration to urban centers, the change in social environment, and the stress of modern life.[41]

There are also personal factors, such as the ability to resist the attractiveness of drugs (particularly against the peers that stimulate consumption) and the ability not to continue with the drug after trying it.

Denial of Risks

A characteristic element of addictions is the denial of their risks. Teens may feel indestructible and might not consider the consequences of their actions, leading them to take dangerous risks with drugs. The person who begins to consume a psychoactive drug does not believe that he will be transform into an addict. Despite the examples of other drug addicts, who are visibly very bad and cannot stop the drug intake, those who "taste" the drug often believe that they will resist the addiction.

The myth about one's ability to resist temptations defies all personal experiences. The addicts believe that they will resist a future temptation to consume, even though they repeatedly fall into that temptation. The myth also resists observations about the adverse results of addictions of friends or family members. Most of those who start using a drug know the difficulties in stopping using them and the adverse effects of this

[38] Why Do Teens Use Drugs? Get Smart About Drugs. DEA Publications, USA, 2021.

[39] Mutie J. Effects of Emotionally Absent Parents on the Behaviour of Adolescents in Select Secondary Schools in Machakos County, Kenya. A Research Project Submitted to the School of Humanities and Social Sciences in Partial Fulfilment of the Requirements for the Award of Master of Arts (Counseling Psychology) of Kenyatta University, Kenya, 2015.

[40] Tween and teen health, Healthy Lifestyle, Mayo Clinic, 2021.

[41] Gagliardi Raul: "Traumatic Situations and Mental Health Disorders in Migrants, Refugees, and Asylum Seekers," in Psychiatry and Neuroscience Vol. IV, Chapter 36. Editors Dr. Pascual Gargiulo and Dr. Humberto Mesones-Arroyo. Ed. Springer, 2021.

consumption. However, the personal myth is more potent. "I will resist the temptation of consumption in the future, while others were not able to do so."

A tragic example occurred in Argentina on February 2, 2022, when adulterated cocaine caused the death of at least 24 people and severe conditions in several dozen who had to be hospitalized and treated with artificial respirators.[42]

At least three of those hospitalized used the same cocaine again when they were discharged from the hospital, and had to be hospitalized again. In these cases, it is evident that the dramatic experience itself was not enough to prevent them from returning to use a drug that put their lives in danger.

Another dramatic example is the consumption of "Paco" (cocaine paste base) or glues in Argentina, which very quickly deteriorates the physical and mental health of the consumers, transforming them into what is called "a dead person in life." This situation does not serve as an example for community members or peers who begin the consumption of drugs. The curiosity or peer pressure to initiate the consumption is stronger than the perceived effect of the self-destruction of the addicts.

These examples show that knowledge about a severe problem is not enough to prevent it. The evident relationships between lung cancer and smoking, traffic accidents and alcoholism, or self-destruction and consumption of drugs are not enough to prevent these psychoactive drugs. The effects of nicotine, alcohol, or cocaine are more potent than knowing about their effects when the drug is tested or should be abandoned in an addiction.

For this reason, it is vital to help children and adolescents to develop "brakes" on the self-destructive behavior characteristic of addictions. The false idea "nothing can happen to me" is one of the entry doors for addictions. The risk culture and the impossibility of building a future are also essential elements of addiction.

Low self-esteem or depression plays against the development of that ability to avoid risky behaviors or self-destructive behaviors. Public education can significantly improve students' self-esteem and help them believe in their importance as responsible and conscious beings.

An element that favors the abuse of drugs is related to the explanatory models used by the addict.[43,44,45] An explanatory model of magical type can facilitate consumption by the acceptance of a myth of superpower; "I am not going to continue using" or "I can stop using drugs when I want to." Another element for understanding the denial of risks is an addict's cognitive bias, a systematic error in thinking that occurs when people are processing and interpreting information and affects their decisions and judgments.[46] This bias determines the addict's attitude not to accept the evidence about the risk of drug abuse. Therefore, talking about the risks is not sufficient for helping the addict avoid consuming the drugs or stopping them.

Consequences of Teen Drug Abuse

The consequences of teen drug use are severe, including an increased risk of serious drug abuse later in life. Other harmful effects are high-risk sexual activity, unsafe sex, and an unplanned pregnancy. There is also a decline in academic performance.[47] Other adverse outcomes are inju-

[42] Tragedia en Argentina: al menos 20 muertos y más de 70 hospitalizados por consumir cocaína envenenada. El Pais. 2022. Online https://elpais.com/internacional/2022-02-02/tragedia-en-argentina-varios-muertos-y-decenas-de-hospitalizados-por-consumir-cocaina-envenenada.html#

[43] Lynch E., Medin D, Explanatory models of illness: A study of within-culture variation. Cogn. Psychol. 53(4):285–309. 2006.

[44] Kleinman, A. Concepts and a Model for the Comparison of Medical Systems as Cultural Systems. Social Science & Medicine 12:85–93.1978.

[45] Kleinman, A. Culture, illness, and care: Clinical lessons from anthropologic and cross-cultural research. Annals of Internal Medicine 88:251–258. 1976.

[46] Cherry K. What Is Cognitive Bias?, Very Well Mind, online, 2022 https://www.verywellmind.com/what-is-a-cognitive-bias-2794963

[47] Mayo Clinical Staff. Teen drug abuse: Help your teen avoid drugs, Healthy Lifestyle, Tween and Teen Health, Mayo Clinic 2021.

ries, criminal justice involvement, school dropout, and death.

Drug use can also complicate or increase the risk of mental health disorders, such as depression and anxiety.

Driving under the influence of any drug can impair a driver's motor skills, putting the driver, passengers, and others on the road at risk.

Looking for money for paying the drug is a high motivation for illegal activities, leading many addicts to prostitution, with the consequent risk of HIV infection or other sexually transmitted infections. Injecting drug use increases the risk of HIV infection when syringes are shared. The relationship between HIV / AIDS is a severe problem in some countries where drug use is one of the biggest causes of HIV contamination.

Students who report ever using prescription drugs without a doctor's prescription are more likely than other students to have been victims of physical or sexual dating violence.[48]

Frequent drug use during adolescence can compromise the development of cognitive ability. For example, consuming marijuana in adolescence can reduce IQ. It is not recovered in adulthood, even if the use of that drug is interrupted.[49]

Violence and Drug Abuse

Individual violence is a phenomenon that causes severe damage to drug addicts, their families, and their environment and can also alter the lives of strangers. The effects of cocaine, methamphetamine, or alcohol as a promoter of violence are well known.

Drugs affect the brain area that controls irrational behavior and thinking, resulting in violent behaviors or suicide attempts.[50]

There is a clear relationship between drug use and violence. One cause is the direct effect of drugs on the consumer, as in the case of cocaine, alcohol, or methamphetamines. Another effect is the consumer's need to obtain money to buy the drug, leading to theft or prostitution. Finally, there is the violence associated with drug trafficking, with thousands of deaths in the struggles to conquer new markets or reprisals to consumers who cannot pay for the drug. Legal substances such as alcohol also engender violent behaviors in addicts.

It is necessary to distinguish between organized violence, characteristic of drug cartels, responsible for hundreds of thousands of murders, and individual violence of those who use drugs, either as a result of the effect of consumption on the central nervous system or as a result of the search for means to obtain the drug.

A study shows that 72% of men and 50% of women who started treatment for their addiction indicated that they had performed various acts of violence, including mugging, assault, and attacking another person with a weapon. In addition, many families of those who initiated the treatments said that the addicts had violent characters when they were under the effect of drugs. Domestic violence is related to the consumption of alcohol or other drugs such as cocaine.

The "Cannibal Drug"

> Police in Florida have warned of a potent new mind-altering drug called 'Cloud Nine' after a homeless man threatened to eat two officers a week after a naked man chewed off most of a homeless man's face before being shot dead. The ecstasy-like drug is part of a new line of over-the-counter "bath salts," a synthetic stimulant usually sold in shops selling drug paraphernalia that pro-

[48] Seyed Mohammad Rasoul Khalkhali S. M. R., Najafi1 K. Ahmadi1 R., Yousefnezhad A.

Hamidi1 A., Ellahi1 M., Amiri A. Afsar Montakhabi1 A., and Zavarmousavi1, M. Domestic Violence in Methamphetamine Psychotic Users, Psychiatric Inpatients, and Healthy People: A Comparative Study. Iran J Med Sci November 2016; Vol 41 No 6.

[49] National Institute of Drug Abuse. 2014 Opus cité.

[50] Hohmann P. Organized Crime vs. Addiction | Misconception, Drugs, and Violence. Delphi. 2019 Online. https://delphihealthgroup.com/blog/drugs-and-violence/

> duces intense hallucinations and sparks erratic, violent behavior.[51]

> Under the effect of Cloud Nine, a young man attacked several police officers and nurses in a health center in the Ibiza town of San Antonio in 2015. A neurologist explains that this drug generates an aggressiveness that reaches extremes in which the addicts mutilate themselves by biting, or they attack each other[52]

Cloud Nine has very long effects over time. Five milligrams of it can last up to 7 days. It is also called flake, or the "cannibal drug." Its scientific name is methylenedioxypyrovalerone.

Among the main effects of this substance are the feeling of euphoria, sexual arousal, and emotional excitement. On the other hand, it can also cause excitation of the nervous system, chills, excessive sweating, continuous vomiting, jaw tension, rapid heartbeat, hypertension, paranoia, anxiety, delusions, and extreme behaviors. In addition, the abuse of Cloud Nine produces a high risk of myocardial infarction or stroke.

This drug is hazardous for those who consume it, who lose the notion of their own body and come not to notice the pain as sharp as a broken bone.

The effects of Cloud Nine on behavior can be watched in videos showing erratic movements, screams, grimaces, or attempts at self-harm, such as throwing himself against a wall. In a video, a drug addict jumps from a great height believing that he can fly.

The people around the person who consumes Cloud Nine are in danger because of the aggressiveness and extreme force of the drug's effect; In some cases, six policemen were necessary to control an addict.

Alcohol and Violence

Alcohol is a psychoactive drug consumed worldwide. It is socially acceptable. Excessive consumption of alcohol can produce high aggressiveness and physical and psychological violence. Alcoholism can destroy the life of addicts and their families.

The increase in violent acts related to the consumption of alcohol is not only the result of its action on the brain. The handling of emotions seems to have a role in the frequency of violent acts committed under the influence of alcohol. The people who suppress their anger when they are sober tend to get drunk more frequently and perform violent acts under the influence of alcohol than those who do not suppress their anger.[53]

An explanation for this phenomenon may be related to some effects of alcohol and other drugs, such as suppressing inhibitions, increasing risky behavior, and reducing self-control. These effects may allow the expression of the contained rage, not expressed when sober. Just as behavior control is a brake on drug or alcohol use, excessive control of negative emotions related to violence can facilitate violent acts when one gets drunk.

A report published by the Drug Abuse Warning Network (DAWN) suggested that approximately 32% of all drug abuse Emergency Department (ED) visits in 2009 involved the use of alcohol. Cocaine was the single most common illicit drug found in these individuals during toxicology screening.[54,55]

---

[51] Miami police warn of 'Cloud Nine' drug after homeless man threatens to eat officers.

France 24. 2012. Online. https://www.france24.com/en/20120607-zombie-cannibal-attacks-spark-miami-police-drug-warning-cloud-nine

[52] Droga caníbal, o cómo una sustancia de diseño causa agresividad, alucinaciones, convulsiones, crisis epilépticas. La Sexta. Spain. 2021 Online https://www.lasexta.com/programas/equipo-investigacion/droga-canibal-como-sustancia-diseno-causa-agresividad-alucinaciones-convulsiones-crisis-epilepticas_2022080562ed369f8d51040001d14685.html

[53] People Who Suppress Anger Become Violent When Drunk Life Science. 2010 Online https://www.livescience.com/6640-people-suppress-anger-violent-drunk.html

[54] Gossop, M. Manning V., and Ridge G, "Concurrent use of alcohol and cocaine: differences in patterns of use and problems among users of crack cocaine and cocaine powder," Alcohol vol. 41, pp. 121–125, 2006.

[55] Apantaku-Olajide T., Darker C. D., and Smyth B. P. Onset of cocaine use: Associated alcohol intoxication and psychosocial characteristics among adolescents in substance abuse treatment. *J. Addict. Med.*, vol. 7,

Cocaine and Violence

In the USA, 29% of crimes are related to the consumption of cocaine. Twenty-three million people use cocaine in the world, a figure only surpassed by the use of marijuana. Cocaine use produces intense euphoria, reduces inhibitions, increases self-confidence, and gives a feeling of invincible and superior intelligence. It also reduces appetite, calms pain, and reduces fatigue. Unfortunately, these effects can lead the addict to have erratic and reckless behavior.

The adverse effects are anxiety, agitation, paranoia (cocaine paranoia), and the promotion of violent behaviors. Cocaine addiction can start first and present physical and mental health risks. It also increases tendencies to violence.

The rage and violence provoked by cocaine are related to its effect on neurotransmitters in the brain's pleasure centers, mainly changes in norepinephrine and Serotonin, which produce hyperactivity, impaired judgment and paranoia.

Research carried out in the United States indicates that the substance most consumed by criminals was cocaine and that 30% of the attackers had used cocaine and alcohol.

Multidrug Abuse

Addicts often use different drugs simultaneously. One of the most frequent and dangerous combinations is cocaine and alcohol, which increases the probability of suicidal or homicidal behavior.

The simultaneous use of these drugs increases the subjective effects of both. In addition, cocaine reduces drunkenness and cognitive and psychomotor deficits caused by alcohol. Alcohol reduces the effects of cocaine after the high. The combination of alcohol and cocaine in the body produces a metabolite called cocaethylene that circulates and has a potentially addictive effect more significant than each of the drugs alone. It increases the risk of sudden death by 18 to 25%, primarily due to its cardiotoxic effects.[56,57,58]

Methamphetamines and Violence

One type of synthetic psychoactive drug frequently used is methamphetamine, produced in large clandestine laboratories in Mexico from which it is transported to the USA. Small quantities for consumption or direct sale by "artisanal" drug traffickers are also produced in the USA. Domestic production has a high risk of explosion. The production of methamphetamine increased significantly in recent years. Methamphetamine use can lead to domestic violence, especially with previous trauma.

The Fentanyl Crisis in the USA

Fentanyl is a synthetic opioid that is 80–100 times stronger than morphine. Pharmaceutical fentanyl was developed for the pain management treatment of cancer patients. It is added to heroin to increase its potency or be disguised as highly potent heroin.

Many users believe that they are purchasing heroin and don't know that they are purchasing fentanyl, which often results in overdose deaths. Clandestinely-produced fentanyl is primarily manufactured in Mexico. Fentanyl produces effects such as relaxation, euphoria, pain relief, sedation, confusion, drowsiness, dizziness, nausea, vomiting, urinary retention, pupillary constriction, and respiratory depression.

Overdose may result in stupor, changes in pupillary size, cold and clammy skin, cyanosis, coma, and respiratory failure leading to death.

pp. 183–188, 2013.

[56] D. S. Harris, E. T. Everhart, J. Mendelson, and R. T. Jones, "The pharmacology of cocaethylene in humans following cocaine and ethanol administration," Drug Alcohol Depend., vol. 72, pp. 169–182, 2003.

[57] Pennings E. J., Leccese A. P., and de Wolff F. A.. Effects of concurrent use of alcohol and cocaine," Addiction, vol. 97, pp. 773–783, 2002.

[58] Pennings E. J., Leccese, A. P. and de Wolff, F. A. Opus cite.

The presence of a triad of symptoms such as coma, pinpoint pupils, and respiratory depression are strongly suggestive of opioid poisoning. Drugs that cause similar effects include other opioids such as morphine, hydrocodone, oxycodone, hydromorphone, methadone, and heroin.

Drug Addiction and Suicide

Different studies have shown that the suicide rate is higher in those addicted to psychoactive drugs than in the rest of the population. For example, research conducted in 2013 indicates that almost 40% of those who committed suicide were drug abusers. The drug most frequently related to suicides is alcohol, followed by antidepressants, benzodiazepines, opiates, and marijuana.[59]

In the USA, suicide is the second leading cause of death for people between 10 and 34 years old. Each day 15,000 teens will attempt suicide.[60]

Suicides are often related to drug use. Postmortem tests carried out on people who committed suicide are very significant. In 2013, 38.2% of those tests were positive for alcohol, 35.3% for antidepressants, 31.3% for benzodiazepines, 26.8% for opiates, and 16.6% for marijuana. Probably, the causes of suicide may be related to the psychological and social effects of drug use, or to the need to use drugs due to depression or other psychological conditions.[61]

[59] Elkins Ch. Substance Abuse and Suicide. A Guide to Understanding the Connection and Reducing Risk. DrugRehab. Online, 2020 https://www.drugrehab.com/guides/suicide-risks/

[60] Morin A. Opus cité.

[61] Substance Abuse and Suicide: A Guide to understanding tge Connection and Reducing Risk. DrugRehab.com, Online. 2013 https://www.drugrehab.com/guides/suicide-risks/

Warning Signs of Teenage Alcohol and Drug Use

Parents, friends, and teachers can recognize drug abuse and help the adolescent stopping it. Behavioral changes and mood changes (euphoria and depression) are frequently the first symptoms of drug use. However, prolonged drug use often has more marked effects and may be accompanied by petty theft and other crimes that the drug addict does to get the money to get high.

Physical signs of drug abuse include red and glazed eyes, lasting cough, health problems, and fatigue. Emotional signs are mainly irritability, poor judgment, and irresponsible behavior.[62]

More permanent psychological changes are low self-esteem, a general lack of interest, and depression. It also frequently starts arguments with the family and breaks the rules. Withdrawing from the family can follow these attitudes.

Frequently, the teenager who starts abusing drugs has difficulties in school, such as discipline problems, many absences, decreased interest, negative attitude, truancy and drop in grades. Abandon studies can result from drug abuse.

The addicted adolescent frequently changes to less conventional music and dress styles and has new friends who are less interested in standard home and school activities.

A meaningful sign is the starting of problems with the law. They can jeopardize the future of the addict.

Parents must consult a physician to rule out the physical causes of the warning signs to understand if their son or daughter has health problems or is starting to consume drugs. A comprehensive evaluation by a child and adolescent psychiatrist or mental health professional is always helpful.

The ability to recognize the signs of drug use in family members, especially parents and hus-

[62] Miami police warn of 'Cloud Nine' drug after homeless man threatens to eat officers. The Telegraph, 14–9—2012. Online, https://www.telegraph.co.uk/news/worldnews/northamerica/usa/9316220/Miami-police-warn-of-Cloud--Nine-drug-after-homeless-man-threatens-to-eat-officers.html

bands, has improved with the appearance of the "home test drugs" that helps identify illegal drugs or prescription drugs with great precision. In the United States, these tests cost the Internet between $ 2 for simple tests (for example, for marijuana in all its forms) and $ 4 for combined tests for marijuana, cocaine, methadone, and opiates. Some tests use urine, and others use hair follicles.

Difficulties in Stopping Addiction

Many people do not understand how or why some adolescents become addicted to drugs. It is often mistakenly assumed that drug addicts have no moral principles or sufficient will and that they could stop using drugs if they were only willing to change their behavior. In reality, drug addiction is a complex problem, and the cessation of drug consumption does not occur with the simple intention or the firm decision to do so. Psychoactive drugs change the brain to encourage compulsive abuse, making it difficult to stop using them, even for those who are willing to do so. Thanks to scientific advances, it is known how drugs work in the brain, allowing that drug addiction to be treated successfully, and helping the drug user stop using drugs and return to a productive life.

Research shows that the best method of ensuring success for most addicts is a combination of behavioral therapy with medications to treat addiction. In addition, sustained recovery and a life without drug abuse can be achieved using approaches designed to address each patient's specific drug abuse pattern in conjunction with any concurrent medical, psychiatric, or social problems.

Drug addiction can be treated successfully like many other chronic diseases with relapses, such as diabetes, asthma, or heart disease. However, like other chronic diseases, it is also common for relapses and for the drug addict to return to drug use. These relapses, however, do not mean that the treatment has failed. Instead, they are a sign that treatment must be reinstated or adjusted, or that an alternative treatment is necessary.

Elements for Preventing Drugs Addiction

Preventing addictions can be done in social, familial, and personal domains. Coordination between these domains is positive for success.

Strategies that can help teens not use drugs are having positive and strong connections with parents, other family members, and school. It is also essential that parents present clear limits, precise discipline, and reduced access to the home of illegal substances.

Two factors must be analyzed: the knowledge about the harmful effects of drugs and the psychological phenomena that make it easier to start using drugs and not stop using them.

Information about drugs can be transmitted using the methods developed by didactics of sciences, adapting the teaching of information to the characteristics of the student (conceptions, learning styles, explanatory models, personal history, and motivation).[63,64] An investigation of these characteristics in the target population will facilitate teaching.

A valuable element of didactics of sciences is the definition of the essential concepts that the student must possess to understand and integrate the related information (structuring concepts). In the case of drug addiction, these concepts are related to the difficulties to stop using the drug (addiction), the adverse effects that drug use produces on a health level, and the living conditions of the addict.

[63]Gagliardi, R. Atti dei Seminari di Didattica delle Scienze della Natura (Ed. Elena Ferrero y Elena Camino), Università degli Studi di Torino, Dipartimenti di Biología Animale, Scienze della Terra, Psicologia, Edition Cooperativa libraria Universitaria, Turin, Italia, 1990.

[64]Gagliardi, R. Le reti concettuali", in "Scuolambientesviluppo: Idee e materiali per l'educazione ambientale", I Libri di Ecole, FNISM - Schole, Turin, Italia, 1989.

Another factor is the difficulty of having correct behavior related to drug abuse prevention. Multiple experiences show that it is not enough to know a phenomenon for having acceptable behavior. Likewise, information is not enough to change a negative behavior or prevent it. For example, many people know the adverse health effects of cigarette smoking and continue smoking.

The problem to solve is how to help adolescents refuse the use of drugs, including legal ones, such as alcohol, tobacco, and pharmaceutical drugs.

Basic Information About Drugs

Psychoactive Substances

Some substances act on the central nervous system and are consumed to obtain pleasant effects and stimulate or calm pain, anxiety, or anguish. Some of these substances produce hallucinations. Others provoke euphoria or despair or intensify or hinder the senses. They are substances that pass the barrier between the blood and the brain, affecting certain brain functions and causing changes in perceptions, mood, consciousness, judgment, emotions, or behavior. They are called "psychoactive," "psycho-pharmaceutical," or "psychotropic drugs." The effects depend on the type of drug, the frequency of consumption, and the untaken amount.

Like alcohol, caffeine, or nicotine, some are accepted by society, and their consumption is allowed with certain restrictions. Others are not accepted socially, and in some cases, their production, sale, or consumption are illegal. Some of these substances are used in religious ceremonies (entheogenic substances). Others can be used as medicines, such as opiates.

Among the psychoactive drugs, we can mention alcohol, amphetamines, barbiturates, benzodiazepines, cannabis (marijuana), cocaine, crack, ecstasy, methaqualone, opioids (heroin, morphine, fentanyl), and "glues." Some are produced from vegetables, such as marijuana, cocaine, morphine, or heroin. In some cases, long transformation processes are required until they can be used. Others are synthesized in laboratories (synthetic psychoactive drugs), such as amphetamines, fentanyl, or ecstasy.

Addiction is a chronic disease of the brain, often with relapses, characterized by compulsive drug seeking and consumption despite the harmful consequences for the addicted person and those around him. While it is true that, in the case of most people, the initial decision to take drugs is voluntary, over time, the changes that occur in the brain of addicted people can affect self-control and hamper their ability to resist the intense impulses of consuming drugs.

Dependence of Drugs

Addiction to certain drugs is difficult to overcome. Addiction is caused by searching for the effects produced by the drug consumed. In some cases, the body becomes accustomed to the drug, and it is necessary to increase the consumption or frequency of consumption for obtaining the same effects. In addition, some drugs, such as heroin, cause very unpleasant sensations when the addict stops using them (withdrawal syndrome).

The dependence produced by drugs can be of two types:

Physical Dependence It occurs when the organism becomes habituated to drugs, and when consumption is interrupted appear physiological disorders (withdrawal syndrome) such as nausea, chills, intense pain in the joints, and depression. The addicts are "forced" by their bodies to consume the drug and the process of abstinence can be long and complicated.

Psychic Dependence It occurs when the drug produces a state of pleasure and euphoria that ceases when the drug's effect ceases. In some cases, the addict experiences a negative emotion that stimulates the repetition of the consumption. For example, abstinence from cocaine can lead to depression. The addict wants to reproduce a pleasant state and returns to consumption. In some very addictive drugs, such as crack, consumption can be done dozens of times daily.

Both physical and psychic dependence transform the life of the addict, who frequently directs his activities to obtaining and consuming drugs, losing his job, failing his studies, losing his friends, committing serious crimes, and making very difficult the life of his family and his friends. In addition, the drug "dominates" the addict and "imposes" increasingly harsh conditions, such as illegal activities to obtain money. As a result, the addict steals, commits other crimes or becomes a prostitute.

Some drugs like crack are very addictive. In general, addiction tends to be faster when the effect of consumption is high and decays fat. In the case of "*paco*" (cocaine pasta base consumed in Argentina), it is possible to consume 10 or 15 doses per day and, in the most severe cases, 100 doses per day can be consumed. Paco is cheap, but its consumption produces very adverse effects on the addict. Other cheap drugs are glues that usually have solvents that produce cancer. Some children or adolescents that consume them are called "dead boys" because they are always somnolent. They die after a few months of high consumption.

What Happens to the Brain When Psychotropic Drugs Are Used?

The adolescent years are a crucial window for both substance use and the development of substance use disorders. Brain systems governing emotion and reward-seeking are fully developed by this time, but circuits governing judgment and self-inhibition are still maturing, causing teenagers to act on impulse, seek new sensations, and be easily swayed by their peers—all of which may draw them to take risks such as trying psychoactive drugs. Moreover, because critical neural circuits are still actively forming, teens' brains are particularly susceptible to being modified by those substances in a lasting way—making the development of a substance use disorder much more likely. The drugs contain substances that infiltrate the brain's communication system, disrupting the sending, receiving, and processing of information between nerve cells. There are at least two ways that drugs can do this: (1) by mimicking the natural chemical messengers of the brain and (2) by stimulating the brain's "reward circuit."

Some drugs like marijuana and heroin have a structure similar to certain neurotransmitters, which the brain naturally produces. This resemblance allows drugs to "cheat" the brain's receptors and activate the nerve cells to send abnormal messages.

Other drugs, such as cocaine or methamphetamine, can cause nerve cells to release excessively high amounts of natural neurotransmitters (mainly dopamine) or block the recycling of these chemicals into the brain, which is necessary to cut the sending and receiving signals between neurons. The result is that dopamine saturates the brain.

Dopamine is a neurotransmitter found in regions of the brain that control movement, emotions, motivation, and pleasurable sensations. Usually, the gratification system responds to natural behaviors related to survival, such as eating or spending time with loved ones), but when overstimulated by psychoactive drugs, it produces euphoric effects. Unfortunately, this reaction initiates a vicious reinforcement cycle that "teaches" people to repeat the drug abuse behavior that caused the gratification.

When a person continues to abuse drugs, the brain adapts to these overwhelming waves of dopamine by producing less dopamine or decreasing the number of dopamine receptors in the reward circuit. The result is a lower impact of dopamine on the gratification circuit, limiting the pleasure that the user can derive from drugs and events in his life that previously caused him pleasure. This decrease in pleasure forces the drug addict to continue abusing drugs to regain pleasure by maintaining the dopamine function. Besides, he frequently needs to consume a more significant amount of the drug to elevate the function of dopamine to its initial average level. This effect is known as tolerance.

Long-term abuse also causes changes in other systems and chemical circuits of the brain. For example, Glutamate is a neurotransmitter that influences the gratification circuit and learning ability. When drug abuse alters the optimal concentration of Glutamate, the brain tries to compensate for this imbalance, which can impair cognitive function. In addition, imaging studies of the brain of drug addicts show changes in areas of the brain essential for judgment, decision-making, learning, memory, and behavior control. All these changes can make the drug addict seek and use drugs compulsively despite knowing the adverse and devastating consequences of his behavior.

There are many ways that a drug can act to enhance (agonize) or reduce (antagonize) a given neurotransmitter. For example, it can increase the production of particular neurotransmitters. It can also interfere with neurotransmitters' reuptake, forcing them to remain in the synapse and interact with receptors longer than usual. An antagonistic drug can interfere with the release of neurotransmitters into the synapse. It can compete with the neurotransmitter for binding to the neurotransmitter's receptor without activating it and blocking the neurotransmitter receptors. An antagonistic drug can also cause neurotransmitters to leak out of their containers in the terminal button, making the neurotransmitter unavailable for release into the synapse. Another effect can be bypassing the neurotransmitter entirely and binding with and activating the neurotransmitter's receptors.[65]

The Key Is Prevention

The results of research sponsored by the National Institue on Drug Abuse of the USA (NIDA) have shown that prevention programs that involve the family, school, community, and the media effectively reduce drug abuse. While many cultural events and factors affect trends in drug abuse, when young people perceive that drug use is harmful, there is a decrease in the tendency to consume them. Therefore, education and community activism are key to helping young people and the general public understand the risks of drug abuse. In addition, teachers, parents, doctors, and other public health professionals must continue to send the message that drug addiction can be avoided if the person never uses drugs.

There Are Solutions

Teen drug use is a severe problem. The solution requires joint actions by the family and society, with educational campaigns on the risks of drug use, support for drug addicts and their families, and adequate treatment in specialized centers.

Addiction is not just an individual or family problem. It is a problem of a society that promotes legal drugs such as sugar, alcohol, and tobacco, allows the production and trafficking of drugs, and in many cases only have repressive policies for addicts.

Importance of the Participation of Teachers in the Prevention of Addictions

The consumption of psychoactive drugs increases and reaches all sectors of society. In many cases, consumption begins in childhood. The effects are severe.

Formal education can play a significant role in the prevention of addictions for several reasons:

- The majority of children go to school. Therefore, the campaigns developed there can reach large sectors of the population.
- The prevention of drug use is related to developing habits and accepting values and attitudes during childhood. Therefore, teachers can significantly influence the prevention of addictions by teaching topics related to psychoactive drugs and promoting habits and attitudes to prevent their consumption.
- The consumption of psychoactive substances is also done in schools. The adverse effects on

[65] How Drugs Affect the Brain. MentalHealth.Net. Online https://www.mentalhelp.net/substance-abuse/how-drugs-affect-the-brain/

learning capacity and the behavior of addicted students increase the problems of students and teachers.

- The daily presence of students in the school facilitates the execution of activities to prevent drug use and its evaluation.
- Information about the harmful effects of psychoactive drugs can be integrated into study programs.
- Students can participate in drug prevention campaigns of other students or other children (prevention between peers). They can also participate in campaigns aimed at their families or neighbors.
- In many cases, teachers have roles that go beyond teaching. Many students perceive them as the only adults who offer them affection and containment.

Preventing addictions at school needs accurate data on the most frequently consumed drugs, the frequency of consumption, and their effects on consumers. Teachers can obtain these data because they are daily with students and can perceive changes in behavior related to consumption. They can also perceive the social and economic changes related to drugs, particularly in the marginalized areas where drug gangs are being set up.

The Fight of Mothers Against Drug Abuse

In Argentina, Spain, the USA, and other countries, mothers of drug addicts build organizations to help their sons. They denounce drug traffic power and government and police corruption. They ask for new policies for helping the thousands of teens destroyed by drugs. They suffer threats, but they continue the fight.

Conclusions

Drug abuse by adolescents is one of the most important problems in many countries, where the consumption of psychoactive drugs frequently starts in childhood and continues during adolescence Recreational consumption can lead to addiction, with serious individual, family, and social consequences that it can cause.

Influence of peers during adolescence, characteristics of the family, and easy access to drugs are factors that promote drug use and difficult the prevent addictions.

Drug addiction can produce negative effects on psychological development and jeopardize the studies. Many of the addicted adolescents change their way of living, becoming violent and committing crimes. The violence related to drug trafficking jeopardizes the lives of adolescent dealers and produces negative effects on addict families and communities.

The health impact of drug use can be very serious, in particular, the thousands of deaths due to overdose. The opioid epidemic in the United States caused nearly 70,000 deaths per year, is an example of the difficulties in dealing with the spread of addictions in the country.

There are no clear solutions to the problem of adolescent drug addiction. Teachers and families can play an important role in the education of adolescents and the development of the brakes of drug use. The action of mothers against drugs is a good possibility for reducing drug abuse. Campaigns for prevention of drug abuse with the participation of teachers and students can also be part of the solution.

49 Early Detection and Treatment Options for Psychosis in Transition from Childhood to Adolescence: A Review About Three Decades of Psychiatric Clinical Experience

Ralph Meyers

Introduction

While schizophrenia is best known for episodes of psychosis, it is also marked by chronic neurocognitive deficits, such as problems with memory and attention. These neurocognitive symptoms are evident prior to the onset of psychosis in the prodromal phase. The findings suggest that these impairments may serve as early warning signs of schizophrenia, as well as potential targets for intervention that could mitigate the onset of the psychotic disorder and significantly improve cognitive function [1].

Impaired working memory and declarative memory turned out to be the key neurocognitive functions that are impaired in the high-risk, prodromal phase prior to the onset of full-blown psychosis. These findings, as reported by Seidman, are in keeping with the experiences of many people with schizophrenia who report sudden difficulties reading, concentrating, or remembering things in the earliest days of the disorder [1].

Drug abuse will have an important impact on either the first onset or the further development, e.g., the prognosis for treatment outcomes (Fig. 49.1).

R. Meyers (✉)
Socialpsychiatric Center for Child and Adolescent Psychiatry, Dorsten, Germany
e-mail: info@meyers-dorsten.com; Dr.Meyers@gmx.de; https://www.meyers-dorsten.com

P. Á. Gargiulo, H. L. Mesones-Arroyo (eds.), *Psychiatry and Neuroscience Update – Vol. V*, https://doi.org/10.1007/978-3-031-72219-6_49

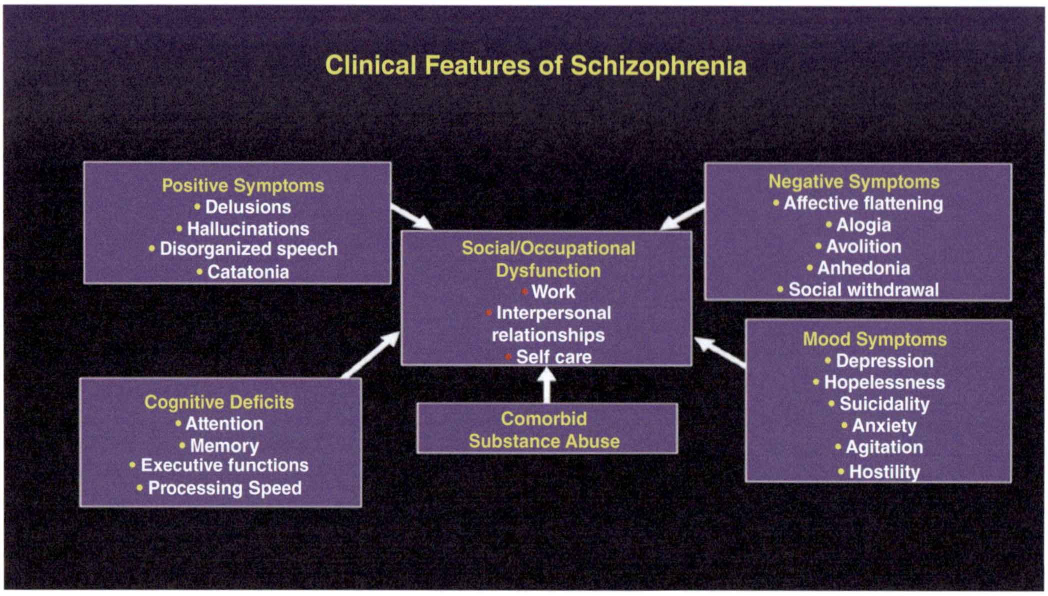

Fig. 49.1 Clinical features of schizophrenia, Best of PSYCH FORUM 2016. Schizophrenia: Preventing Deterioration and Returning to Baseline. Henry A. Nasrallah, MD, Sydney W. Souers Professor, Chair, Department of Psychiatry and Behavioral Neuroscience, Saint Louis University School of Medicine St. Louis, MO. (extract from presentation with authorization by Nasralla) [2]

Early Detection and Treatment Options for Psychosis in Transition from Childhood to Adolescence

As previously mentioned by Seidman, early detection is essential for the later outcome in psychosis. So, in our centre, we focus on a holistic way in anamnesis and diagnosis including neurological, psychiatric, and test psychological assessments for all our patients [1].

Our neurological examination includes motor abilities, checks for persisting preborn reflexes, regarding all kinds of sensory disabilities and hypersensitivities. We also check for generalized internal diseases, and we have a cursory check including the static and orthopaedic state.

Psychiatric evaluation will include the age and mental status and also the cognitive functions, memory, and attention. These have to be objectively measured, and we regularly include the OPATUS CPTa® from age 3 onwards [3–5].

We use a fixed test battery for each developmental stage [3–5]. If there arises the suspicion, there could be a prepsychotic or psychotic disorder behind the symptoms presented, additional examinations and tests will be followed-up.

Quite effective is to check for cognitive basic impairments:

Cognitive Perceptual Basic Disorders [6]

It may be observed more than one of the following 10 basic symptoms within the last 3 months and a first occurrence more than 12 months before:

Thought interference
Compulsive perseveration of contents of consciousness
Urging and chasing thoughts
Mind blocking
Disorder of receptive language
Disorder of discrimination of ideas and perceptions, imagination, and memory ideas
"Subject centrism," self-relationship tendencies
Derealization
Disorders of visual perception
Acoustic perception disorders

Basic Cognitive Disorders [6]

It may be observed more than two of the following nine basic symptoms within the last 3 months:

Impaired ability to split attention
Thought interference
Urging and chasing thoughts
Mind blocking
Disorder of receptive language
Disorder of expressive language
"Subject centrism," self-relationship tendencies
Disturbance of symbol recognition
Captivation through perceptual details

When suspicion continues, this will be accompanied by a deeper anamnesis, using parents and grandparents reports as well.

Case Report: Anna (Age 12)

Anna reported to our clinic with symptoms of distraction, anxiety, and impulsivity. She was the youngest of four siblings, the others aged 19, 23, and 27 years.

What made her diagnosis a lot easier was that the eldest sister aged 27 and the brothers aged 19 and 23 had been previously diagnosed with psychosis some years ago and were still in treatment. The brother aged 19 had been in our clinic with psychosis, aggravated by substance abuse for nearly 2 years. And, of course, the family had been "forewarned": over the past years, they had all developed into experts to recognize the prodromal symptoms.

Anna then quickly got on neuroleptics and we could prevent an acute phase with hallucinations and more.

Case Report: Arthur (Age 17)

Arthur is Anna's brother, 2 years before the case report mentioned above. When he came to our clinic, he showed a lot of active psychotic symptoms with his first episode like hallucinations, derealization, decline in school performance, depression, and anxiety plus impulsivity.

He was still on cannabis and in the early stage of treatment unwilling to part with this abuse, because, as he put it, THC helped him to control his anxiety and gave him subjectively an increase in attention.

Interventions of his elder siblings helped, to get his consent for neuroleptics and to cease using drugs. He attended a psychotherapy group for young adults at our clinic for several years until his follow-up treatment had to be transferred to an adult psychiatrist.

He managed to achieve his high school grade and afterwards started with training to become a nurse. And gratefully, there was no relapse in all this time and he even started with his own family.

But till today, we regard this outcome special, because it does not represent the long way of clinical persuasion it usually takes to get someone discontinuing substance abuse in the early stages of psychosis (first or even second episode).

In our work, intensive counseling is given to inform our patients that their own management of life will have an important impact on their prognosis. If they are willing to take neuroleptics early on and stop substance abuse, they will face a much better outcome.

At this stage, not only to get a better measurement for mental performance, but also to achieve a good compliance, the application of OPATUS CPTa has proven quite successful.

The results are objective measurements of impulsivity, activity, and volatility, and the graphic test result is easily explained and will show either the decline of former skills or the improvement over time, when treated.

Decline of Mental Performance

Mental decline is observed as rapidly deterioration with each episode, even if treatment is given. This explains why early intervention is essential to prevent the amount of mental decline (Fig. 49.2).

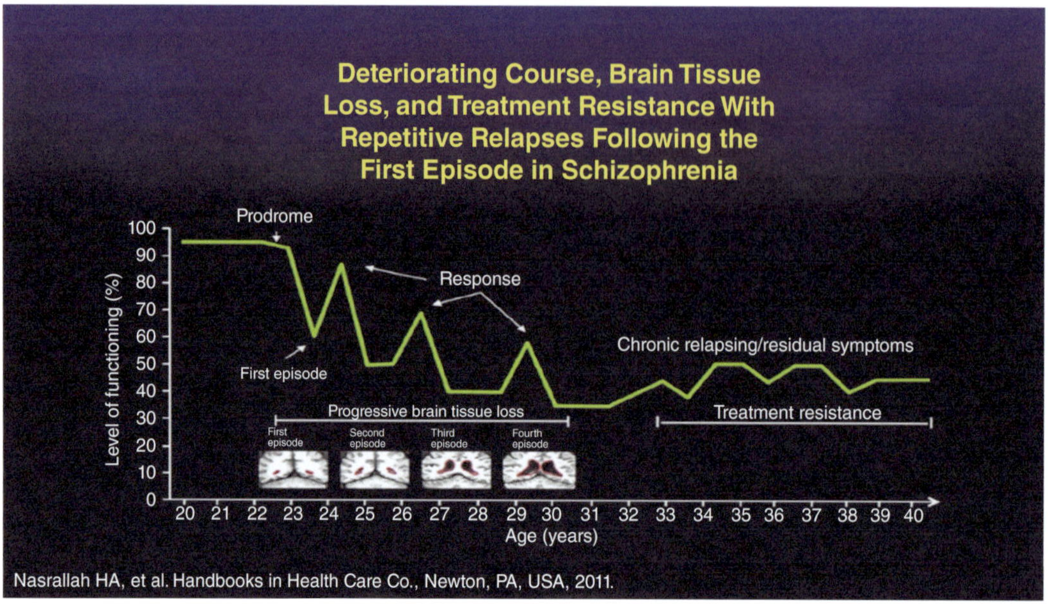

Fig. 49.2 Deteriorating course, brain tissue loss, and treatment resistance with repetitive relapses following the first episode in schizophrenia. (Nasralla et al. [2])

Case Report: George (Age 19)

George was presented by his father with ongoing psychotic derealization, that he tried to dissimulate.

After finishing his exams, he had taken a year abroad in Australia ("work and travel"). In skype and zoom calls, his parents got suspicious of his mental decline and derealization. So, his father decided to fly over and get him home again.

He admitted having tried hallucinogenic mushrooms, LSD, cannabis, ecstasy and legal highs and was not easily persuaded to regard his mental state as declining.

Under the strict control of his parents, it was possible to administer neuroleptics. These medications had an immediate effect in clearing his mind of derealization. It was also possible to improve basic cognitive disorders such as impaired ability to divide attention, thought interference, urgency and pursuit of thoughts, mental blocking, and self-referential tendencies.

However, his attention span was quite affected, as the OPATUS CPTa results shown as follows.

Opatus CPTa in early stage of treatment (3 weeks on aripiprazole 20 mg) (Fig. 49.3). Neurocognitive deficits may be a red flag for psychosis [7]. But there is also the other way round: if you continue to take objective measurements e.g. with a CPTa like the OPATUS test, you may as well show, how the remission is working and how stable this state is.

George recovered fast and wanted to assume personal responsibility again. He then started with study of legal affairs in a town 1.5 h distance to his home town. He was living at a student facility and got involved with drugs again and ceased taking his medication. Four months later, he was presented again with similar symptoms like in his first episode. Starting with aripiprazole again, quickly got him out of the productive phase, but mental decline could be monitored clinically.

However, all our talks about his vulnerability regarding drugs and discontinuation of neuroleptics were not to be held up for long. He was not able to continue with his studies. His father provided him with a training as a commercial clerk at his factory; but in reality, he had to be pushed to rise in the mornings and he was not able to fulfil any difficult task at work.

His situation worsened, when he started using drugs again and discontinued with his medica-

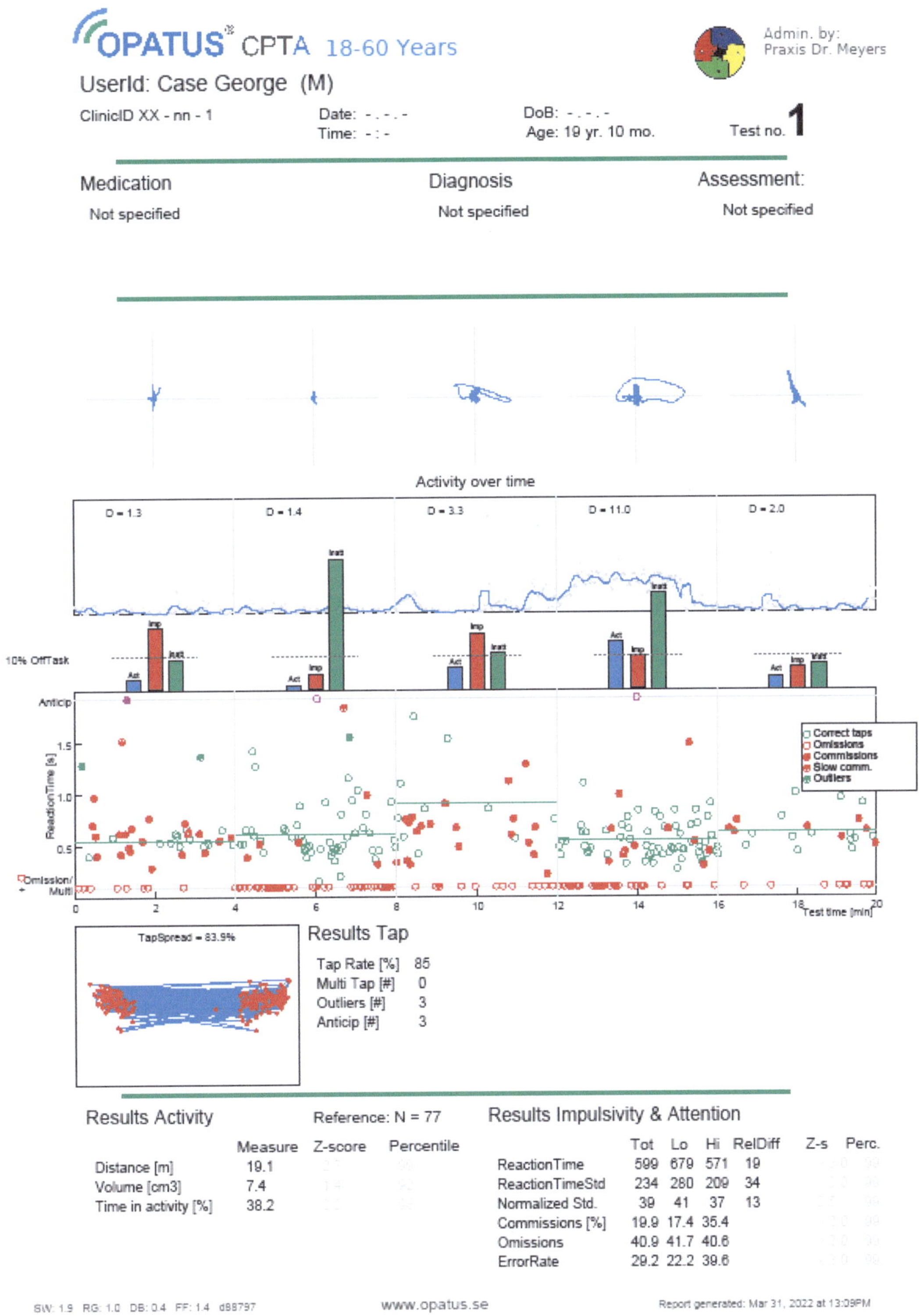

Fig. 49.3 This figure shows George's performance: greens circles are good reactions, red dots represent impulsivity, and red circles stay for omissions. His overall error rate is 29.2%, the blue line in the upper field represents the movement activity, z-scores above 0 are abnormal [4]

tion. He ended with tattoos all over his face, living under guardianship in a therapeutic residential group.

Today, 4 years later, he is willing to maintain drug abstinence and to take his medication. And with intensive support by his family, he is actually studying social work in Spain (his mother has Spanish roots, and the acceptability of his obvious former problems is better than in Germany) and according to his family, he is doing well.

OPATUS CPTa—Objective Measurement for Concentration and Activity [5]

In our clinic, the OPATUS-CPTa test for objective measurement of concentration and activity is an important part of the test packages for all age groups. Its validity has been confirmed in various clinical studies [8–11].

It offers a fast and accurate procedure to support the diagnosis and for progress controls under treatment of ADHD, and it can be used to describe the decline of attention correlating with psychosis as well as shown above.

The OPATUS CPTa is available as an App that runs on Apple devices. It is intended for doctors and scientists in research and therapy. The different versions are adapted for patients from the age of 3 to seniors. Its execution time varies between 8 min for infants, 16 min for children between 6 and 12, and 20 min for older test persons. The complete evaluation including a graphical report is available for professionals.

The test is performed as described below:

The test person holds the iPhone or iPod with both hands. Because the devices can determine their position in space, they pick up the subject's movement pattern. The movement sensor of iPads is less sensitive. They are suitable for presenting the test, but not for conducting it. On the screen, either a yellow or blue triangle points up, down, left, or right and becomes visible in rapid succession. The patient has to press on the screen, when two identical targets follow in time. In the adult version that is shown in our example, there are 4 min intervals of low target phases, followed by high target phases and so on.

The upper section shows movement patterns for each of the four 4 min sections. If the device is held calmly in the hand, the picture is quite closed. The more restless the subject is, the more expansive the scribbles become.

The four individual pictures give a first impression of the movement pattern for each 4 min of the test duration; much more meaningful is the graph below. Here, the movement activity is listed as a function of the total time. The blue line shows the real-time deflections, and the red line is somewhat "softer" because it reflects the values averaged over a certain period of time in each case.

The graph with many dots of different colours gives information about the frequency of errors and thus about the concentration ability. This part is divided into 4 min sections.

- Green circles show the correct reactions.
- Red dots show when the respondent made mistakes.
- The green solid lines parallel to the time axis show the average reaction times for each 4 min segment.
- Purple circles stand for random reactions; they are of course not linked to a reaction time and are therefore all displayed at the same height parallel to the time axis.
- Black crosses on the time axis show when the client pressed twice (so-called multitaps); this is also interpreted as a sign of impulsivity.
- Red circles can be seen on the same axis as the black crosses; they indicate the omission errors. This means that there was no response because the client was dreaming or was distracted.

The four small bar charts above the dot diagram give a quick overview of the reaction patterns:

- The blue column reflects the level of restlessness (data from the blue movement lines).

- The red column shows the measure of impulsivity (data from purple circles and black crosses).
- The green column is the measure of inattention (data from the red circles).

Schizophrenia Risk on Heritability up to 80%

In a complete study by Hilker et al. on schizophrenia involving twins to date, researchers estimate that as much as 79% of schizophrenia risk may be explained by genetic factors [12].

Hany et al. say that risk factors include birthing complications, the season of birth, severe maternal malnutrition, maternal influenza in pregnancy, family history, childhood trauma, social isolation, cannabis use, minority ethnicity, and urbanization. Due to its relative complexity and heterogeneity, the etiology and pathophysiological mechanisms are not fully understood. Despite a low prevalence, schizophrenia's global burden of disease is immense. Over half of the patients have significant comorbidities, both psychiatric and medical, making it one of the leading causes of disability worldwide. The diagnosis correlates with a 20% reduction in life expectancy, with up to 40% of deaths attributed to suicide [13].

Schizophrenia is most likely caused by a combination of genetic and environmental factors, most likely interacting in a "two hit" longitudinal trajectory. This means that early factors, such as certain genetic polymorphisms, can cause increased vulnerability of the brain to environmental factors in late adolescence/young adulthood, such as stress or drugs of abuse. This combination might synergize to cause onset of the illness, whereas either of these "hits" by themselves do not have this effect [14].

Schizophrenia risk has often been conceptualized using a model which requires two hits in order to generate the clinical phenotype-the first as an early priming in a genetically predisposed individual and the second a likely environmental insult. Davis et al. sourced the data from PUBMED. They conclude that the development of schizophrenia may be driven by genetic vulnerability interacting with multiple vulnerability factors including lowered prenatal vitamin D exposure, viral infections, smoking intelligence quotient, social cognition cannabis use, social defeat, nutrition, and childhood trauma. They regard it likely that these genetic risks, environmental risks, and vulnerability factors are cumulative and interactive with each other and with critical periods of neurodevelopmental vulnerability. The development of schizophrenia is regarded to be more complex and nuanced than the binary two-hit model originally proposed nearly 30 years ago. Risk appears influenced by a more complex process involving genetic risk interfacing with multiple potentially interacting hits and vulnerability factors occurring at key periods of neurodevelopmental activity, which culminate in the expression of disease state [15].

Psychotic Disorder and Substance Use

It is well known that drug abuse will have an impact on developing the first psychotic episode. The vulnerability depends on heritability and quality as well as dosage of drugs taken.

Not the number of times a drug is used or the dosage, but the personally in most cases unknown risk of heritability will determine, if a psychotic development will start. Sometimes, in our experience, a single use of hallucinogens may be sufficient to start the first episode.

This leads to our next item, the development of substance abuse and connections with clinically relevant needs to treat.

We give an overview, using Canadian and German statistics.

Canadian Hospitalization Trends, 2006–2015

Between 2006 and 2015, the rate of hospitalizations for cannabis-related mental or behavioral disorders in Canada rose from 2.11 to 5.18 per 1,00,000 (Fig. 49.4).

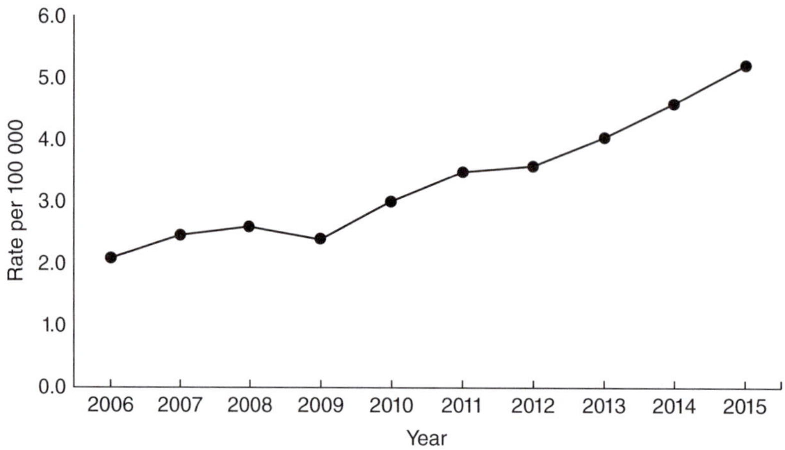

Fig. 49.4 Rate of hospitalizations for cannabis-related mental or behavioral disorder (per 100.000) in Canada (excluding Quebec), 2006–2015. Canadian Institute of Health Information. Hospitalizations were extracted from the Hospital Mental Health Database (HMHDB) for the 10 fiscal years spanning April 2006 to March 2016 (herein referred to as 2006–2015) [16]

Further research is required to investigate the reasons for the increase in hospitalizations for cannabis-related psychotic disorder. The introduction of high-potency cannabinoid products and synthetic cannabinoids into the illicit market is considered as a possible factor in Canada [16].

Incidence of Inpatient Cases with Mental Disorders Due to Use of Cannabinoids in Germany: A Nationwide Evaluation

Quantitative and qualitative changes in cannabinoid use may be associated with changes in the prevalence of cannabinoid-related mental and behavioral disorders and, accordingly, changes the need for medical care.

The study we are presenting here [17] investigated if there are changes in the number of inpatient cases due to cannabinoid-related disorders in Germany. Absolute numbers increased statistically significantly in Germany between 2000 and 2018, and corresponding relative admissions increased considerably (4.8-fold increase when comparing 2000 and 2018). Specifically, absolute numbers with cannabinoid intoxications, dependence syndrome, withdrawal state, psychotic disorders, and residual and late-onset psychotic disorder statistically significantly increased [17].

The Transition from Child and Adolescent Psychiatry to Adult Psychiatry

Working in a clinic for child and adolescent psychiatry, we have to conclude that even if we are able to prevent some outcome of psychosis going chronic, that later on have to be transferred to a clinic for adult psychiatry, if we are able to get an early diagnosis and work with families generating a systemic support net, the willingness and compliance to cease drug abuse, supporting the psychosis to develop into a chronic disorder, is crucial.

In adult psychiatry, an outcome of 50% improvement still is regarded as a positive achievement, like in the early 80 s [18]. And even if specialized residential groups are available, they often deal with patients, that have deteriorated a lot during their history, so the expectations for improvement have to be kept realistically low.

My old professor Hartmut Dziewas described this with the following picture: “Imagine, that your brain is a kind of library, where someone let through a hefty gush of wind, so that all the books got pushed to the ground, out of their primary order. Your task now, after suffering from a psychotic episode is, to get a new sense into what you want to understand or want to express without direct access to the right book or words". This is what the above-mentioned Benner Program is about [19].

Social cognition was shown as a rate limiting factor for both psychosocial outcome and response to psychosocial intervention in schizophrenia. In a randomized controlled trial, a new cognitive-behavioral group treatment for schizophrenic inpatients (the "Training of Emotional Intelligence", TEI) was tested against the well evaluated "Integrated Psychological Therapy Program" (IPT) of Brenner. Within the framework of Salovey's study, the Training of Emotional Intelligence focussed on three domains of deficits in schizophrenia: emotional perception, emotional understanding, and emotional management. In the randomized controlled trial with 41 DSM-IV schizophrenic inpatients, no differences were found in problem-solving and negative symptoms, both posttreatment and in the 12 months-follow-up. Additionally, there was a better outcome in effect decoding capacity posttreatment and a progress in regulation of negative effects in the follow-up. Emotional role taking behavior and social anxiety returned to the baseline level, perhaps by reasons of no "booster sessions" in the follow-up. Unfortunately, in contrast to our hypotheses, we failed to show treatment-specific effects, which may be due to an underpowered statistical testing. There was only one exception of this: While the Integrated Psychological Therapy Program showed a greater reduction of global psychopathology after treatment, the Training of Emotional Intelligence reduced psychopathology in the follow-up more strongly [20, 21].

Conclusions

- Psychosis prediction is based on clinical criteria in terms of risk symptoms and will be supplemented by a multilevel approach that includes neuropsychological, brain-structural, and brain-functional as well as genetic data and biomarkers.
- Specialized early detection centres should be available for diagnostics to assess the risk of psychosis and should be easily accessible and expanded regionally.
- In psychosis prevention, cognitive behavioral therapy-oriented psychotherapeutic interventions have been established as measures of first choice.
- Second-line drugs are antipsychotics of the second generation, especially if the subjective burden of symptoms is high, in order to prevent severe extrapyramidal side effects and massive weight gain.
- The transition from child and adolescent psychiatry to adult psychiatry should be improved.
- Prevention of drug-related relapses should be improved.
- General knowledge about risks of drugs and their effect on brain function as well as the risk to develop a drug induced psychosis should be improved.
- Systemic therapy might help prevent relapses, because a well-connected family or/and peer group may help to get better results.
- Additional objective measurement tools like OPATUS CPTa may help to indicate the grade of cognitive and concentrative decline as well as improvement under therapy.

References

1. Seidman LJ, Shapiro DI, Stone WS, Woodberry KA, Ronzio A, Cornblatt BA, Addington J, Bearden CE, Cadenhead KS, Cannon TD, Mathalon DH, McGlashan TH, Perkins DO, Tsuang MT, Walker EF, Woods SW. Association of neurocognition with Transition to psychosis: baseline functioning in the second phase of the North American Prodrome longitudinal study. JAMA Psychiatry. 2016;73(12):1239–48. https://doi.org/10.1001/jamapsychiatry.2016.2479.
2. Nasrallah HA, Smeltzer DJ. Contemporary diagnosis and management of the patient with schizophrenia. 2nd ed. Newton: Handbooks in Health. Care CO.; 2011.
3. Meyers R. A new approach in diagnostics and therapy of ADHD, Lecture. Dorsten: Sozialpsychiatrisches Centrum; 2018. www.meyers-hamburg.com

4. Meyers R. OPATUS CPTa: new ways in precise diagnostics and therapy support for optimized treatment results in ADHD and other neuropsychiatric disorders, Dorsten. 2022, ISBN13: 979-8847115193.
5. Meyers R. ADHD IS CURABLE: precise diagnosis—optimized outcome, Dorsten. 2022,. ISBN13: 979-8404994049.
6. Gross G, Huber G, Klosterkoetter J, Linz AM. Bonner Skala für die Beurteilung von Basissymptomen (BSABS; Bonn Scale for the Assessment of Basic Symptoms). Berlin: Springer; 1987.
7. Beth Israel Deaconess Medical Center. Neurocognitive deficits may be a red flag for psychosis. Boston. November 02, 2016. https://www.bidmc.org/about-bidmc/news/neurocognitive-deficitis-red-flag-for-psychosis
8. Klosterkoetter J, Mueller H. Chapter 11: Prävention schizophrener und anderer psychotischer Störungen. In: Klosterkoetter J, Maier W, editors. Handbuch präventive Psychiatrie. Stuttgart: Schattauer Verlag; 2017. p. 227–83.
9. Levin C. Mental fatigue—is it objectively measurable? Master thesis. Sweden: The Department of Psychology, Univ. of Gothenburg; 2014.
10. Skau S, Jonsdottir IH, Dahlman AS, Johansson B, Kuhn HG. Exhaustion disorder and altered brain activity in frontal cortex detected with fNIRS. Stress. 2020; https://doi.org/10.1080/10253890.2020.1777972.
11. Skau S, Bunketorp-Käll L, Kuhn HG, Johansson B. Mental Fatigue and Functional Near-Infrared Spectroscopy (fNIRS)—based assessment of cognitive performance after mild traumatic brain injury. Front Hum Neurosci. 2019, Sec. Brain Health and Clinical Neuroscience; https://doi.org/10.3389/fnhum.2019.00145.
12. Hilker R, Helenius D, Fagerlund B, Skytthe A, Christensen K, Werge TM, Nordentoft M, Glenthøj B. Heritability of schizophrenia and schizophrenia Spectrum based on the Nationwide Danish twin register. Biol Psychiatry. 2018;83(6):492–8. https://doi.org/10.1016/j.biopsych.2017.08.017.
13. Hany M, Rehman B, Azhar Y, Chapman J. Schizophrenia. In: StatPearls [Internet]. Treasure Island: StatPearls Publishing; 2023. 2024 Jan–. PMID: 30969686.
14. Klug M, Hill R, Van den Buuse M. 'Two hit' neurodevelopmental mechanisms in schizophrenia: focus on animal models and the role of BDNF. In: Gargiulo PÁ, Mesones Arroyo HL, editors. Psychiatry and neuroscience update, vol. 1. Switzerland: Springer; 2015. p. 335–51. https://doi.org/10.1007/978-3-319-17103-6_24.
15. Davis J, Eyre H, Jacka FN, Dodd S, Dean O, McEwen S, Debnath M, McGrath J, Maes M, Amminger P, McGorry PD, Pantelis C, Berk M. A review of vulnerability and risks for schizophrenia: beyond the two hit hypothesis. Neurosci Biobehav Rev. 2016;65:185–94. https://doi.org/10.1016/j.neubiorev.2016.03.017. Epub 2016 Apr 9. PMID: 27073049; PMCID: PMC4876729
16. Maloney-Hall B, Wallingford SC, Konefal S, Young MM. Psychotic disorder and cannabis use: Canadian hospitalization trends, 2006–2015. Health Promot Chronic Dis Prev Can. 2020;40(5–6):176–83. https://doi.org/10.24095/hpcdp.40.5/6.06. PMID: 32529977; PMCID: PMC7367424
17. Gahr M, Ziller J, Keller F, Muche R, Preuss UW, Schönfeldt-Lecuona C. Incidence of inpatient cases with mental disorders due to use of cannabinoids in Germany: a nationwide evaluation. Eur J Pub Health. 2022;32(2):239–45. https://doi.org/10.1093/eurpub/ckab207.
18. Meyers R. Erfolgsaussichten der ambulanten Behandlung von Suchtkranken mit Apomorphin. [Prospects of success of outpatient treatment of addicts with apomorphine], Medical thesis. Hamburg: University of Hamburg; 1984.
19. Roder V, Brenner HD, Mueller D. Integriertes Psychologisches Therapieprogramm bei schizophren Erkrankten IPT. [Integrated psychological therapy program for schizophrenic patients IPT]. Beltz 9.A., 2019.
20. Roder V, Mueller DR, Mueser KT, Brenner HD. Integrated psychological therapy (IPT) for schizophrenia: is it effective? Schizophr Bull. 2006;32(Suppl 1):S81–93. https://doi.org/10.1093/schbul/sbl021.
21. Vauth R, Joe A, Seitz M, Dreher-Rudolph M, Olbrich H, Stieglitz RD. Differenzielle Kurz- und Langzeitwirkung eines "Trainings Emotionaler Intelligenz" und des "Integrierten Psychologischen Therapieprogramms" für schizophrene Patienten? [Differentiated short- and long-term effects of a "training of emotional intelligence" and of the "integrated psychologic therapy program" for schizophrenic patients?]. Fortschr Neurol Psychiatry. 2001;69(11):518–25. https://doi.org/10.1055/s-2001-18383.

50 Diagnosis and Management of Comorbid ADHD in Patients with Substance Use Disorders

Betsy Busch

Abbreviations

ACC	anterior cingulate cortex
ACDS	Adult ADHD Clinical Diagnostic Scale
ADHD-NOS	attention-deficit/hyperactivity disorder-not otherwise specified
ADHD	attention-deficit/hyperactivity disorder
ADSA	Attention-Deficit Scales for Adults
AMPH(s)	amphetamine(s)
ASPD	antisocial personality disorder
ASRS	Adult ADHD Self-Report Scale
ATX	atomoxetine
AUD(s)	alcohol use disorder
BD	behavioral disinhibition
BDEFS	Barkley Deficits in Executive Functioning Scale
BFIS	Barkley Functional Impairment Scale for Adults
BorPD	borderline personality disorder
BPD	bipolar disorder
BRIEF-A	Behavior Rating Inventory of Executive Function®–Adult Version
CAADID	*Conners' Adult ADHD Diagnostic Interview for DSM-IV*
CAARS	Conners Adult ADHD Rating Scale
CBT	cognitive-behavioral therapy
CD	conduct disorder
CGI-I	Clinical Global Impressions Scale-Improvement
CUD	cocaine use disorder
DA	dopamine
DESR	deficient emotional self-regulation
DIVA	Diagnostic Interview for Adult ADHD
DMN	default mode network
DSM	Diagnostic and Statistical Manual of Mental Disorders
fMRI	functional magnetic resonance imaging
GWAS	genome-wide association study
GXR	guanfacine extended-release
LDX:	lisdexamfetamine
MAS-XR	mixed amphetamine salts, extended-release
MBSR	mindfulness-based stress reduction
MDD	major depressive disorder
MINI-Plus	Mini-International Neuropsychiatric Interview
MPH	methylphenidate

B. Busch (✉)
Tufts University School of Medicine,
Boston, MA, USA
e-mail: betsy.busch@tufts.edu

P. Á. Gargiulo, H. L. Mesones-Arroyo (eds.), *Psychiatry and Neuroscience Update – Vol. V*,
https://doi.org/10.1007/978-3-031-72219-6_50

nAChR(s)	nicotinic acetylcholine receptor(s)
NE	norepinephrine
NMU	nonmedical use
OROS-MPH	osmotic-release oral system™ methylphenidate
OUD	opioid use disorder
PFC	prefrontal cortex
SAD	seasonal affective disorder
StimUD(s)	stimulant use disorder(s)
SNP(s)	single nucleotide polymorphism(s)
SUD(s)	substance use disorder(s)
SUD+ADHD	substance use disorder with comorbid ADHD
WFIRS	Weiss Functional Impairment Rating Scale
WURS	Wender Utah Rating Scale

Introduction

Attention-deficit/hyperactivity disorder (ADHD) is the most common neurodevelopmental disorder of childhood [1]. Its diagnostic criteria are comprised of behaviors reflecting age-inappropriate levels of inattention, hyperactivity, and impulsivity that are pervasive and impairing, and that interfere with normal development and functioning.

ADHD is an important childhood-onset risk factor for substance use disorders (SUDs), and thus, those with SUDs have increased rates of ADHD. The presence of ADHD typically precedes SUD, and if left untreated, ADHD predicts a higher likelihood of alcohol and/or drug dependence in adulthood, greater severity and complexity of SUDs, and earlier adolescent onset of addictive substance use [2–5]. Understanding the problems across the lifespan to which ADHD may have contributed can help the clinician to elicit the historical clues needed to suspect comorbid adult ADHD in those with SUDs. Knowledge of the shared biology between ADHD and SUDs can help explain why the presence of ADHD increases the duration, severity, and chronicity of SUDs, and why this comorbidity also makes the typical course of treatment more complex. Treatment of comorbid ADHD can improve the ultimate outcomes for patients with SUD+ADHD who seek treatment for their SUD.

It is important to understand ADHD as a neurodevelopmental disorder that begins in childhood, but that frequently persists throughout adolescence and, in 70–90% of individuals, continues into adulthood [6, 7]. Severity of ADHD may wax and wane over the years, depending on the intensity of external demands and availability of accommodations, treatment, and support at a given time. At each developmental phase of life, individuals experience new demands from school, jobs, family, and relationships; therefore, the impairments from ADHD manifest differently, across the lifespan. ADHD presents at younger ages than most psychiatric conditions, many of which emerge during adolescence or adulthood; thus, over time, as additional comorbidities become apparent, the patient's clinical presentation and complexity may change further [8]. An appreciation of this evolution can assist the clinician in knowing when to suspect the comorbidity of SUD+ADHD; how to elicit the necessary history to arrive at an understanding of each patient's comorbid diagnoses and, ultimately, how to provide the most successful treatment regimen to patients with SUD+ADHD.

This chapter will:

1. Familiarize the reader with the *prevalence, problems, and correlates of ADHD through the lifespan*, and the typical *developmental sequence from ADHD to recreational substance use to SUD*;
2. Discuss the *neurobiology* of ADHD and its potential areas of neural overlap with SUDs;
3. Review *nonmedical stimulant use/abuse*, including motivations and demographics;
4. Describe the *specific characteristics of ADHD in patients with SUDs*;
5. Describe the *impact of ADHD treatment on adults with ADHD*;
6. Consider findings on the *impact of ADHD pharmacotherapy in adults with comorbid SUD+ADHD*;

7. Describe instruments for *screening and diagnosis* of adult ADHD in patients seeking treatment for SUDs;
8. Discuss specific *pharmacological and non-pharmacological treatment options* for treatment of comorbid ADHD in patients seeking treatment for SUDs; and
9. Address best practices for *prevention of stimulant misuse and diversion.*

A Lifespan Approach to ADHD

ADHD Is a Worldwide Problem

Attention-deficit/hyperactivity disorder, or ADHD, is not new. It was first described clinically in a German textbook in 1775 [9], and again by the British pediatrician, George F. Still, in 1902 [10]. However, ADHD has only been the topic of serious study since about 1980, when diagnostic criteria for "Attention Deficit Disorder" were operationalized for research by the American Psychiatric Association's *Diagnostic and Statistical Manual, third edition* (DSM-III) [11]. The DSM-III was in preparation at the time the World Health Organization's ninth revision of the *International Classification of Disease* (ICD-9) was published in 1978 [12], so the diagnostic criteria for "Attention Deficit Disorder" and the ICD-9's "Hyperkinetic Syndrome of Childhood" were not harmonized at that time.

Because of this non-alignment of diagnostic criteria, most research articles about what we now call ADHD came from the United States, in the 1980s and 1990s. For over two decades, international debate raged about the validity of the diagnosis of ADHD. In fact, ADHD was widely perceived to be "an American condition [13]" or a social construct [14], rather than a valid and impairing neurodevelopmental disorder. However, a huge body of subsequent research has proven these ideas wrong. For example, a meta-analysis of 102 studies found that the worldwide prevalence of ADHD in children and adolescents was approximately 5.3% [15]. Studies that (a) applied the same diagnostic criteria, (b) required that subjects have both ADHD symptoms and significant functional impairment, and (c) used the same sources of information, had reduced variability across many countries. Although some geographic variation was noted, no significant differences in prevalence were noted among studies from North America vs. Europe. An updated version of this meta-analysis, which included 135 studies, found that, despite increasing rates of ADHD recognition, diagnosis, and treatment in children, there has been no evidence of an increase in prevalence worldwide, over the past three decades [16].

Early identification of childhood ADHD and other psychiatric disorders (preferably by age 9 years) [17] and adequate pharmacological and behavioral treatment are of paramount importance. Early identification permits early and sustained treatment during crucial developmental phases of childhood and adolescence. The longitudinal studies of children with ADHD by Biederman and colleagues have shown that early and sustained childhood pharmacotherapy of ADHD can substantially reduce adult rates of psychiatric comorbidity, including major depressive disorder (MDD), multiple anxiety disorders, and conduct disorder (CD) [18, 19]. Childhood pharmacotherapy for ADHD also has been associated with (a) less adult functional impairment, (b) less use of alcohol, cannabis, tobacco, and illicit drugs, and (c) lower risk for later SUD and nicotine dependence [20–24]. Importantly, continued stimulant treatment during adolescence is *not* associated with increased risk for later use of either cocaine or methamphetamine; if anything, ongoing treatment of ADHD through adolescence and into young adulthood may be protective [25]. Much research clearly shows the benefits of early and sustained treatment of ADHD during childhood and throughout adolescence. This evidence should finally refute the false, but widely held, belief that childhood pharmacotherapy for ADHD might increase the risk of later SUD. We must improve our ability to communicate the real benefits of early, sustained pharmacotherapy of childhood ADHD in conversations with our patients and their families.

Prevalence of Adult ADHD and the Problem of Underdiagnosis

The most recent meta-analyses of the prevalence of ADHD using DSM-IV criteria for the diagnosis suggest that ADHD is present in approximately 2.5% of adults [26, 27]. A large population study found a prevalence of adult ADHD of 3.55% when a cut-off of 5/9 DSM-5 criteria was used [28].

Although there is a male preponderance in childhood ADHD, adult ADHD (especially the inattentive presentation) appears to occur in at least as many females as males [28, 29]. The inattentive presentation is the most common among adolescents and adults with ADHD, although some symptoms of hyperactivity (e.g., interrupting others, difficulty waiting, subjective restlessness, or fidgeting) also are commonly present.

Females with ADHD may have less obvious manifestations of hyperactive-impulsive symptoms (e.g., they may talk excessively, or interrupt others). Because these behaviors are minimally disruptive, and perhaps because they are consistent with certain gender stereotypes, such problems among females with ADHD may not be clinically perceived as typical hyperactivity. Other manifestations of hyperactivity (e.g., an inner sense of restlessness) can only be elicited with a careful history. Thus, ADHD in females is more likely to go undiagnosed, unless female patients have prominent externalizing features [30–32].

If left untreated, adult ADHD has a highly morbid course with adverse outcomes. Thus, it is problematic that adult ADHD is still widely under-diagnosed [33, 34] and undertreated [35–37]. In one study, the average age at diagnosis of adults with ADHD was 28 years, despite the fact that this is a disorder with an early childhood onset [38]. Another study found that, even in high-income countries, over 70% of those with adult ADHD received no treatment for any mental health problem. Even more alarming was the fact that *95% of adult ADHD patients received no specific treatment for their ADHD* [36]. In Germany, a country with universal health insurance, the prevalence of ADHD in 18- to 64-year-old adults was estimated to be 4.7%, in one large population study [39]. Yet, the prevalence of German adult patients receiving an ADHD diagnosis was only 0.4% [40], suggesting that 90% of adults with ADHD in Germany remain undiagnosed. Clearly, there is a need for better clinician education regarding the recognition and treatment of ADHD in adults.

There are a variety of reasons for underdiagnosis. Importantly, adolescents and adults with ADHD are known to underestimate the severity of, and impairment from, their ADHD [41, 42]. They often have diminished awareness of the self, and thus, impaired self-appraisal abilities [43, 44]. They also may mis-attribute the impairment from their ADHD symptoms to another disorder. Furthermore, adults may not recall accurately their childhood ADHD symptoms or appreciate the degree of impairment they manifested, decades earlier. Many adults may not have been diagnosed with ADHD during childhood, for a variety of reasons, including lack of clinician awareness, in earlier decades. A recent meta-analysis of prevalence studies worldwide suggests that symptomatic adult ADHD among those who never received a childhood diagnosis may be far more common than previously thought [27]. For all these reasons, many ADHD experts caution that a strict reliance on adult self-reports of childhood and current symptoms and impairment may lead to underdiagnosis of ADHD.

To address these problems with obtaining accurate historical (and current) information, it is recommended that *collateral information on childhood and current ADHD symptoms and impairment be obtained*, when possible, from a parent, spouse, and/or other adult(s) who know(s) the adult patient well. Support from any available past documentation (e.g., school records, performance reviews from work) also can be very helpful in improving diagnostic accuracy, in addition to the information acquired from the patient self-report [37, 45]. Careful history-taking, with a variety of examples of common areas of impairment specific to adults with ADHD [46], is essential. Appreciation of cultural and racial bias also is important. For example, in the United States, ADHD also may be especially under-diagnosed in children and adults from non-white racial and ethnic groups [47, 48].

DSM-5 Changes to the Diagnostic Criteria for ADHD

The current revision of the ADHD diagnostic criteria in DSM-5 [49] includes several important changes relevant to the diagnosis of adult ADHD. These include:

1. Changing the requirement for age-of-onset of symptoms from age 7 to age 12 years [50];
2. Decreasing the number of ADHD symptom criteria required to make the diagnosis from 6/9 to 5/9 inattention and/or hyperactivity/impulsivity criteria, for those ≥17 years of age, and providing patients with adult-relevant examples of the childhood criteria [51, 52];
3. Allowing the diagnosis of ADHD to be made in the presence of a diagnosis of autism spectrum disorder, since these conditions do co-exist frequently [53]; and
4. Eliminating ADHD subtypes, since these do not retain their stability over time [54]. Instead of identifying ADHD subtypes, the predominant ADHD symptoms at the time a patient presents for care are noted, as a descriptor (inattentive, hyperactive-impulsive, or combined presentation).

These changes are consistent with the reclassification of ADHD in DSM-5 as a neurodevelopmental disorder, rather than a disruptive behavioral disorder. They reflect the findings from family and twin studies, genetic and neuroimaging findings that indicate that childhood and persistent adult ADHD have the same neurodevelopmental origins [8, 55, 56]. It has become clear that ADHD is neither merely a transient, "maturational lag," nor a behavioral disorder of childhood that always remits [8]. In fact, a very small group of "late-onset" ADHD patients who never met full childhood criteria for ADHD have been described recently. It is not yet clear whether these individuals are different from others with adult ADHD. Their ADHD impairment typically appeared between ages 12–16 years [57], which may indicate that even an age-of-onset criterion of 12 years is occasionally too stringent [58]. Other features of those with "late-onset" ADHD tend to include: a) the inattentive presentation of ADHD, b) a larger proportion of females, and c) high IQs. Thus, these individuals may represent a small group of bright patients with non-disruptive, subthreshold ADHD, who were able to manage their symptoms by using compensatory strategies to minimize impairment until adolescence or young adulthood, when they finally became unable to keep up with new, age-appropriate, attentional, and executive function demands on their cognition, and they then presented with "adult onset" ADHD [56, 57, 59]. Importantly, even those with ADHD and high IQ can have substantial and impairing executive function deficits [59, 60]. Additional studies will be needed to clarify this "late-onset" group, but clinicians should be aware that adolescents and adults occasionally may present with ADHD without a clear childhood history of ADHD.

One of the relatively new, but important, concepts regarding ADHD and its prevalence is that, although we treat ADHD as a categorical diagnosis, it actually represents the problems of a small fraction of people whose poor attentional, behavioral, and motor control are at the severe, impairing end of a normative continuum of behaviors in the population [61, 62]. Much concern has been expressed about excessive or inflated estimates of the prevalence of ADHD, especially with the DSM-5 changes in the diagnostic criteria [63, 64]. Are we over-diagnosing ADHD? What *should* be the prevalence of ADHD? An analogous situation is found with medical hypertension, which also represents the extreme upper end of a normative distribution of blood pressures. The diagnosis of hypertension, and the decision to treat it, requires cardiologists to define an arbitrary cut-off point for a physiologic measurement that occurs on a continuum. Over the years, as our understanding of hypertension has grown, cardiologists have revised the blood pressure levels that define "hypertension" to include cases that would have been considered "subthreshold" hypertension, in the past. Few would consider this "over-diagnosis" of hypertension, however. Instead, we understand that cardiologists have revised the cut-off point for defining hypertension based on evidence that demonstrates that treating blood pressure to keep it lower than that cut-off point will decrease a person's risk of cardiovascular disease and adverse (and possibly fatal) cardiovascular events [65]. Similarly, the extensive literature on children and adults with ADHD suggests that, rather than arguing over what the prevalence *should* be, or what exact number of DSM criteria must be required for adult ADHD, our approach to the diagnosis of ADHD should instead be *to diagnose and treat this disorder when its symptom severity is sufficient to cause substantial functional impairment.*

The Child with ADHD Grows Up

Until about 50 years ago, ADHD was thought to be a childhood disorder that was outgrown by adolescence. The earliest suggestions that ADHD might persist into adulthood, and adults with ADHD might respond to the same treatment as children with ADHD appeared in the 1970s [66], and the earliest prospectively followed outcomes of young adults who had been diagnosed with ADHD in childhood were described in the 1980s [67]. However, until recent decades, persistence of childhood ADHD into adulthood was thought to be rare [68].

As the child with ADHD becomes an adolescent, the overt appearance of hyperactivity diminishes or transforms into an internal sense of restlessness or impatience. However, symptoms of inattention and impulsivity often remain prominent, causing impairment [69]. In an early follow-up study, Biederman and colleagues [70] demonstrated in boys with childhood ADHD that there was an age-related decline in symptoms throughout adolescence, so that some 18- to 20-year-olds no longer met the full DSM-III-R diagnostic criteria for ADHD, but over 60% of those 18- to 20-year-olds who met fewer criteria than the DSM-III-R threshold for diagnosis of ADHD still struggled with ADHD symptoms and had substantial functional impairment. Few subjects achieved full remission, free of ongoing, ADHD-related dysfunction. Subsequent studies found that the rate of ADHD persistence in adults was far higher, approximately 50–65% [71, 72]. In recent years, the persistence of ADHD in older adults (>65 years) has also been recognized [73, 74]. Most recently, Sibley and colleagues found that ADHD symptoms might wax and wane, over time, but by a mean age of 25 years, *only 9% of subjects followed longitudinally since childhood had experienced true recovery from ADHD symptoms and impairment* [6]. So, as we refine our studies and follow more children with ADHD into adulthood, adult ADHD appears to be a chronic and persistent problem, for most.

By late adolescence and throughout adulthood, individuals are expected to demonstrate competence in a variety of self-regulatory skills that are not developmentally mastered by younger children. These adult self-regulatory tasks are varied, but include: planning; setting priorities and maintaining long-term goals; time management; organization; problem-solving; money management; task completion; meeting deadlines; paying attention to the most salient stimulus; maintaining/shifting attention appropriately; anticipating the consequences of one's actions; using good judgment; retrieving and applying knowledge at the appropriate moment; observing social, behavioral, and pragmatic language conventions when interacting with others; delaying gratification; and regulating/modulating one's emotional responses (see Table 50.1). Problems with emotional over-reactivity, known as "deficient emotional self-regulation (DESR)" or "emotional impulsivity [75, 76]," are a particularly impairing aspect of self-regulation difficulties [77, 78]. Together, the constellation of self-regulation skills listed above is described as "executive functions." Deficits in these executive functions, including difficulty with emotional and attentional self-regulation, are frequently seen in adolescents and adults with ADHD [76, 79–81], and they contribute to severe impairment and reduced quality of life in adults with ADHD symptoms across a variety of life roles, including

Table 50.1 Common executive functioning tasks that may be impaired in patients with ADHD

Selecting and paying attention to the most salient stimulus	Initiating tasks promptly; avoiding procrastination
Maintaining attentional focus; sustaining effort	Estimating accurately how long a task will take to complete
Ignoring irrelevant distractions	Completing long-term projects; meeting deadlines
Shifting attention from task to task	Managing time effectively
Setting priorities appropriately	Regulating processing speed for efficiency and accuracy
Planning	Problem-solving; thinking of multiple solutions to a problem
Applying good judgment	Using working memory when performing complex mental tasks
Reflecting before making important decisions	Remembering to retrieve and apply knowledge at the appropriate time
Anticipating the consequences of one's actions	Monitoring errors
Organizing belongings	Having cognitive flexibility; being able to shift mental set
Organizing thoughts and language (spoken and written)	Managing one's money responsibly; paying bills on time
Maintaining one's own train of thought during conversation	Deferring small, immediate rewards to achieve long-term goals
Observing social and pragmatic language rules in interpersonal interactions: Not interrupting Responding succinctly, so others have a chance to speak Remaining on-topic Expressing reciprocal interest in others Tailoring one's language and behavior to various social situations appropriately	Modulating one's emotional responses: Tolerating minor frustrations and disappointments Tolerating waiting, minor delays Not over-reacting or being too quick to anger Avoiding impulsive aggression and excessive irritability

academic, occupational, and interpersonal functioning [82–87]. In fact, some experts feel that problems with executive functions, although not part of the core DSM-5 diagnostic criteria, are perhaps the most specific predictors of adult ADHD (especially in combination with symptoms of inattention) [88, 89], and that executive function deficits should be considered for inclusion as a core feature, in future versions of ADHD criteria in the DSM [51].

Outcomes of Untreated/Undertreated ADHD: Functional Impairment, Morbidity, and Mortality

Untreated adult ADHD imposes a substantial burden on society. This societal burden is manifested in academic/work under-achievement, decreased productivity and income, higher unemployment rates, poorer physical and mental health, more accidents and injuries, increased medical resource use and costs, more need for public assistance, and greater legal/court involvement, including higher incarceration rates.

Educational and Occupational Impairments The pervasively negative adult outcomes of those with untreated/undertreated ADHD have been extensively documented. Educational and occupational under-achievement is common [90–94]. Graduation rates from high school and college are lower than expected [90]. Compared with non-ADHD peers, adults with ADHD demonstrate more unemployment and underemployment [90]. They change jobs frequently over time (both from being fired and quitting) [95, 96]. Common work-related impairments include procrastination and reduced productivity, absenteeism, irritability and low frustration tolerance, and high rates of workplace injury [97].

Adults with ADHD often manage their finances poorly, make unwise or impulsive financial decisions, and save less money [98–100]. They may be more dependent on financial support from family and/or the welfare system [94]. They demonstrate significant deficits in lifetime earnings, compared to non-ADHD peers with similar educational/occupational achievement [94, 101–103]. Even those adults with ADHD who appear to be functioning adequately at work may have to expend excessive amounts of time and effort to manage their work responsibilities, and this may result in neglect of family, social and other responsibilities, loss of sleep, and poor physical and psychological well-being [104].

Accidents, Injuries, and Premature Death Adolescents and young adults with untreated/undertreated ADHD are at increased risk for motor vehicle accidents [105, 106] and sport-related concussions [107, 108]. Adults with untreated/undertreated ADHD are known to have high rates of motor vehicle (and other) accidents [109–111] and workplace injuries [97]. Adult ADHD has higher than expected mortality rates [112, 113], mostly from accidents [112], substance use disorders [114], and suicide [115–117]. Females with ADHD have high rates of self-harm and suicidality, especially when there is a history of prior physical or sexual maltreatment [118, 119]. The association of ADHD and suicide suggests that *the coexistence of suicidal ideation and impulsivity may be especially dangerous* [120]. The likelihood of premature death in patients with ADHD, especially from unnatural causes (accidents, injuries, SUD, suicide) increases dramatically with an increasing number of comorbidities [113]. Several studies have demonstrated that sustained ADHD medication treatment decreases all these risks substantially [22, 121–124].

Medical Comorbidities Up to 80% of treatment-naïve patients with ADHD have concomitant sleep disorders, and these are strongly associated with more severe ADHD symptoms [125, 126]. Most commonly, patients with ADHD have an extreme evening chronotype (delayed sleep phase disorder), which also may predispose individuals with ADHD to seasonal affective disorder (SAD) [127]. Also common are insomnia (particularly difficulty falling asleep and staying asleep) [128], obstructive sleep apnea, restless legs syndrome, and periodic limb movement disorder [125, 126]. Neuroimaging indicates that ADHD symptoms and sleep disturbances have common neural correlates, including structural differences in the ventral attention system and fronto-striatal circuitry [128].

There is an association between ADHD and obesity [129–131], especially in females with ADHD [132]. Impulsivity may be a particularly important feature in the association with obesity [131]. ADHD also is associated with a higher prevalence of eating disorders, especially binge-eating disorder and bulimia nervosa [133, 134]. Interestingly, patients with ADHD and eating disorders both may have deficits in the perception and regulation of satiety [135, 136].

Recently, adult ADHD, and high genetic risk for ADHD, have been associated with a greater likelihood of a variety of somatic health conditions, including many cardiovascular, metabolic, and autoimmune diseases [137–140]. Not surprisingly, overall *per capita* healthcare utilization and costs are substantially higher for those with ADHD [141].

Social, Personal, and Intimate Relationships Interpersonal interactions, both at work and in the patient's personal life, are often problematic for adults with ADHD. It is difficult for others to sustain a relationship with an individual who demonstrates chronic problems with disorganization, misplacing things, poor planning, failing to remember chores, appointments or obligations, difficulty completing tasks on time, low frustration tolerance, impulsive decisions, irritability, and over-reacting to minor frustrations or disappointments. This is especially true in the context of intimate relationships [142, 143]. Excessive talking and interrupting, or "tuning out" when others talk, can be irritating to others; those with ADHD also are more likely to have a history of bullying and being bullied [144]. Self-esteem and social functioning are reported to be poorer among those with untreated ADHD [145]. More adults with ADHD are divorced or single [39, 82, 83]. Adults with ADHD also report more loneliness than others [146, 147].

Risky sexual behaviors are also notable, and begin early in adolescence [148]. Patients with ADHD are younger at first intercourse, have more sexual partners by age 18 years, and those 12–19 years old with ADHD are more likely to become teenage parents [149–154]. Adults with ADHD are more likely to be victims or perpetrators of sexual or interpersonal violence than population samples [155]. Men and women with ADHD experience more sexual dysfunction than the general population [156, 157].

Being a responsible parent can be especially difficult for adults with ADHD. With their own disorganization and time management difficulties, the additional parental responsibilities of keeping family schedules organized, getting children to and from school/day-care and other activities on time, and supervising/supporting homework can be very difficult for the parent with ADHD. If the parent has low frustration tolerance or emotional dysregulation, they are poorly equipped to demonstrate modulated emotional responses to daily challenges and disappointments, or to use praise and positive reinforcement as their primary tools for discipline and child-rearing. Parents with ADHD may provide inadequate or excessively permissive supervision to children, give inadequate support, are poorer problem-solvers, discipline children inconsistently, over-react to problematic child behaviors, have more negative and critical verbal interactions with their children, and use more corporal punishment [158–160]. If the parent with ADHD has a behaviorally disordered child with ADHD, the situation becomes even more problematic. Among children with ADHD, approximately 20–50% have at least one parent who has ADHD [161, 162].

Parenting problems also exacerbate romantic, relational stresses with partners. Arguing over failing to share parenting responsibilities, forgetfulness, and unreliability may be frequent. This takes a toll on the co-parenting partnership, and may further damage an already-stressed marriage [142].

Behavioral parent training is crucial for parents of children with ADHD, but for parents who have ADHD themselves, and who also have a child who has ADHD, behavioral training often is less than optimally effective [163]. However, the *combination* of teaching parenting skills and pharmacological treatment of parental ADHD has been shown to be helpful in several ways. Pharmacological treatment reduces parental symptoms of ADHD and increases parents' awareness of both their own ADHD symptoms and the child's ADHD symptoms. Behavioral parent training also improves disciplinary consistency, increases parental use of praise and decreases critical comments, and decreases the use of corporal punishment in parents' interactions with their children [164–166].

Legal Problems Adolescents and adults with ADHD have more legal problems than the population at large. Among a large sample of adult ADHD patients in a private, outpatient psychiatric clinic, 24.5% of males and 11.7% of females with ADHD reported that they had a past criminal conviction [167]. These convictions were associated with the presence of emotional dysregulation and more symptoms of hyperactivity impulsivity. Offenses range from dangerous driving (e.g., more speeding citations, license revocations, and personal injury [168, 169]) to being arrested and convicted for both non-violent and violent crimes [170, 171]. There is a younger age of onset of antisocial and criminal involvement, twice the risk of adolescent and adult arrests, and three times the risk of convictions and incarcerations. There also is an increased risk of criminal recidivism [170].

ADHD Among Incarcerated Persons There is a high prevalence of ADHD among incarcerated men and women. A recent meta-analysis found a fivefold increase in the prevalence of ADHD among imprisoned youth (30.1%), and a 10-fold increase in the prevalence of ADHD among adult prisoners (26.2%), compared with population prevalence [172]. A study of incarcerated women found the same elevation in rates of ADHD as those seen in incarcerated men [173].

Prisoners with ADHD have significantly increased risks of comorbid psychiatric disorders, substance use disorders, and suicidality [174]. A history of childhood ADHD and/or current ADHD symptoms appear to be associated with younger age at first arrest, number of offenses, likelihood of re-offending [175], and time to re-offending [176]. In addition, while incarcerated, those with untreated ADHD are likely to have more incidents of verbal or physical aggression, property damage, and self-injury. The more severe the symptoms of ADHD and emotional dysregulation, the more likely such incidents are [167, 177]. These ADHD-related behaviors are often misunderstood [178], and the ADHD is mistakenly left untreated, which increases the potential harms to both the incarcerated individuals and to prison personnel.

Psychiatric Comorbidities Adult ADHD also has very high rates of psychiatric comorbidity (50–80%), and psychiatric comorbidities are bi-directional. Mood disorders, SUDs, and anxiety disorders are the most common comorbidities seen among patients with ADHD [36, 179]. For many common psychiatric disorders, a good "rule-of-thumb" is that comorbid ADHD is present in 10–20% of patients with another psychiatric diagnosis. For patients with SUDs, comorbid ADHD may be present in up to 25% [38] (see Fig. 50.1). The onset of ADHD precedes the onset of almost all other comorbid psychiatric conditions [36].

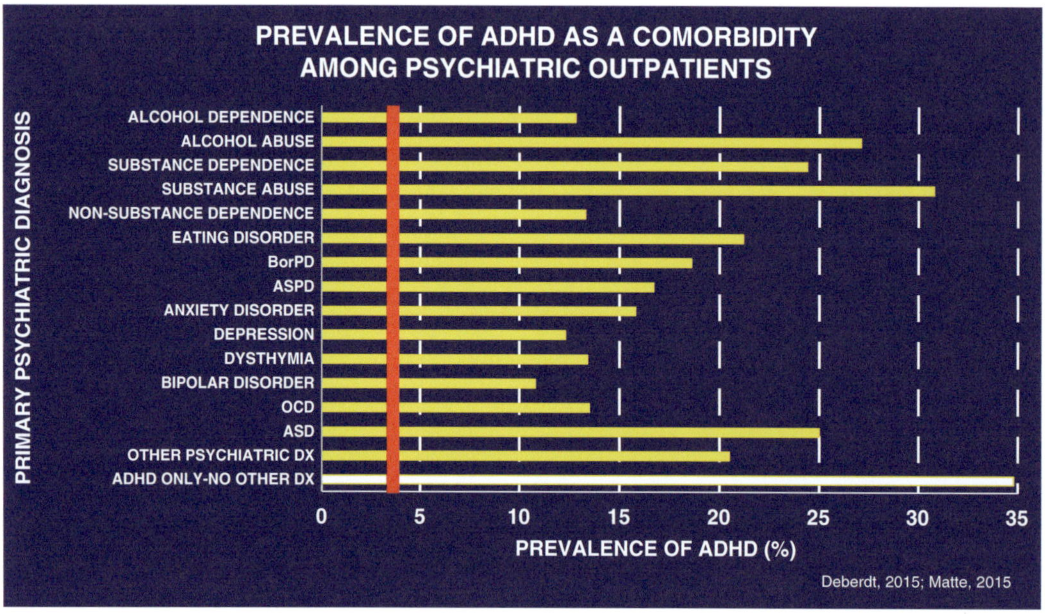

Fig. 50.1 Prevalence of ADHD as a comorbidity among psychiatric outpatients. A total of 1,986 adult, nonpsychotic individuals under outpatient psychiatric treatment were screened with the *Adult ADHD Self-Report Scale* (ASRS); those who screened positive were given a full diagnostic assessment for ADHD with the *Diagnostic Interview for ADHD in Adults, version 2.0* (DIVA-2). The data shown are the prevalence of ADHD in patients under treatment for the specified diagnoses. Fifty-four percent of those diagnosed with ADHD during this study had not been previously diagnosed with ADHD; 67% had not been treated for adult ADHD. Data were obtained from multiple sites across 8 European countries. The vertical red line represents the prevalence of DSM-5-defined ADHD in the general adult population, 3.55%. Abbreviations: *ASD* autism spectrum disorder, *ASPD* antisocial personality disorder; *ASRS Adult ADHD Self-Report Scale*, *BorPD* borderline personality disorder, *DIVA Diagnostic Interview for ADHD in Adults, version 2.0*, *Dx* diagnosis, *OCD* obsessive-compulsive disorder. (Figure adapted from: Deberdt et al. [38] and Matte et al. [28])

Over 15% of individuals with bipolar disorder (BPD) have comorbid ADHD [36]. ADHD is especially common in patients with childhood-onset BPD [180], and ADHD is associated with an earlier onset of the first mood episode among patients with BPD [181–184]. BPD and adolescent hypomania appear to have strong genetic links to comorbid ADHD, especially to the hyperactive-impulsive traits [185].

Another common comorbidity found in adults with ADHD is borderline personality disorder (BorPD). A large, epidemiological study found that those with ADHD had a lifetime rate of BorPD of 33.7%, compared with 5.2%, in the general population [186]. Recently, another large study noted that, in patients with BorPD, stimulants were the only class of medications that were effective in decreasing suicidal behaviors, once again suggesting that the impulsivity associated with ADHD may be a significant risk factor for suicide, in patients with other psychiatric comorbidities [187]. In such vulnerable patients, recognition and treatment of comorbid ADHD may be lifesaving.

A Swedish study of adult patients with ADHD found that over 50% had at least 1 comorbid psychiatric disorder [179]. In that study, the comorbidity of SUD+ADHD comprised just over 15% of adult patients with ADHD [179]. It is common for those with ADHD to have two or three psychiatric comorbidities [36]. Additional psychiatric comorbidities also are common among patients with SUD+ADHD who seek treatment for their SUDs [188]. Women with ADHD have higher rates of premenstrual dysphoric disorder (PMDD), postpartum depression, and postpartum anxiety [189–191].

One of the reasons that adult ADHD may be so significantly under-diagnosed is that adult patients with ADHD may initially seek help for a comorbid condition (e.g., mood or anxiety disorders, SUDs, mania, borderline personality disorder) rather than for ADHD itself. The comorbid condition may mask, or overshadow, the comorbid ADHD, and delay or deter the diagnosis of ADHD [33, 38, 192, 193]. Conversely, the secondary anxiety or demoralization created by ADHD-related chronic under-achievement at school/work, or the overreactions and emotional lability of emotional dysregulation from ADHD, may be misdiagnosed as another psychiatric condition. The literature suggests that misdiagnosis and underdiagnosis are common, and many adults may have their own ADHD considered only after their children receive an ADHD diagnosis [33, 34, 162]. Many patients report struggling to receive appropriate care, and even having to exercise extraordinary levels of self-advocacy to have their ADHD diagnosed and treated effectively [194].

Importantly, undiagnosed, comorbid ADHD may be mistaken for a poor treatment response in a patient's initially diagnosed psychiatric condition, and this misattribution may interfere with the patient's response and/or adherence to a treatment regimen [195–197]. It is especially important to recognize when the problems of ADHD are the antecedent cause of a patient's anxiety and/or depression. Given the high frequency of dysfunction, impairment and premature mortality caused by ADHD, and the availability of effective treatment, it is important to screen all patients with psychiatric conditions for ADHD, and to consider the possibility of comorbid ADHD in patients with another psychiatric condition that appears to be only partially responsive to usual treatment, or treatment resistant [195–198]. In these situations, treatment of the comorbid ADHD may have dramatic benefits.

The Developmental Sequence from ADHD to SUD

It has been known for almost 25 years that youth with ADHD begin using tobacco substantially earlier than their non-ADHD peers. In an early study, 71% of probands with ADHD (versus 27% of those without ADHD) began smoking cigarettes by age 16 years. Psychiatric comorbidity increases the smoking rates, and multiple comorbidities increase the risk of early smoking in a linear fashion [199]. High perceived levels of stress independently increase the likelihood of smoking among those with ADHD [200]. Peer rejection, as well as internalizing problems, have been identified as additional, specific risk factors leading to early initiation of tobacco and marijuana use [201].

A large, longitudinal study of children with and without ADHD found that the median age of first trying a cigarette for those with ADHD was 13.0(±3.2) years vs. 14(±2.6) years for the non-ADHD group. The adolescents with ADHD were more likely than the non-ADHD comparison group to progress to daily smoking, and those who did become daily smokers did so more quickly than their comparison group counterparts. ADHD youth who were smokers also reported more intense withdrawal and craving during periods of abstinence from nicotine than non-ADHD smokers [202]. The presence of ADHD is associated with more subjectively pleasant and reinforcing effects of nicotine [203], and ADHD increases the severity of nicotine addiction in patients seeking treatment for SUDs [204]. The early age-of-onset of nicotine use in pediatric patients with ADHD would imply that *preventive physician conversations about nicotine avoidance should begin by age 9–10 years.*

Cigarette smoking among adolescents with ADHD has been found to increase the likelihood of subsequent substance use and SUD [205–208]. Nicotine dependence severity is associated with cannabis use severity [209]. A recent population study found a strong association between adolescent nicotine use (e-cigarettes and/or smoking) and both cannabis use and binge drinking [210]. Females with a history of childhood ADHD may be at particular risk for nicotine dependence [211]. Importantly, nicotine often is the first addictive substance to which youth are exposed, altering the young brain and making it more vulnerable to later forms of substance use and dependence.

Historically, the adolescent's typical sequence of drug initiation began with tobacco and alcohol use, followed by cannabis and other illicit drugs of abuse [212]. Recently, however, the legalization of cannabis in an increasing number of states in the United States, and the dramatic rise in e-cigarettes as nicotine and cannabis delivery systems [213, 214], as well as the new availability of other, concentrated cannabinoid products for consumption or use [215] have increased concerns about the early use of *both* nicotine and cannabis in those with ADHD [216–221]. Daily cigarette smoking among teens has been largely overtaken by vaping, in recent years. In 2020, almost 20% of American high school students reported current e-cigarette use, and among those who used e-cigarettes, almost 40% of high school students reported using these devices on ≥20 of the past 30 days [222]. Many who vape nicotine in e-cigarettes also use these devices with cannabis [210, 223].

Although there is evidence to the contrary, youth perceive e-cigarettes as safer and less addictive than smoking cigarettes [224]. A recent, longitudinal population study found that adolescents taking stimulants for ADHD at age 18 years had no greater risk of cocaine or methamphetamine use at ages 19–24 years. However, compared with 18-year-olds who never took prescription stimulants for ADHD, adolescents taking stimulants for ADHD at age 18 years who *also* reported cigarette use, binge drinking, or past-year prescription stimulant misuse had about twice the risk for cocaine or methamphetamine use by young adulthood [25]. This suggests that prescription stimulant misuse and untreated ADHD are early behavioral predictors of later stimulant use disorders (StimUDs), and both warrant careful monitoring, follow-up, and intervention, when possible [25].

Unfortunately, adolescents and young adults also appear to be remarkably unconcerned about the risks of early cannabis use [218, 225]. The neuroscience of cannabis effects in youth, however, suggests that even minor exposure to cannabis may be neurotoxic during a sensitive period in adolescence when there is enhanced neuroplasticity, and immature neural networks undergo dramatic changes that are necessary for adult judgment, decision-making, and self-regulation [226–231]. A large, longitudinal study of adolescents found that, after early cannabis use, there was a dose-dependent effect on prefrontal cortical thinning [232].

Early cannabis use is associated with neuropsychological abnormalities. Young cannabis users have amygdala over-reactivity to angry faces, suggesting that early adolescent cannabis use may be associated with elevated sensitivity to threat signals [233]. Amygdala hyper-reactivity to angry faces also predicts cannabis use five years later [234]. Cognitive deficits in decision-making and inhibition were also demonstrated in early marijuana users, when they were tested on the Interference condition of the Stroop Color Word Test (a frontally mediated test of executive function) [235]. Chronic cannabis use is associated with decreased striatal DA release, worsening inattention, and induced anhedonia [236, 237]. Since ADHD is associated with catecholamine deficits, any short-term benefits of cannabis are likely to be outweighed by these longer-term harms.

Many of the variables that make youth with ADHD more likely to try marijuana are non-specific factors that also are known to elevate the risk for developing SUDs. These include genetic predisposition [238], psychiatric comorbidity [5], adverse childhood experiences [239–241], impulsivity [242], abnormal delay discounting [243, 244], excessive risk-taking [245], social isolation [246, 247], substance-using peers [248, 249], and poor coping with stress [250]. Thus, the presence of any of these factors may add cumulative risk to developing a SUD among youth with ADHD.

Early nicotine and cannabis use also may cause problems with gene expression, and derangement of the normal brain changes appropriate for this sensitive period of adolescent development [231, 238]. Such early use of nicotine and/or cannabis may cause changes in brain function that further predispose those with ADHD to the development of a SUD. Thus, both nicotine and cannabis can be considered “gateway” drugs that may facilitate addiction to other drugs, when used by those with still-developing brains [205, 231, 251]. To emphasize the powerful effects of such exposures among youth, it has been demonstrated that younger age at the initiation of substance misuse (ages 12–17 years vs.18–25 years) is associated with more rapid progression to SUD [252]. For patients with ADHD, the risks of early nicotine and cannabis use may be especially great. Those taking stimulants for ADHD at age 18 years who also reported past-year marijuana use had over 4 times the risk of using cocaine or methamphetamine at ages 19–24 years, compared with population controls [25]. Interestingly, the administration of nicotine also is associated with decreased functional connectivity between the anterior insula (thought to send information about physical nicotine/withdrawal effects), the nucleus accumbens (which appraises the motivational relevance of the information), and the dorsal anterior cingulate cortex (which then plans and evaluates goal-directed behavior) [253]. This certainly seems relevant for a population with high risk for later SUDs.

Prevention of nicotine and cannabis use in youth, especially young people with ADHD, may be crucial to the prevention and/or mitigation of all SUDs. Early recognition of ADHD and pharmacological treatment that is sustained throughout childhood appear to reduce early drug exposures and also decrease the overall risks of developing an SUD among youth with ADHD [22, 23].

The Neurobiology of ADHD and SUDs

Many avenues of study have been used to characterize the neurobiology of ADHD. These include studies of genetic risk, neuroanatomic abnormalities, alterations in the functional connectivity of neural networks, and behavioral characteristics. The findings suggest that patients with ADHD have genetic risks and differences in brain structure and function that may predispose them to developing SUDs. Furthermore, these biological abnormalities in patients with ADHD may make the treatment of their SUD+ADHD more complex, and recovery more difficult.

Genetics of ADHD

ADHD is a highly genetic disorder. Among psychiatric disorders, ADHD has exceptionally high heritability, estimated to be 77–88% [254]. Many specific single nucleotide polymorphisms (SNPs) have been identified in association with ADHD through genome-wide association studies (GWAS). Most of these SNPs appear to be common variants, each of which make small contributions to the overall genetic risk of these disorders, while some rare variants also have been identified [255–262]. Overall, genetic vulnerability to ADHD may be comprised of thousands of genetic risk variants. These genetic variants relate to the development of a variety of brain circuits, especially those with connections to the frontal cortex (implicating executive function), and to midbrain dopaminergic neurons (implicating reward processing) [262]. Child and adult ADHD populations share the same genetic variants [263, 264], offering further proof that adult ADHD is the same neurodevelopmental disorder as childhood ADHD. Genes regulating neuronal wiring, neurotransmitter availability, neuronal plasticity, cell adhesion at the blood-brain barrier, and the transcription/regulation of brain-derived neurotrophic factor all have been implicated among the rare copy number variants (CNVs) associated with ADHD [254, 255, 262, 265–267]. ADHD is a familial disorder, further supporting its genetic origins. Relatives of those with ADHD are over five times more likely to have ADHD than relatives of those without ADHD [268].

There appear to be common genetic vulnerabilities between ADHD and SUDs. High polygenic risk scores for ADHD have been shown to predict SUDs [261, 269]. Strong genetic correlations have been noted between problematic alcohol use and both major depressive disorder and ADHD [270]. In family studies, the presence of ADHD alone in probands increased the risk of SUDs in their relatives [271, 272].

Among the SUDs, nicotine use disorder, cannabis use disorder, and alcohol use disorder (AUD) each appear to be approximately 50% heritable [273–275]. Cocaine use disorder (CUD) appears to have a heritability of about 65% [276], which is quite high, among the SUDs. Opiate use disorder (OUD) appears to have moderate heritability; estimates range from 23 to 54% [277]. Recent studies suggest genetic links among different SUDs [278]. Many SUDs appear to be associated with ADHD, high levels of impulsivity, risk-taking and deficient self-regulation [269, 279–282], emphasizing that high genetic risk for ADHD confers added risk for SUDs.

Neuroanatomic Abnormalities

Neuroimaging studies have been helpful in identifying neurodevelopmental decreases in cortical and subcortical volumes in children, adolescents, and adults with ADHD. Findings include smaller overall intracranial volume, smaller cortical surface area, and gray matter reductions [283]. Cortical changes are observed mainly in prefrontal cortex (PFC), insula, and temporal brain regions, and in the dorsal anterior cingulate cortex (ACC) [284–290]. In subcortical structures, smaller volumes have been found in the caudate, putamen, hippocampus, amygdala, and nucleus accumbens of individuals with ADHD [287, 291, 292]. ADHD-related decreases in gray matter volume also have been observed in the cerebellum [293–295]. The differences in brain structure volume and cortical thickness diminish in some studies of adults with ADHD, although frontal, temporal, parietal, striatal, and limbic abnormalities still can be observed in young adults with ADHD [296].

Decreases in gray matter volumes are more prominent in those with severe ADHD symptoms. Smaller gray matter volumes in multiple regions of frontal lobe, cerebellum and temporal lobe have been related to poorer working memory performance [294]. Smaller gray matter volumes in cerebellar regions were associated with more impaired attention [288].

A recent, large study of individuals with 6 different psychiatric disorders (ADHD, autism spectrum disorder, MDD, BPD, obsessive-compulsive disorder, and schizophrenia) helps us to understand how the *genetic risk* for certain psychiatric disorders may explain some of the *anatomical* differences (specifically, cortical thickness and gray matter volumes) associated with those disorders. Common gene expression profiles associated with pyramidal cells, astrocytes, and microglia accounted for much of the group differences in cortical thickness seen on neuroimaging for each of these 6 psychiatric disorders [297]. Further analysis revealed two important gene clusters with abnormal expression and enrichment of disorder-associated genes: a "prenatal" cluster of genes that control the neurodevelopmental processes necessary for correctly guiding axons to their appropriate neuronal connections, and a "postnatal" cluster of genes involved in synaptic plasticity and other synaptic activity. Thus, this study suggests that anatomic abnormalities associated with various psychiatric disorders have largely a genetic etiology [297], and that the genes involved appear to control early brain development.

Delayed Brain Maturation and Its Potential Consequences

Age-related cortical thickening and thinning has been examined in children and adolescents with and without ADHD, as they mature. Various cortical regions of the brain mature at different ages; primary sensory areas mature early, while the poly-modal, higher-order association areas are among the last to mature. Children with ADHD show the same *sequence* of cortical thinning as control children. However, compared with controls, they have extraordinary delays in: a) reaching peak cortical thickness, and then b) initiating normal cortical thinning. The areas of most prominent delay in children and adolescents with ADHD are in the superior and dorsolateral PFC, regions that are particularly important for *attentional control* and *executive functions*. Delays in temporal cortex maturation for those with ADHD are most prominent in areas that, along with the frontal lobes, *integrate and assign salience* to information from lower-order sensory areas into higher-order concepts that influence attention, decision-making, and subsequent actions [298]. Meanwhile, the limbic system, controlling *emotional circuitry* and *reward systems*, matures before those delayed, but crucial, frontotemporal areas. This developmental mismatch between early limbic and late frontal maturation is most exaggerated during adolescence [299]. In adolescents with ADHD, who have delayed maturation of the PFC, the consequences of inadequate cognitive controls in the presence of surging emotions may be especially serious [296]. The delayed developmental sequence of cortical maturation may also have later detrimental effects on myelination, dendritic spine number/thickness, pruning of neurons, atypical functional connectivity, and a host of other processes. Delayed brain maturation may thus be an early manifestation of a cascade of later brain anomalies associated with ADHD.

Circuits, Connectivity, and Network Activation

Patients with ADHD appear to have abnormalities in white matter microstructure, especially in tracts relevant to fronto-striatal and callosal-cingulate networks [300–303], although results have been inconsistent [304, 305]. More important, however, is the almost universal finding of widespread abnormalities in task-related activation and functional connectivity of many white matter tracts throughout the brain in patients with ADHD. These abnormalities are particularly prominent in those tracts that mediate attention, cognitive control, decision-making, error detection, working memory, motivation, delay aversion, and emotional processing [306–311]. There is substantial underactivation of frontoparietal networks, reflecting deficits in executive function (impulse and inhibitory control; working memory; sustained attention; error detection; planning; and time estimation), vigilance and reward processing (Fig. 50.2a, b). Improvements in some of these circuits appear to differentiate ADHD remitters from persisters, both on neurocognitive testing and with event-related potentials on EEG [312], but executive function deficits continue to be seen in both groups [313]. Over-activation is seen in visual and dorsal attention systems and in the default mode network, suggesting difficulty "turning off" these circuits and activating the appropriate task-specific circuits that are required for proper task performance [307]. Visual and dorsal attentional hyperactivation may reflect attempts to compensate for dysfunction in primary frontal attentional networks [306]. Dysfunctions in the prefrontal, medial frontal, and fronto-striatal cortical areas in patients with ADHD also are of particular interest for patients with SUD+ADHD, since these anatomic brain regions, along with the dorsal ACC, are thought to be responsible for so-called "cool," or top-down, cognitive controls, namely, attentional and executive functions that we depend on to for our most rational thinking and behaviors [307, 314, 315].

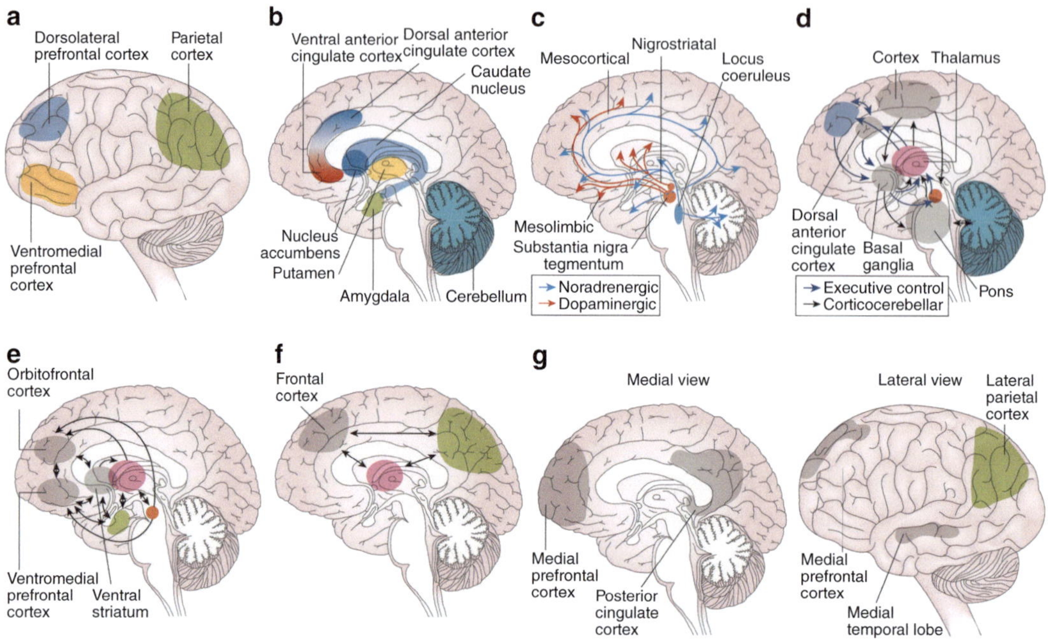

Fig. 50.2 Brain Mechanisms in Attention-Deficit/Hyperactivity Disorder. (**a**) The cortical regions (lateral view) of the brain have a role in attention-deficit/hyperactivity disorder (ADHD). The dorsolateral prefrontal cortex is linked to working memory, the ventromedial prefrontal cortex to complex decision-making and strategic planning, and the parietal cortex to orientation of attention. (**b**) ADHD involves the subcortical structures (medial view) of the brain. The ventral anterior cingulate cortex and the dorsal anterior cingulate cortex subserve affective and cognitive components of executive control. Together with the basal ganglia (comprising the nucleus accumbens, caudate nucleus, and putamen), they form the fronto-striatal circuit. Neuroimaging studies show structural and functional abnormalities in all of these structures in patients with ADHD, extending into the amygdala and cerebellum. (**c**) Neurotransmitter circuits in the brain are involved in ADHD. The dopamine system plays an important part in planning and initiation of motor responses, activation, switching, reaction to novelty, and processing of reward. The noradrenergic system influences arousal modulation, signal-to-noise ratios in cortical areas, state-dependent cognitive processes, and cognitive preparation of urgent stimuli. (**d**) Executive control networks are affected in patients with ADHD. The executive control and corticocerebellar networks coordinate executive functioning, that is, planning, goal-directed behavior, inhibition, working memory, and the flexible adaptation to context. These networks are under-activated and have lower internal functional connectivity in individuals with ADHD compared with individuals without the disorder. (**e**) ADHD involves the reward network. The ventromedial prefrontal cortex, orbitofrontal cortex, and ventral striatum are at the center of the brain network that responds to anticipation and receipt of reward. Other structures involved are the thalamus, the amygdala, and the cell bodies of dopaminergic neurons in the substantia nigra, which, as indicated by the arrows, interact in a complex manner. Behavioral and neural responses to reward are abnormal in ADHD. (**f**) The alerting network is impaired in ADHD. The frontal and parietal cortical areas and the thalamus intensively interact in the alerting network (indicated by the arrows), which supports attentional functioning and is weaker in individuals with ADHD than in controls. (**g**) ADHD involves the default mode network (DMN). The DMN consists of the medial prefrontal cortex and the posterior cingulate cortex (medial view) as well as the lateral parietal cortex and the medial temporal lobe (lateral view). DMN fluctuations are 180 degrees out of phase with fluctuations in networks that become activated during externally oriented tasks, presumably reflecting competition between opposing processes for processing resources. Negative correlations between the DMN and the frontoparietal control network are weaker in patients with ADHD than in people who do not have the disorder. (Reproduced with permission from Faraone et al. [419]).

Deficits in cortical-subcortical structural and functional connectivity have been found in the ventral attention, somatomotor and limbic networks, and in subcortical regions of patients with ADHD [307, 309, 316]. Hypoperfusion of the left putamen, globus pallidus, left amygdala, and hippocampus was correlated with both the inattentive and total diagnostic criteria of ADHD [309, 317] (Fig. 50.2b). Another brain structure of recent interest is the habenula, a modulator of dopamine that has been implicated in reward-driven and aversive behaviors, as well as in ADHD-associated behaviors. Abnormalities of structural connectivity between the prefrontal cortex and the habenula have been documented in individuals with both cocaine and heroin addiction [318]. Children with ADHD have been shown to have reduced functional connectivity between the habenula and the putamen [319]. The habenula also has a significant role in nicotine addiction [320].

Adolescents with ADHD have been found to have abnormal responses (both exaggerated and blunted responses) to reward anticipation in fronto-striatal and ventrostriatal circuits [321, 322]. Among individuals with ADHD who were considered at high risk of developing an SUD (defined as ADHD with disruptive behavior disorders, familial SUD and/or early onset of substance use), there was hyperactivation in the motivation-reward processing brain network during tasks of impulsive choice, emotion processing, and risky decision-making, while during response-inhibition tasks there was aberrant hypoactivation of the inhibitory control brain networks [323]. Interestingly, CD has been associated with abnormalities in the so-called "hot" paralimbic system that is responsible for motivation and reward processing. This paralimbic circuit is comprised the orbitofrontal and ventromedial PFCs, rostral ACC, superior temporal lobes, and the underlying limbic structures, most prominently, the amygdala [307, 312, 315] (Fig. 50.2d, e). Since ADHD with comorbid CD is a strong predictor of SUDs, it may be that the combination of an under-stimulated frontal inhibitory network, co-existing with an over-stimulated motivation-reward processing network, underlies the increased risk for developing SUDs in patients with ADHD [323–325].

It is interesting to note that stimulant treatment of ADHD appears to normalize some of the functional abnormalities in the fronto-cingulate and fronto-striatal circuits seen in neuroimaging of untreated patients with ADHD [326–328]. These network-related normalizations may explain some of the clinical improvements that are the hallmark of stimulant treatment of ADHD

Neurotransmitters

ADHD has been characterized as a deficiency of catecholamine signaling and/or production, since most of the characteristic brain areas implicated in ADHD are mediated by dopamine (DA) in subcortical structures, and by norepinephrine (NE) in the frontal cortex-ACC [329] and the prefrontal-amygdala circuit [260] (Fig. 50.2c). This deficit in catecholamine function may help to explain how stimulant (and some nonstimulant) medications can normalize some abnormal brain activation in patients with ADHD [326, 327, 330–332], and achieve their many therapeutic effects for patients with ADHD. Adolescents with untreated ADHD have been found to have higher striatal dopamine transporter density than control subjects [333], as if the ADHD brain is "hungry" for more catecholamine neurotransmission. When striatal dopamine transporters are occupied by MPH in patients with ADHD, patients demonstrate less impulsive decision-making than in the placebo condition [334]. These observations have led to the theory that some individuals with SUD+ADHD begin their drug misuse as a form of self-medication, especially the early use of nicotine, cannabis, and illicit stimulants (including methamphetamine and cocaine) [335–338]. The "self-medication theory" of substance misuse/abuse has led to clinical trials that report successful treatment of StimUDs with ADHD medications [339–345].

The stimulant medications, methylphenidate (MPH) and amphetamine (AMPH) decrease the pre-synaptic reuptake of DA and NE, increasing the availability of catecholamines at the synapse. AMPHs also increase the vesicular release of pre-synaptic DA [346]. Atomoxetine (ATX), a nonstimulant medication approved for the treatment of ADHD, is a selective NE reuptake inhibitor, and it increases pre-synaptic NE release in the frontal cortex [331]. Viloxazine, a norepinephrine-serotonin modulating agent, also acts as a norepinephrine reuptake inhibitor [347]. The alpha 2(α_2)-adrenergic agonists (i.e., guanfacine and clonidine) activate post-synaptic α_2-adrenergic receptors that are involved in improving signal-to-noise perception [348], and this different mechanism of action is complementary to the actions of catecholamines. Recent genetic studies make it clear that a variety of other neurotransmitter systems and neural processes may play important and varied roles in what is turning out to be a far more complex neurodevelopmental process than just a disorder of catecholamines, and this may permit new therapeutic targets to be identified [320, 349]. Among other neurotransmitters, glutamate [350], GABA [351], nicotinic acetylcholine receptors (nAChRs) [352], and serotonin receptors [353] are other targets for new therapies in ADHD.

The striatal DA increases caused by stimulants are of special concern in patients with SUDs, because of the potential reinforcing effects resulting from blockade of the DA transporters in the nucleus accumbens (Fig. 50.2e). However, the reinforcement effect (drug "likeability") that promotes abuse relates to the *rate* of DA increase, which is determined by the pharmacokinetics of the specific stimulant formulation (in addition to requiring a drug dose large enough to increase DA). A faster rise in DA levels causes more intense reward and reinforcement [354, 355]. Thus, an oral dose of immediate-release MPH (which may reach peak concentration in brain in ≥1 hour) is less reinforcing than the same dose administered intravenously or by insufflation (which produces high concentrations of drug and high DA transporter occupancy within minutes) [356]. In contrast, extended-release formulations of stimulants take several hours to reach peak plasma concentrations and maximum DA transporter occupancy, and have less likeability than immediate-release stimulants [357]. Although these extended-release properties do not eliminate the risks of abuse for prescription stimulants, they diminish them substantially. The prodrugs lisdexamfetamine (LDX) and serdexmethylphenidate (serdexMPH) also decrease the possibility of abuse [358–360] by limiting the rate of prodrug that can be metabolized to active drug. Thus, the ADHD medications that should be used preferentially in adults with SUD+ADHD should be extended-release stimulants, extended-release stimulant-prodrug formulations and nonstimulants.

Environmental Exposures and Psychosocial Influences

A variety of environmental neurotoxins and lived experiences of adversity are associated with a higher risk for, and more severe and persistent, ADHD. In those with high genetic risk for ADHD, environmental exposures magnify risk and the behavioral manifestations of the ADHD phenotype.

Toxic Exposures to Substances of Abuse

Animal studies have shown that prenatal nicotine exposure of both male and female mice can cause powerful, epigenetic changes that affect the expression of important regulatory genes in frontal, striatal, and hippocampal regions of the offspring brain [361]. Maternal exposure to nicotine in mice decreases GABA-producing neurons in the PFC [362], and can cause behavioral impairment in multiple generations of offspring [361, 363, 364]. In humans, maternal and paternal smoking during pregnancy has been associated with an increased risk of ADHD in children [365, 366]. Continuous maternal smoking during pregnancy has been associated with extensive decreases in offspring brain volume, gray and white matter volumes, brain surface area, and gyrification [367]. Even exposure to second-hand smoke during the prenatal and early postnatal period seems to confer risk for offspring ADHD [368–370]. Chronic exposure to nicotine decreases sensitivity to DA and nAChR in the brain, and can activate the endogenous opioid system. Prenatal and early childhood nicotine exposure can alter brain circuits involved in learning, stress, and self-control, which may influence later vulnerability to addiction and dependence [370]. Concurrent maternal use of nicotine and opioids, as well as other substances of abuse, may increase the risk for ADHD in offspring even further [371]. DNA methylation may be one explanation of the association between prenatal substance exposures and offspring neurodevelopmental abnormalities [372, 373].

Alcohol is a well-known teratogen that is known to have adverse effects on fetal development, and many studies find associations between prenatal maternal alcohol consumption and ADHD; however, findings have been inconsistent [374, 375]. The most consistent finding for prenatal alcohol exposure is that it adversely affects emotion regulation [376].

Prenatal cannabis exposure has been associated with higher risks for a variety of poor neurodevelopmental outcomes and psychopathology in children, including poor attention [377] and more sleep problems [378]. Prenatal cocaine and heroin exposures are also known to have associations with deficient attention and poor behavioral self-regulation [379, 380].

Other Environmental Toxins

Prenatal and/or early postnatal exposure to a variety of neurotoxic environmental chemicals and elements have been associated with greater risk of ADHD. These include polychlorinated biphenyls (PCBs) [381, 382], fire-retardant chemicals, known as polybrominated diphenyl esters (PBDEs) and polybrominated biphenyls (PBBs) [383, 384], pesticides [385, 386], and heavy metal exposure, including lead [387, 388], copper, cobalt, and tin [389].

Psychosocial Risk Factors Early exposure to adversity is well-documented as a risk factor for ADHD, and for more severe and persistent ADHD. This includes exposure to a variety of adverse childhood experiences (ACEs) [241] and social determinants of poor health [390, 391], including food insecurity [392, 393], institutionalization [394, 395], child maltreatment [396, 397], other traumatic exposures [398, 399], parental history of mental disorders, and lower parental education and income [390, 400, 401]. Poor family functioning, from the prenatal period onward, has been associated with smaller brain volumes and more problem behaviors in children, by adolescence [115, 402, 403]. These risk factors are dose-dependent, cumulative, and bidirectional. That is, psychosocial adversities are all more common in those with ADHD and they also are associated with higher risks of ADHD in children. In a highly genetic disorder like ADHD, this makes it challenging to distinguish genetic propensity from environmental exposures.

Many of the same environmental exposures discussed above also have associations with elevated risks for SUDs [404–407]. It should be noted, however, that environmental exposures rarely occur in isolation. Those who use one substance of abuse may also be polysubstance users, confounding any association of a single substance with ADHD or SUDs. Those with one psychosocial risk factor are more prone to other harmful exposures or psychosocial risk factors. Untreated ADHD *alone* is a risk factor for nonmedical stimulant use (NMU) and for SUDs [25, 408]. Overriding all, genetic predisposition to ADHD is associated with a host of unfavorable outcomes [409] including those discussed earlier in this section. Few studies have successfully distinguished a single environmental exposure of interest from the potential confounding contributions of other drugs, toxins, or adverse psychosocial exposures, and most studies fail to consider the context of the underlying ADHD and SUD genetic risks. Since environmental exposures may affect biological processes, such as DNA methylation and the modification of gene expression, the literature on environmental risks in ADHD must be considered in context. It can be extremely difficult to separate a single variable of interest from multiple potentially confounding variables, and to distinguish genetic from environmental etiologies. However, it is important to remember that environmental toxins and lived experiences can further dysregulate a genetically vulnerable individual, contributing to the complexity of ADHD [373, 410, 411].

Behaviorally, both ADHD and SUDs have been associated with high levels of impulsivity (sometimes with compulsivity), including impulsive aggression and emotional dysregulation. Disinhibition, sensation seeking, and impulsive decision-making are seen in both ADHD and SUD patients [412]. Poor judgment, delay aversion, weak executive function, and poor self-regulation (especially in unstructured situations) are common clinical features of both disorders. Delay discounting is the tendency to prefer smaller, but immediate, rewards over larger, but delayed, rewards; or to place lower value on deferred rewards. This also appears to be a prominent finding in both ADHD and SUD [98, 243, 413]. Importantly, abnormal stress reactivity has been identified in both ADHD and SUD clinical populations. Both stress over-reactivity (leading to substance use for coping with stressors) and stress under-reactivity (leading to novelty-seeking) appear to contribute to substance use as a final, common pathway [414–416]. When some or all of these behaviors are present, they tend to increase the complexity and chronicity of the course of SUDs and SUD treatment for patients with SUD+ADHD [243, 417, 418].

In summary, the neurobiology of ADHD helps us to understand how those with ADHD enter adolescence and adulthood with impaired attention, impulsivity, and possibly ongoing internal restlessness and fidgetiness, and also with deficient "top-down" behavioral and emotional regulation and inhibition. Because of their genetic attributes and functional neuroanatomy, these individuals make impulsive decisions which often carry high risks. They are less successful educationally and professionally, and have emotional dysregulation, which may lead to poorer interpersonal relationships and fewer social supports, and they are twice as likely to be addicted to nicotine as those without ADHD. They have up to an 80% chance of having at least one comorbid psychiatric disorder, and multiple comorbidities are common. Those with comorbid CD also may have particular over-reactivity in the realms of emotion and reward processing. These behaviors all are associated with atypically delayed development of gray matter, and less efficient white matter tracts. ADHD involves dysfunction in fronto-striato-limbic, fronto-cingulate, fronto-parietal, and fronto-striato-cerebellar circuits. These circuits mediate executive functions and reward processing. ADHD patients have abnormal difficulty "turning off" the default mode network, which prevents them from "turning on" more effective neural circuits appropriate for task performance, when these are needed (Fig. 50.2a, f, g). It is not difficult to see how individuals with this constellation of problems might find themselves using one or more addictive substances to experiment or to self-medicate to alleviate symptoms, and then being more susceptible to problematic substance use, and eventually, struggling with one or more SUDs. The neurobiology of ADHD also helps to explain why patients with comorbid SUD+ADHD have a more complex and difficult course in treatment.

Nonmedical Stimulant Use/Misuse/Abuse

There has been great concern about prescribing stimulant medications, especially for adolescents and young adults with ADHD, because of the risk of nonmedical use (NMU) of stimulants. NMU is typically defined as a) "the use of prescription stimulants, whether obtained by prescription or otherwise, other than in the manner, for the reasons, or for the time period prescribed, or by a person for whom the drug was not prescribed [420]." Stimulant NMU is real, and it requires prescriber awareness, vigilance, and diversion-resistant practice management.

Most of the studies on stimulant diversion and misuse focus on high school and college students, and prescription drug misuse (with any medication class) is more prevalent among young adults than any other age group in the United States [421, 422]. Most adolescents and young adults with ADHD take their stimulant medication as prescribed, and those who do demonstrate later adult outcomes that generally do not differ from population controls in educational attainment or risk for SUDs [25, 423]. However, a substantial minority of 18- to 25-year-olds report NMU of stimulant medications, including those who have a legitimate stimulant prescription for previously diagnosed ADHD [424]. A recent review of studies found that ~50–90% of individuals reporting stimulant NMU obtained stimulants from friends, family, or peers. Up to one-third of these individuals report some misuse of their own prescribed stimulant medication (e.g., taking an extra dose of medication, giving/selling medication to others). Those who engage in NMU report higher levels of ADHD symptoms than those who do not report NMU [425] and have higher risks of binge drinking, nicotine marijuana, and nonmedical opioid use [426]. Yet, even among those who report having ever engaged in stimulant NMU, over 50% appear to be at low risk for serious polysubstance abuse [427]. Despite common perceptions among healthcare professionals, "doctor shopping" for stimulant prescriptions is uncommon [428], and government prescribing registries make such behavior easy to discover.

Misuse of stimulants is predominantly oral, but especially in those with polysubstance use, snorting (intranasal), smoking, and even injection have been reported [425]. Intranasal use of stimulants is associated with more frequent stimulant NMU, more co-use with alcohol, marijuana or cocaine, and more co-occurring SUD [429]. Stimulant misuse during adolescence in those *never* under stimulant treatment for ADHD also is associated with significantly higher odds of cocaine or methamphetamine use by young adulthood [25], suggesting that adolescents engaging in stimulant NMU (especially those using other potentially addictive substances, like nicotine, marijuana, alcohol, and/or illicit drugs) warrant careful assessment for their degree of substance use, education, intervention, and careful follow-up.

Because of extensive publicity and concern, many clinicians are surprised to learn that prescription stimulant NMU is no more common than the NMU of prescription tranquilizers/sedatives or benzodiazepines, and is far less common than NMU of prescription pain relievers [430]. Although most of the research in this area has been based on U.S. samples, concerns about prescription drug abuse, especially opioid abuse, have now been reported in Canada [431] and across the European Union [432].

Motivations for NMU

The overwhelming motivations reported for stimulant NMU among college students are academic in nature, and are cited as the primary reason for NMU in ~50–90% of subjects in over 2 dozen studies [425]. A large U.S. survey found that college students and college graduates cite the motivation of academic/cognitive enhancement *only* at particularly high rates (college = 78.2%; non-college = 63.5%) [433]. Among adults, the primary motivations (in ~40–80%) for NMU are comparable: the desire to be more productive, to enhance work/academic performance, or to help alertness/concentration [434–436]. Interestingly, individuals who self-report stimulant NMU also self-report higher ADHD symptom severity than those not reporting stimulant NMU. One study of college student NMU found that nonmedical stimulant users were 7 times more likely to screen positive for ADHD than non-misusers [335], and some U. S college students *without* ADHD who reported stimulant NMU believed that they were self-medicating their undiagnosed ADHD. Thus, some NMU may stem from undertreated or undiagnosed ADHD [425, 437–439] and highlights the need to screen nonmedical stimulant users for ADHD [429].

Contrary to most students' beliefs, stimulant NMU is *inversely* correlated with grade-point average (GPA). The data suggest that academic struggles and poor grades lead to stimulant NMU, as students become more desperate to improve their academic performance [440]. One longitudinal study used growth curve modeling to demonstrate that alcohol and cannabis use disorders during college may lead to students skipping class, resulting in declining academic performance, and that NMU is associated with this constellation of features [441]. Abuse-related motivations (e.g., to get high; being "hooked"; to modify other drug effects; to experiment), although far less common than attempts to improve academic performance and/or productivity, were cited by 15.5% of the entire population sample in one study, and by 23.6% among those with StimUDs [434]. Among college students, getting "high"; curiosity/experimentation; feeling more comfortable in social situations; enhancing the effects of alcohol; and staying awake while partying were the most common non-academic motivations for NMU [425], but these were far less common than academic/cognitive motivations.

More dangerous misuse does occur, especially among substance-abusing adults, and is an important concern for prescribers. However, *the majority of college student NMU appears to be related to infrequent, episodic attempts at academic performance enhancement* (e.g., taking a peer's Adderall in a therapeutic dosage range to stay up late writing a paper) or brief experimentation [422, 425, 429]. Supporting this thesis, one study found that most college students who engage in oral stimulant NMU do so while they are alone or with just one or two others, rather than while at a party [429]. In these situations, when not mixed with other medications or recreational substances, the greatest medical dangers are for those with undiagnosed vulnerability to cardiac arrhythmias or severe psychiatric illness; in such a situation, stimulant NMU could lead to severe consequences, including hospitalization or death. It should be noted that immediate-release stimulants are generally preferred for oral NMU and by those without SUD, while those with both stimulant NMU and a SUD are more than twice as likely to use stimulants intranasally and to use while at a party [429]. Faraone and colleagues [442] reported that intranasal AMPH users were at greater risk of serious side-effects, hospitalization, and death than those who misused AMPH orally.

Prevalence of NMU

Lifetime estimates of NMU in U.S. high school seniors and college students were 9.5% and 17%, respectively [424, 443]. Less information has been published about adults with stimulant NMU. One U.S. population study (N=102,000) from 2015 to 2016 asked adults about stimulant misuse, using a broad definition ("use in any way that a doctor did not direct you to use them," which included taking stimulants more often, in greater amounts, or for longer than directed). This study estimated that among adults ≥18 years of age, approximately 6.6% of the surveyed adults used prescription stimulants in the past year (with/without NMU), and *more than two-thirds (4.5%) took stimulants without misuse.* However, about one-third of all adult prescription stimulant users had engaged in stimulant NMU at least once in the past year but did not have StimUD; only 3% of adult stimulant users had StimUDs. Among those with any misuse in the past year, approximately 15% had misused stimulants on ≥3 days in the past month. High-frequency misuse was associated with being male, having less education, having other SUDs (past-year cocaine/heroin use disorders; past-year inhalant/prescription sedative/tranquilizer/opioid misuse or use disorder), past-year major depressive episode, being divorced/separated, and having chronic obstructive pulmonary disease (COPD) [434]. The limited data on stimulant NMU in adults over age 50 years suggest that it is much less common than in young adults of high school and college age, and prevalence rates are quite low, overall [434, 444].

Stimulant NMU is associated with high rates of other substance use and SUDs. An analysis of U.S. adults (≥18 years) who reported using ADHD stimulants nonmedically in the past year (N = 6103) in U.S. surveys from 2006 to 2011 found that concurrent problematic use was reported frequently for alcohol (64.2%); marijuana (43.6%); cocaine (10.6%); tranquilizers/sedatives (8.8%); hallucinogens (8.4%); heroin (2.5%); inhalants (2.3%); and pain relievers (2.1%), often in combination [427]. Others also have found that college students who meet diagnostic criteria for SUD are more likely to a) engage in stimulant NMU, b) to use stimulants with alcohol, marijuana, and/or cocaine, c) to endorse motives of "getting high" or increasing the effects of other drugs, d) to report intranasal use of stimulants, and e) to report more frequent lifetime use [429]. With the increased legalization of marijuana and rise in opioid abuse, problematic concurrent use of multiple substances is likely to increase in those with, or at-risk for, SUDs.

U.S. data suggest that AMPH NMU, in particular, has increased over the past 25 years, especially among adolescents and young adults [425], commensurate with the dramatic increase in

AMPH prescriptions for adults with ADHD [445, 446]. Yet, overall prevalence of all stimulant NMU is still quite low, in the context of the use of alcohol, nicotine products, and marijuana [422]. Importantly, a large U.S. study of prescription stimulant NMU among individuals being assessed for treatment of SUD (a group at potentially very high risk for stimulant NMU) found that the prevalence rate for past 30-day stimulant NMU was only 1.3%, far lower than comparable rates for prescription opioids (19.8%) or sedatives (10.6%) [447].

ADHD in Patients with Substance Use Disorders

Childhood ADHD substantially elevates the risk of developing a SUD [448, 449]. When compared to a group without ADHD, individuals with ADHD that persisted to age 18 years had almost a fourfold probability of cannabis dependence and almost twice the likelihood of illicit drug use [450].

Furthermore, among adolescents and adults with SUD, comorbid ADHD predicted 1) an earlier onset of substance use [451]; 2) more rapid progression to substance dependence [452, 453]; 3) polysubstance abuse [454]; and 4) more psychiatric comorbidity, including conduct disorder (CD) and antisocial personality disorder (ASPD) [455–457]. Most importantly for clinicians treating patients with SUDs, those with SUD+ADHD tend to have a more severe and persistent course of SUD [458, 459], with more treatment failures [460] and higher relapse rates after successful treatment [461]. It is in this context that *diagnosis and treatment of comorbid ADHD becomes important as a means of improving treatment outcomes for patients with SUD.*

The varied presentations of adult ADHD, described in Part 1 of this chapter, challenge every clinician's diagnostic skills. However, the high prevalence of ADHD in patients with SUDs makes it clear that one must have a high index of suspicion for ADHD, and screen for it routinely among patients with SUDs. *ADHD is best diagnosed with a careful, longitudinal history.* Therefore, a thorough understanding of commonly reported impairments from ADHD and knowledge of the many ADHD-associated historical features and comorbidities described above can improve the clinician's traditional history-taking among patients seeking treatment for their SUDs. Recognition of these common historical elements and impairments may help to generate a clinical diagnosis of comorbid ADHD in those with chronic problems at work, with family and friends, with other psychiatric disorders, repeated accidents/injuries, and with patterns of substance use. Recognition of ADHD as an antecedent and predictor of poor outcomes may be a crucial step in identifying effective treatments for patients with SUDs. Diagnosis and treatment of ADHD in patients with SUD+ADHD, in the context of a comprehensive SUD treatment program, could help to mitigate years of severe impairment and diminished quality of life.

Prevalence of Substance Use Disorders *Plus* ADHD

ADHD is markedly over-represented in individuals seeking treatment for SUDs, but early estimates of the prevalence of ADHD in SUD patients varied widely, both by country and by assessment method. Even among treatment-seeking patients with SUDs, the use of DSM-5 criteria for ADHD, compared with DSM-IV criteria, does not substantially increase estimates of the prevalence of SUD+ADHD [462].

Over the past 15 years, a worldwide research network, the *International Collaboration on ADHD and Substance Abuse (ICASA)*, has been created to a) investigate the link between ADHD and SUD, b) reduce the proportion of ADHD patients who develop SUD, and c) to improve the detection, diagnosis, and treatment of patients with SUD+ADHD [463]. A comprehensive meta-analysis performed by the ICASA group found that *the prevalence of ADHD in patients with SUDs was 23.1%* [464]. This was followed by a prospective, multi-site assessment of patients referred to inpatient or outpatient treatment programs for those with SUDs in 7 European countries [462]. Patients ages 18–65 years were screened with the Adult ADHD Self-Report Scale (ASRS V 1.1). This is a brief screening questionnaire validated for use in adolescents and adults with ADHD [465, 466], including those with SUD+ADHD [467]. In this large sample (N=3,558) of treatment-seeking adults with SUDs, on average, 40% of subjects screened positive for ADHD. The screening phase was followed by a full diagnostic assessment for ADHD. This study found geographic differences in both comorbid ADHD prevalence (range = 6–33%, average = 14%), with higher prevalence of ADHD in patients from Nordic countries, and lower prevalence among those with alcohol abuse than with other drug abuse [462].

Similar to the ICASA meta-analysis, another recent meta-analysis of treatment-seeking patients with SUDs estimated the prevalence of ADHD to be 21% [468]. A study of general psychiatric outpatients found even higher rates of comorbid ADHD: 24.4% and 30.8% among patients with substance dependence and abuse, respectively, and 12.8% and 27.1% among patients with alcohol dependence and abuse, respectively [38] (see Fig. 50.1).

Underdiagnosis and lack of treatment of ADHD in patients with SUDs is a serious problem. A recent examination of >63 million patients with SUDs who were seen in American hospital emergency departments found that comorbid ADHD was diagnosed in fewer than 1%, not the ~15–25% that would be expected [469]. An international study of treatment-seeking adults with SUD+ADHD found that *only 12% had their ADHD diagnosed and treated as children* [470]. Therefore, the opportunity to diagnose this treatable condition, often for the first time, may present itself when patients seek treatment for their SUDs. From this collection of studies, there is a clear implication for the clinician working with patients who have SUDs: *Instead of expecting to diagnose ADHD in perhaps one in every 25–30 adults in the general population, the clinician can expect to see comorbid ADHD in one in every 4–7 patients seeking treatment for SUDs.*

Clinical Features of Comorbid SUD+ADHD

The SUD+ADHD comorbidity is bi-directional. That is, whichever problem is diagnosed initially, the other diagnosis is likely to be seen more commonly than one would expect from population prevalence estimates. However, symptoms and impairment from ADHD (even if never diagnosed) almost *always* precede substance misuse [36, 470].

Additional psychiatric comorbidities are common in patients with SUD+ADHD. The presence of comorbid ADHD among patients with SUDs also increases the odds of *additional* psychiatric comorbidities. A large, international study of treatment-seeking patients with SUDs demonstrated the added burden of additional comorbidities conferred by the SUD+ADHD comorbidity. Among treatment-seeking patients, SUD+ADHD patients were 4 times more likely also to have a current diagnosis of depression, and 7 times more likely to have a current diagnosis of BorPD, compared with patients who presented with SUD without ADHD [471]. Patients with SUD+ADHD also were four times as likely to have current hypomania and almost three times as likely to have ASPD, compared with those who had SUD without ADHD. Fully 75% of those with SUD+ADHD had at least one additional psychiatric comorbidity (vs. 37% in patients without ADHD), and over 11% had ≥3 psychiatric comorbidities, in addition to their SUD+ADHD [471]. Thus, patients with SUD+ADHD are diagnostically complex and often very ill. They require comprehensive and meticulous psychiatric assessment when they seek treatment. Similarly, their treatment regimens also might need to be more complex than is customary.

Longitudinal, family, twin, and genetic studies all have demonstrated that childhood ADHD increases the risk of all forms of SUD in adults. Subjects with ADHD have an earlier onset of nicotine use, marijuana use, and other substance use [2]. In patients with alcohol use disorder (AUD), the presence of ADHD symptoms, particularly inattentive symptoms and impulsivity, predicted more severe alcohol-related problems [472]. ADHD+AUD also predicted other SUDs, with an earlier age of onset, compared with controls, and any substance use was more likely to progress to dependence [473]. Patients who screen positive for ADHD are twice as likely to report a history of heavy alcohol use, as well as longer histories of AMPH, benzodiazepine, and opioid SUDs [417]. Individuals diagnosed with ADHD prior to age 15 years had over three times the risk of future SUDs [474].

The behavioral cluster of high levels of impulsivity, emotional dysregulation, executive function deficits, and delay discounting is frequently seen, not only in children and adolescents with ADHD, but also among adults with persistent symptoms of ADHD [281, 475–477], sometimes with the additional trait of high novelty-seeking [478]. Often, but not always, accompanied by CD and/or ASPD, this cluster of clinical findings is often described as behavioral disinhibition (BD). BD, along with persistent ADHD, is predictive of SUDs in adults [479] and is seen more in patients with SUDs [418].

Impact of Treatment of Adult ADHD

Longitudinal studies have demonstrated that early and long-term stimulant medication treatment of childhood ADHD, preferably starting by age 9 years, exerts important *protective* effects from many of the negative outcomes of ADHD, including SUDs [17–19, 22, 480–482]. Childhood stimulant treatment substantially ameliorates ADHD and its functional consequences [18]. However, adult ADHD outcomes are not normalized fully [483]. A longitudinal study found that at age 35 years, adolescents with ADHD who took stimulants only as prescribed (without NMU) before age 18 years had achieved educational attainment and had risks of SUD that were comparable to population controls, which is a far better outcome than that seen in most individuals with untreated ADHD [423]. The risks and poor outcomes associated with unrecognized and untreated (or undertreated) ADHD make it a significant public health concern. For ADHD that persists into adulthood, ongoing ADHD pharmacotherapy plus appropriate nonmedical therapies continue to be helpful. Even some anatomic improvements have been observed in adult patients after 3 years of psychostimulant treatment [484].

Several pharmacoepidemiologic studies, including those using within-individual designs, have demonstrated that pharmacotherapy of adult ADHD reduces the "real world" risk of some of the most serious consequences of ADHD, including substantial decreases in motor vehicle accidents [122], criminal behavior [485, 486], depression [487], suicidality [123], early and unplanned pregnancies [153], and substance use [481, 488]. This literature was reviewed recently in detail by Chang et. al. [124]. Stimulants also have been shown to reduce delay discounting and improve activation of brain regions associated with reward processing, under experimental conditions [489, 490]. Such improvements might enable some patients with ADHD to persist toward longer-term goals and make better choices, despite short-term temptations, which could be immensely helpful in the context of treatment for SUDs. Pharmacotherapy for ADHD can improve emotional dysregulation in patients with ADHD [491–493], and can improve executive function [494–497]. These are two additional domains where functional improvements might enhance outcomes in those seeking treatment for their SUD(s).

The long-term impact of stimulant medications for ADHD (beyond 1–2 years) remains controversial [498], but extensive clinical experience, patient reports, and limited scientific literature would suggest that ADHD pharmacotherapy continues to be associated with positive outcomes *throughout* adulthood. However, positive outcomes require ongoing medication adherence, careful dose optimization, regular prescriber monitoring and follow-up, addressing significant medication side-effects, attention to treatment of comorbidities, and appropriate nonmedical treatment of psychological and executive dysfunctions. In light of the extensive publicity in the popular press concerning over-prescribing and addictive potential of stimulants, it is perhaps ironic that one of the greatest problems in ADHD management is poor adherence to pharmacotherapy, despite the fact that ongoing adherence is crucial for optimal outcomes [499–502].

Experienced clinicians have found that *ADHD symptoms need to be reduced by ≥40% to see clinically meaningful improvement* [503]. An improvement of >65% in a functional assessment score has been used as an approximation of "remission" [504]. Thus, *persistent titration of ADHD medication to the optimal tolerated dosage* is of utmost importance for the best functional outcomes [504–506] (see Fig. 50.4). One stimulant medication study in children and adolescents assessed the relationships between a) a quantitative measure of symptom improvement from baseline ratings, b) the change in Clinical Global Improvement (CGI-I), and c) the change in parent rating of the child's functional impairment. On the CGI-I, ratings of much improved and very much improved were associated with approximately 55% and 80% percent improvements in ADHD symptoms and approximately 40% and 70% improvements in functional impairment, respectively [507]. Comparable studies in adult ADHD have not yet been performed, but similar results would be expected, and these data can serve as a useful guide, when gauging each patient's progress.

Although not studied as extensively, combining pharmacotherapy with ADHD-specific CBT appears to improve outcomes for virtually *all* patients with ADHD [508, 509]. Especially in combination with CBT, current ADHD pharmacotherapies have large, beneficial effects on ADHD symptoms. ADHD pharmacotherapy (especially with CBT) appears to be moderately helpful for executive function deficits, and may also help emotional dysregulation [77]. Several CBT programs have been adapted for patients with ADHD by some of the foremost psychologists in the field of ADHD [510–512]. They typically focus on helping patients understand ADHD-related impairments, change maladaptive cognitions, and develop adaptive/coping skills. Most have lessons/modules on a) organizational skills, b) time management, c) interpersonal relationships, d) managing frustration and anger, e) reflective problem-solving, f) moderating impulsivity, and g) sleep hygiene, all of which have been found to help adult patients with ADHD. Thus, multimodal treatment of ADHD is preferred.

Impact of ADHD Pharmacotherapy in Adult SUD+ADHD

This is still a relatively new area of research, and it remains controversial. However, the available research suggests that pharmacotherapy for ADHD: a) improves ADHD symptoms, b) decreases impulsivity, c) may offer modest improvement in emotional dysregulation, and d) may increase the duration of engagement in SUD treatment, with associated decreases in substance use. Most studies suggest that ADHD pharmacotherapy does not treat SUD directly, although there may be direct treatment benefits for those with StimUDs [344]. Prescription stimulant treatment may offer effective and safe agonist substitution for those with StimUDs [338], and such treatment, in robust doses, improves abstinence and decreases drug-related hospitalizations and deaths. As illicit stimulants are increasingly adulterated with synthetic opioids, making them much more likely to cause overdose deaths [513], prescription stimulant treatment actually may save patients' lives.

As discussed in detail below, treatment of ADHD in those seeking treatment for SUDs *does* appear to decrease ADHD symptoms and ADHD-related impairment, which may improve overall functioning in those with SUD+ADHD. Furthermore, ADHD pharmacotherapy appears to offer indirect benefits that make SUD treatment more successful, including better retention in SUD treatment, which is a widely used measure of SUD treatment program success [514]. Some studies have found that ADHD medications also may decrease cravings [515–517].

In patients with OUD and ADHD, treatment of ADHD is associated with better retention in OUD treatment and reductions in illicit substance use [518], and ADHD treatment has been noted to improve retention in buprenorphine treatment for patients with OUD and co-occurring StimUDs [519]. In patients with StimUDs, prescription stimulant treatment, especially lisdexamfetamine (LDX) has been: a) associated with lower all-cause mortality and fewer SUD-related hospitalizations [520], and has been shown to b) promote sustained abstinence, c) decrease illicit stimulant

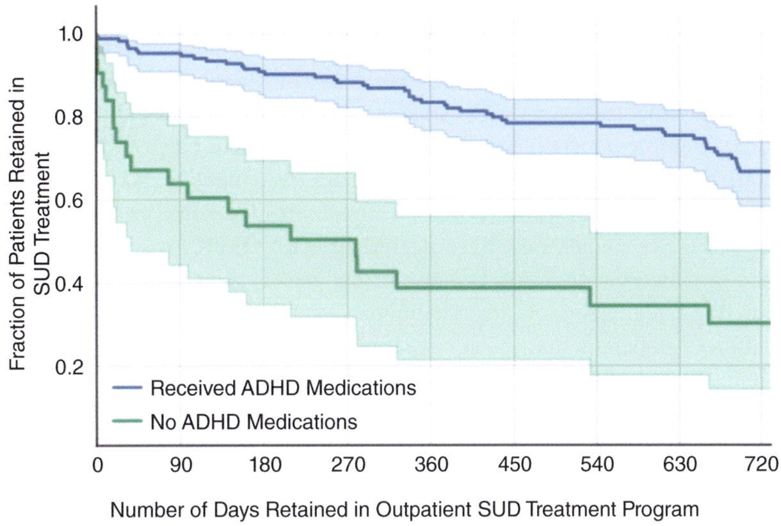

Fig. 50.3 Kaplan-Meier retention curves for ADHD pharmacotherapy versus no ADHD medication. (From Kast et al. [522]. Copyright 2021, Physicians Postgraduate Press. Reprinted by permission)

use, and d) extend the duration of abstinence [344, 521]. A retrospective study of SUD+ADHD patients in an outpatient SUD treatment program demonstrated a robust association between ADHD pharmacotherapy and better short- and longer-term SUD treatment retention [522] (see Fig. 50.3).

In patients with SUD+ADHD, stimulant medications for treating ADHD, that is, methylphenidates (MPHs) and amphetamines (AMPHs), are the most studied, and have had the most success, especially for treatment of StimUDs [339, 340, 343–345, 515, 519, 523–525]. ATX also has shown promising results for improving treatment of SUD+ADHD [343, 526–529]. Newer drugs for ADHD have not yet been studied in patients with SUD+ADHD. They show promise in adults with ADHD [358, 530, 531] or have been shown to be safe in healthy adults [532, 533], but effectiveness has not yet been demonstrated in adults with comorbid SUD+ADHD. Several of these newer drugs are extended-release stimulant prodrugs or nonstimulants with low abuse potential [360, 530, 534]. Pharmacotherapy for ADHD also has been shown to have small-to-medium positive effects on emotional dysregulation [77, 492, 493, 535, 536], which may be helpful for patients with SUD+ADHD. Patients with SUD+ADHD who were treated with robust doses of MPH were even more adherent to their MPH treatment than patients with ADHD only, after 3 years of follow-up [537]. Doses stabilized and no evidence of tolerance was seen, over time. In non-abstinent adolescents and adults with SUD+ADHD, euphoric effects and misuse/diversion of extended-release prescription MPH were not affected by substance use severity [538].

A growing body of literature indicates that one unique aspect of treating ADHD in patients with SUD+ADHD is the beneficial effect of higher-than-typical stimulant doses. A large follow-up study of individuals with ADHD and SUD+ADHD found that, 2 years after initiating MPH treatment, *SUD+ADHD patients required 40% higher MPH doses* than those with ADHD only, that they demonstrated high long-term adherence to MPH treatment, and that they did not develop signs of tolerance to MPH or need ongoing dosage increases [537]. In fact, *higher* MPH dosage showed a linear trend toward better adherence to longer-term ADHD pharmacotherapy, in patients with SUD+ADHD [539]. A small, Swedish study of subjects with SUD+ADHD found that 40% were prescribed daily doses of MPH >180 mg/day [540]. Another small study of cocaine users found that treatment of ADHD with extended-release MPH (up to 90 mg/day) or ATX (1.2 mg./kg./day) improved ADHD symptoms and decreased cocaine use over a mean 7-month follow-up period [343].

The more recent stimulant treatment studies contrast with earlier studies treating ADHD in patients with SUD+ADHD with lower doses of stimulant medication. Older studies showed either no improvement or small improvements in ADHD symptoms, with no apparent impact on SUD outcomes. The lower doses of stimulants used in those studies may have decreased efficacy in patients with SUDs because of the general down-regulation of the dopamine system and lower dopamine transporter availability and occupancy in patients whose use includes cocaine or stimulants as chronic drugs of abuse [334, 541].

Extended-release mixed amphetamine salts (MAS-XR) up to 80 mg/day and extended-release dextroamphetamine up to 110 mg/day have been studied for patients with ADHD and cocaine use disorder (CUD), with improvements in ADHD symptoms, more continuous abstinence from cocaine, decreased marijuana use, and better treatment retention [340, 341, 542]. In a small (N=16), open-label pilot study of LDX, patients with ADHD and CUD were titrated to a maximum of 140 mg/day over 2 weeks, maintained the maximal tolerated dose for 4 weeks, then were tapered and discontinued from LDX. The mean dose of LDX achieved was 118 mg ±40 mg. No participants discontinued medication because of adverse effects, and LDX was safe and generally well-tolerated. During the last 3 weeks of their study participation, 37.5% of the participants were abstinent from cocaine; mean dollars/day spent on cocaine decreased dramatically; and the mean percent of days using was halved from baseline [345]. Another recent, small study of subjects with CUD found that extended-release AMPH reduced subjects' choosing cocaine, under experimental conditions [543]. Importantly, in patients with StimUDs (AMPH or methamphetamine), a recent large, Swedish register study found that the *only* prescribed medications associated with a reduction in all-cause mortality were LDX and MPH. LDX was the only prescription medication that also was associated with a reduction in the risk for SUD-related hospitalizations [520].

For those incarcerated in the criminal justice system, ADHD pharmacotherapy can make the system and its processes fairer and less traumatic. A recent expert consensus report identified current barriers to appropriate recognition and treatment of ADHD in offenders and incarcerated persons, and offers a variety of helpful suggestions for screening, diagnosis, multimodal treatment interventions and liaison between multiple relevant agencies for more smoothly coordinated and expert care [544]. The functional improvements that can result from ADHD treatment may decrease impulsivity and improve emotional dysregulation. Ultimately, these changes would be expected to reduce unwanted behaviors in incarcerated individuals. ADHD treatment could even reduce the duration of an individual's incarceration, because of improved behavior. Continued treatment after release may also contribute positively to community reintegration and employability [545]. A Swedish study treated incarcerated individuals with AMPH dependence + ADHD with OROS-MPH (up to 180 mg/day), starting 2 weeks before their release from prison, and followed them twice weekly, on an outpatient basis. Treatment also included weekly cognitive-behavioral therapy (CBT). The group treated with OROS-MPH had fewer ADHD symptoms, more AMPH-negative urine tests and better retention in SUD treatment, which decreased the risk of relapse to substance use over the 24-week trial [523].

OROS-MPH was the first extended-release product to come to market in the United States in 2000, offering the potential of all-day stimulant coverage from a single morning dose. The National Institute for Health and Clinical Excellence (NICE) guidelines recommend pharmacotherapy as first-line treatment for adult ADHD [546] and identify MPH as the first choice for the treatment of adults. However, a 2018 review and meta-analysis found that AMPH formulations (e.g., LDX) appeared to be the most efficacious ADHD pharmacotherapies for adults, and were as well-tolerated as MPH [547], making them the first choice for adult ADHD pharmacotherapy in the newest European Consensus Statement on the diagnosis and treatment of adult

ADHD [37]. Some ADHD patients respond preferentially to, and/or experience fewer side-effects with, either MPH or AMPH treatments, but it is hard to predict which stimulant will be preferable for an individual patient [548]. Therefore, if a clinical trial of one stimulant (MPH or AMPH) does not produce the optimal response, or if it causes excessive side-effects, it is customary practice to switch to the other stimulant class, for a second clinical trial of stimulants [549].

Screening, Diagnosis, and Treatment of ADHD in Patients with SUDs

Basic Principles of SUD+ADHD Comorbidity in the Context of the Treatment of SUDs

1. ADHD is associated with higher risks for the development of substance use disorders. In patients with ADHD, nicotine and/or other substance use often begin at a very early age and is associated with a shorter interval from the onset of use to severe SUD [208, 452, 550–552]. The prevalence of ADHD among adults with SUD is exceptionally high (up to 1 in 4 patients), compared with ADHD prevalence in the general adult population of about 1 in 25–30 patients [172, 464, 553].
2. Patients with comorbid SUD+ADHD have more chronic patterns of substance use, with more complexity, more psychiatric comorbidity, more polysubstance use, and a markedly reduced quality of life [3, 417, 454, 459, 471, 554]. The patient may be receiving the diagnosis of ADHD for the first time, and many have not previously considered ADHD as a possible explanation for some of their difficulties [552, 555]. Psychoeducation and reinterpretation of prior life events can help patients appreciate the impact of their ADHD, understand ADHD pharmacotherapy, and value treatment adherence.
3. The presence of untreated ADHD has a significant, negative impact on the course of SUD and its treatment [556]. Early diagnosis of comorbid ADHD in patients seeking treatment for SUD is crucially important, since untreated ADHD is associated with poor SUD treatment retention, while treatment of ADHD is associated with improvement in ADHD symptoms, less nicotine withdrawal, and better SUD treatment retention [204, 339, 342, 522, 557–559], ultimately leading to more treatment success. ADHD medications *do not* appear to cause more adverse events in the SUD+ADHD population, compared with adults treated for ADHD alone, and ADHD treatment *does not* worsen SUD [560–563].
4. Recent studies using robust stimulant doses in patients with SUD+ADHD have shown promise [537]. It is important to continue to increase the dose after improvement first appears, titrating until maximal improvement is achieved, with tolerable side-effects [564] (see Fig. 50.4). This may require using doses that are higher than those currently recommended, if there is only a partial response to usual doses [565]. The maximum doses of stimulants that are safe and effective have never been established [565, 566]. If there is no response to therapeutic doses of one medication, a stimulant from the other class (MPH or AMPH) should be tried. Response should be monitored quantitatively, with a diagnostic rating scale, to track the degree of improvement in ADHD symptoms. The goal is to achieve remission of ADHD symptoms (ADHD rating scale scores in the normative range) and substantial improvement of functional impairment. Note that symptoms tend to improve first (within weeks), and functional impairment improves more gradually (within months). In patients with cocaine dependence, pharmacological treatment of ADHD initially produces improvement in ADHD symptoms; abstinence from cocaine may follow within weeks [342].
5. Patients with SUD+ADHD can be challenging to treat, but they can be treated successfully.

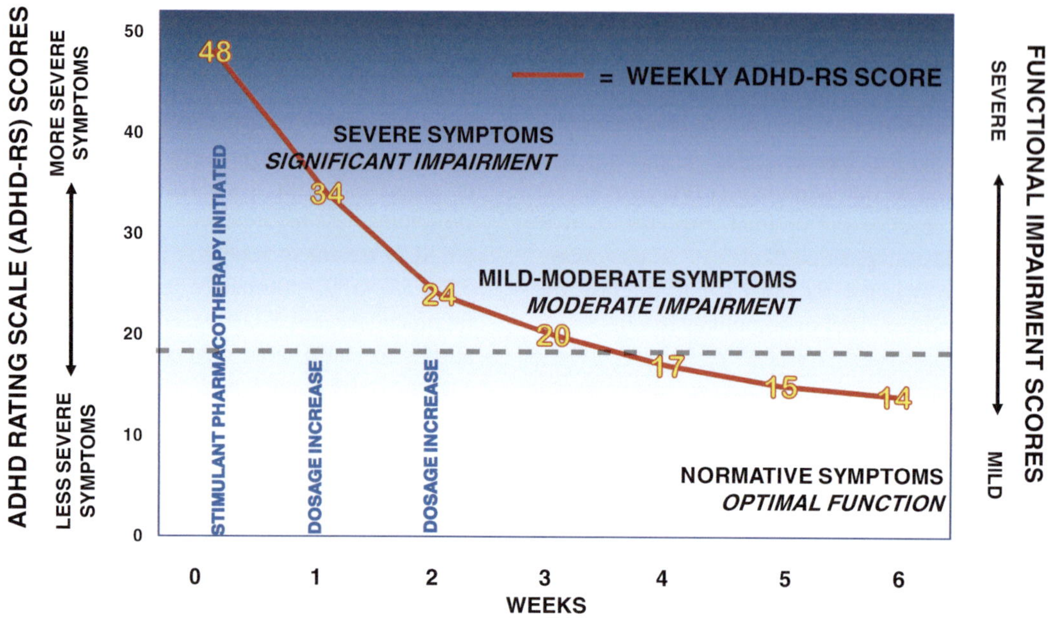

Fig. 50.4 Optimizing symptom reduction and minimizing functional impairment with ADHD pharmacotherapy. ADHD rating scales (ADHD-RS) typically have 18 ADHD symptom items, each rated on a 0–3 scale (0 = minimal; 3 = very frequent). Summary scores thus range from 0 to 52, with higher scores indicating more severe symptoms. By convention, normative scores for each item are ≤1, and scores <18 points are considered in the normative range (below dotted gray line). In this hypothetical example, the patient's baseline ADHD Rating Scale score was 48. Treatment with an extended-release stimulant began at baseline (week 0), and the dosage was titrated upward at week 1 and week 2. By the one-month follow-up visit, the patient's ADHD-RS scores were <18, so patient was maintained at that dosage. Abbreviation: *ADHD-RS* ADHD Rating Scale

There are now several detailed, international consensus statements and quality measures for screening, diagnosing, and treating ADHD in adults [37, 546, 567–570], including specific guidance regarding the presentation and treatment of females with ADHD [31]. Several similarly comprehensive statements address specific considerations when treating patients with SUD+ADHD [544, 552, 571, 572]. Clinicians new to this topic should refer to these documents for their excellent, detailed discussions and recommendations.

Screening for ADHD in Patients with SUDs

All patients seeking treatment for SUDs should be screened for ADHD. Patients seeking treatment for SUDs may not spontaneously mention ADHD symptoms, and therefore, clinicians need to ask specifically, and screen systematically, as part of the standard evaluation of each patient [552]. The *World Health Organization Adult ADHD Self-Report Scale (ASRS)*, version 1.1, is the most widely employed and studied screening tool for individuals with SUD+ADHD [467, 552, 573]. The short version is a 6-item screener, while the long form has 18 items, and is available online. A new version, the *Adult ADHD Self-Report Screening Scale (ASRS) for DSM-5* became available recently. It demonstrates very high sensitivity and specificity in the general population, and high sensitivity and adequate specificity in clinical populations of ADHD patients [574]. This new ASRS is an open-access document, currently the only screener consistent with DSM-5 criteria, and it has better operating characteristics than the original ASRS. Other screening instruments with acceptable sensitivity and specificity in the SUD+ADHD population (using DSM-IV criteria, however) include the

Conners Adult ADHD Rating Scale (CAARS) [575], *Wender Utah Rating Scale (WURS)* [576], *Attention-Deficit Scales for Adults (ADSA)*, and the ADHD module of the *Mini-International Neuropsychiatric Interview MINI-Plus* [577–580]. Adult patients with ADHD are typically accurate reporters, but they have been shown to overestimate their competence and under-report their ADHD impairment on screening, and a knowledgeable informant may frequently rate the patient's ADHD-related impairment as more severe than the patient self-report [42, 581]. Collateral ratings from informants, lower cut-off scores on screening instruments and generous referral for full diagnostic assessment when there is clinical suspicion of ADHD, even with a negative screening score, have been recommended [28, 52, 552, 582–585]. Up to 20% of patients with SUD+ADHD may be missed when a single screener is used, so when possible, the use of two different ADHD screeners also is recommended [552]. Since ADHD is ultimately a clinical diagnosis, patients who are *clinically* suspected of having ADHD from their history, *even if they screen negative*, should be considered candidates for a full diagnostic assessment [552].

Diagnostic Process

The diagnosis of ADHD in patients with SUD should be incorporated into a comprehensive medical-psychiatric examination. Observation, initial history-taking, and screening can begin immediately, and the full diagnostic process should begin as soon as the patient has no serious withdrawal symptoms and when there is no serious intoxication. Although collateral informants/records are desirable, self-report alone is acceptable [586]. Abstinence is not necessary for the diagnostic assessment to begin, since over 95% of those diagnosed with ADHD at intake to an SUD treatment program still meet full criteria for adult ADHD at re-assessment [463, 587].

It is easier to under-diagnose ADHD in the context of SUD, because a clear history may be more difficult to elicit. Adult patients with ADHD often have more difficulties recalling their childhood history of ADHD symptoms, and ADHD may never have been diagnosed during childhood. ADHD-related behaviors can be misattributed to intoxication, withdrawal, or SUD-related life problems at work, school, and with interpersonal/family interactions [588]. Individuals with SUD+ADHD also may under-report both their symptoms and impairment from ADHD, and have limited awareness of the causal relationship between their ADHD symptoms and their functional impairments [582]. It is the clinician's responsibility to clarify in detail the onset, nature, timing, and lifetime course of these problems (when possible, with additional informants), and to differentiate ADHD symptoms from complications of SUD, so that the appropriate treatments can be implemented for the best SUD treatment outcome [552]. When the history provides a high index of suspicion that a patient may have ADHD, a negative screening test may turn out to be inadequately sensitive, and additional probing and clarification may reveal the diagnosis, when it might otherwise have been missed.

Carefully inquire about the onset of ADHD symptoms and substance use (ADHD symptoms almost always precede SUD [36]), and whether ADHD symptoms have persisted even during periods of decreased use/abstinence [569]. Adults with ADHD who seek care for other psychiatric concerns (including SUD) often have developed a variety of compensatory strategies that may mask their ADHD symptoms further [192], and this is especially true for those who are female, high-achieving, have predominantly inattentive ADHD symptoms, and/or have high IQ [56, 59]. These individuals may excel in certain aspects of their lives (e.g., they may have notable educational and career accomplishments or great talent), yet have significant impairment, especially with routine, boring tasks (e.g., paying bills on time, keeping belongings organized, doing chores without reminders) [37, 104, 589]. It also is important to remember that *ADHD symptoms are context-dependent,* so they can vary in different settings. This can be explained as follows: a) It is easier to pay attention to tasks one finds interesting and engaging than to tasks one finds boring or tedious; and b) some tasks (e.g., mowing the lawn, fishing; video games) do not impose a high penalty for inattention, whereas other tasks require sustained attention (e.g., listening to instructions, detailed paperwork). Unfortunately, this appearance of variable attention in different contexts sometimes gives rise to the perception in others that dysfunctional behaviors are volitional, or that an individual "can pay attention when he/she *wants* to pay attention." Such misinterpretations of observed behavior can delay diagnosis and cause substantial harm.

Less frequent, but also important, is avoiding over-diagnosis of ADHD, which can occur if SUD-related symptoms/behaviors are misattributed to ADHD. To distinguish these, remember that ADHD-related symptoms should have been present even in settings and stages of life when substance abuse was not present. ADHD symptoms do not develop acutely; they are present in several domains of life, and the continuity of symptoms from childhood/early adolescence to the present is essential. New situational/environmental stressors or changes in supports (e.g., more demanding job/school, new family responsibilities, fewer supports; or conversely, additional help, more structure, fewer tasks) can contribute to variations in an individual's impairment from ADHD, but ADHD symptoms do not resolve completely, and then re-appear. It also is important not to confuse symptoms from intoxication or severe withdrawal with those of ADHD, which is why evaluation should begin as soon as these potential confounders are no longer present. Finally, re-assessment of ADHD after a period of SUD treatment ascertains the accuracy of the diagnosis and guards against over-diagnosis [587].

The clinician should look for essential elements of classic adult ADHD (for those age ≥17 years), which include:

(a) ≥5 DSM-5 symptoms of inattention and/or impulsivity-hyperactivity have been present for ≥6 months;
(b) several ADHD *symptoms* were present before age 12 years (however, *impairment* before age 12 years is not required).
(c) several symptoms are present in two or more settings, (such as at home/family, school/work; with friends/relatives; or during other activities);
(d) there is clear evidence that the symptoms interfere with, or reduce the quality of, functioning in social or school/work settings (impairment); and
(e) the symptoms cannot be better explained by any other mental disorder, and do not occur only during periods of psychosis [49].

Keep in mind that the DSM criteria for ADHD were normed on ages 8–10 years, and the criteria often need to be adapted to ask equivalent, age-appropriate questions for adults. A few adult examples are given in DSM-5 (e.g., instead of "Runs about or climbs excessively" in children, one can inquire about a sense of extreme restlessness, in adults). Fortunately, many of the diagnostic instruments designed for adults with ADHD take these developmental adjustments into account. There is an age-related decline in hyperactivity with age (which often manifests instead as an internal sense of restlessness), while inattention and impulsivity remain quite impairing, in adults [70]. Most experts recommend that, if the patient's overall presentation is highly consistent with ADHD, and impairment is clinically significant, it is acceptable for adult patients to receive the diagnosis of ADHD if they meet 4 of 9 DSM-inattention and/or impulsivity-hyperactivity criteria [28, 52]. In adults, some suggest a liberal interpretation of the age-of-onset criterion [590, 591]. Some of the complex considerations of specific concern to those making the diagnosis of ADHD in adult patients with SUDs are discussed in more detail elsewhere [552].

When considering impairment, it is particularly important to include in the history how ADHD symptoms affect family life (e.g., marriage, parenting engagement, intimacy, degree of family conflict); occupational history; finances (e.g., paying bills/taxes on time, financial stability, impulsive spending); driving/accident history (e.g., aggressive driving, patience when driving in traffic, history of moving violations, crashes, arrests; and any work-related or other accidents)

[245]. Ask about the strengths and protective factors available to the patient (e.g., high IQ, spouse pays bills and tracks finances, job permits movement and/or a variety of tasks; neighbors can pick up the kids from sports, if patient runs late at work). Collateral history from a family member or close friend can be very helpful, when it can be obtained [584].

A variety of diagnostic semi-structured interviews for ADHD have been developed. Some are available online, for little or no cost, while others are available commercially. Diagnostic instruments that have been validated in patients with SUD+ADHD include the *Diagnostic Interview for ADHD in Adults (DIVA-5 and DIVA 2.0)* [592, 593], the *Conners' Adult ADHD Diagnostic Interview for DSM-IV (CAADID)* [594], and the *Psychiatric Research Interview for Substance and Mental Disorders (PRISM)* [595]. Other commonly used diagnostic instruments for adult ADHD are the *Adult ADHD Clinical Diagnostic Scale (ACDS)* [51], and the *Adult ADHD Investigator Symptom Rating Scale (AISRS)* [596].

Executive function self-report questionnaires appear to be more clinically relevant to impairment from ADHD than neuropsychological measures of executive functioning [597], especially in individuals with antisocial, criminal, and dangerous driving behaviors [598]. Neuropsychological testing is not required to make a diagnosis of ADHD, and *most expert clinicians in this field do not require full neuropsychological testing for the diagnosis of adult ADHD*. Neuropsychological tests appear to measure different constructs from those assessed in executive functioning rating scales [598]. It also is important to note that neuropsychological testing has a very high false-negative rate, so normal scores on neuropsychological tests *do not* rule out the presence of ADHD [599–602]. Neuropsychological deficits also are not helpful in identifying DESR [603]. Untreated ADHD itself worsens neuropsychological performance, and test scores have been shown to improve when ADHD patients are taking MPH [604]. Preferable measures for assessing executive dysfunction and impairment include the *Weiss Functional Impairment Rating Scale (WFIRS)* [605], the *Behavior Rating Inventory of Executive Function®–Adult Version (BRIEF-A)* [606], the *Barkley Deficits in Executive Functioning Scale (BDEFS for Adults)* [607], and the *Barkley Functional Impairment Scale for Adults (BFIS)* [608]. For more details and additional resources, an excellent, comprehensive review of the available screening and diagnostic instruments for adult ADHD was published recently [609].

Neuropsychological testing *may* be useful, later in treatment, to assess learning styles or to develop appropriate workplace accommodations. In that situation, if the diagnosis of ADHD has been made previously and neuropsychological testing is subsequently needed, the results of the testing may be most meaningful if the patient takes their ADHD medication(s) prior to the assessment, so that the medication(s) are actively working during the testing.

In all patients with ADHD, psychiatric comorbidities are common, and this is especially true in the SUD+ADHD population. Thus, a comprehensive psychiatric diagnostic assessment is crucially important for identifying areas of needed treatment, and for determining a rational treatment sequence.

ADHD symptoms overlap with symptoms seen in other psychiatric disorders. Adults with ADHD often have irritability, low frustration tolerance, low self-esteem, negative mood, rejection sensitivity, and fluctuating mood. These symptoms must be differentiated from dysthymia, BPD, and BoPD (although these disorders commonly co-exist with ADHD). Unlike BPD, mood shifts in ADHD are common, brief (lasting a day or less), and mildly dysregulated (often manifesting as over-reacting to minor disappointments or frustrations), but within the normal mood range, rather than the longer and more profound periods of bipolar depression or the extremes of elation, grandiosity, and irritability common in the manic episodes seen in BPD [184, 610–612]. Unlike BoPD, ADHD-related impulsivity, mood dysregulation, rejection sensitivity, and anger tend to be thoughtless and short-lived, without the persistence, driven quality, or poor sense of self that characterize BoPD [315, 613, 614].

Pretreatment medical evaluation should include: a) baseline weight and BMI, b) baseline heart rate and blood pressure, c) history of eating disorders (particularly with vomiting/electrolyte disturbance), d) any history of traumatic brain injury (ADHD symptoms should precede most mild traumatic brain injuries), and e) any prior history of liver damage. In addition, a detailed personal and family cardiac history is essential (e.g., history of cardiac arrhythmias or unexplained syncope; structural cardiac anomalies; cardiomyopathy; or family history of premature, sudden cardiac death). The diagnosis of ADHD, especially in combination with SUD, confers increased risks for cardiovascular disease, and other chronic medical conditions [137]. Elicit information about appetite and typical diet and eating patterns, as well as caffeine consumption (e.g., coffee, tea, sodas, energy drinks and/or caffeine supplements). Ask about all current and past prescription and non-prescription medications, vitamins and supplements, and ask about current and past non-medical use of prescription drugs. Take a careful history of substance use, including nicotine, alcohol, marijuana and other THC-containing products, and illicit substances of abuse. Inquire about somatic complaints and their frequency and severity (e.g., gastrointestinal distress, headaches). Take a careful history about baseline bedtime routines and sleep patterns. Ask about the patient's: a) typical bedtime, b) exposure to light from the use of phones, tablets, laptops, or television in the evening, c) presence of restless leg symptoms when falling asleep, d) sleep latency (duration between turning off the lights and falling asleep), e) number of nighttime awakenings and ease of returning to sleep, f) presence of snoring, g) history of frequent nightmares, h) time of morning awakening, and i) whether the patient feels refreshed in the morning, upon awakening. The detailed baseline information gathered about appetite, sleep, and somatic complaints will be especially useful when evaluating the impact of possible medication adverse events and addressing typical sleep problems associated with ADHD treatments.

Treatment of SUD+ADHD

Treatment of SUD+ADHD should have multiple components, including psychoeducation, pharmacotherapy for each condition (including other comorbidities), peer support, and individual/group cognitive-behavioral therapy. Modules addressing both ADHD and SUD should be integrated into each component of treatment. SUD intervention begins immediately, and ADHD treatment should follow as soon as the patient is stabilized [552].

Generally, when treating patients with psychiatric comorbidities, the most severe and impairing disorders are treated first; additional treatments may be added once the most severe problems are stabilized. For example, in the presence of BPD, pharmacological ADHD treatment should be deferred until the mood is stabilized [37, 615, 616]. Similarly, in hypertensive patients, once blood pressure is controlled, stimulants and/or ATX are safe to use, with ongoing monitoring. A recent study suggested that, in addition to traditional risk factors for cardiovascular disease in patients initiating medications for ADHD, several additional risk factors may include SUD (other than tobacco or alcohol-related), the use of methadone or disulfiram in patients with SUD, mood stabilizers, and antipsychotic medications [617]. Thus, in patients with SUD+ADHD, careful consideration of the patient's entire medication regimen is warranted, along with careful cardiovascular monitoring. As always, these treatment risks must be weighed against the risks of untreated ADHD, which, as discussed earlier, are far from benign, especially in patients with SUDs.

Severe depression and severe anxiety often require treatment before ADHD treatment is initiated, while milder anxiety and mood problems (including mood dysregulation) may respond to ADHD treatment alone; anxiety and mood symptoms can then be re-assessed, and decisions made about need for additional treatment. For those entering SUD treatment, ADHD treatment can be started as soon as abuse is stabilized [37]; abstinence is not usually required, if patients have begun reducing use and are committed to treatment [587]. A recent study demonstrated that pregnant women with ADHD who took ADHD medications had offspring with normal neurodevelopment and growth, which should reassure prescribers when counseling women who would benefit from taking ADHD medications during pregnancy [618].

Specific SUD+ADHD Psychoeducation

It is useful to provide information to patients about the causes of ADHD, adult ADHD symptoms, ADHD-related impairment (including relationships, driving/accidents, emotional dysregulation, and executive function difficulties), treatment options for ADHD, and need for sustained, daily treatment. This information may help patients both to see some of their lifelong difficulties from a new perspective, with less self-blame, and to understand the importance of consistent, long-term, daily pharmacotherapy for ADHD. Where relevant, partners/families should be provided with information and appropriate resources. Information on typical sleep problems associated with ADHD, especially insomnia and delayed sleep phase disorder, can be useful. Several ADHD psychoeducation programs have been evaluated in adults with ADHD [619, 620], and these sessions can be integrated into the psychoeducation programs typically offered for patients in treatment for SUD.

Cognitive-Behavioral Therapy (CBT) for SUD+ADHD and Other Nonmedical Treatments

As mentioned above, there are several excellent CBT-based programs that have been designed for patients with ADHD [510–512]; adding some of these ADHD-specific topics and skills training to the traditional CBT found in SUD treatment programs may be helpful to many patients [508]. Specific skill instruction and practice (e.g., organizational skills, To-Do lists, calendars and reminders, considering alternative choices, interrupting negative thoughts, managing intense emotions) can be very helpful. The first integrated CBT program specifically designed for adults with SUD+ADHD was recently described [621]. Another CBT program for adolescents and adults with ADHD has a separate module on SUD+ADHD [622]. There also is a specific program for those who have a SUD+ADHD plus a history of antisocial or criminal behavior [623]. Some investigators have found that shorter sessions may promote better adherence in patients with short attention spans.

On average, dropout rates for all psychosocial SUD programs appear to be about 30%, with better retention for AUD than other SUDs. Higher dropout rates are also reported for those with more cognitive and executive dysfunction [624, 625]. This is another reason to target ADHD executive function with skills training. The prompt addition of psychosocial-behavioral therapies to buprenorphine treatment for patients with OUD has been shown to lower the risk of premature discontinuation of buprenorphine during the first 6 months of treatment by 30–45% [626].

Adding contingency management (CM) to CBT can enhance treatment participation and abstinence, when implemented in an evidence-based program [624, 627]. A detailed description of the CM program implemented in SUD programs throughout the U.S. Veterans Affairs medical system was recently published, with descriptions of the elements necessary for maximal program effectiveness [628].

Another variety of interventions that have proven helpful, when added to traditional CBT, are mindfulness-based therapies [629–632]. Mindfulness practices have been shown to improve adult ADHD symptoms. Neuroimaging studies have demonstrated that mindfulness may improve ADHD symptoms by activating the DLPFC, improve executive function through activation of the dorsal ACC and striatum, and increase functional connectivity in the cortico-striatal-thalamic circuit [619, 633]. A recent, 8-week trial of school-based mindfulness training in typical 6th graders found that post-training improved performance on a sustained attention task was associated with greater anti-correlation between the activity in the DMN and the right DLPFC [634].

It also is important to address underlying sleep problems associated with ADHD, since impaired sleep worsens ADHD symptoms. Initially, patients should improve sleep hygiene. Since delayed sleep phase disorder is also very common among patients with SUD+ADHD, addressing this condition with low-dose melatonin, bright light therapy, and a gradual adjustment of bedtimes appears to be helpful [635]. Sleep apnea, if present, should be addressed. Lastly, exercise appears to be helpful as an adjunctive treatment in those with ADHD, SUDs, eating disorders, and mood disorders [636–639].

Adjunctive ADHD Pharmacotherapy for Patients with SUD+ADHD

Stabilization and initiation of SUD-related pharmacological and psychological treatments is the most urgent priority for patients seeking treatment for SUDs. Following this initial stabilization, and initiation of the SUD treatment program, assessment for comorbid ADHD should be initiated. If ADHD is diagnosed, and the patient appears committed to harm reduction and engagement in treatment for their SUD(s), the provider and patient may choose to initiate adjunctive ADHD pharmacotherapy as one component of their overall treatment. Keep in mind that the most serious psychiatric comorbidities (e.g., bipolar disorder) should be treated and stabilized prior to ADHD pharmacotherapy.

The general procedures are as follows:

1. Define the symptoms and behaviors to be targeted with ADHD treatment, based on the patient's individual circumstances, burden of impairment, and patient goals. ADHD symptom reduction (e.g., better attentional focus, being more patient, being able to sit through a meal without restlessness), reduced impairment, less impulsive decision-making, and longer SUD treatment engagement may be common considerations. Discuss alternatives to ADHD pharmacotherapy, and potential risks and benefits, including side-effects, and the abuse/addiction potential of stimulant medications, especially immediate-release stimulants.
2. Initiate treatment with *abuse-resistant, extended-release stimulant medication*; OROS-MPH, LDX, and serdexMPH are considered the most abuse-resistant, and extended-release stimulants are preferred over immediate-release preparations. Both OROS-MPH and LDX have shown efficacy in patients with SUD+ADHD [360, 583]. All three formulations have rapid onset (30 min to 2 h), and initial effects can be seen within days to weeks, depending on the titration schedule. The rapid onset of symptom improvement may be an additional source of motivation for patients with SUD+ADHD to remain in treatment. Two recent articles offer extensive discussions of stimulant formulations and how to choose among stimulant preparations, for those who wish to develop additional expertise in this area [640, 641]. Most experts do not require complete abstinence from illicit substances before starting treatment for ADHD, and for individuals with ADHD and StimUDs, ADHD treatment and improvement appear to precede abstinence from cocaine [342].
3. Extended-release stimulants are usually started at low doses, and titrated every 5–7 days, or as tolerated, until there are no further improvements in ADHD symptoms and side-effects are tolerable. Titration typically takes up to 4–6 weeks. Use a quantitative symptom scale to ascertain medication response and symptom reduction, weekly, during titration (see Fig. 50.4). Target doses of MPH for ADHD only can be up to 1.0–1.8 mg/kg/day (depending on formulation and number of doses per day). Doses in this range have been shown to improve treatment efficacy but because of sub-optimal titration, are rarely achieved in all but the most recent of studies in adult patients with ADHD [566, 642]. For AMPHs, daily doses are typically 50% of target MPH doses (~0.5–1.0 mg/kg/day). The recommended starting dose for SerdexMPH/

dexMPH in adults is 39.2 mg/7.8 mg orally, each morning [358, 643]. Experience with patients with SUD+ADHD suggests that titration to higher-than-typical doses may be necessary [524, 537, 540, 552, 568, 571, 583]. Optimizing treatment outcomes beyond the brief discussion in this chapter can be challenging, but there is expert advice to assist caregivers in this effort [505, 644, 645]. Stimulants also can be used with naltrexone, to mitigate stimulant-related euphoria, without altering the efficacy of the treatment for ADHD [646, 647], and naltrexone also may be useful in decreasing craving, in some patients with StimUDs [648]. Patients should be seen for in-person or virtual visits as frequently as needed, weekly, at first, and all patients should be seen for a follow-up visit not more than 1 month after ADHD treatment initiation. With more complex or unstable patients, more frequent follow-up visits, for longer periods, are advised.

4. If stimulant misuse appears to be too great a risk initially, the nonstimulant ATX has little risk of abuse, but takes longer before an initial response may be apparent (4–6 weeks), so it may be better for patients where rapid onset of effect is not essential [649]. In adolescents and adults, ATX is typically started at a dose of 40 mg/day, and gradually increased every 7 days to a daily dose of 80 mg/day; after 2–4 weeks on 80 mg/day, if a partial response is observed, the dose may be increased to a maximum of 100 mg/day. At least partial response should be observed within 4 weeks, or another class of ADHD medication should be initiated. The full effect of ATX can take 4–6 months (or longer) to achieve, and the effect size seen with ATX is lower than effect sizes for stimulants [526, 527, 650, 651]. ATX also may be useful in patients with co-occurring severe anxiety, especially if anxiety has been exacerbated by stimulants.
5. Other nonstimulants, particularly the α_2 adrenergic receptor agonists guanfacine and clonidine, have no abuse potential. However, when used as monotherapy, they have smaller effect sizes than stimulants in adults with ADHD [530, 531]. They have not yet been studied extensively in adults with SUD+ADHD [652]. In children, adolescents and adults, their greatest benefits have been when they are *added to stimulants* adjunctively, to achieve full ADHD symptom remission, better treatment response, to mitigate stimulant side-effects (especially sleep and cardiovascular) or when the highest-tolerated stimulant doses are not sufficient to achieve optimal symptom control and mitigation of impairment [653–657]. They may also be helpful in decreasing symptoms of cannabis withdrawal [658]. Unlike stimulants and atomoxetine, guanfacine and clonidine can cause *decreases* in heart rate and blood pressure, and may offset cardiovascular effects of stimulants, when used in combination. The α_2 adrenergic receptor agonists also promote sleep, when taken in the evenings. In clinical practice, ATX also is used as an adjunct to stimulants, although there are few formal studies addressing combination stimulant-nonstimulant treatments in adults with ADHD [656, 659–661]. ATX and OROS-MPH also have been used adjunctively with SSRIs, for treatment of adults with ADHD and comorbid, partially responsive MDD [662].
6. Viloxazine extended-release (ER) is a nonstimulant, serotonin-norepinephrine modulating agent (SNMA) [347]. It has been classified as a non-controlled substance. The U.S. Food & Drug Administration approved viloxazine ER for treatment of ADHD in adults with ADHD in 2022. Viloxazine is usually started at 200 mg./day and may be titrated every 7–14 days, up to 600 mg/day [531]. Viloxazine has been demonstrated to be safe in healthy adults when co-administered with MPH or LDX and does not affect the corrected QT interval (QTc). In a small study of adults taking viloxazine ER, a partial response within 2–3 weeks predicted a reduction in ADHD symptoms of ≥50% by week 6 of treatment [663]. Other nonstimulants, such as bupropion, have also been used, particularly in combination with stimulants, but occasionally as monotherapy, for comorbid SUD+ADHD and MDD [664].

Bupropion and OUD medications (buprenorphine, naltrexone, methadone) also have been shown to decrease emergency department and hospital admissions for stimulant-related (cocaine, amphetamine) events in patients with OUDs [665].

There are several interesting new drugs in the pharmaceutical development pipeline, including novel, nonstimulant entities, and some stimulants with additional abuse resistance. Prescribers should stay current with new drug releases and the ADHD treatment literature [531, 661, 666, 667].

Once symptoms are optimized, patients should be seen at regular intervals for long-term follow-up. Patients should be seen frequently, until both SUD and ADHD are stabilized. Most patients with ADHD *only* are then seen at least every 3–6 months for another year, but SUD+ADHD patients are likely to require more frequent follow-up and monitoring. Monitor heart rate, blood pressure, and weight at each follow-up visit. Use a validated tool to measure ADHD symptoms at every follow-up visit (with a rating scale from a collateral informant, when possible), and continue to measure symptoms over the long-term, at least annually [609]. Monitor other psychiatric symptoms regularly, over the first year, and at least annually, thereafter.

ADHD Medications: Common Side-Effects and Their Management

Stimulants

Both MPH and AMPH prescription medications have similar side-effects. Common side-effects are typically discomforting and are rarely dangerous, while serious potential side-effects tend to be rare. The most common stimulant side-effects include decreased appetite, sometimes with transient weight loss; difficulty falling asleep; headache; dry mouth; nausea; irritability or anxiety and increases in heart rate (mean increase: 3–6 beats/minute) and blood pressure (mean increase: 2–4 mmHg). These changes are typically not clinically significant in individuals without significant structural or genetic cardiac risk [668]. However, clinically relevant elevations in blood pressure and heart rate can be seen in adults. In patients who are using illicit stimulants, cardiovascular effects of stimulants are additive [525], so careful cardiovascular monitoring is essential. Nevertheless, several major reviews have found *no increase in serious adverse events*, even cardiovascular events, in patients with StimUDs and ADHD, who take prescription stimulants [669–671]. All patients should have heart rate and blood pressure measured prior to initiating treatment, frequently during the initial stages of treatment, and after every dosage change. Monitor heart rate and blood pressure at regular intervals during follow-up. In patients with hypertension, control blood pressure first, and then initiate stimulants, with close monitoring.

Erectile dysfunction and decreased libido have been reported in <5% of patients. Priapism has been reported rarely, as well.

Insomnia is common in untreated patients with ADHD [672]. Both circadian rhythm disorders and seasonal sleep and affective disturbances have been associated with ADHD [127]. Exacerbation of insomnia is commonly an early side-effect of many ADHD medications, especially stimulants [673]. Fortunately, for many patients, the worsening of their pre-existing insomnia is a transient problem that improves over the first weeks of treatment. Insomnia may return to its baseline level, and for many ADHD patients, sleep quality actually may improve, after the first few weeks of treatment [672, 674–676]. A slower stimulant titration schedule, having patients take their medication earlier in the morning, or switching to an extended-release stimulant formulation with a different pharmacokinetic profile may all be useful strategies to consider, if insomnia is persistently bothersome. Sleep disturbances with ADHD should be treated concomitantly with ADHD treatment, since sleep deprivation worsens both inattention and emotional dysregulation, and lowers mental functioning and productivity [677, 678]. Instruction in good sleep hygiene [679–681] is essential. Persistent, severe insomnia may be responsive to adding an evening dose of melatonin 0.5–1.0 mg, guanfacine 2–6 mg, or low-dose mirtazapine 7.5–15.0 mg [635, 682, 683]. Early morning bright light therapy, especially for those with seasonal affective disorder or delayed sleep phase disorder [684, 685], may also help insomnia. Finally, for a minority of patients who find it difficult to quiet their thoughts at night, a supplemental, low dose of stimulant medication may help them get to sleep [37].

Appetite suppression is not as great a problem for adults as it is for children, who need to grow. However, it can be unpleasant, to some adults. Appetite problems may be transient and may improve over the first few weeks of treatment. If not, they usually can be managed by having patients eat high calorie meals when medication effects are least prominent (i.e., in early morning before taking medication and in late evening, after medication has worn off).

Stimulants can precipitate manic or mixed episodes in patients with BPD, especially if mood is poorly stabilized before treatment. After mood stabilization, however, stimulants may be used with careful monitoring, in patients with BPD. Slower titration also may be warranted. If mania emerges, stimulants should be discontinued. Psychosis has been reported, in rare cases.

Other rare and serious stimulant side-effects can include peripheral vasculopathy, including Raynaud's phenomenon. Rashes (ranging from urticaria to Stevens-Johnson syndrome) have been reported but are extremely rare. Stimulants can exacerbate tics, in vulnerable patients.

Clinically significant tachycardia or heart palpitations have been reported, either from stimulants alone, or when stimulants are taken with high doses of caffeine (e.g., energy drinks or supplements). Caution patients to limit their caffeine consumption, and to avoid energy drinks and supplements. There are rare reports of sudden death, myocardial infarction, stroke, and hypertension; *a careful cardiac history is essential*, including family history of sudden death before age 40 or heritable arrhythmias or structural cardiac anomalies. Additional medical/cardiac consultation before stimulant initiation is recommended primarily for those with a concerning cardiac history; it is not routinely indicated. Cochrane systematic reviews of prescription stimulants have shown no additional risk for cardiac or other serious adverse events in those with StimUDs [670, 686]. Do not use stimulants with, or within 14 days of, discontinuation of, MAO inhibitors.

Atomoxetine (ATX)

Common side-effects are usually mild and include small increases in blood pressure (average 2 mm Hg) and heart rate (average 5 bpm). However, approximately 5–10% of adult patients on ATX experienced "potentially clinically important changes in heart rate (≥20 bpm) or blood pressure (>15–20 mmHg) [687]." All patients should have heart rate and blood pressure measured prior to initiating treatment, at follow-up visits and after every dosage change. Monitor heart rate and blood pressure at regular intervals during follow-up. In patients with hypertension, control blood pressure first, and then initiate stimulants, with close monitoring.

Other common side-effects include dry mouth, constipation, decreased appetite or nausea, fatigue or insomnia, sexual dysfunction, and urinary retention or hesitation. ATX can precipitate manic or mixed episodes in patients with BPD, especially if mood is poorly stabilized before treatment. After mood stabilization, however, ATX may be used with careful monitoring, in patients with BPD. Discontinue ATX if mania emerges. ATX is contraindicated in those with narrow-angle glaucoma or a history of pheochromocytoma. There are rare reports of sudden death, myocardial infarction, stroke, and hypertension. A careful cardiac history is essential, including family history of sudden death before age 40 or heritable arrhythmias or structural cardiac anomalies. Additional medical/cardiac consultation before ATX initiation is recommended primarily for those with a concerning cardiac history; it is not routinely indicated.

Raynaud's phenomenon and priapism have been reported rarely. Monitor patients for worsening or emergence of aggression or hostility; this has been reported in patients taking ATX. There is a Black Box warning related to suicidal ideation in children and adolescents early in ATX treatment. However, this is rare and *has not* been noted in adult patients taking ATX [688]. Use with caution in patients with liver disease; rare, reversible hepatobiliary events have been reported [689]. Do not use with, or within 14 days of discontinuation of, MAO inhibitors. Caution patients not to drive or operate machinery until they know how they respond to ATX, since it may induce drowsiness.

Guanfacine and Clonidine

The most common side-effects of α_2 adrenergic agents are sedation, somnolence, dry mouth, constipation, sexual dysfunction, headaches, hypotension, bradycardia, and dizziness. Measure blood pressure and pulse prior to initiation, following dosage increases, and periodically while taking. Titrate gradually, to minimize side-effects, especially sedation and hypotension. Watch for orthostatic hypotension and syncope. Patients should maintain good hydration. Do not discontinue $\alpha2$ adrenergic receptor agonists suddenly, to avoid rebound hypertension. Instead, taper medication over several weeks, before discontinuation. Use with caution in patients with heart block and in those already taking antihypertensive medication. Caution patients not to drive or operate machinery until they know how they respond to α_2 adrenergic receptor agonists.

Viloxazine

Because viloxazine was only recently approved for treatment of adults with ADHD, we have only modest clinical trial data. Common side-effects include insomnia, headache, somnolence, fatigue, nausea, decreased appetite, dry mouth, and constipation. A minority of patients may have clinically relevant elevations in blood pressure and heart rate. All patients should have heart rate and blood pressure measured prior to initiating treatment and after every dosage change. Heart rate and blood pressure should be monitored at regular intervals during follow-up. In patients with hypertension, control blood pressure first, and then initiate stimulants, with close monitoring. Additional medical/cardiac consultation before medication initiation is recommended primarily for those with a concerning cardiac history; it is not routinely indicated.

Because of its noradrenergic activity, viloxazine could precipitate manic or mixed episodes in patients with BPD, especially if mood is poorly stabilized before treatment. After mood stabilization, however, viloxazine may be used with careful monitoring, in patients with BPD. Discontinue viloxazine if mania emerges. Caution patients not to drive or operate machinery until they know how they respond to viloxazine.

Patients should be monitored for the emergence or worsening of suicidal ideation during medication initiation, during the first few months of treatment, and after dosage adjustments. Do not use viloxazine with, or within 14 days of discontinuation of, MAO inhibitors. Dosage modification may be needed, in patients with renal impairment.

Table 50.2 Cytochrome P450 drug-drug potential interactions in treatment of patients with SUD+ADHD

Drug	Substrate	Inhibitor	Inducer	Notes
ADHD medications				
Amphetamine Lisdexamfetamine	2D6	–	–	The pharmacokinetics of amphetamines are generally linear and dose proportional. Few pharmacokinetically based drug-drug interactions have been documented [690]. Metabolized by hydroxylation, with oxidation, de-amination, and renal excretion as alternative metabolic pathways. LDX undergoes hydrolysis to make active d-AMPH and lysine. Do not use with strong 2D6 inhibitors, since in rare cases, this can increase risk of serotonin syndrome. Do not use with MAO inhibitors, or within 14 days after their discontinuation. Limit caffeine intake, as needed. Ethanol can increase AMPH levels [657]. There are 2 case reports of possibly dose-dependent psychosis due to drug-drug interactions between stimulants and disulfiram

(continued)

Table 50.2 (continued)

Drug	Substrate	Inhibitor	Inducer	Notes
Atomoxetine	2C19; 2D6	–	–	Do not use with strong 2D6 inhibitors. Do not use with MAO inhibitors, or within 14 days after their discontinuation. Limit caffeine intake, as needed. ATX can potentiate cardiovascular effects of β_2 agonists and pressor agents. Monitor QTc if ATX is used with buprenorphine
Clonidine	2D6; 1A2; 3A4/5	–	–	Taper dose when discontinuing; do not discontinue abruptly, to avoid rebound hypertension. Do not use with MAO inhibitors, or within 14 days after their discontinuation. Reduce dosage if either renal or hepatic function is impaired
Guanfacine	3A4/5/7	–	–	Reduce dose with strong 3A4/5/7 inhibitors. May increase dose ($\geq$ 8 mg/day) if used with 3A4/5/7 inducers. Taper dose when discontinuing; do not discontinue abruptly, to avoid rebound hypertension. Reduce dosage if either renal or hepatic function is impaired
Methylphenidate Serdexmethylphenidate	–	–	–	The pharmacokinetics of stimulants are generally linear and dose proportional. Few pharmacokinetically based drug-drug interactions have been documented [690]. Hepatic metabolism (CES1-catalyzed de-esterification), no CYP450 enzyme interactions. Consider decreasing MPH dosage if co-administered with CES1 inhibitors. Do not use with MAO inhibitors, or within 14 days after their discontinuation. Ethanol can increase MPH levels [694, 695]
Viloxazine	2D6: 2B15	1A2 2D6 (weak)	2B6	Mostly renally excreted; decrease dosage if renal function is impaired. Multiple metabolic routes, with some metabolism by 2D6. Do not use with MAO inhibitors, or within 14 days after their discontinuation. Limit caffeine intake, as needed. One case report suggests possible inhibition of theophylline metabolism [657]. May be relatively contraindicated for concomitant use with drugs that are 1A2 substrates
SUD medications and drugs of abuse				
Acamprosate	–	–	–	Not metabolized. Excreted as acamprosate in urine
Buprenorphine	2C8; 2C9; 3A4/5/7	–	–	Fewer clinically relevant drug-drug interactions than methadone. Monitor QTc, if used with atomoxetine. No adverse drug-drug interactions have been reported with stimulants [696]
Cocaine	3A4/5/7	2D6 (*in vitro* only)	–	Monitor heart rate and blood pressure when using ADHD medications during cocaine use
Codeine/oxycodone	2D6: 3A4/5/7	–	–	
Disulfiram	–	2E1 (strong)	–	There are 2 case reports of possibly dose-dependent psychosis due to drug-drug interactions between stimulants and disulfiram [697, 698]
Ethanol	2E1	–	–	Ethanol can increase AMPH levels [657]
Fentanyl	3A4/5/7	–	–	
Methadone	2B6; 2C19; 2D6: 3A4/5/7	2D6 (?)	–	No adverse drug-drug interactions have been reported with stimulants [696]
Naltrexone	–	–	–	Undergoes first pass metabolism in liver; no CYP450 enzymes involved. Can be used with stimulants [646].
Nicotine	–	–	1A2; 2B6	
Varenicline	–	–	–	

Drug-Drug Interactions Several excellent and comprehensive reviews have been written on drug-drug interactions relevant to ADHD treatments [657, 690] and medications used for treatment of various substance use disorders [691–693]. A comprehensive table of drug-drug interactions related to cytochrome P450 enzymes is also published online by Indiana University [688]. Table 50.2 summarizes some of the most common, clinically relevant, drug-drug interactions for patients in treatment for SUD+ADHD, with a focus on cytochrome P450 interactions.

Prescriber Practices That Can Prevent Stimulant NMU

Clinicians should employ several routine practices to discourage stimulant diversion and NMU. Patient education, clinical assessment of patient diversion/NMU risks, and employment of diversion-resistant prescribing and record-keeping are all important measures that should be standard prescriber practices.

Patient education about stimulant diversion/NMU, especially in adolescents and young adults, is important to prevent diversion and discourage NMU. Students who engage in stimulant NMU often believe that NMU is more widespread among their peers than current data would suggest. Compared with non-users, young people who misuse stimulants perceive that stimulant NMU is not as frowned upon by peers as cocaine or nonmedical opioid use, and often believe that the risks of stimulant NMU are modest. Most college students indicate that stimulants for NMU are easy to obtain [248, 699]. Peer pressure from being asked to share or sell one's prescription stimulant medication is often cited as the main reason for diversion [700], and thus, advising patients to limit disclosure to peers that they take prescription stimulants, and teaching students how to say "no" to peers' requests to divert their medication appear to be helpful practices [701, 702]. Furthermore, many young people who engage in stimulant NMU believe stimulants enhance academic performance and focus, although little evidence supports this belief, absent a diagnosis of ADHD [335, 703]. A trusted prescriber challenging unrealistic expectations for performance enhancement may reduce adolescent/young adult patients' NMU [704].

Molina et al. [705] have demonstrated that among high school students, the likelihood of diversion is increased with older age, stimulant treatment disclosure to peers, a patient's permissive attitude about stimulant NMU, peer norms favorable to stimulant NMU, and perceived low probability of negative consequences from diversion. Primary care providers often feel ill-prepared to educate patients about diversion prevention and to discourage nonmedical use, despite their concerns about patients' stimulant diversion and NMU [706, 707]. In a recent study, primary care providers treating college students with stimulants for ADHD attended a one-hour training on strategies aimed at reducing stimulant diversion. Areas of training included: brief patient education and counseling (e.g., negative consequences of diversion), enhancing diversion prevention strategies, and effective medication monitoring. Provider training resulted in high provider satisfaction; pre- and post-intervention patient surveys demonstrated: (1) reduction in college students' intention to share, sell, or trade stimulants, (2) decreased student disclosure to peers that they use stimulants, and (3) decreases in the number of times students were asked to divert their medications [702]. Teaching individuals how to decline requests for diversion, limited peer disclosure of prescription stimulant use, safe storage practices, and discussion of medical, academic and legal risks of diversion all appear to be effective educational measures.

In addition to patient education, the prescriber's own diversion-resistant/abuse-resistant medication prescribing practices are of utmost importance. Familiarity with several extended-release stimulant and nonstimulant medications and their various formulations and pharmacokinetic patterns is essential for choosing a medication that best suits each patient's individual schedule and needs [640, 641, 645]. Assessment of comorbidities, including past and current substance use/abuse, and overall level of functioning, can assist the prescriber in determining an individual's risk for stimulant diversion/abuse. Treat the most impairing comorbid(y/ies) first, and initiate ADHD treatment after those other conditions are stabilized.

Prescription of extended-release medication is preferable for better adherence, and for reduced abuse/diversion liability, compared with immediate-release stimulants [247, 248]. Rates of NMU for extended-release stimulants are actually remarkably low (<2 per 100,000 stimulant prescriptions), compared with other commonly misused classes of prescription drugs [435]. Nonstimulant medications (e.g., atomoxetine or viloxazine) also are an option and may be preferred in patients with active substance abuse, although nonstimulants have smaller effect sizes than those of stimulants [708], and take longer to demonstrate a therapeutic effect. Lisdexamfetamine, OROS-MPH, and a recently approved combination of the prodrug serdexmethylphenidate/d-MPH (Azstarys®, Corium LLC) are three widely-available extended-release stimulants with particularly abuse-resistant properties [360, 545], and other options and drugs in development show promise [647, 666, 709]. Repeated, quantitative assessments of symptom burden and functioning, both at diagnosis and regularly throughout treatment, are essential for guiding medication choice, dosage optimization, and long-term management.

Clear instructions to patients to take stimulant medications as prescribed, and not to change timing, dosage or medication without prior discussion with the prescriber, are important. Taking stimulants "as-needed" should be discouraged. ADHD impairments affect patients' judgment, safety, and functioning throughout the day, and therefore, the *default* prescription practice should be every-day, all-day, extended-release ADHD medication coverage [97, 99, 122, 123, 487, 710–712], including the hours when the patient is driving. Patients should both be advised not to use other substances of abuse concurrently, and must be educated about stimulants' potential for increasing risks of substance abuse/misuse [713]. In those with active SUD, whether to require illicit substance abstinence is controversial. Most clinicians feel that some substance use is not an absolute contraindication to beginning medical treatment, but substance use should be stabilized, and patients should be committed to SUD treatment [587, 463, 569].

Careful, ongoing assessment of patient response to treatment is essential. Typically, dosage titration to maximal improvement in symptoms and function (and preferably full remission, if possible) is the goal [714], unless adverse events limit tolerability. Extended-release stimulants once or twice daily are more convenient, improve adherence, and may decrease the risk of diversion/NMU, compared with immediate-release preparations [435, 447]. Beginning with a low dose, stimulant titration can occur every 3–7 days, over 4–6 weeks, with close monitoring, since there are marked individual differences in tolerability and optimal dosage. Slower titration may be indicated, if side-effects are prominent. Prescribers should be explicit about when patients should call for advice, and brief, frequent, telephone, and/or video check-ins during the initial titration period can be helpful. Patients with ADHD without SUD should have a follow-up visit within 4 weeks of medication initiation, and patients with SUD+ADHD should be seen at even more frequent intervals, with even closer monitoring by telephone, for patients who are being treated in an outpatient program. Close follow-up with both quantitative assessment of symptoms (e.g., an ADHD symptom screening instrument) and careful assessment of ongoing comorbidities and level of function (preferably with information from both the patient and a collateral contact), is essential [609] (see Fig. 50.4).

Prescribers need to maintain an active, working relationship with their patients with ADHD, with follow-up visits at least monthly, until good symptom control has been achieved, and not less than every 3–6 months thereafter. Instructions regarding prescription refill requests, and how the prescriber handles early requests for stimulant refills (including requests for "lost" medication) should be explicit. Systems that alert the prescriber if refills are being requested prematurely (suggesting NMU or diversion), or, conversely, if refills are not being requested regularly (suggesting inconsistent stimulant adherence), may be helpful. When concerns about diversion or NMU are elevated, abuse-resistant, extended-release stimulant prescriptions should be written for a limited number of doses at a time, with close monitoring, or a switch to a nonstimulant medication may be indicated. State/national databases that track controlled substance prescriptions should be checked before writing each prescription, to ascertain that there is only one prescriber, and that other prescriptions with abuse potential are not being filled without that prescriber's knowledge. Good record-keeping, with details of advice given, prescription dates, medication doses and times, and number of doses prescribed, is essential. And, of course, prescribers must be familiar with local and national regulations and laws concerning all aspects of controlled substance prescribing [569]. It may not be possible to prevent all NMU, but these practices can discourage diversion, alert the prescriber to signs of possible NMU, and are considered diversion-resistant/abuse-resistant prescribing routines.

Conclusion

ADHD is a common comorbidity in adults seeking treatment for SUDs. The clinician is likely to encounter ADHD in approximately 15–25% of SUD patients. Patients with SUD+ADHD have a typical historical pattern, and a careful and detailed history is the most important diagnostic tool available to the clinician. The symptoms of ADHD should almost always antedate the onset of SUD, and ADHD symptoms persist, even during periods of abstinence or reduced substance use. There are many neurobiological features common to both ADHD and SUD, and the co-occurrence of the disorders creates a more severe clinical condition. By the time patients with SUD+ADHD present for SUD treatment, they often have greater SUD severity, more comorbidities, and greater complexity than patients with SUD without ADHD. They are often impulsive, have emotional dysregulation, and are harder to retain in SUD treatment programs.

For those in SUD treatment who have SUD+ADHD, the current best practices involve combining psychoeducation, CBT, appropriate medications for the patient's particular SUD, and adjunctive ADHD pharmacotherapy. Clinicians should prescribe abuse-resistant, sustained-release, or long-acting ADHD medications, using clinical strategies that help to prevent stimulant diversion/abuse. Together, these practices allow ADHD pharmacotherapies to be used with high levels of safety [715]. With careful selection, most ADHD pharmacotherapies can be used in conjunction with the pharmacotherapies used to treat SUDs. In addition, nonmedical treatment aimed at the patient's skill-building and developing compensatory strategies to minimize impairment from ADHD should be integrated into the conventional CBT and nonmedical therapies commonly used in programs treating SUDs.

There are a variety of resources available to assist clinicians in developing expertise in the treatment of patients with SUD+ADHD. Clinical expertise is crucial to address treatment challenges and promote better outcomes in patients with SUD+ADHD. Our knowledge and dissemination of the best practices for treatment of patients with SUD+ADHD has expanded exponentially, over the past decade. There is new energy focused on translating basic biological discoveries into clinically relevant interventions. New medications, with novel mechanisms of action, are in development. Innovative, nonmedical treatment modalities, including therapeutic video games and a variety of neuromodulatory interventions, show promise, but are not yet developed or tested enough to recommend for adults with SUD+ADHD. The clinical and research challenges are great, but much progress has been made, and our patients with SUD+ADHD will continue to be the beneficiaries of each new discovery.

References

1. Subcommittee on Attention-Deficit/Hyperactivity D, Steering Committee on Quality I, Management, Wolraich M, Brown L, Brown RT, DuPaul G,

Earls M, Feldman HM, Ganiats TG, Kaplanek B, Meyer B, Perrin J, Pierce K, Reiff M, Stein MT, Visser S. ADHD: Clinical practice guideline for the diagnosis, evaluation, and treatment of attention-deficit/hyperactivity disorder in children and adolescents. Pediatrics 2011;128(5):1007–22.
2. Wilens TE, Martelon M, Joshi G, Bateman C, Fried R, Petty C, Biederman J. Does ADHD predict substance-use disorders? A 10-year follow-up study of young adults with ADHD. J Am Acad Child Adolesc Psychiatry. 2011;50(6):543–53.
3. Icick R, Moggi F, Slobodin O, Dom G, Mathys F, van den Brink W, Levin FR, Blankers M, Kaye S, Demetrovics Z, van de Glind G, Velez-Pastrana MC, Schellekens ASA, ICASA Group. Attention deficit/hyperactivity disorder and global severity profiles in treatment-seeking patients with substance use disorders. Eur Addict Res 2020;26(4–5):201–10.
4. Molina BSG, Howard AL, Swanson JM, Stehli A, Mitchell JT, Kennedy TM, Epstein JN, Arnold LE, Hechtman L, Vitiello B, Hoza B. Substance use through adolescence into early adulthood after childhood-diagnosed ADHD: findings from the MTA longitudinal study. J Child Psychol Psychiatry. 2018;59(6):692–702.
5. Lee SS, Humphreys KL, Flory K, Liu R, Glass K. Prospective association of childhood attention-deficit/hyperactivity disorder (ADHD) and substance use and abuse/dependence: a meta-analytic review. Clin Psychol Rev. 2011;31(3):328–41.
6. Sibley MH, Arnold LE, Swanson JM, Hechtman LT, Kennedy TM, Owens E, BSG M, Jensen PS, Hinshaw SP, Roy A, Chronis-Tuscano A, Newcorn JH, Rohde LA, MTA Cooperative Group. Variable patterns of remission from ADHD in the Multimodal Treatment Study of ADHD. Am J Psychiatry. 2022;179(2):142–51.
7. Kaye S, Ramos-Quiroga JA, van de Glind G, Levin FR, Faraone SV, Allsop S, Degenhardt L, Moggi F, Barta C, Konstenius M, Franck J, Skutle A, Bu ET, Koeter MWJ, Demetrovics Z, Kapitany-Foveny M, Schoevers RA, van Emmerik-van Oortmerssen K, Carpentier PJ, Dom G, Verspreet S, Crunelle CL, Young JT, Carruthers S, Cassar J, Fatseas M, Auriacombe M, Johnson B, Dunn M, Slobodin O, van den Brink W. Persistence and subtype stability of ADHD among substance use disorder treatment seekers. J Atten Disord. 2019;23(12):1438–53.
8. Thapar A, Riglin L. The importance of a developmental perspective in psychiatry: what do recent genetic-epidemiological findings show? Mol Psychiatry. 2020;25(8):1631–9.
9. Barkley RA, Peters H. The earliest reference to ADHD in the medical literature? Melchior Adam Weikard's description in 1775 of "attention deficit" (Mangel der Aufmerksamkeit, Attentio Volubilis). J Atten Disord. 2012;16(8):623–30.
10. Still GF. The Goulstonian lectures on some abnormal psychical conditions in children. Lancet. 1902;159(4102):1008–13.
11. American Psychiatric Association. Diagnostic and Statistical Manual of Mental Disorders, 3rd edition (DSM-III). 3rd ed. American Psychiatric Association Press; 1980.
12. World Health Organization. Mental Disorders: Glossary and Guide to their Classification in Accordance with the Ninth Revision of the International Classification of Diseases (ICD-9). Geneva: WHO (World Health Organization); 1978.
13. Faraone SV. The worldwide prevalence of ADHD: is it an American condition? World J Psychiatry. 2003;2(2):104–13.
14. Timimi S, Taylor E. ADHD is best understood as a cultural construct. Br J Psychiatry. 2004;184(1):8–9.
15. Polanczyk G, de Lima MS, Horta BL, Biederman J, Rohde LA. The worldwide prevalence of ADHD: a systematic review and metaregression analysis. Am J Psychiatry. 2007;164(6):942–8.
16. Polanczyk GV, Willcutt EG, Salum GA, Kieling C, Rohde LA. ADHD prevalence estimates across three decades: an updated systematic review and meta-regression analysis. Int J Epidemiol. 2014;43(2):434–42.
17. McCabe SE, Dickinson K, West BT, Wilens TE. Age of onset, duration, and type of medication therapy for attention-deficit/hyperactivity disorder and substance use during adolescence: a multi-cohort national study. J Am Acad Child Adolesc Psychiatry. 2016;55(6):479–86.
18. Uchida M, Spencer TJ, Faraone SV, Biederman J. Adult outcome of ADHD: an overview of results from the MGH longitudinal family studies of pediatrically and psychiatrically referred youth with and without ADHD of both sexes. J Atten Disord. 2018;22(6):523–34.
19. Biederman J, DiSalvo M, Fried R, Woodworth KY, Biederman I, Faraone SV. Quantifying the protective effects of stimulants on functional outcomes in attention-deficit/hyperactivity disorder: a focus on number needed to treat statistic and sex effects. J Adolesc Health. 2019;65(6):784–9.
20. Coetzee C, Schellekens AFA, Truter I, Meyer A. Effect of past pharmacotherapy for attention-deficit/hyperactivity disorder on substance use disorder. Eur Addict Res. 2023;29(1):9–18.
21. Groenman AP, Oosterlaan J, Rommelse NN, Franke B, Greven CU, Hoekstra PJ, Hartman CA, Luman M, Roeyers H, Oades RD, Sergeant JA, Buitelaar JK, Faraone SV. Stimulant treatment for attention-deficit hyperactivity disorder and risk of developing substance use disorder. Br J Psychiatry. 2013;203(2):112–9.
22. Boland H, DiSalvo M, Fried R, Woodworth KY, Wilens T, Faraone SV, Biederman J. A literature review and meta-analysis on the effects of ADHD medications on functional outcomes. J Psychiatr Res. 2020;123:21–30.
23. Wilens TE, Woodward DW, Ko JD, Berger AF, Burke C, Yule AM. The impact of pharmacotherapy of childhood-onset psychiatric dis-

orders on the development of substance use disorders. J Child Adolesc Psychopharmacol. 2022;32(4):200–14.
24. Groenman AP, Schweren LJS, Weeda W, Luman M, Noordermeer SDS, Heslenfeld DJ, Franke B, Faraone SV, Rommelse N, Hartman CA, Hoekstra PJ, Buitelaar J, Oosterlaan J. Stimulant treatment profiles predicting co-occurring substance use disorders in individuals with attention-deficit/hyperactivity disorder. Eur Child Adolesc Psychiatry. 2019;28(9):1213–22.
25. McCabe SE, Schulenberg JE, Wilens TE, Schepis TS, McCabe VV, Veliz PT. Cocaine or methamphetamine use during young adulthood following stimulant use for attention-deficit/hyperactivity disorder during adolescence. JAMA Netw Open. 2023;6(7):e2322650.
26. Simon V, Czobor P, Balint S, Meszaros A, Bitter I. Prevalence and correlates of adult attention-deficit hyperactivity disorder: meta-analysis. Br J Psychiatry. 2009;194(3):204–11.
27. Song P, Zha M, Yang Q, Zhang Y, Li X, Rudan I. The prevalence of adult attention-deficit hyperactivity disorder: a global systematic review and meta-analysis. J Glob Health. 2021;11:04009.
28. Matte B, Anselmi L, Salum GA, Kieling C, Goncalves H, Menezes A, Grevet EH, Rohde LA. ADHD in DSM-5: a field trial in a large, representative sample of 18- to 19-year-old adults. Psychol Med. 2015;45(2):361–73.
29. Hinshaw SP, Nguyen PT, O'Grady SM, Rosenthal EA. Annual research review: attention-deficit/hyperactivity disorder in girls and women: underrepresentation, longitudinal processes, and key directions. J Child Psychol Psychiatry. 2022;63(4):484–96.
30. Mowlem FD, Rosenqvist MA, Martin J, Lichtenstein P, Asherson P, Larsson H. Sex differences in predicting ADHD clinical diagnosis and pharmacological treatment. Eur Child Adolesc Psychiatry. 2019;28(4):481–9.
31. Young S, Adamo N, Asgeirsdottir BB, Branney P, Beckett M, Colley W, Cubbin S, Deeley Q, Farrag E, Gudjonsson G, Hill P, Hollingdale J, Kilic O, Lloyd T, Mason P, Paliokosta E, Perecherla S, Sedgwick J, Skirrow C, Tierney K, van Rensburg K, Woodhouse E. Females with ADHD: an expert consensus statement taking a lifespan approach providing guidance for the identification and treatment of attention-deficit/ hyperactivity disorder in girls and women. BMC Psychiatry. 2020;20(1):404.
32. Skoglund C, Sundstrom Poromaa I, Leksell D, Ekholm Selling K, Cars T, Giacobini M, Young S, Kopp KH. Time after time: failure to identify and support females with ADHD - a Swedish population register study. J Child Psychol Psychiatry. 2023;65(6):832–44.
33. Ginsberg Y, Quintero J, Anand E, Casillas M, Upadhyaya HP. Underdiagnosis of attention-deficit/ hyperactivity disorder in adult patients: a review of the literature. Prim Care Companion CNS Disord. 2014;16(3):PCC.13r01600.
34. Oliva F, Malandrone F, Mirabella S, Ferreri P, di Girolamo G, Maina G. Diagnostic delay in ADHD: duration of untreated illness and its socio-demographic and clinical predictors in a sample of adult outpatients. Early Interv Psychiatry. 2021;15(4):957–65.
35. Fayyad J, De Graaf R, Kessler R, Alonso J, Angermeyer M, Demyttenaere K, De Girolamo G, Haro JM, Karam EG, Lara C, Lepine JP, Ormel J, Posada-Villa J, Zaslavsky AM, Jin R. Cross-national prevalence and correlates of adult attention-deficit hyperactivity disorder. Br J Psychiatry. 2007;190:402–9.
36. Fayyad J, Sampson NA, Hwang I, Adamowski T, Aguilar-Gaxiola S, Al-Hamzawi A, Andrade LH, Borges G, de Girolamo G, Florescu S, Gureje O, Haro JM, Hu C, Karam EG, Lee S, Navarro-Mateu F, O'Neill S, Pennell BE, Piazza M, Posada-Villa J, Ten Have M, Torres Y, Xavier M, Zaslavsky AM, Kessler RC, WHO World Mental Health Survey Collaborators. The descriptive epidemiology of DSM-IV adult ADHD in the World Health Organization world mental health surveys. Atten Defic Hyperact Disord. 2017;9(1):47–65.
37. Kooij JJS, Bijlenga D, Salerno L, Jaeschke R, Bitter I, Balazs J, Thome J, Dom G, Kasper S, Nunes Filipe C, Stes S, Mohr P, Leppamaki S, Casas M, Bobes J, McCarthy JM, Richarte V, Kjems Philipsen A, Pehlivanidis A, Niemela A, Styr B, Semerci B, Bolea-Alamanac B, Edvinsson D, Baeyens D, Wynchank D, Sobanski E, Philipsen A, McNicholas F, Caci H, Mihailescu I, Manor I, Dobrescu I, Saito T, Krause J, Fayyad J, Ramos-Quiroga JA, Foeken K, Rad F, Adamou M, Ohlmeier M, Fitzgerald M, Gill M, Lensing M, Motavalli Mukaddes N, Brudkiewicz P, Gustafsson P, Tani P, Oswald P, Carpentier PJ, De Rossi P, Delorme R, Markovska Simoska S, Pallanti S, Young S, Bejerot S, Lehtonen T, Kustow J, Muller-Sedgwick U, Hirvikoski T, Pironti V, Ginsberg Y, Felegyhazy Z, Garcia-Portilla MP, Asherson P. Updated European consensus statement on diagnosis and treatment of adult ADHD. Eur Psychiatry. 2019;56:14–34.
38. Deberdt W, Thome J, Lebrec J, Kraemer S, Fregenal I, Ramos-Quiroga JA, Arif M. Prevalence of ADHD in nonpsychotic adult psychiatric care (ADPSYC): a multinational cross-sectional study in Europe. BMC Psychiatry. 2015;15:242.
39. de Zwaan M, Gruss B, Muller A, Graap H, Martin A, Glaesmer H, Hilbert A, Philipsen A. The estimated prevalence and correlates of adult ADHD in a German community sample. Eur Arch Psychiatry Clin Neurosci. 2012;262(1):79–86.
40. Bachmann CJ, Philipsen A, Hoffmann F. ADHD in Germany: trends in diagnosis and pharmacotherapy. Dtsch Arztebl Int. 2017;114(9):141–8.
41. Dopfner M, Mandler J, Breuer D, Schurmann S, Dose C, Walter D, von Wirth E. Children with

attention-deficit/hyperactivity disorder grown up: an 18-year follow-up after multimodal treatment. J Atten Disord. 2021;25(13):1801–17.
42. Morstedt B, Corbisiero S, Bitto H, Stieglitz RD. Attention-deficit/hyperactivity disorder (ADHD) in adulthood: concordance and differences between self- and informant perspectives on symptoms and functional impairment. PLoS One. 2015;10(11):e0141342.
43. Barkley RA, Fischer M, Smallish L, Fletcher K. The persistence of attention-deficit/hyperactivity disorder into young adulthood as a function of reporting source and definition of disorder. J Abnorm Psychol. 2002;111(2):279–89.
44. Butzbach M, Fuermaier ABM, Aschenbrenner S, Weisbrod M, Tucha L, Tucha O. Metacognition, psychopathology and daily functioning in adult ADHD. J Clin Exp Neuropsychol. 2021;43(4):384–98.
45. Sibley MH, Mitchell JT, Becker SP. Method of adult diagnosis influences estimated persistence of childhood ADHD: a systematic review of longitudinal studies. Lancet Psychiatry. 2016;3(12):1157–65.
46. Spencer TJ, Adler LA, Meihua Q, Saylor KE, Brown TE, Holdnack JA, Schuh KJ, Trzepacz PT, Kelsey DK. Validation of the Adult ADHD Investigator Symptom Rating Scale (AISRS). J Atten Disord. 2010;14(1):57–68.
47. Chung W, Jiang SF, Paksarian D, Nikolaidis A, Castellanos FX, Merikangas KR, Milham MP. Trends in the prevalence and incidence of attention-deficit/hyperactivity disorder among adults and children of different racial and ethnic groups. JAMA Netw Open. 2019;2(11):e1914344.
48. Cenat JM, Blais-Rochette C, Morse C, Vandette MP, Noorishad PG, Kogan C, Ndengeyingoma A, Labelle PR. Prevalence and risk factors associated with attention-deficit/hyperactivity disorder among US Black individuals: a systematic review and meta-analysis. JAMA Psychiatry. 2021;78(1):21–8.
49. American Psychiatric Association. Diagnostic and Statistical Manual of Mental Disorders. 5th ed. Arlington: American Psychiatric Publishing, Inc.; 2013.
50. Polanczyk G, Caspi A, Houts R, Kollins SH, Rohde LA, Moffitt TE. Implications of extending the ADHD age-of-onset criterion to age 12: results from a prospectively studied birth cohort. J Am Acad Child Adolesc Psychiatry. 2010;49(3):210–6.
51. Kessler RC, Green JG, Adler LA, Barkley RA, Chatterji S, Faraone SV, Finkelman M, Greenhill LL, Gruber MJ, Jewell M, Russo LJ, Sampson NA, Van Brunt DL. Structure and diagnosis of adult attention-deficit/hyperactivity disorder: analysis of expanded symptom criteria from the Adult ADHD Clinical Diagnostic Scale. Arch Gen Psychiatry. 2010;67(11):1168–78.
52. Kooij JJS, Buitelaar JK, van den Oord EJ, Furer JW, Rijnders CA, Hodiamont PP. Internal and external validity of attention-deficit hyperactivity disorder in a population-based sample of adults. Psychol Med. 2005;35(6):817–27.
53. Joshi G, Faraone SV, Wozniak J, Tarko L, Fried R, Galdo M, Furtak SL, Biederman J. Symptom profile of ADHD in youth with high-functioning autism spectrum disorder: a comparative study in psychiatrically referred populations. J Atten Disord. 2017;21(10):846–55.
54. Valo S, Tannock R. Diagnostic instability of DSM-IV ADHD subtypes: effects of informant source, instrumentation, and methods for combining symptom reports. J Clin Child Adolesc Psychol. 2010;39(6):749–60.
55. Bonvicini C, Faraone SV, Scassellati C. Common and specific genes and peripheral biomarkers in children and adults with attention-deficit/hyperactivity disorder. World J Biol Psychiatry. 2018;19(2):80–100.
56. Breda V, Rohde LA, Menezes AMB, Anselmi L, Caye A, Rovaris DL, Vitola ES, Bau CHD, Grevet EH. The neurodevelopmental nature of attention-deficit hyperactivity disorder in adults. Br J Psychiatry. 2021;218(1):43–50.
57. Asherson P, Agnew-Blais J. Annual research review: does late-onset attention-deficit/hyperactivity disorder exist? J Child Psychol Psychiatry. 2019;60(4):333–52.
58. Faraone SV, Biederman J, Spencer T, Mick E, Murray K, Petty C, Adamson JJ, Monuteaux MC. Diagnosing adult attention deficit hyperactivity disorder: are late onset and subthreshold diagnoses valid? Am J Psychiatry. 2006;163(10):1720–9.
59. Milioni AL, Chaim TM, Cavallet M, de Oliveira NM, Annes M, Dos Santos B, Louza M, da Silva MA, Miguel CS, Serpa MH, Zanetti MV, Busatto G, Cunha PJ. High IQ may "mask" the diagnosis of ADHD by compensating for deficits in executive functions in treatment-naive adults with ADHD. J Atten Disord. 2017;21(6):455–64.
60. Antshel KM, Faraone SV, Maglione K, Doyle AE, Fried R, Seidman LJ, Biederman J. Executive functioning in high-IQ adults with ADHD. Psychol Med. 2010;40(11):1909–18.
61. Heidbreder R. ADHD symptomatology is best conceptualized as a spectrum: a dimensional versus unitary approach to diagnosis. Atten Defic Hyperact Disord. 2015;7(4):249–69.
62. Larsson H, Anckarsater H, Rastam M, Chang Z, Lichtenstein P. Childhood attention-deficit hyperactivity disorder as an extreme of a continuous trait: a quantitative genetic study of 8,500 twin pairs. J Child Psychol Psychiatry. 2012;53(1):73–80.
63. Batstra L, Frances A. Holding the line against diagnostic inflation in psychiatry. Psychother Psychosom. 2012;81(1):5–10.
64. Fabiano F, Haslam N. Diagnostic inflation in the DSM: a meta-analysis of changes in the stringency of psychiatric diagnosis from DSM-III to DSM-5. Clin Psychol Rev. 2020;80:101889.
65. Whelton PK, Carey RM, Aronow WS, Casey DE Jr, Collins KJ, Dennison Himmelfarb C, DePalma SM,

Gidding S, Jamerson KA, Jones DW, MacLaughlin EJ, Muntner P, Ovbiagele B, Smith SC Jr, Spencer CC, Stafford RS, Taler SJ, Thomas RJ, Williams KA Sr, Williamson JD, Wright JT Jr. 2017 ACC/AHA/AAPA/ABC/ACPM/AGS/APhA/ASH/ASPC/NMA/PCNA guideline for the prevention, detection, evaluation, and management of high blood pressure in adults: a report of the American College of Cardiology/American Heart Association Task Force on Clinical Practice Guidelines. Hypertension. 2018;71(6):e13–e115.

66. Wood DR, Reimherr FW, Wender PH, Johnson GE. Diagnosis and treatment of minimal brain dysfunction in adults: a preliminary report. Arch Gen Psychiatry. 1976;33(12):1453–60.
67. Weiss G, Hechtman L, Milroy T, Perlman T. Psychiatric status of hyperactives as adults: a controlled prospective 15-year follow-up of 63 hyperactive children. J Am Acad Child Psychiatry. 1985;24(2):211–20.
68. Hill JC, Schoener EP. Age-dependent decline of attention deficit hyperactivity disorder. Am J Psychiatry. 1996;153(9):1143–6.
69. Wilens TE, Biederman J, Faraone SV, Martelon M, Westerberg D, Spencer TJ. Presenting ADHD symptoms, subtypes, and comorbid disorders in clinically referred adults with ADHD. J Clin Psychiatry. 2009;70(11):1557–62.
70. Biederman J, Mick E, Faraone SV. Age-dependent decline of symptoms of attention deficit hyperactivity disorder: impact of remission definition and symptom type. Am J Psychiatry. 2000;157(5):816–8.
71. Faraone SV, Biederman J, Mick E. The age-dependent decline of attention deficit hyperactivity disorder: a meta-analysis of follow-up studies. Psychol Med. 2006;36(2):159–65.
72. Roy A, Hechtman L, Arnold LE, Sibley MH, Molina BS, Swanson JM, Howard AL, MTA Cooperative Group. Childhood factors affecting persistence and desistence of attention-deficit/hyperactivity disorder symptoms in adulthood: results from the MTA. J Am Acad Child Adolesc Psychiatry. 2016;55(11):937–44.e4.
73. Michielsen M, de Kruif J, Comijs HC, van Mierlo S, Semeijn EJ, Beekman ATF, Deeg DJH, Kooij JJS. The burden of ADHD in older adults: a qualitative study. J Atten Disord. 2018;22(6):591–600.
74. Goodman DW, Mitchell S, Rhodewalt L, Surman CB. Clinical presentation, diagnosis and treatment of attention-deficit hyperactivity disorder (ADHD) in older adults: a review of the evidence and its implications for clinical care. Drugs Aging. 2016;33(1):27–36.
75. Barkley RA, Fischer M. The unique contribution of emotional impulsiveness to impairment in major life activities in hyperactive children as adults. J Am Acad Child Adolesc Psychiatry. 2010;49(5):503–13.
76. Weibel S, Bicego F, Muller S, Martz E, Costache ME, Kraemer C, Bertschy G, Lopez R, Weiner L. Two facets of emotion dysregulation are core symptomatic domains in adult ADHD: results from the SR-WRAADDS, a broad symptom self-report questionnaire. J Atten Disord. 2022;26(5):767–78.
77. Faraone SV, Rostain AL, Blader J, Busch B, Childress AC, Connor DF, Newcorn JH. Practitioner review: emotional dysregulation in attention-deficit/hyperactivity disorder - implications for clinical recognition and intervention. J Child Psychol Psychiatry. 2019;60(2):133–50.
78. Reimherr FW, Roesler M, Marchant BK, Gift TE, Retz W, Philipp-Wiegmann F, Reimherr ML. Types of adult attention-deficit/hyperactivity disorder: a replication analysis. J Clin Psychiatry. 2020;81(2):19m13077.
79. Van den Driessche C, Bastian M, Peyre H, Stordeur C, Acquaviva E, Bahadori S, Delorme R, Sackur J. Attentional lapses in attention-deficit/hyperactivity disorder: blank rather than wandering thoughts. Psychol Sci. 2017;28(10):1375–86.
80. Durand G, Arbone IS. Exploring the relationship between ADHD, its common comorbidities, and their relationship to organizational skills. Peer J. 2022;10:e12836.
81. Barkley RA. Differential diagnosis of adults with ADHD: the role of executive function and self-regulation. J Clin Psychiatry. 2010;71(7):e17.
82. Surman CB, Biederman J, Spencer T, Miller CA, McDermott KM, Faraone SV. Understanding deficient emotional self-regulation in adults with attention deficit hyperactivity disorder: a controlled study. Atten Defic Hyperact Disord. 2013;5(3):273–81.
83. Skirrow C, Asherson P. Emotional lability, comorbidity and impairment in adults with attention-deficit hyperactivity disorder. J Affect Disord. 2013;147(1–3):80–6.
84. Silverstein MJ, Faraone SV, Leon T, Biederman J, Spencer TJ, Adler L, editors. The influence of ADHD symptoms and executive function deficits on global impairment and quality of life. Association for Behavioral and Cognitive Therapies Annual Convention. Washington, D.C., 2018.
85. Hui XG, Chua ACK, Singh H. Variable attention stimulus trait (VAST) spectrum traits: a brief discussion on attentional control & emotional regulation in attention deficit-hyperactivity disorder (ADHD). Asian J Interdiscipl Res. 2023;6(2):9–16.
86. Biederman J, Lanier J, DiSalvo M, Noyes E, Fried R, Woodworth KY, Biederman I, Faraone SV. Clinical correlates of mind wandering in adults with ADHD. J Psychiatr Res. 2019;117:15–23.
87. Biederman J, DiSalvo M, Woodworth KY, Fried R, Uchida M, Biederman I, Spencer TJ, Surman C, Faraone SV. Toward operationalizing deficient emotional self-regulation in newly referred adults with ADHD: a receiver operator characteristic curve analysis. Eur Psychiatry. 2020;63(1):e21.
88. Adler LA, Faraone SV, Spencer TJ, Berglund P, Alperin S, Kessler RC. The structure of

adult ADHD. Int J Methods Psychiatr Res. 2017;26(1):e1555.
89. Silverstein MJ, Faraone SV, Leon TL, Biederman J, Spencer TJ, Adler LA. The relationship between executive function deficits and DSM-5-defined ADHD symptoms. J Atten Disord. 2020;24(1):41–51.
90. Biederman J, Petty CR, Fried R, Kaiser R, Dolan CR, Schoenfeld S, Doyle AE, Seidman LJ, Faraone SV. Educational and occupational underattainment in adults with attention-deficit/hyperactivity disorder: a controlled study. J Clin Psychiatry. 2008;69(8):1217–22.
91. de Graaf R, Kessler RC, Fayyad J, ten Have M, Alonso J, Angermeyer M, Borges G, Demyttenaere K, Gasquet I, de Girolamo G, Haro JM, Jin R, Karam EG, Ormel J, Posada-Villa J. The prevalence and effects of adult attention-deficit/hyperactivity disorder (ADHD) on the performance of workers: results from the WHO World Mental Health Survey Initiative. Occup Environ Med. 2008;65(12):835–42.
92. Fredriksen M, Dahl AA, Martinsen EW, Klungsoyr O, Faraone SV, Peleikis DE. Childhood and persistent ADHD symptoms associated with educational failure and long-term occupational disability in adult ADHD. Atten Defic Hyperact Disord. 2014;6(2):87–99.
93. Erskine HE, Norman RE, Ferrari AJ, Chan GC, Copeland WE, Whiteford HA, Scott JG. Long-term outcomes of attention-deficit/hyperactivity disorder and conduct disorder: a systematic review and meta-analysis. J Am Acad Child Adolesc Psychiatry. 2016;55(10):841–50.
94. Altszuler AR, Page TF, Gnagy EM, Coxe S, Arrieta A, Molina BS, Pelham WE Jr. Financial dependence of young adults with childhood ADHD. J Abnorm Child Psychol. 2016;44(6):1217–29.
95. Biederman J, Faraone SV, Spencer TJ, Mick E, Monuteaux MC, Aleardi M. Functional impairments in adults with self-reports of diagnosed ADHD: a controlled study of 1001 adults in the community. J Clin Psychiatry. 2006;67(4):524–40.
96. Hechtman L, Swanson JM, Sibley MH, Stehli A, Owens EB, Mitchell JT, Arnold LE, Molina BS, Hinshaw SP, Jensen PS, Abikoff HB, Perez Algorta G, Howard AL, Hoza B, Etcovitch J, Houssais S, Lakes KD, Nichols JQ, MTA Cooperative Group . Functional adult outcomes 16 years after childhood diagnosis of attention-deficit/hyperactivity disorder: MTA results. J Am Acad Child Adolesc Psychiatry. 2016;55(11):945–52.e2.
97. Kupper T, Haavik J, Drexler H, Ramos-Quiroga JA, Wermelskirchen D, Prutz C, Schauble B. The negative impact of attention-deficit/hyperactivity disorder on occupational health in adults and adolescents. Int Arch Occup Environ Health. 2012;85(8):837–47.
98. Beauchaine TP, Ben-David I, Sela A. Attention-deficit/hyperactivity disorder, delay discounting, and risky financial behaviors: a preliminary analysis of self-report data. PLoS One. 2017;12(5):e0176933.
99. Bangma DF, Tucha L, Fuermaier ABM, Tucha O, Koerts J. Financial decision-making in a community sample of adults with and without current symptoms of ADHD. PLoS One. 2020;15(10):e0239343.
100. Koerts J, Bangma DF, Fuermaier ABM, Mette C, Tucha L, Tucha O. Financial judgment determination in adults with ADHD. J Neural Transm (Vienna). 2021;128(7):969–79.
101. Daley D, Jacobsen RH, Lange AM, Sorensen A, Walldorf J. The economic burden of adult attention deficit hyperactivity disorder: a sibling comparison cost analysis. Eur Psychiatry. 2019;61:41–8.
102. Vergunst F, Commisso M, Geoffroy MC, Temcheff C, Poirier M, Park J, Vitaro F, Tremblay R, Cote S, Orri M. Association of childhood externalizing, internalizing, and comorbid symptoms with long-term economic and social outcomes. JAMA Netw Open. 2023;6(1):e2249568.
103. Koepp AE, Watts TW, Gershoff ET, Ahmed SF, Davis-Kean P, Duncan GJ, Kuhfeld M, Vandell DL. Attention and behavior problems in childhood predict adult financial status, health, and criminal activity: a conceptual replication and extension of Moffitt et al. (2011) using cohorts from the United States and the United Kingdom. Dev Psychol. 2023;59(8):1389–406.
104. Asherson P, Akehurst R, Kooij JJS, Huss M, Beusterien K, Sasane R, Gholizadeh S, Hodgkins P. Under diagnosis of adult ADHD: cultural influences and societal burden. J Atten Disord. 2012;16(5 Suppl):20S–38S.
105. Curry AE, Yerys BE, Metzger KB, Carey ME, Power TJ. Traffic crashes, violations, and suspensions among young drivers with ADHD. Pediatrics. 2019;143(6):e20182305.
106. Sobanski E, Sabljic D, Alm B, Skopp G, Kettler N, Mattern R, Strohbeck-Kuhner P. Driving-related risks and impact of methylphenidate treatment on driving in adults with attention-deficit/hyperactivity disorder (ADHD). J Neural Transm (Vienna). 2008;115(2):347–56.
107. Nelson LD, Guskiewicz KM, Marshall SW, Hammeke T, Barr W, Randolph C, McCrea MA. Multiple self-reported concussions are more prevalent in athletes with ADHD and learning disability. Clin J Sport Med. 2016;26(2):120–7.
108. Chang C, Putukian M, Aerni G, Diamond A, Hong G, Ingram Y, Reardon CL, Wolanin A. Mental health issues and psychological factors in athletes: detection, management, effect on performance and prevention: American Medical Society for Sports Medicine Position Statement-Executive Summary. Br J Sports Med. 2020;54(4):216–20.
109. Kittel-Schneider S, Wolff S, Queiser K, Wessendorf L, Meier AM, Verdenhalven M, Brunkhorst-Kanaan N, Grimm O, McNeill R, Grabow S, Reimertz C, Nau C, Klos M, Reif A. Prevalence of ADHD in accident victims: results of the PRADA study. J Clin Med. 2019;8(10):1643.

110. Bron TI, Bijlenga D, Breuk M, Michielsen M, Beekman ATF, Kooij JJS. Risk factors for adverse driving outcomes in Dutch adults with ADHD and controls. Accid Anal Prev. 2018;111:338–44.
111. Brunkhorst-Kanaan N, Libutzki B, Reif A, Larsson H, McNeill RV, Kittel-Schneider S. ADHD and accidents over the life span - a systematic review. Neurosci Biobehav Rev. 2021;125:582–91.
112. Dalsgaard S, Ostergaard SD, Leckman JF, Mortensen PB, Pedersen MG. Mortality in children, adolescents, and adults with attention deficit hyperactivity disorder: a nationwide cohort study. Lancet. 2015;385(9983):2190–6.
113. Sun S, Kuja-Halkola R, Faraone SV, D'Onofrio BM, Dalsgaard S, Chang Z, Larsson H. Association of psychiatric comorbidity with the risk of premature death among children and adults with attention-deficit/hyperactivity disorder. JAMA Psychiatry. 2019;76(11):1141–9.
114. Weye N, Momen NC, Christensen MK, Iburg KM, Dalsgaard S, Laursen TM, Mortensen PB, Santomauro DF, Scott JG, Whiteford HA, McGrath JJ, Plana-Ripoll O. Association of specific mental disorders with premature mortality in the Danish population using alternative measurement methods. JAMA Netw Open. 2020;3(6):e206646.
115. Nigg JT. Attention-deficit/hyperactivity disorder and adverse health outcomes. Clin Psychol Rev. 2013;33(2):215–28.
116. Chronis-Tuscano A, Molina BS, Pelham WE, Applegate B, Dahlke A, Overmyer M, Lahey BB. Very early predictors of adolescent depression and suicide attempts in children with attention-deficit/hyperactivity disorder. Arch Gen Psychiatry. 2010;67(10):1044–51.
117. Stickley A, Tachimori H, Inoue Y, Shinkai T, Yoshimura R, Nakamura J, Morita G, Nishii S, Tokutsu Y, Otsuka Y, Egashira K, Inoue M, Kubo T, Tesen H, Takashima N, Tominaga H, Koyanagi A, Kamio Y. Attention-deficit/hyperactivity disorder symptoms and suicidal behavior in adult psychiatric outpatients. Psychiatry Clin Neurosci. 2018;72(9):713–22.
118. Hinshaw SP, Owens EB, Zalecki C, Huggins SP, Montenegro-Nevado AJ, Schrodek E, Swanson EN. Prospective follow-up of girls with attention-deficit/hyperactivity disorder into early adulthood: continuing impairment includes elevated risk for suicide attempts and self-injury. J Consult Clin Psychol. 2012;80(6):1041–51.
119. Beauchaine TP, Hinshaw SP, Bridge JA. Nonsuicidal self-injury and suicidal behaviors in girls: the case for targeted prevention in preadolescence. Clin Psychol Sci. 2019;7(4):643–67.
120. Chen VC, Chan HL, Wu SI, Lee M, Lu ML, Liang HY, Dewey ME, Stewart R, Lee CT. Attention-deficit/hyperactivity disorder and mortality risk in Taiwan. JAMA Netw Open. 2019;2(8):e198714.
121. Biederman J, Fried R, Hammerness P, Surman C, Mehler B, Petty CR, Faraone SV, Miller C, Bourgeois M, Meller B, Godfrey KM, Reimer B. The effects of lisdexamfetamine dimesylate on the driving performance of young adults with ADHD: a randomized, double-blind, placebo-controlled study using a validated driving simulator paradigm. J Psychiatr Res. 2012;46(4):484–91.
122. Chang Z, Quinn PD, Hur K, Gibbons RD, Sjolander A, Larsson H, D'Onofrio BM. Association between medication use for attention-deficit/hyperactivity disorder and risk of motor vehicle crashes. JAMA Psychiatry. 2017;74(6):597–603.
123. Chang Z, Quinn PD, O'Reilly L, Sjolander A, Hur K, Gibbons R, Larsson H, D'Onofrio BM. Medication for attention-deficit/hyperactivity disorder and risk for suicide attempts. Biol Psychiatry. 2020;88(6):452–8.
124. Chang Z, Ghirardi L, Quinn PD, Asherson P, D'Onofrio BM, Larsson H. Risks and benefits of attention-deficit/hyperactivity disorder medication on behavioral and neuropsychiatric outcomes: a qualitative review of pharmacoepidemiology studies using linked prescription databases. Biol Psychiatry. 2019;86(5):335–43.
125. Vogel SWN, Bijlenga D, Benjamins JS, Beekman ATF, Kooij JJS, Van Someren EJW. Attention deficit hyperactivity disorder symptom severity and sleep problems in adult participants of The Netherlands sleep registry. Sleep Med. 2017;40:94–102.
126. Bijlenga D, Vollebregt MA, Kooij JJS, Arns M. The role of the circadian system in the etiology and pathophysiology of ADHD: time to redefine ADHD? Atten Defic Hyperact Disord. 2019;11(1):5–19.
127. Wynchank DS, Bijlenga D, Lamers F, Bron TI, Winthorst WH, Vogel SW, Penninx BW, Beekman AT, Kooij JJS. ADHD, circadian rhythms and seasonality. J Psychiatr Res. 2016;81:87–94.
128. Shen C, Luo Q, Chamberlain SR, Morgan S, Romero-Garcia R, Du J, Zhao X, Touchette E, Montplaisir J, Vitaro F, Boivin M, Tremblay RE, Zhao XM, Robaey P, Feng J, Sahakian BJ. What is the link between attention-deficit/hyperactivity disorder and sleep disturbance? A multimodal examination of longitudinal relationships and brain structure using large-scale population-based cohorts. Biol Psychiatry. 2020;88(6):459–69.
129. Hanc T, Cortese S. Attention deficit/hyperactivity-disorder and obesity: a review and model of current hypotheses explaining their comorbidity. Neurosci Biobehav Rev. 2018;92:16–28.
130. Khalife N, Kantomaa M, Glover V, Tammelin T, Laitinen J, Ebeling H, Hurtig T, Jarvelin MR, Rodriguez A. Childhood attention-deficit/hyperactivity disorder symptoms are risk factors for obesity and physical inactivity in adolescence. J Am Acad Child Adolesc Psychiatry. 2014;53(4):425–36.
131. Barker ED, Ing A, Biondo F, Jia T, Pingault JB, Du Rietz E, Zhang Y, Ruggeri B, Banaschewski T, Hohmann S, ALW B, Bromberg U, Buchel C, Quinlan EB, Sounga-Barke E, Bowling AB, Desrivieres S, Flor H, Frouin V, Garavan H,

Asherson P, Gowland P, Heinz A, Ittermann B, Martinot JL, Martinot MP, Nees F, Papadopoulos-Orfanos D, Poustka L, Smolka MN, Vetter NC, Walter H, Whelan R, Schumann G, IMAGEN Consortium. Do ADHD-impulsivity and BMI have shared polygenic and neural correlates? Mol Psychiatry. 2021;26(3):1019–28.
132. Cortese S, Faraone SV, Bernardi S, Wang S, Blanco C. Adult attention-deficit hyperactivity disorder and obesity: epidemiological study. Br J Psychiatry. 2013;203(1):24–34.
133. Yao S, Kuja-Halkola R, Martin J, Lu Y, Lichtenstein P, Norring C, Birgegard A, Yilmaz Z, Hubel C, Watson H, Baker J, Almqvist C, Eating Disorders Working Group of the Psychiatric Genomics Consortium, Thornton LM, Magnusson PK, Bulik CM, Larsson H. Associations between attention-deficit/hyperactivity disorder and various eating disorders: a Swedish nationwide population study using multiple genetically informative approaches. Biol Psychiatry. 2019;86(8):577–86.
134. El Ayoubi H, Barrault S, Gateau A, Cortese S, Frammery J, Mollat E, Bonnet-Brilhault F, Grall-Bronnec M, Ballon N, Brunault P. Adult attention-deficit/hyperactivity disorder among alcohol use disorder inpatients is associated with food addiction and binge eating, but not BMI. Appetite. 2022;168:105665.
135. Martin E, Dourish CT, Higgs S. Interoceptive accuracy mediates the longitudinal relationship between attention deficit hyperactivity disorder (ADHD) inattentive symptoms and disordered eating in a community sample. Physiol Behav. 2023;268:114220.
136. Schneider E, Martin E, Rotshtein P, Qureshi KL, Chamberlain SR, Spetter MS, Dourish CT, Higgs S. The effects of lisdexamfetamine dimesylate on eating behaviour and homeostatic, reward and cognitive processes in women with binge-eating symptoms: an experimental medicine study. Transl Psychiatry. 2022;12(1):9.
137. Li L, Chang Z, Sun J, Garcia-Argibay M, Du Rietz E, Dobrosavljevic M, Brikell I, Jernberg T, Solmi M, Cortese S, Larsson H. Attention-deficit/hyperactivity disorder as a risk factor for cardiovascular diseases: a nationwide population-based cohort study. World Psychiatry. 2022;21(3):452–9.
138. Garcia-Argibay M, du Rietz E, Lu Y, Martin J, Haan E, Lehto K, Bergen SE, Lichtenstein P, Larsson H, Brikell I. The role of ADHD genetic risk in mid-to-late life somatic health conditions. Transl Psychiatry. 2022;12(1):152.
139. Kittel-Schneider S, Arteaga-Henriquez G, Vasquez AA, Asherson P, Banaschewski T, Brikell I, Buitelaar J, Cormand B, Faraone SV, Freitag CM, Ginsberg Y, Haavik J, Hartman CA, Kuntsi J, Larsson H, Matura S, McNeill RV, Ramos-Quiroga JA, Ribases M, Romanos M, Vainieri I, Franke B, Reif A. Non-mental diseases associated with ADHD across the lifespan: fidgety Philipp and Pippi Longstocking at risk of multimorbidity? Neurosci Biobehav Rev. 2022;132:1157–80.
140. Garcia-Argibay M, Li L, Du Rietz E, Zhang L, Yao H, Jendle J, Ramos-Quiroga JA, Ribases M, Chang Z, Brikell I, Cortese S, Larsson H. The association between type 2 diabetes and attention- deficit/hyperactivity disorder: a systematic review, meta-analysis, and population-based sibling study. Neurosci Biobehav Rev. 2023;147:105076.
141. Garcia-Argibay M, Pandya E, Ahnemark E, Werner-Kiechle T, Andersson LM, Larsson H, Du Rietz E. Healthcare utilization and costs of psychiatric and somatic comorbidities associated with newly diagnosed adult ADHD. Acta Psychiatr Scand. 2021;144(1):50–9.
142. Wymbs BT, Canu WH, Sacchetti GM, Ranson LM. Adult ADHD and romantic relationships: what we know and what we can do to help. J Marital Fam Ther. 2021;47(3):664–81.
143. VanderDrift LE, Antshel KM, Olszewski AK. Inattention and hyperactivity-impulsivity: their detrimental effect on romantic relationship maintenance. J Atten Disord. 2019;23(9):985–94.
144. Simmons JA, Antshel KM. Bullying and depression in youth with ADHD: a systematic review. Child Youth Care Forum. 2020;50(3):379–414.
145. Harpin V, Mazzone L, Raynaud JP, Kahle J, Hodgkins P. Long-term outcomes of ADHD: a systematic review of self-esteem and social function. J Atten Disord. 2016;20(4):295–305.
146. Stickley A, Koyanagi A, Takahashi H, Ruchkin V, Kamio Y. Attention-deficit/hyperactivity disorder symptoms and loneliness among adults in the general population. Res Dev Disabil. 2017;62:115–23.
147. Michielsen M, Comijs HC, Aartsen MJ, Semeijn EJ, Beekman AT, Deeg DJ. The relationships between ADHD and social functioning and participation in older adults in a population-based study. J Attent Disord. 2015;19(5):368–79.
148. Young S, Klassen LJ, Reitmeier SD, Matheson JD, Gudjonsson GH. Let's talk about sex... And ADHD: findings from an anonymous online survey. Int J Environ Res Public Health. 2023;20(3):2037.
149. Ostergaard SD. Teenage parenthood and birth rates for individuals with and without attention-deficit/hyperactivity disorder: a nationwide cohort study. J Am Acad Child Adolesc Psychiatry. 2017;56(7):578–84.
150. Skoglund C, Kopp Kallner H, Skalkidou A, Wikstrom AK, Lundin C, Hesselman S, Wikman A, Sundstrom PI. Association of attention-deficit/hyperactivity disorder with teenage birth among women and girls in Sweden. JAMA Netw Open. 2019;2(10):e1912463.
151. Owens EB, Hinshaw SP. Adolescent mediators of unplanned pregnancy among women with and without childhood ADHD. J Clin Child Adolesc Psychol. 2020;49(2):229–38.
152. Meinzer MC, LeMoine KA, Howard AL, Stehli A, Arnold LE, Hechtman L, Hinshaw SP, Molina BSG, Murray DW, Sibley MH, Swanson JM, Tamm L,

Chronis-Tuscano A. Childhood ADHD and involvement in early pregnancy: mechanisms of risk. J Atten Disord. 2020;24(14):1955–65.
153. Hua MH, Huang KL, Hsu JW, Bai YM, Su TP, Tsai SJ, Li CT, Lin WC, Chen TJ, Chen MH. Early pregnancy risk among adolescents with ADHD: a nationwide longitudinal study. J Atten Disord. 2021;25(9):1199–206.
154. Flory K, Molina BS, Pelham WE Jr, Gnagy E, Smith B. Childhood ADHD predicts risky sexual behavior in young adulthood. J Clin Child Adolesc Psychol. 2006;35(4):571–7.
155. Arrondo G, Osorio A, Magallon S, Lopez-Del Burgo C, Cortese S. Attention-deficit/hyperactivity disorder as a risk factor for being involved in intimate partner violence and sexual violence: a systematic review and meta-analysis. Psychol Med. 2023;1-10
156. Bijlenga D, Vroege JA, Stammen AJM, Breuk M, Boonstra AM, van der Rhee K, Kooij JJS. Prevalence of sexual dysfunctions and other sexual disorders in adults with attention-deficit/hyperactivity disorder compared to the general population. Atten Defic Hyperact Disord. 2018;10(1):87–96.
157. Soldati L, Bianchi-Demicheli F, Schockaert P, Kohl J, Bolmont M, Hasler R, Perroud N. Sexual function, sexual dysfunctions, and ADHD: a systematic literature review. J Sex Med. 2020;17(9):1653–64.
158. Chronis-Tuscano A, Seymour KE, Stein MA, Jones HA, Jiles CD, Rooney ME, Conlon CJ, Efron LA, Wagner SA, Pian J, Robb AS. Efficacy of osmotic-release oral system (OROS) methylphenidate for mothers with attention-deficit/hyperactivity disorder (ADHD): preliminary report of effects on ADHD symptoms and parenting. J Clin Psychiatry. 2008;69(12):1938–47.
159. Johnston C, Mash EJ, Miller N, Ninowski JE. Parenting in adults with attention-deficit/hyperactivity disorder (ADHD). Clin Psychol Rev. 2012;32(4):215–28.
160. Chronis-Tuscano A. The relation between maternal ADHD symptoms & improvement in child behavior following brief behavioral parent training is mediated by change in negative parenting. J Abnorm Child Psychol 2011;39(7):1047–57.
161. Starck M, Grunwald J, Schlarb AA. Occurrence of ADHD in parents of ADHD children in a clinical sample. Neuropsychiatr Dis Treat. 2016;12:581–8.
162. Insa Pineda I, Huguet Miguel A, Chamorro Fernandez M, Espadas Tejerina M, Gonzalez CLG, Alda JA. ADHD symptoms, academic and social difficulties in parents of children with ADHD. Psychiatry. 2020;83(3):231–43.
163. Sonuga-Barke EJ, Daley D, Thompson M. Does maternal ADHD reduce the effectiveness of parent training for preschool children's ADHD? J Am Acad Child Adolesc Psychiatry. 2002;41(6):696–702.
164. Chronis-Tuscano A, French W, Strickland J, Sasser T, Gonzalez ENS, Whitlock KB, Stein MA. Acute effects of parent stimulant medication versus behavioral parent training on mothers' ADHD, parenting behavior, and at-risk children. J Clin Psychiatry. 2020;81(5):19m13173.
165. Waxmonsky JG, Waschbusch DA, Babinski DE, Humphrey HH, Alfonso A, Crum KI, Bernstein M, Slavec J, Augustus JN, Pelham WE. Does pharmacological treatment of ADHD in adults enhance parenting performance? Results of a double-blind randomized trial. CNS Drugs. 2014;28(7):665–77.
166. Babinski DE, Waxmonsky JG, Waschbusch DA, Humphery H, Pelham WE Jr. Parent-reported improvements in family functioning in a randomized controlled trial of lisdexamfetamine for treatment of parental attention-deficit/hyperactivity disorder. J Child Adolesc Psychopharmacol. 2017;27(3):250–7.
167. Anker E, Ginsberg Y, Heir T. Prevalence of criminal convictions in Norwegian adult ADHD outpatients and associations with ADHD symptom severity and emotional dysregulation. BMC Psychiatry. 2021;21(1):226.
168. Barkley RA, Cox D. A review of driving risks and impairments associated with attention-deficit/hyperactivity disorder and the effects of stimulant medication on driving performance. J Saf Res. 2007;38(1):113–28.
169. Fuermaier AB, Tucha L, Evans BL, Koerts J, de Waard D, Brookhuis K, Aschenbrenner S, Thome J, Lange KW, Tucha O. Driving and attention deficit hyperactivity disorder. J Neural Transm (Vienna). 2017;124(Suppl 1):55–67.
170. Mohr-Jensen C, Steinhausen HC. A meta-analysis and systematic review of the risks associated with childhood attention-deficit hyperactivity disorder on long-term outcome of arrests, convictions, and incarcerations. Clin Psychol Rev. 2016;48:32–42.
171. Dalsgaard S, Mortensen PB, Frydenberg M, Thomsen PH. Long-term criminal outcome of children with attention deficit hyperactivity disorder. Crim Behav Ment Health. 2013;23(2):86–98.
172. Young S, Moss D, Sedgwick O, Fridman M, Hodgkins P. A meta-analysis of the prevalence of attention deficit hyperactivity disorder in incarcerated populations. Psychol Med. 2015;45(2):247–58.
173. Konstenius M, Larsson H, Lundholm L, Philips B, van de Glind G, Jayaram-Lindstrom N, Franck J. An epidemiological study of ADHD, substance use, and comorbid problems in incarcerated women in Sweden. J Atten Disord. 2015;19(1):44–52.
174. Velez-Pastrana MC, Gonzalez RA, Ramos-Fernandez A, Ramirez Padilla RR, Levin FR, Albizu GC. Attention deficit hyperactivity disorder in prisoners: increased substance use disorder severity and psychiatric comorbidity. Eur Addict Res. 2020;26(4–5):179–90.
175. Roman-Ithier JC, Gonzalez RA, Velez-Pastrana MC, Gonzalez-Tejera GM, Albizu-Garcia CE. Attention deficit hyperactivity disorder symptoms, type of offending and recidivism in a prison population: the role of substance dependence. Crim Behav Ment Health. 2017;27(5):443–56.

176. Philipp-Wiegmann F, Rosler M, Clasen O, Zinnow T, Retz-Junginger P, Retz W. ADHD modulates the course of delinquency: a 15-year follow-up study of young incarcerated man. Eur Arch Psychiatry Clin Neurosci. 2018;268(4):391–9.
177. Young S, Gudjonsson GH, Wells J, Asherson P, Theobald D, Oliver B, Scott C, Mooney A. Attention deficit hyperactivity disorder and critical incidents in a Scottish prison population. Personal Individual Differen. 2009;46(3):265–9.
178. Young S, Cocallis K. ADHD and offending. J Neural Transm (Vienna). 2021;128(7):1009–19.
179. Polyzoi M, Ahnemark E, Medin E, Ginsberg Y. Estimated prevalence and incidence of diagnosed ADHD and health care utilization in adults in Sweden—a longitudinal population-based register study. Neuropsychiatr Dis Treat. 2018;14:1149–61.
180. Fahrendorff AM, Pagsberg AK, Kessing LV, Maigaard K. Psychiatric comorbidity in patients with pediatric bipolar disorder—a systematic review. Acta Psychiatr Scand. 2023;148(2):110–32.
181. Geller B, Tillman R, Bolhofner K, Zimerman B, Strauss NA, Kaufmann P. Controlled, blindly rated, direct-interview family study of a prepubertal and early-adolescent bipolar I disorder phenotype: morbid risk, age at onset, and comorbidity. Arch Gen Psychiatry. 2006;63(10):1130–8.
182. Etain B, Lajnef M, Loftus J, Henry C, Raust A, Gard S, Kahn JP, Leboyer M, Scott J, Bellivier F. Association between childhood dimensions of attention deficit hyperactivity disorder and adulthood clinical severity of bipolar disorders. Aust N Z J Psychiatry. 2017;51(4):382–92.
183. Schiweck C, Arteaga-Henriquez G, Aichholzer M, Edwin Thanarajah S, Vargas-Caceres S, Matura S, Grimm O, Haavik J, Kittel-Schneider S, Ramos-Quiroga JA, Faraone SV, Reif A. Comorbidity of ADHD and adult bipolar disorder: a systematic review and meta-analysis. Neurosci Biobehav Rev. 2021;124:100–23.
184. Badrfam R, Zandifar A, Barkhori Mehni M, Farid M, Rahiminejad F. Comorbidity of adult ADHD and substance use disorder in a sample of inpatients bipolar disorder in Iran. BMC Psychiatry. 2022;22(1):480.
185. O'Connell KS, Shadrin A, Bahrami S, Smeland OB, Bettella F, Frei O, Krull F, Askeland RB, Walters GB, Daviethsdottir K, Haraldsdottir GS, Guethmundsson OO, Stefansson H, Fan CC, Steen NE, Reichborn-Kjennerud T, Dale AM, Stefansson K, Djurovic S, Andreassen OA. Identification of genetic overlap and novel risk loci for attention-deficit/hyperactivity disorder and bipolar disorder. Mol Psychiatry. 2021;26(8):4055–65.
186. Bernardi S, Faraone SV, Cortese S, Kerridge BT, Pallanti S, Wang S, Blanco C. The lifetime impact of attention deficit hyperactivity disorder: results from the National Epidemiologic Survey on Alcohol and Related Conditions (NESARC). Psychol Med. 2012;42(4):875–87.
187. Lieslehto J, Tiihonen J, Lahteenvuo M, Mittendorfer-Rutz E, Tanskanen A, Taipale H. Comparative effectiveness of pharmacotherapies for the risk of attempted or completed suicide among persons with borderline personality disorder. JAMA Netw Open. 2023;6(6):e2317130.
188. Brynte C, Aeschlimann M, Barta C, Begeman AHA, Backer A, Crunelle CL, Daigre C, De Fuentes-Merillas L, Demetrovics Z, Dom G, Lopez LG, Icick R, Johnson B, Joostens P, Kapitany-Foveny M, Karsinti E, Kiefer F, Konstenius M, Levin FR, Luderer M, Markus W, Matthys F, Moggi F, Palma-Alvarez RF, Paraskevopoulou M, Ramos-Quiroga JA, Schellekens A, Soravia LM, Therribout N, Thomas A, van de Glind G, van Kernebeek MW, Vollstadt-Klein S, Vorspan F, van den Brink W, Franck J. The clinical course of comorbid substance use disorder and attention deficit/hyperactivity disorder: protocol and clinical characteristics of the INCAS study. BMC Psychiatry. 2022;22(1):625.
189. Dorani F, Bijlenga D, Beekman ATF, van Someren EJW, Kooij JJS. Prevalence of hormone-related mood disorder symptoms in women with ADHD. J Psychiatr Res. 2021;133:10–5.
190. Andersson A, Garcia-Argibay M, Viktorin A, Ghirardi L, Butwicka A, Skoglund C, Bang Madsen K, D'Onofrio BM, Lichtenstein P, Tuvblad C, Larsson H. Depression and anxiety disorders during the postpartum period in women diagnosed with attention deficit hyperactivity disorder. J Affect Disord. 2023;325:817–23.
191. Jaholkowski P, Shadrin AA, Jangmo A, Frei E, Tesfaye M, Hindley GFL, Haram M, Rahman Z, Athanasiu L, Bakken NR, Holen B, Fominykh V, Kutrolli G, Parekh P, Parker N, Rodevand L, Birkenaes V, Djurovic S, Frei O, O'Connell KS, Smeland OB, Tesli M, Andreassen OA. Associations between symptoms of premenstrual disorders and polygenic liability for major psychiatric disorders. JAMA Psychiatry. 2023;80(7):738–42.
192. Barkley RA, Brown TE. Unrecognized attention-deficit/hyperactivity disorder in adults presenting with other psychiatric disorders. CNS Spectr. 2008;13(11):977–84.
193. Libutzki B, May M, Gleitz M, Karus M, Neukirch B, Hartman CA, Reif A. Disease burden and direct medical costs of incident adult ADHD: a retrospective longitudinal analysis based on German statutory health insurance claims data. Eur Psychiatry. 2020;63(1):e86.
194. Matheson L, Asherson P, Wong IC, Hodgkins P, Setyawan J, Sasane R, Clifford S. Adult ADHD patient experiences of impairment, service provision and clinical management in England: a qualitative study. BMC Health Serv Res. 2013;13:184.

195. Chen MH, Pan TL, Hsu JW, Huang KL, Su TP, Li CT, Lin WC, Tsai SJ, Chang WH, Chen TJ, Bai YM. Attention-deficit hyperactivity disorder comorbidity and antidepressant resistance among patients with major depression: a nationwide longitudinal study. Eur Neuropsychopharmacol. 2016;26(11):1760–7.
196. Powell V, Agha SS, Jones RB, Eyre O, Stephens A, Weavers B, Lennon J, Allardyce J, Potter R, Smith D, Thapar A, Rice F. ADHD in adults with recurrent depression. J Affect Disord. 2021;295:1153–60.
197. Sternat T, Fotinos K, Fine A, Epstein I, Katzman MA. Low hedonic tone and attention-deficit hyperactivity disorder: risk factors for treatment resistance in depressed adults. Neuropsychiatr Dis Treat. 2018;14:2379–87.
198. Golubchik P, Kodesh A, Weizman A. Attention-deficit/hyperactivity disorder and comorbid subsyndromal depression: what is the impact of methylphenidate on mood? Clin Neuropharmacol. 2013;36(5):141–5.
199. Milberger S, Biederman J, Faraone SV, Chen L, Jones J. ADHD is associated with early initiation of cigarette smoking in children and adolescents. J Am Acad Child Adolesc Psychiatry. 1997;36(1):37–44.
200. Galera C, Salla J, Montagni I, Hanne-Poujade S, Salamon R, Grondin O, Guichard E, Bouvard MP, Tzourio C, Michel G. Stress, attention deficit hyperactivity disorder (ADHD) symptoms and tobacco smoking: the i-share study. Eur Psychiatry. 2017;45:221–6.
201. Vitulano ML, Fite PJ, Hopko DR, Lochman J, Wells K, Asif I. Evaluation of underlying mechanisms in the link between childhood ADHD symptoms and risk for early initiation of substance use. Psychol Addict Behav. 2014;28(3):816–27.
202. Rhodes JD, Pelham WE, Gnagy EM, Shiffman S, Derefinko KJ, Molina BS. Cigarette smoking and ADHD: an examination of prognostically relevant smoking behaviors among adolescents and young adults. Psychol Addict Behav. 2016;30(5):588–600.
203. Kollins SH, Sweitzer MM, McClernon FJ, Perkins KA. Increased subjective and reinforcing effects of initial nicotine exposure in young adults with attention deficit hyperactivity disorder (ADHD) compared to matched peers: results from an experimental model of first-time tobacco use. Neuropsychopharmacology. 2020;45(5):851–6.
204. Sanchez-Garcia NC, Gonzalez RA, Ramos-Quiroga JA, van den Brink W, Luderer M, Blankers M, Grau-Lopez L, Levin FR, Kaye S, Demetrovics Z, van de Glind G, Schellekens A, Velez-Pastrana MC, the Ig. Attention deficit hyperactivity disorder increases nicotine addiction severity in adults seeking treatment for substance use disorders: the role of personality disorders. Eur Addict Res. 2020;26(4–5):191–200.
205. Biederman J, Monuteaux MC, Mick E, Wilens TE, Fontanella JA, Poetzl KM, Kirk T, Masse J, Faraone SV. Is cigarette smoking a gateway to alcohol and illicit drug use disorders? A study of youths with and without attention deficit hyperactivity disorder. Biol Psychiatry. 2006;59(3):258–64.
206. de Los P, Cobos J, Sinol N, Puerta C, Cantillano V, Lopez Zurita C, Trujols J. Features and prevalence of patients with probable adult attention deficit hyperactivity disorder who request treatment for cocaine use disorders. Psychiatry Res. 2011;185(1–2):205–10.
207. Crean RD, Crane NA, Mason BJ. An evidence based review of acute and long-term effects of cannabis use on executive cognitive functions. J Addict Med. 2011;5(1):1–8.
208. Biederman J, Petty CR, Hammerness P, Batchelder H, Faraone SV. Cigarette smoking as a risk factor for other substance misuse: 10-year study of individuals with and without attention-deficit hyperactivity disorder. Br J Psychiatry. 2012;201(3):207–14.
209. Dierker L, Braymiller J, Rose J, Goodwin R, Selya A. Nicotine dependence predicts cannabis use disorder symptoms among adolescents and young adults. Drug Alcohol Depend. 2018;187:212–20.
210. Kreski NT, Ankrum H, Cerda M, Chen Q, Hasin D, Martins SS, Olfson M, Keyes KM. Nicotine vaping and co-occurring substance use among adolescents in the United States from 2017-2019. Subst Use Misuse. 2023;58(9):1075–9.
211. Elkins IJ, Saunders GRB, Malone SM, Keyes MA, Samek DR, McGue M, Iacono WG. Increased risk of smoking in female adolescents who had childhood ADHD. Am J Psychiatry. 2018;175(1):63–70.
212. Degenhardt L, Chiu WT, Conway K, Dierker L, Glantz M, Kalaydjian A, Merikangas K, Sampson N, Swendsen J, Kessler RC. Does the 'gateway' matter? Associations between the order of drug use initiation and the development of drug dependence in the national comorbidity study replication. Psychol Med. 2009;39(1):157–67.
213. Cullen KA, Gentzke AS, Sawdey MD, Chang JT, Anic GM, Wang TW, Creamer MR, Jamal A, Ambrose BK, King BA. E-cigarette use among youth in the United States, 2019. JAMA. 2019;322(21):2095–103.
214. Chadi N, Schroeder R, Jensen JW, Levy S. Association between electronic cigarette use and marijuana use among adolescents and young adults: a systematic review and meta-analysis. JAMA Pediatr. 2019;173(10):e192574.
215. Struble CA, Ellis JD, Lundahl LH. Beyond the bud: emerging methods of cannabis consumption for youth. Pediatr Clin N Am. 2019;66(6):1087–97.
216. Bidwell LC, Henry EA, Willcutt EG, Kinnear MK, Ito TA. Childhood and current ADHD symptom dimensions are associated with more severe cannabis outcomes in college students. Drug Alcohol Depend. 2014;135:88–94.
217. Dvorsky MR, Langberg JM. Cigarette and e-cigarette use and social perceptions over the transition to college: the role of ADHD symptoms. Psychol Addict Behav. 2019;33(3):318–30.
218. Wadsworth E, Hammond D. Differences in patterns of cannabis use among youth: prevalence, percep-

tions of harm and driving under the influence in the USA where non-medical cannabis markets have been established, proposed and prohibited. Drug Alcohol Rev. 2018;37(7):903–11.
219. Bierhoff J, Haardorfer R, Windle M, Berg CJ. Psychological risk factors for alcohol, cannabis, and various tobacco use among young adults: a longitudinal analysis. Subst Use Misuse. 2019;54(8):1365–75.
220. Han B, Compton WM, Blanco C, Jones CM. Time since first cannabis use and 12-month prevalence of cannabis use disorder among youth and emerging adults in the United States. Addiction. 2019;114(4):698–707.
221. Dernbach MR, Gray KM, Borich A, Seery E, Russo SB, Lewis ET 3rd, Gwynette MF. Prescribing stimulants for children and adolescents with attention-deficit/hyperactivity disorder and co-occurring cannabis use: considerations for managing a clinical dilemma. J Am Acad Child Adolesc Psychiatry. 2023;62(8):842–6.
222. Wang TW, Neff LJ, Park-Lee E, Ren C, Cullen KA, King BA. E-cigarette use among middle and high school students—United States, 2020. MMWR Morb Mortal Wkly Rep. 2020;69(37):1310–2.
223. Sun R, Mendez D, Warner KE. Evaluation of self-reported cannabis vaping among US youth and young adults who use e-cigarettes. JAMA Pediatr. 2022;176(4):417–9.
224. Amrock SM, Lee L, Weitzman M. Perceptions of e-cigarettes and noncigarette tobacco products among US youth. Pediatrics. 2016;138(5):e20154306.
225. Chambers J, Keyhani S, Ling PM, Hoggatt KJ, Hasin D, Nguyen N, Woods A, Ryder A, Cohen BE. Perceptions of safety of daily cannabis vs tobacco smoking and secondhand smoke exposure, 2017–2021. JAMA Netw Open. 2023;6(8):e2328691.
226. Morin JG, Afzali MH, Bourque J, Stewart SH, Seguin JR, O'Leary-Barrett M, Conrod PJ. A population-based analysis of the relationship between substance use and adolescent cognitive development. Am J Psychiatry. 2019;176(2):98–106.
227. Orr C, Spechler P, Cao Z, Albaugh M, Chaarani B, Mackey S, D'Souza D, Allgaier N, Banaschewski T, Bokde ALW, Bromberg U, Buchel C, Burke Quinlan E, Conrod P, Desrivieres S, Flor H, Frouin V, Gowland P, Heinz A, Ittermann B, Martinot JL, Martinot MP, Nees F, Papadopoulos Orfanos D, Paus T, Poustka L, Millenet S, Frohner JH, Radhakrishnan R, Smolka MN, Walter H, Whelan R, Schumann G, Potter A, Garavan H. Grey matter volume differences associated with extremely low levels of cannabis use in adolescence. J Neurosci. 2019;39(10):1817–27.
228. Brumback T, Castro N, Jacobus J, Tapert S. Effects of marijuana use on brain structure and function: neuroimaging findings from a neurodevelopmental perspective. Int Rev Neurobiol. 2016;129:33–65.
229. Jefsen OH, Erlangsen A, Nordentoft M, Hjorthoj C. Cannabis use disorder and subsequent risk of psychotic and nonpsychotic unipolar depression and bipolar disorder. JAMA Psychiatry. 2023;80(8):803–10.
230. Volkow ND, Koob GF, McLellan AT. Neurobiologic advances from the brain disease model of Addiction. N Engl J Med. 2016;374(4):363–71.
231. Williams AR. Cannabis as a gateway drug for opioid use disorder. J Law Med Ethics. 2020;48(2):268–74.
232. Albaugh MD, Ottino-Gonzalez J, Sidwell A, Lepage C, Juliano A, Owens MM, Chaarani B, Spechler P, Fontaine N, Rioux P, Lewis L, Jeon S, Evans A, D'Souza D, Radhakrishnan R, Banaschewski T, Bokde ALW, Quinlan EB, Conrod P, Desrivieres S, Flor H, Grigis A, Gowland P, Heinz A, Ittermann B, Martinot JL, Paillere Martinot ML, Nees F, Papadopoulos Orfanos D, Paus T, Poustka L, Millenet S, Frohner JH, Smolka MN, Walter H, Whelan R, Schumann G, Potter A, Garavan H, IMAGEN Consortium. Association of cannabis use during adolescence with neurodevelopment. JAMA Psychiatry 2021;78(9):1–11.
233. Spechler PA, Orr CA, Chaarani B, Kan KJ, Mackey S, Morton A, Snowe MP, Hudson KE, Althoff RR, Higgins ST, Cattrell A, Flor H, Nees F, Banaschewski T, ALW B, Whelan R, Buchel C, Bromberg U, Conrod P, Frouin V, Papadopoulos D, Gallinat J, Heinz A, Walter H, Ittermann B, Gowland P, Paus T, Poustka L, Martinot JL, Artiges E, Smolka MN, Schumann G, Garavan H, IMAGEN Consortium. Cannabis use in early adolescence: evidence of amygdala hypersensitivity to signals of threat. Dev Cogn Neurosci. 2015;16(63–70):63–70.
234. Spechler PA, Chaarani B, Orr C, Albaugh MD, Fontaine NR, Higgins ST, Banaschewski T, Bokde ALW, Quinlan EB, Desrivieres S, Flor H, Grigis A, Gowland P, Heinz A, Ittermann B, Artiges E, Martinot MP, Nees F, Orfanos DP, Paus T, Poustka L, Hohmann S, Frohner JH, Smolka MN, Walter H, Whelan R, Schumann G, Garavan H. Longitudinal associations between amygdala reactivity and cannabis use in a large sample of adolescents. Psychopharmacology. 2020;237(11):3447–58.
235. Sagar KA, Dahlgren MK, Gonenc A, Racine MT, Dreman MW, Gruber SA. The impact of initiation: Early onset marijuana smokers demonstrate altered Stroop performance and brain activation. Dev Cogn Neurosci. 2015;16:84–92.
236. van de Giessen E, Weinstein JJ, Cassidy CM, Haney M, Dong Z, Ghazzaoui R, Ojeil N, Kegeles LS, Xu X, Vadhan NP, Volkow ND, Slifstein M, Abi-Dargham A. Deficits in striatal dopamine release in cannabis dependence. Mol Psychiatry. 2017;22(1):68–75.
237. Blum K, Khalsa J, Cadet JL, Baron D, Bowirrat A, Boyett B, Lott L, Brewer R, Gondre-Lewis M, Bunt G, Kazmi S, Gold MS. Cannabis-induced hypodopaminergic anhedonia and cognitive decline in humans: embracing putative induction of dopamine homeostasis. Front Psych. 2021;12:623403.
238. Pasman JA, Verweij KJH, Gerring Z, Stringer S, Sanchez-Roige S, Treur JL, Abdellaoui A, Nivard

MG, Baselmans BML, Ong JS, Ip HF, van der Zee MD, Bartels M, Day FR, Fontanillas P, Elson SL, 23andMe Research Team, de Wit H, Davis LK, MacKillop J, Substance Use Disorders Working Group of the Psychiatric Genomics Consortium, International Cannabis Consortium, Derringer JL, Branje SJT, Hartman CA, Heath AC, van Lier PAC, Madden PAF, Magi R, Meeus W, Montgomery GW, Oldehinkel AJ, Pausova Z, Ramos-Quiroga JA, Paus T, Ribases M, Kaprio J, Boks MPM, Bell JT, Spector TD, Gelernter J, Boomsma DI, Martin NG, MacGregor S, Perry JRB, Palmer AA, Posthuma D, Munafo MR, Gillespie NA, Derks EM, Vink JM. GWAS of lifetime cannabis use reveals new risk loci, genetic overlap with psychiatric traits, and a causal influence of schizophrenia. Nat Neurosci. 2018;21(9):1161–1170.

239. Shin SH, McDonald SE, Conley D. Patterns of adverse childhood experiences and substance use among young adults: a latent class analysis. Addict Behav. 2018;78:187–92.
240. Tang S, Ports KA, Zhang K, Lin HC. Adverse childhood experiences, internalizing/externalizing symptoms, and associated prescription opioid misuse: a mediation analysis. Prev Med. 2020;134:106034.
241. Brown NM, Brown SN, Briggs RD, German M, Belamarich PF, Oyeku SO. Associations between adverse childhood experiences and ADHD diagnosis and severity. Acad Pediatr. 2017;17(4):349–55.
242. Miranda A, Colomer C, Berenguer C, Rosello R, Rosello B. Substance use in young adults with ADHD: comorbidity and symptoms of inattention and hyperactivity/impulsivity. Int J Clin Health Psychol. 2016;16(2):157–65.
243. Mitchell SH. Linking delay discounting and substance use disorders: genotypes and phenotypes. Perspect Behav Sci. 2019;42(3):419–32.
244. Levitt EE, Oshri A, Amlung M, Ray LA, Sanchez-Roige S, Palmer AA, MacKillop J. Evaluation of delay discounting as a transdiagnostic research domain criteria indicator in 1388 general community adults. Psychol Med. 2023;53(4):1649–57.
245. Kaye S, Gilsenan J, Young JT, Carruthers S, Allsop S, Degenhardt L, van de Glind G, van den Brink W. Risk behaviours among substance use disorder treatment seekers with and without adult ADHD symptoms. Drug Alcohol Depend. 2014;144:70–7.
246. Oncioiu SI, Orri M, Boivin M, Geoffroy MC, Arseneault L, Brendgen M, Vitaro F, Navarro MC, Galera C, Tremblay RE, Cote SM. Early childhood factors associated with peer victimization trajectories from 6 to 17 years of age. Pediatrics. 2020;145(5):e20192654.
247. Fogleman ND, Slaughter KE, Rosen PJ, Leaberry KD, Walerius DM. Emotion regulation accounts for the relation between ADHD and peer victimization. J Child Fam Stud. 2018;28(9):2429–42.
248. Kollath-Cattano C, Hatteberg SJ, Kooper A. Illicit drug use among college students: the role of social norms and risk perceptions. Addict Behav. 2020;105:106289.
249. Kennedy TM, Walther CAP, Pedersen SL, McKone KMP, Gnagy EM, Pelham WE Jr, Molina BSG. Beers with peers: childhood ADHD and risk for correlated change in perceived peer and personal alcohol use across young adulthood. Alcohol Clin Exp Res. 2020;44(11):2350–60.
250. Chaplin TM, Niehaus C, Goncalves SF. Stress reactivity and the developmental psychopathology of adolescent substance use. Neurobiol Stress. 2018;9:133–9.
251. Kandel ER, Kandel DB. Shattuck Lecture. A molecular basis for nicotine as a gateway drug. N Engl J Med 2014;371(10):932–943.
252. Volkow ND, Han B, Einstein EB, Compton WM. Prevalence of substance use disorders by time since first substance use among young people in the US. JAMA Pediatr. 2021;175(6):640–3.
253. Perry RN, Schlagintweit HE, Darredeau C, Helmick C, Newman AJ, Good KP, Barrett SP. The impacts of actual and perceived nicotine administration on insula functional connectivity with the anterior cingulate cortex and nucleus accumbens. J Psychopharmacol. 2019;33(12):1600–9.
254. Faraone SV, Larsson H. Genetics of attention deficit hyperactivity disorder. Mol Psychiatry. 2019;24(4):562–75.
255. Harich B, van der Voet M, Klein M, Cizek P, Fenckova M, Schenck A, Franke B. From rare copy number variants to biological processes in ADHD. Am J Psychiatry. 2020;177(9):855–66.
256. Demontis D, Walters RK, Martin J, Mattheisen M, Als TD, Agerbo E, Baldursson G, Belliveau R, Bybjerg-Grauholm J, Baekvad-Hansen M, Cerrato F, Chambert K, Churchhouse C, Dumont A, Eriksson N, Gandal M, Goldstein JI, Grasby KL, Grove J, Gudmundsson OO, Hansen CS, Hauberg ME, Hollegaard MV, Howrigan DP, Huang H, Maller JB, Martin AR, Martin NG, Moran J, Pallesen J, Palmer DS, Pedersen CB, Pedersen MG, Poterba T, Poulsen JB, Ripke S, Robinson EB, Satterstrom FK, Stefansson H, Stevens C, Turley P, Walters GB, Won H, Wright MJ, ADHD Working Group of the Psychiatric Genomics Consortium (PGC), Early Lifecourse & Genetic Epidemiology (EAGLE) Consortium, 23andMe Research Team, Andreassen OA, Asherson P, Burton CL, Boomsma DI, Cormand B, Dalsgaard S, Franke B, Gelernter J, Geschwind D, Hakonarson H, Haavik J, Kranzler HR, Kuntsi J, Langley K, Lesch KP, Middeldorp C, Reif A, Rohde LA, Roussos P, Schachar R, Sklar P, EJS S-B, Sullivan PF, Thapar A, Tung JY, Waldman ID, Medland SE, Stefansson K, Nordentoft M, Hougaard DM, Werge T, Mors O, Mortensen PB, Daly MJ, Faraone SV, Borglum AD, Neale BM. Discovery of the first genome-wide significant risk loci for attention deficit/hyperactivity disorder. Nat Genet. 2019;51(1):63–75.

257. Andrade A, Brennecke A, Mallat S, Brown J, Gomez-Rivadeneira J, Czepiel N, Londrigan L. Genetic associations between voltage-gated calcium channels and psychiatric disorders. Int J Mol Sci. 2019;20(14):3537.
258. Treur JL, Demontis D, Smith GD, Sallis H, Richardson TG, Wiers RW, Borglum AD, Verweij KJH, Munafo MR. Investigating causality between liability to ADHD and substance use, and liability to substance use and ADHD risk, using Mendelian randomization. Addict Biol. 2021;26(1):e12849.
259. Thapar A. ADHD: progressing from genetic discoveries to biological insights. Am J Psychiatry. 2020;177(9):802–4.
260. Liu L, Zhao Q, Yu X, Xu D, Li H, Ji N, Wu Z, Cheng J, Su Y, Cao Q, Sun L, Qian Q, Wang Y. Monoaminergic genetic variants, prefrontal cortex-amygdala circuit, and emotional symptoms in children with ADHD: exploration based on the gene-brain-behavior relationship. J Atten Disord. 2021;25(9):1272–83.
261. Du Rietz E, Coleman J, Glanville K, Choi SW, O'Reilly PF, Kuntsi J. Association of polygenic risk for attention-deficit/hyperactivity disorder with co-occurring traits and disorders. Biol Psychiatry Cogn Neurosci Neuroimaging. 2018;3(7):635–43.
262. Demontis D, Walters GB, Athanasiadis G, Walters R, Therrien K, Farajzadeh L, Voloudakis G, Bendl J, Zeng B, Zhang W, Grove J, Als TD, Duan J, Satterstrom FK, Bybjerg-Grauholm J, Bækved-Hansen M, Gudmundsson OO, Magnusson SH, Baldursson G, Davidsdottir K, Haraldsdottir GS, Nielsen TT, Agerbo E, Hoffman GE, Dalsgaard S, Martin J, Ribasés M, Boomsma DI, Artigas MS, Mota NR, Howrigan D, Medland SE, Zayats T, Manikandan V, Nordentoft M, Mors O, Hougaard DM, Mortensen PB, Daly MJ, Faraone SV, Stefansson H, Roussos P, Franke B, Werge T, Neale BM, Stefansson K, Børglum AD. Genome-wide analyses of ADHD identify 27 risk loci, refine the genetic architecture and implicate several cognitive domains. Nat Genet. 2023;55(2):198–208.
263. Rovira P, Demontis D. Shared genetic background between children and adults with attention deficit/hyperactivity disorder. Neuropsychopharmacology. 2020; 45(10):1617–26.
264. Franke B, Faraone SV, Asherson P, Buitelaar J, Bau CH, Ramos-Quiroga JA, Mick E, Grevet EH, Johansson S, Haavik J, Lesch KP, Cormand B, Reif A, International Multicentre Persistent ADHD Collaboration. The genetics of attention deficit/hyperactivity disorder in adults, a review. Mol Psychiatry. 2012;17(10):960–87.
265. Grimm O, Kranz TM, Reif A. Genetics of ADHD: what should the clinician know? Curr Psychiatry Rep. 2020;22(4):18.
266. Sonderby IE, Ching CRK, Thomopoulos SI, van der Meer D, Sun D, Villalon-Reina JE, Agartz I, Amunts K, Arango C, Armstrong NJ, Ayesa-Arriola R, Bakker G, Bassett AS, Boomsma DI, Bulow R, Butcher NJ, Calhoun VD, Caspers S, Chow EWC, Cichon S, Ciufolini S, Craig MC, Crespo-Facorro B, Cunningham AC, Dale AM, Dazzan P, de Zubicaray GI, Djurovic S, Doherty JL, Donohoe G, Draganski B, Durdle CA, Ehrlich S, Emanuel BS, Espeseth T, Fisher SE, Ge T, Glahn DC, Grabe HJ, Gur RE, Gutman BA, Haavik J, Haberg AK, Hansen LA, Hashimoto R, Hibar DP, Holmes AJ, Hottenga JJ, Hulshoff Pol HE, Jalbrzikowski M, Knowles EEM, Kushan L, Linden DEJ, Liu J, Lundervold AJ, Martin-Brevet S, Martinez K, Mather KA, Mathias SR, McDonald-McGinn DM, McRae AF, Medland SE, Moberget T, Modenato C, Monereo Sanchez J, Moreau CA, Muhleisen TW, Paus T, Pausova Z, Prieto C, Ragothaman A, Reinbold CS, Reis Marques T, Repetto GM, Reymond A, Roalf DR, Rodriguez-Herreros B, Rucker JJ, Sachdev PS, Schmitt JE, Schofield PR, Silva AI, Stefansson H, Stein DJ, Tamnes CK, Tordesillas-Gutierrez D, Ulfarsson MO, Vajdi A, van 't Ent D, van den Bree MBM, Vassos E, Vazquez-Bourgon J, Vila-Rodriguez F, Walters GB, Wen W, Westlye LT, Wittfeld K, Zackai EH, Stefansson K, Jacquemont S, Thompson PM, Bearden CE, Andreassen OA, ENIGMA-CNV Working Group, ENIGMA 22q11.2 Deletion Syndrome Working Group. Effects of copy number variations on brain structure and risk for psychiatric illness: Large-scale studies from the ENIGMA working groups on CNVs. Hum Brain Mapp. 2022;43(1):300–328.
267. Kim HJ, Kim SY, Kim GE, Jin HJ. Association between genetic polymorphisms of synaptophysin (SYP) gene and attention deficit hyperactivity disorder in Korean subjects. Genes Genomics. 2023;45(9):1097–105.
268. Biederman J, Faraone SV, Keenan K, Benjamin J, Krifcher B, Moore C, Sprich-Buckminster S, Ugaglia K, Jellinek MS, Steingard R, et al. Further evidence for family-genetic risk factors in attention deficit hyperactivity disorder. Patterns of comorbidity in probands and relatives psychiatrically and pediatrically referred samples. Arch Gen Psychiatry. 1992;49(9):728–38.
269. Wimberley T, Agerbo E, Horsdal HT, Ottosen C, Brikell I, Als TD, Demontis D, Borglum AD, Nordentoft M, Mors O, Werge T, Hougaard D, Bybjerg-Grauholm J, Hansen MB, Mortensen PB, Thapar A, Riglin L, Langley K, Dalsgaard S. Genetic liability to ADHD and substance use disorders in individuals with ADHD. Addiction. 2020;115(7):1368–77.
270. Zhou H, Sealock JM, Sanchez-Roige S, Clarke TK, Levey DF, Cheng Z, Li B, Polimanti R, Kember RL, Smith RV, Thygesen JH, Morgan MY, Atkinson SR, Thursz MR, Nyegaard M, Mattheisen M, Borglum AD, Johnson EC, Justice AC, Palmer AA, McQuillin A, Davis LK, Edenberg HJ, Agrawal A, Kranzler HR, Gelernter J. Genome-wide meta-analysis of problematic alcohol use in 435,563 individuals

yields insights into biology and relationships with other traits. Nat Neurosci. 2020;23(7):809–18.

271. Yule AM, Martelon M, Faraone SV, Carrellas N, Wilens TE, Biederman J. Examining the association between attention deficit hyperactivity disorder and substance use disorders: a familial risk analysis. J Psychiatr Res. 2017;85:49–55.

272. Skoglund C, Chen Q, Franck J, Lichtenstein P, Larsson H. Attention-deficit/hyperactivity disorder and risk for substance use disorders in relatives. Biol Psychiatry. 2015;77(10):880–6.

273. Verweij KJ, Zietsch BP, Lynskey MT, Medland SE, Neale MC, Martin NG, Boomsma DI, Vink JM. Genetic and environmental influences on cannabis use initiation and problematic use: a meta-analysis of twin studies. Addiction. 2010;105(3):417–30.

274. Verhulst B, Neale MC, Kendler KS. The heritability of alcohol use disorders: a meta-analysis of twin and adoption studies. Psychol Med. 2015;45(5):1061–72.

275. Deak JD, Johnson EC. Genetics of substance use disorders: a review. Psychol Med. 2021;51(13):2189–200.

276. Sun J, Kranzler HR, Gelernter J, Bi J. A genome-wide association study of cocaine use disorder accounting for phenotypic heterogeneity and gene-environment interaction. J Psychiatry Neurosci. 2020;45(1):34–44.

277. Crist RC, Reiner BC, Berrettini WH. A review of opioid addiction genetics. Curr Opin Psychol. 2019;27:31–5.

278. Hatoum AS, Colbert SMC, Johnson EC, Huggett SB, Deak JD, Pathak GA, Jennings MV, Paul SE, Karcher NR, Hansen I, Baranger DAA, Edwards A, Grotzinger AD, Tucker-Drob EM, Kranzler H, Davis LK, Sanchez-Roige S, Polimanti R, Gelernter J, Edenberg HJ, Bogdan R, Agrawal A. Multivariate genome-wide association meta-analysis of over 1 million subjects identifies loci underlying multiple substance use disorders. Nat Ment Health. 2023;1(3):210–223.

279. Egan TE, Dawson AE, Wymbs BT. Substance use in undergraduate students with histories of attention-deficit/hyperactivity disorder (ADHD): the role of impulsivity. Subst Use Misuse. 2017;52(10):1375–86.

280. Cservenka A, Ray LA. Self-reported attentional and motor impulsivity are related to age at first methamphetamine use. Addict Behav. 2017;65:7–12.

281. Sousa NO, Grevet EH, Salgado CA, Silva KL, Victor MM, Karam RG, Vitola ES, Picon FA, Zeni GD, Rohde LA, Belmonte-de-Abreu P, Bau CH. Smoking and ADHD: an evaluation of self medication and behavioral disinhibition models based on comorbidity and personality patterns. J Psychiatr Res. 2011;45(6):829–34.

282. Cavicchioli M, Ogliari A, Movalli M, Maffei C. Persistent deficits in self-regulation as a mediator between childhood attention-deficit/hyperactivity disorder symptoms and substance use disorders. Subst Use Misuse. 2022;57(12):1837–53.

283. Boedhoe PSW, van Rooij D, Hoogman M, Twisk JWR, Schmaal L, Abe Y, Alonso P, Ameis SH, Anikin A, Anticevic A, Arango C, Arnold PD, Asherson P, Assogna F, Auzias G, Banaschewski T, Baranov A, Batistuzzo MC, Baumeister S, Baur-Streubel R, Behrmann M, Bellgrove MA, Benedetti F, Beucke JC, Biederman J, Bollettini I, Bose A, Bralten J, Bramati IE, Brandeis D, Brem S, Brennan BP, Busatto GF, Calderoni S, Calvo A, Calvo R, Castellanos FX, Cercignani M, Chaim-Avancini TM, Chantiluke KC, Cheng Y, Cho KIK, Christakou A, Coghill D, Conzelmann A, Cubillo AI, Dale AM, Dallaspezia S, Daly E, Denys D, Deruelle C, Di Martino A, Dinstein I, Doyle AE, Durston S, Earl EA, Ecker C, Ehrlich S, Ely BA, Epstein JN, Ethofer T, Fair DA, Fallgatter AJ, Faraone SV, Fedor J, Feng X, Feusner JD, Fitzgerald J, Fitzgerald KD, Fouche JP, Freitag CM, Fridgeirsson EA, Frodl T, Gabel MC, Gallagher L, Gogberashvili T, Gori I, Gruner P, Gursel DA, Haar S, Haavik J, Hall GB, Harrison NA, Hartman CA, Heslenfeld DJ, Hirano Y, Hoekstra PJ, Hoexter MQ, Hohmann S, Hovik MF, Hu H, Huyser C, Jahanshad N, Jalbrzikowski M, James A, Janssen J, Jaspers-Fayer F, Jernigan TL, Kapilushniy D, Kardatzki B, Karkashadze G, Kathmann N, Kaufmann C, Kelly C, Khadka S, King JA, Koch K, Kohls G, Konrad K, Kuno M, Kuntsi J, Kvale G, Kwon JS, Lazaro L, Lera-Miguel S, Lesch KP, Hoekstra L, Liu Y, Lochner C, Louza MR, Luna B, Lundervold AJ, Malpas CB, Marques P, Marsh R, Martinez-Zalacain I, Mataix-Cols D, Mattos P, McCarthy H, McGrath J, Mehta MA, Menchon JM, Mennes M, Martinho MM, Moreira PS, Morer A, Morgado P, Muratori F, Murphy CM, Murphy DGM, Nakagawa A, Nakamae T, Nakao T, Namazova-Baranova L, Narayanaswamy JC, Nicolau R, Nigg JT, Novotny SE, Nurmi EL, Weiss EO, O'Gorman Tuura RL, O'Hearn K, O'Neill J, Oosterlaan J, Oranje B, Paloyelis Y, Parellada M, Pauli P, Perriello C, Piacentini J, Piras F, Piras F, Plessen KJ, Puig O, Ramos-Quiroga JA, Reddy YCJ, Reif A, Reneman L, Retico A, Rosa PGP, Rubia K, Rus OG, Sakai Y, Schrantee A, Schwarz L, Schweren LJS, Seitz J, Shaw P, Shook D, Silk TJ, Simpson HB, Skokauskas N, Soliva Vila JC, Solovieva A, Soreni N, Soriano-Mas C, Spalletta G, Stern ER, Stevens MC, Stewart SE, Sudre G, Szeszko PR, Tamm L, Taylor MJ, Tolin DF, Tosetti M, Tovar-Moll F, Tsuchiyagaito A, van Erp TGM, van Wingen GA, Vance A, Venkatasubramanian G, Vilarroya O, Vives-Gilabert Y, von Polier GG, Walitza S, Wallace GL, Wang Z, Wolfers T, Yoncheva YN, Yun JY, Zanetti MV, Zhou F, Ziegler GC, Zierhut KC, Zwiers MP, ENIGMA ADHD Working Group, ENIGMA ASD Working Group, ENIGMA OCD Working Group, Thompson PM, Stein DJ, Buitelaar J, Franke B, van den Heuvel OA. Subcortical brain volume, regional cortical thickness, and cortical surface area across

disorders: findings from the ENIGMA ADHD, ASD, and OCD Working Groups. Am J Psychiatry. 2020;177(9):834–43.

284. Hoogman M, Muetzel R, Guimaraes JP, Shumskaya E, Mennes M, Zwiers MP, Jahanshad N, Sudre G, Wolfers T, Earl EA, Soliva Vila JC, Vives-Gilabert Y, Khadka S, Novotny SE, Hartman CA, Heslenfeld DJ, Schweren LJS, Ambrosino S, Oranje B, de Zeeuw P, Chaim-Avancini TM, Rosa PGP, Zanetti MV, Malpas CB, Kohls G, von Polier GG, Seitz J, Biederman J, Doyle AE, Dale AM, van Erp TGM, Epstein JN, Jernigan TL, Baur-Streubel R, Ziegler GC, Zierhut KC, Schrantee A, Hovik MF, Lundervold AJ, Kelly C, McCarthy H, Skokauskas N, O'Gorman Tuura RL, Calvo A, Lera-Miguel S, Nicolau R, Chantiluke KC, Christakou A, Vance A, Cercignani M, Gabel MC, Asherson P, Baumeister S, Brandeis D, Hohmann S, Bramati IE, Tovar-Moll F, Fallgatter AJ, Kardatzki B, Schwarz L, Anikin A, Baranov A, Gogberashvili T, Kapilushniy D, Solovieva A, El Marroun H, White T, Karkashadze G, Namazova-Baranova L, Ethofer T, Mattos P, Banaschewski T, Coghill D, Plessen KJ, Kuntsi J, Mehta MA, Paloyelis Y, Harrison NA, Bellgrove MA, Silk TJ, Cubillo AI, Rubia K, Lazaro L, Brem S, Walitza S, Frodl T, Zentis M, Castellanos FX, Yoncheva YN, Haavik J, Reneman L, Conzelmann A, Lesch KP, Pauli P, Reif A, Tamm L, Konrad K, Oberwelland Weiss E, Busatto GF, Louza MR, Durston S, Hoekstra PJ, Oosterlaan J, Stevens MC, Ramos-Quiroga JA, Vilarroya O, Fair DA, Nigg JT, Thompson PM, Buitelaar JK, Faraone SV, Shaw P, Tiemeier H, Bralten J, Franke B. Brain imaging of the cortex in ADHD: a coordinated analysis of large-scale clinical and population-based samples. Am J Psychiatry. 2019;176(7):531–42.

285. Kasparek T, Theiner P, Filova A. Neurobiology of ADHD from childhood to adulthood: findings of imaging methods. J Atten Disord. 2015;19(11):931–43.

286. Bledsoe JC, Semrud-Clikeman M, Pliszka SR. Anterior cingulate cortex and symptom severity in attention-deficit/hyperactivity disorder. J Abnorm Psychol. 2013;122(2):558–65.

287. Cupertino RB, Soheili-Nezhad S, Grevet EH, Bandeira CE, Picon FA, Tavares MEA, Naaijen J, van Rooij D, Akkermans S, Vitola ES, Zwiers MP, Rovaris DL, Hoekstra PJ, Breda V, Oosterlaan J, Hartman CA, Beckmann CF, Buitelaar JK, Franke B, Bau CHD, Sprooten E. Reduced fronto-striatal volume in attention-deficit/hyperactivity disorder in two cohorts across the lifespan. Neuroimage Clin. 2020;28:102403.

288. Bonath B, Tegelbeckers J, Wilke M, Flechtner HH, Krauel K. Regional Gray matter volume differences between adolescents with ADHD and typically developing controls: further evidence for anterior cingulate involvement. J Atten Disord. 2018;22(7):627–38.

289. Lopez-Larson MP, King JB, Terry J, McGlade EC, Yurgelun-Todd D. Reduced insular volume in attention deficit hyperactivity disorder. Psychiatry Res. 2012;204(1):32–9.

290. Bralten J, Greven CU, Franke B, Mennes M, Zwiers MP, Rommelse NN, Hartman C, van der Meer D, O'Dwyer L, Oosterlaan J, Hoekstra PJ, Heslenfeld D, Arias-Vasquez A, Buitelaar JK. Voxel-based morphometry analysis reveals frontal brain differences in participants with ADHD and their unaffected siblings. J Psychiatry Neurosci. 2016;41(4):272–9.

291. Hoogman M, Bralten J, Hibar DP, Mennes M, Zwiers MP, Schweren LSJ, van Hulzen KJE, Medland SE, Shumskaya E, Jahanshad N, Zeeuw P, Szekely E, Sudre G, Wolfers T, Onnink AMH, Dammers JT, Mostert JC, Vives-Gilabert Y, Kohls G, Oberwelland E, Seitz J, Schulte-Ruther M, Ambrosino S, Doyle AE, Hovik MF, Dramsdahl M, Tamm L, van Erp TGM, Dale A, Schork A, Conzelmann A, Zierhut K, Baur R, McCarthy H, Yoncheva YN, Cubillo A, Chantiluke K, Mehta MA, Paloyelis Y, Hohmann S, Baumeister S, Bramati I, Mattos P, Tovar-Moll F, Douglas P, Banaschewski T, Brandeis D, Kuntsi J, Asherson P, Rubia K, Kelly C, Martino AD, Milham MP, Castellanos FX, Frodl T, Zentis M, Lesch KP, Reif A, Pauli P, Jernigan TL, Haavik J, Plessen KJ, Lundervold AJ, Hugdahl K, Seidman LJ, Biederman J, Rommelse N, Heslenfeld DJ, Hartman CA, Hoekstra PJ, Oosterlaan J, Polier GV, Konrad K, Vilarroya O, Ramos-Quiroga JA, Soliva JC, Durston S, Buitelaar JK, Faraone SV, Shaw P, Thompson PM, Franke B. Subcortical brain volume differences in participants with attention deficit hyperactivity disorder in children and adults: a cross-sectional mega-analysis. Lancet Psychiatry. 2017;4(4):310–9.

292. Greven CU, Bralten J, Mennes M, O'Dwyer L, van Hulzen KJ, Rommelse N, Schweren LJ, Hoekstra PJ, Hartman CA, Heslenfeld D, Oosterlaan J, Faraone SV, Franke B, Zwiers MP, Arias-Vasquez A, Buitelaar JK. Developmentally stable whole-brain volume reductions and developmentally sensitive caudate and putamen volume alterations in those with attention-deficit/hyperactivity disorder and their unaffected siblings. JAMA Psychiatry. 2015;72(5):490–9.

293. Makris N, Liang L, Biederman J, Valera EM, Brown AB, Petty C, Spencer TJ, Faraone SV, Seidman LJ. Toward defining the neural substrates of ADHD: a controlled structural MRI study in medication-naive adults. J Atten Disord. 2015;19(11):944–53.

294. Duan K, Chen J, Calhoun VD, Lin D, Jiang W, Franke B, Buitelaar JK, Hoogman M, Arias-Vasquez A, Turner JA, Liu J. Neural correlates of cognitive function and symptoms in attention-deficit/hyperactivity disorder in adults. Neuroimage Clin. 2018;19:374–83.

295. Jiang W, Duan K, Rootes-Murdy K, Hoekstra PJ, Hartman CA, Oosterlaan J, Heslenfeld D, Franke B, Buitelaar J, Arias-Vasquez A, Liu J, Turner JA. Structural brain alterations and their association

with cognitive function and symptoms in attention-deficit/hyperactivity disorder families. Neuroimage Clin. 2020;27:102273.

296. Gehricke JG, Kruggel F, Thampipop T, Alejo SD, Tatos E, Fallon J, Muftuler LT. The brain anatomy of attention-deficit/hyperactivity disorder in young adults - a magnetic resonance imaging study. PLoS One. 2017;12(4):e0175433.

297. Writing Committee for the Attention-Deficit/Hyperactivity Disorder, Autism Spectrum Disorder, Bipolar Disorder, Major Depressive Disorder, Obsessive-Compulsive Disorder and Schizophrenia ENIGMA Working Groups, Patel Y, Parker N, Shin J, Howard D, French L, Thomopoulos SI, Pozzi E, Abe Y, Abe C, Anticevic A, Alda M, Aleman A, Alloza C, Alonso-Lana S, Ameis SH, Anagnostou E, McIntosh AA, Arango C, Arnold PD, Asherson P, Assogna F, Auzias G, Ayesa-Arriola R, Bakker G, Banaj N, Banaschewski T, Bandeira CE, Baranov A, Bargallo N, Bau CHD, Baumeister S, Baune BT, Bellgrove MA, Benedetti F, Bertolino A, Boedhoe PSW, Boks M, Bollettini I, Del Mar Bonnin C, Borgers T, Borgwardt S, Brandeis D, Brennan BP, Bruggemann JM, Bulow R, Busatto GF, Calderoni S, Calhoun VD, Calvo R, Canales-Rodriguez EJ, Cannon DM, Carr VJ, Cascella N, Cercignani M, Chaim-Avancini TM, Christakou A, Coghill D, Conzelmann A, Crespo-Facorro B, Cubillo AI, Cullen KR, Cupertino RB, Daly E, Dannlowski U, Davey CG, Denys D, Deruelle C, Di Giorgio A, Dickie EW, Dima D, Dohm K, Ehrlich S, Ely BA, Erwin-Grabner T, Ethofer T, Fair DA, Fallgatter AJ, Faraone SV, Fatjo-Vilas M, Fedor JM, Fitzgerald KD, Ford JM, Frodl T, Fu CHY, Fullerton JM, Gabel MC, Glahn DC, Roberts G, Gogberashvili T, Goikolea JM, Gotlib IH, Goya-Maldonado R, Grabe HJ, Green MJ, Grevet EH, Groenewold NA, Grotegerd D, Gruber O, Gruner P, Guerrero-Pedraza A, Gur RE, Gur RC, Haar S, Haarman BCM, Haavik J, Hahn T, Hajek T, Harrison BJ, Harrison NA, Hartman CA, Whalley HC, Heslenfeld DJ, Hibar DP, Hilland E, Hirano Y, Ho TC, Hoekstra PJ, Hoekstra L, Hohmann S, Hong LE, Hoschl C, Hovik MF, Howells FM, Nenadic I, Jalbrzikowski M, James AC, Janssen J, Jaspers-Fayer F, Xu J, Jonassen R, Karkashadze G, King JA, Kircher T, Kirschner M, Koch K, Kochunov P, Kohls G, Konrad K, Kramer B, Krug A, Kuntsi J, Kwon JS, Landen M, Landro NI, Lazaro L, Lebedeva IS, Leehr EJ, Lera-Miguel S, Lesch KP, Lochner C, Louza MR, Luna B, Lundervold AJ, MacMaster FP, Maglanoc LA, Malpas CB, Portella MJ, Marsh R, Martyn FM, Mataix-Cols D, Mathalon DH, McCarthy H, McDonald C, McPhilemy G, Meinert S, Menchon JM, Minuzzi L, Mitchell PB, Moreno C, Morgado P, Muratori F, Murphy CM, Murphy D, Mwangi B, Nabulsi L, Nakagawa A, Nakamae T, Namazova L, Narayanaswamy J, Jahanshad N, Nguyen DD, Nicolau R, O'Gorman Tuura RL, O'Hearn K, Oosterlaan J, Opel N, Ophoff RA, Oranje B, Garcia de la Foz VO, Overs BJ, Paloyelis Y, Pantelis C, Parellada M, Pauli P, Pico-Perez M, Picon FA, Piras F, Piras F, Plessen KJ, Pomarol-Clotet E, Preda A, Puig O, Quide Y, Radua J, Ramos-Quiroga JA, Rasser PE, Rauer L, Reddy J, Redlich R, Reif A, Reneman L, Repple J, Retico A, Richarte V, Richter A, Rosa PGP, Rubia KK, Hashimoto R, Sacchet MD, Salvador R, Santonja J, Sarink K, Sarro S, Satterthwaite TD, Sawa A, Schall U, Schofield PR, Schrantee A, Seitz J, Serpa MH, Setien-Suero E, Shaw P, Shook D, Silk TJ, Sim K, Simon S, Simpson HB, Singh A, Skoch A, Skokauskas N, Soares JC, Soreni N, Soriano-Mas C, Spalletta G, Spaniel F, Lawrie SM, Stern ER, Stewart SE, Takayanagi Y, Temmingh HS, Tolin DF, Tomecek D, Tordesillas-Gutierrez D, Tosetti M, Uhlmann A, van Amelsvoort T, van der Wee NJA, van der Werff SJA, van Haren NEM, van Wingen GA, Vance A, Vazquez-Bourgon J, Vecchio D, Venkatasubramanian G, Vieta E, Vilarroya O, Vives-Gilabert Y, Voineskos AN, Volzke H, von Polier GG, Walton E, Weickert TW, Weickert CS, Weideman AS, Wittfeld K, Wolf DH, Wu MJ, Yang TT, Yang K, Yoncheva Y, Yun JY, Cheng Y, Zanetti MV, Ziegler GC, Franke B, Hoogman M, Buitelaar JK, van Rooij D, Andreassen OA, Ching CRK, Veltman DJ, Schmaal L, Stein DJ, van den Heuvel OA, Turner JA, van Erp TGM, Pausova Z, Thompson PM, Paus T. Virtual histology of cortical thickness and shared neurobiology in 6 psychiatric disorders. JAMA Psychiatry. 2021;78(1):47–63.

298. Shaw P, Eckstrand K, Sharp W, Blumenthal J, Lerch JP, Greenstein D, Clasen L, Evans A, Giedd J, Rapoport JL. Attention-deficit/hyperactivity disorder is characterized by a delay in cortical maturation. Proc Natl Acad Sci USA. 2007;104(49):19649–54.

299. Konrad K, Firk C, Uhlhaas PJ. Brain development during adolescence: neuroscientific insights into this developmental period. Dtsch Arztebl Int. 2013;110(25):425–31.

300. Liston C, Malter Cohen M, Teslovich T, Levenson D, Casey BJ. Atypical prefrontal connectivity in attention-deficit/hyperactivity disorder: pathway to disease or pathological end point? Biol Psychiatry. 2011;69(12):1168–77.

301. van Ewijk H, Heslenfeld DJ, Zwiers MP, Faraone SV, Luman M, Hartman CA, Hoekstra PJ, Franke B, Buitelaar JK, Oosterlaan J. Different mechanisms of white matter abnormalities in attention-deficit/hyperactivity disorder: a diffusion tensor imaging study. J Am Acad Child Adolesc Psychiatry. 2014;53(7):790–9.e3.

302. Wu YH, Gau SS, Lo YC, Tseng WY. White matter tract integrity of frontostriatal circuit in attention deficit hyperactivity disorder: association with attention performance and symptoms. Hum Brain Mapp. 2014;35(1):199–212.

303. Hung Y, Uchida M, Gaillard SL, Woodworth H, Kelberman C, Capella J, Kadlec K, Goncalves M, Ghosh S, Yendiki A, Chai XJ, Hirshfeld-Becker DR, Whitfield-Gabrieli S, Gabrieli JDE, Biederman

J. Cingulum-Callosal white-matter microstructure associated with emotional dysregulation in children: a diffusion tensor imaging study. Neuroimage Clin. 2020;27:102266.
304. Aoki Y, Cortese S, Castellanos FX. Research review: diffusion tensor imaging studies of attention-deficit/hyperactivity disorder: meta-analyses and reflections on head motion. J Child Psychol Psychiatry. 2018;59(3):193–202.
305. Gagnon A, Descoteaux M, Bocti C, Takser L. Better characterization of attention and hyperactivity/impulsivity in children with ADHD: the key to understanding the underlying white matter microstructure. Psychiatry Res Neuroimaging. 2022;327:111568.
306. Cortese S, Kelly C, Chabernaud C, Proal E, Di Martino A, Milham MP, Castellanos FX. Toward systems neuroscience of ADHD: a meta-analysis of 55 fMRI studies. Am J Psychiatry. 2012;169(10):1038–55.
307. Rubia K. Cognitive neuroscience of attention deficit hyperactivity disorder (ADHD) and its clinical translation. Front Hum Neurosci. 2018;12:100.
308. Gao Y, Shuai D, Bu X, Hu X, Tang S, Zhang L, Li H, Hu X, Lu L, Gong Q, Huang X. Impairments of large-scale functional networks in attention-deficit/hyperactivity disorder: a meta-analysis of resting-state functional connectivity. Psychol Med. 2019;49(15):2475–85.
309. Broulidakis MJ, Golm D, Cortese S, Fairchild G, Sonuga-Barke E. Default mode network connectivity and attention-deficit/hyperactivity disorder in adolescence: associations with delay aversion and temporal discounting, but not mind wandering. Int J Psychophysiol. 2022;173:38–44.
310. Musella KE, Weyandt LL. Attention-deficit hyperactivity disorder and youth's emotion dysregulation: a systematic review of fMRI studies. Appl Neuropsychol Child. 2023;12(4):353–66.
311. Wolf RC, Plichta MM, Sambataro F, Fallgatter AJ, Jacob C, Lesch KP, Herrmann MJ, Schonfeldt-Lecuona C, Connemann BJ, Gron G, Vasic N. Regional brain activation changes and abnormal functional connectivity of the ventrolateral prefrontal cortex during working memory processing in adults with attention-deficit/hyperactivity disorder. Hum Brain Mapp. 2009;30(7):2252–66.
312. Michelini G, Kitsune GL, Cheung CH, Brandeis D, Banaschewski T, Asherson P, McLoughlin G, Kuntsi J. Attention-deficit/hyperactivity disorder remission is linked to better neurophysiological error detection and attention-vigilance processes. Biol Psychiatry. 2016;80(12):923–32.
313. Gordon CT, Hinshaw SP. Executive functions in girls with and without childhood ADHD followed through emerging adulthood: developmental trajectories. J Clin Child Adolesc Psychol. 2020;49(4):509–23.
314. Rubia K. "cool" inferior frontostriatal dysfunction in attention-deficit/hyperactivity disorder versus "hot" ventromedial orbitofrontal-limbic dysfunction in conduct disorder: a review. Biol Psychiatry. 2011;69(12):e69–87.
315. Petrovic P, Castellanos FX. Top-down dysregulation-from ADHD to emotional instability. Front Behav Neurosci. 2016;10:70.
316. Ohnishi T, Toda W, Itagaki S, Sato A, Matsumoto J, Ito H, Ishii S, Miura I, Yabe H. Disrupted structural connectivity and less efficient network system in patients with the treatment-naive adult attention-deficit/hyperactivity disorder. Front Psych. 2023;14:1093522.
317. Tan YW, Liu L, Wang YF, Li HM, Pan MR, Zhao MJ, Huang F, Wang YF, He Y, Liao XH, Qian QJ. Alterations of cerebral perfusion and functional brain connectivity in medication-naive male adults with attention-deficit/hyperactivity disorder. CNS Neurosci Ther. 2020;26(2):197–206.
318. King SG, Gaudreault PO, Malaker P, Kim JW, Alia-Klein N, Xu J, Goldstein RZ. Prefrontal-habenular microstructural impairments in human cocaine and heroin addiction. Neuron. 2022;110(22):3820–32.e4.
319. Arfuso M, Salas R, Castellanos FX, Krain RA. Evidence of altered habenular intrinsic functional connectivity in pediatric ADHD. J Atten Disord. 2021;25(5):749–57.
320. Volkow ND, Boyle M. Neuroscience of Addiction: relevance to prevention and treatment. Am J Psychiatry. 2018;175(8):729–40.
321. von Rhein D, Cools R, Zwiers MP, van der Schaaf M, Franke B, Luman M, Oosterlaan J, Heslenfeld DJ, Hoekstra PJ, Hartman CA, Faraone SV, van Rooij D, van Dongen EV, Lojowska M, Mennes M, Buitelaar J. Increased neural responses to reward in adolescents and young adults with attention-deficit/hyperactivity disorder and their unaffected siblings. J Am Acad Child Adolesc Psychiatry. 2015;54(5):394–402.
322. Buchel C, Peters J, Banaschewski T, Bokde AL, Bromberg U, Conrod PJ, Flor H, Papadopoulos D, Garavan H, Gowland P, Heinz A, Walter H, Ittermann B, Mann K, Martinot JL, Paillere-Martinot ML, Nees F, Paus T, Pausova Z, Poustka L, Rietschel M, Robbins TW, Smolka MN, Gallinat J, Schumann G, Knutson B, IMAGEN Consortium. Blunted ventral striatal responses to anticipated rewards foreshadow problematic drug use in novelty-seeking adolescents. Nat Commun. 2017;8:14140.
323. Adisetiyo V, Gray KM. Neuroimaging the neural correlates of increased risk for substance use disorders in attention-deficit/hyperactivity disorder-a systematic review. Am J Addict. 2017;26(2):99–111.
324. Kwon E, Hummer T, Andrews KD, Finn P, Aalsma M, Bailey A, Hanquier J, Wang T, Hulvershorn L. Functional connectivity in frontostriatal networks differentiate offspring of parents with substance use disorders from other high-risk youth. Drug Alcohol Depend. 2021;219:108498.
325. Anker E, Haavik J, Heir T. Alcohol and drug use disorders in adult attention-deficit/hyperactivity

disorder: prevalence and associations with attention-deficit/hyperactivity disorder symptom severity and emotional dysregulation. World J Psychiatry. 2020;10(9):202–11.
326. Rubia K, Halari R, Mohammad AM, Taylor E, Brammer M. Methylphenidate normalizes frontocingulate underactivation during error processing in attention-deficit/hyperactivity disorder. Biol Psychiatry. 2011;70(3):255–62.
327. Rubia K, Halari R, Cubillo A, Smith AB, Mohammad AM, Brammer M, Taylor E. Methylphenidate normalizes fronto-striatal underactivation during interference inhibition in medication-naive boys with attention-deficit hyperactivity disorder. Neuropsychopharmacology. 2011;36(8):1575–86.
328. Spencer TJ, Brown A, Seidman LJ, Valera EM, Makris N, Lomedico A, Faraone SV, Biederman J. Effect of psychostimulants on brain structure and function in ADHD: a qualitative literature review of magnetic resonance imaging-based neuroimaging studies. J Clin Psychiatry. 2013;74(9):902–17.
329. Sigurdardottir HL, Kranz GS, Rami-Mark C, James GM, Vanicek T, Gryglewski G, Berroteran-Infante N, Kautzky A, Hienert M, Traub-Weidinger T, Mitterhauser M, Wadsak W, Hartmann AM, Hacker M, Rujescu D, Kasper S, Lanzenberger R. Association of norepinephrine transporter methylation with in vivo NET expression and hyperactivity-impulsivity symptoms in ADHD measured with PET. Mol Psychiatry. 2021;26(3):1009–18.
330. Yang Z, Kelly C, Castellanos FX, Leon T, Milham MP, Adler LA. Neural correlates of symptom improvement following stimulant treatment in adults with attention-deficit/hyperactivity disorder. J Child Adolesc Psychopharmacol. 2016;26(6):527–36.
331. Kowalczyk OS, Cubillo AI, Smith A, Barrett N, Giampietro V, Brammer M, Simmons A, Rubia K. Methylphenidate and atomoxetine normalise fronto-parietal underactivation during sustained attention in ADHD adolescents. Eur Neuropsychopharmacol. 2019;29(10):1102–16.
332. Czerniak SM, Sikoglu EM, King JA, Kennedy DN, Mick E, Frazier J, Moore CM. Areas of the brain modulated by single-dose methylphenidate treatment in youth with ADHD during task-based fMRI: a systematic review. Harv Rev Psychiatry. 2013;21(3):151–62.
333. Silva N Jr, Szobot CM, Shih MC, Hoexter MQ, Anselmi CE, Pechansky F, Bressan RA, Rohde LA. Searching for a neurobiological basis for self-medication theory in ADHD comorbid with substance use disorders: an in vivo study of dopamine transporters using (99m)Tc-TRODAT-1 SPECT. Clin Nucl Med. 2014;39(2):e129–34.
334. Crunelle CL, van den Brink W, Dom G, Booij J. Dopamine transporter occupancy by methylphenidate and impulsivity in adult ADHD. Br J Psychiatry. 2014;204(6):486–7.
335. Peterkin AL, Crone CC, Sheridan MJ, Wise TN. Cognitive performance enhancement: misuse or self-treatment? J Atten Disord. 2011;15(4):263–8.
336. Gudjonsson GH, Sigurdsson JF, Sigfusdottir ID, Young S. An epidemiological study of ADHD symptoms among young persons and the relationship with cigarette smoking, alcohol consumption and illicit drug use. J Child Psychol Psychiatry. 2012;53(3):304–12.
337. Gujska JH, Silczuk A, Madejek R, Szulc A. Exploring the link between attention-deficit hyperactivity disorder and cannabis use disorders: a review. Med Sci Monit. 2023;29:e939749.
338. Carli G, Cavicchioli M, Martini AL, Bruscoli M, Manfredi A, Presotto L, Mazzeo C, Sestini S, Perani D. Neurobiological dysfunctional substrates for the self-medication hypothesis in adult individuals with attention-deficit hyperactivity disorder and cocaine use disorder: a Fluorine-18-Fluorodeoxyglucose positron emission tomography study. Brain Connect. 2023;13(7):370–82.
339. Mariani JJ, Khantzian EJ, Levin FR. The self-medication hypothesis and psychostimulant treatment of cocaine dependence: an update. Am J Addict. 2014;23(2):189–93.
340. Levin FR, Mariani JJ, Specker S, Mooney M, Mahony A, Brooks DJ, Babb D, Bai Y, Eberly LE, Nunes EV, Grabowski J. Extended-release mixed amphetamine salts vs placebo for comorbid adult attention-deficit/hyperactivity disorder and cocaine use disorder: a randomized clinical trial. JAMA Psychiatry. 2015;72(6):593–602.
341. Notzon DP, Mariani JJ, Pavlicova M, Glass A, Mahony AL, Brooks DJ, Grabowski J, Levin FR. Mixed-amphetamine salts increase abstinence from marijuana in patients with co-occurring attention-deficit/hyperactivity disorder and cocaine dependence. Am J Addict. 2016;25(8):666–72.
342. Levin FR, Choi CJ, Pavlicova M, Mariani JJ, Mahony A, Brooks DJ, Nunes EV, Grabowski J. How treatment improvement in ADHD and cocaine dependence are related to one another: a secondary analysis. Drug Alcohol Depend. 2018;188:135–40.
343. Manni C, Cipollone G, Pallucchini A, Maremmani AGI, Perugi G, Maremmani I. Remarkable reduction of cocaine use in dual disorder (adult attention deficit hyperactive disorder/cocaine use disorder) patients treated with medications for ADHD. Int J Environ Res Public Health. 2019;16(20):3911.
344. Tardelli VS, Bisaga A, Arcadepani FB, Gerra G, Levin FR, Fidalgo TM. Prescription psychostimulants for the treatment of stimulant use disorder: a systematic review and meta-analysis. Psychopharmacology. 2020;237(8):2233–55.
345. Mariani JJ, Choi CJ, Pavlicova M, Mahony AL, Brooks DJ, Grabowski J, Levin FR. Open-label pilot study of lisdexamfetamine for cocaine use disorder. Am J Drug Alcohol Abuse. 2021;47(3):402–9.

346. Faraone SV. The pharmacology of amphetamine and methylphenidate: relevance to the neurobiology of attention-deficit/hyperactivity disorder and other psychiatric comorbidities. Neurosci Biobehav Rev. 2018;87:255–70.
347. Yu C, Garcia-Olivares J, Candler S, Schwabe S, Maletic V. New insights into the mechanism of action of viloxazine: serotonin and norepinephrine modulating properties. J Exp Pharmacol. 2020;12:285–300.
348. Arnsten AF. The use of α-2A adrenergic agonists for the treatment of attention-deficit/hyperactivity disorder. Expert Rev Neurother 2010;10(10):1595–1605.
349. Hegvik TA, Waloen K, Pandey SK, Faraone SV, Haavik J, Zayats T. Druggable genome in attention deficit/hyperactivity disorder and its co-morbid conditions. New avenues for treatment. Mol Psychiatry. 2021;26(8):4004–15.
350. Huang X, Wang M, Zhang Q, Chen X, Wu J. The role of glutamate receptors in attention-deficit/hyperactivity disorder: from physiology to disease. Am J Med Genet B Neuropsychiatr Genet. 2019;180(4):272–86.
351. Sharp BM. Basolateral amygdala and stress-induced hyperexcitability affect motivated behaviors and addiction. Transl Psychiatry. 2017;7(8):e1194.
352. Potter AS, Schaubhut G, Shipman M. Targeting the nicotinic cholinergic system to treat attention-deficit/hyperactivity disorder: rationale and progress to date. CNS Drugs. 2014;28(12):1103–13.
353. Groenman AP, Greven CU, van Donkelaar MM, Schellekens A, van Hulzen KJ, Rommelse N, Hartman CA, Hoekstra PJ, Luman M, Franke B, Faraone SV, Oosterlaan J, Buitelaar JK. Dopamine and serotonin genetic risk scores predicting substance and nicotine use in attention deficit/hyperactivity disorder. Addict Biol. 2016;21(4):915–23.
354. Volkow ND, Fowler JS, Wang GJ, Swanson JM, Telang F. Dopamine in drug abuse and addiction: results of imaging studies and treatment implications. Arch Neurol. 2007;64(11):1575–9.
355. Volkow ND, Swanson JM. Variables that affect the clinical use and abuse of methylphenidate in the treatment of ADHD. Am J Psychiatry. 2003;160(11):1909–18.
356. Volkow ND, Wang GJ, Fowler JS, Gatley SJ, Logan J, Ding YS, Hitzemann R, Pappas N. Dopamine transporter occupancies in the human brain induced by therapeutic doses of oral methylphenidate. Am J Psychiatry. 1998;155(10):1325–31.
357. Spencer TJ, Biederman J, Ciccone PE, Madras BK, Dougherty DD, Bonab AA, Livni E, Parasrampuria DA, Fischman AJ. PET study examining pharmacokinetics, detection and likeability, and dopamine transporter receptor occupancy of short- and long-acting oral methylphenidate. Am J Psychiatry. 2006;163(3):387–95.
358. Barnhardt EA, Narayanan AR, Coury DL. Evaluating serdexmethylphenidate and dexmethylphenidate capsules as a once-daily treatment option for ADHD. Expert Opin Pharmacother. 2023;24(11):1215–9.
359. Jasinski DR, Krishnan S. Abuse liability and safety of oral lisdexamfetamine dimesylate in individuals with a history of stimulant abuse. J Psychopharmacol. 2009;23(4):419–27.
360. Shram MJ, Setnik B, Webster L, Guenther S, Mickle TC, Braeckman R, Kanski J, Martin A, Kelsh D, Vince BD, Barrett AC. Oral, intranasal, and intravenous abuse potential of serdexmethylphenidate, a novel prodrug of d-methylphenidate. Curr Med Res Opin. 2022;38(7):1237–50.
361. Buck JM, O'Neill HC, Stitzel JA. Developmental nicotine exposure engenders intergenerational downregulation and aberrant posttranslational modification of cardinal epigenetic factors in the frontal cortices, striata, and hippocampi of adolescent mice. Epigenetics Chromatin. 2020;13(1):13.
362. Martin MM, McCarthy DM, Schatschneider C, Trupiano MX, Jones SK, Kalluri A, Bhide PG. Effects of developmental nicotine exposure on frontal cortical GABA-to-non-GABA neuron ratio and novelty-seeking behavior. Cereb Cortex. 2020;30(3):1830–42.
363. McCarthy DM, Morgan TJ Jr, Lowe SE, Williamson MJ, Spencer TJ, Biederman J, Bhide PG. Nicotine exposure of male mice produces behavioral impairment in multiple generations of descendants. PLoS Biol. 2018;16(10):e2006497.
364. Zhu J, Lee KP, Spencer TJ, Biederman J, Bhide PG. Transgenerational transmission of hyperactivity in a mouse model of ADHD. J Neurosci. 2014;34(8):2768–73.
365. Zhu JL, Olsen J, Liew Z, Li J, Niclasen J, Obel C. Parental smoking during pregnancy and ADHD in children: the Danish national birth cohort. Pediatrics. 2014;134(2):e382–8.
366. Huang L, Wang Y, Zhang L, Zheng Z, Zhu T, Qu Y, Mu D. Maternal smoking and attention-deficit/hyperactivity disorder in offspring: a meta-analysis. Pediatrics. 2018;141(1):e20172465.
367. Zou R, Boer OD, Felix JF, Muetzel RL, Franken IHA, Cecil CAM, El Marroun H. Association of maternal tobacco use during pregnancy with preadolescent brain morphology among offspring. JAMA Netw Open. 2022;5(8):e2224701.
368. Biederman J, Fitzgerald M, Spencer TJ, Bhide PG, McCarthy DM, Woodworth KY, Saunders A, Faraone SV. Is paternal smoking at conception a risk for ADHD? A controlled study in youth with and without ADHD. J Atten Disord. 2020;24(11):1493–6.
369. Lin LZ, Xu SL, Wu QZ, Zhou Y, Ma HM, Chen DH, Chen GB, Yu HY, Yang BY, Zeng XW, Hu LW, Dong GH. Association of prenatal, early postnatal, or current exposure to secondhand smoke with Attention-Deficit/Hyperactivity Disorder symptoms in children. JAMA Netw Open. 2021;4(5):e2110931.
370. McGrath-Morrow SA, Gorzkowski J, Groner JA, Rule AM, Wilson K, Tanski SE, Collaco JM,

Klein JD. The effects of nicotine on development. Pediatrics. 2020;145(3):e20191346.
371. Garrison-Desany HM, Hong X, Maher BS, Beaty TH, Wang G, Pearson C, Liang L, Wang X, Ladd-Acosta C. Individual and combined association between prenatal polysubstance exposure and childhood risk of attention-deficit/hyperactivity disorder. JAMA Netw Open. 2022;5(3):e221957.
372. Knopik VS, Marceau K, Bidwell LC, Rolan E. Prenatal substance exposure and offspring development: does DNA methylation play a role? Neurotoxicol Teratol. 2019;71:50–63.
373. Neumann A, Walton E, Alemany S, Cecil C, Gonzalez JR, Jima DD, Lahti J, Tuominen ST, Barker ED, Binder E, Caramaschi D, Carracedo A, Czamara D, Evandt J, Felix JF, Fuemmeler BF, Gutzkow KB, Hoyo C, Julvez J, Kajantie E, Laivuori H, Maguire R, Maitre L, Murphy SK, Murcia M, Villa PM, Sharp G, Sunyer J, Raikkonen K, Bakermans-Kranenburg M, MV IJ, Guxens M, Relton CL, Tiemeier H. Association between DNA methylation and ADHD symptoms from birth to school age: a prospective meta-analysis. Transl Psychiatry. 2020;10(1):398.
374. Pagnin D, Zamboni Grecco ML, Furtado EF. Prenatal alcohol use as a risk for attention-deficit/hyperactivity disorder. Eur Arch Psychiatry Clin Neurosci. 2019;269(6):681–7.
375. Yolton K, Cornelius M, Ornoy A, McGough J, Makris S, Schantz S. Exposure to neurotoxicants and the development of attention deficit hyperactivity disorder and its related behaviors in childhood. Neurotoxicol Teratol. 2014;44:30–45.
376. Chu JTW, McCormack J, Marsh S, Wells A, Wilson H, Bullen C. Impact of prenatal alcohol exposure on neurodevelopmental outcomes: a systematic review. Health Psychol Behav Med. 2022;10(1):973–1002.
377. Paul SE, Hatoum AS, Fine JD, Johnson EC, Hansen I, Karcher NR, Moreau AL, Bondy E, Qu Y, Carter EB, Rogers CE, Agrawal A, Barch DM, Bogdan R. Associations between prenatal cannabis exposure and childhood outcomes: results from the ABCD study. JAMA Psychiatry. 2021;78(1):64–76.
378. Winiger EA, Hewitt JK. Prenatal cannabis exposure and sleep outcomes in children 9-10 years of age in the adolescent brain cognitive development (SM) study. Sleep Health. 2020;6(6):787–9.
379. Ackerman JP, Riggins T, Black MM. A review of the effects of prenatal cocaine exposure among school-aged children. Pediatrics. 2010;125(3):554–65.
380. Ornoy A. The impact of intrauterine exposure versus postnatal environment in neurodevelopmental toxicity: long-term neurobehavioral studies in children at risk for developmental disorders. Toxicol Lett. 2003;140–141:171–81.
381. Pessah IN, Lein PJ, Seegal RF, Sagiv SK. Neurotoxicity of polychlorinated biphenyls and related organohalogens. Acta Neuropathol. 2019;138(3):363–87.
382. Sussman TJ, Baker BH, Wakhloo AJ, Gillet V, Abdelouahab N, Whittingstall K, Lepage JF, St-Cyr L, Boivin A, Gagnon A, Baccarelli AA, Takser L, Posner J. The relationship between persistent organic pollutants and attention deficit hyperactivity disorder phenotypes: evidence from task-based neural activity in an observational study of a community sample of Canadian mother-child dyads. Environ Res. 2022;206:112593.
383. Park S, Cowell W, Margolis AE, Sjodin A, Jones R, Rauh V, Wang S, Herbstman JB. Prenatal exposure to polybrominated diphenyl ethers and inattention/hyperactivity symptoms in mid to late adolescents. Front. Epidemiol. 2023;3:1061234.
384. Choi G, Keil AP, Richardson DB, Daniels JL, Hoffman K, Villanger GD, Sakhi AK, Thomsen C, Reichborn-Kjennerud T, Aase H, Engel SM. Pregnancy exposure to organophosphate esters and the risk of attention-deficit hyperactivity disorder in the Norwegian mother, father and child cohort study. Environ Int. 2021;154:106549.
385. Xu Y, Yang X, Chen D, Xu Y, Lan L, Zhao S, Liu Q, Snijders AM, Xia Y. Maternal exposure to pesticides and autism or attention-deficit/hyperactivity disorders in offspring: a meta-analysis. Chemosphere. 2023;313:137459.
386. Lee KS, Lim YH, Lee YA, Shin CH, Kim BN, Hong YC, Kim JI. The association of prenatal and childhood pyrethroid pesticide exposure with school-age ADHD traits. Environ Int. 2022;161:107124.
387. Froehlich TE, Lanphear BP, Auinger P, Hornung R, Epstein JN, Braun J, Kahn RS. Association of tobacco and lead exposures with attention-deficit/hyperactivity disorder. Pediatrics. 2009;124(6):e1054–63.
388. Nigg JT, Nikolas M, Mark Knottnerus G, Cavanagh K, Friderici K. Confirmation and extension of association of blood lead with attention-deficit/hyperactivity disorder (ADHD) and ADHD symptom domains at population-typical exposure levels. J Child Psychol Psychiatry. 2010;51(1):58–65.
389. Li Y, Cha C, Lv X, Liu J, He J, Pang Q, Meng L, Kuang H, Fan R. Association between 10 urinary heavy metal exposure and attention deficit hyperactivity disorder for children. Environ Sci Pollut Res Int. 2020;27(25):31233–42.
390. Ostergaard SD, Larsen JT, Dalsgaard S, Wilens TE, Mortensen PB, Agerbo E, Mors O, Petersen L. Predicting ADHD by assessment of Rutter's Indicators of Adversity in infancy. PLoS One. 2016;11(6):e0157352.
391. Zhang N, Gao M, Yu J, Zhang Q, Wang W, Zhou C, Liu L, Sun T, Liao X, Wang J. Understanding the association between adverse childhood experiences and subsequent attention deficit hyperactivity disorder: a systematic review and meta-analysis of observational studies. Brain Behav. 2022;12(10):e32748.
392. Lu S, Perez L, Leslein A, Hatsu I. The relationship between food insecurity and symptoms of attention-deficit hyperactivity disorder in children: a summary of the literature. Nutrients. 2019;11(3):659.

393. Anderson KK, Clemens KK, Le B, Zhang L, Comeau J, Tarasuk V, Shariff SZ. Household food insecurity and health service use for mental and substance use disorders among children and adolescents in Ontario, Canada. CMAJ. 2023;195(28):E948–55.
394. Golm D, Sarkar S, Mackes NK, Fairchild G, Mehta MA, Rutter M, ERA Young Adult Follow Up Study Team, Sonuga-Barke EJ. The impact of childhood deprivation on adult neuropsychological functioning is associated with ADHD symptom persistence. Psychol Med. 2021;51(15):2675–84.
395. Sonuga-Barke EJS, Kennedy M, Kumsta R, Knights N, Golm D, Rutter M, Maughan B, Schlotz W, Kreppner J. Child-to-adult neurodevelopmental and mental health trajectories after early life deprivation: the young adult follow-up of the longitudinal English and Romanian adoptees study. Lancet. 2017;389(10078):1539–48.
396. Golm D, Brandt V. The longitudinal association between infant negative emotionality, childhood maltreatment, and ADHD symptoms: a secondary analysis of data from the fragile families and child wellbeing study. Dev Psychopathol. 2024;36(3):1231–8.
397. Claussen AH, Holbrook JR, Hutchins HJ, Robinson LR, Bloomfield J, Meng L, Bitsko RH, O'Masta B, Cerles A, Maher B, Rush M, Kaminski JW. All in the family? A systematic review and meta-analysis of parenting and family environment as risk factors for attention-deficit/hyperactivity disorder (ADHD) in children. Prev Sci. 2022;25(Suppl 2):1–23.
398. Luderer M, Reinhard I, Richter A, Kiefer F, Weber T. ADHD is associated with a higher risk for traumatic events, self-reported PTSD, and a higher severity of PTSD symptoms in alcohol-dependent patients. Eur Addict Res. 2020;26(4–5):245–53.
399. Bolstad I, Lien L, Bramness JG. ADHD symptoms as risk factor for PTSD in inpatients treated for alcohol use disorder. Psychiatry Res. 2021;300:113904.
400. Ostergaard SD, Trabjerg BB, Als TD, Climent CA, Prive F, Vilhjalmsson BJ, Baekvad-Hansen M, Bybjerg-Grauholm J, Hougaard DM, Nordentoft M, Werge T, Demontis D, Mortensen PB, Borglum AD, Mors O, Agerbo E. Polygenic risk score, psychosocial environment and the risk of attention-deficit/hyperactivity disorder. Transl Psychiatry. 2020;10(1):335.
401. Russell AE, Ford T, Williams R, Russell G. The association between socioeconomic disadvantage and attention deficit/hyperactivity disorder (ADHD): a systematic review. Child Psychiatry Hum Dev. 2016;47(3):440–58.
402. Xerxa Y, Delaney SW, Rescorla LA, Hillegers MHJ, White T, Verhulst FC, Muetzel RL, Tiemeier H. Association of poor family functioning from pregnancy onward with preadolescent behavior and subcortical brain development. JAMA Psychiatry. 2021;78(1):29–37.
403. Sigfusdottir ID, Asgeirsdottir BB, Hall HA, Sigurdsson JF, Young S, Gudjonsson GH. An epidemiological study of ADHD and conduct disorder: does family conflict moderate the association? Soc Psychiatry Psychiatr Epidemiol. 2017;52(4):457–64.
404. McNair LF, Kohlmeier KA. Prenatal nicotine is associated with reduced AMPA and NMDA receptor-mediated rises in calcium within the laterodorsal tegmentum: a pontine nucleus involved in addiction processes. J Dev Orig Health Dis. 2015;6(3):225–41.
405. Rogers CJ, Forster M, Sussman S, Steinberg J, Barrington-Trimis JL, Grigsby TJ, Unger JB. The impact of childhood trauma on problematic alcohol and drug use trajectories and the moderating role of social support. Int J Environ Res Public Health. 2023;20(4):2829.
406. Winter JJ, Rodriguez-Acevedo KL, Dittrich M, Heller EA. Early life adversity: epigenetic regulation underlying drug addiction susceptibility. Mol Cell Neurosci. 2023;125:103825.
407. Slobodin O, Blankers M, Kapitany-Foveny M, Kaye S, Berger I, Johnson B, Demetrovics Z, van den Brink W, van de Glind G. Differential diagnosis in patients with substance use disorder and/or attention-deficit/hyperactivity disorder using continuous performance test. Eur Addict Res. 2020;26(3):151–62.
408. Capusan AJ, Bendtsen P, Marteinsdottir I, Larsson H. Comorbidity of adult ADHD and its subtypes with substance use disorder in a large population-based epidemiological study. J Atten Disord. 2019;23(12):1416–26.
409. Ajnakina O, Murray R, Wimberley MT, Dalsgaard S, Steptoe A. Mapping relationships between polygenic propensity for ADHD and difficulties across multiple life domains in the general population: evidence from the English Longitudinal Study of Ageing. European Neuropsychopharmacology. 2022;63:e100.
410. Cabana-Dominguez J, Soler Artigas M, Arribas L, Alemany S, Vilar-Ribo L, Llonga N, Fadeuilhe C, Corrales M, Richarte V, Ramos-Quiroga JA, Ribases M. Comprehensive analysis of omics data identifies relevant gene networks for attention-deficit/hyperactivity disorder (ADHD). Transl Psychiatry. 2022;12(1):409.
411. McNeill RV, Palladino VS, Brunkhorst-Kanaan N, Grimm O, Reif A, Kittel-Schneider S. Expression of the adult ADHD-associated gene ADGRL3 is dysregulated by risk variants and environmental risk factors. World J Biol Psychiatry. 2021;22(5):335–49.
412. Ortal S, van de Glind G, Johan F, Itai B, Nir Y, Iliyan I, van den Brink W. The role of different aspects of impulsivity as independent risk factors for substance use disorders in patients with ADHD: a review. Curr Drug Abuse Rev. 2015;8(2):119–33.
413. Paloyelis Y, Asherson P, Mehta MA, Faraone SV, Kuntsi J. DAT1 and COMT effects on delay discounting and trait impulsivity in male adolescents with attention deficit/hyperactivity disorder and

healthy controls. Neuropsychopharmacology. 2010;35(12):2414–26.

414. Barra S, Grub A, Roesler M, Retz-Junginger P, Philipp F, Retz W. The role of stress coping strategies for life impairments in ADHD. J Neural Transm (Vienna). 2021;128(7):981–92.
415. Heshmati M, Christoffel DJ, LeClair K, Cathomas F, Golden SA, Aleyasin H, Turecki G, Friedman AK, Han MH, Menard C, Russo SJ. Depression and social defeat stress are associated with inhibitory synaptic changes in the nucleus accumbens. J Neurosci. 2020;40(32):6228–33.
416. Kreek MJ, Nielsen DA, Butelman ER, LaForge KS. Genetic influences on impulsivity, risk taking, stress responsivity and vulnerability to drug abuse and addiction. Nat Neurosci. 2005;8(11):1450–7.
417. Young JT, Carruthers S, Kaye S, Allsop S, Gilsenan J, Degenhardt L, van de Glind G, van den Brink W, Preen D. Comorbid attention deficit hyperactivity disorder and substance use disorder complexity and chronicity in treatment-seeking adults. Drug Alcohol Rev. 2015;34(6):683–93.
418. MacKillop J, Amlung MT, Few LR, Ray LA, Sweet LH, Munafo MR. Delayed reward discounting and addictive behavior: a meta-analysis. Psychopharmacology. 2011;216(3):305–21.
419. Faraone SV, Asherson P, Banaschewski T, Biederman J, Buitelaar JK, Ramos-Quiroga JA, Rohde LA, Sonuga-Barke EJ, Tannock R, Franke B. Attention-deficit/hyperactivity disorder. Nat Rev Dis Primers. 2015;1:15020.
420. United Nations Office on Drugs and Crime. The nonmedical use of prescription drugs - Policy Direction Issues. 2011. Available from: https://www.unodc.org/documents/drug-prevention-and-treatment/nonmedical-use-prescription-drugs.pdf
421. McCabe SE, Arterberry BJ, Dickinson K, Evans-Polce RJ, Ford JA, Ryan JE, Schepis TS. Assessment of changes in alcohol and marijuana abstinence, co-use, and use disorders among US young adults from 2002 to 2018. JAMA Pediatr. 2021;175(1):64–72.
422. Schulenberg J, Johnston L, O'Malley P, Bachman J, Miech R, Patrick M. Monitoring the Future national survey results on drug use, 1975–2018: volume II: College students and adults ages 19–60. Ann Arbor: Institute for Social Research, The University of Michigan; 2019.
423. McCabe SE, Veliz P, Wilens TE, Schulenberg JE. Adolescents' prescription stimulant use and adult functional outcomes: a national prospective study. J Am Acad Child Adolesc Psychiatry. 2017;56(3):226–33.e4.
424. McCabe SE, West BT. Medical and nonmedical use of prescription stimulants: results from a national multicohort study. J Am Acad Child Adolesc Psychiatry. 2013;52(12):1272–80.
425. Faraone SV, Rostain AL, Montano CB, Mason O, Antshel KM, Newcorn JH. Systematic review: nonmedical use of prescription stimulants: risk factors, outcomes, and risk reduction strategies. J Am Acad Child Adolesc Psychiatry. 2020;59(1):100–12.
426. Teter CJ, DiRaimo CG, West BT, Schepis TS, McCabe SE. Nonmedical use of prescription stimulants among US high school students to help study: results from a national survey. J Pharm Pract. 2020;33(1):38–47.
427. Chen LY, Crum RM, Martins SS, Kaufmann CN, Strain EC, Mojtabai R. Patterns of concurrent substance use among nonmedical ADHD stimulant users: results from the National Survey on Drug Use and Health. Drug Alcohol Depend. 2014;142:86–90.
428. Hulme S, Bright D, Nielsen S. The source and diversion of pharmaceutical drugs for non-medical use: a systematic review and meta-analysis. Drug Alcohol Depend. 2018;186:242–56.
429. Wilens TE, Martelon M, Yule A, Kaminski TA, Burke C, Schepis TS, McCabe SE. Disentangling the social context of nonmedical use of prescription stimulants in college students. Am J Addict. 2020;29(6):476–84.
430. National Institute on Drug Abuse. What is the scope of prescription drug misuse in the United States? 2023, December 14. Available from: https://nida.nih.gov/publications/research-reports/misuse-prescription-drugs/what-scope-prescription-drug-misuse.
431. Fischer B, Argento E. Prescription opioid related misuse, harms, diversion and interventions in Canada: a review. Pain Physician. 2012;15(3 Suppl):ES191-203.
432. European Monitoring Centre for Drugs and Drug Addiction. Fentanils and Synthetic Cannabinoids: Driving Greater Complexity into the Drug Situation. An Update from the EU Early Warning System. Luxembourg: Publications Office of the European Union; 2018.
433. Schepis TS, Ford JA, Wilens TE, Teter CJ, McCabe SE. Differences in prescription stimulant misuse motives across adolescents and young adults in the United States. J Clin Psychiatry. 2020;81(6):20m13302.
434. Compton WM, Han B, Blanco C, Johnson K, Jones CM. Prevalence and correlates of prescription stimulant use, misuse, use disorders, and motivations for misuse among adults in the United States. Am J Psychiatry. 2018;175(8):741–55.
435. Cassidy TA, Varughese S, Russo L, Budman SH, Eaton TA, Butler SF. Nonmedical use and diversion of ADHD stimulants among U.S. adults ages 18-49: a national internet survey. J Atten Disord. 2015;19(7):630–40.
436. Novak SP, Kroutil LA, Williams RL, Van Brunt DL. The nonmedical use of prescription ADHD medications: results from a national internet panel. Subst Abuse Treat Prev Policy. 2007;2:32.
437. Advokat CD, Guidry D, Martino L. Licit and illicit use of medications for attention-deficit hyperactivity disorder in undergraduate college students. J Am Coll Heal. 2008;56(6):601–6.

438. DeSantis AD, Webb EM, Noar SM. Illicit use of prescription ADHD medications on a college campus: a multimethodological approach. J Am Coll Heal. 2008;57(3):315–24.
439. Benson K, Woodlief DT, Flory K, Siceloff ER, Coleman K, Lamont A. Is ADHD, independent of ODD, associated with whether and why college students misuse stimulant medication? Experim Clin Psychopharmacol. 2018;26(5):476–87.
440. Garnier-Dykstra LM, Caldeira KM, Vincent KB, O'Grady KE, Arria AM. Nonmedical use of prescription stimulants during college: four-year trends in exposure opportunity, use, motives, and sources. J Am Coll Heal. 2012;60(3):226–34.
441. Arria AM, Wilcox HC, Caldeira KM, Vincent KB, Garnier-Dykstra LM, O'Grady KE. Dispelling the myth of "smart drugs": cannabis and alcohol use problems predict nonmedical use of prescription stimulants for studying. Addict Behav. 2013;38(3):1643–50.
442. Faraone SV, Hess J, Wilens T. Prevalence and consequences of the nonmedical use of amphetamine among persons calling poison control Centers. J Atten Disord. 2019;23(11):1219–28.
443. Benson K, Flory K, Humphreys KL, Lee SS. Misuse of stimulant medication among college students: a comprehensive review and meta-analysis. Clin Child Fam Psychol Rev. 2015;18(1):50–76.
444. Schepis TS, Klare DL, Ford JA, McCabe SE. Prescription drug misuse: taking a lifespan perspective. Subst Abuse. 2020;14:1178221820909352.
445. Piper BJ, Ogden CL, Simoyan OM, Chung DY, Caggiano JF, Nichols SD, McCall KL. Trends in use of prescription stimulants in the United States and territories, 2006 to 2016. PLoS One. 2018;13(11):e0206100.
446. Morkem R, Patten S, Queenan J, Barber D. Recent trends in the prescribing of ADHD medications in Canadian primary care. J Atten Disord. 2020;24(2):301–8.
447. Cassidy TA, McNaughton EC, Varughese S, Russo L, Zulueta M, Butler SF. Nonmedical use of prescription ADHD stimulant medications among adults in a substance abuse treatment population: early findings from the NAVIPPRO surveillance system. J Atten Disord. 2015;19(4):275–83.
448. Charach A, Yeung E, Climans T, Lillie E. Childhood attention-deficit/hyperactivity disorder and future substance use disorders: comparative meta-analyses. J Am Acad Child Adolesc Psychiatry. 2011;50(1):9–21.
449. Fuller-Thomson E, Lewis DA, Agbeyaka S. Attention-Deficit/Hyperactivity Disorder and alcohol and other substance use disorders in young adulthood: findings from a Canadian nationally representative survey. Alcohol Alcohol. 2022;57(3):385–95.
450. Agnew-Blais JC, Polanczyk GV, Danese A, Wertz J, Moffitt TE, Arseneault L. Young adult mental health and functional outcomes among individuals with remitted, persistent and late-onset ADHD. Br J Psychiatry. 2018;213(3):526–34.
451. Gonzalez RA, Velez-Pastrana MC, Blankers M, Backer A, Konstenius M, Holtmann M, Levin FR, Noack M, Kaye S, Demetrovics Z, van de Glind G, van den Brink W, Schellekens A, ICASA Group. Onset and severity of early disruptive behavioral disorders in treatment-seeking Substance Use Disorder patients with and without Attention-Deficit/Hyperactivity Disorder. Eur Addict Res. 2020;26(4–5):211–22.
452. Sullivan MA, Rudnik-Levin F. Attention deficit/hyperactivity disorder and substance abuse. Diagnostic and therapeutic considerations. Ann N Y Acad Sci. 2001;931:251–70.
453. Wilens TE. Impact of ADHD and its treatment on substance abuse in adults. J Clin Psychiatry. 2004;65(Suppl 3):38–45.
454. Fatseas M, Hurmic H, Serre F, Debrabant R, Daulouede JP, Denis C, Auriacombe M. Addiction severity pattern associated with adult and childhood attention deficit hyperactivity disorder (ADHD) in patients with addictions. Psychiatry Res. 2016;246:656–62.
455. Erskine HE, Ferrari AJ, Polanczyk GV, Moffitt TE, Murray CJ, Vos T, Whiteford HA, Scott JG. The global burden of conduct disorder and attention-deficit/hyperactivity disorder in 2010. J Child Psychol Psychiatry. 2014;55(4):328–36.
456. Mannuzza S, Klein RG, Bessler A, Malloy P, LaPadula M. Adult outcome of hyperactive boys. Educational achievement, occupational rank, and psychiatric status. Arch Gen Psychiatry. 1993;50(7):565–76.
457. Biederman J, Wilens T, Mick E, Milberger S, Spencer TJ, Faraone SV. Psychoactive substance use disorders in adults with attention deficit hyperactivity disorder (ADHD): effects of ADHD and psychiatric comorbidity. Am J Psychiatry. 1995;152(11):1652–8.
458. Estevez-Lamorte N, Foster S, Eich-Hochli D, Moggi F, Gmel G, Mohler-Kuo M. Adult attention-deficit/hyperactivity disorder, risky substance use and substance use disorders: a follow-up study among young men. Eur Arch Psychiatry Clin Neurosci. 2019;269(6):667–79.
459. Wilens TE, Biederman J, Mick E. Does ADHD affect the course of substance abuse? Findings from a sample of adults with and without ADHD. Am J Addict. 1998;7(2):156–63.
460. McAweeney M, Rogers NL, Huddleston C, Moore D, Gentile JP. Symptom prevalence of ADHD in a community residential substance abuse treatment program. J Atten Disord. 2010;13(6):601–8.
461. Carroll KM, Rounsaville BJ. History and significance of childhood attention deficit disorder in treatment-seeking cocaine abusers. Compr Psychiatry. 1993;34(2):75–82.
462. van de Glind G, van Emmerik-van Oortmerssen K, Carpentier PJ, Levin FR, Koeter MW, Barta C, Kaye

S, Skutle A, Franck J, Konstenius M, Bu ET, Moggi F, Dom G, Demetrovics Z, Fatseas M, Schillinger A, Kapitany-Foveny M, Verspreet S, Seitz A, Johnson B, Faraone SV, Ramos-Quiroga JA, Allsop S, Carruthers S, Schoevers RA, IASP Research Group, van den Brink W. The international ADHD in substance use disorders prevalence (IASP) study: background, methods and study population. Int J Methods Psychiatr Res. 2013;22(3):232–44.
463. Van de Glind G, Brynte C, Skutle A, Kaye S, Konstenius M, Levin F, Mathys F, Demetrovics Z, Moggi F, Ramos-Quiroga JA, Schellekens A, Crunelle C, Dom G, van den Brink W, Franck J. The International Collaboration on ADHD and Substance Abuse (ICASA): mission, results, and future activities. Eur Addict Res. 2020;26(4–5):173–8.
464. van Emmerik-van Oortmerssen K, van de Glind G, van den Brink W, Smit F, Crunelle CL, Swets M, Schoevers RA. Prevalence of attention-deficit hyperactivity disorder in substance use disorder patients: a meta-analysis and meta-regression analysis. Drug Alcohol Depend. 2012;122(1–2):11–9.
465. Adler LA, Spencer T, Faraone SV, Kessler RC, Howes MJ, Biederman J, Secnik K. Validity of pilot adult ADHD self- report scale (ASRS) to rate adult ADHD symptoms. Ann Clin Psychiatry. 2006;18(3):145–8.
466. Green JG, DeYoung G, Wogan ME, Wolf EJ, Lane KL, Adler LA. Evidence for the reliability and preliminary validity of the Adult ADHD Self-Report Scale v1.1 (ASRS v1.1) screener in an adolescent community sample. Int J Methods Psychiatr Res. 2019;28(1):e1751.
467. van de Glind G, van den Brink W, Koeter MW, Carpentier PJ, van Emmerik-van Oortmerssen K, Kaye S, Skutle A, Bu ET, Franck J, Konstenius M, Moggi F, Dom G, Verspreet S, Demetrovics Z, Kapitany-Foveny M, Fatseas M, Auriacombe M, Schillinger A, Seitz A, Johnson B, Faraone SV, Ramos-Quiroga JA, Casas M, Allsop S, Carruthers S, Barta C, Schoevers RA, IASP Research Group, Levin FR. Validity of the adult ADHD self-report scale (ASRS) as a screener for adult ADHD in treatment seeking substance use disorder patients. Drug Alcohol Depend. 2013;132(3):587–96.
468. Rohner H, Gaspar N, Philipsen A, Schulze M. Prevalence of attention deficit hyperactivity disorder (ADHD) among substance use disorder (SUD) populations: meta-analysis. Int J Environ Res Public Health. 2023;20(2):1275.
469. Hale EW, Coyle TD. Under-documented or under-recognized? Comorbid ADHD in emergency department patients with addictive disorders. J Atten Disord. 2023;27(3):270–2.
470. Skutle A, Bu ETH, Jellestad FK, van Emmerik-van Oortmerssen K, Dom G, Verspreet S, Carpentier PJ, Ramos-Quiroga JA, Franck J, Konstenius M, Kaye S, Demetrovics Z, Barta C, Fatseas M, Auriacombe M, Johnson B, Faraone SV, Levin FR, Allsop S, Carruthers S, Schoevers RA, Koeter MWJ, van den Brink W, Moggi F, Moller M, van de Glind G. Early developmental, temperamental and educational problems in 'substance use disorder' patients with and without ADHD. Does ADHD make a difference? Addict Behav Rep. 2015;2:13–8.
471. van Emmerik-van Oortmerssen K, van de Glind G, Koeter MW, Allsop S, Auriacombe M, Barta C, Bu ET, Burren Y, Carpentier PJ, Carruthers S, Casas M, Demetrovics Z, Dom G, Faraone SV, Fatseas M, Franck J, Johnson B, Kapitany-Foveny M, Kaye S, Konstenius M, Levin FR, Moggi F, Moller M, Ramos-Quiroga JA, Schillinger A, Skutle A, Verspreet S, IASP Research Group, van den Brink W, Schoevers RA Psychiatric comorbidity in treatment-seeking substance use disorder patients with and without attention deficit hyperactivity disorder: results of the IASP study. Addiction 2014;109(2):262–72.
472. Bozkurt M, Evren C, Umut G, Evren B. Relationship of attention-deficit/hyperactivity disorder symptom severity with severity of alcohol-related problems in a sample of inpatients with alcohol use disorder. Neuropsychiatr Dis Treat. 2016;12:1661–7.
473. Biederman J, Wilens TE, Mick E, Faraone SV, Spencer T. Does attention-deficit hyperactivity disorder impact the developmental course of drug and alcohol abuse and dependence? Biol Psychiatry. 1998;44(4):269–73.
474. Sundquist J, Ohlsson H, Sundquist K, Kendler KS. Attention-deficit/hyperactivity disorder and risk for drug use disorder: a population-based follow-up and co-relative study. Psychol Med. 2015;45(5):977–83.
475. Sadeh N, Spielberg JM, Logue MW, Hayes JP, Wolf EJ, McGlinchey RE, Milberg WP, Schichman SA, Stone A, Miller MW. Linking genes, circuits, and behavior: network connectivity as a novel endophenotype of externalizing. Psychol Med. 2019;49(11):1905–13.
476. Rooney M, Chronis-Tuscano AM, Huggins S. Disinhibition mediates the relationship between ADHD and problematic alcohol use in college students. J Atten Disord. 2015;19(4):313–27.
477. Levitt E, Sanchez-Roige S, Palmer AA, MacKillop J. Steep discounting of future rewards as an impulsivity phenotype: a concise review. Curr Top Behav Neurosci. 2020;47:113–38.
478. Young SE, Friedman NP, Miyake A, Willcutt EG, Corley RP, Haberstick BC, Hewitt JK. Behavioral disinhibition: liability for externalizing spectrum disorders and its genetic and environmental relation to response inhibition across adolescence. J Abnorm Psychol. 2009;118(1):117–30.
479. Kozak K, Lucatch AM, Lowe DJE, Balodis IM, MacKillop J, George TP. The neurobiology of impulsivity and substance use disorders: implications for treatment. Ann N Y Acad Sci. 2019;1451(1):71–91.
480. Dalsgaard S, Mortensen PB, Frydenberg M, Thomsen PH. ADHD, stimulant treatment in childhood and subsequent substance abuse in adulthood -

a naturalistic long-term follow-up study. Addict Behav. 2014;39(1):325–8.
481. Chang Z, Lichtenstein P, Halldner L, D'Onofrio B, Serlachius E, Fazel S, Langstrom N, Larsson H. Stimulant ADHD medication and risk for substance abuse. J Child Psychol Psychiatry. 2014;55(8):878–85.
482. Rasmussen K, Palmstierna T, Levander S. Differences in psychiatric problems and criminality between individuals treated with central stimulants before and after adulthood. J Atten Disord. 2019;23(2):173–80.
483. Shaw M, Hodgkins P, Caci H, Young S, Kahle J, Woods AG, Arnold LE. A systematic review and analysis of long-term outcomes in attention deficit hyperactivity disorder: effects of treatment and non-treatment. BMC Med. 2012;10(1):99.
484. Pretus C, Ramos-Quiroga JA, Richarte V, Corrales M, Picado M, Carmona S, Vilarroya O. Time and psychostimulants: opposing long-term structural effects in the adult ADHD brain. A longitudinal MR study. Eur Neuropsychopharmacol. 2017;27(12):1238–47.
485. Lichtenstein P, Halldner L, Zetterqvist J, Sjolander A, Serlachius E, Fazel S, Langstrom N, Larsson H. Medication for attention deficit-hyperactivity disorder and criminality. N Engl J Med. 2012;367(21):2006–14.
486. Mohr-Jensen C, Muller Bisgaard C, Boldsen SK, Steinhausen HC. Attention-deficit/hyperactivity disorder in childhood and adolescence and the risk of crime in young adulthood in a Danish nationwide study. J Am Acad Child Adolesc Psychiatry. 2019;58(4):443–52.
487. Chang Z, D'Onofrio BM, Quinn PD, Lichtenstein P, Larsson H. Medication for attention-deficit/hyperactivity disorder and risk for depression: a nationwide longitudinal cohort study. Biol Psychiatry. 2016;80(12):916–22.
488. Quinn PD, Chang Z, Hur K, Gibbons RD, Lahey BB, Rickert ME, Sjolander A, Lichtenstein P, Larsson H, D'Onofrio BM. ADHD medication and substance-related problems. Am J Psychiatry. 2017;174(9):877–85.
489. Shiels K, Hawk LW, Reynolds B, Mazzullo RJ, Rhodes JD, Pelham WE, Waxmonsky JG, Gangloff BP. Effects of methylphenidate on discounting of delayed rewards in attention deficit/hyperactivity disorder. Exp Clin Psychopharmacol. 2009;17(5):291–301.
490. Newcorn JH, Ivanov I, Krone B, Li X, Duhoux S, White S, Schulz KP, Bedard AV, Pedraza J, Adler L, Blair RJ. Neurobiological basis of reinforcement-based decision making in adults with ADHD treated with lisdexamfetamine dimesylate: preliminary findings and implications for mechanisms influencing clinical improvement. J Psychiatr Res. 2023;170:19–26.
491. Surman CBH, Walsh DM. Do treatments for adult ADHD improve emotional behavior? A systematic review and analysis. J Atten Disord. 2022;26(14):1822–32.
492. Moukhtarian TR, Cooper RE, Vassos E, Moran P, Asherson P. Effects of stimulants and atomoxetine on emotional lability in adults: a systematic review and meta-analysis. Eur Psychiatry. 2017;44:198–207.
493. Lenzi F, Cortese S, Harris J, Masi G. Pharmacotherapy of emotional dysregulation in adults with ADHD: a systematic review and meta-analysis. Neurosci Biobehav Rev. 2018;84:359–67.
494. Surman CBH, Walsh DM. Do ADHD treatments improve executive behavior beyond core ADHD symptoms in adults? Evidence from systematic analysis of clinical trials. J Clin Pharmacol. 2023;63(6):640–53.
495. Adler LA, Solanto M, Escobar R, Lipsius S, Upadhyaya H. Executive functioning outcomes over 6 months of atomoxetine for adults with ADHD: relationship to maintenance of response and relapse over the subsequent 6 months after treatment. J Atten Disord. 2020;24(3):363–72.
496. Weisler R, Ginsberg L, Dirks B, Deas P, Adeyi B, Adler LA. Treatment with lisdexamfetamine dimesylate improves self- and informant-rated executive function behaviors and clinician- and informant-rated ADHD symptoms in adults: data from a randomized, double-blind, placebo-controlled study. J Atten Disord. 2017;21(14):1198–207.
497. Brown TE, Chen J, Robertson B. Improved executive function in adults diagnosed with attention-deficit/ hyperactivity disorder as measured by the Brown Attention-Deficit Disorder Scale following treatment with SHP465 mixed amphetamine salts extended-release: post hoc analyses from 2 randomized, placebo-controlled studies. J Atten Disord. 2022;26(2):256–66.
498. Cortese S. Debate: are stimulant medications for attention-deficit/hyperactivity disorder effective in the long term? J Am Acad Child Adolesc Psychiatry. 2019;58(10):936.
499. Bijlenga D, Kulcu S, van Gellecum T, Eryigit Z, Kooij JJS. Persistence and adherence to psychostimulants, and psychological well-being up to 3 years after specialized treatment of adult attention-deficit/hyperactivity disorder: a naturalistic follow-up study. J Clin Psychopharmacol. 2017;37(6):689–96.
500. Biederman J, Fried R, DiSalvo M, Woodworth KY, Biederman I, Noyes E, Faraone SV, Perlis RH. A novel text message intervention to improve adherence to stimulants in adults with attention deficit/hyperactivity disorder. J Clin Psychopharmacol. 2019;39(4):351–6.
501. Gajria K, Lu M, Sikirica V, Greven P, Zhong Y, Qin P, Xie J. Adherence, persistence, and medication discontinuation in patients with attention-deficit/hyperactivity disorder - a systematic literature review. Neuropsychiatr Dis Treat. 2014;10:1543–69.
502. Rao K, Carpenter DM, Campbell CI. Attention-deficit/hyperactivity disorder medication adherence in the transition to adulthood: associated adverse

outcomes for females and other disparities. J Adolesc Health. 2021;69(5):806–14.
503. Weiss M, Childress A, Nordbrock E, Adjei AL, Kupper RJ, Mattingly G. Characteristics of ADHD symptom response/remission in a clinical trial of methylphenidate extended release. J Clin Med. 2019;8(4):461.
504. Weiss MD, McBride NM, Craig S, Jensen P. Conceptual review of measuring functional impairment: findings from the Weiss Functional Impairment Rating Scale. Evid Based Ment Health. 2018;21(4):155–64.
505. Mattingly GW, Anderson RH. Optimizing outcomes in ADHD treatment: from clinical targets to novel delivery systems. CNS Spectr. 2016;21(S1):45–59.
506. Nagai T, Kurihara T, Koya H, Nakano Y, Sugisawa S, Sambe T, Kishimoto K, Kogo M, Ota H, Iwanami A, Uchida N. Identification of factors associated with the efficacy of atomoxetine in adult attention-deficit/hyperactivity disorder. Neuropsychopharmacol Rep. 2022;42(3):249–55.
507. Nasser A, Kosheleff AR, Hull JT, Liranso T, Qin P, Busse GD, O'Neal W, Fava M, Faraone SV, Rubin J. Translating Attention-Deficit/Hyperactivity Disorder Rating Scale-5 and Weiss Functional Impairment Rating Scale-Parent Effectiveness Scores into Clinical Global Impressions clinical significance levels in four randomized clinical trials of SPN-812 (Viloxazine Extended-Release) in children and adolescents with attention-deficit/hyperactivity disorder. J Child Adolesc Psychopharmacol. 2021;31(3):214–26.
508. Knouse LE, Teller J, Brooks MA. Meta-analysis of cognitive-behavioral treatments for adult ADHD. J Consult Clin Psychol. 2017;85(7):737–50.
509. Pan MR, Huang F, Zhao MJ, Wang YF, Qian QJ. A comparison of efficacy between cognitive behavioral therapy (CBT) and CBT combined with medication in adults with attention-deficit/hyperactivity disorder (ADHD). Psychiatry Res. 2019;279:23–33.
510. Safren SA, Sprich SE, Perlman CA, Otto MW. Mastering Your Adult ADHD: A Cognitive-Behavioral Treatment Program, Therapist Guide. 2nd ed. Barlow DH, editor. New York: Oxford University Press; 2017.
511. Solanto MV. Cognitive-Behavioral Therapy for Adult ADHD: Targeting Executive Dysfunction. New York: The Guilford Press; 2011.
512. Ramsay JR, Rostain AL. Cognitive-Behavioral Therapy for Adult ADHD: An Integrative Psychosocial and Medical Approach. New York: Routledge; 2007.
513. Ciccarone D. The rise of illicit fentanyls, stimulants and the fourth wave of the opioid overdose crisis. Curr Opin Psychiatry. 2021;34(4):344–50.
514. Dacosta-Sanchez D, Gonzalez-Ponce BM, Fernandez-Calderon F, Sanchez-Garcia M, Lozano OM. Retention in treatment and therapeutic adherence: how are these associated with therapeutic success? An analysis using real-world data. Int J Methods Psychiatr Res. 2022;31(4):e1929.
515. Acheson LS, Ezard N, Lintzeris N, Dunlop A, Brett J, Rodgers C, Gill A, Christmass M, McKetin R, Farrell M, Shoptaw S, Siefried KJ. Lisdexamfetamine for the treatment of acute methamphetamine withdrawal: a pilot feasibility and safety trial. Drug Alcohol Depend. 2022;241:109692.
516. Wilens TE, Adler LA, Tanaka Y, Xiao F, D'Souza DN, Gutkin SW, Upadhyaya HP. Correlates of alcohol use in adults with ADHD and comorbid alcohol use disorders: exploratory analysis of a placebo-controlled trial of atomoxetine. Curr Med Res Opin. 2011;27(12):2309–20.
517. Rezaei F, Emami M, Zahed S, Morabbi MJ, Farahzadi M, Akhondzadeh S. Sustained-release methylphenidate in methamphetamine dependence treatment: a double-blind and placebo-controlled trial. Daru. 2015;23(1):2.
518. Ramey OL, Bonny AE, Silva Almodovar A, Nahata MC. Gaps in evidence-based treatment of concurrent attention deficit hyperactivity disorder and opioid use disorder: a scoping review. Ann Pharmacother. 2023;57(8):978–90.
519. Tardelli V, Xu KY, Bisaga A, Levin FR, Fidalgo TM, Grucza RA. Prescription amphetamines in people with opioid use disorder and co-occurring psychostimulant use disorder initiating buprenorphine: an analysis of treatment retention and overdose risk. BMJ Ment. Health. 2023;26(1):e300728
520. Heikkinen M, Taipale H, Tanskanen A, Mittendorfer-Rutz E, Lahteenvuo M, Tiihonen J. Association of pharmacological treatments and hospitalization and death in individuals with amphetamine use disorders in a Swedish nationwide cohort of 13,965 patients. JAMA Psychiatry. 2023;80(1):31–9.
521. Bisaga A, Tardelli VS, Gerra G, Busse A, Campello G, Kashino W, Saenz E, Fidalgo TM. Continuing increase in stimulant dependence - time to implement medical treatment. Can J Psychiatr. 2022;67(7):507–11.
522. Kast KA, Rao V, Wilens TE. Pharmacotherapy for attention-deficit/hyperactivity disorder and retention in outpatient substance use disorder treatment: a retrospective cohort study. J Clin Psychiatry. 2021;82(2):20m13598.
523. Konstenius M, Jayaram-Lindstrom N, Guterstam J, Beck O, Philips B, Franck J. Methylphenidate for attention deficit hyperactivity disorder and drug relapse in criminal offenders with substance dependence: a 24-week randomized placebo-controlled trial. Addiction. 2014;109(3):440–9.
524. Ezard N, Clifford B, Dunlop A, Bruno R, Carr A, Liu Z, Siefried KJ, Lintzeris N. Safety and tolerability of oral lisdexamfetamine in adults with methamphetamine dependence: a phase-2 dose-escalation study. BMJ Open. 2021;11(5):e044696.
525. Collins SL, Levin FR, Foltin RW, Kleber HD, Evans SM. Response to cocaine, alone and in combination with methylphenidate, in cocaine

abusers with ADHD. Drug Alcohol Depend. 2006;82(2):158–67.

526. Wilens TE, Adler LA, Weiss MD, Michelson D, Ramsey JL, Moore RJ, Renard D, Brady KT, Trzepacz PT, Schuh LM, Ahrbecker LM, Levine LR, Atomoxetine ADHD-SUD Study Group. Atomoxetine treatment of adults with ADHD and comorbid alcohol use disorders. Drug Alcohol Depend. 2008;96(1–2):145–54.
527. Thurstone C, Riggs PD, Salomonsen-Sautel S, Mikulich-Gilbertson SK. Randomized, controlled trial of atomoxetine for attention-deficit/hyperactivity disorder in adolescents with substance use disorder. J Am Acad Child Adolesc Psychiatry. 2010;49(6):573–82.
528. Schottenfeld RS, Chawarski MC, Sofuoglu M, Chooi WT, Zaharim NM, MA MY, Ahmad I, Syed Jaapar SZ, Vicknasingam BK. Atomoxetine for amphetamine-type stimulant dependence during buprenorphine treatment: a randomized controlled trial. Drug Alcohol Depend. 2018;186:130–7.
529. Benegal V, Viswanath B, Narayanaswamy JC, Jose SP, Chakraborty V, Sankar D, Kandavel T, Kesavan M. The efficacy of atomoxetine as adjunctive treatment for co-morbid substance use disorders and externalizing symptoms. Asian J Psychiatr. 2013;6(6):544–7.
530. Iwanami A, Saito K, Fujiwara M, Okutsu D, Ichikawa H. Efficacy and safety of guanfacine extended-release in the treatment of attention-deficit/hyperactivity disorder in adults: results of a randomized, double-blind, placebo-controlled study. J Clin Psychiatry. 2020;81(3):19m12979.
531. Radonjic NV, Bellato A, Khoury NM, Cortese S, Faraone SV. Nonstimulant medications for attention-deficit/hyperactivity disorder (ADHD) in adults: systematic review and meta-analysis. CNS Drugs. 2023;37(5):381–97.
532. Faison SL, Fry N, Adewole T, Odebo O, Wang Z, Maletic V, Nasser A. Pharmacokinetics of coadministered viloxazine extended-release (SPN-812) and methylphenidate in healthy adults. J Clin Psychopharmacol. 2021;41(2):155–62.
533. Faison SL, Fry N, Adewole T, Odebo O, Schwabe S, Wang Z, Maletic V, Nasser A. Pharmacokinetics of coadministered viloxazine extended-release (SPN-812) and lisdexamfetamine in healthy adults. Clin Drug Investig. 2021;41(2):149–59.
534. Nasser A, Hull JT, Chaturvedi SA, Liranso T, Odebo O, Kosheleff AR, Fry N, Cutler AJ, Rubin J, Schwabe S, Childress A. A phase III, randomized, double-blind, placebo-controlled trial assessing the efficacy and safety of viloxazine extended-release capsules in adults with attention-deficit/hyperactivity disorder. CNS Drugs. 2022;36(8):897–915.
535. Adler LA, Silverstein MJ. Emotional dysregulation in adult ADHD. Psychiatr Ann. 2018;48(7):318–22.
536. Adler LA, Dirks B, Deas PF, Raychaudhuri A, Dauphin MR, Lasser RA, Weisler RH. Lisdexamfetamine dimesylate in adults with attention-deficit/ hyperactivity disorder who report clinically significant impairment in executive function: results from a randomized, double-blind, placebo-controlled study. J Clin Psychiatry. 2013;74(7):694–702.
537. Skoglund C, Brandt L, D'Onofrio B, Larsson H, Franck J. Methylphenidate doses in attention deficit/hyperactivity disorder and comorbid substance use disorders. Eur Neuropsychopharmacol. 2017;27(11):1144–52.
538. Winhusen TM, Lewis DF, Riggs PD, Davies RD, Adler LA, Sonne S, Somoza EC. Subjective effects, misuse, and adverse effects of osmotic-release methylphenidate treatment in adolescent substance abusers with attention-deficit/hyperactivity disorder. J Child Adolesc Psychopharmacol. 2011;21(5):455–63.
539. Skoglund C, Brandt L, Almqvist C, D'Onofrio BM, Konstenius M, Franck J, Larsson H. Factors associated with adherence to methylphenidate treatment in adult patients with attention-deficit/hyperactivity disorder and substance use disorders. J Clin Psychopharmacol. 2016;36(3):222–8.
540. Arvidsson M, Franck J, Ackehed G, Pettersson Bergstrand M, Ekstrom L, Rosenborg S, Dahl ML. Plasma concentrations of methylphenidate enantiomers in adults with ADHD and substance use disorder, with focus on high doses and relationship to carboxylesterase activity. Basic Clin Pharmacol Toxicol. 2022;130(4):492–500.
541. Ashok AH, Mizuno Y, Volkow ND, Howes OD. Association of stimulant use with dopaminergic alterations in users of cocaine, amphetamine, or methamphetamine: a systematic review and meta-analysis. JAMA Psychiatry. 2017;74(5):511–9.
542. Longo M, Wickes W, Smout M, Harrison S, Cahill S, White JM. Randomized controlled trial of dexamphetamine maintenance for the treatment of methamphetamine dependence. Addiction. 2010;105(1):146–54.
543. Lile JA, Johnson AR, Banks ML, Hatton KW, Hays LR, Nicholson KL, Poklis JL, Rayapati AO, Rush CR, Stoops WW, Negus SS. Pharmacological validation of a translational model of cocaine use disorder: effects of d-amphetamine maintenance on choice between intravenous cocaine and a nondrug alternative in humans and rhesus monkeys. Exp Clin Psychopharmacol. 2020;28(2):169–80.
544. Young S, Gudjonsson G, Chitsabesan P, Colley B, Farrag E, Forrester A, Hollingdale J, Kim K, Lewis A, Maginn S, Mason P, Ryan S, Smith J, Woodhouse E, Asherson P. Identification and treatment of offenders with attention-deficit/hyperactivity disorder in the prison population: a practical approach based upon expert consensus. BMC Psychiatry. 2018;18(1):281.
545. Scott DA, Gignac M, Kronfli RN, Ocana A, Lorberg GW. Expert opinion and recommendations for the management of attention-deficit/hyperactivity disorder in correctional facilities. J Correct Health Care. 2016;22(1):46–61.

546. National Institute for Health and Care Excellence. Attention Deficit Hyperactivity Disorder: Diagnosis and Management. National Institute for Health and Care Excellence (NICE); 2018.
547. Cortese S, Adamo N, Del Giovane C, Mohr-Jensen C, Hayes AJ, Carucci S, Atkinson LZ, Tessari L, Banaschewski T, Coghill D, Hollis C, Simonoff E, Zuddas A, Barbui C, Purgato M, Steinhausen HC, Shokraneh F, Xia J, Cipriani A. Comparative efficacy and tolerability of medications for attention-deficit hyperactivity disorder in children, adolescents, and adults: a systematic review and network meta-analysis. Lancet Psychiatry. 2018;5(9):727–38.
548. Biederman J, DiSalvo M, Green A, Woodworth KY, Gilfix T, Law C, Gabrieli J, Faraone SV. Rates of switching stimulants in consecutively referred medication naive adults with ADHD. Acta Psychiatr Scand. 2021;144(6):626–34.
549. Kolar D, Keller A, Golfinopoulos M, Cumyn L, Syer C, Hechtman L. Treatment of adults with attention-deficit/hyperactivity disorder. Neuropsychiatr Dis Treat. 2008;4(2):389–403.
550. Wilens TE. A sobering fact: ADHD leads to substance abuse. J Am Acad Child Adolesc Psychiatry. 2011;50(1):6–8.
551. Kollins SH, McClernon FJ, Fuemmeler BF. Association between smoking and attention-deficit/hyperactivity disorder symptoms in a population-based sample of young adults. Arch Gen Psychiatry. 2005;62(10):1142–7.
552. Crunelle CL, van den Brink W, Moggi F, Konstenius M, Franck J, Levin FR, van de Glind G, Demetrovics Z, Coetzee C, Luderer M, Schellekens A, ICASA Consensus Group, Matthys F. International consensus statement on screening, diagnosis and treatment of substance use disorder patients with comorbid attention deficit/hyperactivity disorder. Eur Addict Res 2018;24(1):43–51.
553. van de Glind G, Konstenius M, MWJ K, van Emmerik-van Oortmerssen K, Carpentier PJ, Kaye S, Degenhardt L, Skutle A, Franck J, Bu ET, Moggi F, Dom G, Verspreet S, Demetrovics Z, Kapitany-Foveny M, Fatseas M, Auriacombe M, Schillinger A, Moller M, Johnson B, Faraone SV, Ramos-Quiroga JA, Casas M, Allsop S, Carruthers S, Schoevers RA, Wallhed S, Barta C, Alleman P, IASP Research Group, Levin FR, van den Brink W. Variability in the prevalence of adult ADHD in treatment seeking substance use disorder patients: results from an international multi-center study exploring DSM-IV and DSM-5 criteria. Drug Alcohol Depend. 2014;134:158–66.
554. Kronenberg LM, Goossens PJ, van Etten DM, van Achterberg T, van den Brink W. Need for care and life satisfaction in adult substance use disorder patients with and without attention deficit hyperactivity disorder (ADHD) or autism spectrum disorder (ASD). Perspect Psychiatr Care. 2015;51(1):4–15.
555. Dakwar E, Levin FR, Olfson M, Wang S, Kerridge B, Blanco C. First treatment contact for ADHD: predictors of and gender differences in treatment seeking. Psychiatr Serv. 2014;65(12):1465–73.
556. Schellekens AFA, van den Brink W, Kiefer F, Goudriaan AE. Often overlooked and ignored, but do not underestimate its relevance: ADHD in Addiction - Addiction in ADHD. Eur Addict Res. 2020;26(4–5):169–72.
557. Carpentier PJ, Levin FR. Pharmacological treatment of ADHD in addicted patients: what does the literature tell us? Harv Rev Psychiatry. 2017;25(2):50–64.
558. Daigre C, Rodriguez L, Roncero C, Palma-Alvarez RF, Perea-Ortueta M, Sorribes-Puertas M, Martinez-Luna N, Ros-Cucurull E, Ramos-Quiroga JA, Grau-Lopez L. Treatment retention and abstinence of patients with substance use disorders according to addiction severity and psychiatry comorbidity: a six-month follow-up study in an outpatient unit. Addict Behav. 2021;117:106832.
559. Riggs PD, Winhusen T, Davies RD, Leimberger JD, Mikulich-Gilbertson S, Klein C, Macdonald M, Lohman M, Bailey GL, Haynes L, Jaffee WB, Haminton N, Hodgkins C, Whitmore E, Trello-Rishel K, Tamm L, Acosta MC, Royer-Malvestuto C, Subramaniam G, Fishman M, Holmes BW, Kaye ME, Vargo MA, Woody GE, Nunes EV, Liu D. Randomized controlled trial of osmotic-release methylphenidate with cognitive-behavioral therapy in adolescents with attention-deficit/hyperactivity disorder and substance use disorders. J Am Acad Child Adolesc Psychiatry. 2011;50(9):903–14.
560. Kollins SH, Youcha S, Lasser R, Thase ME. Lisdexamfetamine dimesylate for the treatment of attention deficit hyperactivity disorder in adults with a history of depression or history of substance use disorder. Innov Clin Neurosci. 2011;8(2):28–32.
561. Herbrink M, Nuijten M, Nuijen B, Huitema ADR, Beijnen JH, Hendriks VM, Blanken P, Janmohamed A, van den Brink W. Pharmacokinetics of sustained-release oral dexamphetamine sulfate in cocaine and heroin-dependent patients. J Clin Psychopharmacol. 2018;38(3):212–7.
562. Krishnan S, Moncrief S. An evaluation of the cytochrome p450 inhibition potential of lisdexamfetamine in human liver microsomes. Drug Metab Dispos. 2007;35(1):180–4.
563. Klassen LJ, Bilkey TS, Katzman MA, Chokka P. Comorbid attention deficit/hyperactivity disorder and substance use disorder: treatment considerations. Curr Drug Abuse Rev. 2012;5(3):190–8.
564. Ermer JC, Adeyi BA, Pucci ML. Pharmacokinetic variability of long-acting stimulants in the treatment of children and adults with attention-deficit hyperactivity disorder. CNS Drugs. 2010;24(12):1009–25.
565. Cortese S. Evidence-based prescribing of medications for ADHD: where are we in 2023? Expert Opin Pharmacother. 2023;24(4):425–34.
566. Ching C, Eslick GD, Poulton AS. Evaluation of methylphenidate safety and maximum-dose titration rationale in attention-deficit/hyperactivity disorder: a meta-analysis. JAMA Pediatr. 2019;173(7):630–9.

567. Kooij JJS, Bejerot S, Blackwell A, Caci H, Casas-Brugue M, Carpentier PJ, Edvinsson D, Fayyad J, Foeken K, Fitzgerald M, Gaillac V, Ginsberg Y, Henry C, Krause J, Lensing MB, Manor I, Niederhofer H, Nunes-Filipe C, Ohlmeier MD, Oswald P, Pallanti S, Pehlivanidis A, Ramos-Quiroga JA, Rastam M, Ryffel-Rawak D, Stes S, Asherson P. European consensus statement on diagnosis and treatment of adult ADHD: the European Network Adult ADHD. BMC Psychiatry. 2010;10:67.
568. Faraone SV, Banaschewski T, Coghill D, Zheng Y, Biederman J, Bellgrove MA, Newcorn JH, Gignac M, Al Saud NM, Manor I, Rohde LA, Yang L, Cortese S, Almagor D, Stein MA, Albatti TH, Aljoudi HF, Alqahtani MMJ, Asherson P, Atwoli L, Bolte S, Buitelaar JK, Crunelle CL, Daley D, Dalsgaard S, Dopfner M, Espinet S, Fitzgerald M, Franke B, Gerlach M, Haavik J, Hartman CA, Hartung CM, Hinshaw SP, Hoekstra PJ, Hollis C, Kollins SH, Kooij JJS, Kuntsi J, Larsson H, Li T, Liu J, Merzon E, Mattingly G, Mattos P, McCarthy S, Mikami AY, Molina BSG, Nigg JT, Purper-Ouakil D, Omigbodun OO, Polanczyk GV, Pollak Y, Poulton AS, Rajkumar RP, Reding A, Reif A, Rubia K, Rucklidge J, Romanos M, Ramos-Quiroga JA, Schellekens A, Scheres A, Schoeman R, Schweitzer JB, Shah H, Solanto MV, Sonuga-Barke E, Soutullo C, Steinhausen HC, Swanson JM, Thapar A, Tripp G, van de Glind G, van den Brink W, Van der Oord S, Venter A, Vitiello B, Walitza S, Wang Y. The World Federation of ADHD international consensus statement: 208 evidence-based conclusions about the disorder. Neurosci Biobehav Rev. 2021;128:789–818.
569. Faraone SV, Silverstein MJ, Antshel K, Biederman J, Goodman DW, Mason O, Nierenberg AA, Rostain A, Stein MA, Adler LA. The Adult ADHD Quality Measures Initiative. J Atten Disord. 2019;23(10):1063–78.
570. Bellgrove MA; Australian ADHD Guideline Development Group. Australian Evidence-Based Clinical Guidelines for Attention Deficit Hyperactivity Disorder (ADHD). Melbourne, Australia, Australasian ADHD Professionals Association (AADPA), 2022. Available at: https://adhdguideline.aadpa.com.au.
571. Ozgen H, Spijkerman R, Noack M, Holtmann M, Schellekens ASA, van de Glind G, Banaschewski T, Barta C, Begeman A, Casas M, Crunelle CL, Daigre Blanco C, Dalsgaard S, Demetrovics Z, den Boer J, Dom G, Eapen V, Faraone SV, Franck J, Gonzalez RA, Grau-Lopez L, Groenman AP, Hemphala M, Icick R, Johnson B, Kaess M, Kapitany-Foveny M, Kasinathan JG, Kaye SS, Kiefer F, Konstenius M, Levin FR, Luderer M, Martinotti G, Matthys FIA, Meszaros G, Moggi F, Munasur-Naidoo AP, Post M, Rabinovitz S, Ramos-Quiroga JA, Sala R, Shafi A, Slobodin O, Staal WG, Thomasius R, Truter I, van Kernebeek MW, Velez-Pastrana MC, Vollstadt-Klein S, Vorspan F, Young JT, Yule A, van den Brink W, Hendriks V. International consensus statement for the screening, diagnosis, and treatment of adolescents with concurrent attention-deficit/hyperactivity disorder and substance use disorder. Eur Addict Res. 2020;26(4–5):223–32.
572. Young S, Woodhouse E. Assessment and treatment of substance use in adults with ADHD: a psychological approach. J Neural Transm (Vienna). 2021;128(7):1099–108.
573. van der Burg D, Crunelle CL, Matthys F, van den Brink W. Diagnosis and treatment of patients with comorbid substance use disorder and adult attention-deficit and hyperactivity disorder: a review of recent publications. Curr Opin Psychiatry. 2019;32(4):300–6.
574. Ustun B, Adler LA, Rudin C, Faraone SV, Spencer TJ, Berglund P, Gruber MJ, Kessler RC. The World Health Organization Adult Attention-Deficit/Hyperactivity Disorder Self-Report Screening Scale for DSM-5. JAMA Psychiatry. 2017;74(5):520–7.
575. Conners CK, Erhardt D. Conners' Adult ADHD Rating Scales (CAARS). 1998. Available from: https://www.wpspublish.com/caars-conners-adult-adhd-rating-scales.
576. Gift TE, Reimherr ML, Marchant BK, Steans TA, Reimherr FW. Wender Utah Rating Scale: psychometrics, clinical utility and implications regarding the elements of ADHD. J Psychiatr Res. 2021;135:181–8.
577. Palma-Alvarez RF, Barta C, Carpentier PJ, Carruthers S, Crunelle CL, Demetrovics Z, Dom G, Faraone SV, Franck J, Johnson B, Kapitany-Foveny M, Kaye S, Konstenius M, Matthys F, Moggi F, Moller M, Schellekens A, Skutle A, van de Glind G, van Emmerik-van Oortmerssen K, Verspreet S, Schoevers RA, Wallhed S, Levin FR, Grau-Lopez L, Casas M, van den Brink W, Ramos-Quiroga JA, IASP Research Group. Validity of the ADHD module of the Mini International Neuropsychiatric Interview PLUS for screening of adult ADHD in treatment seeking substance use disorder patients: ADHD screening with MINI-Plus. Rev Psiquiatr Salud Ment (Engl Ed). 2020;16(1):11–15.
578. Dakwar E, Mahony A, Pavlicova M, Glass A, Brooks D, Mariani JJ, Grabowski J, Levin FR. The utility of attention-deficit/hyperactivity disorder screening instruments in individuals seeking treatment for substance use disorders. J Clin Psychiatry. 2012;73(11):e1372–8.
579. Daigre C, Roncero C, Rodriguez-Cintas L, Ortega L, Lligona A, Fuentes S, Perez-Pazos J, Martinez-Luna N, Casas M. Adult ADHD screening in alcohol-dependent patients using the Wender-Utah Rating Scale and the Adult ADHD Self-Report Scale. J Atten Disord. 2015;19(4):328–34.
580. Brevik EJ, Lundervold AJ, Haavik J, Posserud MB. Validity and accuracy of the Adult Attention-Deficit/Hyperactivity Disorder (ADHD) Self-Report Scale (ASRS) and the Wender Utah Rating Scale (WURS) symptom checklists in

discriminating between adults with and without ADHD. Brain Behav. 2020;10(6):e01605.
581. Kooij JJS, Marije Boonstra A, Swinkels SH, Bekker EM, de Noord I, Buitelaar JK. Reliability, validity, and utility of instruments for self-report and informant report concerning symptoms of ADHD in adult patients. J Atten Disord. 2008;11(4):445–58.
582. Luderer M, Kaplan-Wickel N, Richter A, Reinhard I, Kiefer F, Weber T. Screening for adult attention-deficit/hyperactivity disorder in alcohol dependent patients: underreporting of ADHD symptoms in self-report scales. Drug Alcohol Depend. 2019;195:52–8.
583. Young S, Abbasian C, Al-Attar Z, Branney P, Colley B, Cortese S, Cubbin S, Deeley Q, Gudjonsson GH, Hill P, Hollingdale J, Jenden S, Johnson J, Judge D, Lewis A, Mason P, Mukherjee R, Nutt D, Roberts J, Robinson F, Woodhouse E, Cocallis K. Identification and treatment of individuals with attention-deficit/hyperactivity disorder and substance use disorder: an expert consensus statement. World J Psychiatry. 2023;13(3):84–112.
584. Sibley MH. Empirically-informed guidelines for first-time adult ADHD diagnosis. J Clin Exp Neuropsychol. 2021;43(4):340–51.
585. Anbarasan D, Kitchin M, Adler LA. Screening for adult ADHD. Curr Psychiatry Rep. 2020;22(12):72.
586. Silverstein MJ, Faraone SV, Alperin S, Biederman J, Spencer TJ, Adler LA. How informative are self-reported adult attention-deficit/hyperactivity disorder symptoms? An examination of the agreement between the Adult Attention-Deficit/Hyperactivity Disorder Self-Report Scale V1.1 and Adult Attention-Deficit/Hyperactivity Disorder Investigator Symptom Rating Scale. J Child Adolesc Psychopharmacol. 2018;28(5):339–49.
587. van Emmerik-van Oortmerssen K, Vedel E, Kramer FJ, Koeter MW, Schoevers RA, van den Brink W. Diagnosing ADHD during active substance use: feasible or flawed? Drug Alcohol Depend. 2017;180:371–5.
588. Levin FR, Upadhyaya HP. Diagnosing ADHD in adults with substance use disorder: DSM-IV criteria and differential diagnosis. J Clin Psychiatry. 2007;68(7):e18.
589. Torralva T, Gleichgerrcht E, Lischinsky A, Roca M, Manes F. "ecological" and highly demanding executive tasks detect real-life deficits in high-functioning adult ADHD patients. J Atten Disord. 2013;17(1):11–9.
590. Sharma MJ, Lavoie S, Callahan BL. A call for research on the validity of the age-of-onset criterion application in older adults being evaluated for ADHD: a review of the literature in clinical and cognitive psychology. Am J Geriatr Psychiatry. 2021;29(7):669–78.
591. Chandra S, Biederman J, Faraone SV. Assessing the validity of the age at onset criterion for diagnosing ADHD in DSM-5. J Atten Disord. 2021;25(2):143–53.
592. Kooij JJS, Franken MH. Diagnostic Interview of ADHD in Adults, Version 2.0 (DIVA). The Hague: DIVA Foundation; 2010. Available from: https://www.divacenter.eu
593. Kooij JJS, Franken MH, Bron TI. Diagnostic Interview of ADHD in Adults for DSM-5 (DIVA-5). The Hague: DIVA Foundation; 2019. Available from: www.divacenter.eu
594. Epstein JE, Johnson DE, Conners CK. Conners' Adult ADHD Diagnostic Interview for DSM-IV (CAADID): technical manual. Toronto: Multi-Health Systems Inc. (MHS); 2001.
595. Ramos-Quiroga JA, Diaz-Digon L, Comin M, Bosch R, Palomar G, Chalita JP, Roncero C, Nogueira M, Torrens M, Casas M. Criteria and concurrent validity of adult ADHD section of the Psychiatry Research Interview for Substance and Mental Disorders. J Atten Disord. 2015;19(12):999–1006.
596. Silverstein MJ, Faraone SV, Alperin S, Leon TL, Biederman J, Spencer TJ, Adler LA. Validation of the expanded versions of the Adult ADHD Self-Report Scale v1.1 Symptom Checklist and the Adult ADHD Investigator Symptom Rating Scale. J Atten Disord. 2019;23(10):1101–10.
597. Barkley RA, Fischer M. Predicting impairment in major life activities and occupational functioning in hyperactive children as adults: self-reported executive function (EF) deficits versus EF tests. Dev Neuropsychol. 2011;36(2):137–61.
598. Barkley RA, Murphy KR. The nature of executive function (EF) deficits in daily life activities in adults with ADHD and their relationship to performance on EF tests. J Psychopathol Behav Assess. 2011;33(2):137–58.
599. Planton M, Lemesle B, Cousineau M, Carlier J, Milongo-Rigal E, Carle-Toulemonde G, Salles J, Pariente J. The role of neuropsychological assessment in adults with attention deficit/hyperactivity disorders. Rev Neurol (Paris). 2021;177(4):341–8.
600. Guo N, Fuermaier ABM, Koerts J, Mueller BW, Diers K, Mross A, Mette C, Tucha L, Tucha O. Neuropsychological functioning of individuals at clinical evaluation of adult ADHD. J Neural Transm (Vienna). 2021;128(7):877–91.
601. Pettersson R, Soderstrom S, Nilsson KW. Diagnosing ADHD in adults: an examination of the discriminative validity of neuropsychological tests and diagnostic assessment instruments. J Atten Disord. 2018;22(11):1019–31.
602. Arrondo G, Mulraney M, Iturmendi-Sabater I, Musullulu H, Gambra L, Niculcea T, Banaschewski T, Simonoff E, Dopfner M, Hinshaw SP, Coghill D, Cortese S. Systematic review and meta-analysis: clinical utility of continuous performance tests for the identification of attention-deficit/hyperactivity disorder. J Am Acad Child Adolesc Psychiatry. 2023;63(2):154–171.
603. Surman CB, Biederman J, Spencer T, Miller CA, Petty CR, Faraone SV. Neuropsychological deficits are not predictive of deficient emotional self-

regulation in adults with ADHD. J Atten Disord. 2015;19(12):1046–53.
604. LeBlond E, Smith-Paine J, Riemersma JJ, Horn PS, Wade SL, Kurowski BG. Influence of methylphenidate on long-term neuropsychological and everyday executive functioning after traumatic brain injury in children with secondary attention problems. J Int Neuropsychol Soc. 2019;25(7):740–9.
605. Weiss MD. Weiss Functional Impairment Rating Scale (WFIRS). Vancouver: University of British Columbia; 2011. Available from: http://www.shared-care.ca/files/Weiss_Functional_Impairment_Self-Report.pdf.
606. Roth RM, Isquith PK, Gioia GA. Behavior Rating Inventory of Executive Function®–Adult Version (BRIEF-A). PAR. Available from: https://www.parinc.com/products/BRIEF2A.
607. Barkley RA. Barkley Deficits in Executive Functioning Scale (BDEFS for Adults). New York. 2011. Available from: https://www.guilford.com/books/Barkley-Deficits-Executive-Functioning-Scale-BDEFS-Adults/Russell-Barkley/9781606239346.
608. Barkley RA. Barkley Functional Impairment Scale for Adults (BFIS for Adults). New York: Guilford Press; 2011. Available from: https://www.guilford.com/books/Barkley-Functional-Impairment-Scale-BFIS-for-Adults/Russell-Barkley/9781609182199.
609. Ramsay JR. Assessment and monitoring of treatment response in adult ADHD patients: current perspectives. Neuropsychiatr Dis Treat. 2017;13:221–32.
610. Pendergast LL, Youngstrom EA, Merkitch KG, Moore KA, Black CL, Abramson LY, Alloy LB. Differentiating bipolar disorder from unipolar depression and ADHD: the utility of the general behavior inventory. Psychol Assess. 2014;26(1):195–206.
611. Kitsune GL, Kuntsi J, Costello H, Frangou S, Hosang GM, McLoughlin G, Asherson P. Delineating ADHD and bipolar disorder: a comparison of clinical profiles in adult women. J Affect Disord. 2016;192:125–33.
612. Nierenberg AA, Miyahara S, Spencer T, Wisniewski SR, Otto MW, Simon N, Pollack MH, Ostacher MJ, Yan L, Siegel R, Sachs GS, Investigators S-B. Clinical and diagnostic implications of lifetime attention-deficit/hyperactivity disorder comorbidity in adults with bipolar disorder: data from the first 1000 STEP-BD participants. Biol Psychiatry. 2005;57(11):1467–73.
613. Moukhtarian TR, Mintah RS, Moran P, Asherson P. Emotion dysregulation in attention-deficit/hyperactivity disorder and borderline personality disorder. Borderline Personal Disord Emot Dysregul. 2018;5:9.
614. Leichsenring F, Heim N, Leweke F, Spitzer C, Steinert C, Kernberg OF. Borderline Personality Disorder: A Review. JAMA. 2023;329(8):670–9.
615. Comparelli A, Polidori L, Sarli G, Pistollato A, Pompili M. Differentiation and comorbidity of bipolar disorder and attention deficit and hyperactivity disorder in children, adolescents, and adults: a clinical and nosological perspective. Front Psych. 2022;13:949375.
616. Perugi G, Vannucchi G. The use of stimulants and atomoxetine in adults with comorbid ADHD and bipolar disorder. Expert Opin Pharmacother. 2015;16(14):2193–204.
617. Dobrosavljevic M, Fazel S, Du Rietz E, Li L, Zhang L, Chang Z, Jernberg T, Faraone SV, Jendle J, Chen Q, Brikell I, Larsson H. Risk prediction model for cardiovascular diseases in adults initiating pharmacological treatment for attention-deficit/hyperactivity disorder. Evid Based Ment Health. 2022;25(4):185–90.
618. Bang Madsen K, Robakis TK, Liu X, Momen N, Larsson H, Dreier JW, Kildegaard H, Groth JB, Newcorn JH, Hove Thomsen P, Munk-Olsen T, Bergink V. In utero exposure to ADHD medication and long-term offspring outcomes. Mol Psychiatry. 2023;28(4):1739–46.
619. Bachmann K, Lam AP, Soros P, Kanat M, Hoxhaj E, Matthies S, Feige B, Muller H, Ozyurt J, Thiel CM, Philipsen A. Effects of mindfulness and psychoeducation on working memory in adult ADHD: a randomised, controlled fMRI study. Behav Res Ther. 2018;106:47–56.
620. Hirvikoski T, Lindstrom T, Carlsson J, Waaler E, Jokinen J, Bolte S. Psychoeducational groups for adults with ADHD and their significant others (PEGASUS): a pragmatic multicenter and randomized controlled trial. Eur Psychiatry. 2017;44:141–52.
621. van Emmerik-van Oortmerssen K, Vedel E, Kramer FJ, Blankers M, Dekker JJM, van den Brink W, Schoevers RA. Integrated cognitive behavioral therapy for ADHD in adult substance use disorder patients: results of a randomized clinical trial. Drug Alcohol Depend. 2019;197:28–36.
622. Young S, Bramham J. Cognitive-Behavioral Therapy for ADHD in Adolescents and Adults: A Psychological Guide to Practice (2nd edition). Malden: Wiley; 2012.
623. Young SJ, Ross RR. R&R2 for ADHD Youths and Adults: A Prosocial Competence Training Program. Ottawa: Cognitive Centre of Canada; 2007.
624. van Emmerik-van Oortmerssen K, Blankers M, Vedel E, Kramer F, Goudriaan AE, van den Brink W, Schoevers RA. Prediction of drop-out and outcome in integrated cognitive behavioral therapy for ADHD and SUD: results from a randomized clinical trial. Addict Behav. 2020;103:106228.
625. Lappan SN, Brown AW, Hendricks PS. Dropout rates of in-person psychosocial substance use disorder treatments: a systematic review and meta-analysis. Addiction. 2020;115(2):201–17.
626. Samples H, Williams AR, Crystal S, Olfson M. Psychosocial and behavioral therapy in con-

junction with medication for opioid use disorder: patterns, predictors, and association with buprenorphine treatment outcomes. J Subst Abus Treat. 2022;139:108774.
627. Petry NM, Martin B, Cooney JL, Kranzler HR. Give them prizes, and they will come: contingency management for treatment of alcohol dependence. J Consult Clin Psychol. 2000;68(2):250–7.
628. Rash CJ, DePhilippis D. Considerations for implementing contingency management in substance abuse treatment clinics: the Veterans Affairs Initiative as a model. Perspect Behav Sci. 2019;42(3):479–99.
629. Zylowska L, Mitchell JT. Mindfulness for Adult ADHD: A Clinician's Guide. New York: The Guilford Press; 2020.
630. Oliva F, Malandrone F, di Girolamo G, Mirabella S, Colombi N, Carletto S, Ostacoli L. The efficacy of mindfulness-based interventions in attention-deficit/hyperactivity disorder beyond core symptoms: a systematic review, meta-analysis, and meta-regression. J Affect Disord. 2021;292:475–86.
631. Garland EL, Hanley AW, Nakamura Y, Barrett JW, Baker AK, Reese SE, Riquino MR, Froeliger B, Donaldson GW. Mindfulness-oriented recovery enhancement vs supportive group therapy for co-occurring opioid misuse and chronic pain in primary care: a randomized clinical trial. JAMA Intern Med. 2022;182(4):407–17.
632. Janssen L, Kan CC, Carpentier PJ, Sizoo B, Hepark S, Schellekens MPJ, Donders ART, Buitelaar JK, Speckens AEM. Mindfulness-based cognitive therapy v. treatment as usual in adults with ADHD: a multicentre, single-blind, randomised controlled trial. Psychol Med. 2019;49(1):55–65.
633. Gu Y, Zhu Y, Brown KW. Mindfulness and attention deficit hyperactivity disorder: a neuropsychological perspective. J Nerv Ment Dis. 2021;209(11):796–801.
634. Bauer CCC, Rozenkrantz L, Caballero C, Nieto-Castanon A, Scherer E, West MR, Mrazek M, Phillips DT, Gabrieli JDE, Whitfield-Gabrieli S. Mindfulness training preserves sustained attention and resting state anticorrelation between default-mode network and dorsolateral prefrontal cortex: a randomized controlled trial. Hum Brain Mapp. 2020;41(18):5356–69.
635. van Andel E, Bijlenga D, Vogel SWN, Beekman ATF, Kooij JJS. Effects of chronotherapy on circadian rhythm and ADHD symptoms in adults with attention-deficit/hyperactivity disorder and delayed sleep phase syndrome: a randomized clinical trial. Chronobiol Int. 2021;38(2):260–9.
636. Ashdown-Franks G, Firth J, Carney R, Carvalho AF, Hallgren M, Koyanagi A, Rosenbaum S, Schuch FB, Smith L, Solmi M, Vancampfort D, Stubbs B. Exercise as medicine for mental and substance use disorders: a meta-review of the benefits for neuropsychiatric and cognitive outcomes. Sports Med. 2020;50(1):151–70.
637. Sung MC, Ku B, Leung W, MacDonald M. The effect of physical activity interventions on executive function among people with neurodevelopmental disorders: a meta-analysis. J Autism Dev Disord. 2022;52(3):1030–50.
638. Mehren A, Reichert M, Coghill D, Muller HHO, Braun N, Philipsen A. Physical exercise in attention deficit hyperactivity disorder - evidence and implications for the treatment of borderline personality disorder. Borderline Personal Disord Emot Dysregul. 2020;7:1.
639. Vysniauske R, Verburgh L, Oosterlaan J, Molendijk ML. The effects of physical exercise on functional outcomes in the treatment of ADHD: a meta-analysis. J Atten Disord. 2020;24(5):644–54.
640. Childress AC. Novel formulations of ADHD medications: stimulant selection and management. Focus (Am Psychiatr Publ). 2021;19(1):31–8.
641. Mattingly GW, Young J. A clinician's guide for navigating the world of attention deficit hyperactivity disorder medications. CNS Spectr. 2021;26(2):104–14.
642. Franke B, Michelini G, Asherson P, Banaschewski T, Bilbow A, Buitelaar JK, Cormand B, Faraone SV, Ginsberg Y, Haavik J, Kuntsi J, Larsson H, Lesch KP, Ramos-Quiroga JA, Rethelyi JM, Ribases M, Reif A. Live fast, die young? A review on the developmental trajectories of ADHD across the lifespan. Eur Neuropsychopharmacol. 2018;28(10):1059–88.
643. Corium I. Prescribing information for AZSTARYS (serdexmethylphenidate and dexmethylphenidate) capsules, for oral use, CII. 2021.
644. Weiss M, Childress A, Mattingly G, Nordbrock E, Kupper RJ, Adjei AL. Relationship between symptomatic and functional improvement and remission in a treatment response to stimulant trial. J Child Adolesc Psychopharmacol. 2018;28(8):521–9.
645. Cambron-Mellott MJ, Mikl J, Matos JE, Erensen JG, Beusterien K, Cataldo MJ, Hallissey B, Mattingly GW. Adult patient preferences for long-acting ADHD treatments: a discrete choice experiment. Patient Prefer Adherence. 2021;15:1061–73.
646. Spencer TJ, Bhide P, Zhu J, Faraone SV, Fitzgerald M, Yule AM, Uchida M, Spencer AE, Hall AM, Koster AJ, Biederman J. Opiate antagonists do not interfere with the clinical benefits of stimulants in ADHD: a double-blind, placebo-controlled trial of the mixed opioid receptor antagonist naltrexone. J Clin Psychiatry. 2018;79(1):16m11012.
647. Spencer TJ, Bhide P, Zhu J, Faraone SV, Fitzgerald M, Yule AM, Uchida M, Spencer AE, Hall AM, Koster AJ, Feinberg L, Kassabian S, Storch B, Biederman J. The mixed opioid receptor antagonist naltrexone mitigates stimulant-induced euphoria: a double-blind, placebo-controlled trial of naltrexone. J Clin Psychiatry. 2018;79(2):17m11609.
648. Jayaram-Lindstrom N, Hammarberg A, Beck O, Franck J. Naltrexone for the treatment of amphetamine dependence: a random-

ized, placebo-controlled trial. Am J Psychiatry. 2008;165(11):1442–8.
649. Camporeale A, Porsdal V, De Bruyckere K, Tanaka Y, Upadhyaya H, Deix C, Deberdt W. Safety and tolerability of atomoxetine in treatment of attention deficit hyperactivity disorder in adult patients: an integrated analysis of 15 clinical trials. J Psychopharmacol. 2015;29(1):3–14.
650. Newcorn JH, Sutton VK, Weiss MD, Sumner CR. Clinical responses to atomoxetine in attention-deficit/hyperactivity disorder: the integrated data exploratory analysis (IDEA) study. J Am Acad Child Adolesc Psychiatry. 2009;48(5):511–8.
651. Childress AC. A critical appraisal of atomoxetine in the management of ADHD. Ther Clin Risk Manag. 2016;12:27–39.
652. Newcorn JH, Huss M, Connor DF, Hervas A, Werner-Kiechle T, Robertson B. Efficacy of guanfacine extended release in children and adolescents with attention-deficit/hyperactivity disorder and comorbid oppositional defiant disorder. J Dev Behav Pediatr. 2020;41(7):565–70.
653. Wilens TE, Bukstein O, Brams M, Cutler AJ, Childress A, Rugino T, Lyne A, Grannis K, Youcha S. A controlled trial of extended-release guanfacine and psychostimulants for attention-deficit/hyperactivity disorder. J Am Acad Child Adolesc Psychiatry. 2012;51(1):74–85 e2.
654. Cutler AJ, Brams M, Bukstein O, Mattingly G, McBurnett K, White C, Rubin J. Response/remission with guanfacine extended-release and psychostimulants in children and adolescents with attention-deficit/hyperactivity disorder. J Am Acad Child Adolesc Psychiatry. 2014;53(10):1092–101.
655. Adler LA, Reingold LS, Morrill MS, Wilens TE. Combination pharmacotherapy for adult ADHD. Curr Psychiatry Rep. 2006;8(5):409–15.
656. Butterfield ME, Saal J, Young B, Young JL. Supplementary guanfacine hydrochloride as a treatment of attention deficit hyperactivity disorder in adults: a double blind, placebo-controlled study. Psychiatry Res. 2016;236:136–41.
657. Schoretsanitis G, de Leon J, Eap CB, Kane JM, Paulzen M. Clinically significant drug-drug interactions with agents for attention-deficit/hyperactivity disorder. CNS Drugs. 2019;33(12):1201–22.
658. Haney M, Cooper ZD, Bedi G, Herrmann E, Comer SD, Reed SC, Foltin RW, Levin FR. Guanfacine decreases symptoms of cannabis withdrawal in daily cannabis smokers. Addict Biol. 2019;24(4):707–16.
659. Bahn GH, Seo K. Combined medication with stimulants and non-stimulants for attention-deficit/hyperactivity disorder. Clin Psychopharmacol Neurosci. 2021;19(4):705–11.
660. Ozbaran B, Kose S, Yuzuguldu O, Atar B, Aydin C. Combined methylphenidate and atomoxetine pharmacotherapy in attention deficit hyperactivity disorder. World J Biol Psychiatry. 2015;16(8):619–24.
661. Newcorn JH, Krone B, Dittmann RW. Nonstimulant treatments for ADHD. Child Adolesc Psychiatr Clin N Am. 2022;31(3):417–35.
662. Shim SH, Woo YS, Kim JS, Heo IS, Yoon HJ, Sung HM, Lee J, Bahk WM. Comparison between atomoxetine and OROS methylphenidate as an adjunctive to SSRIs in attention-deficit/hyperactivity disorder adults with comorbid partially responsive major depressive disorder: a head-to-head, 12-week, randomized, rater-blinded clinical trial. Clin Psychopharmacol Neurosci. 2022;20(1):143–53.
663. Faraone SV, Gomeni R, Hull JT, Chaturvedi SA, Busse GD, Melyan Z, O'Neal W, Rubin J, Nasser A. Predicting efficacy of viloxazine extended-release treatment in adults with ADHD using an early change in ADHD symptoms: machine learning post hoc analysis of a Phase 3 clinical trial. Psychiatry Res. 2022;318:114922.
664. Solhkhah R, Wilens TE, Daly J, Prince JB, Van Patten SL, Biederman J. Bupropion SR for the treatment of substance-abusing outpatient adolescents with attention-deficit/hyperactivity disorder and mood disorders. J Child Adolesc Psychopharmacol. 2005;15(5):777–86.
665. Xu KY, Mintz CM, Presnall N, Bierut LJ, Grucza RA. Association of Bupropion, naltrexone, and opioid agonist treatment with stimulant-related admissions among people with opioid use disorder: a case-crossover analysis. J Clin Psychiatry. 2022;83(4):21m14112.
666. Childress AC, Beltran N, Supnet C, Weiss MD. Reviewing the role of emerging therapies in the ADHD armamentarium. Expert Opin Emerg Drugs. 2021;26(1):1–16.
667. Cortese S, D'Acunto G, Konofal E, Masi G, Vitiello B. New formulations of methylphenidate for the treatment of attention-deficit/hyperactivity disorder: pharmacokinetics, efficacy, and tolerability. CNS Drugs. 2017;31(2):149–60.
668. Zhang L, Yao H, Li L, Du Rietz E, Andell P, Garcia-Argibay M, D'Onofrio BM, Cortese S, Larsson H, Chang Z. Risk of cardiovascular diseases associated with medications used in attention-deficit/hyperactivity disorder: a systematic review and meta-analysis. JAMA Netw Open. 2022;5(11):e2243597.
669. Castells X, Cunill R, Perez-Mana C, Vidal X, Capella D. Psychostimulant drugs for cocaine dependence. Cochrane Database Syst Rev. 2016;9(9):CD007380.
670. Perez-Mana C, Castells X, Torrens M, Capella D, Farre M. Efficacy of psychostimulant drugs for amphetamine abuse or dependence. Cochrane Database Syst Rev 2013(9):CD009695.
671. Bhatt M, Zielinski L, Baker-Beal L, Bhatnagar N, Mouravska N, Laplante P, Worster A, Thabane L, Samaan Z. Efficacy and safety of psychostimulants for amphetamine and methamphetamine use disorders: a systematic review and meta-analysis. Syst Rev. 2016;5(1):189.
672. Brevik EJ, Lundervold AJ, Halmoy A, Posserud MB, Instanes JT, Bjorvatn B, Haavik J. Prevalence

and clinical correlates of insomnia in adults with attention-deficit hyperactivity disorder. Acta Psychiatr Scand. 2017;136(2):220–7.
673. Wynchank D, Bijlenga D, Beekman AT, Kooij JJS, Penninx BW. Adult attention-deficit/hyperactivity disorder (ADHD) and insomnia: an update of the literature. Curr Psychiatry Rep. 2017;19(12):98.
674. Low AM, Vangkilde S, le Sommer J, Fagerlund B, Glenthoj B, Jepsen JRM, Habekost T. Effects of methylphenidate on subjective sleep parameters in adults with ADHD: a prospective, non-randomized, non-blinded 6-week trial. Nord J Psychiatry. 2023;77(1):102–7.
675. Cataldo M, Donnelly G, Cutler AJ, Childress A, Mikl J, Bhaskar S, Waxmonsky J. Analysis of daily sleep diary measures from multilayer extended-release methylphenidate (PRC-063) studies in children and adults with ADHD. J Atten Disord. 2022;26(14):1870–81.
676. Mattingly GW, Childress AC, Cutler AJ, Estrada J, Corliss M. Serdexmethylphenidate/dexmethylphenidate effects on sleep in children with attention-deficit/hyperactivity disorder. Front Psych. 2023;14:1193455.
677. Sanabra M, Gomez-Hinojosa T, Grau N, Alda JA. Deficient emotional self-regulation and sleep problems in ADHD with and without pharmacological treatment. J Atten Disord. 2022;26(3):426–33.
678. van Andel E, Ten Have M, Bijlenga D, Beekman ATF, de Graaf R, Kooij JJS. Combined impact of ADHD and insomnia symptoms on quality of life, productivity, and health care use in the general population. Psychol Med. 2022;52(1):36–47.
679. Kwon SJ, Kim Y, Kwak Y. Influence of smartphone addiction and poor sleep quality on attention-deficit hyperactivity disorder symptoms in university students: a cross-sectional study. J Am Coll Health. 2022;70(1):209–15.
680. Spadola CE, Rottapel RE, Zhou ES, Chen JT, Guo N, Khalsa SBS, Redline S, Bertisch SM. A sleep hygiene and yoga intervention conducted in affordable housing communities: pilot study results and lessons for a future trial. Complement Ther Clin Pract. 2020;39:101121.
681. Wong KF, Perini F, Lin J, Goldstein M, Ong JL, Lo J, Ong JC, Doshi K, Lim J. Dissociable changes in sleep architecture with mindfulness and sleep hygiene intervention in older adults: secondary and exploratory analysis of polysomnography data from the mindfulness sleep therapy (MIST) trial. Sleep Health. 2022;8(4):364–72.
682. Cortese S, Brown TE, Corkum P, Gruber R, O'Brien LM, Stein M, Weiss M, Owens J. Assessment and management of sleep problems in youths with attention-deficit/hyperactivity disorder. J Am Acad Child Adolesc Psychiatry. 2013;52(8):784–96.
683. Wilens TE, Spencer TJ, Swanson JM, Connor DF, Cantwell D. Combining methylphenidate and clonidine: a clinically sound medication option. J Am Acad Child Adolesc Psychiatry 1999;38(5):614–9.
684. Schwartz RS, Olds J. The psychiatry of light. Harv Rev Psychiatry. 2015;23(3):188–94.
685. Surman CBH, Walsh DM. Managing sleep in adults with ADHD: from science to pragmatic approaches. Brain Sci. 2021;11(10):1361.
686. Cunill R, Castells X, Gonzalez-Pinto A, Arrojo M, Bernardo M, Saiz PA, Florez G, Torrens M, Tirado-Munoz J, Fonseca F, Arranz B, Garriga M, Goikolea JM, Zorrilla I, Becona E, Lopez A, San L. Clinical practice guideline on pharmacological and psychological management of adult patients with attention deficit and hyperactivity disorder and comorbid substance use. Adicciones. 2022;34(2):168–78.
687. Strattera (package insert). Lilly USA, LLC. Indianapolis; 2022.
688. Flockhart DA, Thacker D, McDonald C, Desta Z. The Flockhart cytochrome P450 drug-drug interaction table. Indianapolis: Division of Clinical Pharmacology, Indiana University School of Medicine; 2021. Available from: https://drug-interactions.medicine.iu.edu/MainTable.aspx.
689. Bangs ME, Jin L, Zhang S, Desaiah D, Allen AJ, Read HA, Regev A, Wernicke JF. Hepatic events associated with atomoxetine treatment for attention-deficit hyperactivity disorder. Drug Saf. 2008;31(4):345–54.
690. Markowitz JS, Melchert PW. The pharmacokinetics and pharmacogenomics of psychostimulants. Child Adolesc Psychiatr Clin N Am. 2022;31(3):393–416.
691. Berger O, Rector K, Meredith J, Sebaaly J. Evaluation of drug-drug interactions in hospitalized patients on medications for OUD. Ment Health Clin. 2021;11(4):231–7.
692. Abbott KL, Flannery PC, Gill KS, Boothe DM, Dhanasekaran M, Mani S, Pondugula SR. Adverse pharmacokinetic interactions between illicit substances and clinical drugs. Drug Metab Rev. 2020;52(1):44–65.
693. Guerzoni S, Pellesi L, Pini LA, Caputo F. Drug-drug interactions in the treatment for alcohol use disorders: a comprehensive review. Pharmacol Res. 2018;133:65–76.
694. Patrick KS, Straughn AB, Minhinnett RR, Yeatts SD, Herrin AE, DeVane CL, Malcolm R, Janis GC, Markowitz JS. Influence of ethanol and gender on methylphenidate pharmacokinetics and pharmacodynamics. Clin Pharmacol Ther. 2007;81(3):346–53.
695. Patrick KS, Straughn AB, Reeves OT 3rd, Bernstein H, Bell GH, Anderson ER, Malcolm RJ. Differential influences of ethanol on early exposure to racemic methylphenidate compared with dexmethylphenidate in humans. Drug Metab Dispos. 2013;41(1):197–205.
696. McCance-Katz EF, Sullivan LE, Nallani S. Drug interactions of clinical importance among the opioids, methadone and buprenorphine, and other frequently prescribed medications: a review. Am J Addict. 2010;19(1):4–16.

697. Grau-Lopez L, Roncero C, Navarro MC, Casas M. Psychosis induced by the interaction between disulfiram and methylphenidate may be dose dependent. Subst Abus. 2012;33(2):186–8.
698. Spiegel DR, McCroskey A, Puaa K, Meeker G, Hartman L, Hudson J, Hung YC. A case of disulfiram-induced psychosis in a previously asymptomatic patient maintained on mixed amphetamine salts: a review of the literature and possible pathophysiological explanations. Clin Neuropharmacol. 2016;39(5):272–5.
699. Hadler N, Strome A, Waselewski M, Herbert K, Harper C, Chang T. Perspectives of US adolescents on diverted stimulant use. J Pediatr. 2021;235:190–5.
700. Holt LJ, Marut PN, Schepis TS. Pursued for their prescription: exposure to compliance-gaining strategies predicts stimulant diversion in emerging adults. Psychol Addict Behav. 2018;32(1):122–31.
701. Holt LJ, Schepis TS, Looby A, Marsh E, Marut P, Feinn R. How to say "no" most effectively: evaluating resistance strategies for prescription stimulant diversion to inform preventive interventions. J Am Coll Health. 2020;68(8):872–82.
702. Molina BSG, Kipp HL, Joseph HM, Engster SA, Harty SC, Dawkins M, Lindstrom RA, Bauer DJ, Bangalore SS. Stimulant diversion risk among college students treated for ADHD: primary care provider prevention training. Acad Pediatr. 2020;20(1):119–27.
703. Arria AM, Caldeira KM, Vincent KB, O'Grady KE, Cimini MD, Geisner IM, Fossos-Wong N, Kilmer JR, Larimer ME. Do college students improve their grades by using prescription stimulants nonmedically? Addict Behav. 2017;65:245–9.
704. Holt LJ, Looby A. Factors that differentiate prescription stimulant misusers from those at-risk for misuse: expectancies, perceived safety, and diversion. Subst Use Misuse. 2018;53(7):1068–75.
705. Molina BSG, Joseph HM, Kipp HL, Lindstrom RA, Pedersen SL, Kolko DJ, Bauer DJ, Subramaniam GA. Adolescents treated for attention-deficit/hyperactivity disorder in pediatric primary care: characterizing risk for stimulant diversion. J Dev Behav Pediatr. 2021;42(7):540–52.
706. Loskutova NY, Waterman J, Callen E, Staton EW, Bullard E, Shields J. Knowledge, attitudes, and practice patterns of health professionals toward medical and non-medical stimulant use by young adults. J Am Board Fam Med. 2020;33(1):59–70.
707. Adler LA, Farahbakhshian S, Romero B, Flood E, Doll H. Healthcare provider perspectives on diagnosing and treating adults with attention-deficit/hyperactivity disorder. Postgrad Med. 2019;131(7):461–72.
708. Faraone SV, Glatt SJ. A comparison of the efficacy of medications for adult attention-deficit/hyperactivity disorder using meta-analysis of effect sizes. J Clin Psychiatry. 2010;71(6):754–63.
709. Faraone SV, Childress A, Caras S, Arnold VK, Montano CB, Sarkis EH, Cutler AJ, Young JL. A Randomized, Double-Blind, Placebo-Controlled Trial to Evaluate the Efficacy and Safety of AR19, a Manipulation-Resistant Formulation of Amphetamine Sulfate, in Adults With Attention-Deficit/Hyperactivity Disorder. J Clin Psychiatry. 2021;82(5):21m13927.
710. Dekkers TJ, Agelink van Rentergem JA, Huizenga HM, Raber H, Shoham R, Popma A, Pollak Y. Decision-making deficits in ADHD are not related to risk seeking but to suboptimal decision-making: meta-analytical and novel experimental evidence. J Atten Disord. 2021;25(4):486–501.
711. Fuermaier ABM, Tucha L, Butzbach M, Weisbrod M, Aschenbrenner S, Tucha O. ADHD at the workplace: ADHD symptoms, diagnostic status, and work-related functioning. J Neural Transm (Vienna). 2021;128(7):1021–31.
712. Cox DJ, Davis M, Mikami AY, Singh H, Merkel RL, Burket R. Long-acting methylphenidate reduces collision rates of young adult drivers with attention-deficit/hyperactivity disorder. J Clin Psychopharmacol. 2012;32(2):225–30.
713. Arria AM, DuPont RL. Prescription stimulant use and misuse: implications for responsible prescribing practices. Am J Psychiatry. 2018;175(8):707–8.
714. Ramos-Quiroga JA, Casas M. Achieving remission as a routine goal of pharmacotherapy in attention-deficit hyperactivity disorder. CNS Drugs. 2011;25(1):17–36.
715. Chamakalayil S, Strasser J, Vogel M, Brand S, Walter M, Dursteler KM. Methylphenidate for attention-deficit and hyperactivity disorder in adult patients with substance use disorders: good clinical practice. Front Psych. 2020;11:540837.

51 From Stigma to Therapy: The Evolution of Psychiatry in Substance Use Disorders

Claudia Sagheddu, Giuseppe Virdis, and Miriam Melis

Introduction—A Historical Perspective

Search for the causes of drug addiction has gone through different stages over time. These have been influenced by both cultural and social processes as well as by different interpretative models. Changes of social, medical, scientific and political perception of the phenomenon of drug dependence has been considered as a privileged subject of study in various disciplines, ranging from socio-anthropology to epistemology. In the 1970s, the use of drugs spread as sociocultural and political phenomena often assigned with "positive" connotations. Particularly, it was regarded as a political or even a spiritual phenomenon characterizing the protest and the emancipation of those times. However, in the 1980s', as the cultural context profoundly changed, abuse of alcohol and of any drug has been perceived as a deviance, which resulted in social marginalization and moral condemnation. This highlights how the perspective of this phenomenon can be strongly conditioned by contingent factors, which are influenced by social changes, and therefore, can be judgmental. As the perspective changed within few decades, the same phenomenon that was first framed as a non-negative or even as a functional distinctive trait, it turned subsequently into as a morally deplorable deviance, to reach finally the status of a brain disease deserving a medical treatment at the end of the twentieth century [1].

C. Sagheddu · M. Melis (✉)
Division of Neuroscience and Clinical Pharmacology, Department of Biomedical Sciences, University of Cagliari, Cagliari, Italy
e-mail: claudiasagheddu@unica.it; myriam@unica.it

G. Virdis
Liceo Scientifico Statale "Pitagora", Selargius, Italy
e-mail: giuseppe.virdis@liceopitagoraselargius.edu.it

Interpretative Models in Psychology

Over time, the different interpretative models have revealed both the strengths and the limitations related to their partial perspective. For this reason, nowadays, a "circular interpretation" prevails in the field as opposed to a unilateral approach. Drug dependence relies on psychological factors associated with the personality of the individual, being social and biological underpinnings relevant for pleasure, tolerance, and abstinence. Hence, the understanding of drug use shall consider individual's personal history and the relationships one is involved into at a given time in life [2].

The many and heterogeneous theories of the psychology of addiction and drug abuse can be largely attributed to the so-called "*disease*" and "*adaptive*" interpretative paradigms. According to an interpretative medical concept, the theories attributable to the "*disease*" paradigm refer to

P. Á. Gargiulo, H. L. Mesones-Arroyo (eds.), *Psychiatry and Neuroscience Update – Vol. V*,
https://doi.org/10.1007/978-3-031-72219-6_51

addiction as a direct exposure to the substance, or as an individual predisposition to the disease based on biological and/or psychological risk factors. Among these theories, the physiological ones [3] focus on neurobiological modifications triggered by pharmacological properties of drugs of abuse (as will be discussed later). Therefore, altered metabolic processes in SUDs can be counteracted mainly by drugs blocking these effects (i.e., antagonists) or by other pharmacological tools and nonpharmacological methodologies (e.g., transcranial magnetic stimulation, TMS) to reinstate the patient's well-being.

An experimental psychologist perspective, such as the reinforcement theories, also represents a reductionist paradigm [4], because it refers to the addictive state as the mere association between taking drugs and stimulus-response. Finally, the Freudian theory posits that drug addicts are victims of an obsession on the oral phase. Those psychodynamic theories established in the 1960s also fall within this interpretative model.

The "*adaptive*" paradigm is a synthesis of various psychiatric, sociological, and psychological theories. This considers that one individual begins the use of addictive substances because of several factors, such as cognitive, emotional, subjective, and occasional, beside the personality trait, which reveals a dysfunctional response to the exposure to stressful situations. These theories do not exclude biological factors, but highlight the interactions with other factors of psychological, interpersonal, and social origin.

Among the main theories belonging to this paradigm, there are the psychodynamic ones. These latter posit that drug addiction is an aberrant and unsuccessful attempt to heal profound discomforts/traumas occurred early in life and usually related to the relationship with the caregiver. According to Bergeret [5], any personality trait that is neurotic, psychotic, or depressed would result *per se* in addictive behaviors. On the other hand, Cancrini [6] proposed that drug addiction is a coping strategy against intolerable suffering and describes the phenomenon in four different types: type A, tied to traumatic episodes such as bereavement and separation; type B, related to self-identification problems arising during adolescence; type C, as a self-medication to control preexisting mental disorders; and type D, as a feature of sociopathic personality disorders associated with problematic family context.

Reversing the Paradigm in Neuropsychiatry: From Personality Disorder to Brain Disease

In the second half of the eighteenth century, the pioneer psychiatrists Pinel and Rush proposed that alcoholism was a medical disease and, as such, the patient (i.e., the alcoholic) deserved a treatment rather than being treated as an individual with a bad habit and a loss of willpower [7]. Nonetheless, social stigma for drug addicts continues until contemporary times. In 1952, the first edition of the *Diagnostic and statistical manual of mental disorders* (DSM-I) described alcoholism and drug addiction as an expression of sociopathic disturbance of the personality arising from having experienced adverse events. In the most recent edition, the DSM-5 [8] defines drug addiction as a pattern of "cognitive, behavioral, and physiological symptoms indicating that the individual continues using the substance despite significant substance-related problems" [8]. This latest definition describes the disorder as a *continuum* from use-abuse to dependence. This also served as the motivation that led to the novel diagnostic term introduced in the DSM-5, where the term *addiction* is replaced with *substance use disorder* (SUD) [8].

This new perspective in clinical psychiatry has also been crucial towards the cultural eradication of stigma over addicts. According to the World Health Organization (WHO), and based on modern scientific psychiatry, SUD is nowadays conceptualized as a chronic and recurrent neuropsychiatric disease. Upon an acute drug intake, the reward is followed by emotional discomfort (i.e., dysphoria), which serves as a motivational driving force towards compulsive behaviors. Consequently, the relapse results from a loss of self-restraint to drug seeking. Additionally, the DSM-5 introduced nondrug-related behavioral compulsions (i.e., behavioral addictions), such as pathological gambling and compulsive buying/shopping, based on the substantial converging evidence from preclinical and clinical studies showing that SUD and behavioral addictions share similar stages ranging from habit formation to dysphoric responses, as well as neurobiological and genetic factors contributing to mental illness [9].

Neurobiological Mechanisms Underlying SUDs and Behavioral Addictions

Nowadays, SUD as a whole is described as a spiraling distress syndrome that manifests with four common stages: binge-intoxication, preoccupation-anticipation, withdrawal-negative affect, and craving-anticipation. Each stage involves emotional and behavioral neuroplastic alterations, which in turn facilitate the reoccurrence of drug use, i.e., the relapse [10, 11].

Diverse substances of abuse and behavioral compulsions share biopsychological mechanisms, which have been elucidated by modeling the pathology in experimental animals and by using neuroimaging technologies in humans [12]. Metanalysis studies of the human brain structure have recently confirmed a lower subcortical volume and cortical thickness in subjects addicted to discrete substances as compared with nondependent individuals [13], thus revealing a general detrimental drug effect.

Drug consumption stimulates dopamine neurotransmission in the mesolimbic reward system, i.e., the projection from the midbrain ventral tegmental area (VTA) to the ventral striatum. This is considered the first step underlying positive reinforcing effects, which promote the behavior and the effort to obtain the drug. However, once the status of dependence is established, dopamine release and dopamine receptor levels are diminished, which mirror alterations of reward/aversion processing. In addition, decreased serotonin levels in the prefrontal cortex (PFC) induce imbalances within frontostriatal control, thus leading to detrimental changes in salience attribution, cognitive flexibility and behavioral compulsivity. In the cerebral cortex, the insula has also been involved in decision-making and emotional processing, keys in both behavioral and drug dependence [14, 15]. As a result, both the negative affective state and the emergence of lack of control facilitate the occurrence of the relapse after a period of withdrawal.

Besides the neural circuits and the neurotransmitters, several neuromodulators have been proven crucial in various brain regions involved in SUD and at different stages of the whole spectrum of the disease. Among these, the endocannabinoids (ECBs), such as anandamide and 2-acyl-glycerol, are lipid signaling molecules involved in diverse forms of synaptic plasticity and metaplasticity in reward brain regions [16]. The cannabinoid receptor type 1 (CB1) is both the target of Δ^9-Tetrahydrocannabinol (THC) present in Cannabis and a modulator of the mesocorticolimbic circuit. Additionally, altered G-protein-coupled signaling downstream from CB1 is involved in the effects of diverse drugs of abuse, such as alcohol [17], nicotine [18], and cocaine [19]. Fatty acid amide hydrolase (FAAH) is a major degrading enzyme responsible for the regulation of the levels of ECB and related lipid molecules [20]. Accordingly, a wide body of preclinical evidence avails novel pharmacological strategies exploiting the ECB system (and its related lipids) as potentially clinically candidates to counteract drug-induced dopamine system maladaptations contributing to the risk of relapse [21, 22].

Individual Vulnerability for Behavioral Addictions and SUDs

Discrete social and biological determinants influence the transition from substance abuse to loss of control towards dependence. The understanding of the biological reasons for only a small proportion of drug users to become addicted is still elusive. Significant progress has been made in the past decades that demonstrated the important roles of sex, genetic background, the stage of brain development, as well as of environmental factors and their impact on epigenetic mechanisms on this transition [23]. However, the comprehension of the complexity of the interplay among these different factors is still a challenge.

Individual genetic differences in the dopamine [24] and ECB system [25] have been shown to be either a protecting or a predicting determinant. For instance, dopamine D2 receptor levels in reward brain regions have been correlated with drug abuse, being higher and lower levels a protective and risk factor, respectively [26]. Different variants of triplets throughout the CB1 receptor genomic sequence have been associated with enhanced individual vulnerability to SUDs [27, 28]. Similarly, specific gene polymorphisms of FAAH enzyme are related with increased reward processing in the brain, thereby identified as marker for susceptibility to drug abuse [28–33]. In experimental preclinical models of drug dependence, discrete environmental factors have been shown to impact on addictive behaviors. As an example, food deprivation and environmental enrichment are positively or negatively reinforcing the acquisition and the maintenance of drug taking, respectively.

External influences operate *inter alia* onto epigenetic processes, i.e., changing the state of the chromatin by acetylation and methylation or by means of noncoding RNAs in neural and nonneural brain cells that are involved in distinct stages of SUDs [34]. Among environmental factors having an impact towards the manifestation of addictive disorders, perinatal exposure to drugs of abuse is worth to be mentioned, being fetal life an extremely sensitive window for brain development. Increasing evidence indicates that drugs impact onto neural development both directly and indirectly by affecting also the ECB system [35, 36]. Finally, along with early exposure to substances of abuse, gender is another critical variable in the increased susceptibility to the development of SUDs later in life [37, 38].

Therapeutic Approach for Behavioral Dependence and SUDs

In psychiatry, a dual diagnosis, which is the cooccurrence of a mental health disorder with SUD, is common rather than exceptional. In fact, between one-third and a half of the people accessing mental health services have coexisting SUD and a psychiatric disorder. For instance, the prevalence of patients affected with schizophrenia or other severe psychotic disorders and developing a SUDs, typically tobacco dependence, is about 50% [39]. Vice versa, the development of a psychiatric condition can also be secondary to or parallel to SUD and/or a behavioral addiction. Because of its biological complexity along with its social implications, SUD treatment requires interventions that cannot be curtailed to psychiatric practice. Psychological and psychosocial approaches, such as therapeutic communities, are all useful and flexible means for individual recovery and rehabilitation. Hence, pharmacological therapy, which is mainly aimed at managing negative state/painful symptoms and at preventing withdrawal and stress driven relapse, must be associated and followed by psychotherapy and other social assistance.

Nonpharmacological Therapies: Psychotherapeutic Approach

The most used approach in psychotherapy is the *cognitive-behavioral therapy* (CBT) [40], which regards SUD as a learned dysfunctional behavior that has to be replaced with wellbeing-aimed behaviors, rather than considering remote and unconscious causes [41, 42]. The fundamental assumption of the CBT model is that drug dependence is "learned" behavior tied to classical and operative conditioning. Therefore, SUD emerges in a given environmental context. Key elements of CBT are a functional analysis of the context, the thoughts, and the emotions associated to the consumption of addicting substances and the acquisition of new skills and learned behaviors to move towards healthier and functional ones.

On one hand, treatments similar to CBT are the *motivational interview* (MI) and the *dialectical-behavioral therapy* (DBT). DBT, developed by Linehan for the treatment of borderline personality disorder (BPD) [43, 44], has also proven to be effective in the treatment of behavioral addictions and SUDs [45, 46]. DBT is characterized by a specific attention to the patient's quality of life.

On the other hand, the psychodynamic psychotherapeutic approach is paradigmatically focus to unconscious aspects and differs from the CBT. This therapy is particularly oriented to long-lasting changes in patients by helping them to develop an inner awareness that reveals previously inaccessible emotional contents. Consequently, this rises the ability to manage difficult emotions related to past trauma.

Nonpharmacological Therapies: Transcranial Magnetic Stimulation

Over the past decade, transcranial magnetic stimulation (TMS) has been drawing attention as a promising nonpharmacological and noninvasive technique to treat several neuropathological conditions, including SUD [47]. The accurate position of the coil nearby the skull together with precise protocols for delivering magnetic pulses—that is the combination of timing and modulation of the electric field—proved to impact onto brain activity with minimal side effects. Similarly to physiological memory and learning processes, the drug-induced memory trace, also termed "*drug engram,*" relies upon molecular mechanisms of neuroplasticity [48]. Therapies based on TMS aim at remodeling brain circuit plasticity and function. Accordingly, TMS enables changes in emotional discomfort and misconducts associated with behavioral addiction and SUD by helping addicts to quit or delay relapses. The insula is probably one of the main brain targets of TMS for the successful treatment of SUD. Indeed, both preclinical and clinical evidence suggests that TMS aimed at this cortical area is an aid to the therapy of SUD [49]. Finally, yet importantly, a patented TMS device has received the first FDA clearance for smoking cessation based on the positive results showing its safety and efficacy in a multicenter, double-blind, sham controlled clinical trial [50].

Pharmacological Therapies

Current knowledge built upon both molecular and brain imaging studies, along with those collected from psychologists and psychiatrists, converge into an interdisciplinary-oriented approach where pharmacological and nonpharmacological interventions are combined to improve the clinical outcome. In this respect, the pharmacotherapies would help to restore those physiological functions in neuronal circuits that are disrupted by drug use, thus supporting the individual in the engagement of healthy behaviors. Based upon distinct mechanisms, several approved pharmacological therapies are currently available for diverse SUDs [51, 52]. In particular, naltrexone/acamprosate, nicotine replacement/bupropion/varenicline, and methadone/buprenorphine/lofexidine are approved for the treatment of alcohol, tobacco, and opioid use disorder, respectively. Unfortunately, these pharmacotherapies result ineffective in a significant number of patients seeking for medical aid, thereby suggesting the need for additional molecular investigations to address such a clinical challenge [53, 54].

Novel Pharmacological Approaches from Preclinical Studies

The further understanding of drug-induced molecular, cellular, and circuit adaptations arising from chronic drug exposure can be exploited for the development of novel pharmacotherapies. Given that ECBs play a pivotal role in the mesocorticolimbic dopamine system [55], the modulation of this system represents an opportunity to restore the physiology of the reward/aversion processes. Accordingly, CB1 neutral antagonists and negative allosteric modulators (NAM) are promising medications for SUD. In particular, CB1 neutral antagonists might be effective for opioid use disorder but also for cocaine, cannabis, nicotine, methamphetamine, and alcohol [56–60]. In contrast, the efficacy of NAMs of CB1 appears specific for the drug and to be curtailed to cannabis use disorder [61] or cocaine and methamphetamine [62]. Alternatively, indirect CB1 agonists, drugs aimed at increasing ECBs and ECB-like system through inhibition of degrading enzymes (e.g., FAAH) appear nowadays as the preferred drug pipelines for targeting this system. This rationale stems from the evidence that these drugs would interfere with the ECB system only at synapses where there is a phasic activation, and this might lead to fewer side effects. FAAH inhibitors, particularly, appear to be the most promising against nicotine and cocaine dependence [63–66].

References

1. Rodríguez ME. The psychiatrist at the Centre of the opioid crisis. Nature. 2020;580(7802):178–81.
2. Ravenna M. Psicologia delle tossicodipendenze—Il Mulino Editore; 1997.
3. Dole VP, Nyswander ME. Heroin addiction-a metabolic disease. Arch Intern Med. 1967;120(1):19–24.
4. Olds J, Milner P. Positive reinforcement produced by electrical stimulation of septal area and other regions of rat brain. J Comp Physiol Psychol. 1954;47(6):419–27.
5. Bergeret J. Toxicomanie et personnalité. Presses universitaires de France. 1986.127 p.
6. Cancrini L. Quei temerari sulle macchine volanti. Studio sulle terapie dei tossicomani. 1982.
7. Nathan PE, Conrad M, Skinstad AH. History of the concept of addiction. Annu Rev Clin Psychol. 2016;12:29–51.
8. Psychiatry.org—DSM. https://www.psychiatry.org:443/psychiatrists/practice/dsm
9. Figee M, Pattij T, Willuhn I, Luigjes J, van den Brink W, Goudriaan A, et al. Compulsivity in obsessive-compulsive disorder and addictions. J Eur Coll Neuropsychopharmacol. 2016;26(5):856–68.
10. Koob GF, Le Moal M. Drug abuse: hedonic homeostatic dysregulation. Science. 1997;278(5335):52–8.
11. Koob GF, Le Moal M. Drug addiction, dysregulation of reward, and allostasis. Neuropsychopharmacology. 2001;24(2):97–129.
12. Kalivas PW, Volkow ND. The neural basis of addiction: a pathology of motivation and choice. Am J Psychiatry. 2005;162(8):1403–13.
13. Mackey S, Allgaier N, Chaarani B, Spechler P, Orr C, Bunn J, et al. Mega-analysis of gray matter volume in substance dependence: general and substance-specific regional effects. Am J Psychiatry. 2019;176(2):119–28.
14. Koob GF, Volkow ND. Neurocircuitry of addiction. Neuropsychopharmacology. 2010;35(1):217–38.
15. Koob GF, Volkow ND. Neurobiology of addiction: a neurocircuitry analysis. Lancet Psychiatry. 2016;3(8):760–73.
16. Sagheddu C, Muntoni AL, Pistis M, Melis M. Endocannabinoid signaling in motivation, reward, and addiction: influences on Mesocorticolimbic dopamine function. Int Rev Neurobiol. 2015;125:257–302.
17. Hungund BL, Basavarajappa BS. Role of endocannabinoids and cannabinoid CB1 receptors in alcohol-related behaviors. Ann N Y Acad Sci. 2004;1025:515–27.
18. Castañé A, Berrendero F, Maldonado R. The role of the cannabinoid system in nicotine addiction. Pharmacol Biochem Behav. 2005;81(2):381–6.
19. Arnold JC. The role of endocannabinoid transmission in cocaine addiction. Pharmacol Biochem Behav. 2005;81(2):396–406.
20. Pistis M, Melis M. From surface to nuclear receptors: the endocannabinoid family extends its assets. Curr Med Chem. 2010;17(14):1450–67.
21. Sagheddu C, Torres LH, Marcourakis T, Pistis M. Endocannabinoid-like lipid neuromodulators in the regulation of dopamine signaling: relevance for drug addiction. Front Synaptic Neurosci. 2020;12:588660.
22. Luján MÁ, Cheer JF, Melis M. Choosing the right drug: status and future of endocannabinoid research for the prevention of drug-seeking reinstatement. Curr Opin Pharmacol. 2021;56:29–38.
23. Sagheddu C, Melis M. Individual differences and vulnerability to drug addiction: a focus on the endocannabinoid system. CNS Neurol Disord Drug Targets. 2015;14(4):502–17.
24. Volkow ND, Fowler JS, Wang GJ, Baler R, Telang F. Imaging dopamine's role in drug abuse and addiction. Neuropharmacology. 2009;56(Suppl 1):3–8.
25. Parsons LH, Hurd YL. Endocannabinoid signalling in reward and addiction. Nat Rev Neurosci Ottobre. 2015;16(10):579–94.
26. Gorwood P, Le Strat Y, Ramoz N, Dubertret C, Moalic JM, Simonneau M. Genetics of dopamine receptors and drug addiction. Hum Genet. 2012;131(6):803–22.
27. Benyamina A, Kebir O, Blecha L, Reynaud M, Krebs MO. CNR1 gene polymorphisms in addictive disorders: a systematic review and a meta-analysis. Addict Biol. 2011;16(1):1–6.
28. Proudnikov D, Kroslak T, Sipe JC, Randesi M, Li D, Hamon S, et al. Association of polymorphisms of the cannabinoid receptor (CNR1) and fatty acid amide hydrolase (FAAH) genes with heroin addiction: impact of long repeats of CNR1. Pharmacogenomics J. 2010;10(3):232–42.
29. Hungund BL, Szakall I, Adam A, Basavarajappa BS, Vadasz C. Cannabinoid CB1 receptor knockout mice exhibit markedly reduced voluntary alcohol consumption and lack alcohol-induced dopamine release in the nucleus accumbens. J Neurochem. 2003;84(4):698–704.
30. Chiang KP, Gerber AL, Sipe JC, Cravatt BF. Reduced cellular expression and activity of the P129T mutant of human fatty acid amide hydrolase: evidence for a link between defects in the endocannabinoid system and problem drug use. Hum Mol Genet. 2004;13(18):2113–9.
31. Palmer RHC, McGeary JE, Knopik VS, Bidwell LC, Metrik JM. CNR1 and FAAH variation and affective states induced by marijuana smoking. Am J Drug Alcohol Abuse. 2019;45(5):514–26.
32. Hindocha C, Freeman TP, Schafer G, Gardner C, Bloomfield MAP, Bramon E, et al. Acute effects of cannabinoids on addiction endophenotypes are moderated by genes encoding the CB1 receptor and FAAH enzyme. Addict Biol. 2020;25(3):e12762.
33. Zhang W, Liu H, Deng XD, Ma Y, Liu Y. FAAH levels and its genetic polymorphism association with susceptibility to methamphetamine dependence. Ann Hum Genet. 2020;84(3):259–70.
34. Beayno A, El Hayek S, Noufi P, Tarabay Y, Shamseddeen W. The role of epigenetics in addiction: clinical overview and recent updates. Methods Mol Biol. 2019;2011:609–31.

35. Scheyer AF, Melis M, Trezza V, Manzoni OJJ. Consequences of perinatal cannabis exposure. Trends Neurosci. 2019;42(12):871–84.
36. Hurd YL, Manzoni OJ, Pletnikov MV, Lee FS, Bhattacharyya S, Melis M. Cannabis and the developing brain: insights into its long-lasting effects. J Neurosci. 2019;39(42):8250–8.
37. Fattore L, Melis M. Sex differences in impulsive and compulsive behaviors: a focus on drug addiction. Addict Biol. 2016;21(5):1043–51.
38. Traccis F, Frau R, Melis M. Gender differences in the outcome of offspring prenatally exposed to drugs of abuse. Front Behav Neurosci. 2020;14:72.
39. Regier DA, Farmer ME, Rae DS, Locke BZ, Keith SJ, Judd LL, et al. Comorbidity of mental disorders with alcohol and other drug abuse. Results from the epidemiologic catchment area (ECA) study. JAMA. 1990;264(19):2511–8.
40. An H, He RH, Zheng YR, Tao R. Cognitive-behavioral therapy. Adv Exp Med Biol. 2017;1010:321–9.
41. Carroll KM, Kiluk BD. Cognitive behavioral interventions for alcohol and drug use disorders: through the stage model and back again. J Soc Psychol Addict Behav. 2017;31(8):847–61.
42. Majeed MH, Sudak DM. Cognitive behavioral therapy for chronic pain-one therapeutic approach for the opioid epidemic. J Psychiatr Pract. 2017;23(6):409–14.
43. Rizvi SL, Linehan MM. Dialectical behavior therapy for personality disorders. Curr Psychiatry Rep. 2001;3(1):64–9.
44. Koerner K, Linehan MM. Research on dialectical behavior therapy for patients with borderline personality disorder. Psychiatr Clin North Am. 2000;23(1):151–67.
45. Parmar A, Kaloiya G. Comorbidity of personality disorder among substance use disorder patients: a narrative review. Indian J Psychol Med. 2018;40(6):517–27.
46. Riegler A, Bumb JM, Wisch C, Schuster R, Reinhard I, Hoffmann S, et al. Does the augmentation of trauma informed hatha yoga increase the effect of dialectical behavior therapy for substance use disorders on psychopathological strain of patients with borderline personality disorder and comorbid substance use disorder? Results of a quasi-experimental study. Eur Addict Res. 2022;1–8.
47. Diana M, Raij T, Melis M, Nummenmaa A, Leggio L, Bonci A. Rehabilitating the addicted brain with transcranial magnetic stimulation. Nat Rev Neurosci. 2017;18(11):685–93.
48. Mahoney JJ, Hanlon CA, Marshalek PJ, Rezai AR, Krinke L. Transcranial magnetic stimulation, deep brain stimulation, and other forms of neuromodulation for substance use disorders: review of modalities and implications for treatment. J Neurol Sci. 2020;418:117149.
49. Ibrahim C, Rubin-Kahana DS, Pushparaj A, Musiol M, Blumberger DM, Daskalakis ZJ, et al. The insula: a brain stimulation target for the treatment of addiction. Front Pharmacol. 2019;10:720.
50. Zangen A, Moshe H, Martinez D, Barnea-Ygael N, Vapnik T, Bystritsky A, et al. Repetitive transcranial magnetic stimulation for smoking cessation: a pivotal multicenter double-blind randomized controlled trial. World Psychiatry. 2021;20(3):397–404.
51. Forray A, Sofuoglu M. Future pharmacological treatments for substance use disorders. Br J Clin Pharmacol. 2014;77(2):382–400.
52. Carton L, Nourredine M, Rolland B. Pharmacotherapy of substance use disorders in the neuroscience-based nomenclature (NbN). Therapie. 2021;76(2):127–36.
53. Klein JW. Pharmacotherapy for substance use disorders. Med Clin North Am. 2016;100(4):891–910.
54. Volkow ND, Boyle M. Neuroscience of addiction: relevance to prevention and treatment. Am J Psychiatry. 2018;175(8):729–40.
55. Melis M, Pistis M. Hub and switches: endocannabinoid signalling in midbrain dopamine neurons. Philos Trans R Soc Lond Ser B Biol Sci. 2012;367(1607):3276–85.
56. Rasmussen EB, Hillman C. Naloxone and rimonabant reduce the reinforcing properties of exercise in rats. Exp Clin Psychopharmacol. 2011;19(6):389–400.
57. Gueye AB, Pryslawsky Y, Trigo JM, Poulia N, Delis F, Antoniou K, et al. The CB1 neutral antagonist AM4113 retains the therapeutic efficacy of the inverse agonist Rimonabant for nicotine dependence and weight loss with better psychiatric tolerability. Int J Neuropsychopharmacol. 2016;19(12):pyw068.
58. Schindler CW, Redhi GH, Vemuri K, Makriyannis A, Le Foll B, Bergman J, et al. Blockade of nicotine and cannabinoid reinforcement and relapse by a cannabinoid CB1-receptor neutral antagonist AM4113 and inverse agonist Rimonabant in squirrel monkeys. Neuropsychopharmacology. 2016;41(9):2283–93.
59. Balla A, Dong B, Shilpa BM, Vemuri K, Makriyannis A, Pandey SC, et al. Cannabinoid-1 receptor neutral antagonist reduces binge-like alcohol consumption and alcohol-induced accumbal dopaminergic signaling. Neuropharmacology. 2018;131:200–8.
60. He XH, Jordan CJ, Vemuri K, Bi GH, Zhan J, Gardner EL, et al. Cannabinoid CB1 receptor neutral antagonist AM4113 inhibits heroin self-administration without depressive side effects in rats. Acta Pharmacol Sin. 2019;40(3):365–73.
61. Vallée M, Vitiello S, Bellocchio L, Hébert-Chatelain E, Monlezun S, Martin-Garcia E, et al. Pregnenolone can protect the brain from cannabis intoxication. Science. 2014;343(6166):94–8.
62. Jing L, Qiu Y, Zhang Y, Li JX. Effects of the cannabinoid CB1 receptor allosteric modulator ORG 27569 on reinstatement of cocaine- and methamphetamine-seeking behavior in rats. Drug Alcohol Depend. 2014;143:251–6.
63. Adamczyk P, McCreary AC, Przegalinski E, Mierzejewski P, Bienkowski P, Filip M. The effects of fatty acid amide hydrolase inhibitors on maintenance of cocaine and food self-administration and on reinstatement of cocaine-seeking and food-taking behav-

ior in rats. J Physiol Pharmacol Off J Pol Physiol Soc. 2009;60(3):119–25.
64. Justinova Z, Panlilio LV, Moreno-Sanz G, Redhi GH, Auber A, Secci ME, et al. Effects of fatty acid amide hydrolase (FAAH) inhibitors in non-human primate models of nicotine reward and relapse. Neuropsychopharmacology. 2015;40(9):2185–97.
65. Scherma M, Muntoni AL, Melis M, Fattore L, Fadda P, Fratta W, et al. Interactions between the endocannabinoid and nicotinic cholinergic systems: preclinical evidence and therapeutic perspectives. Psychopharmacology. 2016;233(10):1765–77.
66. Forget B, Guranda M, Gamaleddin I, Goldberg SR, Le Foll B. Attenuation of cue-induced reinstatement of nicotine seeking by URB597 through cannabinoid CB1 receptor in rats. Psychopharmacology. 2016;233(10):1823–8.

52 Addiction as a Rigid Disposition Towards Akratic Actions

Javier Bernacer, Julia Velez-Ramos, and Jose Ignacio Murillo

Introduction

West and Brown define addiction as "a chronic condition involving a repeated powerful motivation to engage in a rewarding behavior, acquired as a result of engaging in that behavior, that has significant potential for unintended harm. Someone is addicted to something to the extent that they experience this repeated powerful motivation" [1, pp. 15–16]. Behavioral addictions, such as gambling, pornography, video games, or social networks, are on the rise in the twenty-first century, but substance addiction is still massive. According to the World Health Organization, 35 million people suffer from drug use disorders, and about half a million died during the last year due to drug use.

This chapter primarily aims to contribute to a comprehensive substance addiction framework by focusing on some aspects of its phenomenology. Specifically, we will present addiction as a sort of rigid disposition that tends toward akratic actions, that is, actions that contradict one's own better judgment. Each element associated with this conceptualization will be clarified throughout the text. First, the most relevant theories of addiction will be summarized. We will point to a shift between most of the theories that originated in the twentieth century, which viewed addiction as an uncontrollable behavior of the person, and more recent proposals suggesting that addictive behaviors are deliberative, voluntary, and intentional. Among them, Heather's hypothesis of addiction as akratic behavior will be used to introduce the notion of akrasia.

Next, the philosophical concept of akrasia and its application to substance addiction will be explained. Therein, Plato and Aristotle criticized their master Socrates, who assumed that knowing the truth inevitably leads to acting according to the truth. Like their philosophical schools, their responses followed different paths, but they agreed on the capacity of human agents to act against one's ideal of behavior. Aristotle used the term *akrasia* and the concept of practical reason, which is crucial for his ethics. Why is the notion of akrasia important in the context of substance addiction? According to most recent frameworks, the addicted person is aware that their consump-

J. Bernacer (✉)
Mind-Brain Group, Institute for Culture and Society (ICS), University of Navarra, Pamplona, Spain

International Center for Neuroscience and Ethics (CINET), Fundación Tatiana, Madrid, Spain
e-mail: jbernacer@unav.es

J. Velez-Ramos
Departamento de Historia del Derecho y Filosofía Jurídica, Moral y Política, University of Salamanca, Salamanca, Spain
e-mail: juvra@usal.es

J. I. Murillo
Mind-Brain Group, Institute for Culture and Society (ICS), University of Navarra, Pamplona, Spain
e-mail: jimurillo@unav.es

P. Á. Gargiulo, H. L. Mesones-Arroyo (eds.), *Psychiatry and Neuroscience Update – Vol. V*,
https://doi.org/10.1007/978-3-031-72219-6_52

tion goes against their good; in fact, they usually withdraw for some time but eventually relapse and, in so doing, act against their own better judgment. Thus, they are akratics. After explaining Heather's hypothesis on addiction as akrasia, we will go deeper into the philosophical foundations of the term through the works of Alfred Mele and Amelie Rorty. Interestingly, both stress that, even though "akratic" is an adjective that can be applied to individual actions, "akrasia" is better understood as a character trait or disposition.

In the next section, we will summarize our interpretation of habit as a disposition based on Aristotelian philosophy and applied to psychology and neuroscience. As many authors suggest (see, for example, [2]), habit is a two-sided phenomenon that can be considered *good* or *bad*. We propose that good habits are goal-directed, flexible dispositions that allow for the establishment of increasingly complex goals and an enhanced conscious experience of behavior. Conversely, bad habits are rigid routines progressively disengaged from goals, mere automatisms akin to stimulus-response pairs. We claim that distinguishing between good (cognitively enriched) and bad (cognitively impoverished) habits depends on the cognitive enrichment of the actions through which habits are acquired. Hence, addiction is a bad habit.

Finally, we discuss the connection between addiction, akrasia, and habits in dialogue with other proposals. We contend that addiction is a bad (rigid) habit that tends toward akratic actions in the context of substance consumption. Disagreeing with Heather's hypothesis and the general interpretation of akrasia as an entirely free and intentional behavior, we instead suggest that addiction and akrasia are bad habits and, therefore, are progressively disengaged from the agent's deliberation and tend to become uncontrollable.

In conclusion, our proposal can be used to shed light on the complex phenomenon of substance addiction by clarifying its relationship with automaticity and by stressing the importance of the cognitive enrichment of actions for the distinction between good and bad habits.

Theories of Addiction

Over the last century, addiction has been a hot research topic in psychology and related fields of knowledge. Consequently, several theories and models have been proposed to explain the process itself, as well as why certain *objects* –not just substances but also activities such as gambling– are easier to get addicted to or why specific individuals are more susceptible to becoming addicts, or the environmental factors that are relevant for making addiction more likely, or which of these factors are relevant to recovery and relapse, etc. [3]. In this section, we will summarize the main theories of substance addiction. Further information can be found in Ramirez-Castillo [4].

Most classical theories on addiction view the related process as "something that happens" to the person, an occurrence that escapes their control. In most cases, initial consumption of the addictive substance is voluntary, but it eventually becomes a harmful behavior alien to the person's will. Within these theories, we distinguish those built upon learning frameworks from those based on individual traits that make some people vulnerable to addiction, and those that emphasize neurobiology and the dopamine system. Then, more recent theories will be introduced, presenting addiction as a goal-directed, voluntary, and free behavior of the agent. These hypotheses include the view of addiction as akrasia, which will be explained in detail in the following section.

First, we will briefly summarize the relevant learning-based theories. Among them, the most popular correspond to Skinner's operant conditioning, Wikler's classical conditioning, and Bandura's social learning theory. The first [5] states that the probability of occurrence of a particular behavior is mediated by its consequences. In the case of addictive substance consumption, the first steps are characterized by negative reinforcement (e.g., the nausea associated with heroin, alcohol's bitter taste) that, if consumption is maintained, progressively loses its negative value until it disappears. At that point, the substance becomes a positive reinforcement that alleviates a craving. Environmental and social factors are unconditioned stimuli at the beginning. Still, they end up acting as conditioned stimuli: their mere presence leads the person to seek and consume the drug in question.

The second learning theory [6] was inspired by the finding that opiate consumers undergoing group therapy experienced abstinence symptoms during their treatment. These emotional responses were termed conditioned abstinence. Once again, social and environmental factors are viewed as conditioned stimuli that may produce a response (consumption) when the drug has already lost its reinforcing effects. In the context of this theory, this is called "conditioned tolerance," and it has a strong influence on cravings and abstinence syndrome. Conditioned tolerance may be chemical (derived from the drug itself) or behavioral (related to social and environmental factors). Interestingly, when a saline solution was administered instead of the drug in the same social setting where the person with an addiction usually consumed, the effect and the addict's emotional state were similar to actual drug consumption. This was considered a placebo effect for drug consumption.

Finally, Bandura's social learning theory [7] proposes that addictive behavior is based on interpersonal and individual beliefs and expectations towards self-medication, as well as on the social environment and behavioral models gleaned from close acquaintances. Therefore, the factors explaining addictive behavior are related to the motives of consumption, its meaning to the addicted person, and the expected efficacy of alternative behaviors. A person with a structured social context that precludes them from repeating consumption will probably dodge addiction; otherwise, self-control is at stake, and addiction is likely to occur.

After this brief outline of learning theories, we will now summarize those based on some individuals' susceptibility to developing an addictive disorder. The vulnerability hypothesis [8] suggests that, whereas initial consumption of a substance is associated with social and environmental factors, some character and personality traits (such as disinhibition, sensation seeking, or preexistent mental disorders) are critical to the development of a substance abuse disorder. Similarly, the "gateway drug" hypothesis highlights sporadic consumption of nicotine during infancy or early adolescence as an initial step to developing an addiction to illicit drugs. Khantzian's self-medication hypothesis [9] emphasizes the adverse physiological and emotional symptoms experienced by people with addiction before the development of a substance-use disorder. Thus, drug consumption is initially carried out to alleviate those negative symptoms, and it eventually becomes an incontrollable behavioral pattern. For example, opiate consumption may be used to mitigate rage, shame, or solitude, whereas cocaine may increase frustration tolerance and self-esteem and decrease boredom. However, dual pathology (i.e., the coexistence of addiction and a mental health disorder) does not appear in every addiction patient, and not every patient with a psychological disorder turns to drug consumption.

Another set of theories relies on neurobiological findings rather than on social or psychological factors. For example, Wise and Bozarth [10] proposed the "psychomotor stimulant theory of addiction," according to which positive reinforcers activate the dopaminergic reward system, which eventually gets imbalanced and causes physical dependence. This theory was built upon animal research, testing how different drugs commonly activated the dopaminergic system. When applied to humans, the authors admit the importance of social context in the addiction process and relapse. The opponent-process theory [11, 12] assumes that the brain balances affective states through homeostatic systems. When consuming addictive substances, the affective state of the person results from two opposite emotional processes. Throughout the process of addiction, a negative emotional state will progressively replace the initial positive feeling. Since the latter eventually becomes more potent than the former, consumption is gradually increased to overcome the negative affective state, resulting in augmented substance dependence. Similarly, Koob and Le Moal proposed the motivational theory of addiction based on neuroadaptation and allostasis

[13]. Like Wise and Bozarth's theory, they start from dysregulation of the dopaminergic reward system, which leads to neural adaptations to recover balance and homeostasis—a process they term allostasis. This theory successfully explains the neurobiology of addiction consolidation and relapse, although why a person initiates consumption remains unclear.

The two final "classical theories" (that is, those that see addiction as an uncontrollable behavior of the person) mentioned here also rely on impairment of the dopaminergic system. From a psychological point of view, both involve transfer from a goal-directed and pleasurable situation (initial consumption of the drug) to harmful and compulsive behavior. Robinson and Berridge proposed the incentive-sensitization theory of addiction [14]. They distinguished two key concepts such as the incentive value of the drug, which is related to "wanting" the substance, and the hedonic value of the drug, which is associated with "liking" the substance. Thus, in the addiction process, the person initially "likes" the drug but experiences a progressive transfer toward just "wanting" the drug, even though the hedonic value decreases.

Everitt and Robbins' theory of habits and compulsions [15] is another influential theory that combines neurobiological and behavioral features. It is inspired by Anthony Dickinson's [16] sharp distinction between the concepts of action and habit, which will be explained in depth further on (in the section entitled "Good and bad habits"). In short, an action is a goal-directed behavior that the agent fully controls, whereas a habit is an automatic, ateleological, and rigid behavior unconsciously carried out by the agent. According to Everitt and Robbins, addiction consists of a transition from a voluntary action—the recreational consumption of a drug—to a stimulus-response habit, which eventually becomes compulsive drug-seeking behavior. From a neuroanatomical perspective, this transition is associated with enhanced activity in the dorsal striatum compared with the ventral striatum and prefrontal cortex.

In recent years, new theories of addiction have been proposed. Regarding the "classical" theories outlined above, the new ones differentiate themselves by presenting addictive behavior as part of a deliberative context. Among them, we will briefly explain Hogarth's view of addiction as an excessive goal-directed drug choice under negative affect, Graham's interpretation of addiction and responsibility for self, and, finally, Heather's proposal regarding the relationship between addiction and akrasia, which will be explained in detail in the next section.

Hogarth argues that drug seeking and consumption should be considered a goal-directed action [17]. This theory is framed in the context of value-based decision making, which is part of the broader field of behavioral economics. According to it, agents choose the most valued option among the ones available at a particular time. Valuation is subjective; that is, personal preferences modulate the objective value of the expected reward. In the context of addiction, Hogarth proposes that a person with addiction seeks and consumes a drug because it is highly valued concerning alternative options. In his opinion, human studies preferentially support this theory over habit and compulsion theories [15] because the subjective value applied to the drug correlates with dependence severity, psychiatric symptoms, and stress induction, which is not the case within the habit/compulsion framework. Besides, drug choice is goal-directed because decision-related parameters modulate it.

Graham's primary goal is to prove that addiction is a mental disorder but not a brain illness. Arguments related to the latter goal—i.e., denying that addiction is a brain disease—will not be discussed here since it is tangential to the scope of this chapter. The idea of addiction as a mental illness is justified by presenting it as an inability to take responsibility for oneself. According to Graham, this is the case of "compulsive behavior" understood in a particular way:

> In light of the notions of reflective self-evaluation and responsibility for self, another way of understanding the category of compulsive behavior suggests itself. This is not the notion of behavior under physically external or motivationally by-passed control. Not the notion of repetitively dangerous behavior. Not that of behavior driven by essentially insatiable cravings or irresistible desires. But of

> behavior that contravenes an agent's efforts to take responsibility of self –a self understood as an historical person, when lucid, who prudently takes account of their future [18, p. 191].

Hence, the person with an addiction can evaluate the available options—which can be simplified as consuming versus not consuming—but, at a certain point, long-term goals are obscured by the more accessible and immediate option of consuming. Even though within this framework, Graham considers the addict's behavior "a-rational," some capacity to decide is preserved: this is why nearly all addicts try to withdraw at some point and are even successful, at least for a while [18, p. 179].

In short, recent theories on addiction stress that this disease does not entail a kind of deterministic behavior towards drug consumption; instead, the person with an addiction can weigh available options, with consumption as one of them. Heather's interpretation of addiction as akrasia is a more assertive stance in this sense since consumption, by definition, is a deliberate and free choice. This hypothesis and an explanation of akratic actions will be developed in the following section.

Akrasia and Addiction

According to Heather, the ancient concept of akrasia must underlie a proper theory of addiction [19]. He defines addiction as a "repeated and continuing failure to refrain from or radically reduce a behavior that gives short-term rewards but longer-term punishments despite prior resolutions to do so" [19, p. 3]. Importantly, this definition implies that addiction only applies to instances in which the person intends to change their behavior. Thus, according to Heather, someone who repeatedly consumes a harmful substance but does not express or feel the intention to withdraw should not be considered an addict; rather, this would be a case of "potential addiction." The definition of akrasia that Heather accepts corresponds to acting against one's better judgment. Some equivalent terms are incontinence and weakness of will, and the ancient antonym is *enkrateia*, which Heather translates as self-control. He accepts Alfred Mele's definition of akrasia as follows:

> An action A is a strict incontinent action if and only if it is performed intentionally and freely and, at the time at which it is performed, its agent consciously holds a judgment to the effect that there is good and sufficient reason for his not performing an A at that time [20, p. 7].

Thus, this kind of action is free and deliberate, albeit it goes against one's better judgment (and therefore "irrational" for some authors, such as Heather). Moreover, the agent recognizes that said action goes against their better judgment. In a nutshell, addiction is seen as an extreme case of akrasia, and Heather comes up with a dual-system theory of addiction. This pathological condition arises because of the competition between two opposing mental systems such as reflective and impulsive. Obviously, in the case of akratic actions (and addiction), the latter dominates the former. Revisiting ancient Greek myths, Heather sees the advantage of interpreting addiction as an extreme case of akrasia in "that it is thereby possible to navigate a course between the *scylla* of compulsion and the *charybdis* of free choice" [19, p. 1]. Like some of the recent hypotheses of addiction outlined above, this is formulated against the interpretation of addiction as a compulsive or automatic behavior: the patient freely decides to consume the substance, even though, at some point, they resolve to quit. This is why akrasia, in contemporary analyses, has also been termed weakness of will. However, as we explain below, we argue against this translation because Aristotle, the first thinker to systematically discuss the term, did not recognize the faculty of the will as it is understood in contemporary philosophy. In line with diverse authors, the concept of will was fully developed after Augustine following stoic precedents [21–24]. Consequently, considering akrasia as weakness of will may be too distant from its original meaning.

Amélie Rorty explained in depth the origins of the concept of akrasia (see, for example, [25]). The problem of akrasia arose when Socrates' two most influential students, namely Plato and

Aristotle, confronted their master on his declaration that "to know the good is to do the good." Both philosophers, each with his own method, found this Socratic idea nonsensical; they could easily exemplify and, at least to some extent, explain actions against one's better judgment. Plato crucially emphasizes that cognitive functions can direct and even motivate actions without any further element; thus, if knowledge is true, actions should be directed towards better judgment. But how is it then possible to act against one's better judgment? According to Santas' interpretation of Plato ([26], as cited in Rorty, 1970), an agent always acts according to their strongest desires, which could contradict the evaluation of the action in question and its consequences. Thus, there are three elements such as evaluation, desire, and action. In Platonic philosophy, the words *epithymia* and *boulesis* have been translated as "appetite" or "desire." Following Rorty's interpretation, their main difference is that the object of the former is the satisfaction of a sensitive need, whereas that of the latter is a good grasped by reason. More importantly, the satisfaction of *epithymia* must be immediate –although *thymos* allows it to be delayed–but *bouleseis* can be prospective. Thus, akrasia is possible when the immediate satisfaction of an *epithymia* overcomes *logos*' better judgment involved in *boulesis*. Note that this interpretation is not far from Heather's dual systems theory of addiction.

On the other hand, Aristotelian philosophy introduces a concept that allows for a deeper understanding of akrasia, i.e., practical reason. For Aristotle, behavior (*ethos*) involves character, habits, emotions, and knowledge, all orchestrated by practical wisdom (*phronesis*) to act towards a good. He does not distinguish between mere desires and judgments, as Plato did. Instead, he sees actions as a *combination* of desire and thought (*oretikos nous* and *orexis dianoetike*) ([27], 1139b 3–5). Below, we follow Rorty's reading of Aristotle when she highlights the importance of habit in moral action:

> One does not become moral simply by learning to reason as the moral man reasons; one must also acquire the habit of acting as the moral man acts, from deliberation, on the basis of one's active knowledge, and not merely after deliberation, 'repeating one's knowledge as an actor repeats his lines'" [25, p. 57].

Since behavior entails character, desires, emotions, and habits, moral misbehavior (such as akrasia) may be due to failures in any of these aspects. Significantly, Aristotle clarifies that one should not be considered an akratic person for just one single akratic behavior; in other words, the virtuous person may also act akratically at some point. The akratic person, however, behaves akratically on similar occasions under similar circumstances. This is essential for our argument because akrasia is a habitual behavior rather than a label for a particular action. Rorty also suggests this connection when she states, "*Akrasia* involves a special kind of second-order habit, a habit of actualizing other sorts of habits, or a habit of making action-guiding knowledge actually guides action" [25, p. 58]. In turn, in the conclusion of her analysis, she formulates two possible types of akrasia: (1) an agent unaware of the real consequences of their action, that is, their knowledge was inaccurate; (2) when the agent is not in the habit of following their deliberations, that is, not used to "acting rationally."

In our view, essential nuances notwithstanding and following a deeper analysis of the concept of habit in Aristotle, the second type of akrasia is relevant for a better understanding of addiction. In the following section, we will summarize our interpretation of this matter, pinpointing the interplay between dispositions, flexibility, goals, and the cognitive enrichment of behavior.

Good Habits and Bad Habits

Several years ago, our research group started to adapt the Aristotelian notion of habit for its study in current psychology and neuroscience (see, for example, [28]). We were motivated to demonstrate that the most common view of habit in neuroscience, mainly developed in light of animal research, applies to part of human behavior but not to all types of habits that humans can develop. In short, the standard view of habit in neuroscience is based on Anthony Dickinson's outstanding experiments on rodents (see, for example, [16]), after which habits began to be considered automatic, rigid, and unconscious behaviors. Crucially, according to this view, habits are opposed to goal-directed actions and are, therefore, ateleological routines. This view was based upon William James' description of habit; for him, habits are a fundamental part of human behavior because they automatize our performance to save mental energy, so to speak [29]. As in any other aspect of human life, habits may go astray, and thus behavioral "errors" arise, such as slips-of-action [30], compulsions [31], or addiction. In turn, two of Dickinson's colleagues in Cambridge –Trevor Robbins and Barry Everitt– were inspired by his research to develop the compulsion theory of addiction mentioned above [15]. Therefore, in neuroscience, the term "habit" refers to a rigid sequence of movements that, once started, keeps going until completion without conscious supervision or control on the part of the agent. In some sense, it is similar to a stimulus-response pairing.

However, we contend that humans can perform activities resulting from acquired habits flexibly and consciously. As exemplified by Aristotle, the ability to play a musical instrument is a habit that can only be acquired through practice [27]; if correctly acquired, the agent's performance and overall experience—including technical skill and enjoyment—will increasingly improve. We have argued elsewhere [32] that the exercise of consciousness is even enhanced in this type of habit. Based on our previous description [28], this applies to a technical habit. Moreover, according to Aristotle, ethical virtues are the highest kind of habits that humans can develop; they result in *knowing how to act*. The ruler of ethical or behavioral habits is *phronesis*, i.e., the perfection of practical reason, as mentioned in Rorty's account of akrasia. Additionally, theoretical or intellectual habits are related to understanding the internal coherence of a field of knowledge, such as geometry. Crucially, in all three cases, habits are not necessarily just routines but may also be a particular type of learning. To recognize this dual aspect of habit, we coined the terms habit-as-learning and habit-as-routine.

More generally, a habit is an acquired disposition that inclines or enables behavior towards particular types of actions. Thus, habits are not behaviors per se but dispositions, tendencies, inclinations, or behavioral patterns. An agent may be lazy, temperate, or an expert pianist, and therefore, their behavior will probably be unenergetic, moderate, or provide an exquisite performance, respectively. However, under certain circumstances or just out of chance, they can *possibly* act promptly, impulsively, or in a flawed manner. Actions –or behaviors– are the expression of habits. Furthermore, habits are acquired through actions, "for the things we have to learn before we can do them, we learn by doing them" [27]. Thus, the relationship between habits and actions is circular: actions configure habits, which make possible and facilitate actions.

When Anthony Dickinson operationalized William James' view of habit for experimental psychology, teleology was the critical point differentiating "actions" and "habits" (as termed in [16], and subsequently in most neuroscientific studies); while actions are goal-directed behaviors, habits are performed irrespective of a behavior's goal. This was empirically supported when "habituated" rodents kept pressing a lever in exchange for water, even when they were sated or poisoned with a toxic substance: they just had the habit of pressing the lever. Considering this experiment, it was only a matter of time before researchers interpreted human substance addiction under this umbrella. Interestingly, goal-directedness was also a crucial topic for Aristotle in his extensive study of habits; in fact, the pursuit of the good is the central topic of Aristotelian ethics ("the good has rightly been declared to be that at which all things aim" [27]), and good habits are dispositions that aid agents in achieving goods more efficiently, more promptly, and with increased enjoyment. Moreover, the agent can pursue further and better goals through good habits.

Another crucial topic on habit acquisition and the performance of its related actions corresponds to "cognitive enrichment:" From our point of view, cognitive enrichment refers to the proper understanding of the actions through which a habit is acquired. In turn, this is the decisive factor for acquiring either a good (i.e., flexible, teleological, cognitively enriched) or a bad (i.e., rigid, routine-like, ateleological, cognitively impoverished) habit. For example, a technical habit such as guitar playing can be acquired through cognitively enriched actions, meaning that the novice player understands the internal coherence of scales, harmonies, and tonalities and knows how they are implemented in the instrument; on the other hand, one can also learn how to play the guitar by just paying attention to finger movements and learning popular songs by heart through repetition. From our point of view, the former type of acquisition leads to flexible performance open to improvisation, whereas the latter is restricted to a rigid performance of well-learned songs. This does not mean that the latter is a "bad musician," but that their habit is unquestionably a routine instead of a flexible type of learning.

To sum up, a good habit is a cognitively enriched disposition acquired through cognitively enriched actions, which allow the agent to perform increasingly flexible and goal-directed behaviors related to that habit; conversely, a bad habit is a cognitively impoverished disposition acquired through cognitively impoverished actions, which restrict the agent to rigid and ateleological routines.

Different accounts of substance addiction have viewed it as a bad habit. For example, Ramirez-Vizcaya and Froese [33] explain habits from the paradigm of 4e (embodied, embedded, extended, and enactive) cognition and define them as "self-sustaining networks of bodily, neural, and interactional processes that become a source of normativity for an agent, in such a way that the preservation of her habitual identities guides much of her perceptions, thoughts, and behaviors" [33, p. 7]. Since bad habits go against the organism's other sources of normativity that lead to well-being, they specifically consider a bad habit as something "whose expression, while positive for its own continued self-maintenance, is negative for a person's well-being because it consistently overrules the expression of other situationally relevant actions and habits" (p. 8).

Other views from psychology stress the distinctive feature of bad habits as going against the person's well-being [34]. Still, some experts on the neuroscience of habits do not define bad habits, even though it is an important topic in their research [35]. In other cases, habits are called "unwanted behavior" [36, 37]. Other authors assume that substance addiction is a case of bad habit [38] but do not clarify whether this is due to its automatic performance, being harmful to the organism, or even if there are other types of bad habits. Our Aristotelian framework allows for a more comprehensive understanding by considering that intellectual, technical, and moral habits can also be good or bad since these habits need not have an effect on the health of the organism and, therefore, could abstain from being categorized as good or bad according to the explanations mentioned above.

In the last section of this chapter, we will show how addiction can be interpreted as a habit-as-routine (i.e., bad habit) that disposes the agent towards akratic actions. In turn, akrasia itself is a habit that inclines toward performing akratic actions, that is, actions that depart from the good use of practical reason. In our opinion, this is due to the main feature associated with bad habits, namely being cognitively impoverished.

Addiction as a Bad Habit Towards Akratic Actions

So far, the key issues for understanding addiction as a bad habit towards akratic actions are as follows: (1) habits are dispositions, not actual behaviors; (2) good habits are flexible and cognitively enriched dispositions acquired through cognitively enriched actions; (3) conversely, bad habits are rigid and cognitively impoverished dispositions acquired through cognitively impoverished actions; (4) akrasia is a disposition towards actions without proper exercise of practical reason; and (5) addiction is a rigid disposition towards akratic actions because of cognitive impoverishment.

The first point is, in principle, unquestionable since the vast majority of research on habits, irrespective of its primary field, assumes that habits are dispositions of behavior. However, in some experimental approaches, especially those involving experiments on rodents, it is unclear whether habits are understood as a tendency/disposition or a particular behavior. When Dickinson identifies habits with a sort of ateleological stimulus-response pair, and establishes the criteria for distinguishing habits from actions (insisting on the behavior even though the reward is omitted or devalued) [16], habits seem like a type of behavior, rather than an acquired disposition that leads to this behavior. When this model is applied to addiction [39], the behavior of the addicted rodent or human is explained as "S-R [stimulus-response] habits" (p. 134) or "habitual S-R drug-seeking" (p. 134) or a "compulsive habit under the control of the S-R process" (p. 131). Interestingly, it also mentions a "propensity to relapse" (p. 134), which seems synonymous with a "disposition" to relapse. One straightforward way of clarifying this issue comes by assuming that Dickinson's proposal (defining habit after observing behavior) is a way to detect when a specific type of behavior is *a consequence of* an acquired habit; hence, the habit is not precisely the ateleological behavior, but such ateleological behavior is a reliable indicator of the presence of a disposition. This may seem obvious, but conceptually, it is important to stress that a habit is an acquired behavioral and/or cognitive trait rather than an actual behavior.

Categorizing habits as good or bad based on cognitive enrichment criteria has been discussed elsewhere (for example, [28, 40]). Our point here is that an adequate understanding of actions, together with a strong sense of agency (that is, when the agent feels fully responsible for the action), lead to a habit where the agent is fully aware of how, when and why actions related to that habit should be performed. In turn, this is associated with a flexible performance that enhances the promptness, efficiency, enjoyment of actions, and conscious experience while performing them [32]. In all, cognitively enriched actions lead to good habits that dispose toward cognitively enriched actions.

Conversely, bad habits are acquired through cognitively impoverished actions, which are multifaceted; there are many reasons why an action could have this attribute. For instance, when an action is not goal-directed, or at least when its real goal is unknown. Considering this, it would be easier for a disposition to be disengaged from a behavioral aim, resulting in ateleological, rigid instrumental conditioning. Another possibility, in the case of technical habits (such as playing a musical instrument), is found in the agent paying exclusive attention to bodily movements (for example, finger movements), disregarding the cognitive aspects of those movements. In this case, the "how to" of acting would be covered, but not the "when" and "why" a pianist may move her fingers quickly and accurately. The pianist will not be a virtuoso if his/her performance, from a holistic point of view, is not truly excellent. Lisboa and collaborators [41] argued that playing from memory makes this kind of performance possible. According to these authors –with Lisboa, an expert cellist, standing in as a "subject" of research– interpreting a piece comes with important milestones that they term "performance cues," defined as "thoughts and feelings they [performers] want to convey to the audience along with the actions that produce the musical sounds" (p. 521). The authors also stress the importance of attention, expressive timing, error monitoring, and musical goals, pinpointing the role of consciousness, flexibility, and teleology in these technical habits. From our point of view, these attributes could be generalized to intellectual and behavioral (ethical) habits. On the other side of the coin, bad habits have opposing characteristics, and addiction is thus viewed as a bad habit not just because it goes against the agent's general well-being or because it is an unwanted behavior. Addiction is a bad habit primarily because it is a rigid and ateleological routine that weakens the ability of the agent to control their behavior to their good, and this is due to its cognitive impoverishment.

Akrasia should be understood as a behavioral disposition that is the consequence of bad habits:

as the just person is disposed to perform just actions, the akratic person is disposed to perform akratic actions. In other words, "akratic" can be an adjective for actions and persons. As Mele states, "Akrasia, strictly speaking, is not a type of action but a trait of character" [42, p. 3]. Indirectly, Rorty seems to support this view by understanding akrasia as a type of habit –a disposition not to follow practical wisdom– and by primarily considering virtue and vice character attributes (p. 57). Interestingly, Rorty also defines akrasia as a "regional" character trait, claiming it can only affect specific actions. Following our arguments in the section "Akrasia and addiction," the akratic person is disposed to perform actions against practical reason.

At first sight, our view of akrasia as a habitual disposition seems to contain a contradictory element: the leading authors on akrasia mentioned in this chapter (Rorty, Mele, and Heather) insist that the intentional, free, and conscious nature of the akratic action is defining, and it is unclear whether actions associated with a habit can be considered intentional and deliberate. As we have explained in the previous lines, good habits are out of the question: since they are cognitively enriched and enhance performance, attention, consciousness, and teleology, their associated actions are intentional and deliberate. In the case of bad habits, the opposite attributes lead to rigid routines, where intentionality and the ability to deliberate are impaired. Hence, is akrasia a good or a bad habit, or could it be good or bad depending on how it has been acquired? Since akratic actions go against practical reason, the disposition they establish must be a bad habit because an action contradictory to *phronesis* cannot be cognitively enriched. Therefore, akratic actions performed by an akratic person are progressively more automatic and less conscious and deliberate. The contradiction between akrasia and deliberation appears in Rorty, Mele, and Heather's proposals because they define akratic action in both a "positive" and a "negative" sense: an action contrary to one's own better judgment. In other words, it is an action in which the agent deliberately *does not do* the best possible action but rather an alternative one.

The open question thus remains: does the akratic person intentionally and deliberatively undertake the akratic action, or do they intentionally and deliberatively undertake *whichever action* other than the most appropriate one? In the latter case, the agent deliberately decides not to do an action, but that does not imply that the action performed is entirely intentional or deliberate. For example, Peter knows he should go to the gym but stays home watching TV. It is unimportant whether Peter intentionally and deliberatively performs the action of watching TV. The key issue is that Peter has decided not to go to the gym (i.e., he has decided to act against his better judgment); watching TV is the most straightforward alternative. Suppose a habit is established after this behavior; focusing on its habitual akratic aspect, we should assume that Peter's decision to not go to the gym would be increasingly automatic and, therefore, less intentional. The original intention was to go to the gym rather than stay home watching TV. Thus, the latter was never an entirely intentional action.

Finally, following this train of thought, addiction can be considered a bad (rigid) habit towards akratic actions, that is, actions that go against a good exercise of practical reason. About the relationship between akrasia (incontinence) and habits, Vigo writes the following:

> The internal dissociation of *ethos* and an ideal life, which is characteristic of the incontinent person, proceeds, at bottom, from the fact that the incontinent person has not successfully transformed their ideal life into an *ethos*, that is through the corresponding process of habituation. To the extent that *ethos* constitutes the reality of a certain life project, one might say that the incontinent person provides an especially clear example of a life project that is deficiently realized. The incontinent person possesses a life ideal conforming to reason, but only in the way of a yearning devoid of actuality in their person reality, since this ideal is not supported by a consolidated combination of habitual dispositions of character (…) The incontinent person produces, in fact, the same type of actions as the intemperate, that is to say, by immoderately pursuing bodily pleasure, but does this in contrast to their own *proairesis* ([43], pp. 158–159).

As Graham clearly explained [18], and as included in all the frameworks outlined above, the crucial point for distinguishing substance addiction from recreational drug use is found in the addicted person's unrealizable will to withdraw. There is a "positive" action against one's own better judgment (consuming), and a "negative" action dictated by one's judgment (refraining from consumption). In other words, there is an akratic action and the alternative inaction (or doing any other non-akratic alternative). A rigid habit is then progressively established and the akratic action is easier and faster to carry out. In our view, the akratic action is also done less deliberatively and intentionally: the intention is to withdraw, but the automatic behavior is to relapse.

From this perspective, viewing the *phronetic* action as "negative" (i.e., as inaction) and the akratic action as "positive" (i.e., as an action), it is clear why most therapies for overcoming addiction do not focus on withdrawal per se, but instead on substituting consumption for alternative behavior. Our view seems to go against Heather's definition of addiction as a free and intentionally irrational (i.e., akratic) action. Once again, we believe that this is due to erroneous identification of a disposition (in this case, addiction) and its realization (in this case, the akratic action of consuming the substance). As it is clear to most authors, the problem is not consumption itself but rather consumption by an addicted person: while recreational consumption may involve severe health, social, and legal problems, it differs from addiction. Hence, consumption is the external expression of the core problem, which is the rigid habit of addiction. Adding akrasia into the equation shows that consumption is an akratic action that unveils the agent's rigid disposition to act akratically.

We endorse Rorty's idea of akrasia being "regional," affecting some aspects of the agent's behavior and sparing others. According to this, substance addiction would be a disposition towards akratic actions related to substance consumption. However, we would like to stress that when this habit progressively grows, precisely because it goes against *phronesis*, it invades other aspects of the addicted person. This is why the most severe cases of addiction are catastrophic for the person as a whole.

Conclusions

In this chapter, we have proposed an interpretation of addiction as a disposition that tends toward akratic actions. Most previous research interprets addiction as a disposition, although analysis of experimental work sometimes misleadingly identifies addiction with the actual behavior of consumption. Moreover, specific hypotheses propose that akrasia should be a foundational term for correctly understanding human substance addiction. Accordingly, a person acts akratically when acting freely and intentionally against their better judgment. Although it is widely recognized that akrasia is a character trait or disposition, there is again some interpretative confusion when dealing with akrasia and akratic actions.

From our perspective, akratic actions should not be considered entirely deliberate and intentional because a rigid (bad) habit comes into conflict with the ability to deliberate. Bad habits are cognitively impoverished dispositions and, therefore, they are rigid, automatic, and ateleological. Since akrasia is a disposition acquired after akratic actions, which by definition go against practical reason, we suggested that akrasia is a cognitively impoverished (bad) habit. Therefore, its associated actions cannot be considered entirely intentional or deliberate. This framework, in our opinion, explains more adequately certain aspects of substance addiction and its treatment, in particular, why the therapeutic objective of substituting consumption for a healthier alternative is more successful than just seeking withdrawal.

Acknowledgements This work received support from Funciva, Proeduca Summa, and Fundación Tatiana Pérez de Guzmán el Bueno.

References

1. West R, Brown J. Theory of Addiction. Addiction Press. Chichester: Wiley Blackwell; 2013.
2. Carlisle C. On habit. Oxon: Routledge; 2014.
3. West R. Theories of addiction. Addiction. 2001;96(1):3–13.
4. Ramirez-Castillo D. Adicción, Personalidad y Tolerancia a la Frustración: un estudio neuropsicológico en sujetos adscritos a Proyecto Hombre. University of Navarra; 2017.
5. Skinner B. The behavior of organisms: an experimental analysis. New York: Appleton-Century; 1938.
6. Wikler A, Haertzen CA, Chessick RD, Hill HE, Pescor FT. Reaction time ("mental set") in control and chronic schizophrenic subjects and in postaddicts under placebo, LSD-25, morphine, pentobarbital and amphetamine. Psychopharmacologia [Internet]. 1965;7(6):423–43. Available from: http://www.ncbi.nlm.nih.gov/pubmed/5319301
7. Bandura A. Self-efficacy: toward a unifying theory of behavioral change. Psychol Rev [Internet]. 1977;84(2):191–215. Available from: http://www.ncbi.nlm.nih.gov/pubmed/847061
8. Glantz M, Pickens R. Vulnerability to drug abuse. American Psychological Association; 1992.
9. Khantzian EJ. The self-medication hypothesis of addictive disorders: focus on heroin and cocaine dependence. Am J Psychiatry [Internet]. 1985;142(11):1259–64. Available from: http://www.ncbi.nlm.nih.gov/pubmed/3904487
10. Wise RA, Bozarth MA. A psychomotor stimulant theory of addiction. Psychol Rev [Internet]. 1987 Oct;94(4):469–92. Available from: http://www.ncbi.nlm.nih.gov/pubmed/3317472
11. Solomon RL, Corbit JD. An opponent-process theory of motivation. I. Temporal dynamics of affect. Psychol Rev [Internet]. 1974 Mar;81(2):119–45. Available from: http://www.ncbi.nlm.nih.gov/pubmed/4817611
12. Koob GF, Stinus L, Le Moal M, Bloom FE. Opponent process theory of motivation: neurobiological evidence from studies of opiate dependence. Neurosci Biobehav Rev [Internet]. 1989;13(2–3):135–40. Available from: http://www.ncbi.nlm.nih.gov/pubmed/2682399
13. Koob GF, Le Moal M. Drug abuse: hedonic homeostatic dysregulation. Science [Internet]. 1997;278(5335):52–8. Available from: http://www.ncbi.nlm.nih.gov/pubmed/9311926
14. Robinson TE, Berridge KC. The neural basis of drug craving: an incentive-sensitization theory of addiction. Brain Res Rev. 1993;18(3):247–91.
15. Everitt BJ, Robbins TW. Drug addiction: updating actions to habits to compulsions ten years on. Annu Rev Psychol [Internet]. 2016;67(1):23–50. Available from: http://www.annualreviews.org/doi/10.1146/annurev-psych-122414-033457
16. Dickinson A. Actions and habits: the development of behavioural autonomy. Philos Trans R Soc B Biol Sci [Internet]. 1985;308(1135):67–78. Available from: http://rstb.royalsocietypublishing.org/cgi/doi/10.1098/rstb.1985.0010
17. Hogarth L. Addiction is driven by excessive goal-directed drug choice under negative affect: translational critique of habit and compulsion theory. Neuropsychopharmacology [Internet]. 2020;45(5):720–35. https://doi.org/10.1038/s41386-020-0600-8.
18. Graham G. The disordered mind. An introduction to philosophy of mind and mental illness. 2nd ed. Oxon: Routledge; 2013.
19. Heather N. The concept of akrasia as the foundation for a dual systems theory of addiction. Behav Brain Res. 2020;390(May)
20. Mele AR. Irrationality. Oxford: Oxford University Press; 1987.
21. Dihle A. The theory of will in classical antiquity. Berkeley: University of California Press; 1982.
22. Garcia-Valiño J. La génesis del concepto de voluntad en occidente. Un estudio de las fuentes griegas y cristianas de Tomás de Aquino. Pamplona: EUNSA; 2019.
23. Frede M. A free will: origins of the notion in ancient thought. Oakland: University of California Press; 2011.
24. Inwood B. The will in Seneca the Younger. Class Philol. 2000;95(1):44–60.
25. Rorty A. Plato and Aristotle on belief, habit, and "Akrasia". Am Philos Q [Internet]. 1970;7(1):50–61. Available from: http://www.jstor.org/stable/20009333
26. Santas G. Plato's protagoras and explanations of weakness. Philos Rev. 1966;75(1):3–33.
27. Aristotle. Nicomachean ethics. Cambridge: Harvard University Press; 2014.
28. Bernacer J, Murillo JI. The Aristotelian conception of habit and its contribution to human neuroscience. Front Hum Neurosci. 2014:8(November).
29. James W. Principles of psychology [Internet]. Toronto: An Internet Resource developed by Chrisopher Green; 1890. Available from: http://psychclassics.yorku.ca/James/Principles/prin4.htm
30. Gillan CM, Papmeyer M, Morein-Zamir S, Sahakian BJ, Fineberg NA, Robbins TW, et al. Disruption in the balance between goal-directed behavior and habit learning in obsessive-compulsive disorder. Am J Psychiatry. 2011;168(7):718–26.
31. De Wit S, Dickinson A. Associative theories of goal-directed behaviour: a case for animal-human translational models. Psychol Res. 2009;73(4):463–76.
32. Bernacer J, Murillo JI. Habits and the integration of conscious and non-conscious human actions. In: Before consciousness. Exeter: Imprint Academic; 2017.

33. Ramírez-Vizcaya S, Froese T. The enactive approach to habits: new concepts for the cognitive science of bad habits and addiction. Front Psychol. 2019;10(FEB)
34. Wood W. Good habits, bad habits. New York: Farrar, Straus and Giroux; 2019.
35. Graybiel A, Smith K. Good habits, bad habits. Sci Am. 2014;310(6):38–43.
36. Graybiel AM. Habits, rituals, and the evaluative brain. Annu Rev Neurosci [Internet]. 2008;31(1):359–87. Available from: http://www.annualreviews.org/doi/10.1146/annurev.neuro.29.051605.112851
37. Quinn JM, Pascoe A, Wood W, Neal DT. Can ' t control yourself ? Monitor those bad habits. 2010;
38. Robbins TW, Everitt BJ. Drug addiction: bad habits add up. Nature [Internet]. 1999;398(6728):567–70. Available from: http://www.ncbi.nlm.nih.gov/pubmed/10217139
39. Everitt BJ, Dickinson A, Robbins TW. The neuropsychological basis of addictive behaviour. Brain Res Rev. 2001;36(2–3):129–38.
40. Bernacer J. An integrative understanding of habit to explore its neural correlates. J Conscious Stud. 2018;7–8:112–34.
41. Lisboa T, Demos AP, Chaffin R. Training thought and action for virtuoso performance. 2018;
42. Mele AR. Akratics and addicts. Am Philos Q. 2002;39(2):153–67.
43. Vigo A. Action, reason and truth. Studies in Aristotle's conception of practical rationality. Louvain-La Neuve: Peeters; 2016.

53 Attachment and Its Relationship with Pornography's Addiction

María Contreras, José Víctor Orón, and Francisco Güell

Introduction

Sexuality is the result of interactions between biological, psychological, cultural, ethical, spiritual, and brain structures. The sexual dimension goes beyond the purely biological and is influenced by various factors [1]. According to scientific data, human beings are so marked by sexuality that it is a factor that characterizes their lives and is among the main elements of adult relationships [2]. Sexuality is also of vital importance in the organization of family systems, in the social structure and for the health and well-being of families, and by extension, of society [3]. In the last half-century, technological advances have led to societies dominated by the media [4]. In the 1990s, the Internet arrived to the majority of households, bringing with it digitized pornographic content, making it accessible, anonymous, and affordable, which professionals refer to as AAA. Pornography affects its consumers, relationships, family, and society, and is very likely to become addictive, which could manifest itself in a public health problem.

Young people today commonly consume pornography and their consumption is especially on the rise in countries that have unrestricted access to the Internet [5]. As mentioned, it is accessible from anywhere, unlimited and anonymous. The latest study conducted in the United States indicates that 46% of adult men and 16% of adult women under 40 admit to having used pornography in the last week [6]. Recent studies, carried out in other countries, such as Australia, have published similar results [7]. Addiction to pornography has been around for many years and its prevalence seems to be increasing [8].

This is currently a worldwide problem. As we will see later, addiction to pornography generates personal discomfort, as well as feelings of shame and guilt, which affect people's social life and intimate relationships. Despite increasing consumption, there is discussion in the scientific world about the origin and conceptualization of the harmful consumption of pornography [8]. Different terms have been used, such as sexual addiction, sexual compulsivity, sexual fixation, uncontrolled sexual behavior, and hypersexuality, to describe behavior that continues to be controversial [9].

"Sexual addiction" is the most frequently used term. The DSM V considered including this concept with a new psychiatric diagnosis under the term hypersexual disorder. Hypersexual disorder

M. Contreras
Mind-Brain Group, ICS, University of Navarra, Pamplona, Spain

Faculty of Education and Psychology, University of Navarra, Pamplona, Spain
e-mail: mcontreras.3@unav.es

J. V. Orón · F. Güell (✉)
Mind-Brain Group, ICS, University of Navarra, Pamplona, Spain
e-mail: fguell@unav.es

P. Á. Gargiulo, H. L. Mesones-Arroyo (eds.), *Psychiatry and Neuroscience Update – Vol. V*,
https://doi.org/10.1007/978-3-031-72219-6_53

includes addiction to pornography as one of its symptoms; they are not separate entities since empirical studies are lacking [10]. The DSM V working group proposed some criteria (see Table 53.1) but, at the end, the Hypersexual disorder it was not included, not even in Section III as something that needs further research [11].

On the other hand, the ICD-11 (International Classification of Diseases from the World Health Organization) has classified what is commonly known as sexual addiction as Compulsive Sexual Behavior [12]. It defines this behavior as a persistent pattern of failure to control sexual desires or intense and continual sexual impulses that result in repetitive sexual behavior. The acceptance of this disorder has led to the emergence of different opinions since there are many who doubt that it is an independent diagnostic entity, a comorbid symptom or a type of addiction, and others who doubt that it is a psychological disorder.

While debate continues, there is clear evidence that many people consider their own consumption of pornography a problem [13] since they face serious consequences when carrying out this type of behavior [14], such as interpersonal conflicts, difficulties at work, mental health problems [8], feelings of guilt and shame, social isolation, family problems or even legal problems [15], and feelings of loneliness [3]. Certainly, many people turn to psychotherapy to treat their own addiction. Although the APA does not consider it a proper entity to include in its classification, there are an increasing number of mental health professionals who encounter this type of problem in their practices.

Today, scientific studies and research are needed on the conceptualization, epidemiology, psychopathology, phenomenology, physiopathology, evaluation, treatment, and prevention of the harmful consumption of pornography [9].

In this chapter, we will address the origin of this behavior from the perspective of attachment.

Origin

Some have attempted to present models from a different scientific perspective to explain the nature of out-of-control sexual behaviors and thoughts. Currently, there are a variety of theories regarding the origin of this addiction, including psychobiological theory [15], attachment theory [16], increased sexual desire [17], and multimodal theories [18].

Table 53.1 DSM-V proposed criteria for hypersexual disorder (proposed, NOT APROVED)

A. Over a period of at least 6 months, recurrent and intense sexual fantasies, sexual urges, and sexual behavior in association with four or more of the following five criteria:
1. Excessive time is consumed by sexual fantasies and urges, and by planning for and engaging in sexual behavior.
2. Repetitively engaging in these sexual fantasies, urges, and behavior in response to dysphoric mood states (e.g., anxiety, depression, boredom, and irritability).
3. Repetitively engaging in sexual fantasies, urges, and behavior in response to stressful life events.
4. Repetitive but unsuccessful efforts to control or significantly reduce these sexual fantasies, urges, and behavior.
5. Repetitively engaging in sexual behavior while disregarding the risk for physical or emotional harm to self or others.
B. There is clinically significant personal distress or impairment in social, occupational, or other important areas of functioning associated with the frequency and intensity of these sexual fantasies, urges, and behavior.
C. These sexual fantasies, urges, and behavior are not due to direct physiological effects of exogenous substances (e.g., drugs of abuse or medications), a cooccurring general medical condition, or to manic episodes.
D. The person is at least 18 years of age. Specify if masturbation, pornography, sexual behavior with consenting adults, cybersex, telephone sex, and strip clubs.

Reproduced with permission of Reid & Kafka, 2014 [11]

Some authors have proposed two types of patients who have a problem with pornography, according to its psychological origin [19]:

- Patients with pathology in Axis 1 and symptomatology of out-of-control sexual behavior [20]:
  - ADHD: Impulsive symptoms: Out-of-control sexual behavior activates as an excessive response to stress in people with impaired impulse control and with difficulty in delaying gratification [21].
  - OCD: Compulsive symptoms: When resisting an obsessive thought involving sexual content, obsessive impulses emerge, urging one to carry out certain acts that can be deemed compulsions. These compulsions are fulfilled to reduce anxiety and not so much to obtain genital stimulation [22].
  - Addictive symptomatology: Out-of-control consumption of pornography can be considered an addiction since it shares features with chemical addictions. Out-of-control consumption persists for a long period of time, at least 12 months, and occurs with excessive frequency and intensity. Patients report that they suffer a loss of control over said behavior due to the duration, frequency, intensity, and risk associated with it [23].
- Patients with pornography consumption problems that do not present any Axis I pathologies develop their out-of-control sexual behavior as a habit [20] without clear psychopathological components at the base of their behaviors. With the emergence of the Internet, the prevalence of this second type of patient profile has increased due to unrestricted access to pornography that new technologies permit. These people have a problem with pornography due to repeated, frequent, and prolonged exposure to pornographic images [24], causing the brain to release dopamine and form an addiction.

It is important to explore and understand the emotional and cognitive processes that influence the psychological process of pornography addiction [25]. Although there is still little scientific literature on the subject, one recent research line hypothesizes that the origin of pornography addiction may be rooted in attachment [26], which affords one the ability to interpret social relationships. Different attachment styles are formed with this capacity that influences interpersonal relationships, including aspects like falling in love, attraction, choosing a partner, and also sexuality [23].

In fact, some authors posit that the development of an addiction to pornography is based on interpersonal difficulties with one's main attachment figs. [27]. It is likely that people with pornography addiction exhibit this behavior to alleviate certain unresolved conflicts that have to do with affection early on in their lives. In addition, the theory of attachment posits that difficulties in forming a secure attachment with others are associated with intimacy problems [28], a key variable for living out a healthy and enriching sexuality in adulthood.

What Is Attachment? The Relationship Between Attachment and Sexuality

Bowlby proposed the original attachment theory, which has its roots in psychoanalysis, arguing that babies are born biologically prepared to create emotional bonds with their main caregivers, i.e., their principle attachment figures, in the interest of survival. Attachment is defined as a special bond with emotional intensity between two people, and is a necessary condition for the development of psychological health. According to this theory, the relationship style that develops in early childhood is contiguous with adulthood, such that one's childhood attachment style continues to manifest itself in adulthood. Therefore, during childhood and adolescent development, an attachment style forms that shapes the way one relates and establishes intimate relationships in adulthood. Adolescence represents a time of change, growth, and transformation, taking a leap from the immaturity of childhood to the physical, psychosocial, and sexual maturity that must be achieved in adulthood [29].

The attachment theory argues that the type of attachment that emerges, and certain early experiences that alter one's affective bond with one's main attachment figure, affects personal and social life, professional relationships, the regulation of stress, physical health, and mental and cognitive development. In addition, those who develop a secure attachment during childhood can form healthy relationships in adolescence and adulthood [30]. As a result of different attachment experiences, each person ends up shaping their own style. This style translates into a way of acting, feeling, and thinking that transcends all attachment relationships, friendship, love relationships, and many other aspects of life [31].

Although not all authors [32] agree on the typologies they present [33], after about 40 years of study, the different classifications coincide in important ways, especially along dimensions like "degree of trust/mistrust," "security/anxiety," and "privacy/exhibition."

In the mid-twentieth century, Mary Ainsworth classified three main types of attachment in adulthood [34], that is, secure attachment, anxious insecure attachment, and avoidant insecure attachment.

- People who feel safe in social relationships exercise secure attachment. They trust others and are confident and open. For these people, it is easy to establish intimacy with others; they are also comfortable with privacy, and can act autonomously without incident. They are not usually worried about abandonment or about someone being too attached to them. A low level of dependence and a low level of avoidance characterize them.
- Insecure-anxious attachment corresponds to people who believe that others are reluctant to get close to them. They are often worried about and fear being abandoned, focusing their attention on signs that could imply abandonment or distancing. They may even think that others do not want to be with them. These people want to be very close to others, usually causing rejection that leads to anger. A high level of dependency and low level of avoidance characterize them, as they align themselves with other people and lose their autonomy.
- Insecure-avoidant attachment is found in people who are themselves uncomfortable in intimate relationships with others. They tend not to trust people and are afraid of intimacy. When a person becomes intimate with them, they get nervous, deactivating the emotional connection. These people tend to avoid relationships by having difficulties with empathy, which makes them appear as cold. They have low levels of dependence and high levels of avoidance.

Some authors have studied the relationship between these attachment styles and sexual behavior and relationships [35] and have found the following characteristics:

- From the affective-sexual point of view, adults with secure attachment tend to have more positive experiences with sexuality and greater satisfaction in this area. They tend to feel comfortable with their sexuality, they are open to sexual exploration, they do not practice promiscuous behaviors [36], they enjoy intimacy, are not compulsive or controlling with their partners, have more stable and satisfactory relationships, experience more love, passion and positive emotions with their intimate partner, and enjoy physical contact outside sexual behavior itself [37].
- Adults with anxious attachment tend to interpret the sexual experience ambivalently [38]. These individuals tend to engage in sexual behaviors in order to reduce their own insecurity and to establish an intense closeness with another person (i.e., achieve emotional inti-

macy) [39]. In the same way, they tend to experience intrusive thoughts during the sex. Anxious people see the sexual relationship as a means for bringing out caring behaviors in their partner, with an eye on avoiding abandonment [40].

- Adults with avoidance attachment tend to distance themselves from sexual activities, initiate their sexual life later, have more casual sex (relationships where intimacy is nonexistent), respond aversely to sex and be uncomfortable with closeness. Similarly, studies have found that males with this attachment style tended to experience less sexual desire in their relationships. In addition, these people are motivated by exercising control over their partner or reducing stress, while promoting union with and the pleasure of their partner is not among their main motivations [41].

Certainly, sexuality converges on attachment. To experience a healthy sexuality and obtain sexual satisfaction, emotional, psychological, and physical proximity are required. These factors create intimacy, that is, a space that allows privileged, verbal, and nonverbal communication. The type of attachment plays an important role in the experience of intimacy. In order for intimacy to be safely shared, one needs a structured self that depends, among other things, on one's attachment style, which is a consequence of the quality of one's emotional history. People with secure attachment feel comfortable and do not perceive this space as threatening; they are not on the defensive. Insecure people endure the intimate space and tend to perceive it as threatening and dangerous since they can be abandoned. A fear of rejection and abandonment activates their defenses and tends to encourage isolation.

People with avoidance attachment try to avoid the intimate space through defensive strategies, separating erotic desire from emotional involvement [42], a principal characteristic of pornography since it displays sexual scenes devoid of emotion.

Origin of Pornography Addiction from the Perspective of Attachment

As mentioned, some mental health professionals believe that addiction to pornography is a disorder rooted in attachment [43], which is a highly intense emotional bond between two people and is configured in the first months of life between an infant and her main caregiver. The development and quality of early relationships are very important in emotional, social, personality, and mental health development. One of the etiological factors related to attachment and pornography addiction is the failure to configure an adequate attachment with one's main caregiver [43]. Clinical professionals who treat this symptomatology confirm that many of their patients have developed an insecure attachment style starting from their childhood and feel they have an inability to love and feel loved [44]. For Bowlby, secure attachment with a caregiver is necessary for healthy independence and intimacy; the "I" needs an adequate bond with the main caregiver for healthy growth and development [45].

Some authors have studied the relationship of inadequate care from a main caregiver (where the child does not have basic needs covered) and addiction to pornography. Other authors have studied the relationship between trauma (physical, emotional, or sexual) in childhood and its impact on addiction and pornography [46]. Thus, the development of an insecure attachment can be rooted in traumatic experiences in early childhood or in difficulties with main attachment figures during development [47].

According to these authors, these childhood events are translated into an insecure attachment, which manifests itself in social isolation from peers and in difficulties relating to people of the opposite sex.

The most prevalent type of attachment in this type of patient is insecure avoidant attachment [48]. Due to its characteristics, its correlation with pornography addiction is more obvious, and thus has been studied the most. When the perpetrator of trauma is very close, such as a father, an uncle, or a grandparent, the ability to establish intimate relationships of trust is damaged, which limits the development of adaptive strategies.

People with an avoidant insecure attachment style are characterized by a desire for intimacy and emotional connection with people, but at the same time, they feel unable to be intimate with a person for fear of rejection, abandonment, or hurting them. In addition, they do not possess certain social skills necessary to connect emotionally [49] with those around them.

People with this attachment style are characterized by an independent attitude that is, in the end, a defense mechanism in hopes of avoiding the pain that rejection from a main attachment figure and failure to satisfy basic needs can cause [50]. For this reason, they develop a feeling of loneliness typical of people addicted to pornography. Loneliness is characterized by dissatisfaction produced by a lack of proximity, love, and security from a main attachment fig. [51]. This feeling can, on the one hand, hinder the development of intimacy during adulthood [52] and, on the other hand, consumption of pornography presents itself as a strategy to dissuade loneliness [53]. Bowlby suggests that this type of sexual behavior results when an adult does not have a secure base from which he can relate in a healthy and safe way, nor a family of origin in which he feels welcomed [54]. This leads to a sense of uprootedness accompanied by a sense of loneliness. Other authors understand that this loneliness occurs in two ways, namely, through the absence of a main attachment figure and because of scarce relationships with others [55].

In short, people with this type of attachment may be more likely to develop feelings of loneliness and, therefore, mental health problems and social isolation. Certain situations of emotional deprivation or loneliness can activate erotic desire and lead to autoerotic behaviors through the consumption of pornography.

Another factor to bear in mind when studying the origin of pornographic addiction from the perspective of attachment is sexual desire. Due to its own configuration, sexual desire can be activated due to psychological or environmental stimuli and can be self-focused. In people with an avoidant attachment style, as already mentioned, the feeling of loneliness is an activating factor of sexual desire. Self-focused sexual desire serves the needs of the self and contributes to the structuring of a consolidated self-characterized by security. Some people with insecure avoidance attachment feel more secure and comfortable with autoerotic behaviors, such as masturbation, which accompanies the consumption of pornography. They tend to focus more on the expectation of abandonment or loss; therefore, autoerotism appears as a protected space where no one can enter. It represents a way of accessing sexual satisfaction while avoiding the fear of intimacy [56], thus compensating for a lack of emotional satisfaction in social relationships, and searching for contact and affection from an attachment figure through pornography [57].

Pornography consumption can become a "means" of feeling safe and making human connection free of threat, even though it is through a screen [58]. This type of "virtual" relationship, although it is not relational, can make the consumer feel part of a community, giving him a sense of security. It is a way of compensating for an inability to establish social bonds and dissatisfaction based on a lack of care and affection [59].

From the point of view of interpersonal relationships, a person with addiction to pornography will find it very difficult to establish a secure attachment with another person within a healthy and real relationship. This difficulty entails suffering and incites feelings of sadness and loneliness, making the addict more likely to consume as a reaction to the desire to connect emotionally with a real person. Pornographic content does not show any kind of affective bond. Consequently, on the one hand, the consumer feels comfortable because he is not required to share in an intimate space and, on the other hand, it provokes a predisposition toward a lack of emotional connection with real people. Feeling increasingly insecure in interpersonal relationships promotes a search for security through the consumption of pornography. This feedback loop leads to more frequent consumption with the risk of forming an addictive behavior.

The consumption of pornography also harms insecure attachment avoidant people that have a romantic partner. They often consume more pornography because it represents a mechanism for disconnecting from their partner since, for them, it can be difficult and uncomfortable to meet demands for physical proximity and intimacy [16], a space in which they feel uncomfortable and that they actively avoid. The consumption of pornography has been associated with less satisfaction in interpersonal relationships for people who report little intimacy with their partners [60].

In addition, studies show that people who are avoidant and addicted to pornography tend to attract partners with an anxious attachment style. For these couples, the person with anxious attachment is usually less satisfied with the relationship [61], and, in particular, with their sexual life [38], and is characterized by immature emotional development and high levels of anxiety when it comes to emotionally connecting with their partner. The person with avoidant attachment does not feel comfortable with their partner's anxious and demanding attitude, and manages this anguish, anxiety, and loneliness through the consumption of pornography.

The Clinical Perspective

Twenty years ago and before, the consumption of pornography was considered a moral question rather than a mental health problem [62]. The prevalence of this sexual behavior has changed many clinical professionals' minds about the need to emphasize and taking into account the magnitude of this problem from a clinical perspective [63].

Some authors suggest the need to evaluate and explore a patient's attachment style in psychotherapy [64]. Few have studied it as a predisposing factor toward developing an addiction to pornography. Leedes and Carnes were the first researchers to take into account the concept of attachment from the clinical perspective. They conceptualized addiction to sex as a clinical diagnosis in which addiction to pornography is a symptom and is a relational problem in which the person has problems interacting with and relating to others. For these authors, although the inability to establish attachment relationships may not be sufficient to explain the origin of this problem, they believe it is important to take it into account [18].

In what follows, we will present factors that need to be evaluated, treated, and repaired in an attachment relationship between the patient the psychotherapist within the framework of psychotherapy [42]:

- Inappropriate care towards the child by main attachment figures.
- Extreme responses from main caregivers, whether above or below the emotional threshold, in the face of a situation of anguish on the part of the child.
- Insensitive, irresponsible, or severe reactions when communicating thoughts and emotions.
- A restrictive family system that is distant and cold when attending to family members' needs.
- Caregiver behavior that is too uninhibited or too inhibited.
- Controlling responses to the expression of emotions, especially negative emotions.
- Sexual, physical, and emotional abuse.

In addition, Carnes considers this type of addiction a deficit in the capacity to become intimate with a real person, the main difficulty of people with avoidant attachment [18]. People who are unable to identify, understand, express, or address their emotional needs often use sexual behavior as a substitute. These relational problems should be evaluated and resolved in therapy with patients who have this type of pathology so that they can establish a secure attachment with their therapist and enjoy solid support, thereby becoming capable of intimacy.

Using Cassidy's theory of attachment and intimacy [64], therapists and patients can work on attachment relationships in adulthood if the patient suffers from insecure avoidance attachment. Harmful sexual expressions such as the consumption of pornography can be an obstacle in the work of repairing attachment, thus a person's sexual health can improve by working on attachment and restoring it.

In short, one can work on his attachment style and on evaluating and restoring one's capacity for intimacy in attachment relationships, and thus gain greater satisfaction in interpersonal relationships and quality of life.

Some authors [17] even propose, on the one hand, that a deficiency in forming appropriate attachment relationships is a necessary element for defining addiction to pornography and, on the other hand, that any theory involving excessive sexual behavior should focus first on processes of attachment rather than on behavior.

More generally, in therapy, psychotherapists should focus on their relationship with the patient diagnosed with pornography addiction. The interpersonal relationship that is generated between them corresponds to the "place" where the wounds related to the patient's affective history open up and a variety of emotions arise. For this type of patient, it is of vital importance that a secure attachment is established between them to recover from addiction. Through psychotherapy, the therapist can be a healthy model for establishing a relationship of intimacy. From this secure basis created within the framework of therapy, the patient feels better prepared to analyze his past and present experiences [65] and express feelings related to situations that have caused suffering.

From the therapeutic framework of attachment and throughout the recovery process, patients can begin to trust themselves and leave behind self-blame and self-punishment; they can also express emotions, as well as reaffirm and connect with people around them. When patients identify the wounds of their past and the origin of their difficulties with adult attachment relationships, they are able to integrate the personal, social, physical, and spiritual aspects of their sexuality. Recovery is then aimed towards a positive attitude regarding sexuality and away from limiting addiction to pornography [66].

References

1. Cano A, Contreras M, Neuropsicología de la sexualidad. [Neuropsychology of sexuality]. Eunsa. Pamplona. Spain: Navarra; 2014. p. 2014.
2. Cassidy J, Shaver PR. Handbook of attachment: theory, research, and clinical applications (2nd and 3rd ed). New York: Guilford; 2016.
3. Butler MH, Pereyra SA, Draper TW, Leonhardt ND, Skinner KB. Pornography use and loneliness: a bidirectional recursive model and pilot investigation. J Sex Marital Ther. 2018;44(2):127–37.
4. Zeifman D, Hazan C. Pair bonds as attachments: reevaluating the evidence. In: The Handbook of Attachment. 2008:436–55.
5. Vasey PL, Abild M. A billion wicked thoughts: what the internet tells us about sexual relationships. Arch Sex Behav [Internet]. 2013;42(6):1101–3. Available from: http://link.springer.com/10.1007/s10508-013-0170-5
6. Regnerus M, Gordon D, Price J. Documenting pornography use in America: a comparative analysis of methodological approaches. J Sex Res. 2016;53(7):873–81.
7. Rissel C, Richters J, de Visser RO, McKee A, Yeung A, Caruana T. A profile of pornography users in Australia: findings from the second Australian study of health and relationships. J Sex Res. 2017;54(2):227–40.
8. Chiclana C, Contreras M, Carriles S, Rama V. Adicción al sexo ¿patología independiente o síntoma comórbido? Cuad Med psicosomática y Psiquiatr enlace. 2015;115:19–26.
9. Turner D, Schöttle D, Bradford J, Briken P. Assessment methods and management of hypersexuality and paraphilic disorders. Curr Opin Psychiatry. 2014;27:413–22.
10. George M, Maheshwari S, Chandran S, Rao SS, SM J, Rao TSS. Psychosocial intervention for sexual addiction. Indian J Psychiatry [Internet]. 2018;60:S510–3. Available from: http://ezproxy.staffs.ac.uk/login?url=http://search.ebscohost.com/login.aspx?direct=true&db=rzh&AN=131557681&site=ehost-live
11. Reid RC, Kafka MP. Controversies about hypersexual disorder and the DSM-5. Curr Sex Heal Rep [Internet]. 2014;6(4):259–64. Available from: http://link.springer.com/10.1007/s11930-014-0031-9
12. WHO. WHO | International Classification of Diseases, 11th Revision (ICD-11). WHO; 2018.
13. Gola M, Lewczuk K, Skorko M. What matters: quantity or quality of pornography use? Psychological and behavioral factors of seeking treatment for problematic pornography use. J Sex Med. 2016;13(5):815–24.
14. Gola M, Potenza MN. Paroxetine treatment of problematic pornography use: a case series. J Behav Addict [Internet]. 2016;5(3):529–32. Available from: http://www.akademiai.com/doi/abs/10.1556/2006.5.2016.046
15. Gola M, Wordecha M, Marchewka A, Sescousse G. Visual sexual stimuli—cue or reward? A perspective for interpreting brain imaging findings on human sexual behaviors. Front Hum Neurosci [Internet]. 2016;10. Available from: http://journal.frontiersin.org/Article/10.3389/fnhum.2016.00402/abstract
16. Zapf JL, Greiner J, Carroll J. Attachment styles and male sex addiction. Sex Addict Compul. 2008;15(2):158–75.

17. Leedes R. The three most important criteria in diagnosing sexual addictions: obsession, obsession, and obsession. Sex Addict Compul. 2001;8(3–4):215–26.
18. Carnes P, Delmonico DL, Griffin E. In the shadows of the net: breaking free of compulsive online sexual behavior. 2nd ed; 2007.
19. Chiclana Actis C, Contreras Chicote M, Carriles Cervera S, Rama VD. Adicción al sexo ¿patología independiente o síntoma comórbido? Cuad Med psicosomática y Psiquiatr enlace, ISSN 1695-4238. 2015;115(115):19–26.
20. Chiclana C. Atrapados en el sexo. Córdoba: Editorial Almuzara; 2013.
21. Bőthe B, Tóth-Király I, Potenza MN, Griffiths MD, Orosz G, Demetrovics Z. Revisiting the role of impulsivity and compulsivity in problematic sexual behaviors. J Sex Res [Internet]. 2018; [cited 2018 Dec 10];1–14. Available from: http://www.ncbi.nlm.nih.gov/pubmed/29913087
22. Blum AW, Chamberlain SR, Grant JE. Quality of life of young adults with non-paraphilic problematic sexual behaviors: an exploratory study. Addict Behav Rep [Internet]. 2018;8(March):164–9. https://doi.org/10.1016/j.abrep.2018.10.003.
23. Blum K, Badgaiyan RD, Gold MS. Hypersexuality addiction and withdrawal: phenomenology, neurogenetics and epigenetics. Cureus [Internet]. 2015;7759. Available from: http://www.cureus.com/articles/3046-hypersexuality-addiction-and-withdrawal-phenomenology-neurogenetics-and-epigenetics
24. Bancroft J, Vukadinovic Z. Sexual addiction, sexual compulsivity, sexual impulsivity, or what? Toward a theoretical model. J Sex Res. 2004;41:225–34.
25. Riemersma J, Sytsma M. A new generation of sexual addiction. Sex Addict Compul. 2013;20(4):306–22.
26. Hall P. A biopsychosocial view of sex addiction. Sex Relatsh Ther. 2011;26(3):217–28.
27. Monacis L, de Palo V, Griffiths MD, Sinatra M. Social networking addiction, attachment style, and validation of the Italian version of the Bergen social media addiction scale. J Behav Addict [Internet]. 2017;6(2):178–86. Available from: http://www.akademiai.com/doi/abs/10.1556/2006.6.2017.023
28. Bárcenas I, Contreras M, Trigo E, Chiclana C. Literature review: attachment style and hypersexual disorder. J Sex Med [Internet]. 2017;14(5):e280. Available from: http://rave.ohiolink.edu/ejournals/article/347685289
29. Gilliland R, Blue Star J, Hansen B, Carpenter B. Relationship attachment styles in a sample of hypersexual patients. J Sex Marital Ther. 2015;41(6):581–92.
30. El BJ. Apego y la pérdida, Biblioteca de Psicología Profunda, vol. 2. Barcelona: Paidós; 1998.
31. Zacarés J, Iborra A, Tomás J, Serra E. El desarrollo de la identidad en la adolescencia y adultez emergente. An Psicol [Internet]. 1984;25(2):326–9. Available from: http://www.redalyc.org/html/167/16712958014/
32. Uytun MC, Oztop DB, Esel E, Adam D. Evaluating the attachment behaviour in during puberty and adulthood. J Psychiatry Neurol Sci. 2013;26(2):177–89.
33. López F, Etxeberría I, Fuentes M, Ortiz M. Desarrollo afectivo y social. Madrid: Ediciones Pirámide; 2005.
34. Ainsworth MDS, Blehar MC, Waters E, Wall SN. Patterns of attachment: a psychological study of the strange situation. Patterns of attachment: a psychological study of the strange situation; 2015. 1–417 p
35. Fraley RC, Shaver PR. Airport separations: a naturalistic study of adult attachment dynamics in separating couples. J Pers Soc Psychol [Internet]. 1998;75(5):1198–212. Available from: http://doi.apa.org/getdoi.cfm?doi=10.1037/0022-3514.75.5.1198
36. Bowlby J, Ainsworth MDS. Child care and the growth of love. Biblioteca de psicología y psicoanálisis. London: Penguin; 1965.
37. Jacobson SM. The attachment, caregiving, and sexual systems relationship to conflict communication in adult pair-bond relationships. Dissertation. Madison: University of Wisconsin; 2008.
38. Butzer B, Campbell L. Adult attachment, sexual satisfaction, and relationship satisfaction: a study of married couples. Pers Relatsh [Internet]. 2008; [cited 2018 Dec 12];15(1):141–54. Available from: http://doi.wiley.com/10.1111/j.1475-6811.2007.00189.x
39. Gómez-zapiain J, Ortiz M, Gómez-Lope J. Experiencia sexual, estilos de apego y tipos de cuidados de pareja. An Psicol. 2011;27:447–56.
40. Strait JG, Sandberg JG, Larson JH, Harper JM. The relationship between family-of-origin experiences and sexual satisfaction in married couples. J Fam Ther. 2015;37(3):361–85.
41. Gómez-Zapiain J. Apego y sexualidad. Madrid: Alianza Editorial; 2009.
42. Harris J. Does attachment theory apply to working with pornographic addiction in men? Auckland University of Technology; 2005.
43. Katehakis A. Affective neuroscience and the treatment of sexual addiction. Sex Addict Compul. 2009;16(1):1–31.
44. Guigliamo J. Out of control sexual behavior: a qualitative investigation. Sex Addict Compul. 2006;13(4):361–75.
45. Bowlby J. The making and breaking of affectional bonds: aetiology and psychopathology in the light of attachment theory. Br J Psychiatry. 1977;130:201–10.
46. Weiss R. Loneliness: the experience of emotional and social isolation. Massachussets: MIT Press; 1973.
47. Seinfeld J. Containing rage, terror, and despair: an object relations approach to psychotherapy. New Jersey: Jason Aronson Inc; 1996.
48. Leedes RA. Fantasy and the internal working models held toward "comfortable interpersonal attachments" shape sexual desire: a theory applied to persons with hypersexuality [Internet]. ProQuest Dissertations and Theses. 1999; Available from: http://search.proquest.com.ezproxy.library.yorku.ca/docview/304533593?accountid=15182%5Cn http://sfx.scholarsportal.info/

york?url_ver=Z39.88-2004&rft_val_fmt=info:ofi/fmt:kev:mtx:dissertation&genre=dissertations+&+theses&sid=ProQ:ProQuest+Dissertations+&+Theses+Global&atitle=&title=Fantasy+and+the+internal+working+models+held+toward+%22comfortable+interpersonal+attachments%22+shape+sexual+desire:+A+theory+applied+to+persons+with+hypersexuality&issn=&date=1999-01-01&volume=&issue=&spage=&au=Leedes,+Richa

49. Earle RH, Dillon D, Jecmen D. Systemic approach to the treatment of sex offenders. Sex Addict Compul. 1998;5(1):49–61.
50. Efrati Y, Amichai-Hamburger Y. The use of online pornography as compensation for loneliness and lack of social ties among Israeli adolescents. Psychol Rep [Internet]. 2018:003329411879758. Available from: http://journals.sagepub.com/doi/10.1177/0033294118797580
51. Timberlake D, Meyer D, Hitchings S, Oakley A, Stoltzfus L, Aguirre S, et al. Sexually compulsive behaviors: implications for attachment, early life stressors, and religiosity. Sex Addict Compul. 2016;23(4):361–73.
52. Berlin LJ, Cassidy J, Belsky J. Loneliness in young children and infant-mother attachment: a longitudinal study loneliness in young children a longitudinal study. Source Merrill-Palmer Q Merrill-Palmer Q. 1995.
53. Mikulincer M, Shaver PR. Attachment in adulthood, second edition: structure, dynamics, and change. New York: Guilford; 2016. p. 690.
54. Erickson RJ. The importance of authenticity for self and society. Symb Interact [Internet]. 1995;18(2):121–44. Available from: http://doi.wiley.com/10.1525/si.1995.18.2.121
55. Cooper M, Lebo RA. Assessment and treatment of sexual compulsivity: a multi-modal perspective. J Soc Work Pract Addict. 2001;1(2):61–74.
56. Szymanski DM, Stewart-Richardson DN. Psychological, relational, and sexual correlates of pornography use on young adult heterosexual men in romantic relationships. J Mens Stud [Internet]. 2014;22(1):64–82. Available from: http://men.sagepub.com/lookup/doi/10.3149/jms.2201.64
57. Reid RC, Woolley SR. Using emotionally focused therapy for couples to resolve attachment ruptures created by hypersexual behavior. Sex Addict Compul. 2006;13(2–3):219–39.
58. Laaser M, Smalley G (Foreword), Carnes P (Foreword). Healing the wounds of sexual addiction. Michigan: Zondervan, Grand Rapids; 2004.
59. Miner MH, Robinson BE, Knight RA, Berg D, Romine RS, Netland J. Understanding sexual perpetration against children: effects of attachment style, interpersonal involvement, and hypersexuality. Sex Abus J Res Treat. 2010;22(1):58–77.
60. Veit M, Štulhofer A, Hald GM. Sexually explicit media use and relationship satisfaction: a moderating role of emotional intimacy? Sex Relatsh Ther. 2017;32(1):58–74.
61. Stackert RA, Bursik K. Why am I unsatisfied? Adult attachment style, gendered irrational relationship beliefs, and young adult romantic relationship satisfaction. Pers Individ Dif. 2003;34(8):1419–29.
62. Wolfe JL. Assessment and treatment of compulsive sex/love behavior. J Ration Emot Cogn Behav Ther. 2000;18(4):235–46.
63. Carnes PJ. Contrary to love. Minneapolis: CompCare Publishers; 1989.
64. Cassidy J. Truth, lies, and intimacy: an attachment perspective. Attach Hum Dev. 2001;3(2):121–55.
65. Parish M, Eagle MN. Attachment to the therapist, vol. 20. Psychoanal Psychol; 2003. p. 271–86.
66. Manley G, Koehler J. Sexual behavior disorders: proposed new classification in the DSM-V. Sex Addict Compul. 2001;8(3–4):253–65.

Correction to: Psychiatry and Neuroscience Update – Vol. V

Pascual Ángel Gargiulo
and Humberto Luis Mesones-Arroyo

Correction to:
P. Á. Gargiulo, H. L. Mesones-Arroyo (eds.), *Psychiatry and Neuroscience Update – Vol. V*, https://doi.org/10.1007/978-3-031-72219-6

This book was recently published. The editor affiliations are to be updated as listed below for the following book components:

Current Affiliation of Editors

Pascual Ángel Gargiulo
Laboratory of Neurosciences and Experimental Psychology. Area of Pharmacology
Department of Pathology, Faculty of Medical Sciences
Universidad Nacional de Cuyo
Guayamallén, Mendoza, Argentina

Humberto Luis Mesones-Arroyo
Cátedra de Psicopatología. Facultad de Humanidades y Ciencias Económicas
Pontificia Universidad Católica Argentina (UCA), Filial Mendoza
Mendoza, Argentina

Affiliation to be updated:

Pascual Ángel Gargiulo

Laboratory of Neurosciences and Experimental Psychology, Latin American Technological Corporation Foundation (FUCOTEL), Cathedra of Psychopathology, Catholic University of Argentina, Area of Pharmacology, Department of Pathology, National University of Cuyo, CONICET, Guaymallén, Mendoza, Argentina

---

The updated version of this book can be found at https://doi.org/10.1007/978-3-031-72219-6

P. Á. Gargiulo, H. L. Mesones-Arroyo (eds.), *Psychiatry and Neuroscience Update – Vol. V*,
https://doi.org/10.1007/978-3-031-72219-6_54

Humberto Luis Mesones-Arroyo

Laboratory of Neurosciences and Experimental Psychology, Latin American Technological Corporation Foundation (FUCOTEL), Cathedra of Psychopathology, Catholic University of Argentina, Area of Pharmacology, Department of Pathology, National University of Cuyo, CONICET, Guaymallén, Mendoza, Argentina

The editor affiliations are to be updated in the following portions of the book:
Title/CR Page
List of Contributors
Chapter 3 Opener
Chapter 10 Opener
Chapter 29 Opener
Chapter 30 Opener
Chapter 34 Opener
Chapter 35 Opener
Chapter 37 Opener
Chapter 38 Opener

Index

P. Á. Gargiulo, H. L. Mesones-Arroyo (eds.), *Psychiatry and Neuroscience Update – Vol. V*,
https://doi.org/10.1007/978-3-031-72219-6

D

O

P

Q

R

MIX
Papier aus verantwortungsvollen Quellen
Paper from responsible sources
FSC® C105338

If you have any concerns about our products,
you can contact us on
ProductSafety@springernature.com

In case Publisher is established outside the EU,
the EU authorized representative is:
Springer Nature Customer Service Center GmbH
Europaplatz 3, 69115 Heidelberg, Germany

Printed by Libri Plureos GmbH
in Hamburg, Germany